Nelson Yuan-sheng Kiang

# Congenital Anomalies of the Ear, Nose, and Throat

# CONGENITAL ANOMALIES OF THE EAR, NOSE, AND THROAT

Edited by

TED L. TEWFIK, M.D.

*Associate Professor of Otolaryngology*
*McGill University*
*Clinical Director of Otolaryngology*
*Montreal Children's Hospital*
*Montreal, Québec, Canada*

VAZKEN M. DER KALOUSTIAN, M.D.

*Professor of Pediatrics and Human Genetics*
*McGill University*
*Director, The F. Clarke Fraser Clinical Genetics Unit*
*Montreal Children's Hospital*
*Montreal, Québec, Canada*

New York Oxford
OXFORD UNIVERSITY PRESS
1997

Oxford University Press

Oxford New York
Athens Auckland Bangkok Bogota Bombay Buenos Aires
Calcutta Cape Town Dar es Salaam Delhi Florence Hong Kong
Istanbul Karachi Kuala Lumpur Madras Madrid Melbourne
Mexico City Nairobi Paris Singapore Taipei Tokyo Toronto

and associated companies in
Berlin Ibadan



Published by Oxford University Press, Inc.
198 Madison Avenue, New York, New York 10016

Oxford is a registered trademark of Oxford University Press



Library of Congress Cataloging-in-Publication Data
Congenital anomalies of the ear, nose, and throat/
edited by Ted L. Tewfik, Vazken M. Der Kaloustian.
p. cm. Includes bibliographical references and index.
ISBN 0-19-507784-9 (alk. paper)
1. Ear—Abnormalities—Genetic aspects.
2. Nose—Abnormalities—Genetic aspects.
3. Throat—Abnormalities—Genetic aspects.
I. Tewfik, Ted L., 1946– II. Der Kaloustian, Vazken M., 1937– .
[DNLM: 1. Ear abnormalities. 2. Nose—abnormalities.
3. Pharynx—abnormalities.
WV 101 C749 1997] RF122.C66 1997
617.5′1043—dc20 DNLM/DLC for Library of Congress 96-24705

1 3 5 7 9 8 6 4 2

Printed in the United States of America
on acid-free paper

*To our families*

# Foreword

The past few decades have seen an extraordinary growth in knowledge of gene structure and function, and how detectable alterations in genes result in metabolic or structural disorders. In particular, the recent revelations of how genes are involved in development and its errors have been astounding. This means that those who deal with the diagnosis and management of developmental disorders need to know about the new insights into developmental pathology, about the significance of family history, and about where genetic testing can be helpful in diagnosis, either post-or prenatally. On the other hand, those involved in genetic counselling need to know, not only about the genetics of those disorders, but about their developmental origins, natural history, and effectiveness of treatment. The two groups will, no doubt, increasingly overlap.

This unique volume is a veritable buffet of informational preparations that will appeal to a wide variety of tastes. Herein a stellar team of gnostic chefs have prepared a wealth of dishes that both groups will find intellectually tasty and nutritional, as well as some that will appeal to the more peculiar (in the good sense) tastes of teratologists, epidemiologists, syndromologists, or surgeons. As with any good buffet, not every dish will appeal to everyone, but everyone will find lots of goodies to suit their own tastes.

Read, mark, learn, and inwardly digest!

*F. Clarke Fraser, O.C., Ph.D., M.D., FRS(C)*
*Molson Emeritus Professor of Human Genetics*
*McGill University*
*Montreal, Québec, Canada*
*Spring 1997*

# Preface

The practicing specialist dealing with the ear, nose, and bucco-pharyngeal region is now confronted relatively more frequently with problems related to congenital anomalies since the treatment of infections and neoplasms has become more effective. Moreover, the spectacular advances in basic and clinical genetics during the past two decades have brought the congenital malformations and inherited disorders to the forefront of medical attention and care. The elucidation of the genetic code, the mapping and cloning of an increasing number of genes, recent advances in DNA techniques of screening and prenatal diagnosis, and the accomplishments of the Human Genome Project allow us to have not only a better understanding of pathogenetic and pathophysiologic mechanisms, but also more effective clinical management.

Most of the books published on this subject have considered issues from the viewpoint of either the basic scientist, the clinical geneticist, or the surgeon. The aim of *Congenital Anomalies of the Ear, Nose, and Throat* is to take a multidisciplinary approach to these problems since they are multifaceted and require the input of specialists with varied backgrounds and expertise. Thus, as we have multidisciplinary clinics for the effective study and treatment of specific anomalies such as the cleft palate, we have tried to make this a multidisciplinary book for a thorough approach to many of these conditions. Moreover, we have stressed not only the accurate description of clinical manifestations, but also their etiologic heterogeneity, their developmental pathogenesis, and their treatments and outcomes. In this effort, we had the invaluable collaboration of our colleagues, the authors of the various chapters, who contributed their expertise in the various fields of developmental biology, genetics, otolaryngology, and surgery.

The first section of the book provides general information on the principles of medical genetics and dysmorphology, anatomical landmarks, teratogenic mechanisms, epidemiologic data, and techniques and approaches to prenatal diagnosis. These chapters are intended to help the reader to understand better the concepts and terminology used throughout the book. The following sections cover anomalies of specific organs. These sections are organized in a consistent way to explain the embryology of the region, describe the major congenital anomalies and their treatments and provide extensive tables of syndromes associated with these anomalies. The classification of the diseases presented some difficulties. To make the book easier for clinicians to use, we divided the conditions according to their presenting signs rather than the pathogenetic or pathophysiologic mechanisms. As a syndrome may have several presenting signs, it could be discussed under different headings. We decided to classify diseases, whenever possible, according to the most striking or most frequent sign. Despite our efforts, a few overlaps and repetitions among the chapters were unavoidable.

This book is not limited in its content to the organs mentioned in the title. It covers anomalies of the mouth, the lips, the palate, the pharynx, the larynx and even some conditions involving the esophagus, the trachea, and their surrounding vessels. Surgical approaches are discussed for different groups of conditions that are either relatively more frequent or present particular problems. The same broad approach is taken in the last section on "Selected Syndromes and Conditions" where various clinical entities are discussed in more detail. Most of these were chosen because either they are relatively common or recent and important information about their pathogenetic mechanisms is available.

In preparing the book, we drew upon many sources of information. Other than the most recent papers on specific issues, the following publications and reference texts were most valuable: *Syndromes of the Head and Neck* by R.J. Gorlin, M.M. Cohen, Jr., and L.S. Levin; *Hereditary Hearing Loss and Its Syndromes* by R.J. Gorlin, H.V. Toriello, and M.M. Cohen, Jr.; *Human Malformations and Related Anomalies,* edited by R.E. Stevenson, J.G. Hall, and R.M. Goodman; *Smith's Recognizable Patterns of Human Malformation,* by K.L. Jones; *Birth Defects Encyclopedia,* edited by M.-L. Buyse; *Pathology of the Ear* by H.F. Schuknecht; *Pediatric Otolarygology,* edited by C.D. Bluestone, and *Mendelian Inheritance in Man,* by V.A. McKusick. Other main references for parts of our book were *Thompson and Thompson's Genetics in Medicine,* by M.W. Thompson, R.R. McInnes, and H.F. Willard; *Nora and Fraser's Medical Genetics: Principles and Practice,* by J.J. Nora, F.C. Fraser, J. Bear, C.R. Greenberg, D. Patterson, and D. Warburton; *The Metabolic and Molecular Bases of Inherited Disease,* edited by C.R. Scriver, A.L. Beaudet, W.S. Sly, and D. Valle. We are indebted to POSSUM (Pictures of Standard Syndromes and Undiagnosed Malformations, Melbourne, Australia) and LDDB (London Dysmorphology Database, London, United Kingdom)—the two computerized diagnostic databases that provided us with a lot of information for the preparation of the tables.

*Congenital Anomalies of the Ear, Nose, and Throat* aims to serve not only otolaryngologists, clinical geneticists, and plastic surgeons, but also pediatricians, internists, general surgeons, and physicians in family practice.

*Montreal*
*1997*

T.L.T.
V.M.D.K.

### References


1. Bluestone CD, Stool SE, Kenna MA: Pediatric Otolaryngology, 3rd ed. WB Saunders, Philadelphia, 1996.
2. Buyse M-L (ed): Birth Defects Encyclopedia, Blackwell, Cambridge, 1990.

3. Gorlin RJ, Cohen MM Jr, Levin LS: Syndromes of the Head and Neck, 3rd ed. Oxford University Press, New York, 1990.
4. Gorlin RJ, Toriello HV, Cohen MM Jr: Hereditary Hearing Loss and its Syndromes, Oxford University Press, New York, 1995.
5. Jones KL: Smith's Recognizable Patterns of Human Malformation, 5th ed. WB Saunders Co, Philadelphia, 1996.
6. McKusick VA: Mendelian Inheritance in Man, 11th ed. The Johns Hopkins University Press, Baltimore, 1994.
7. Nora JJ, Fraser FC, Bear J, Greenberg CR, Patterson D, Warburton D: Nora and Fraser's Medical Genetics, 4th ed. Lea & Febiger, Philadelphia, 1994.
8. Schuknecht HF: Pathology of the Ear, 2nd ed. Lea & Febiger, Philadelphia, 1993.
9. Scriver CR, Beaudet AL, Sly WS, Valle D (eds): The Metabolic and Molecular Bases of Inherited Disease, 7th ed. McGraw-Hill Inc, New York, 1995.
10. Stevenson RE, Hall JG, Goodman RM: Human Malformations and Related Anomalies. Oxford University Press, New York, 1993.
11. Thompson MW, McInnes RR, Willard HF: Thompson and Thompson's Genetics in Medicine, 5th ed. WB Saunders Co, Philadelphia, 1991.

# Contents

## Part IV The Mouth, Palate, and Pharynx



## Part V The Cranium and Face



## Part VI The Neck



## Part VII The Larynx



## Part VIII The Esophagus



## Part IX Selected Syndromes and Conditions

# Acknowledgments

We are indebted to many whose help made this book possible. In particular, we wish to express our thanks to Dr. F. Clarke Fraser for his encouragement and advice; Dr. Patrice Eydoux for his assistance in preparing the addendum on the chromosomal map; Dr. Ahmad Teebi for his help in the description of certain syndromes; Ms. Joanna Amberger and Dr. Victor McKusick for providing information about the confirmed genes and their chromosomal distribution; Dr. Patricia Howard-Peebles for her advice on the diagrammatic representation of the karyotypes.

We want to express our gratitude to Dr. Malcolm C. Johnston for his exceptional help and understanding in certain difficult situations.

We are particularly indebted to Ms. Irene Ferko for her invaluable dedication, meticulous and hard work, patience, and high degree of competence in preparing the whole manuscript of this book at different stages of its production.

The secretarial assistance of Ms. Susan Laurie and Ms. Gaby Stanischewski is greatly appreciated.

The kind and highly professional support of the staff members of the Audiovisual Department and the Medical Library at the Montreal Children's Hospital is gratefully acknowledged.

Part of this work was supported by the Musto Foundation.

Finally, throughout the different phases of the production of this book we have benefited from the counsel of Mr. Jeffrey House and Ms. Nancy Wolitzer of Oxford University Press.

T.L.T.
V.M.D.K.

# Contributors


JUDITH E. ALLANSON, M.D.
*Professor of Pediatrics*
*University of Ottawa*
*Children's Hospital of Eastern Ontario*
*Ottawa, Ontario, Canada*

PATRICK BROOKHOUSER, M.D.
*Father Flanagan Professor and Chairman*
*Department of Otolaryngology and Human Communication*
*Creighton University School of Medicine*
*Director, Boys Town National Research Hospital*
*Omaha, Nebraska*

ROBIN T. COTTON, M.D.
*Professor of Otolaryngology and Maxillofacial Surgery*
*University of Cincinnati*
*Director of Otolaryngology and Maxillofacial Surgery*
*Children's Hospital Medical Center*
*Cincinnati, Ohio*

EUGENE DANIELS, PH.D.
*Associate Professor of Anatomy and Cell Biology*
*McGill University*
*Montreal, Québec, Canada*

VAZKEN M. DER KALOUSTIAN, M.D.
*Professor of Pediatrics and Human Genetics*
*McGill University*
*Director, The F. Clarke Fraser Clinical Genetics Unit*
*Montreal Children's Hospital*
*Montreal, Québec, Canada*

TASSOS DIONISOPOULOS, M.D.
*Assistant Professor of Surgery*
*McGill University*
*Sir Mortimer B. Davis Jewish General Hospital*
*Montreal, Québec, Canada*

J. DAVID ERICKSON, PH.D., D.D.S.
*Chief, Birth Defects and Genetic Diseases Branch*
*Centers for Disease Control and Prevention*
*Atlanta, Georgia*

PATRICE EYDOUX, M.D.
*Associate Professor of Human Genetics, Pathology and Pediatrics*
*McGill University*
*Director, Prenatal Diagnosis Program*
*Montreal Children's Hospital*
*Montreal, Québec, Canada*

SAUL FRENKIEL, M.D.
*Associate Professor of Otolaryngology*
*McGill University*
*Director of Otolaryngology—Head and Neck Surgery*
*Sir Mortimer B. Davis Jewish General Hospital*
*Montreal, Québec, Canada*

THOMAS J. GAMPPER, M.D.
*Assistant Professor of Plastic Surgery*
*University of Virginia*
*University of Virginia Health Center*
*Charlottesville, Virginia*

ROBERT GORLIN, D.D.S., D.SC.
*Regents' Professor Emeritus*
*Department of Oral Sciences*
*University of Minnesota*
*Minneapolis, Minnesota*

LEWIS B. HOLMES, M.D.
*Professor of Pediatrics*
*Harvard Medical School*
*Chief, Genetics and Teratology Unit*
*Massachusetts General Hospital*
*Boston, Massachusetts*

MALCOLM C. JOHNSTON, D.D.S.
*Professor of Orthodontics*
*Professor of Cell Biology and Anatomy*
*University of North Carolina at Chapel Hill*
*Chapel Hill, North Carolina*

DANIEL J. KELLEY, M.D.
*Chief Resident*
*Department of Otolaryngology and Maxillofacial Surgery*
*University of Cincinnati*
*Children's Hospital Medical Center*
*Cincinnati, Ohio*

SAMIR KHALIFÉ, M.D.
*Associate Professor of Obstetrics and Gynecology*
*McGill University*
*Royal Victoria Hospital*
*Montreal, Québec, Canada*

MUIN J. KHOURY, M.D., PH.D.
*Chief, Epidemiology and Genetics Section*
*Birth Defects and Genetic Diseases Branch*
*Centers for Disease Control and Prevention*
*Atlanta, Georgia*

JEAN-MARTIN LABERGE, M.D.
*Associate Professor of Surgery*
*McGill University*
*Director of Pediatric General Surgery*
*Montreal Children's Hospital*
*Montreal, Québec, Canada*

EDWARD J. LAMMER, M.D.
*Director, Department of Medical Genetics*
*Director, Craniofacial Anomalies Center*
*Children's Hospital*
*Oakland, California*

M-LUCIE LESSARD, M.D.
*Assistant Professor of Surgery*
*McGill University*
*Royal Victoria Hospital and*
*Shriners Hospital for Children*
*Montreal, Québec, Canada*

KANT Y. K. LIN, M.D.
*Assistant Professor of Plastic Surgery*
*University of Virginia*
*University of Virginia Health Center*
*Charlottesville, Virginia*

JOHN J. MANOUKIAN, M.D.
*Associate Professor of Otolaryngology*
*McGill University*
*Montreal Children's Hospital*
*Montreal, Québec, Canada*

JOHN B. MULLIKEN, M.D.
*Associate Professor of Surgery*
*Harvard Medical School*
*Boston Children's Hospital*
*Boston, Massachusetts*

CHARLES MYER III, M.D.
*Professor of Otolaryngology and Maxillofacial Surgery*
*University of Cincinnati*
*Children's Hospital Medical Center*
*Cincinnati, Ohio*

LUONG T. NGUYEN, M.D.
*Associate Professor of Surgery*
*McGill University*
*Montreal Children's Hospital,*
*Montreal, Québec, Canada*

RICHARD S. OLNEY, M.D.
*Medical Epidemiologist*
*Birth Defects and Genetic Diseases Branch*
*Centers for Disease Control and Prevention*
*Atlanta, Georgia*

ROBERT S. SHAPIRO, M.D.
*Associate Professor of Otolaryngology*
*McGill University*
*Montreal Children's Hospital*
*Montreal, Québec, Canada*

MELVIN D. SCHLOSS, M.D.
*Professor and Chairman of Otolaryngology*
*McGill University*
*Director of Otolaryngology*
*Montreal Children's Hospital*
*Montreal, Québec, Canada*

HAROLD C. SLAVKIN, D.D.S.
*Director, National Institute of Dental Research*
*National Institute of Arthritis and Musculoskeletal*
*and Skin Diseases*
*National Institutes of Health*
*Bethesda, Maryland*

ANDRÉ K. TAN, M.D.
*Assistant Professor of Otolaryngology*
*Queen's University*
*Kingston General Hospital*
*Kingston, Ontario, Canada*

AHMAD S. TEEBI, M.D.
*Associate Professor of Pediatrics and Human Genetics*
*McGill University*
*Montreal Children's Hospital*
*Montreal, Québec, Canada*

TED L. TEWFIK, M.D.
*Associate Professor of Otolaryngolgy*
*McGill University*
*Clinical Director of Otolaryngology*
*Montreal Children's Hospital*
*Montreal, Québec, Canada*

J. PAUL WILLGING, M.D.
*Assistant Professor of Otolaryngology and Maxillofacial Surgery*
*University of Cincinnati*
*Children's Hospital Medical Center*
*Cincinnati, Ohio*

H. BRUCE WILLIAMS, M.D.
*Professor of Surgery*
*McGill University*
*Surgeon-in-Chief*
*Montreal Children's Hospital*
*Montreal, Québec, Canada*

ROBERT L. WILLIAMS, M.D., Ph.D.
*Associate Professor of Radiology and Pediatrics*
*McGill University*
*Montreal Children's Hospital*
*Montreal, Québec, Canada*

ANTHONY ZEITOUNI, M.D.
*Assistant Professor of Otolaryngology*
*McGill University*
*Royal Victoria Hospital*
*Montreal, Québec, Canada*

# I

# GENERAL THEMES

# 1

# Introduction to Medical Genetics and Dysmorphology

VAZKEN M. DER KALOUSTIAN

This introductory chapter presents basic information to acquaint the nongeneticist reader with the fields of medical genetics and dysmorphology, the definition of certain terms, the concepts and mechanisms involved in pathogenesis, and the attitudes and approaches in counseling and prevention.

## Molecular genetics

Molecular genetics has made giant strides in the past five decades. The detailed structure of DNA (deoxyribonucleic acid) was elucidated, the genetic code was deciphered, the nature of the gene was clarified, and many of the intricacies of its functions were explained. A multitude of "nature's errors" in the genetic material were studied, leading to better understanding of the pathogenesis of hereditary disorders and genetic–environmental interactions.

### Structure of DNA

Genetic information is encoded in DNA. This is a macromolecule found predominantly in the nucleus but also in the mitochondria. It is composed of a sugar (deoxyribose), a phosphate, and a base. There are four types of bases in DNA: two purines (adenine [A] and guanine [G]) and two pyrimidines (thymine [T] and cytosine [C]) (Fig. 1–1). The DNA molecule has the shape of a double helix (Fig. 1–2), alternating ribose and phosphate molecules from backbones of the helices.[135,136] The bases project from them and pair by hydrogen bonds: A pairs with T, and G pairs with C. DNA serves (a) to transmit the hereditary message to somatic and germ cells and (b) to synthesise proteins and modulate cell metabolism according to an inherited code or in response to varying environmental conditions.[129]

### Structure and expression of the gene

The *gene* is a hereditary unit. It is a specific sequence of DNA found on a chromosome (nuclear or mitochondrial) that is required for the synthesis of a functional product, which may be an RNA molecule or a polypeptide. These products are involved in the performance and regulation of metabolic mechanisms or the establishment of anatomic structures.[127] There were 4,577 gene loci presented as "confirmed" (asterisked) entries in McKusick's catalog, *Mendelian Inheritance in Man.*[85] Mutated genes are responsible, individually or in groups, for an important portion of human dysmorphology and disturbance in homeostasis. They produce 63% of the conditions described in Jones' *Smith's Recognizable Patterns of Human Malformations.*[62]

The expression of genetic information in proteins involves the *transcription* (nucleic acid → nucleic acid) of the genetic message from DNA to RNA (ribonuleic acid) and its *translation* (nucleic acid → protein) from RNA to protein (Fig. 1–4).[93]

On a single DNA helix, each sequence of three bases (triplet) codes for a specific amino acid, although the amino acid in question may be coded by different triplets. These triplets are the *codons.* The sequence of triplets on the DNA helix determines the sequence of amino acids in a polypeptide chain.[128] A gene is also composed of coding sequences, or *exons,* separated by intervening sequences, or *introns* (Fig. 1–3).

RNA is a nucleic acid similar in its structure to DNA but different in three major respects: (1) the sugar is ribose instead of deoxyribose , (2) the fourth base is uracil instead of thymine, and (3) it is single stranded, except for transfer RNA which coils on itself. There are three main types of RNA: *messenger RNA* (mRNA), *transfer RNA* (tRNA), and *ribosomal RNA* (rRNA). mRNA is transcribed by the enzyme RNA polymerase using one of the DNA strands as a template. Transcription continues through both the intron and exon portions of the gene.[128]

The primary transcript is processed in three different ways: (1) addition of a "CAP" structure to the 5′ end of the RNA and cleavage of the 3′ end; (2) addition of a poly A tail at the 3′ end; and (3) splicing of the primary RNA transcript to excise the introns. The fully processed mRNA is then transported to the cytoplasm, where protein synthesis occurs (Fig. 1–4).[128]

In the cytoplasm, mRNA binds to *ribosomes,* which are structures composed of ribosomal RNA and proteins. They are the site of protein synthesis to which amino acids are transferred by a special type of RNA, called *transfer RNA.* Each amino acid is transferred by its own specific tRNA. The various tRNA–amino acid molecules bind to triplet codons on the mRNA. The binding is guided by the complementary base sequence between the mRNA codons and anticodons on the tRNA molecules (Fig. 1–5). Thus the sequences of bases in DNA dictate the sequences of amino acids in polypeptides. These in turn determine the structure of the resulting protein and consequently the phenotype of the individual and the characteristics of the species.[128] Translation of a processed mRNA is always initiated by a "START" (or initiator, AUG) codon. It ends when a "STOP" (UGA, UAA, UAG) codon is encountered in the same reading frame as the initiator codon. The completed polypeptide is then released from the ribosome, which may then begin the synthesis of another polypeptide.[128]

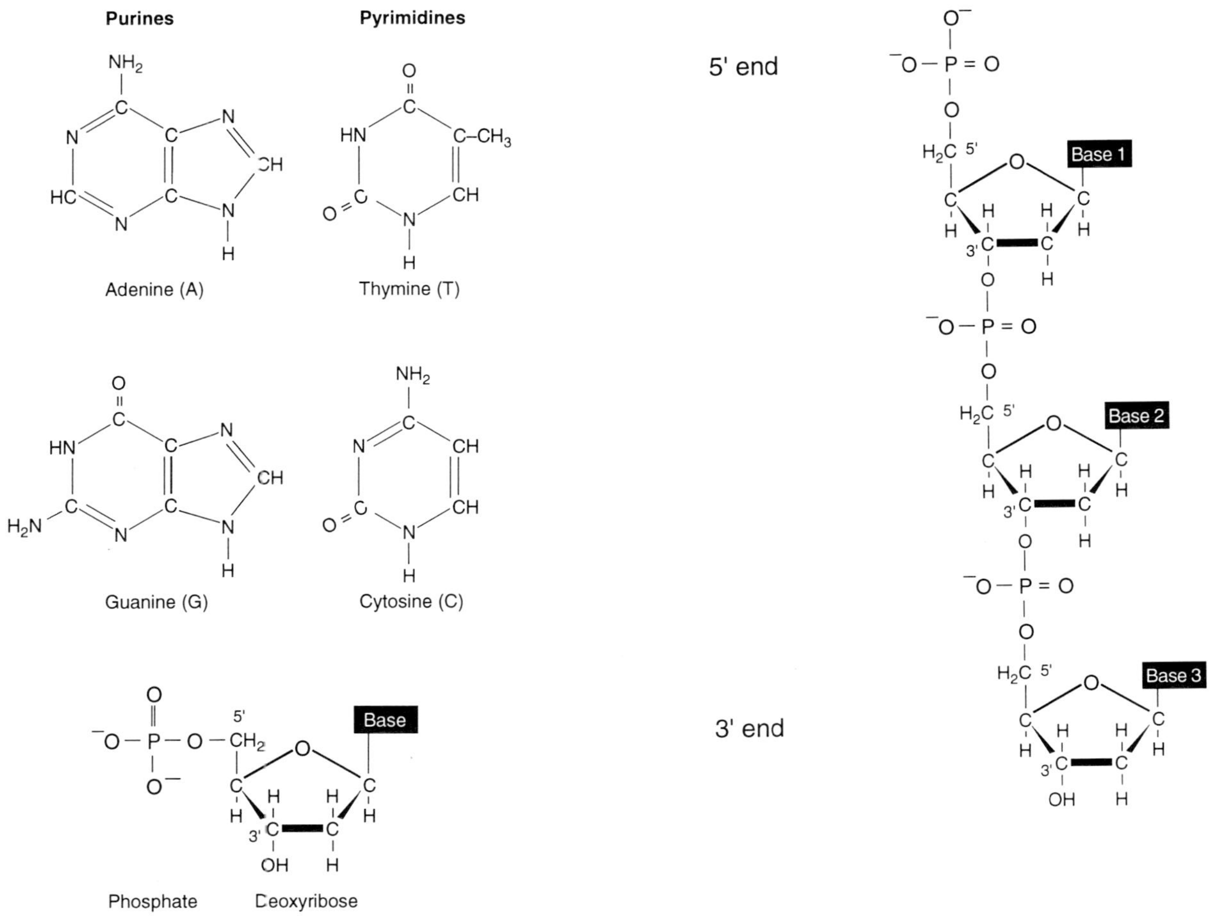


**Fig. 1–1.** A: The four bases of DNA and the general structure of a nucleotide. B: A portion of a DNA polynucleotide chain, showing the 3′–5′ phosphodiester bonds that link adjacent nucleotides. (A and B modified from Thompson et al., *Genetics in Medicine,* 5th ed., WB Saunders, Philadelphia, 1991, pp. 13–30,[127] with permission.)

A gene also has adjacent nucleotide sequences that are required for its proper expression. At the upstream flanking region (the 5' end of the gene) (Fig. 1–3) lies a *promoter* region. This region has sequences responsible for the proper initiation of transcription, thus playing an important role in regulation. The promoter consists of a series of relatively short functional elements that react with specific proteins. One important sequence in the ß-globin gene is the *TATA box* (actually ATAAT), rich in adenines and thymines and approximately 25 to 30 base pairs upstream to the start site of transcription (Fig. 1–3).[128] A second region, the *CAT box* (actually CCAAT), is farther upstream. These sequences, as well as the CACCC sequences even farther upstream, are important for normal gene expression. They are more typical of *tissue-specific* genes than *housekeeping genes* the promoters of which often lack the CAT and TATA boxes and are located in regions called *CG* (or CpG) *islands,* which have a high concentration of the dinucleotide 5′-CG-3′.[128]

## Mutations and disease

The term *mutation* is generally used for changes either in the chromosomal structure (cytogenetically detectable or not) or in the DNA at the level of the base pairs. The latter type of change is called a *point mutation* when it involves a single base pair or a *submicroscopic deletion* when a small portion of the DNA is absent. Not all mutations produce disease. Many represent normal genetic differences or polymorphisms.[122] Alternative forms of the same gene are called *alleles.*

Point mutations are “mistakes” in the replication of the genetic material preceding cell division. The frequencies of these errors may be increased by chemical or physical agents (e.g., X-rays, ultraviolet [UV] light) or by viruses. They may also be associated with advanced paternal age (e.g., achondroplasia,[65] Apert syndrome,[66] or Crouzon syndrome).[69]

Certain mutations may produce changes in structural proteins and result in disorders such as Marfan syndrome (fibrillin gene)[2] or Williams syndrome (elastin gene).[91] Others produce disturbances in circulating transport proteins such as hemoglobin, lipoproteins, and other plasma proteins.[94]

A number of diseases result from defects in membrane transport, involving carrier substances. Certain mutations involve genes coding for receptors, such as those of the fibroblast growth factor receptors (FGFRs), which have recently been found to be responsible for different types of craniosynostoses.[23,84] Mutations also produce changes in enzymes, which may cause metabolic derangements. These may result in the inadequate synthesis of important hormones (e.g., congenital adrenal hyperplasia),[94] the accumulation of toxic substances (e.g., phenylketonuria),[94] or the production of syndromes (e.g., Smith-Lemli-Opitz syndrome associated with inadequate synthesis of 7–dehydrocholesterol reductase).[132] Finally, muta-

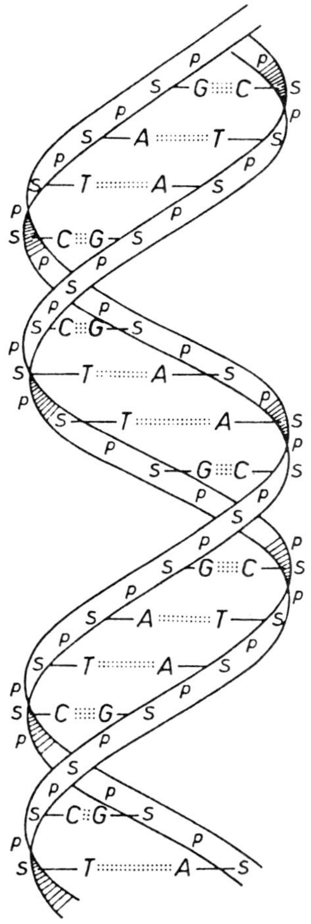


**Fig. 1–2.** The double helix. (From Der Kaloustian and Kurban, *Genetic Diseases of the Skin,* Springer-Verlag, 1979, pp. 1–6,[29] with permission.)

tions may involve developmental genes (e.g., HOX and PAX; see Homeotic genes).

Lysosomal storage diseases (e.g., Hurler syndrome or MPHI), peroxisomal diseases (e.g., chondrodysplasia punctata, rhizomelic form),[78] mitochondrial diseases (e.g., Kearns-Sayre syndrome),[108] and disorders involving homeobox genes (e.g., Waardenburg syndrome),[71] have been elucidated in recent years. Thus, the concept of *inherited metabolic disorder* has become much broader than it was, as the three volumes of the 1995 edition of *The Metabolic and Molecular Bases of Inherited Disease* testify.[119]

Two of the most important recent advances in the understanding of development and the pathogenesis of congenital anomalies and birth defects are concerned with the respective roles of homeotic genes and fibroblast growth factor receptors.

## Homeotic genes

*Homeotic genes,* long since recognized as controlling segmentation in *Drosophila,* have recently been found to be involved in orienting the very early mammalian embryo in gastrulation and in coordinating the formation of specific structures from segments or subsegments. Most of these regulatory genes have a common or very similar segment, or *box.* Their product seems to be involved in binding to specific DNA segments, thus controlling transcription from DNA to mRNA. Much of this research was carried out by Edward Lewis, Christiane Nüesslein-Volhard, and Eric Wieschaus, who received the Nobel Prize for medicine in 1995 for their extensive studies of homeotic genes.

Three types of control box genes have been transmitted through evolution and identified in *Drosophila,* mice and humans: human homeobox *(HOX),* paired-box *(PAX),* and pituitary-specific *(POU)* genes.[32,43,74,83,99,142] These are transcriptional control genes associated with early post-implantation processes including neurulation, as well as branchial arch and limb formation.

*HOX* genes all contain a 183 bp region that encodes a 61 amino acid–binding domain. This domain is present in several classes of homeotic developmental control genes, each controlling the specification of different body segments.

Four major clusters of homeobox-containing genes, A, B, C, and D, have been found in humans (Fig. 1–6). The individual gene loci are designated numerically according to their physical location (3′ to 5′) within a given gene cluster. This scheme assumes that each cluster will have 13 gene loci. The human *HOX* A through D clusters map respectively to chromosomes 7p, 17q, 12q, and 2q. The classes of homeobox genes display colinearity and functional hierarchy.[32] Colinearity implies that there is a correlation between the physical order of genes along the chromosome and their expression and function along the anteroposterior axis of the embryo.[74] Functional hierarchy implies the importance of one gene in superseding the effect of another one. The general tendency is that anterior homeotic products are suppressed by posterior homeotic products.

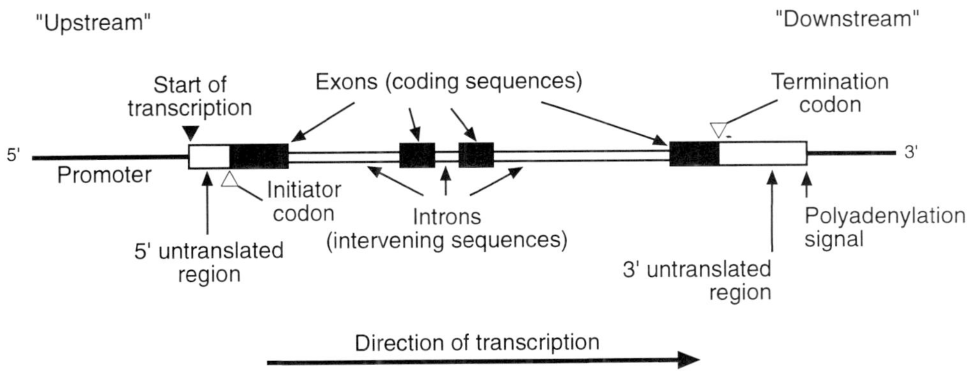


**Fig. 1–3.** General structure of a typical human gene. (Modified from Thompson et al., *Genetics in Medicine,* 5th ed., WB Saunders, Philadelphia, 1991, pp. 13–30,[127] with permission.)

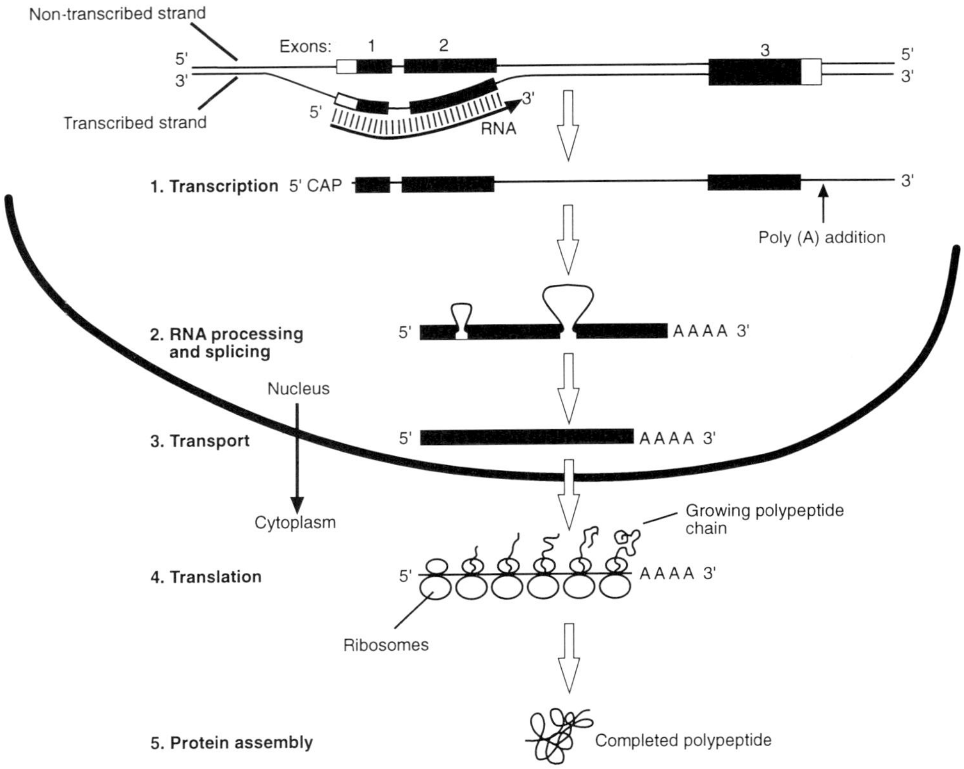


**Fig. 1–4.** Transfer of information from DNA to RNA to protein for a hypothetical gene with three exons and two introns. (Modified from Thompson et al., *Genetics in Medicine,* 5th ed., WB Saunders, Philadelphia, 1991, pp. 13–30,[127] with permission.)

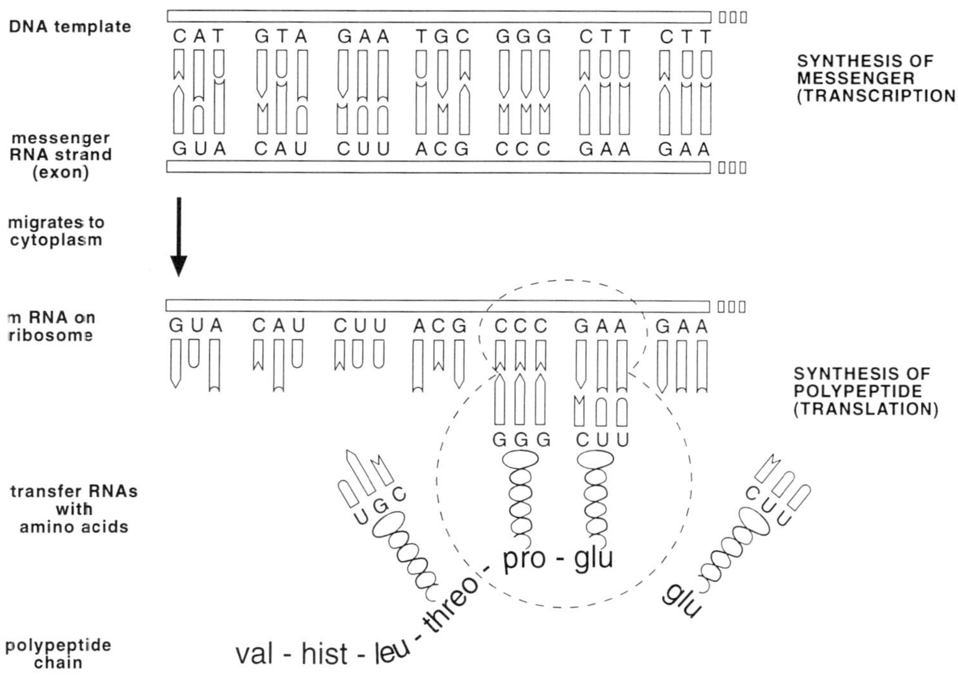


**Fig. 1–5.** Synthesis of a polypeptide with a sequence of amino acids corresponding to a sequence of nucleotide triplets in DNA. (Modified from Nora et al., *Medical Genetics: Principles and Practice,* 4th ed. Lea and Febiger, Philadelphia, 1994, pp. 68–90,[92] with permission.)

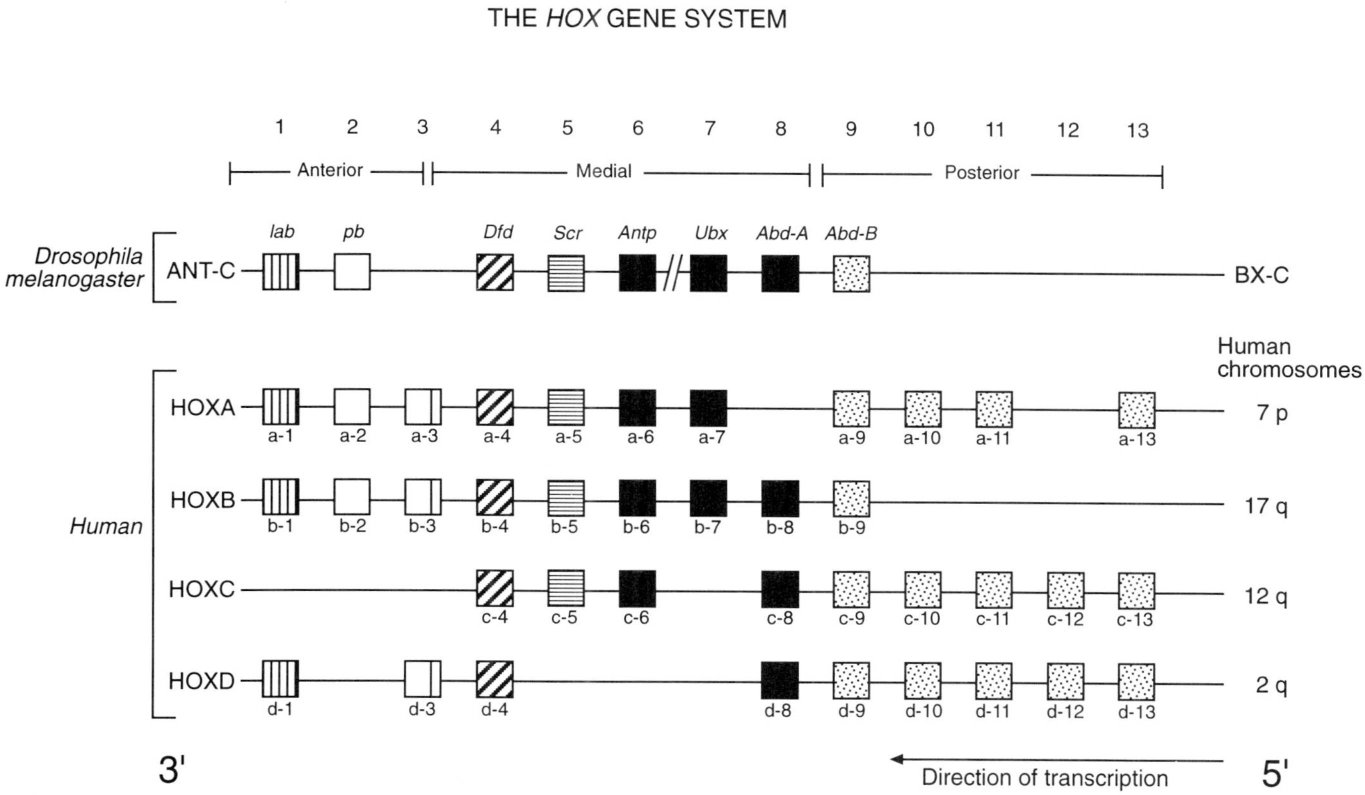


**Fig. 1–6.** Chromosomal organization of *HOX* clusters. The diagram shows the structural organization of the *Drosophila* and human networks and their phylogenetic correspondence. All *HOX* genes are transcribed 5′→3′ from right to left. Genes are represented by boxes. No attempt was made to represent physical distance. (Modified from Duboule and Morata, Trends Genet 10:358–364, 1994,[32] and Ruddle et al., Annu Rev Genet 22:423–442, 1994,[111] with permission.)

*HOX* genes are involved in the embryonic development of the face and the ear. A mutation in the homeodomain of the human *HOX* gene *MSX2* is responsible for craniosynostosis of the Boston type.[60] *HOX* genes are also involved in the pathogenetic mechanisms of certain teratogens, for example, isotretinoin (see Chapters 4, 6, and 14).

*PAX* genes consist of a highly conserved DNA sequence of 384 base pairs. Unlike the *HOX* genes, *PAX* genes are not arranged in clusters but are each located on a different chromosome. This suggests that they act singularly and not in combination, as do the *HOX* genes.[123,124] Nine human *PAX* genes have been identified (Fig. 1–7).[124] *PAX* genes have a fundamental role in specification of embryonic development as well as roles in the pathogenesis of cancer and mendelian syndromes.

Several human phenotypes are known to be caused by mutations in three *PAX* genes. A mutation in *PAX2* (10q25) produces optic nerve colobomas, renal anomalies, and vesicoureteral reflux.[112] *PAX3* (2q35) is responsible for Waardenburg syndrome (WS) types 1 and 3,[6] and *PAX6* (11p13) mutations cause aniridia[56] and autosomal dominant keratitis.[87]

Different tissues show differential sensitivity to reduced *PAX* gene dosage. This is clear in the pathogenesis of WS types 1 and 3. Almost all affected persons have dystopia canthorum. About two-thirds show some pigmentary disturbance of the eyes, hair, and skin, and have some degree of deafness. These reflect faulty differentiation or migration of melanocyte precursors from the neural crest.[103] Very few *PAX3* heterozygotes have neural tube defects and a very few have contractures or hypoplasia of the upper limbs, termed *WS type 3*. It is thus hypothesized that, whereas with 100% effective *PAX3* dosage there is normal development, with dosage reduced by <50%, dystopia canthorum is evident, with 50%, patchy failure of melanocytes is noted and, with >50%, limb muscle defects and neural tube defects are produced. However, there is little correlation between specific *PAX3* mutations and particular clinical phenotypes.[96a]

Mutations are detected more frequently in *PAX* genes than in *HOX* genes. This may be because homozygosity is required in *HOX* mutations before a phenotype is noted. On the other hand, phenotypic manifestations of mutations in *PAX* genes are the effects of heterozygous dosage when only one copy has been mutated.[97]

### The Fibroblast Growth Factor Receptor (FGFR) Genes

*Fibroblast growth factors* (FGF) are heparin-binding polypeptides. They play a fundamental role in many important processes including regulation of mitogenesis for cells of ectodermal, mesodermal, and endodermal origin; in many other normal physiological processes of embryonic and fetal development; in neovascularization; and in responses to wounding.[84] The FGF gene family is comprised of nine members.

FGFs transduce signals to the cytoplasm through a family of transmembrane receptor tyrosine kinases, the FGF receptors. FGFRs are activated by ligand binding and phosphorylate their

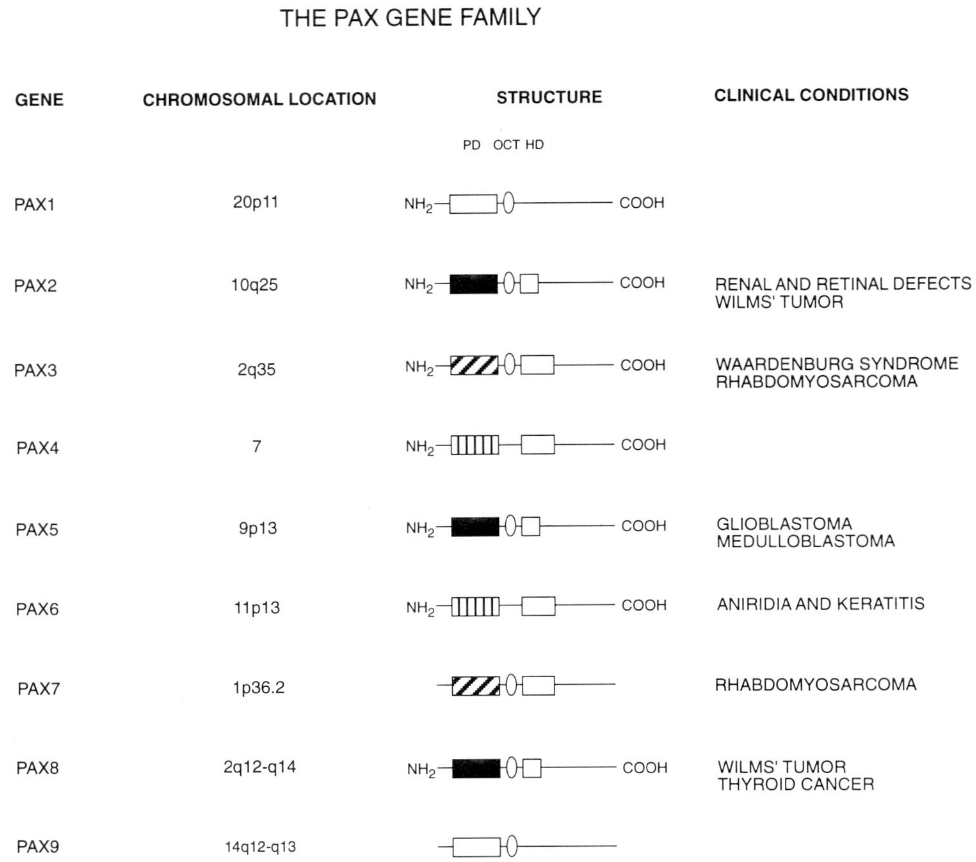


**Fig. 1–7.** The *PAX* gene family. The nine *PAX* genes are divided into four classes according to their structure. Class I genes (*PAX* 1 and 9) have no homeodomain. They are not expressed in the central nervous system. Class II genes (*PAX* 3 and 7) are the earliest *PAX* genes to be expressed in the developing embryo. Class III genes (*PAX* 2, 5, and 8) have a small homeodomain. In addition to their role in embryogenesis, they appear to be influential in a number of diverse cancers. Class IV genes (*PAX* 4 and 6) lack the octapeptide region. (Modified from Stuart and Gruss, Hum Mol Genet 4:1717–1720, 1995,[124] with permission.)

intracellular tyrosine residues. Four FGFRs are known.[97] All of them have three extracellular immunoglobulin-like domains. They are designated immunoglobulin-like loops I–III in the order of their increasing proximity to the plasma membrane (Fig. 1–8).[97]

Human mutations producing various syndromes that manifest skeletal anomalies have been found in *FGFR1, FGFR2,* and *FGFR3* genes, which are located at chromosome sites 8p11.2–p12, 10q25.3–q26, and 4p16, respectively.[23] Mutation in exon 5 of *FGFR1* produces Pfeiffer syndrome.[113] Different mutations in exon 9 of the *FGFR2* gene produce Crouzon syndrome,[59] Pfeiffer syndrome,[76,113] or Jackson-Weiss syndrome.[59] A mutation in exon 7 of *FGFR2* causes Apert syndrome.[141] *FGFR2* mutations may also produce Beare-Stevenson cutis gyrata syndrome.[101a] Mutations of *FGFR3* are responsible for achondroplasia, hypochondroplasia, thanatophoric dwarfism and Crouzon syndrome with acanthosis nigricans.[7,85a,97,109a] The gene of craniosynostosis Adelaide type is localized to 4p16.[58]

Two important observations have been made regarding *FGFR* genes: (1) a specific phenotype may be produced by mutations in various *FGFR* genes (e.g., Pfeiffer syndrome); and (2) the same point mutation may be responsible for different phenotypes (e.g., Pfeiffer, Crouzon, and Jackson-Weiss syndromes).[97]

## Inheritance in humans

The human genome is estimated to contain 60,000 to 70,000 genes.[36] The Human Genome Project aims at completing the mapping and sequencing of all the genes by the year 2005.[137] By September 1996, 5,230 confirmed gene loci had been identified (Online Mendelian Inheritance in Man, OMIM), and 4,073 of them had been mapped to one of the chromosomes (Table 1–1). Around 30% of the total loci identified are linked to congenital anomalies or morphologic features.[85]

Inheritance of traits and disorders may be monogenic, multigenic, or the result of the transmission of an abnormal chromosome (e.g., a deletion or a duplication). The expression of specific genes is influenced by other genes or environmental conditions. Beside the classical mendelian patterns of inheritance, several nonclassical patterns of inheritance have been discovered and studied in recent years. These will be discussed later in this chapter.

## Single gene inheritance

### Classical patterns

Single genes are usually inherited according to one of the following mendelian patterns: autosomal dominant, autosomal recessive, X-linked dominant, or X-linked recessive. These patterns may be apparent in pedigrees, the proper drawing of which is the first step in the study of inherited diseases in families. They should be included in all case histories in which a familial disease is suspected. They are also essential for linkage studies, gene mapping, genetic counseling, and prenatal diagnosis. The symbols commonly used are standard and generally accepted (Figs. 1–9, 1–10, 1–11).

A person is *homozygous* for a certain gene when both alleles at the same locus are identical. *Heterozygosity* implies the presence of two different alleles. Usually the term is used for situations when one of the alleles bears a pathogenic mutation.

In either case, there is no absolute distinction between dominant and recessive genes. By definition, a *recessive* gene has no detectable expression in a heterozygote under the conditions of study and analysis. Diseases due to deficiency of enzymatic activity behave as recessives because, in the heterozygous situation, the amount of enzymatic activity produced by the unaffected allele allows a normal metabolic function. When the gene codes for an abnormal structural protein, the mutant allele acts usually, though not always, as a *dominant*. In that case, the cells of the heterozygote carry the mutant gene and synthesize a mixture of the structurally normal and abnormal proteins. As a result of changes in the physical properties of the protein, heterozygotes may show phenotypic abnormalities. Marfan syndrome behaves as a dominant with a defect in the structural gene fibrillin.[2]

The following are the characteristics of *autosomal dominant* inheritance (Fig. 1–12):

1. At least one of the parents of an affected person is also affected, except when the penetrance is reduced or the trait arises by a new mutation or when there is germ-line mosaicism. The trait appears in every generation. There is no skipping except when the penetrance is reduced (see Penetrance).
2. An affected person heterozygous for the trait has an equal chance of transmitting the mutant or the normal allele to each child.
3. Males and females can have and transmit the trait equally. By

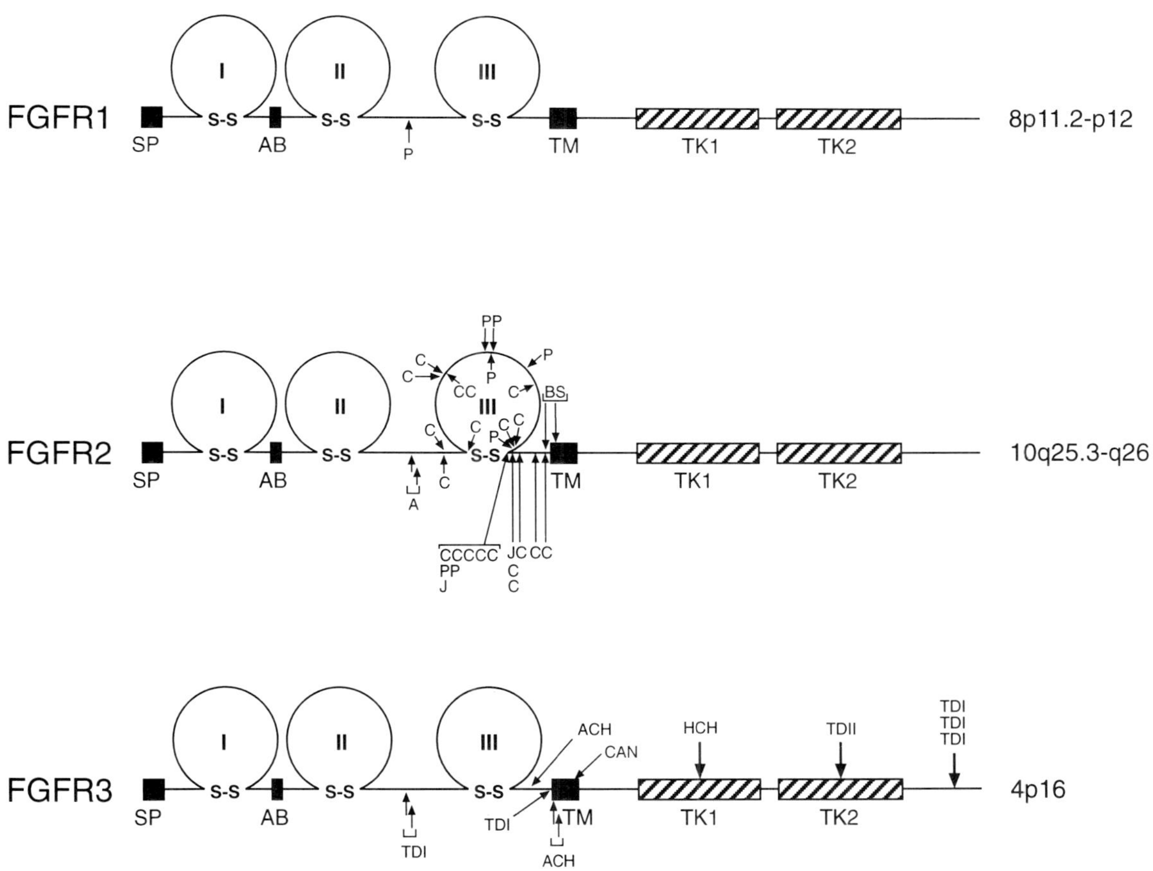


**Fig. 1–8.** Human mutations in fibroblast growth factor receptors (FGFRs). The structure of human FGFRs is shown with the location of the mutations. Each mutation site is indicated by one arrow, and the number of disease symbols at the same locus indicates the number of different amino acid changes at the same residue. SP = signal peptide; AB = acidic box; I, II, and III = immunoglobulin-like domains; S-S = disulfide bond; TM = transmembrane domain; TK1 and TK2 = tyrosine kinase domain; ACH = achondroplasia; TDI = thanatophoric dysplasia type 1; TDII = thanatophoric dysplasia type 2; HCH = hypochondroplasia; A = Apert syndrome; C = Crouzon syndrome; CAN = Crouzon syndrome with acanthosis nigricans; J = Jackson-Weiss syndrome; P = Pfeiffer syndrome; BS = Beare-Stevenson cutis gyrata syndrome.[101a] (Modified from Park et al., Am J Hum Genet 57:748–754, 1995,[97] with permission.)

**Table 1–1.** Number of genes assigned to each human chromosome

| Chromosome number | Number of genes assigned |
|---|---|
| 1 | 395 |
| 2 | 223 |
| 3 | 171 |
| 4 | 164 |
| 5 | 152 |
| 6 | 228 |
| 7 | 175 |
| 8 | 111 |
| 9 | 152 |
| 10 | 117 |
| 11 | 245 |
| 12 | 211 |
| 13 | 50 |
| 14 | 124 |
| 15 | 100 |
| 16 | 148 |
| 17 | 221 |
| 18 | 60 |
| 19 | 219 |
| 20 | 74 |
| 21 | 51 |
| 22 | 82 |
| X | 257 |
| Y | 18 |
| Mitochondrial | 60 |
| Total | 3808 |

Online Mendelian Inheritance in Man, OMIM (TM). Center for Medical Genetics, Johns Hopkins University (Baltimore, MD) and National Center for Biotechnology Information, National Library of Medicine (Bethesda, MD), 1996. World Wide Web URL:http://www3.ncbi.nlm.nih.gov/omim/.

September 1996, 4,934 confirmed autosomal genes had been identified (Online Mendelian Inheritance in Man, OMIM).

Two traits are said to be *codominant* when their genes are allelic and are both expressed in a heterozygote individual. For example, in a person with blood group AB, genes for both groups A and B are expressed.

The following are the characteristics of *autosomal recessive* inheritance (Fig. 1–13):

1. The parents are heterozygous and phenotypically normal, and the trait appears only in the children who are homozygous for the mutant gene.
2. Statistically, one-fourth of the children of heterozygous parents are affected and thus there is a 25% risk at each pregnancy.
3. Males and females have equal chance of being affected.

When an individual carries two different mutated alleles at the same locus, the condition is called a *genetic compound.* In consanguineous marriages both partners have a higher risk of being carriers of the same rare recessive gene. Thus the children who are products of consanguineous marriages run an increased risk of being affected with autosomal recessively inherited conditions. This risk may be increased by 100-fold. However, in absolute terms, this increase is close to 1%.[93]

*X-linked recessive inheritance* (Fig. 1–14) occurs when the mutant gene is on the X chromosome. It has the following characteristics:

1. The trait is much more common in males than in females. Females have two X chromosomes and males have only one. All males carrying the X-linked gene express the trait. Females are affected when they are homozygous and in certain rare heterozygous cases, as an effect of the Lyon hypothesis, when a high percentage of cells have random inactivation of the X chromosome carrying the normal allele.
2. An affected man passes his X-linked gene to all of his daughters who become carriers but not affected. He does not transmit it to any of his sons.
3. A carrier woman passes her X-linked gene to half of her sons who manifest the trait and to half of her daughters who become carriers.

*X-linked dominant inheritance* (Fig. 1–15) has the following characteristics:

1. Affected men transmit the trait to all of their daughters, who then display the clinical manifestations of that particular condition. They transmit the gene to none of their sons.
2. Heterozygous women are affected. They transmit the trait to half of their sons and half of their daughters.

By September 1996, 270 confirmed X-linked genes had been identified (Online Mendelian Inheritance in Man, OMIM).

*Y-linked genes* occur only in males. They are transmitted to all the sons and none of the daughters. There are very few genes known to be definitely on the Y chromosome. By September 1996, 19 confirmed Y-linked genes had been identified (Online Mendelian Inheritance in Man, OMIM).

## Penetrance

Certain traits may be modified by other genes and by environmental factors to such an extent, that they may not be recognizable either clinically or by laboratory tests, even though the gene causing the trait is present. In such cases, the gene or trait is said to have *incomplete* or *reduced penetrance.* Thus, certain autosomal dominant traits with reduced penetrance may skip a generation.

## Expressivity

This term indicates the variation in expression of a phenotype that a gene may have. In clinical medicine, a certain gene with variable expressivity may produce mild, moderate, or severe disease. A *forme fruste* is an extremely mild and clinically insignificant expression of a condition. Variable expressivity and formes frustes are noted especially in autosomal dominant inheritance. For example, certain patients with cleidocranial dysostosis may not be identified clinically and are diagnosed in retrospect by special radiographic testing when other, more affected members of their families are detected.[20]

## Pleiotropy

Pleiotropy is the occurrence of multiple phenotypic effects of a mutant gene or gene pair. For example, the primary defect in Hurler syndrome is the specific deficiency of $\alpha$-L-iduronidase, with accumulation of the substrate in the lyzosome. Secondary effects are mental retardation, craniofacial anomalies, dysostosis multiplex, corneal opacification, and hepatosplenomegaly.[67]

Instructions:
— Key should contain all information relevant to interpretation of pedigree (e.g., define shading)
— For clinical (non-published) pedigrees, include:
 a) family names/initials, when appropriate
 b) name and title of person recording pedigree
 c) historian (person relaying family history information)
 d) date of intake/update
— Recommended order of information placed below symbol (below to lower right, if necessary):
 a) age/date of birth or age at death
 b) evaluation (see Figure 5)
 c) pedigree number (e.g., I-1, I-2, I-3)

| | Male | Female | Sex Unknown | Comments |
|---|---|---|---|---|
| 1. Individual | b. 1925 | 30 y | 4 mo | Assign gender by phenotype. |
| 2. Affected individual | | | | Key/legend used to define shading or other fill (e.g., hatches, dots, etc.). |
| | | | | With ≥2 conditions, the individual's symbol should be partitioned accordingly, each segment shaded with a different fill and defined in legend. |
| 3. Multiple individuals, number known | 5 | 5 | 5 | Number of siblings written inside symbol. (Affected individuals should not be grouped.) |
| 4. Multiple individuals, number unknown | n | n | n | "n" used in place of "?" mark. |
| 5a. Deceased individual | d. 35 y | d. 4 mo | | Use of cross (†) may be confused with symbol for evaluated positive (+). If known, write "d." with age at death below symbol. |
| 5b. Stillbirth (SB) | SB 28 wk | SB 30 wk | SB 34 wk | Birth of a dead child with gestational age noted. |
| 6. Pregnancy (P) | P LMP: 7/1/94 | P 20 wk | P | Gestational age and karyotype (if known) below symbol. Light shading can be used for affected and defined in key/legend. |
| 7a. Proband | P | P | P P | First affected family member coming to medical attention. |
| 7b. Consultand | | | Individual(s) seeking genetic counseling/testing. | |

**A**

Instructions:
— Symbols are smaller than standard ones and individual's line is shorter. (Even if sex is known, triangles are preferred to a small square/circle; symbol may be mistaken for symbols 1, 2, and 5a/5b of Figure 1, particularly on hand drawn pedigrees.)
— If gender and gestational age known, write below symbol in that order.

| | Male | Female | Sex Unknown | Comments |
|---|---|---|---|---|
| 1. Spontaneous abortion (SAB) | male | female | ECT | If ectopic pregnancy, write ECT below symbol. |
| 2. Affected SAB | male | female | 16 wk | If gestational age known, write below symbol. Key/legend used to define shading. |
| 3. Termination of pregnancy (TOP) | male | female | | Other abbreviations (e.g., TAB, VTOP, Ab) not used for sake of consistency. |
| 4. Affected TOP | male | female | | Key/legend used to define shading. |

**B**

**Fig. 1–9.** A: Common pedigree symbols, definitions, and abbreviations. B: Pedigree symbols and abbreviations for pregnancies not carried to term. (A and B from Bennett et al., Am J Hum Genet 56:745–752, 1995,[8] with permission.)

### Heterogeneity

A condition is causally heterogeneous when multiple causes result in the same effect. Genetic heterogeneity of a disease may result in confusing pedigrees. Thus, inherited congenital neurosensory deafness in different families may be the result of two autosomal recessive genes at two different loci. The children of two deaf individuals, each being homozygous for a recessive trait at a different locus, may all have normal hearing because they will be heterozygous for two separate loci.

The craniosynostoses are also genetically heterogeneous. Thus, Pfeiffer syndrome may be due to mutations of *FGFR1* (fibroblast growth factor receptor 1) on chromosome 8 (8p11.2–p12) or *FGFR2* on chromosome 10 (10q25.3–q26).[113]

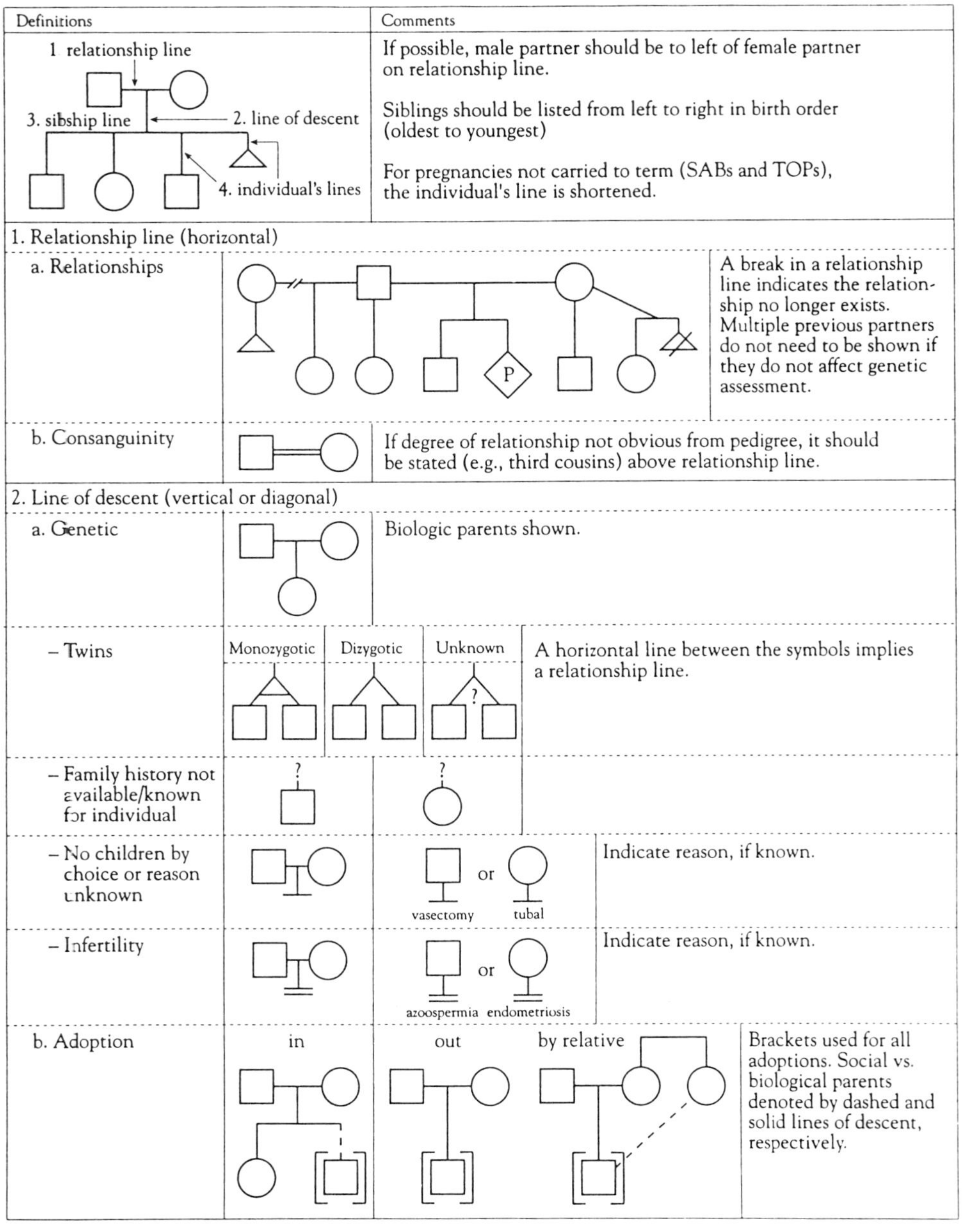


**A**

**Fig. 1–10.** A: Pedigree line definitions. B: Symbols and definitions used in reproductive technologies and adoption. (A and B from Bennett et al., Am J Hum Genet 56:745–752, 1995,[8] with permission.)

Moreover, many malformations are pathogenetically heterogeneous, separate mechanisms being responsible for the same effect. Robin sequence is an example of this. It is commonly present in Stickler syndrome which is a single gene autosomal dominant condition. Alternatively, it may be due to predominantly environmental conditions in utero, such as oligohydramnios, in which case the chin is compressed against the sternum, thus restricting mandibular growth and impacting the tongue between the palatal shelves.[24]

## Nonclassical patterns

Other than the classical mendelian patterns of single gene inheritance, certain conditions follow nonclassical mechanisms of genetic transmission or expression: mitochondrial inheritance, mosaicism, genomic imprinting and uniparental disomy, and triplet repeats.[95]

### Mitochondrial inheritance

Mitochondrial DNA (mtDNA) in humans has been completely sequenced.

When a cell divides, the mitochondria carrying the normal and abnormal mtDNA are distributed randomly in the daughter cells which may therefore contain different proportions of normal and mutant mtDNA. Thus, pedigrees of mitochondrial disorders are characterized by variability of expression and reduced penetrance of the specific mutation.

Mitochondrial inheritance is also characterized by transmission of the condition only through women, while the offspring

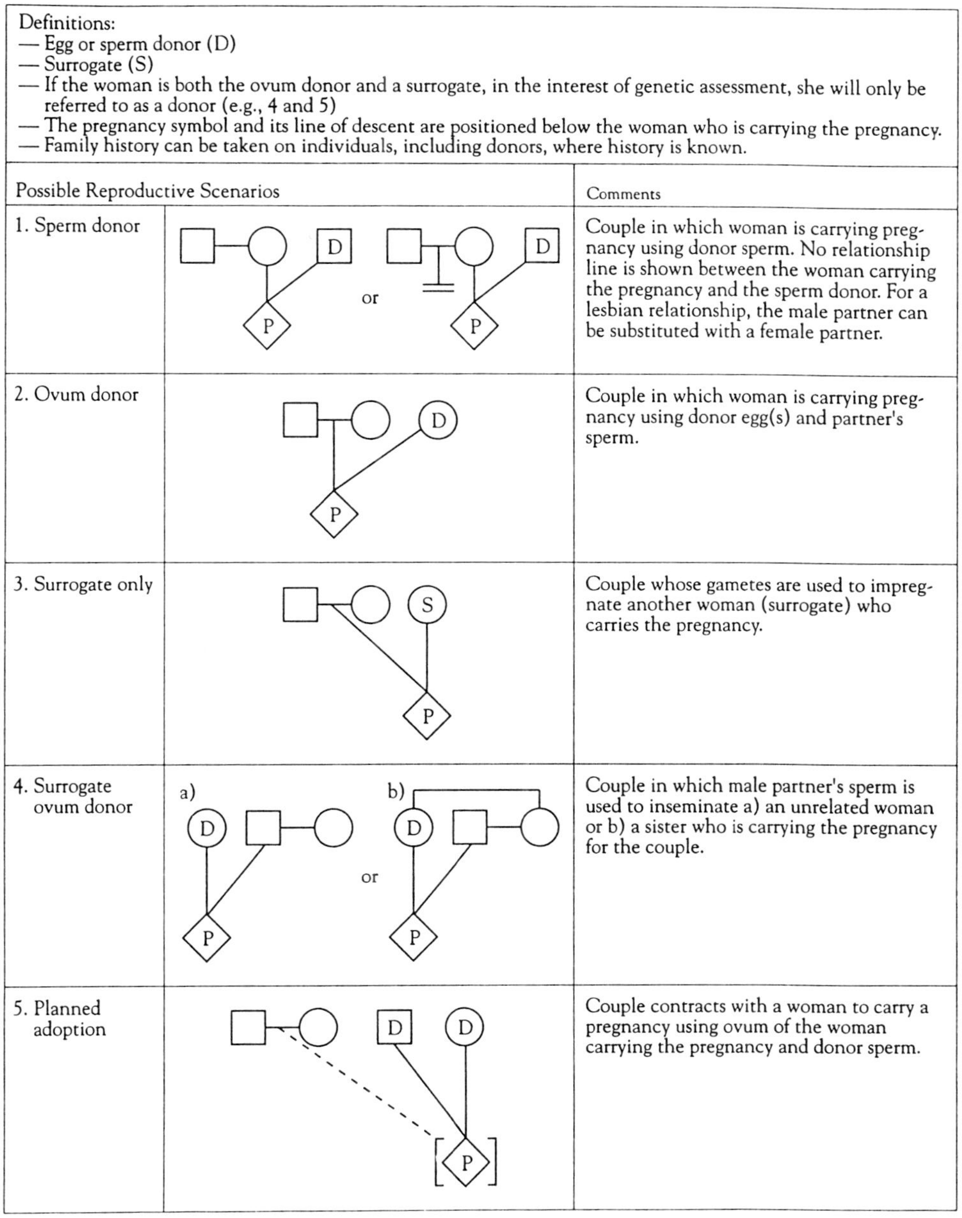


**B**

of male patients are unaffected. This is because the ovum has a large number of mitochondria in its cytoplasm, while the sperm contain few mitochondria , which are usually not transmitted to the offspring (Fig. 1–16).[22,95] By September 1996, 60 mitochondrial genes and traits had been identified. (Online Mendelian Inheritance in Man, OMIM).

## Mosaicism

*Somatic mosaicism.* In somatic mosaicism, more than one genetically different cell lines are present in an individual's somatic cells. After the formation of the zygote and during the development of the embryo, a mutation may occur in a cell, which may give rise to a lineage. If the mutation is pathogenic, parts of an individual's body may be affected, thus expressing localized manifestations of a certain condition, e.g., segmental neurofibromatosis 1 (NF1), affecting only one part of the body.[102] Proteus syndrome is considered to be another form of somatic cell mosaicism, where only certain cell lines in the body contain the mutation and manifest disease. All conditions manifesting somatic mosaicism only, without involvement of the germ line, are sporadic.[118]

*Germ-line mosaicism.* In some sibships, an autosomal dominant condition with high penetrance may occur in siblings, while the parents are unaffected. In such situations, it is thought that the gonads of either one of the parents may have germ-line mosaicism with the original normal parental cell line as well as a cell line carrying the new mutation responsible for that particular condition. Examples of these may happen in families with more than one child affected with achondroplasia, pseudoachondroplasia,[51] osteogenesis imperfecta,[25] or Crouzon

Instructions:

— Evaluation (E) is used to represent clinical and/or test information on the pedigree.
  a. E is to be defined in key/legend.
  b. If more than one evaluation, use subscript ($E_1$, $E_2$, $E_3$) and define in key. May be written side by side or below each other depending on available space.
  c. Test results should be put in parentheses or defined in key/legend.
  d. If results of exam/family study/testing not documented or unavailable, may use a question mark (e.g., E?).

— Documented evaluation (*)
  a. Asterisk is placed next to lower right edge of symbol.
  b. Use *only* if examined/evaluated by you or *your* research/clinical team or if the outside evaluation has been personally reviewed and verified.

— A symbol is shaded only when an individual is clinically symptomatic.

— For linkage studies, haplotype information is written below the individual. The haplotype of interest should be on left and appropriately highlighted.

— Repetitive sequences, trinucleotides and expansion numbers are written with affected allele first and placed in parentheses.

— If mutation known, identify and place in parentheses.

— Recommended order of information:
  1) age/date of birth or age at death
  2) evaluation information
  3) pedigree number (e.g., I-1, I-2, I-3)

| Definition | Symbol | Scenario | Example |
|---|---|---|---|
| 1. Documented evaluation (*) | * | Woman with normal physical exam and negative fragile X chromosome study (normal phenotype and negative test result). | * E – |
| 2. Obligate carrier (will not manifest disease). | | Woman with normal physical exam and premutation for fragile X (normal phenotype and positive test result). | * E+(100n/35n) |
| 3. Asymptomatic/presymptomatic carrier (clinically unaffected at this time but could later exhibit symptoms) | | Man age 25 with normal physical exam and positive DNA test for Huntington disease (symbol filled in if/when symptoms develop). | 25 y * E+(45n/18n) |
| 4. Uninformative study (u) | Eu | Man age 25 with normal physical exam and uninformative DNA test for Huntington disease ($E_1$) and negative brain MRI study ($E_2$). | 25 y * $E_1$u(36n/18n) $E_2$– |
| 5. Affected individual with positive evaluation (E+) | E+ | Individual with cystic fibrosis and positive mutation study, although only one mutation has currently been identified. | E+(ΔF508) Eu * E+(ΔF508/u) |
| | | 18 week male fetus with abnormalities on ultrasound and a trisomy 18 karyotype. | P 18 wk * E+(tri 18) |

**Fig. 1–11.** Pedigree symbolization of genetic evaluation and testing information. (From Bennett et al., Am J Hum Genet 56:745–752,[8] 1995 with permission.)

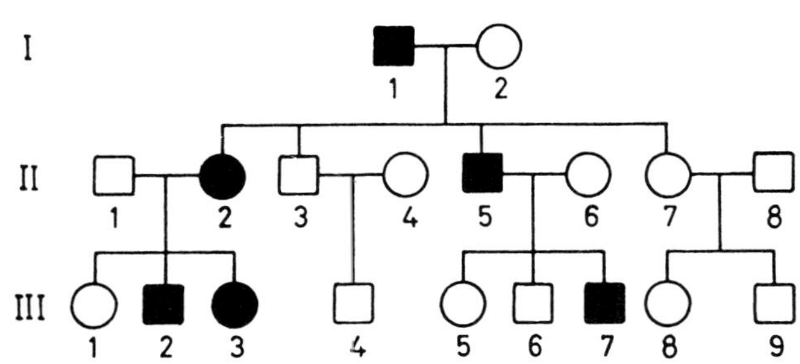


**Fig. 1–12.** Stereotype pedigree of autosomal dominant inheritance. (From Der Kaloustian and Kurban, *Genetic Diseases of the Skin*, Springer-Verlag, Berlin, 1979, pp. 1–16,[29] with permission.)

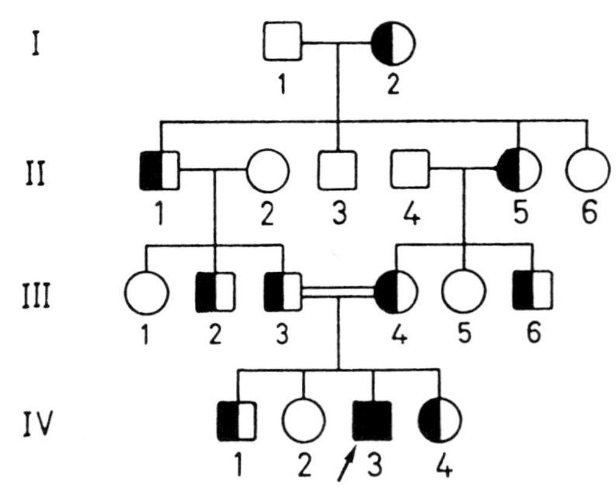


**Fig. 1–13.** Stereotype pedigree of autosomal recessive inheritance. (From Der Kaloustian and Kurban, *Genetic Diseases of the Skin*, Springer-Verlag, Berlin, 1979, pp. 1–16,[29] with permission.)

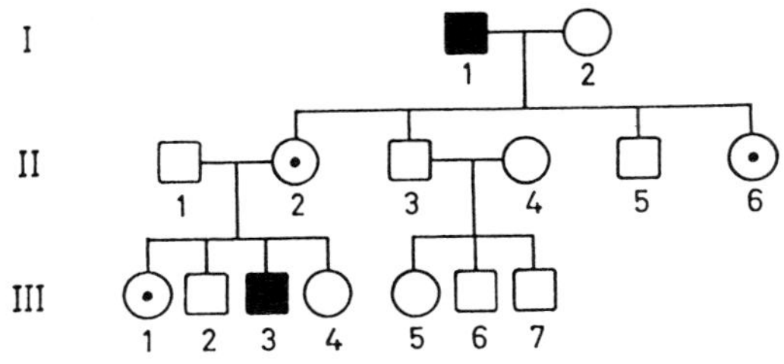


**Fig. 1–14.** Stereotype pedigree of X-linked recessive inheritance. (From Der Kaloustian and Kurban, *Genetic Diseases of the Skin,* Springer Verlag, Berlin, 1979 pp. 1–16,[29] with permission.)

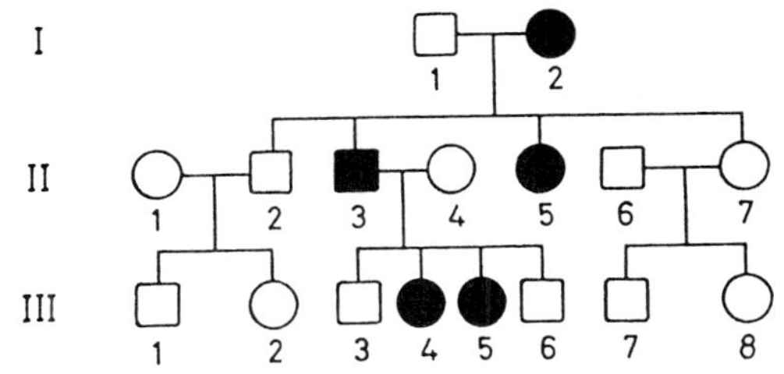


**Fig. 1–15.** Stereotype pedigree of X-linked dominant inheritance. (From Der Kaloustian and Kurban, *Genetic Diseases of the Skin,* Springer Verlag, Berlin, 1979, pp. 1–16,[29] with permission.)

syndrome, while the parents are normal. It is thus important, when counseling families with a child affected with one of these conditions (and probably others with autosomal dominant inheritance), to inform them that the recurrence risk is very low but not negligible. These families should be offered appropriate prenatal diagnostic tests.

## Genomic imprinting

According to the principles of mendelian inheritance, a child receives one set of genes from the father and another from the mother. Until recently, it was assumed that both the paternal and the maternal genes are expressed in the child. Thus, in autosomal recessively inherited metabolic disorders, it had been accepted that each normal gene provides information for half of the normal amount of the enzyme, so that heterozygotes for severe mutations have approximately 50% of the enzymatic activity of normals.

We now know that some genes are normally inactivated when transmitted by the father, while others are inactivated when transmitted by the mother. This process of different expression of genes according to their parental origin is called *imprinting* and may influence the manifestation of specific disorders.[105] Well-documented examples of imprinting are Prader-Willi syndrome (PWS),[30,37] Angelman syndrome (AS), and Beckwith-Wiedemann syndrome (BWS).[105]

In Prader-Willi and Angelman syndromes, there may be deletion of a segment of the long arm of one of the #15 chromosomes (15q11–q13). While in Prader-Willi syndrome the deleted chromosome is of paternal origin, in Angelman syndrome it is of maternal origin. Thus, it is thought that the specific gene responsible for Prader-Willi syndrome is normally inactivated in the maternally inherited chromosome and active in the one that is paternally inherited. With deletion of the 15q11–q13 in the paternally inherited chromosome, the active allele is lost and this causes Prader-Willi syndrome. The reverse is true for Angelman syndrome, where the active gene is on the maternal chromosome (Fig. 1–17). The genes for PWS and AS have not been identified yet, although there are many proposals for candidate genes.[16,46,73,117a,134]

A subset of patients with AS and PWS have apparently normal chromosomes of biparental origin, but abnormal DNA methylation at several loci within the chromosomal region of 15q11–q13. An inherited microdeletion has been identified in certain AS and PWS families. The deletions probably affect a single genetic element that is termed the 15q11–q13 *imprinting center* (IC). Mutations of the imprinting center may be transmitted silently through the germ-line of one sex, but appear to block the resetting of the imprint in the germ line of the opposite sex.[17,35a]

In certain patients with AS or PWS, no 15q11–q13 deletion is identified. It has been found, however, that in the patients with AS, both chromosome 15s are of paternal origin, thus lacking the maternal (active) allele, while in the patients with PWS, both chromosome 15s are of maternal origin, thus lack-

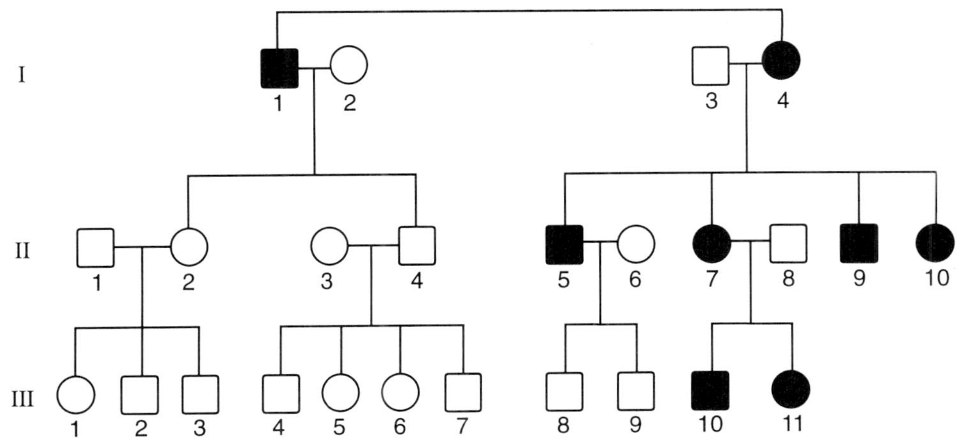


**Fig. 1–16.** Stereotype pedigree of mitochondrial inheritance. (From Thompson et al., *Genetics in Medicine,* 5th ed., WB Saunders, Philadelphia, 1991, pp. 89,[129] with permission.)

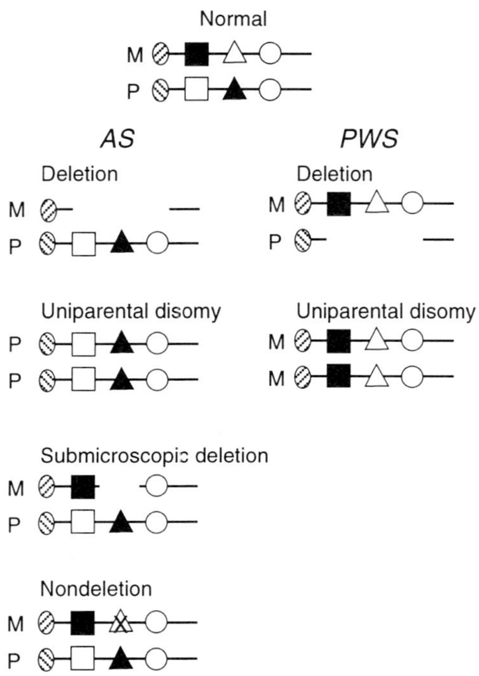


**Fig. 1–17.** Model for gene activity of 15q11-q13 loci in normal individuals and in individuals with Angelman syndrome (AS) or Prader-Willi syndrome (PWS): Hatched ovals denote chromosome 15 centromeres, with different directions of hatching indicating maternal (M) or paternal (P) origin of the centromere. Open symbols indicate active genes; shaded symbols indicate inactive or hypoactive genes. Triangles indicate genes preferentially active on maternal chromosomes (type I); squares indicate genes preferentially active on paternal chromosomes (type II); and circles indicate genes active to equal extents on maternal and paternal chromosomes (type III). Mechanisms that can give rise to Angelman syndrome include maternally inherited visible or submicroscopic deletions that remove type I genes, paternal uniparental disomy, or mutation in type I gene(s). Mechanisms that can lead to Prader-Willi syndrome include paternal deletions that involve type II genes or maternal uniparental disomy. (From Wagstaff et al., Nat Genet 1:291–294, 1992,[134] with permission.)

ing the paternal (active) allele. This situation, where both chromosomes of the same pair are from the same parent, is called *uniparental disomy* (Fig. 1–17).[90]

Whereas Prader-Willi syndrome and Angelman syndrome result from the lack of active gene(s) (of maternal origin in Angelman syndrome and of paternal origin in Prader-Willi syndrome), in Beckwith-Wiedemann syndrome, the disorder is due to the duplication of an active gene.[75] The gene for BWS is on chromosome 11p15 and is related to the one that codes for insulin growth factor 2 (IGF2), which seems to play a role predominantly during fetal development.[106,116] The paternally inherited allele is normally active and the maternally inherited one is inactive. In patients with BWS, one of three types of genetic mechanisms may be present. The gene on the paternally inherited chromosome is duplicated, or there is uniparental disomy, with both chromosomes 11 being of paternal origin. There may also be a mutation on the maternally inherited chromosome 11, derepressing the gene and thus allowing again the expression of a doubledose.[140] Recently it has been suggested that there may be more than one locus involved in the pathogenesis of BWS.[104,139]

### Uniparental disomy

Uniparental disomy is not limited to imprinted genes and may involve other loci on the autosomes or sex chromosomes (e.g., the case of a female with cystic fibrosis and short stature who was found to have two identical copies of most or all of her maternal chromosome 7, or the case of a father-to-son transmission of hemophilia A, in which an affected boy inherited both his X and Y chromosomes from his father and no sex chromosomes from his mother).[120]

### Triplet repeats

Most genes are considered to be transmitted unaltered through the generations of a family. However, certain genes have been recently found to undergo a specific pattern of changes in successive generations. These changes involve a gradually increasing (or occasionally decreasing) number of triplet repeats.

The prototype of this group of diseases is the fragile-X syndrome where the repeats are those of the CGG triplet at the 5′ untranslated region of the *FMR-1* gene (Fig. 1–18). Normally, between 6 and 60 CGG repeats are present. Expansion to more than 200 repeats is seen in affected, fully expressing males. When the CGG repeats are in the range between 60 and 200, they constitute premutations, which are meiotically unstable and may undergo either expansion or reduction in triplet repeat size.[109,110,143] The phenotypically normal males are referred to as *transmitting males*. In a pedigree where transmitting males are identified, it is expected that the newer generations may have affected, fully expressing males. This phenomenon is called *anticipation*. There are several other conditions known to be associated with CTG or CAG repeats (e.g., myotonic dystrophy, Huntington disease, Kennedy disease, and androgen receptor defect).

## Polygenic and multifactorial inheritance

Polygenic inheritance (also called quantitative) is difficult to analyze. In this type of inheritance, the variability with respect to a given trait follows a normal distribution. These characteristics are called *continuous traits*. Examples of these are head circumference, height, and interpupillary distance.[122] However, even though the distribution is continuous, a threshold effect for certain phenotypic manifestations or congenital anomalies may make it appear discontinuous (Fig. 1–19).[18,39] On the other hand, the term *multifactorial causation* connotes a combined genetic and environmental etiology.[40,107] Several of the more common human congenital anomalies, especially the neural tube defects and cleft lip and palate, are included among these traits.[41]

The characteristics expected in multifactorial causation are as follows:

1. The disorder is familial but without a distinctive pattern of inheritance.
2. The risk to first-degree relatives is approximately the square root of the population risk.
3. For common threshold disorders the risk for first degree relatives is usually between 2 and 5%. The risk is about one-fourth that for second-degree relatives and one-tenth as high for third-degree relatives.
4. The recurrence risk is higher when more than one family member is affected. It is about double after the birth of a second affected first-degree relative.

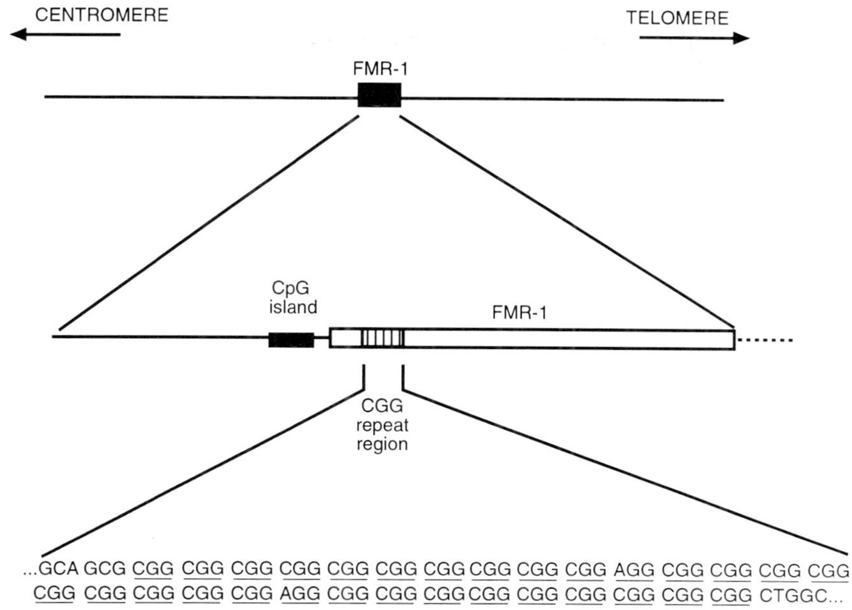


**Fig. 1–18.** The gene of familial mental retardation 1 (FMR-1). Note the CGG repeat region with 28 CGGs, interrupted on two occasions by AGG triplets. (Modified from Tarleton and Saul, J Pediatr 122:169–185, 1993,[126] with permission.)

5. The more severe the malformation is in the index case, the greater is the recurrence risk.
6. The recurrence risk increases if the index case is of the sex less frequently affected in that particular condition.
7. The recurrence risk is increased when the parents are consanguineous.

The genes and environmental factors involved in conditions of multifactorial causation do not have to be a large number. Nutritional variations are suspected to be strong environmental contributors prenatally.[122] In this respect, pre- and periconceptional supplementation of folic acid may reduce the incidence of neural tube defects, both in the isolated form[88] and the forms associated with other anomalies, and perhaps also in other malformations.[69a]

### Contiguous gene syndromes

*Contiguous gene syndromes* (CGS) are "a group of clinically recognizable disorders characterized by a deletion or a duplication of a chromosomal segment spanning multiple disease genes, each independently contributing to the phenotype."[79]

Contiguous gene syndromes are also termed *segmental aneusomy,* resulting from gene dosage imbalance at certain parts of the chromosomes. These syndromes provide approaches and hypotheses to explain phenotypic variability of clinical conditions, which should not be necessarily attributed to the variation in expressivity of a single gene. However, these phenotypes may have different components, each of which may be caused by the absence of a separate gene, as part of the microdeletion. Consequently, it is possible that mutations may occur in any single gene in a contiguous gene complex, producing a specific phenotypic manifestation, without disturbing the functions of the adjacent genes.[122] This pathogenetic mechanism has been strongly suggested recently in the case of the DiGeorge syndrome.[4,15,47] Examples of conditions that possibly have this etiologic mechanism are the tricho-rhino-pharyngeal syndrome with exostoses,[77] the WAGR syndrome (**W**ilms tumor, **A**niridia, **G**enital anomalies, **R**etardation),[89] DiGeorge syndrome,[47] Prader-Willi syndrome,[73] Angelman syndrome[134] and others (Table 1–2).[79,80,115]

## The human chromosomes

### Classification and techniques

The normal human chromosomal number of 46 (instead of the 48 previously assumed) was established by Tjio and Levan in 1956.[13,133] Of the 46 chromosomes in human cells, 44 are au-

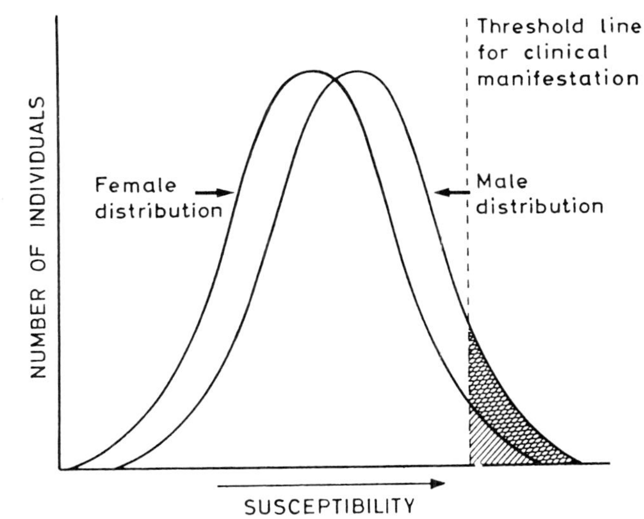


**Fig. 1–19.** Curve of multifactorial inheritance. Note quasicontinuous variation. (From Der Kaloustian and Kurban, *Genetic Diseases of the Skin,* Springer-Verlag, 1979, pp. 1–16,[29] with permission.)

**Table 1–2.** Cytogenetic and molecular findings in autosomal contiguous gene syndromes (CGS)

| Chromosome region | CGS | Cytogenetic deletion/ duplication | Molecular deletion/ duplication | Uniparental disomy |
|---|---|---|---|---|
| 7q11.23 | Williams | 2 cases | >99% | — |
| 8q24.1 | Langer-Giedion | 75% | >90% | — |
| 11p13 | WAGR | >90% | >90% | — |
| 11p15.5 | Beckwith-Wiedemann | 15 cases | — | 25% |
| 15q11-q13 | Prader-Willi | 70% | 70% | 20–25% |
| | Angelman | 85% | 85% | <5% |
| 16p13.3 | Alpha thalassemia with mental retardation | — | — | — |
| 16p13.3 | Rubinstein-Taybi | 0% | 25% | — |
| 17p13.3 | Miller-Dieker | 50% | >90% | — |
| | Isolated lissencephaly | 0% | ~33% | — |
| 17p11.2 | Smith-Magenis | 100% | 100% | — |
| 20p11.23-p12.2 | Alagille | 16 cases | — | — |
| 22q11.2 | DiGeorge | ~33% | >90% | — |
| | Velo-cardio-facial | 3 cases | >90% | — |

*Three cases with balanced translocation
Modified from Ledbetter and Ballabio,[79] with permission

tosomes and 2 are sex chromosomes. The autosomes constitute 22 homologous pairs. The sex chromosomes are two Xs in normal females and an X and a Y in normal males. Each pair of autosomes is serially numbered from 1 to 22, more or less in descending order of length, and grouped according to the position of the centromere. The chromosomes are described as *metacentric, submetacentric,* or *acrocentric,* depending on whether the centromere is at the center of the chromosome, near the center, or near the end, respectively. The acrocentric chromosomes (except the Y) possess small terminal projections known as *satellite bodies.*

From 1970 on, a more accurate identification of human chromosomes was facilitated by several banding techniques: *Q banding* (quinacrine fluorescence),[19] *C banding* (centromeric banding),[3] *R banding* (reverse banding),[33] and *G banding* (Giemsa banding).[125] Q and G banding patterns are essentially the same. R banding patterns are the reverse of those of G banding. C banding demonstrates mainly the centromeric area with its polymorphisms. These techniques allow identification of each human chromosome individually, since each chromosome has a specific banding pattern. The Giemsa or G banding technique is the one mostly used because it provides the necessary general information to distinguish individual chromosomes and particular areas of each chromosome, and it facilitates the identification of chromosomal aberrations. All four banding methods (Q, C, R, and G) are helpful under different circumstances and complementary in the information that they provide.

*High-resolution banding* (prophase or prometaphase banding) is a more detailed G or R banding technique and is attained when the chromosomes are prepared at an early stage of mitosis and are still in a relatively uncondensed state. This is not a routine procedure. It is resorted to when a specific, subtle, structural chromosomal abnormality is suspected. Whereas standard metaphase preparations show about 400 bands, high-resolution banding reveals 550–850 or more bands in a haploid set (Figs. 1–20, 1–21).[127]

The *International System of Human Chromosome Nomenclature* is the standardized numbering system for all chromosome bands (Fig. 1–22). According to this system, the short and long arms are designated *p* and *q* respectively. The arms are divided numerically into larger regions and then into subregions or bands. The regions and bands are numbered, proceeding from the centromere to the distal part of the arm.[92]

*Fluorescence in situ hybridization* (FISH) is a method based on the hybridization of a single-strand DNA sequence (probe) with its complementary strand on a particular chromosome. It allows the direct localization of a given DNA sequence on a chromosome. *Centromere probes* recognize the repetitive sequences of each chromosome in the centromeric region. *Painting probes* identify sequences specific to each chromosome. *Unique-sequence probes* recognize a particular locus. Besides the primary use for refined gene mapping, FISH is a powerful and complementary tool for the identification of small chromosomal anomalies not revealed by routine karyotype analysis or even prophase banding, e.g., submicroscopic deletion, duplication, or translocation. This method is now used routinely to diagnose certain patients with DiGeorge or Velo-cardio-facial syndrome (22q11 deletions) (Fig. 1–23),[28,31,50] Williams syndrome (deletion of the elastin gene),[35,91] as well as Prader-Willi and Angelman syndromes. It is important to note that DNA analysis cannot distinguish between a normal karyotype and one in which a balanced rearrangement has occurred. This may be diagnosed by karyotype analysis for larger rearrangements and FISH studies for submicroscopic ones. In certain cases of deletions or trisomies, the diagnosis may be confirmed by testing interphase cells, without resorting to cultures.[14,72,100]

*Chromosome painting* is another fluorescence technique, used to establish the origin of a marker chromosome or the site where a small chromosomal piece may be translocated.[61]

Human chromosome analysis can be performed directly on dividing cells or after their culture. Direct techniques involve the bone marrow, gonadal tissue (for meiotic studies),

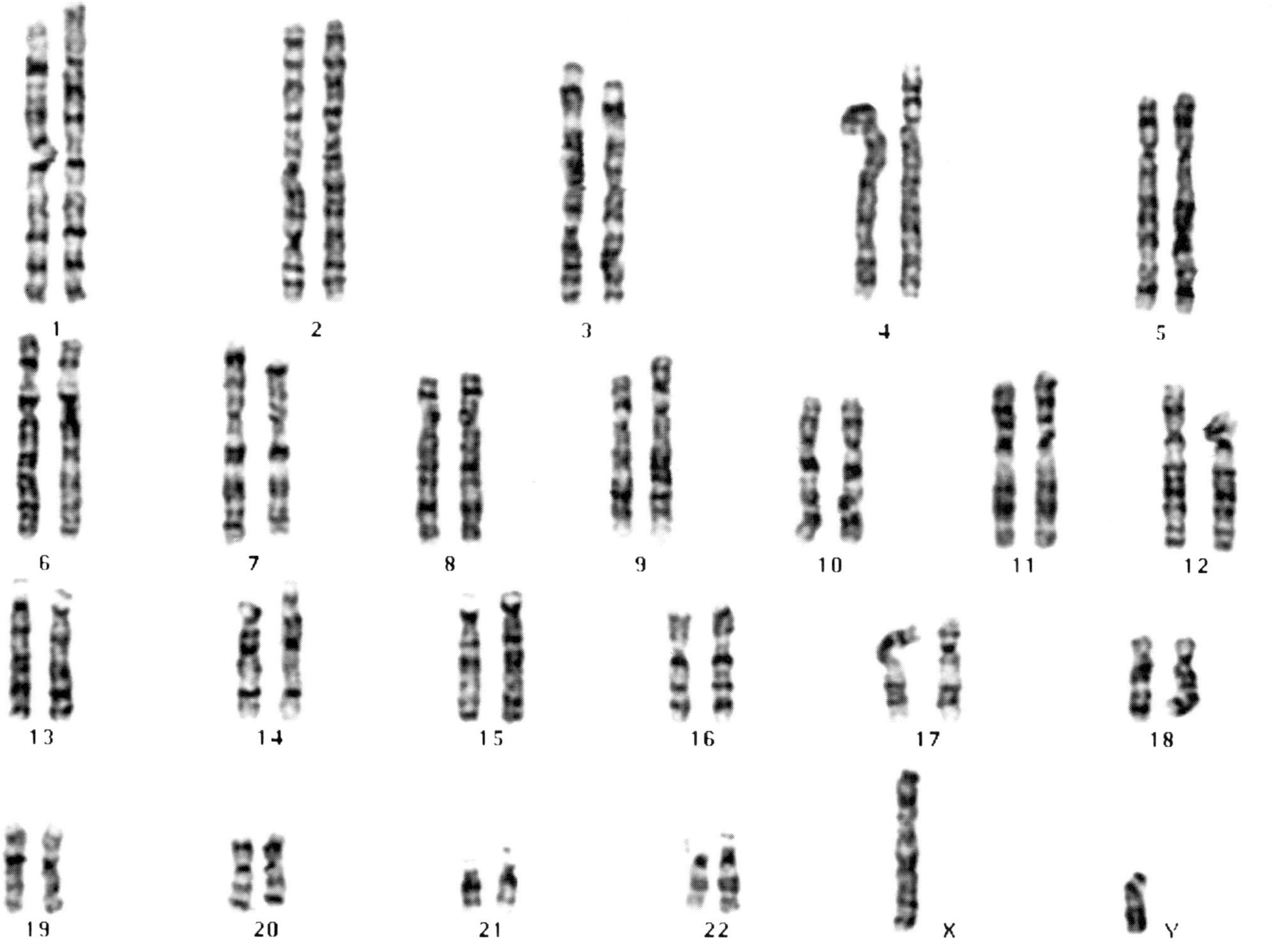


**Fig. 1–20.** Human karyotype with high-resolution G-banding technique. (Courtesy of Dr. P. Eydoux.)

cells from chorionic villus samples obtained for prenatal diagnosis, or other material such as peritoneal and pleural effusions, cerebrospinal fluid, and cells from various solid tumors. Culture techniques involve mainly lymphocytes, bone marrow cells, cells from chorionic villus samples, amniocytes, skin, and less so, the testis, ovary, and most fetal tissues.[12,48,53,86]

Peripheral blood is easily accessible and thus represents the most convenient material for human chromosomal analysis. Lymphocytes, with appropriate stimulation, grow and divide rapidly in culture. Since the technique is relatively easy and reliable, it is used for routine karyotyping.[55] Permanent cell lines can also be established from lymphocytes using special methods.[130] Skin biopsies, which are also easily accessible, provide long-term multiplication of fibroblasts for many generations. In many laboratories, both lymphocyte and fibroblast permanent lines are stored in liquid nitrogen in special repositories. They are thus available to be used at later dates for chromosomal, biochemical, histochemical, or molecular studies[55,130] (Table 1–3).

### Chromosomal aberrations

The prevalence of chromosomal anomalies in live-born infants is more than 1%. About half of live-born affected individuals have autosomal anomalies and half have sex chromosomal anomalies.[101]

The association of a numerical chromosomal aberration with a syndrome was first described in 1959,[81] when it was demonstrated that children with Down syndrome have 47 chromosomes in each somatic cell instead of the normal 46. The most important mechanism leading to a numerical aberration is *nondisjunction.* This represents failure of chromosomes to pair or failure of chromosomes or sister chromatids to disjoin at anaphase either in mitotic division or in the first or second meiotic divisions. Other syndromes resulting from abnormalities of chromosome number include trisomy 13, trisomy 18, Turner syndrome (XO), Klinefelter syndrome (XXY), or the XXX syndrome. When nondisjunction occurs more than once in gametogenesis, the zygote may be XXXY, XXXX, XXYY, XXXXX, or XXXXY. Although monosomy X Turner syndrome is relatively common, absence of the X in a male is lethal. Autosomal monosomies are also generally considered to be lethal, with some rare exceptions.[27,52] If nondisjunction occurs during an early cleavage division of the zygote, the offspring will have two or more lines of cells with different chromosomal numbers (mosaicism). Depending on the percentage of cells with the abnormal chromosomal number, a patient may have more severe or milder manifestations of a syndrome.

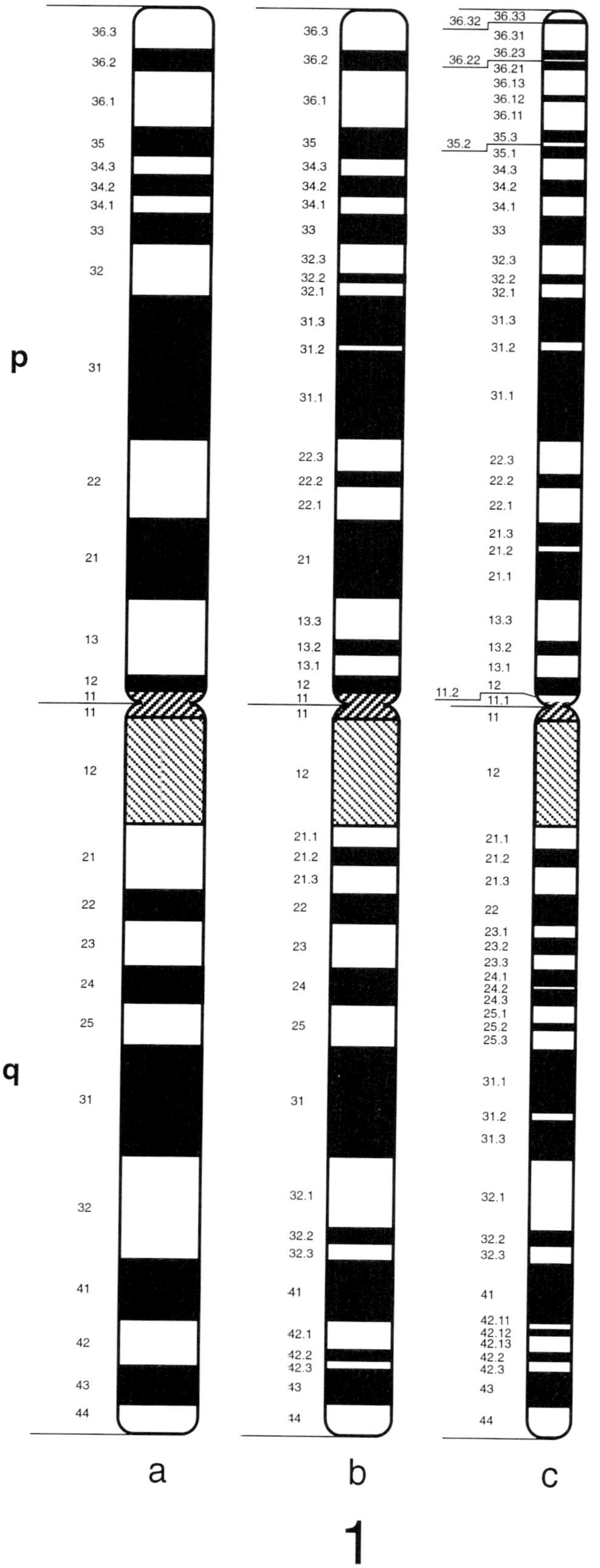


**Fig. 1–21.** G-banding pattern for normal human chromosome 1 with three different degrees of condensation. a: a karyotype of 400 bands in 23 chromosomes; b: a karyotype of approximately 550 bands; and c: a karyotype of approximately 850 bands. p and q = arms of chromosome. (From Harnden and Klinger, eds., *ISCN: an International System for Human Cytogenetic Nomenclature,* Basel, Karger, 1985[57] with permission.)

Aberrations of chromosome structure include deletions, inversions, translocations, isochromosomes, dicentrics, acentrics, and rings. A *deletion* is the loss of a portion of a chromosome, either terminal or interstitial. An *inversion* occurs when there are two breaks on the same chromosome, followed by the inversion of the segment upon reunion. An inversion may be paracentric (with the breaks on the same arm) or pericentric (with the breaks on opposite sides of the centromere). *Translocations* involve the breaking of a segment of a chromosome with transfer to another chromosome. *Reciprocal translocations* involve the exchange of segments between two nonhomologous chromosomes. *Robertsonian translocations* (centric fusion) are a special type of translocation in which the breaks occur at the centromeres of the acrocentric chromosomes and whole arms of chromosomes are joined. An *isochromosome* is an abnormal chromosome with two arms of equal length and bearing the same loci in reverse sequence. It results from transverse rather than longitudinal splitting of the centromere. A *dicentric* chromosome and an *acentric* fragment may be formed by a single crossover in a paracentric inversion. However, they can also

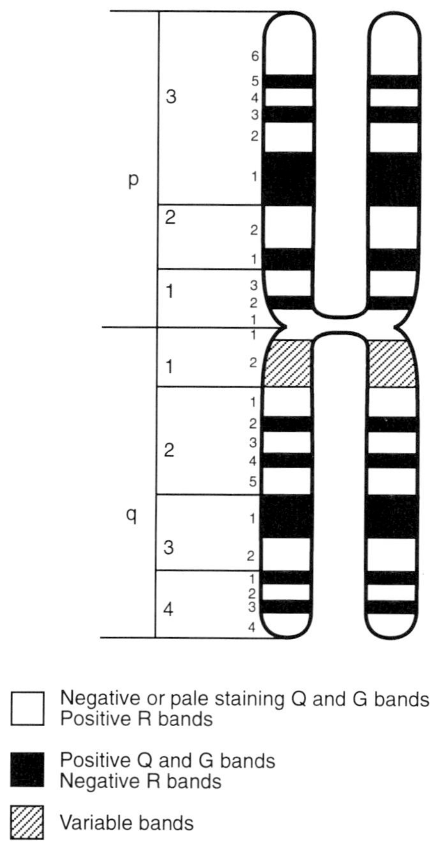


**Fig. 1–22.** Standard numbering system of chromosome bands. The arms, designated as *p* and *q,* are first divided into regions, then into subregions or bands, according to a sort of decimal system. At higher resolution, single bands can be seen to break up into multiple finer bands. The regions and bands are numbered, proceeding from the proximal arm (near the centromere) to the distal arm (near the telomere). It must be noted that band 1q32 is not band 32 on the long arm of chromosome 1; it is the second band in region 3 of the long arm (and should be read as "q three two" and not "q thirty-two". (From Nora et al., *Medical Genetics: Principles and Practices,* 4th ed., Lea and Febiger, Philadelphia, 1994, pp. 10–34,[93] with permission.)

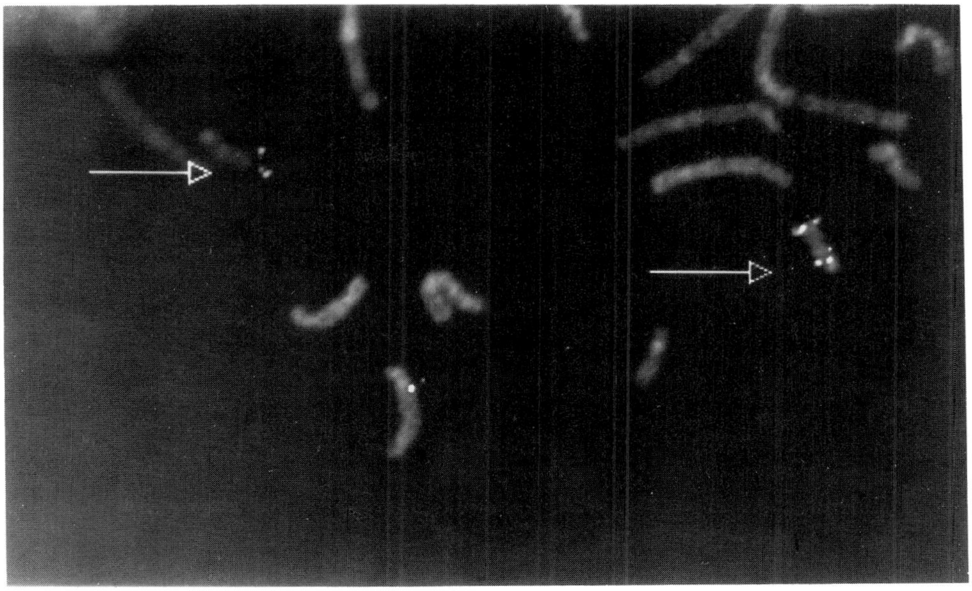

**Fig. 1–23.** Fluorescence in situ hybridization (FISH) in a karyotype of a patient with DiGeorge syndrome (DGS). Note the two sites of fluorescence (DGS-specific site and control) in normal chromosome 22 (arrow on the right). The fluorescence of the DGS-specific site is absent in the abnormal chromosome 22 (arrow on the left). (Courtesy of Dr. P. Eydoux.)

arise in other ways. A *ring* chromosome results from terminal deletions of both arms with reunion of the ends carrying the centromere.[131] Separation of centromeres (chromosome puffs), primarily involving the acrocentric chromosomes and chromosomes 1, 9, and 16, have been found in patients with Roberts syndrome (SC phocomelia) and Baller-Gerold syndrome.[98] *Fragile sites* are nonstaining gaps that are seen at characteristic regions of various chromosomes. These are mostly normal heritable variants. The only fragile sites that are clinically significant are on the long arm of the X chromosome (Xq). One of them, at Xq27.3, results in the fragile X syndrome.[109,110] Fragile sites are best visualized (Fig. 1–24) by special techniques involving particular culture media.[127]

Unbalanced chromosomal aberrations (i.e., those resulting in an excess or lack of chromosomal material) are responsible for many dysmorphogenetic syndromes and conditions associated with mental retardation. Chromosomal breaks may also produce syndromes associated with immunodeficiency and predisposing to neoplastic changes, for examples Fanconi pancytopenia,[5,45] Bloom syndrome,[10] ataxia telangiectasia,[11,114] and Nijmegen breakage syndrome.[21,28a,138] Microdeletion syndromes involving very small parts of chromosomes are usually not detectable even by high-resolution banding techniques and require FISH (e.g., Prader-Willi syndrome, Angelman syndrome, DiGeorge syndrome). Finally, chromosomal aberrations are present in a high percentage of human abortions[70] and are associated with many neoplasms.[131]

Although we know little about the genetic and environmental factors causing or predisposing to chromosomal aberrations, it is clear that late maternal age,[54] genes that increase chromosomal instability in somatic cells,[44] radiation,[9] and chemicals[9] may be involved in their pathogenesis.

Karyotypes are represented by abbreviations based on a report of the Standing Committee of Human Cytogenetic Nomenclature (Table 1–3).[57]

### Assignment of genes to human chromosomes

The assignment of a gene locus to either the X or the Y chromosome may be achieved by studying pedigrees that reveal a specific pattern of inheritance. The assignment of loci to autosomes and their mapping[85] is more complicated. Presently, with the availablility of numerous molecular markers for each human chromosome, the assignment of gene loci to specific chromosomes has become relatively simpler and more rapid.[96] Fluorescence in situ hybridization may also help to situate and clarify the sequence of genes or markers on a chromosome. By October 1995, 3405 genes had been assigned to specific chromosomes (Table 1–1) (VA McKusick, personal communication).

## Genetic and environmental interactions

Phenotypes are the result of the interaction of "nature" and "nurture," the genes and the environment. Specific environmental factors, or teratogens, may be responsible for certain pathologic conditions. Issues related to these and their pathogenesis are discussed in detail in Chapter 4.

## Dysmorphology

*Dysmorphology* is the study of recognizable morphologic abnormalities, their etiology, and their developmental pathogenesis. Individual physical findings may fall within the range of "normal" human variation. However, the extremes of this variation (arbitrarily defined as $<$ 2d centile or $>$ 98th centile) may represent "abnormality" or inadequate function (e.g., microcephaly, macrocephaly, low-set ears, and telecanthus). Assessment of individual morphologic findings thus depends fre-

**Table 1–3.** Some abbreviations used for description of chromosomes and their abnormalities and representative examples

| Abbreviation | Meaning | Example | Condition |
|---|---|---|---|
| | | 46,XX | Normal female karyotype |
| | | 46,XY | Normal male karyotype |
| cen | Centromere | | |
| del | Deletion | 46,XX,del(5p) | Female with cri du chat syndrome due to deletion of part of short arm of one chromosome 5 |
| der | Derivative chromosome | der(1) | Translocation chromosome derived from chromosme 1 and containing centromere of chromosome 1 |
| dic | Dicentric chromosome | dic(X;Y) | Translocation chromosome containing centromeres from both X and Y chromosomes |
| dup | Duplication | | |
| fra | Fragile site | 46,Y,fra(X)(q27.3) | Male with fragile X chromosome |
| i | Isochromosome | 46,X,i(Xq) | Female with isochromosome for long arm of X chromosome |
| ins | Insertion | | |
| inv | Inversion | inv(3)(p25q21) | Pericentric inversion of chromosome 3 |
| mar | Marker chromosome | 47,XX, + mar | Female with an extra, unidentified chromosome |
| mat | Maternal origin | 47,XY, + der(1)mat | Male with additional der(1) translocation chromosome inherited from his mother |
| p | Short arm of chromosome | | |
| pat | Paternal origin | | |
| q | Long arm of chromosome | | |
| r | Ring chromosome | 46,X,r(X) | Female with ring X chromosome |
| rcp | Reciprocal translocation | | |
| rob | Robertsonian translocation | | |
| t | Translocation | 46,XX,t(2;8)(q21;p13) | Female with balanced translocation between chromosome 2 and chromosome 8, with breaks in 2q21 and 8p13 |
| ter | Terminus | 46,X,Xq-(pter→q21:) | Female with partial deletion of long arm from Xq21 to Xqter (nomenclature shows portion of the chromosome that is present) |
| + | Gain of | 47,XX, + 21 | Female with trisomy 21 |
| − | Loss of | 45,XX, − 14, − 21, + t(14q21q) | Normal female carrier of a Robertsonian translocation between long arms of chromosomes 14 and 21; karyotype is missing a normal 14 and a normal 21 |
| | | 4p − | Chromosome 4 with a portion of short arm deleted |
| : | Break | 5qter→5p15: | Deleted chromosome 5 in patient with cri du chat syndrome, with a deletion breakpoint in band p15 |
| :: | Break and join | 2pter→2q21::8p13→8pter | Description of der(2) portion of t(2;8) |
| / | Mosaicism | 46,XX/47,XX, + 8 | Female with two populations of cells, one with a normal karyotype and one with trisomy 8 |

From Thompson et al.[131] with permission

quently on measurements and the interpretation of "normality" or "abnormality", based on the norms established by growth charts (see Chapter 2). Moreover, morphologic findings that individually are not always considered as dysmorphic (e.g., myopia, deafness, high-arched palate, micrognathia) may collectively indicate the presence of a dysmorphic entity (e.g., Stickler syndrome).[64]

Fifty-eight percent of abnormal phenotypes affect more than a single system. Although no system is spared, the nervous system, musculoskeletal system, eye, and integument are most frequently involved, followed by craniofacial anomalies (Fig. 1–25).[26]

### Alterations of form or structure

Congenital anomalies may be properly classified if they are well defined. The emphasis on definition is dictated by an intricate relationship between terminology and nosology. The following definitions have been recommended by an international working group in 1982.[121]

A *malformation* (Fig. 1–26) is "a morphologic defect of an organ, part of an organ, or larger region of the body resulting from an intrinsically abnormal developmental process." Malformations may result from a variety of aberrant developmental mechanisms at the molecular, cellular, or tissue level (Table

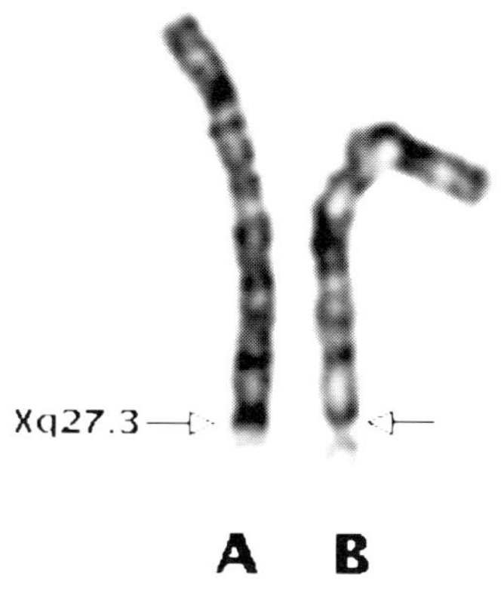


**Fig. 1–24.** The fragile site on the X chromosome. The chromosome on the left (A) is normal. The one on the right (B) has the fragile site, indicated by the arrow. (Courtesy of Dr. P. Eydoux.)

1–4).[49] They usually have their origin before the 10th week of gestation. A *major malformation* is defined as one that presents significant medical or psychologic problems (e.g., holoprosencephaly, arhinia). A *minor malformation* does not generally require medical intervention (e.g., clinodactyly, posteriorly angulated ears). Minor defects may be normal variations. The presence of more than two minor anomalies increases the possibility of the presence of an associated major defect and may help in diagnosing a significant dysmorphic condition.[82,117]

It is generally considered that most malformations are developmental field defects. A *developmental field* is "a region or a part of an embryo which responds as a coordinated unit to embryonic interaction and results in complex or multiple anatomic structures." A *single* developmental field may generate monotopic or polytopic field defects. A *monotopic* field defect represents localized anomalies. For example, a disturbance of prechordial mesoderm may produce clinical anomalies ranging from an isolated coloboma of the iris to the full pattern of alobar holoprosencephaly with cyclopia, proboscis, cleft lip/palate, etc.[121] *Polytopic* defects are considered by some to present a pattern of less closely contiguous anomalies as a result of long-distance inductive relationships (e.g., ear, branchial cleft, and renal anomalies in the BOR syndrome)[42] or the findings in the Shprintzen (velo-cardio-facial) syndrome.[63]

A *disruption* (Fig. 1–25) is "a morphogenetic defect of an organ, part of an organ, or a larger region of the body resulting from the extrinsic breakdown of, or an interference with, an originally normal developmental process." The extrinsic factor may be an infection, teratogen, or trauma (see Chapter 4). One of the most commonly observed disruptions results from early amnion rupture and pressure of *amniotic bands* on different parts of the body, producing such anomalies as amputations or clefts. Disruptions secondary to extrinsic factors usually have a negligible recurrence risk.

A *deformation* (Fig. 1–25) is "an abnormal form, shape, or position of a part of the body caused by mechanical forces." Examples of deformation are micrognathia or facial asymmetry. In general, deformations due to the mechanical forces of uterine constraint may resolve spontaneously and have a very low rate of recurrence in future pregnancies.

A *dysplasia* is an abnormal organization of cells into tissues and its morphologic results. The present use of the term is broad and applies to all abnormalities of histogenesis and not only those with neoplastic potential. For instance, Marfan syndrome and osteogenesis imperfecta are dysplasias because the abnormalities in each condition can be reduced to a defect in connective tissue, fibrilin, and collagen repectively.[121]

### Patterns of morphologic defects

Multiple anomalies in a given patient may have the same cause or pathogenesis, or they may occur together on a statistical basis or by chance alone.[121] Thus patterns of morphologic defects may represent a syndrome, a sequence, or an association.

A *sequence* is "a pattern of multiple anomalies from a single known or presumed prior anomaly or mechanical factor." The original factor or anomaly may give rise to a cascade of secondary problems in subsequent morphogenesis. Thus, in Robin sequence, severe micrognathia may be responsible for pressure of the embryonal tongue against the forming palate, resulting in inadequate closure of the palatal shelves and consequently, a cleft palate.

A *syndrome* is "a pattern of multiple anomalies thought to be pathogenetically related and not known to represent a single sequence or a polytopic field defect." With increasing knowledge in this area, a syndrome may turn out to represent a polytopic field defect or a sequence. The term syndrome often implies a single cause and should be used when the different anomalies are thought to be pathologically related (e.g., Stickler syndrome, Smith-Lemli-Opitz syndrome).

An *association* is "a nonrandom occurrence in two or more

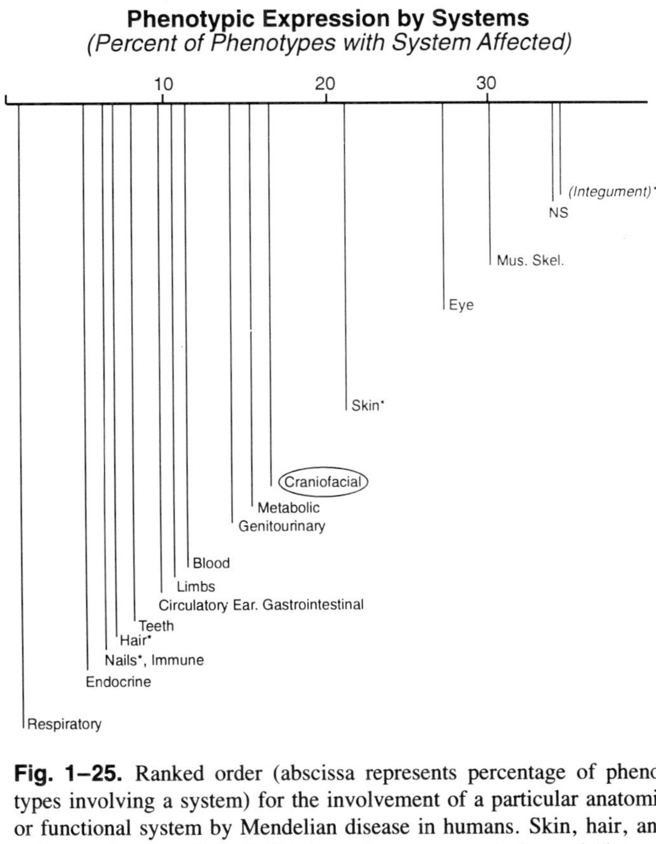


**Fig. 1–25.** Ranked order (abscissa represents percentage of phenotypes involving a system) for the involvement of a particular anatomic or functional system by Mendelian disease in humans. Skin, hair, and nails are shown both individually and as a group designated "integument." Mus. Skel. = musculoskeletal, NS = nervous system. Note the importance of craniofacial anomalies. (Modified from Costa et al., Am J Med Genet 21:231–242 1985,[26] with permission.)

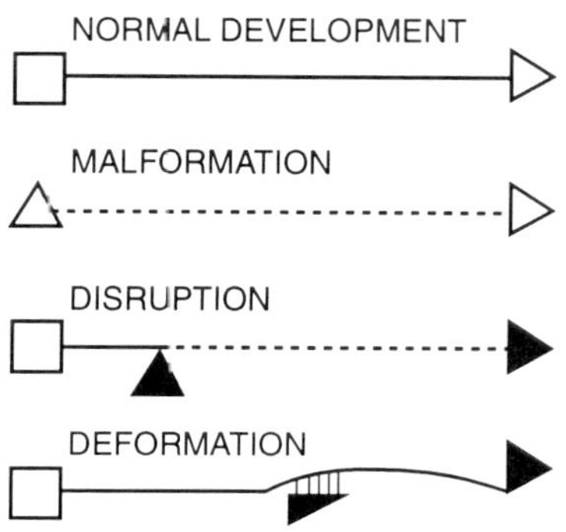


**Fig.1–26.** Diagrammatic representation of processes leading to malformation, disruption, and deformation. (From Spranger et al., J Pediatr 100:160–165 1982,[121] with permission.)

individuals of multiple anomalies not known to be a polytopic field defect, sequence or syndrome." Examples are the VACTERL association[68] or the CHARGE association.[34]

## Prevention and treatment of congenital anomalies

### Prevention

#### Genetic counseling

The American Society of Human Genetics has adopted the following definition of genetic counseling.[1,38] "Genetic counseling is a communication process which deals with the human problems associated with the occurrence, or the risk of occurrence, of a genetic disorder in a family. This process involves an attempt by one or more appropriately trained persons to help the individual or family

1. to comprehend the medical facts, including the diagnosis, the probable course of the disorder, and the available management;
2. to appreciate the way heredity contributes to the disorder, and the risk of recurrence in specified relatives;
3. to understand the options for dealing with the risks of recurrence;
4. to choose the course of action which seems appropriate to them in view of their risk, their family goals, and their ethical and religious standards, and to act in accordance with that decision; and
5. to make the best possible adjustment to the disorder in an affected family member and/or to the risk of recurrence of that disorder."

**Table 1–4.** Malformations resulting from specific aberrant developmental mechanisms

| Mechanism | Malformation |
|---|---|
| Deficient proliferation | Digital hypoplasia, microtia |
| Excess proliferation | Pachyonychia congenita |
| Aberrant differentiation | Hemangiomas, streak gonads |
| Aberrant migration | Lissencephaly, hypertelorism |
| Failure of induction | Biliary atresia |
| Failure of programmed cell death | Imperforate anus, syndactyly |
| Failure of tissue fusion | Cleft lip and palate, cleft earlobe |
| Premature fusion | Craniosynostosis |

After Graham and Teebi,[49] with permission

Proper counseling requires accurate diagnosis and thorough knowledge of the disease or anomaly in question, since certain phenotypes may be due to environmental causes, but may mimic specific genetic diseases. These are known as *phenocopies*. For example, fetal alcohol syndrome (environmental cause) may mimic Dubowitz syndrome (genetic cause, with autosomal recessive inheritance).

Counseling also requires adequate knowledge of the pattern of inheritance of diseases determined by a single gene. Certain conditions are heterogeneous and may have more than one pattern of inheritance (e.g., the Ehlers-Danlos syndrome). In the case of multifactorial conditions, statistical data of the recurrence risks must be available.

Ideally, genetic counseling should be nondirective and provided by clinical geneticists or genetic counselors in a tertiary health care set-up. However, if specialists in a certain field (e.g., an otolaryngologist) are reasonably well versed in the principles of genetics and up to date in their own field of specialty, counseling about the more common and well-established conditions may be provided away from the major tertiary health care center or a university hospital.

In the case of parents who are heterozygous for an autosomal recessive gene, artificial insemination by donor may be resorted to, using sperm from a person known not to be a carrier of the specific gene. In certain cases the possiblity of adoption may also be considered.

#### Pharmacologic modalities

As mentioned above, treatment with folic acid in the pre- and periconceptional period may reduce the risks of neural tube defects. However, pharmacological therapeutic modalities are relatively limited in number in genetic diseases.

#### Prenatal diagnosis

Prenatal diagnosis is possible mainly with the relatively new methods of detailed ultrasonography, amniocentesis, chorionic villus sampling, and, in special cases, cordocentesis or fetoscopy (see Chapter 5).

#### Preimplantation diagnosis

The techniques of preimplantation diagnosis are still experimental and limited to very few conditions. They are not applied in routine clinical medicine.

### Treatment

Patients with genetic diseases or significant congenital anomalies require a lot of understanding and moral support because of the chronic nature of their condition. Many of the inborn errors of metabolism are treated with special diets and vitamins. In the case of anomalies of the ear, nose, and throat, the main treatment modality seems to be surgical (e.g., plastic surgery of craniofacial anomalies, repair of cleft palate and cleft lip, and treatment of tracheoesophageal fistula).

## Conclusion

It is obviously impossible to cover all aspects of medical genetics in an introductory chapter. It is important, however, to use the different concepts presented here in the approach to patients with congenital anomalies of the ear, nose, and throat. Specific anomalies may occur independently or may be parts of syndromes. They may also have risks of recurrence in future pregnancies. Considering that areas of expertise may overlap in the management of certain conditions (e.g. cleft lip/palate or craniofacial anomalies), a "team approach" is indicated, with a close collaboration between pediatricians, family physicians, clinical geneticists, otolaryngologists, and plastic surgeons.

## References


1. Ad Hoc Committee on Genetic Counseling: Report to the American Society of Human Genetics. Am J Hum Genet 27:240–242, 1975.
2. Aoyama T, Francke U, Gasner C, Furthmayr H: Fibrillin abnormalities and prognosis in Marfan syndrome and related disorders. Am J Med Genet 58:169–176, 1995.
3. Arrighi FE, Hsu TC: Localization of heterochromatin in human chromosomes. Cytogenetics 10:81–86, 1971.
4. Aubry M, Demczuk S, Desmaze C, Aikem M, Aurias A, Julien A, Julien J-P, Rouleau GA: Isolation of a zinc finger gene consistently deleted in DiGeorge syndrome. Hum Mol Genet 2:1583–1587, 1993.
5. Auerbach AD, Rogatko A, Schroeder-Kurth TM: International Fanconi Anemia Registry: relation of clinical symptoms to diepoxybutane sensitivity. Blood 73:391–396, 1989.
6. Baldwin CT, Hoth CF, Macina RA, Milunsky A: Mutations in PAX3 that cause Waardenburg syndrome type I: ten new mutations and review of the literature. Am J Med Genet 58:115–122, 1995.
7. Bellus GA, Hefferon TW, Ortiz de Luna RI, Hecht JT, Horton WA, Machado M, Kaitila I, McIntosh I, Francomano CA: Achondroplasia is defined by recurrent G380R mutations of FGFR3. Am J Hum Genet 56:368–373, 1995.
8. Bennett RL, Steinhaus KA, Uhrich SB, O'Sullivan CK, Resta RG, Lochner-Doyle D, Markel DS, Vincent V, Hamanishi J: Recommendations for standardized human pedigree nomenclature. Am J Hum Genet 56:745–752, 1995.
9. Bloom AD: Induced chromosomal aberrations in man. In: Advances in Human Genetics, Vol. 3. Harris 4, K Hirschhorn, eds. Plenum Press, New York, 1972, pp 99–172.
10. Bloom D: The syndrome of congenital telangiectatic erythema and stunted growth: observations and studies. J Pediatr 68:103–113, 1966.
11. Boder E: Ataxia-telangiectasia: an overview. In: Ataxia-telangiectasia: Genetics, Neuropathology, and Immunology of a Degenerative Disease of Childhood, RA Gatti, M Swift, eds. Alan R Liss, New York, 1985, pp 1–63.
12. Boehm CS: Prenatal diagnosis and carrier detection by DNA analysis. Prog Med Genet 7:143–179, 1988.
13. Book JA, Chu EHY, Ford CE, Fraccaro M, Harnden DG, Hsu TC, Hungerford DA, Jacobs PA, Lejeune J, Levan A, Makino S, Puck TT, Robinson A, Tjio JH, Catcheside DG, Muller HJ, Stern C: A proposed standard system of nomenclature of human mitotic chromosomes. Am J Hum Genet 12:384–388, 1960.
14. Breuning MH, Dauwerse HG, Fugazza G, Saris JJ, Sprint L, Wijnen H, Tommerup N, van der Hagen CB, Imaizumi K, Kuroki Y, et al: Rubinstein-Taybi syndrome caused by submicroscopic deletions within 16p13.3. Am J Hum Genet 52:249–254, 1993.
15. Budarf ML, Collins J, Gong W, Roe B, Wang Z, Bailey LC, Sellinger B, Michaud D, Driscoll DA, Emanuel BS: Cloning a balanced translocation associated with DiGeorge syndrome and identification of a disrupted candidate gene. Nat Genet 10:269–278, 1995.
16. Buiting K, Dittrich B, Groß S, Greger V, Lalande M, Robinson W, Mutirangura A, Ledbetter D, Horsthemke B: Molecular definition of the Prader-Willi syndrome chromosome region and orientation of the SNRPN gene. Hum Mol Genet 2:1991–1994, 1993.
17. Buiting K, Saitoh S, Groß S, Dittrich B, Schwartz S, Nicholls RD, Horsthemke B: Inherited microdeletions in the Angelman and Prader-Willi syndromes define an imprinting centre on human chromosome 15. Nat Genet 9:395–400, 1995.
18. Carter CO: Genetics of common disorders. Br Med Bull 25:52–57, 1969.
19. Caspersson T, Lomakka G, Zech L: The 24 fluorescence patterns of the human metaphase chromosomes—distinguishing characters and variability. Hereditas 67:89–102, 1972.
20. Chitayat D, Hodgkinson KA, Azouz EM: Intrafamilial variability in cleidocranial dysplasia: a three generation family. Am J Med Genet 42:298–303, 1992.
21. Chrzanowska KH, Kleijer WJ, Krajewska-Walasek M, Bialecka M, Gutkowska A, Goryluk-Kozakiewicz B, Michalkiewicz J, Stachowski J, Gregorek H, Lyson-Wolciechowska G, Janowicz W, Jozwiak S: Eleven Polish patients with microcephaly, immunodeficiency and chromosomal instability: the Nijmegen breakage syndrome. Am J Med Genet 57:462–471, 1995.
22. Clarke LA: Mitochondrial disorders in pediatrics. Clinical, biochemical and genetic implications. Pediatr Clin North Am 39:319–334, 1992.
23. Cohen MM Jr: Craniosynostoses: Phenotypic/molecular correlations. Am J Med Genet 56:334–339, 1995.
24. Cohen MM Jr: Syndrome delineation and heterogeneity. In: Hereditary Hearing Loss and its Syndromes, RJ Gorlin, HV Toriello, MM Cohen, Jr, eds. Oxford University Press, New York, 1995, pp 5–8.
25. Cohn DH, Starman BJ, Blumberg B, Byers PH: Recurrence of lethal osteogenesis imperfecta due to parental mosaicism in a human type I collagen gene (Col 1A1). Am J Hum Genet 46:591–601, 1990.
26. Costa T, Scriver CR, Childs B: The effect of mendelian disease on human health: a measurement. Am J Med Genet 21:231–242, 1985.
27. DeCicco F, Steele MW, Pan S, Park SC: Monosomy of chromosome No.22: a case report. J Pediatr 83:836–838, 1973.
28. Demczuk S, Desmaze C, Aikem M, Prieur M, Ledeist F, Sanson M, Rouleau G, Thomas G, Aurias A: Molecular cytogenetic analysis of a series of 23 DiGeorge syndrome patients by fluorescence *in situ* hybridization. Ann Génét 37:60–65, 1994.

28a. Der Kaloustian VM, Kleijer W, Booth A, Auerbach AD, Mazer B, Elliott AM, Abish S, Usher R, Walters G, Vekemans M, Eydoux P: Possible new variant of Nijmegen breakage syndrome. Am J. Med Genet 65:21–26, 1996.

29. Der Kaloustian VM, Kurban AK: Genetic Diseases of the Skin. Springer-Verlag, Berlin, 1979, pp 1–16.
30. Dittrich B, Buiting K, Groß S, Horsthemke B: Characterization of a methylation imprint in the Prader-Willi syndrome chromosome region. Hum Mol Genet 2:1995–1999, 1993.
31. Driscoll DA, Salvin J, Sellinger B, Budarf ML, McDonald-McGinn DM, Zackai EH, Emanuel BS: Prevalence of 22q11 microdeletions in DiGeorge and velocardiofacial syndromes: implications for genetic counselling and prenatal diagnosis. J Med Genet 30:813–817, 1993.
32. Duboule D, Morata G: Colinearity and functional hierarchy among genes of the homeotic complexes. Trends Genet 10:358–364, 1994.
33. Dutrillaux B, Lejeune J: Sur une nouvelle technique d'analyse du caryotype humain. C R Acad Sci [D] (Paris) 272:2638–2640, 1971.
34. Escobar LF, Weaver DD: Charge association. In: Birth Defects Encyclopedia, ML Buyse, ed. Blackwell, Cambridge, 1990, pp 308–309.
35. Ewart AK, Morris CA, Atkinson D, Jin W, Sternes K, Spallone P, Stock AD, Leppert M, Keating MT: Hemizygosity at the elastin locus in a developmental disorder, Williams syndrome. Nat Genet 5:11–16, 1993.

35a. Ferguson-Smith AC: Imprinting moves to the centre. Nat Genet 14:119–121, 1996.

36. Fields C, Adams MD, White O, Venter JC: How many genes in the human genome. Nat Genet 7:345–346, 1994.
37. Francke U: Prader-Willi syndrome: chromosomal and gene aberrations. Growth Genet Horm, 10:4–7, 1994.
38. Fraser FC: Genetic counseling. Am J Hum Genet 26:636–661, 1974.
39. Fraser FC: The multifactorial/threshold concept—uses and misuses. Teratology 14:267–280, 1976.
40. Fraser FC: Interactions and multiple causes. In: Handbook of Teratology, Vol. I, JG Wilson, FC Fraser, eds. Plenum Press, New York, 1977, p 445.
41. Fraser FC: The William Allan Memorial Award Address: evolution of a palatable multifactorial threshold model. Am J Hum Genet 32:796–813, 1980.
42. Fraser FC: Branchio-oto-renal dysplasia. In: Birth Defects Encyclopedia. ML Buyse, ed. Blackwell, Cambridge, 1990, pp 243–244.
43. Gehring WJ, Qian YQ, Billeter M, Furukubo-Tokunaga K, Schier AF, Resendez-Perez D, Affolter M, Otting G, Wüthrich K: Homeodomain-DNA recognition. Cell 78:211–223, 1994.
44. German J: Some genes which increase chromosome instability in somatic cells and predispose to cancer. In: Progress in Medical Genetics, Vol. 8, AG Steinberg, AG Bearn, eds. Grune and Stratton, New York, 1972, pp 61–101.
45. Giampietro PF, Adler-Brecher B, Verlander PC, Pavlakis SG, Davis JG, Auerbach AD: The need for more accurate and timely diagnosis

in Fanconi Anemia: a report from the International Fanconi Anemia Registry. Pediatrics 91:1116–1120, 1993.
46. Glenn CC, Porter KA, Jong MTC, Nicholls RD, Driscoll DJ: Functional imprinting and epigenetic modification of the human SNRPN gene. Hum Mol Genet 2:2001–2005, 1993.
47. Glover TW: CATCHing a break on 22. Nat Genet 10:257–258, 1995.
48. Goldberg JD, Golbus MS: Chorionic villus sampling. Adv Hum Genet 17:1–25, 1988.
49. Graham GE, Teebi AS: An approach to the dysmorphic infant or child. In: Textbook of Clinical Pediatrics, HA Harfi, AA El Zouki, eds. Chapman and Hall, London (in press).
50. Greenberg F: DiGeorge syndrome: an historical review of clinical and cytogenetic features. J Med Genet 30:803–806, 1993.
51. Hall JG, Dorst JP, Rotta J, McKusick VA: Gonadal mosaicism in pseudoachondroplasia. Am J Med Genet 28:143–151, 1987.
52. Halloran KH, Breg WR, Mahoney MJ: 21 monosomy in a retarded female infant. J Med Genet 11:386–389, 1974.
53. Hamerton JL: Human Cytogenetics, Vol I. Academic Press, New York, 1971, pp 14–25.
54. Hamerton JL: Human Cytogenetics, Vol I. Academic Press, New York, 1971, pp 197–200.
55. Hamerton JL: Human Cytogenetics, Vol I. Academic Press, New York, 1971, pp 290–309.
56. Hanson IM, Seawright A, Hardman K, Hodgson S, Zaletayev D, Fekete G, van Heyningen V: PAX6 mutations in aniridia. Hum Mol Genet 2:915–920, 1993.
57. Harnden DG, Klinger HP, eds. ISCN: An International System for Human Cytogenetic Nomenclature, Published in collaboration with Cytogenet Cell Genet, Basel, Karger, 1985.
58. Hollway GE, Phillips HA, Adès LC, Haan EA, Mulley JC: Localization of craniosynostosis Adelaide type to 4p16. Hum Mol Genet 4:681–683, 1995.
59. Jabs EW, Li X, Scott AF, Meyers G, Chen W, Eccles M, Mao JI, Charnas LR, Jackson CE, Jaye M: Jackson-Weiss and Crouzon syndromes are allelic with mutations in fibroblast growth factor receptor 2. Nat Genet 8:275–279, 1994.
60. Jabs EW, Müller U, Li X, Ma L, Luo W, Haworth IS, Klisak I, Sparkes R, Warman ML, Mulliken JB, Snead ML, Maxson R: A mutation in the homeodomain of the human MSX2 gene in a family affected with autosomal dominant craniosynostosis. Cell 75:443–450, 1993.
61. Jalal SM, Law ME, Christensen ER, Spurbeck JL, Dewald GW: Method for sequential staining of GTL-banded metaphases with fluorescent-labeled chromosome-specific paint probes. Am J Med Genet 46:98–103, 1993.
62. Jones KL: Smith's Recognizable Patterns of Human Malformation, 5th ed. WB Saunders, Philadelphia, 1996.
63. Jones KL: Smith's Recognizable Patterns of Human Malformation, 5th ed. WB Saunders, Philadelphia, 1996, pp 266–267.
64. Jones KL: Smith's Recognizable Patterns of Human Malformation, 5th ed. WB Saunders, Philadelphia, 1996, pp 282–285.
65. Jones KL: Smith's Recognizable Patterns of Human Malformation, 5th ed. WB Saunders, Philadelphia, 1996, pp 348–351.
66. Jones KL: Smith's Recognizable Patterns of Human Malformation, 5th ed. WB Saunders, Philadelphia, 1996, pp 418–419.
67. Jones KL: Smith's Recognizable Patterns of Human Malformation, 5th ed. WB Saunders, Philadelphia, 1996, pp 456–457.
68. Jones KL: Smith's Recognizable Patterns of Human Malformation, 5th ed. WB Saunders, Philadelphia, 1996, pp 664–665.
69. Jones KL, Smith DW, Harvey MAS, Hall BD, Quan L: Older paternal age and fresh gene mutations: data on additional disorders. J Pediatr 86:84–88, 1975.
69a. Khoury MJ, Shaw GM, Moore CA, Lammer EJ, Mulinare J: Does periconceptional multivitamin use reduce the risk of neural tube defects associated with other birth defects? Data from two population-based case-control studies. Am J Med Genet 61:30–36, 1996.
70. Khudr G: Cytogenetics of habitual abortion. A review. Obstet Gynecol Surv 29:290–310, 1974.
71. King RA, Hearing VJ, Creel DJ, Oetting WS: Albinism. In: The Metabolic and Molecular Bases of Inherited Disease, 7th ed, CR Scriver, AL Beaudet, WS Sly, D Valle, eds. McGraw-Hill, New York, 1995, pp 4353–4392.
72. Klinger K, Landes G, Shook D, Harvey R, Lopez L, Locke P, Lerner T, Osathanondh R, Leverone B, Houseal T, et al: Rapid detection of chromosome aneuploidies in uncultured amniocytes by using fluorescence in situ hybridization (FISH). Am J Hum Genet 51:55–65, 1992.
73. Knoll JHM, Nicholls RD, Magenis RE, Graham JM Jr, Lalande M, Latt SA: Angelman and Prader-Willi syndromes share a common chromosome 15 deletion but differ in parental origin of the deletion. Am J Med Genet 32:285–290, 1989.
74. Krumlauf R: *Hox* genes in vertebrate development. Cell 78:191–201, 1994.
75. Kubota T, Saitoh S, Matsumoto T, Narahara K, Fukushima Y, Jinno Y, Niikawa N: Excess functional copy allele at chromosomal region 11p15 may cause Wiedemann-Beckwith (EMG) syndrome. Am J Med Genet 49:378–383, 1994.
76. Lajeunie E, Ma HW, Bonaventure J, Munnich A, Le Merrer M, Renier D: FGFR2 mutations in Pfeiffer syndrome. Nat Genet 9:108, 1995.
77. Langer LO Jr, Krassikoff N, Laxova R, Scheer-Williams M, Lutter LD, Gorlin RJ, Jennings CG, Day DW: The tricho-rhino-phalangeal syndrome with exostoses (or Langer-Giedion syndrome): four additional patients without mental retardation and review of the literature. Am J Med Genet 19:81–111, 1984.
78. Lazarow PB, Moser HW: Disorders of peroxisome biosynthesis. In: The Metabolic and Molecular Bases of Inherited Disease, 7th ed, CR Scriver, AL Beaudet, WS Sly, D Valle, eds. McGraw-Hill, New York, 1995, pp 2287–2324.
79. Ledbetter DH, Ballabio A: Molecular cytogenetics of contiguous gene syndromes: mechanisms and consequences of gene dosage imbalance. In: The Metabolic and Molecular Bases of Inherited Diseases, 7th ed, CR Scriver, AL Beaudet, WS Sly, D Valle, eds. McGraw-Hill, New York, 1995, pp 811–839.
80. Ledbetter DH, Ledbetter SA, van Tuinen P, Summers KM, Robinson TJ, Nakamura Y, Wolff R, White R, Barker DF, Wallace MR et al: Molecular dissection of a contiguous gene syndrome: frequent submicroscopic deletions, evolutionary conserved sequences, and a hypomethylated "island" in the Miller-Dieker chromosome region. Proc Natl Acad Sci USA 86:5136–5140, 1989.
81. Lejeune J, Gautier M, Turpin R: Etude des chromosomes somatiques de neuf enfants mongoliens. C R Acad Sci [D] (Paris) 248:1721–1722, 1959.
82. Leppig KA, Werler MM, Cann CI, Cook CA, Holmes LB: Predictive value of minor anomalies. I. Association with major malformations. J Pediatr 110:531–537, 1987.
83. Mansouri A, Stoykova A, Gruss P: Pax genes in development. J Cell Sci 18:35–42, 1994.
84. Mason IJ: The ins and outs of fibroblast growth factors. Cell 78:547–552, 1994.
85. McKusick VA: Mendelian Inheritance in Man, A Catalog of Human Genes and Genetic Disorders, 11th ed. Johns Hopkins University Press, Baltimore, 1994.
85a. Meyers GA, Orlow SJ, Munro IR, Przylepa KA, Jabs EW: Fibroblast growth factor receptor 3 *(FGFR 3)* transmembrane mutation in Crouzon syndrome with acanthosis nigricans. Nat Genet 11:462–464, 1995.
86. Milunsky A (ed): Genetic Disorders of the Fetus: Diagnosis, Prevention, and Treatment, 3rd ed. Plenum Press, New York, 1992.
87. Mirzayans F, Pearce WG, MacDonald IM, Walter MA: Mutation of the PAX6 gene in patients with autosomal dominant keratitis. Am J Hum Genet 57:539–548, 1995.
88. [MRC] Medical Research Council Vitamin Study Research Group: Prevention of neural tube defects: results of the Medical Research Council Vitamin Study. Lancet 338:131–137, 1991.
89. Narahara K, Kikkawa K, Kimira S, Kimoto H, Ogata M, Kasai R, Hamawaki M, Matsuoka K: Regional mapping of catalase and Wilms tumor—aniridia, genitourinary abnormalities, and mental retardation triad loci to the chromosome segment 11p1305→1306. Hum Genet 66:181–185, 1984.
90. Nicholls RD, Knoll JHM, Butler MG, Karam S, Lalande M: Genetic imprinting suggested by maternal heterodisomy in non-deletion Prader-Willi syndrome. Nature 342:281–285,1989.
91. Nickerson E, Greenberg F, Keating MT, McCaskill C, Shaffer LG: Deletions of the elastin gene at 7q11.23 in ~90% of patients with Williams syndrome. Am J Hum Genet 56:1156–1161, 1995.
92. Nora JJ, Fraser FC, Bear J, Greenberg CR, Patterson D, Warburton D: Medical Genetics: Principles and Practice, 4th ed. Lea & Febiger, Philadelphia, 1994, pp 10–34.
93. Nora JJ, Fraser FC, Bear J, Greenberg CR, Patterson D, Warburton D: Medical Genetics: Principles and Practice, 4th ed. Lea & Febiger, Philadelphia, 1994, pp 68–90.
94. Nora JJ, Fraser FC, Bear J, Greenberg CR, Patterson D, Warburton

D: Medical Genetics: Principles and Practice, 4th ed. Lea & Febiger, Philadelphia, 1994, pp 91–121.
95. Nora JJ, Fraser FC, Bear J, Greenberg CR, Patterson D, Warburton D: Medical Genetics: Principles and Practice, 4th ed. Lea & Febiger, Philadelphia, 1994, pp 280–287.
96. Ott J: Analysis of Human Genetic Linkage. Johns Hopkins University Press, Baltimore, 1985.
96a. Pandya A, Xia X-J, Landa BL, Arnos KS, Israel J, Lloyd J, James AL, Diehl SR, Blanton SH, Nance WE: Phenotypic variation in Waardenburg syndrome: mutational heterogeneity, modifier genes or polygenic background? Hum Mol Genet 5:497–502, 1996.
97. Park W-J, Bellus GA, Jabs EW: Mutations in fibroblast growth factor receptors: phenotypic consequences during eukaryotic development. Am J Hum Genet 57:748–754, 1995.
98. Parry DM, Mulvihill JJ, Tsai SE, Kaiser-Kupfer MI, Cowan JM: SC phocomelia syndrome, premature centromere separation, and congenital cranial nerve paralysis in two sisters, one with malignant melanoma. Am J Med Genet 24:653–672, 1986.
99. Pierpont JW, Erickson RP: Facts on *PAX*. Am J Hum Genet 52:451–454, 1993.
100. Pinkel D, Landegent J, Collins C, Fuscoe J, Segraves R, Lucas J, Gray J: Fluorescence in situ hybridization with human chromosome-specific libraries. Detection of trisomy 21 and translocations of chromosome 4. Proc Natl Acad Sci USA 85:9138–9142, 1988.
101. Polani PE: Autosomal imbalance and its syndromes, excluding Down's. Br Med Bull 25:81–93, 1969.
101a. Przylepa KA, Paznekas W, Zhang M, Golabi M, Bias W, Bamshad MJ, Carey JC, Hall BD, Stevenson R, Orlow SJ, Cohen MM Jr, Jabs EW: Fibroblast growth factor receptor 2 mutations in Beare-Stevenson cutis gyrata syndrome. Nat Genet 13:492–494, 1996.
102. Rawlings CE 3rd, Wilkins RH, Cook WA, Burger PC: Segmental neurofibromatosis. Neurosurgery 20:946–949, 1987.
103. Read AP: Pax genes—*Paired* feet in three camps. Nat Genet 9:333–334, 1995.
104. Redeker E, Alders M, Hoovers JM, Richard CW 3rd, Westerveld A, Mannens M: Physical mapping of 3 candidate tumor genes relative to Beckwith-Wiedemann syndrome associated breakpoints at 11p15.3. Cytogenet Cell Genet 68:222–225, 1995.
105. Reik W: Genomic imprinting and genetic disorders in man. Trends Genet 5:331–336, 1989.
106. Reik W, Brown KW, Slatter RE, Sartori P, Elliott M, Maher ER: Allelic methylation of *H19* and *IGF2* in the Beckwith-Wiedemann syndrome. Hum Mol Genet 3:1297–1301, 1994.
107. Roberts JAF: Multifactorial inheritance in relation to normal and abnormal human traits. Br Med Bull 17:241–246, 1961.
108. Robinson BH: Lactic acidemia (disorders of pyruvate carboxylase, pyruvate dehydrogenase). In: The Metabolic and Molecular Bases of Inherited Disease, 7th ed, CR Scriver, AL Beaudet, WS Sly, D Valle, eds. McGraw-Hill, New York, 1995, pp 1479–1499.
109. Rousseau F: The fragile X syndrome: implications of molecular genetics for the clinical syndrome. Eur J Clin Invest 24:1–10, 1994.
109a. Rousseau F, El Ghouzzi V, Delezoide AL, Legeai-Mallet L, Le Merrer M, Munnich A, Bonaventure J: Missense *FGFR3* mutations create cysteine residues in thanatophoric dwarfism type I (TD1). Hum Mol Genet **5**:509–512, 1996.
110. Rousseau F, Heitz D, Tarleton J, MacPherson J, Malmgren H, Dahl N, Barnicoat A, Mathew C, Mornet E, Tejeda I, Maddalena A, Spiegel R, Schinzel A, Marcos JAG, Schorderet DF, Schaap T, Maccioni L, Russo S, Jacobs PA: A multicenter study on genotype-phenotype correlations in the fragile X syndrome, using direct diagnosis with probe StB12.3: the first 2,253 cases. Am J Hum Genet 55:225–237, 1994.
111. Ruddle FH, Bartels JL, Bentley KL, Kappen C, Murtha MT, Pendleton JW: Evolution of *HOX* genes. Annu Rev Genet 28:423–442, 1994.
112. Sanyanusin P, Schimmenti LA, McNoe LA, Ward TA, Pierpont MEM, Sullivan MJ, Dobyns WB, Eccles MR: Mutation of the PAX2 gene in a family with optic nerve colobomas, renal anomalies and vesicoureteral reflux. Nat Genet 9:358–363, 1995.
113. Schell U, Hehr A, Feldman GJ, Robin NH, Zackai EH, de Die-Smulders C, Viskochil DH, Stewart JM, Wolff G, Ohashi H, Price RA, Cohen MM Jr, Muenke M: Mutations in *FGFR1* and *FGFR2* cause familial and sporadic Pfeiffer syndrome. Hum Mol Genet 4:323–328, 1995.
114. Scheres JMJC, Hustinx TWJ, Weemaes CMR: Chromosome 7 in ataxia telangiectasia. J Pediatr 97:440–441, 1980.
115. Schmickel RD: Contiguous gene syndromes: a component of recognizable syndromes. J Pediatr 109:231–241, 1986.
116. Schneid H, Le Bouc Y: Insulin-like growth factor 2 and growth. Growth Genet Horm 10:1–4, 1994.
117. Schroer RJ, Stevenson RE: An approach to postnatal diagnosis. In Human Malformations and Related Anomalies Vol I. RE Stevenson, JG Hall, RM Goodman, eds. Oxford University Press, New York, 1993, pp 209–218.
117a. Schulze A. Hansen C, Skakkebaek NE, Brøndum-Nielsen K, Ledbetter DH, Tommerup N: Exclusion of *SNRPN* as a major determinant of Prader-Willi syndrome by a translocation breakpoint, Nat Genet **12**:452–454, 1996.
118. Schwartz CE, Brown AM, Der Kaloustian VM, McGill JJ, Saul SA: DNA fingerprinting: the utilization of minisatellite probes to detect a somatic mutation in the Proteus syndrome. In: DNA Fingerprinting: Approaches and Applications, T Burke, G Dolf, AJ Jeffreys, R Wolff, eds. Springer-Verlag, New York, 1991, pp 95–105.
119. Scriver CR, Beaudet AL, Sly WS, Valle D (eds): The Metabolic and Molecular Bases of Inherited Disease, 7th ed. McGraw-Hill, New York, 1995.
120. Spence JE, Perciaccante RG, Greig GM, Willard HF, Ledbetter DH, Hejtmancik JF, Pollack MS, O'Brien WE, Beaudet AL: Uniparental disomy as a mechanism for human genetic disease. Am J Hum Genet 42:217–226, 1988.
121. Spranger J, Benirschke K, Hall JG, Lenz W, Lowry RB, Opitz JM, Pinsky L, Schwarzacher HG, Smith DW: Errors of morphogenesis: concepts and terms. J Pediatr 100:160–165, 1982.
122. Stevenson RE: The genetic basis of human anomalies. In: Human Malformations and Related Anomalies, Vol I, RE Stevenson, JG Hall, RM Goodman eds. Oxford University Press, New York, 1993, pp 115–135.
123. Strachan T, Read AP: PAX genes. Curr Opin Genet Dev 4:427–438, 1994.
124. Stuart ET, Gruss P: PAX genes: what's new in developmental biology and cancer? Hum Mol Genet 4:1717–1720, 1995.
125. Sumner AT, Evans HJ, Buckland RA: New technique for distinguishing between human chromosomes. Nat New Biol 232:31–32, 1971.
126. Tarleton JC, Saul RA: Molecular genetic advances in fragile X syndrome. J Pediatr 122:169–185, 1993.
127. Thompson MW, McInnes RR, Willard HF: Genetics in Medicine, 5th ed. WB Saunders, Philadelphia, 1991, pp 13–30.
128. Thompson MW, McInnes RR, Willard HF: Genetics in Medicine, 5th ed. WB Saunders, Philadelphia, 1991, pp 31–51.
129. Thompson MW, McInnes RR, Willard HF: Genetics in Medicine, 5th ed. WB Saunders, Philadelphia, 1991, p 89.
130. Thompson MW, McInnes RR, Willard HF: Genetics in Medicine, 5th ed. WB Saunders, Philadelphia, 1991, pp 167–199.
131. Thompson MW, McInnes RR, Willard HF: Genetics in Medicine, 5th ed. WB Saunders, Philadelphia, 1991, pp 201–229.
132. Tint GS, Irons M, Elias ER, Batta AK, Frieden R, Chen TS, Salen G: Defective cholesterol biosynthesis associated with the Smith-Lemli-Opitz syndrome. N Engl J Med 330:107–113, 1994.
133. Tjio JH, Levan A: The chromosome number of man. Hereditas 42:1–6, 1956.
134. Wagstaff J, Knoll JHM, Glatt KA, Shugart YY, Sommer A, Lalande M: Maternal but not paternal transmission of 15q11–13–linked nondeletion Angelman syndrome leads to phenotypic expression. Nat Genet 1:291–294, 1992.
135. Watson JD, Crick FHC: A structure of deoxyribose nucleic acid. Nature 171:737–738, 1953.
136. Watson JD, Hopkins NH, Roberts JW, Steitz JA, Weiner AM, et al: Molecular Biology of the Gene, 4th ed Benjamin/Cummings, Menlo Park, 1987.
137. Watson JD, Jordan E: The Human Genome Program at the National Institutes of Health. Genomics 5:654–656, 1989.
138. Weemaes CMR, Hustinx TWJ, Scheres JMJC, van Munster PJJ, Bakkeren JAJ, Taalman RDFM: A new chromosomal instability disorder: the Nijmegen breakage syndrome. Acta Paediatr Scand 70:557–564, 1981.
139. Weksberg R: Wiedemann-Beckwith syndrome: genomic imprinting revisited. Am J Med Genet 52:235–236, 1994.
140. Weksberg R, Shen DR, Fei YL, Song QL, Squire J: Disruption of insulin-like growth factor 2 imprinting in Beckwith-Wiedemann syndrome. Nat Genet 5:143–150, 1993.
141. Wilkie AOM, Slaney SF, Oldridge M, Poole MD, Ashworth GJ, Hockley AD, Hayward RD, David DJ, Pulleyn LJ, Rutland P, Mal-

colm S, Winter RM, Reardon W: Apert syndrome results from localized mutations of FGFR2 and is allelic with Crouzon syndrome. Nat Genet 9:165–172, 1995.

142. Wilson GN: Relevance of the genetics of embryologic development. Growth Genet Horm 9:1–5, 1993.

143. Zhong N, Yang W, Dobkin C, Brown WT: Fragile X gene instability: anchoring AGGs and linked microsatellites. Am J Hum Genet 57:351–361, 1995.

# 2

# Subjective Evaluation and Physical Measurement of the Head and Face

JUDITH E. ALLANSON

To define properly what is different in the individual with unusual craniofacial features is a challenge, and yet appropriate definition, description, and measurement of such features can be of great value. Evaluation of the craniofacies must include an impression of the overall *gestalt* of the face, both at rest and during movement such as crying, smiling, and frowning. Since the shape of the face and its relative proportions change significantly with age, in both normal and dysmorphic individuals, this evolution of facial phenotype must be taken into account. Detailed measurement of the craniofacies provides objective data which are complementary to an assessment of gestalt. Although there are more than one hundred dimensions for which norms are available, a small subset will provide adequate documentation of appearance for the practicing clinician.

Measurement of the craniofacies requires only a few standard instruments: sliding and spreading calipers and a tape measure. The tape measure should ideally be made of cloth and should not be well worn. In addition, a modified protractor and an instrument to determine ear location are useful, but not essential. In general, when measuring between two soft tissue landmarks, the hard tips of the caliper should touch but not press significantly on the skin surface. In contrast, when measuring between bony landmarks, the blunt points of the caliper should be pressed against the bony surface. When measuring circumference, length, or width of the head, one must be certain that the metric tape or the tips of the caliper are sufficiently pressed against the skull in order to eliminate the effect of thick hair cover.

Accurate measurement requires correct use of the instrument and knowledge of the peculiarities of the landmark. For this reason, detailed explanations of measurement techniques and associated pitfalls are provided. The most common palpable landmarks of the craniofacies are shown in Figure 2–1. These landmarks are defined in the text.

Alternative approaches to craniofacial measurement have been developed using photoanthropometry, cephalometry, and craniofacial pattern profiles. The details are outside the scope of this text, but interested readers should refer to the excellent papers of Garn et al, 1984; McNamara, 1984; Saksena et al, 1987; and Ward, 1989.[7,11,17,21]

An approach to measurement of the craniofacies must include comparison with head circumference and height, in addition to age. For example, inner and outer canthal distances on the 50th percentile, in the presence of microcephaly, would, in fact, be abnormal. Various indices comparing two craniofacial measurements are available in the dental and anthropological literature. Few have been included in this text, but references are found at the end of this chapter.[4,5]

## Skull

The shape of the head is closely related to the bony structures of the skull and to the shape of the underlying brain. Alterations in head shape may be the result of unusual brain growth, but they may also reflect a number of other factors, such as premature synostosis of cranial sutures or unusual intrauterine mechanical forces. Abnormal planes of muscle pull, for example, in torticollis, can cause asymmetric skull growth. Dolichocephaly or scaphocephaly (long, narrow head) is a postural deformation of the head associated with intrauterine breech position or prematurity. It generally resolves during infancy with no apparent residual impairment.

Five major sutures are present in the calvaria (Fig. 2–2). Three—the coronal, lambdoidal, and squamosal—are paired, and two—the sagittal and metopic—are single. Cranial growth normally proceeds in a direction perpendicular to each of the major sutures. Increased length of the skull in comparison to width (dolichocephaly or scaphocephaly) and the converse (brachycephaly) can be normal variants. However, both can also occur because of premature synostosis of cranial sutures, where skull growth at right angles to the fused suture is inhibited and accompanied by compensatory expansion at other patent sutural sites. Head shape depends on which sutures are prematurely synostosed, the order in which they synostose, and the time at which they synostose. The earlier the synostosis occurs, the more dramatic the effect on subsequent cranial growth and development. Premature closure of the cranial sutures can occur in isolation or as part of a syndrome, in association with other clinical anomalies.

A description of skull shape should include a comment on length and width, and on the prominence of various parts of the skull. An assessment of symmetry is also important.

Measurement of head length (Fig. 2–3) is generally performed using spreading calipers. Measurement between the glabella (the most prominent point on the frontal bone, above the root of the nose, between the eyebrows) and the opisthocranion (the most prominent portion of the occiput, close to the midline, on the posterior rim of the foramen magnum) will provide the maximum dimension of the sagittal axis of the skull. These landmarks are also critical for measurement of head circumference. Alterations in skull shape will produce marked variation in this measurement and in head length and width. Dolichocephaly increases, while brachycephaly reduces, head length.

Head width (Fig. 2–4) is the maximum biparietal diameter, and is measured between the most lateral points of the parietal bones (eurion) on each side of the head. Spreading calipers once again give most accurate measurements. The head should

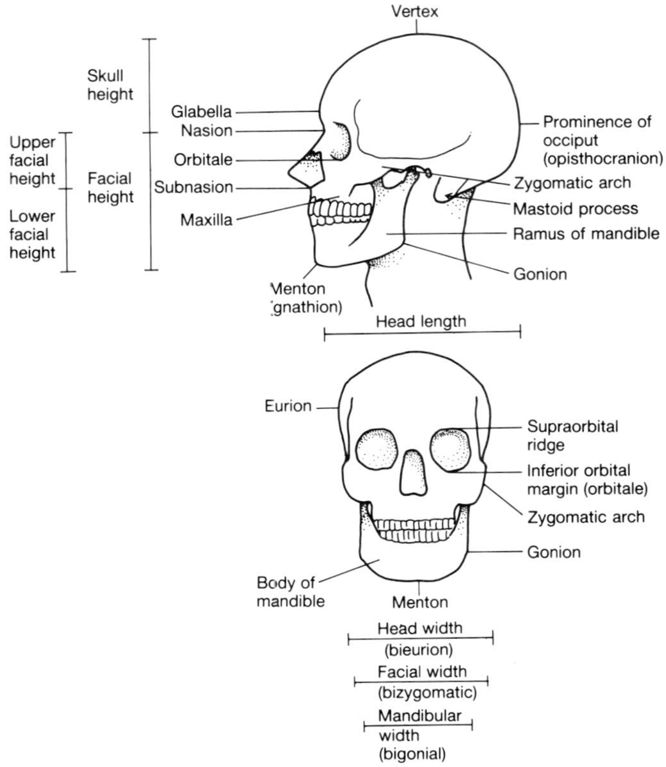


**Fig 2–1.** Palpable landmarks of craniofacies. (From Hall et al., eds., *Handbook of Normal Physical Measurements.* Oxford University Press, 1989, p. 93, with permission.)[7b]

be held erect in the resting position with the eyes looking straight ahead. Caliper tips should be firmly applied to the skull to eliminate the effect of thick hair cover.

Cephalic index (CI) is the ratio of head width expressed as a percentage of head length. In the "normal" head the CI is 76 to 80.9%. In dolichocephaly the CI is less than 75.9%, while in brachycephaly the CI exceeds 81%.

## Head circumference

Head circumference is the maximum circumference of the head and is measured from the glabella to the opisthocranion. These landmarks have been defined in the context of head length. A tape measure must be used. It is recommended that the head circumference measurement be repeated, after completely removing the tape from the head, to ensure accuracy. Thick hair or braids can get in the way when measuring head circumference and can lead to falsely elevated values. If the head has an unusual shape it may be difficult to palpate the landmarks. In the case of craniosynostosis or an unusual head shape, head circumference measurements can give false impressions of micro- or macrocephaly. In these situations, head length and width are more useful parameters.

Although height and weight charts after birth are quite different for North American and northern European populations, head circumference growth data after birth are not. For this reason, combined figures are presented (Figs. 2–5, 2–6).

Examination of the skull should be completed by an assessment of fontanelles. This evaluation can provide information about the rate of development and ossification of the calvaria, which may be altered in a wide variety of disorders affecting morphogenesis. In order to utilize fontanelle size and patency as a clue to altered morphogenesis, it is necessary to have normal age-related standards. Figure 2–2 combination outlines the constant and accessory fontanelles present at birth. The most common accessory fontanelle is the parietal or sagittal fontanelle, otherwise known as a third fontanelle. This is found in 6% of infants and may be more common in infants with Down syndrome. The metopic fontanelle is actually an extremely long anterior arm of the anterior fontanelle which, in the process of closure, becomes separated from the anterior fontanelle. A metopic fontanelle has been reported in association with craniofacial dysostosis, cleidocranial dysostosis, spina bifida occulta and meningomyelocele. It can also occur as an isolated finding. An increased incidence of open metopic fontanelles is found in infants with congenital rubella syndrome, Down syndrome, cleft lip, with or without cleft palate, and widened sutures.

With increasing age, the fontanelles and sutures become smaller and narrower due to the ingrowth of bone into these remnants of the fetal membranous and cartilaginous skull. There is considerable variation in the velocity of this process in different individuals, and on the two sides of the same skull. The anterior fontanelle usually is reduced to fingertip size by the first half of the second year. The posterior fontanelle may close during the last 2 months before birth, or the first 2 months after birth. The anterolateral fontanelles disappear during the first 3 months of life and the posterolateral fontanelles during the second year of life. The metopic suture begins to close in

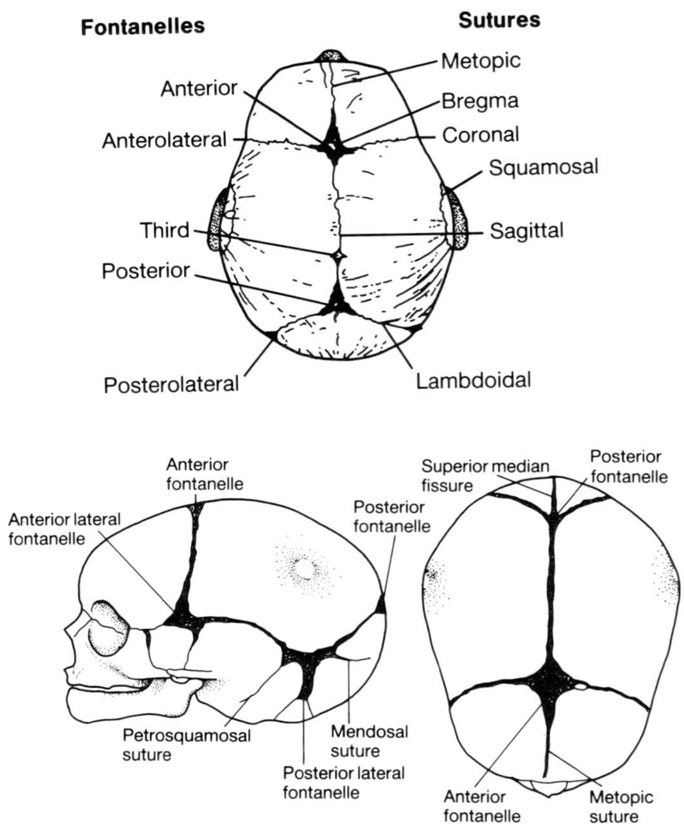


**Fig. 2–2.** a: Normal fontanelle and suture landmarks. (From Pruzansky, ASHA 8:62–94, 1973,[15] with permission.) b: Cranium at birth. (From Caffey, *J. Caffey's Pediatric X-ray Diagnosis,* 7th ed., Year Book publishers, Chicago, 1978,[1] with permission.)

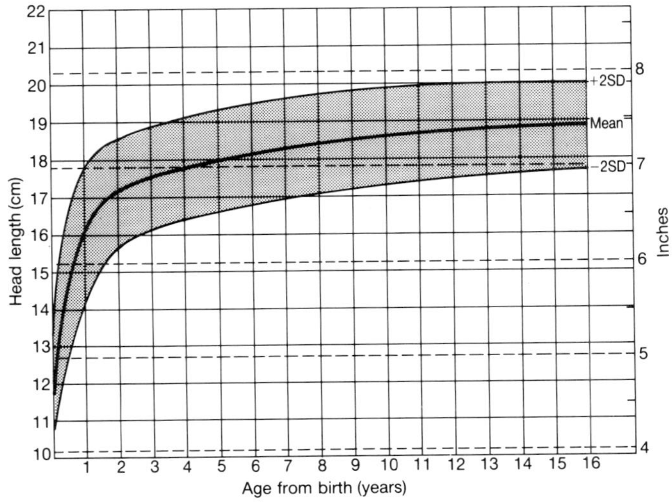


**Fig. 2–3.** Head length, both sexes, birth to 16 years. (From Feingold and Bossert, Birth Defects 10:1–6, 1974,[6] and Farkas, *Anthropometry of the Head and Face in Medicine,* Elsevier, New York, 1981,[4] with permission.)

the second year and is usually completely obliterated during the third year. It persists throughout life in about 10% of individuals. The great sutures of the vault (coronal, lambdoidal, and sagittal) normally persist throughout infancy and childhood and do not completely close before the 30th year.

By comparing fontanelle measurements with age-related norms, the clinician should be able to identify those individuals either having an abnormally large or small fontanelle for their age. The presence of an unusually large fontanelle, without increased intracranial pressure, can be a valuable clue in the recognition of a variety of pathological disorders. An unusually small anterior fontanelle for one's age may be a secondary feature in disorders which affect brain growth such as primary microcephaly, or may be due to craniosynostosis, accelerated osseous maturation secondary to maternal hyperthyroidism, or infantile hyperthyroidism. Occasionally, numerous large and small accessory ossification centers may be seen within the sutures. These so-called wormian bones can be mistaken for multiple fracture fragments, but they are present in normal healthy individuals. However, wormian bones can be associated with inherited disorders such as osteogenesis imperfecta.

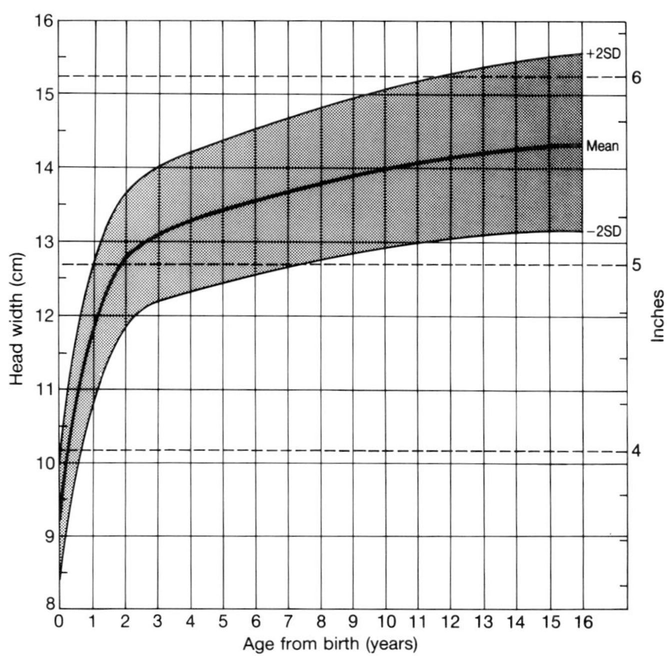


**Fig. 2–4.** Head width, both sexes, birth to 16 years. (From Feingold and Bossert, Birth Defects 10:1–6, 1974,[6] with permission.)

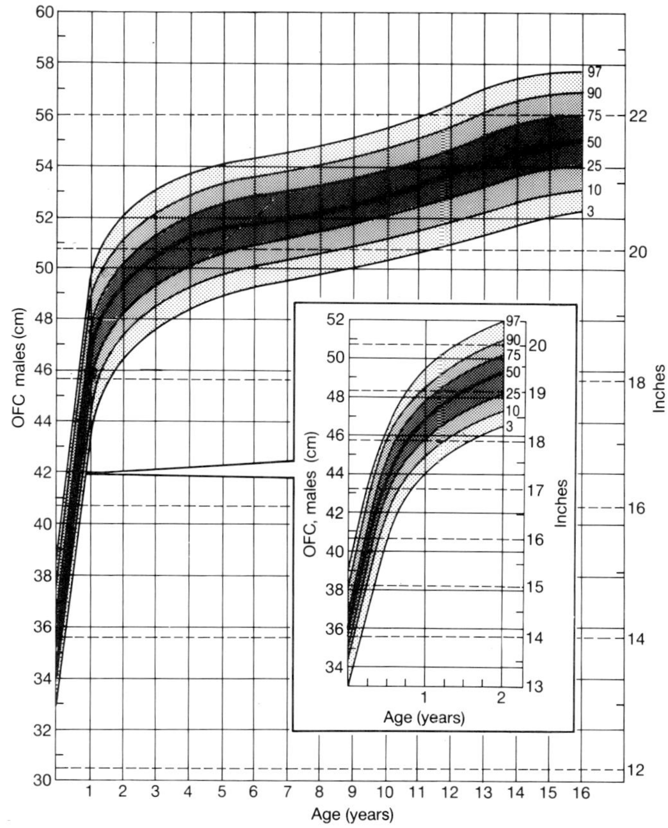


**Fig. 2–5.** Head circumference, males, birth to 16 years. (From Nellhaus, Pediatrics 41:106–114, 1968,[12] and Tanner, *Textbook of Pediatrics,* Churchill Livingston, Edinburgh, 1978,[19] with permission.)

Anterior fontanelle size (Fig. 2–7) is defined as the sum of the longitudinal and transverse diameters of the anterior fontanelle along the sagittal and coronal sutures. To define size, the index finger should be placed as far as possible into each of the four corners of the anterior fontanelle. These four positions may be marked directly or on a piece of white paper pressed firmly over the fontanelle. The four points are joined to form a quadrilateral and the sum of the longitudinal and transverse diameters can be measured. Spreading calipers, tape measure, or ruler may be used. The examiner looks down on the skull vault from above with the head held erect. However, the infant may lie prone or supine with the skull, again, viewed from above. Occasionally, when the sagittal suture is widely patent and communicating with the posterior fontanelle, definition of landmarks is more difficult.

The posterior fontanelle is a triangular structure. Its length is measured from the anterior corner to the midpoint on a line connecting the two posterolateral margins created by the occipital bone (Fig. 2–8). Spreading calipers or a tape measure can be used. Head positioning is identical to that used in measure-

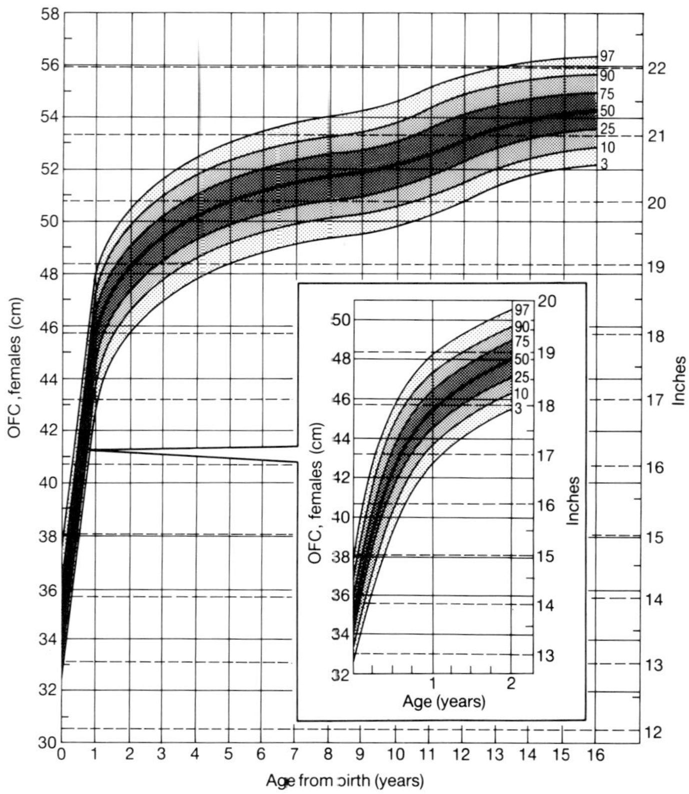


**Fig. 2–6.** Head circumference, females, birth to 16 years. (From Nellhaus, Pediatrics 41:106–114, 1968,[12] and Tanner, *Textbook of Pediatrics,* Churchill Livingston, Edinburgh, 1978,[19] with permission.)

ment of the anterior fontanelle. Only about 3% of normal newborn infants have a posterior fontanelle that measures more than 2 cm. If the sagittal suture is widely patent, the anterior border of the posterior fontanelle may be difficult to distinguish.

Ethnic differences in size of the anterior and posterior fontanelles have been recognized and comparison measurements are available (Fig. 2–8).

## Face

Upper facial height, which also represents nasal height, is the distance from the root of the nose (nasion) to the base of the nose (subnasion) (Fig. 2–9). Sliding calipers are the most accurate tool. Difficulties with this measurement may be encountered if the nasal tip is long or pointed down, masking the subnasion, or if a prominent nasal bridge distorts the position of the nasion.

Lower facial height (Fig. 2–10) is the distance from the base of the nose (subnasion) to the lowest median landmark on the lower border of the mandible (menton or gnathion). The menton is identified by palpation and is identical to the bony gnathion. Sliding calipers should ideally be used. The mouth should be closed with the teeth in occlusion. This measurement can also be obtained from a lateral radiograph, although one should remember that cephalometric data do not take into account soft tissue dimensions. However, the data from both cephalometric and anthropometric sources are surprisingly similar and have been combined in Figure 2–10.

Total facial height (Fig. 2–11) is the combination of upper and lower facial height, representing the distance from the nasion to the gnathion. This measurement is useful in calculating the length-to-width ratio of the face (facial index).

Facial width (Fig. 2–12) is the maximal distance between the most lateral points on the zygomatic arches (zygion). These points are located by palpation, using spreading calipers, with the head held in the resting position and the eyes looking straight ahead. When the zygomatic arches are defective, for example, in first and second branchial arch syndromes, distorted measurements will be produced. In this situation cephalometric assessment is preferable.

Facial index (Fig. 2–13) utilizes the previous two measurements—facial height and width—and provides a numerical estimate of face shape.

## Eyes

Examination of the eye should include a review of periorbital structures. Are the supraorbital brows prominent, pugilistic, heavy, or hypoplastic? Is there periorbital edema? Is pigmentation excessive? Are the eyes deep set or prominent? Are there deep creases under the eyes? Spacing of the eyes is discussed

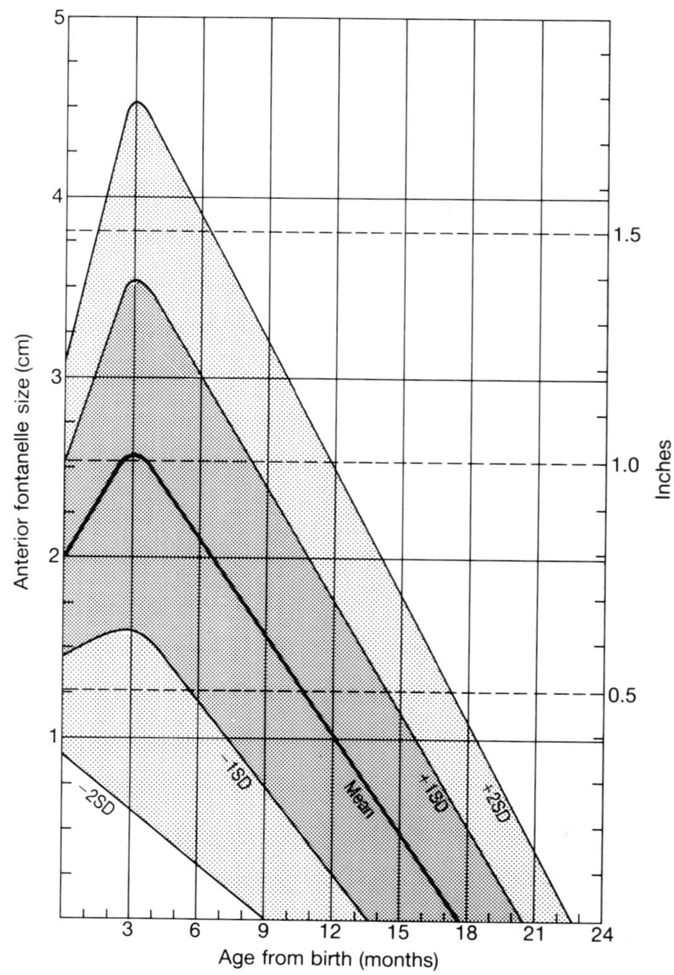


**Fig. 2–7.** Anterior fontanelle size (sum of longitudinal and transverse diameters). (From Popich and Smith, J Pediatr 80:749–752, 1972,[14] with permission.)

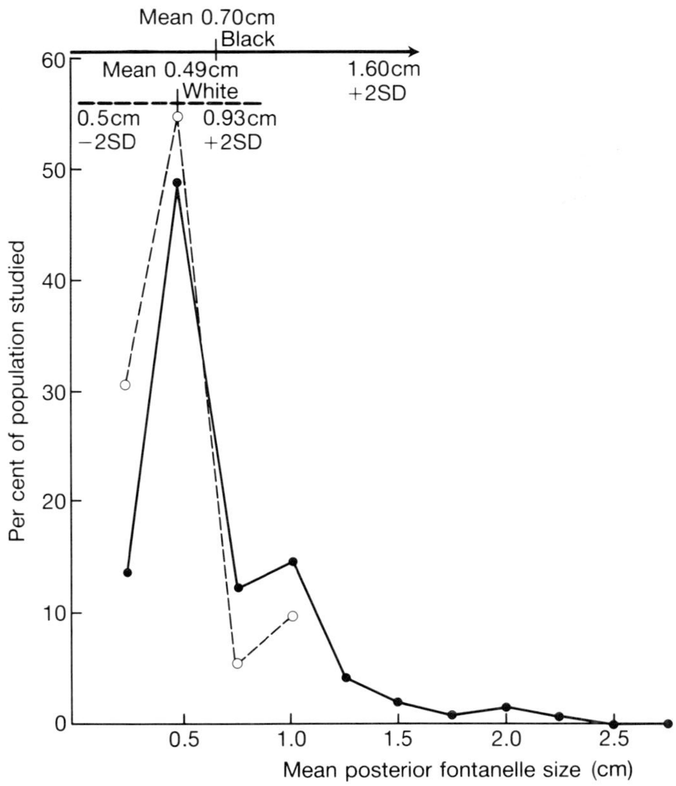


**Fig. 2–8.** Comparison of posterior fontanelle size in Black and White populations, both sexes, at birth. (From Faix, J Pediatr 100:304–306, 1982,[3] with permission.)

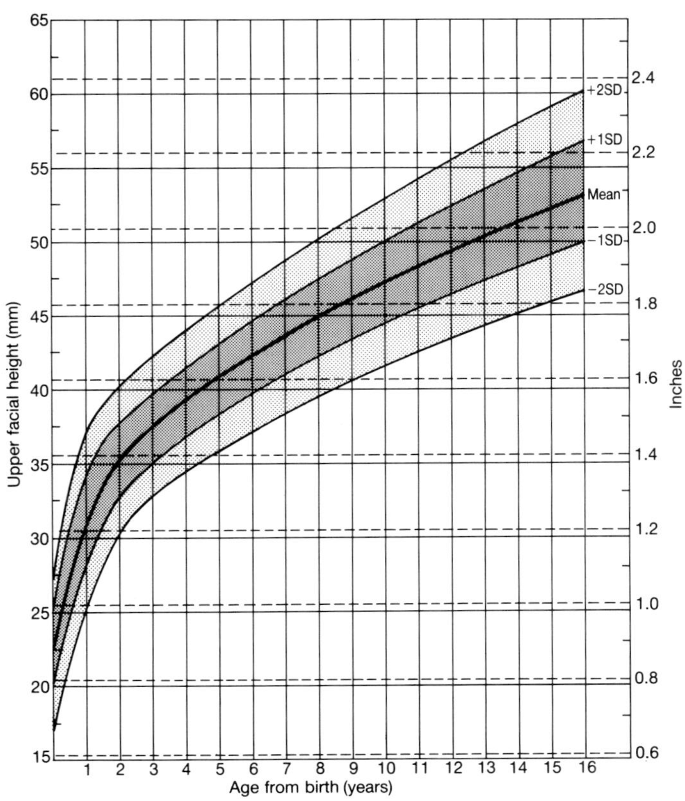


**Fig. 2–9.** Upper facial height, both sexes, birth to 16 years. (From Farkas, *Anthropometry of the Head and Face in Medicine,* Elsevier, New York, 1981,[4] and Goodman and Gorlin, *Atlas of the Face in Genetic Disorders,* 2nd ed., CV Mosby Co, St Louis, 1977,[7a] with permission.)

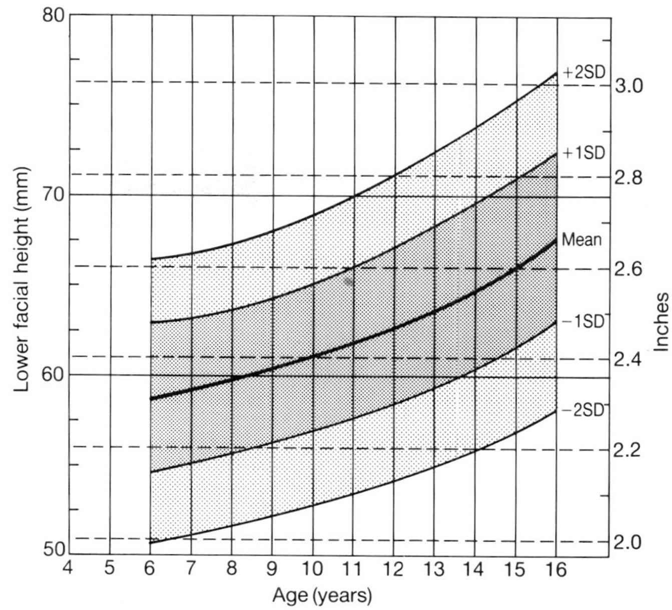


**Fig. 2–10.** Lower facial height, both sexes, 6 to 16 years. (From Saksena et al., Clinical Atlas of Roentgenocephalometry in Norma Lateralis, Alan R Liss, New York, 1987,[17] McNamara, Am J Orthod 86:449–469, 1984,[11] and Farkas, *Anthropometry of the Head and Face in Medicine,* Elsevier, New York, 1981,[4] with permission.)

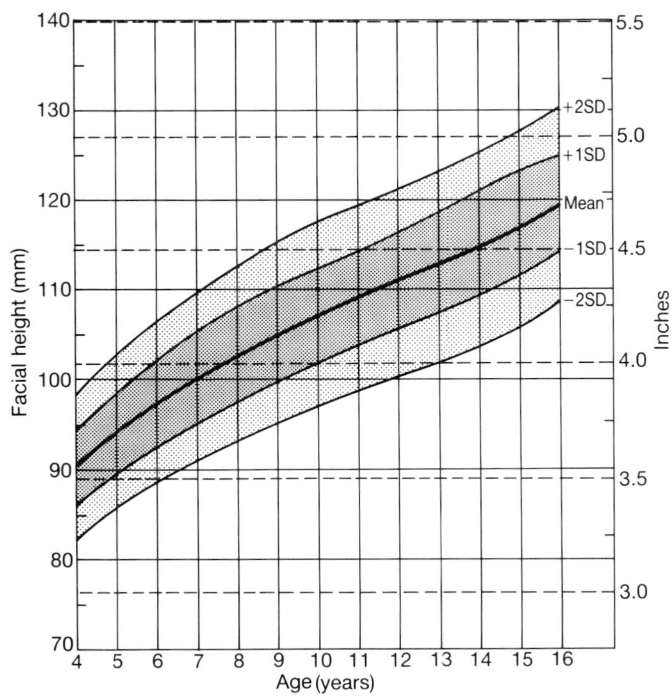


**Fig. 2–11.** Facial height, both sexes, 4 to 16 years. (From Farkas, *Anthropometry of the Head and Face in Medicine,* Elsevier, New York, 1981,[4] and Saksena et al., *Clinical Atlas of Roentgenocephalometry in Norma Lateralis,* Alan R Liss, New York, 1987,[17] with permission.)

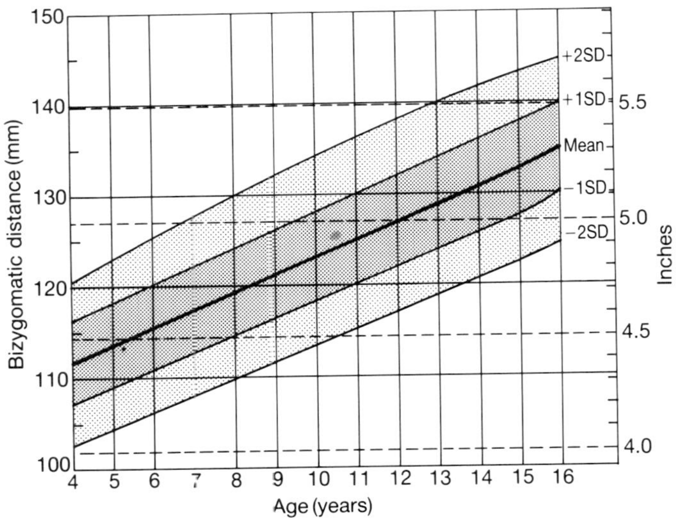


**Fig. 2–12.** Bizygomatic distance, both sexes, 4 to 16 years (From Farkas, *Anthropometry of the Head and Face in Medicine,* Elsevier, New York, 1981,[4] by permission.)

in greater detail in the measurement section, but it is important to note that a clinical impression of eye spacing is often disconsonant with actual measurement. The clinican may be misled by the width of the face, the form of the glabellar area, the presence of epicanthal folds, or the width and shape of the nasal bridge. For this reason, measurement is of great importance. Remember that spacing of the eyes must be compared to head circumference for valid interpretation.

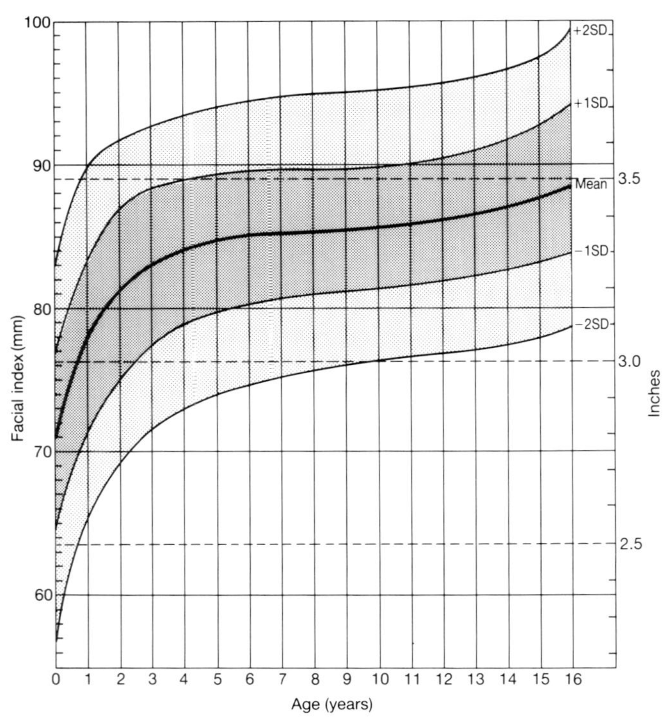


**Fig. 2–13.** Facial index, both sexes, birth to 16 years. (From Feingold and Bossert, Birth Defects 10:1–6, 1974,[6] and Farkas and Munro, *Anthropometric Facial Proportions in Medicine,* Charles C Thomas, Springfield, 1987,[5] with permission.)

True ocular hypertelorism, or wide spacing of the eyes, occurs with an increased interpupillary distance or increased bony interorbital distance (Fig. 2–14). Lateral displacement of the inner canthi and lacrimal puncta (primary telecanthus) may lead to a false impression of widely spaced eyes. A rough, clinical impression of lateral displacement of the lacrimal puncta can be obtained by seating the individual directly in front of the observer and drawing an imaginary vertical line through the inferior lacrimal point. If this line cuts the iris, there is lateral displacement of the inner canthus. The most accurate measurement of eye spacing is radiographic measurement of the bony interorbital distance.

Evaluation of the eyelid includes an assessment of length of the palpebral fissure, which may be reduced in several dysmorphic syndromes, including Dubowitz syndrome and fetal alcohol embryopathy. The width of the palpebral fissure, which is the degree of opening of the eye, may also vary and may be asymmetric. Frank ptosis or drooping of the eyelid is generally caused by weakness of levator palpebrae superioris. However, disinsertion of this muscle is an alternative cause. Ptosis is frequently found in association with Smith-Lemli-Opitz, Noonan and Freeman-Sheldon syndromes. Obliquity of the palpebral fissure varies considerably. One refers to upward slanting palpebral fissures (mongoloid slant) if the lateral margin is superior to the medial margin, and downward slanting palpebral fissures (antimongoloid slant) if the lateral margin is inferior to the medial margin. A defect of the eyelid (coloboma) is characterized by a small notch in the upper or lower eyelid.

An epicanthal fold is a lateral extension of the skin of the nasal bridge down over the inner canthus, covering the inner angle of the orbital fissure. The upper end of the fold can begin at the eyebrow, at the skin of the upper lid, or at the tarsal fold. Epicanthal folds are common in infancy, when associated with normal depression of the nasal root. However, only 3% of Caucasians between 12 and 25 years of age have epicanthal folds, as one might expect, given that the root of the nose becomes more prominent with age. Epicanthal folds are seen more frequently in Down syndrome.

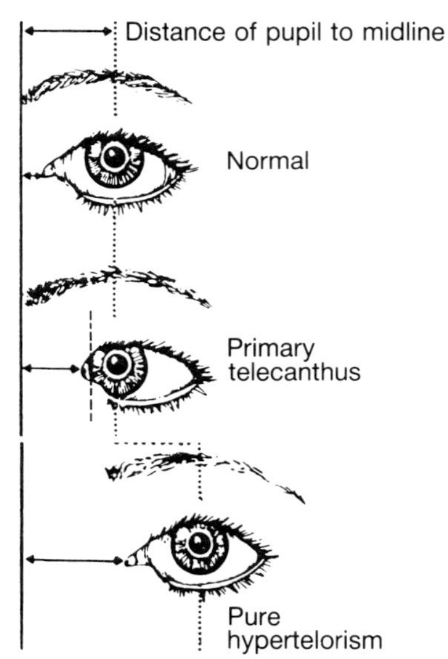


**Fig. 2–14.** Comparison of telecanthus and ocular hypertelorism. (From Pashayan et al., Am J Dis Child 125:389–393, 1973,[13] with permission.)

The thickness and length of the eyelashes should be evaluated. Eyelashes are ingrown in entropion and everted in ectropion. Distichiasis is the term used for a double row of eyelashes: one row in the normal position, the other behind it and located at the site of the openings of the meibomian glands. These glands are consequently hypoplastic or absent.

The configuration of the eyebrows is also useful in syndrome diagnosis. Evaluation should include position, shape, hair texture, and distribution. A medial flair is seen in association with Williams syndrome, a diamond shape in Noonan syndrome. Eyebrows which grow together over the nasal root are termed synophrys and are seen in de Lange syndrome. Fullness of the lateral aspect of the brow may be found in Noonan syndrome, Williams syndrome, and myxedema.

Many anomalies of iris color and structure are also found. Unilateral or patchy hypopigmentation can occur producing heterochromia iridis. A prominent pattern of the iris stroma radiating out from the pupil, known as stellate iris, may be found in Williams syndrome. Brushfield spots, elevated white or light yellow iris nodules, may be associated with peripheral iris hypoplasia in Down syndrome. Lisch nodules are small, grey-tan hamartomata of the iris and are seen in neurofibromatosis. Colobomas can also occur in the iris, giving the pupil a keyhole appearance. The gap or notch may be limited to the iris or may extend deeper to involve the ciliary body and retina.

Variation in size and shape of the pupil should be described. Pupil size varies under ordinary conditions in proportion to the amount of light let into the inner eye. Pupillary asymmetry (anisocoria) may be congenital or may result from a disturbance either locally or in the neural pathways. Irregularly shaped pupils occur secondary to infection, trauma, and neurological disease.

The cornea may vary in size and shape. Microcornea consists of a reduction in size of the corneal diameter to 10 mm or less, usually in association with growth failure of the anterior segment of the eye and incomplete development of the angle. Approximately 20% of patients with microcornea will develop glaucoma in later life. Megalocornea is present if the corneal diameter is 13 to 18 mm. If the anomaly is limited to the anterior portion of the globe, visual acuity can be normal. Megalocornea frequently is associated with subluxation of the lens, cataract, enlargement of the ciliary ring, and noticeable iridodonesis, which is a shimmering of the iris when the eye is moved rapidly from side to side in the presence of a dislocated or absent lens. Keratoconus is an obtuse conical shape to the cornea, with the vertex in or near the corneal centre. It produces abnormal refraction and is seen with an increased frequency in Down syndrome. It may be associated with retinitis pigmentosa or Alport syndrome. The cornea can appear cloudy in various storage disorders, particularly the mucopolysaccharidoses. Corneal clouding is best appreciated from the side of the eye or through a slit lamp. Kayser-Fleischer rings are areas of greenish-yellow pigmentation in Descemet's membrane at the corneal periphery, seen in Wilson disease.

Abnormalities of the conjunctiva include telangiectasia, which are dilatations of the capillary vessels and minute arteries forming a variety of angiomas and pterygia, which are patches of thickened conjunctiva, usually fan-shaped, with the apex toward the pupil. The sclerae are generally white but may be blue-gray in the neonate and in disorders such as osteogenesis imperfecta.

The inner canthal (IC) distance (Figs. 2–15, 2–16) is measured from the innermost corner of one eye to the innermost

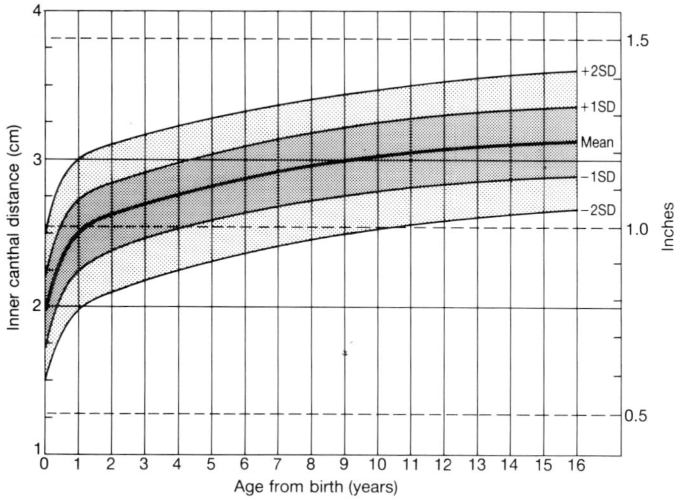


**Fig. 2–15.** Inner canthal distance, both sexes, birth to 16 years. (From Laestadius et al., J Pediatr 74:465–468, 1969,[10] and Feingold and Bossert, Birth Defects 10:1–6, 1974,[6] with permission.)

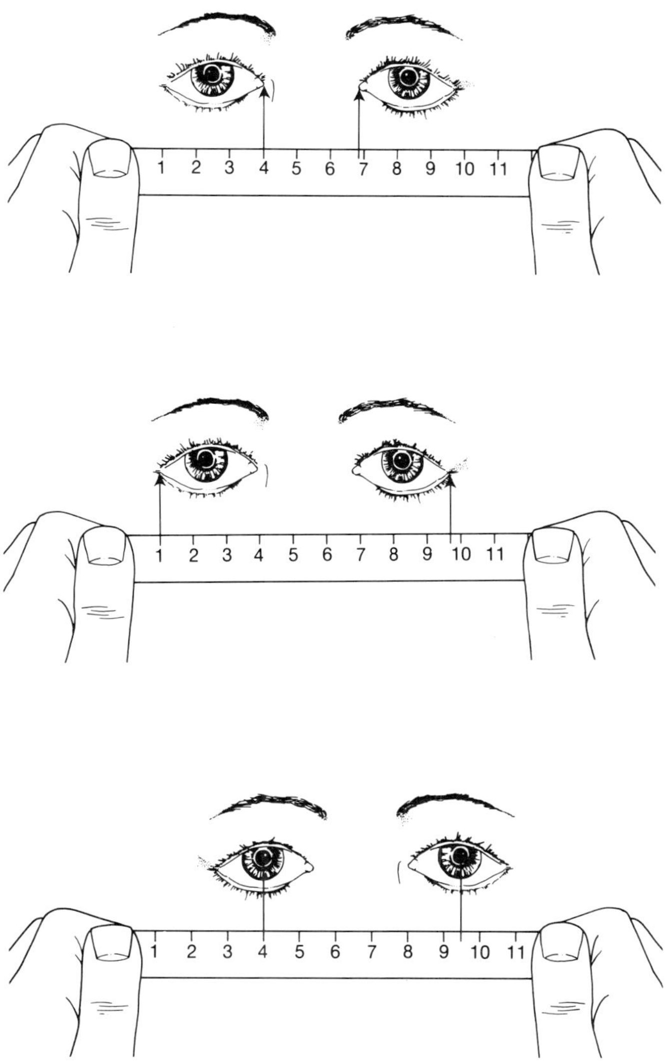

**Fig. 2–16.** Measurements of (a) inner canthal, (b) outer canthal, and (c) interpupillary distances. (From Hall et al., *Handbook of Normal Physical Measurements*. Oxford University Press, 1989[7b].)

corner of the other eye, in a straight line avoiding curvature of the nose. A graduated transparent ruler or blunt tipped sliding calipers are most accurate. However, a tape measure can be used.

The outer canthal (OC) distance (Figs. 2–16, 2–17) is measured from the most lateral corner of one eye to the most lateral corner of the other eye, in a straight line avoiding the curvature of the face. Similarly, a graduated transparent ruler or blunt-tipped sliding calipers are most accurate, but a tape measure may be used. If the eyes are not fully opened, or in the presence of ptosis, definition of the outer canthus may be difficult.

The interpupillary distance (Figs. 2–16, 2–18) is the distance between the centers of the pupils of the two eyes. A graduated transparent ruler should be used and is preferable to the use of a tape measure. This is clearly not an easy task in the infant or young child since the eyes must be fixed to obtain an accurate measurement. As an alternative, Feingold and Bossert,[6] by means of multiple linear regression techniques, have suggested the use of the following formula; IP = 0.17 + 0.59 IC + 0.41 OC. Interpupillary distance measurement is critical in order to distinguish true hypertelorism from telecanthus or lateral displacement of the lacrimal puncta.

Measurement of bony interorbital distance can only be accomplished from Xrays. It is mentioned in this text because it is the most accurate measurement of eye spacing. Measurement must be taken at the level of the junction between the medial angular process of the frontal bone and the maxillary and lacrimal bones (the dacrion). Additional information regarding this technique can be found in the References section.[2,8]

Palpebral fissure length is the distance between the inner and outer canthus of one eye (Fig. 2–19). Measurement should be taken with a graduated transparent ruler or blunt-tipped sliding calipers. Asymmetry of palpebral fissure length is common and occurs in up to 30% of the general population. It is rarely in excess of 1 mm. Additional ethnic variation occurs (Fig. 2–20).[9,20]

The obliquity, inclination, or slant of the palpebral fissures is the angle of slant of the palpebral fissure from the horizontal (Figs. 2–21, 2–22). The assessment of slant cannot be made unless the eye is open and relaxed since the outer canthus is

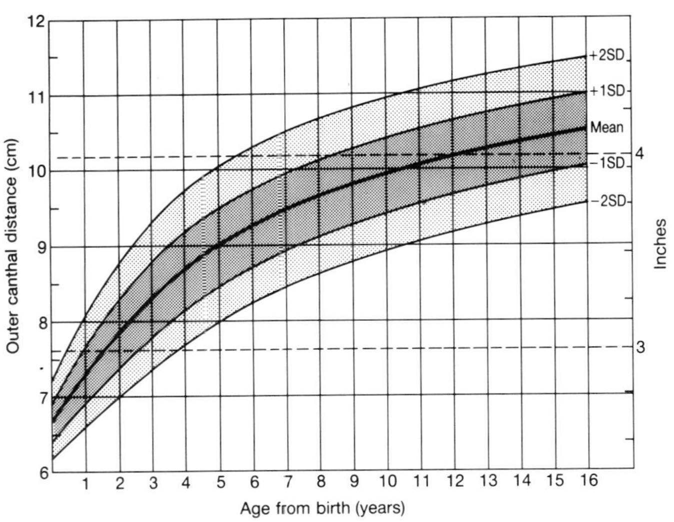


**Fig. 2–17.** Outer canthal distance, both sexes, birth to 16 years. (From Laestadius et al., J Pediatr 74:465–468, 1969,[10] and Feingold and Bossert, Birth Defects 10:1–6, 1974,[6] with permission.)

lower than the inner canthus when the eye is closed. Epicanthal folds will obscure the exact position of the inner canthus. Ectropion or lateral supraorbital fullness may create a false illusion of downward slanting palpebral fissures. Accurate measurement of obliquity necessitates a comparison between two lines. One line connects the inner canthus and outer canthus of the eye, the second line is defined by the Frankfurt horizontal (a line connecting the lowest point of the lower margin of each orbit, identified by palpation [the orbitale], and the highest point on the upper margin of the cutaneous external auditory meatus [the porion]). A commercial angle meter, protractor, or goniometer is a useful instrument for this measurement. One edge is placed along the Frankfurt horizontal, the other straight side follows the line between the canthi of each eye. Alternatively, a rough angle meter or protractor can easily be made on firm transparent material such as X-ray film. A horizontal line on this device is aligned with the Frankfurt horizontal and the angle of obliquity of the fissure is read according to the position of the line joining the canthi. A rough estimate of the horizontal line can be made by joining a line between the two inner canthi and extending this laterally. However, this is less accurate than the use of the Frankfurt horizontal. In clinical practice, an estimation of obliquity of the palpebral fissure can be made by assessing the face with the observer seated in front of the individual with the eyes open and relaxed. The relationship of lateral margin to medial margin of the eye will allow comment of upward slant, level fissure, or downward slant.

## External Ear

The external ear, or pinna, is a complex and extremely variable structure, partly because of its development from 6 auricular hillocks, but also because of the impact of 3 external auricular muscles and 6 intrinsic muscles. A protruding or cupped pinna is usually the consequence of a defect in the posterior auricular muscle. A "lop ear" is secondary to a defect of the superior auricular muscle. Abnormalities of the intrinsic ear muscles may lead to abnormal ear creases and anatomy, for example, a prominent antihelix or the crumpled ear of Beals syndrome. Absence of the superior crus of the antihelix is correlated with an increased risk for deafness. Ears are almost as distinctive as fingerprints, and much has been written about the variation in form, size, and position. The main anatomic landmarks are noted in Figure 2–23.

Subjective evaluation of the ear should include an assessment of the preauricular region, where one should look for skin appendages, fistulae, and pits; the tragus, where one should look at the size in proportion to the size of the ear; the external auditory meatus; the shape of each ear and its symmetry; whether the lobe is free or attached; the anterior and posterior surface of each ear or helix; position and rotation of the ear; and the relative positions of the tragi to see whether or not they are at the same level. Discrepant growth of the ear can occur secondary to pressure phenomena either in utero or after birth. The frequency of missing or attached earlobes varies with the ethnic group studied, but in Caucasians it averages 20 to 25%. Clinically, any patient with a malformed external ear should always be evaluated for hearing loss and abnormalities of the urinary tract.

Complete absence of the auricle, or anotia, is extremely rare. In microtia, vestiges of the external ear are present and a graded classification is applied. In cryptotia there is abnormal

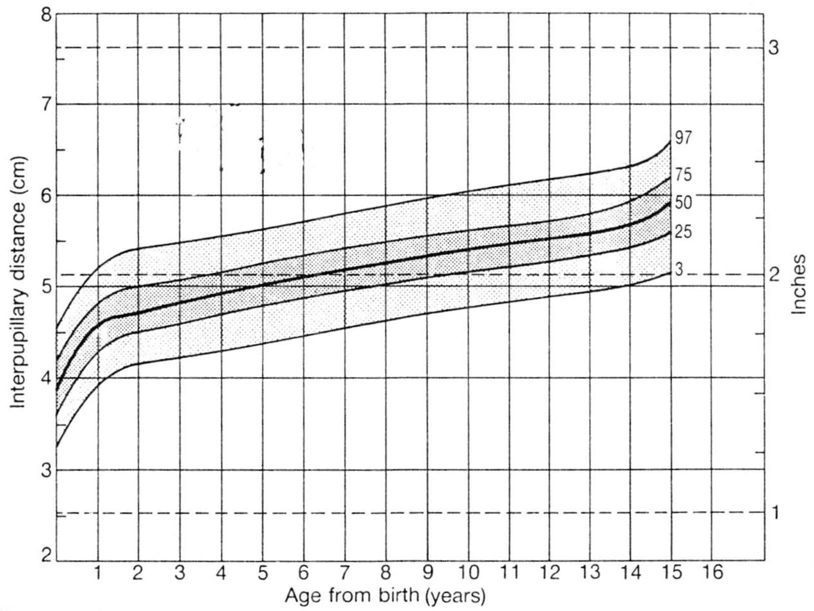


**Fig. 2–18.** Interpupillary distance, birth to 16 years. (From Feingold and Bossert, Birth Defects, 10:1–6, 1974,[6] with permission.)

adherence of the upper part of the auricle to the head, as the skin of the postauricular region directly joins the skin of the upper portion of the auricle. Cryptotia is attributed to the persistence of fetal attachment of the auricle to the underlying skin. Diagonal ear lobe creases may be more common in patients with coronary artery disease. Identical creases are seen in Beckwith-Wiedemann syndrome. In this latter condition there may also be scored grooves or notches on the posterior aspect of the superior helix or lobe.

Variations in ear position and rotation are discussed in detail in subsequent sections of this chapter. Subjective assessment of ear position and rotation is extremely imprecise and influenced by the patient's head position, and the size of the cranial vault, neck, and mandible.

Auricular appendages or tags are relatively common and result from the development of accessory auricular hillocks. They are usually anterior to the auricle, more often unilateral than bilateral. The appendages consist of skin but may also contain cartilage. They vary greatly in size and may be sessile or pedunculated. The most frequent location is the line of junction of the mandibular and hyoid arches. Less frequently they occur in the line of junction of the mandibular and maxillary processes on the cheek between the auricle and the angle of the mouth. Appendages in this area are more often associated with microtia or oblique facial fissures.

Ear length (Figs. 2–24, 2–25) is the maximum distance from the superior aspect of the outer rim of the helix to the most inferior border of the ear lobe or pinna. Measurement is best accomplished with a tape measure, transparent calibrated ruler, or sliding calipers. Small ears have been found to be a consistent clinical characteristic of Down syndrome. The ear is one of the few organs which continues to grow during adulthood. It is mainly an increase in length, since width changes little after 10 years of age. The ear is generally longer in males than in females. If the superior aspect of the helix is folded over, it is not appropriate to unfold it to measure length.

Ear width (Figs. 2–25, 2–26) is measured transversely from

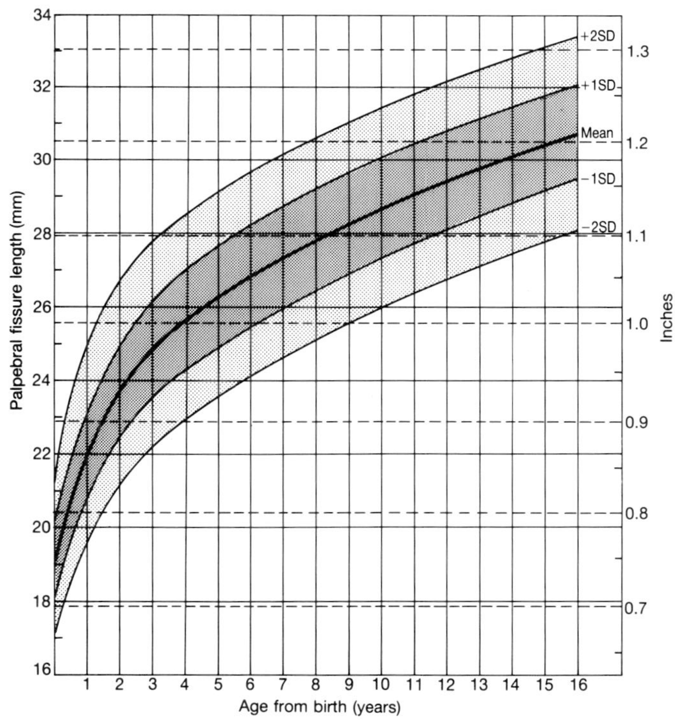


**Fig. 2–19.** Palpebral fissure length, both sexes, birth to 16 years. (From Farkas, *Anthropometry of the Head and Face in Medicine*, Elsevier, New York, 1981,[4] Laestadius et al., J Pediatr 79:465–468, 1969,[10] and Thomas et al., J Pediatr 111:267–268, 1987,[20] with permission.)

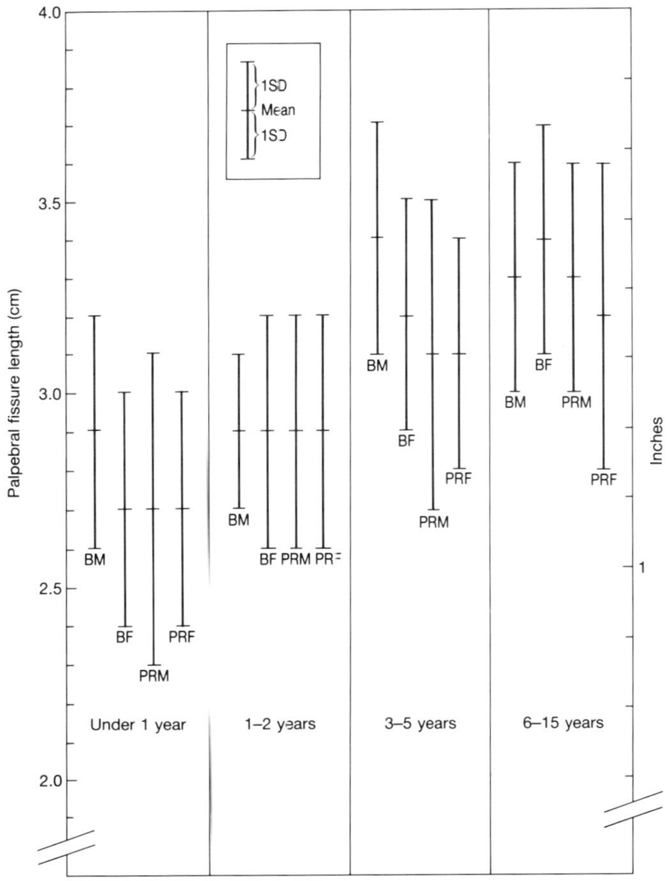


**Fig. 2–20.** Palpebral fissure length, ethnic differences in Black and Hispanic children. (BM black male; BF, black female; PRM, Puerto Rican male; PRF, Puerto Rican female). (From Iosub et al., Pediatrics 75:318–320, 1985,[9] with permission.)

the anterior base of the tragus, which can be palpated, through the region of the external auditory canal to the margin of the helical rim at its widest point. A tape measure, calibrated transparent ruler, or sliding calipers may be used. It is critical that this measurement be taken in the transverse dimension, otherwise a falsely elevated value will be obtained. With cupped or protuberant ears, the most accurate measurement is obtained with the ear pressed firmly against the head.

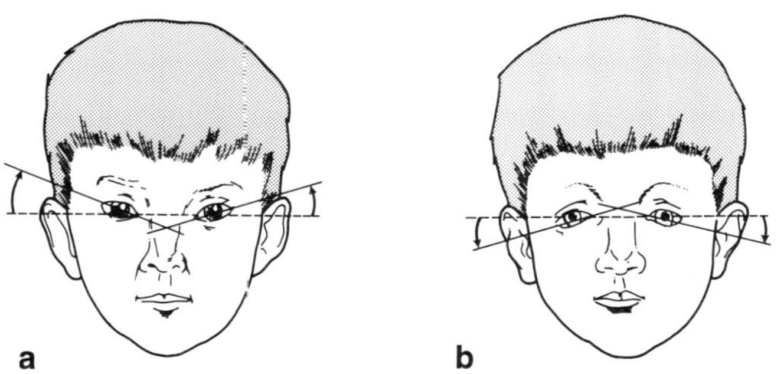


**Fig. 2–21.** Slant of the palpebral fissure: (a) upward and (b) downward. (From Hall et al., *Handbook of Normal Physical Measurements*. Oxford University Press, 1989,[7b] with permission.)

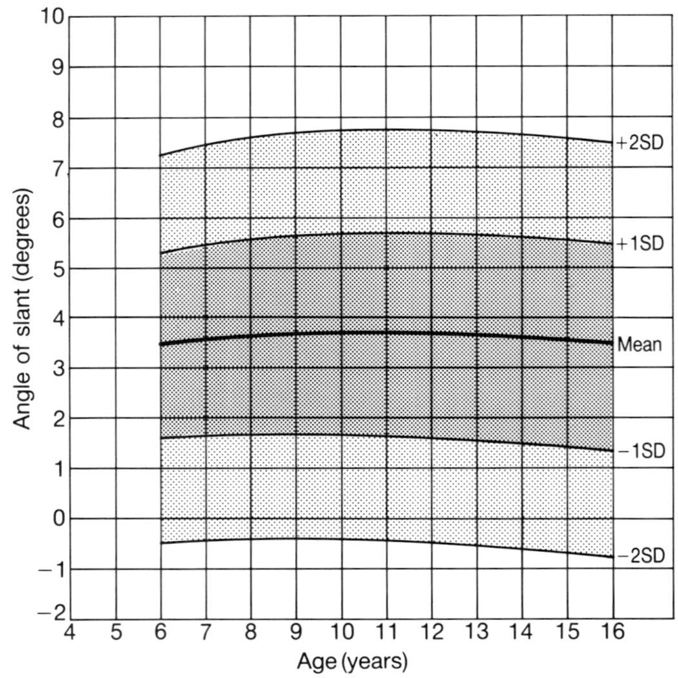


**Fig. 2–22.** Palpebral fissure inclination, both sexes, 6 to 18 years. (From Farkas, *Anthropometry of the Head and Face in Medicine*, Elsevier, New York, 1981,[4] with permission.)

Protrusion of each ear is most accurately measured as the angle subtended from the posterior aspect of the pinna to the mastoid plane of the skull. Using a transparent protractor, the zero mark of the protractor is placed above the point of attachment of the helix in the temporal region and its straight side is pressed against the subject's head. The extent of the protrusion is indicated on the curved side of the protractor. Norms are available in Farkas (1981).[4] Alternatively, a linear

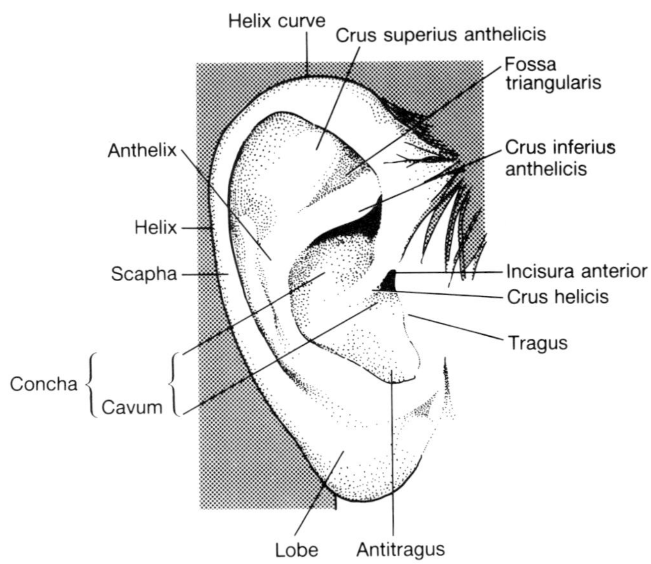


**Fig. 2–23.** Landmarks of the external ear. (From Hall et al., *Handbook of Normal Physical Measurements*. Oxford University Press, 1989, p. 161,[7b] with permission.)

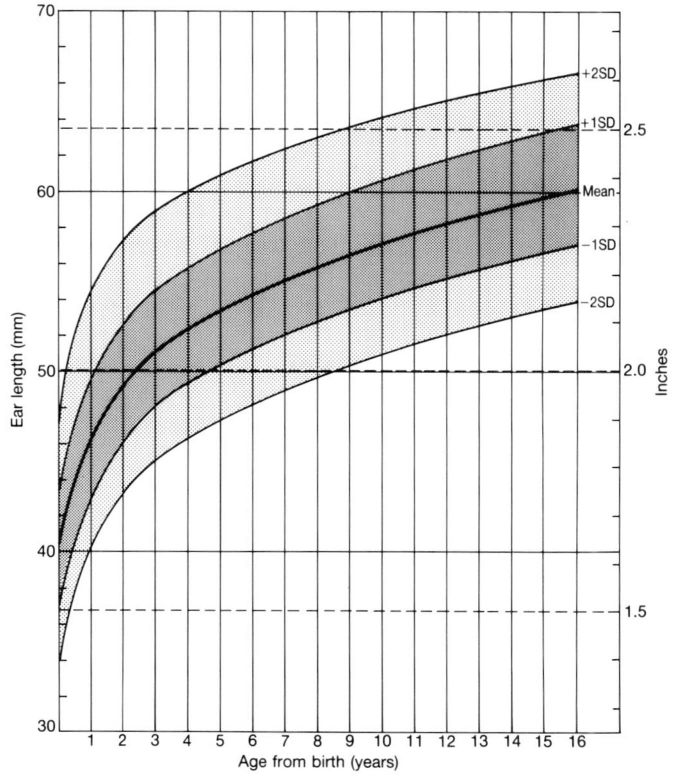


**Fig. 2–24.** Ear length, both sexes, birth to 16 years. (From Farkas, 1981,[4] *Anthropometry of the Head and Neck in Medicine,* Elsevier, New York, and Feingold and Bossert, Birth Defects 10:1–6, 1974,[6] with permission).

measurement can be made with a tape measure, calipers, or transparent ruler. If the greatest linear distance between the external ear and the temporal region of the skull is more than 2 cm, excessive protrusion is considered to be present. In order to ascertain the maximum angle or maximum distance, several measurements of ear protrusion are suggested. Generally, ear protrusion indicates weakness of the posterior auricular muscles.

Subjective evaluation of ear position and rotation is open to marked misinterpretation. Ear position is defined as the location of the superior attachment of the pinna, and four methods to determine position are available (Fig. 2–27). The one preferred by this author is shown in Figure 2–27a. All methods have their advantages and disadvantages. The author advises any reader to become comfortable with one method and use it consistently. One can draw an imaginary line between the outer canthus of the eye and the most prominent part of the occiput (Fig. 2–27a). The superior attachment of the pinna should be on or above this line. This method is probably the one most consistently used.

Alternatively, one can draw an imaginary line through the inner and outer canthi and extend that line posteriorly (Fig. 2–27b). The superior attachment of the pinna should lie on or above that line. This method clearly depends on obliquity of the palpebral fissures. Thirdly, one can draw an imaginary line between both inner canthi and extend that line posteriorly (Fig. 2–27c). Anthropologists determine the position of the ear according to a proposal by Leiber. Details are found in Farkas (1981).[4] For the first three methods, one can use a tape measure, flexible transparent ruler, or graduated piece of X-ray film to determine the horizontal plane.

The landmarks used to determine ear position are among the most controversial in clinical dysmorphology. Although this author prefers to use the superior attachment of the pinna as a landmark, other dysmorphologists and anthropologists may assess ear position based on the level of porion (Fig. 2–27d). Subjective impression of ear placement is clearly influenced by the position of the person's head, relative to that of the ob-

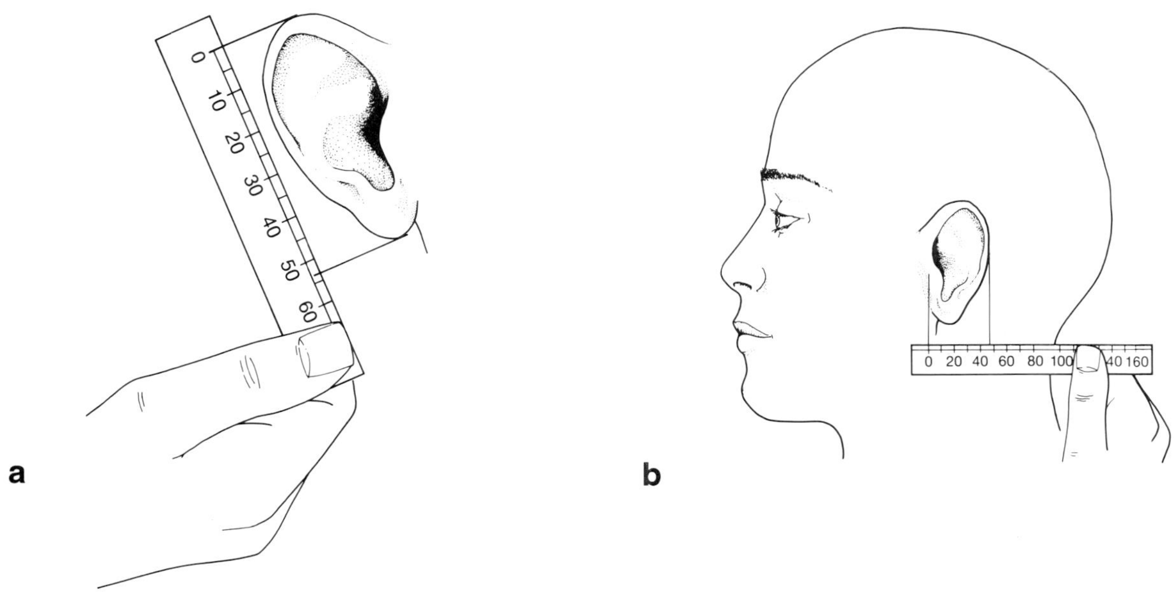


**Fig. 2–25.** Measurement of ear size: (a) length and (b) width. (From Hall et al., *Handbook of Normal Physical Measurements.* Oxford University Press, 1989, pp. 163,[7b] with permission.)

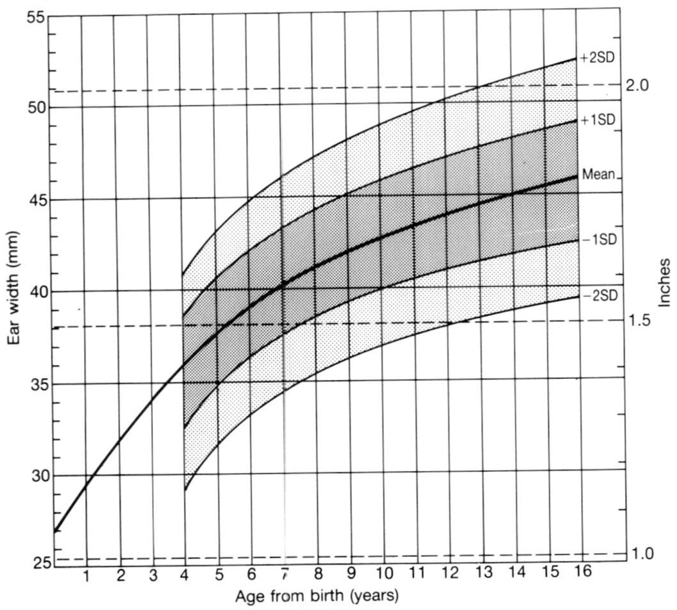


**Fig. 2–26.** Ear width, both sexes, birth to 16 years. (From Farkas, *Anthropometry of the Head and Neck in Medicine,* Elsevier, New York, 1981,[4] and Goodman and Gorlin, *Atlas of the Face in Genetic Disorders,* 2nd ed., CV Mosby Co, St Louis, 1977,[7a] with permission.)

server. In the lateral view, ear position seems to be judged in relation to the vertex above, and the chin and level of the tip of the shoulder below. A high ratio between these distances gives the impression of low-set ears, which may explain why the ears of a small infant appear to be set lower than those of an older child. The infant's neck and mandible are relatively small compared to the cranium. The inclination or rotation of the auricle also affects the observer's impression of ear level. The ears look lower set when the auricles are tilted posteriorly.

Ear rotation (Fig. 2–28) is strictly defined as rotation of the median longitudinal axis of the external auricle. Such inclination from the vertical is measured by placing the long side of an angle meter along the line connecting the two most remote points of the medial axis of the ear, the landmarks used in measurement of ear length. The vertical axis is then established in one of two ways. First, and most accurately, the vertical is a line perpendicular to the Frankfurt horizontal plane. Alternatively, the vertical axis can be estimated by imagining a line perpendicular to a line connecting the outer canthus of the eye and the most prominent part of the occiput. In clinical practice this latter method is most often used. The angle of rotation is the angle subtended between the median longitudinal axis of the ear and the vertical axis. Normal rotation is between 17 and 22 degrees.

## Nose

The nose is remarkable in its variability in profile, frontal plane, and undersurface, as illustrated in Figure 2–29. Details of the soft tissue and bony landmarks are available in references at the end of this chapter. A qualitative assessment of the nose should include the nasofrontal angle: is it normal, flat, or deep; the nasal root protrusion: is it average, high, or low; the nasal bridge: is it high, low, broad, beaky, or bulbous; the nasal tip: is it normal, flat, or bifid; the shape of each nasal ala: is it normal, slightly flat, markedly flat, angled slightly, or markedly; the nasal alar configuration: is it cleft, hypoplastic, hypertrophic, is there a coloboma; and the size and type of the nostrils: are they symmetric or asymmetric, and what type are they according to the Topinard classification.[7a] Attempts to quantify changes in nose shape with age have rarely been documented. However, it is well known that the nasal root is depressed in the infant and young child, associated with a

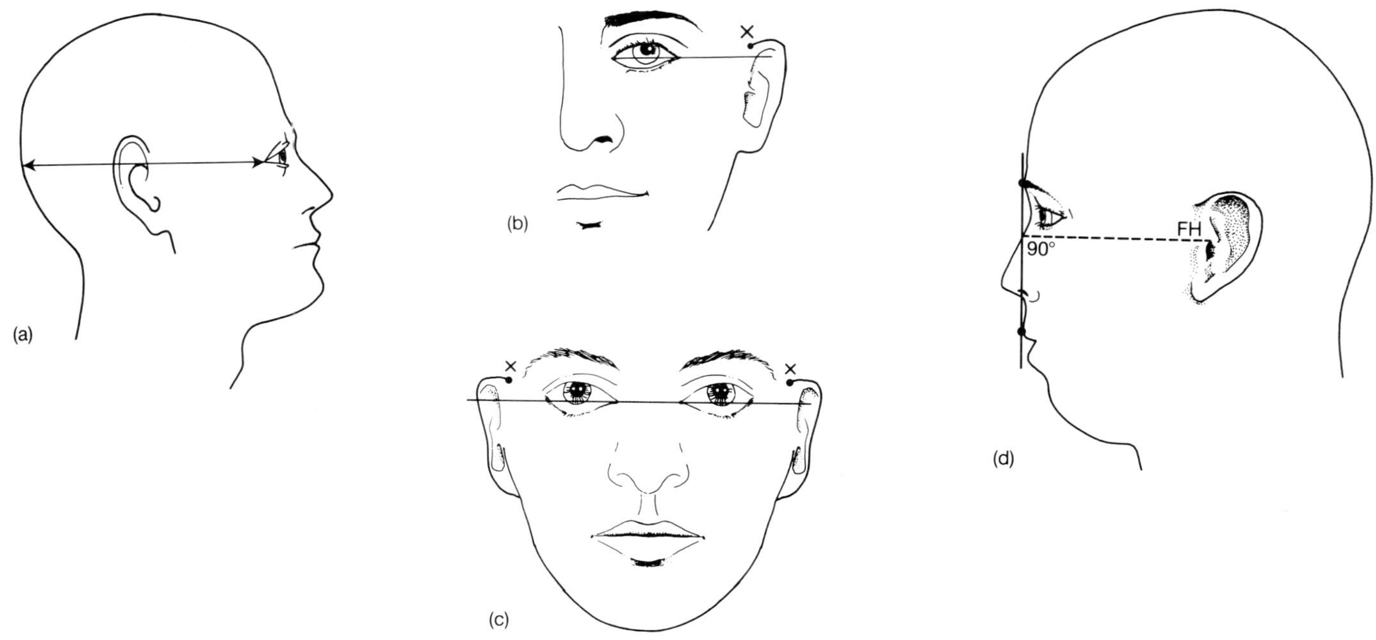


**Fig. 2–27.** Determination of ear position by four methods (a–d). (From Hall et al., *Handbook of Normal Physical Measurements.* Oxford University Press, 1989, pp. 170, 171,[7b] with permission.)

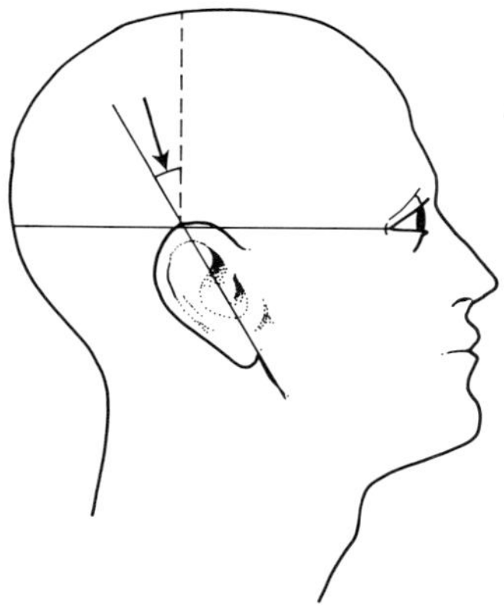

**Fig. 2–28.** Determination of ear angulation. (From Hall et al., *Handbook of Normal Physical Measurements.* Oxford University Press, 1989, p. 174,[7b] with permission.)

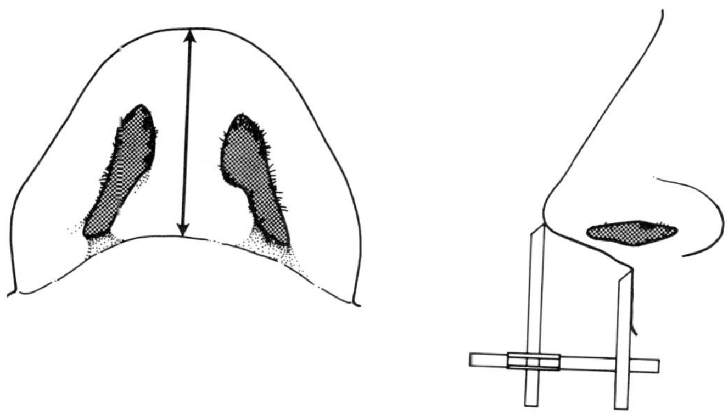

**Fig. 2–30.** Measurement of nasal protrusion. (From Hall et al., *Handbook of Normal Physical Measurements.* Oxford University Press, 1989, p. 182,[7b] with permission.)

scooped-out nasal bridge. With increasing age, the nasal bridge rises, producing a more prominent root. Nostril type also varies with age.

Most nasal measurements are soft tissue measurements. However, many alternatives are available from radiographs. These will not be described in detail here and the interested reader is referred to the literature cited at the end of this chapter.[7,11,17]

Horizontal measurements of the nose, particularly width of the nasal root and the interalar distance, provide information about midline development of the face in the same way that the measurements of eye spacing reflect midline development. The nasal tip may be broad, grooved, cleft, or actually bifid with increasing width of the nose. A bifid nose results when the medial nasal prominences do not merge completely. In this situation, the nostrils are widely separate and the nasal bridge is bifid. This type of malformation may be part of a spectrum known as frontonasal dysplasia.

Nasal height has been mentioned in the context of upper facial height and the reader is referred to that section. Unlike most vertical facial dimensions, nasal height continues to increase throughout life.

Nasal protrusion (Figs. 2–30, 2–31) is measured from the tip of the nose (pronasale) to the deepest concavity at the base of the nose in the midline (subnasion). Sliding calipers are most accurate. However, a transparent graduated ruler can be substituted. This dimension can be assessed from below the nose or from the side. It is important to remember that this dimension is a linear dimension made in a straight line and not along the surface of the nasal septum following its curve to the tip.

Interalar distance, or width of the nasal base, is the distance between the most lateral aspect of the alae nasi (Fig. 2–32). It is best measured with sliding calipers, although a transparent calibrated ruler or tape measure can be substituted. The nostrils should be held in the position of rest when this measurement is taken since some individuals can voluntarily flare their nostrils. There is tremendous variation both within and between ethnic groups in the interalar distance. This distance, like most facial widths, continues to increase with age, mainly due to soft tissue changes.

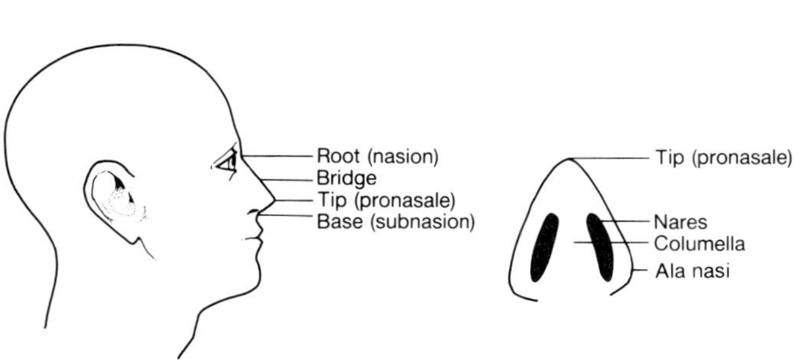


**Fig. 2–29.** Major landmarks of the nose. (From Hall et al., *Handbook of Normal Physical Measurements.* Oxford University Press, 1989, p. 176,[7b] with permission.)

## Philtrum

The philtrum, or vertical groove in the central part of the upper lip, extends from the base of the nose to the superior aspect of the vermilion border of the upper lip. In some individuals, this structure is poorly demarcated, while in others, the cutaneous elevations that mark its lateral borders or pillars are easily discernible. The enclosed area is usually depressed. The philtral margins or pillars may be parallel or divergent. Although ade-

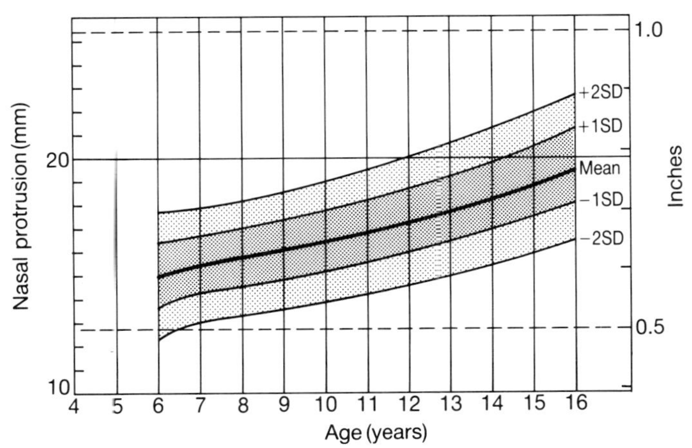


**Fig. 2–31.** Nasal protrusion, both sexes, 6 to 16 years. (From Farkas, *Anthropometry of the Head and Face in Medicine,* Elsevier, New York, 1981,[4] with permission.)

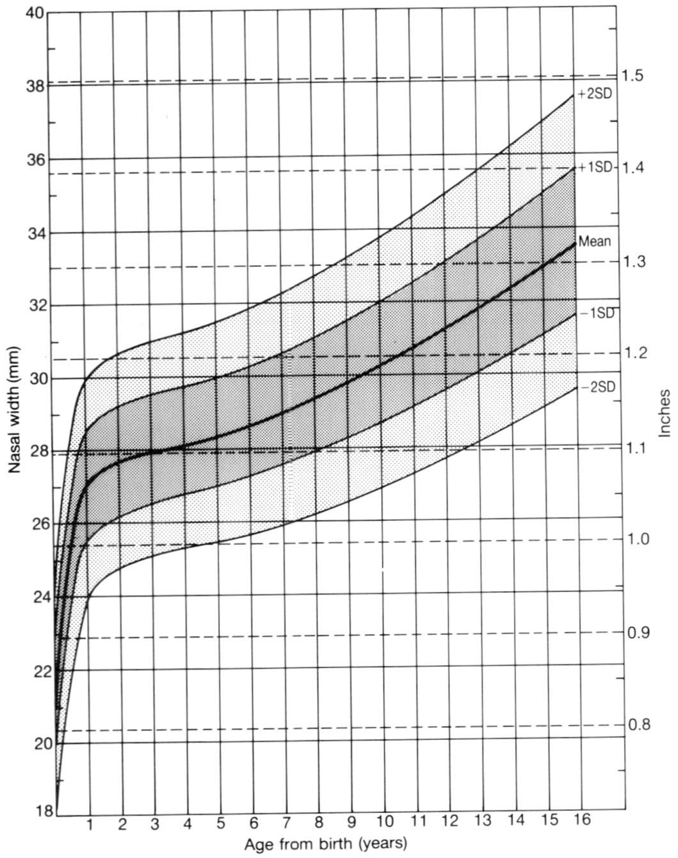


**Fig. 2–32.** Interalar distance (nasal width), both sexes, birth to 16 years. (From Farkas, *Anthropometry of the Head and Face in Medicine,* Elsevier, New York, 1981,[4] and Goodman and Gorlin, *Atlas of the Face in Genetic Disorders,* 2nd ed., CV Mosby Co, St Louis, 1977,[7a] with permission.)

quate graphs are available for philtral lengths, normal philtral width has been of little concern to the clinician. However, increasing width and flattening are subjectively established in fetal alcohol syndrome and Cornelia de Lange syndrome.

Clefts involving the upper lip, with or without cleft palate, occur about once in 1,000 births, but their frequency varies widely among ethnic groups. Sixty to eighty percent of affected infants are males. The clefts vary from small notches of the vermilion border of the lip to larger divisions that extend into the floor of the nostril and through the alveolar part of the maxilla. Cleft lip can be either unilateral or bilateral. In bilateral cases the defects may be similar or dissimilar with varying degrees on each side. Median cleft lip is an extremely rare defect of the upper lip caused by a mesodermal deficiency which results in partial or complete failure of the medial nasal prominences to merge and form the intermaxillary segment. The presence of median cleft lip should alert the observer to look for other midline abnormalities of the brain, including holoprosencephaly.

Other unusual types of facial cleft may occur, but each is individually rare. Clefts of the lower lip and mandible are also rare. The lip may be cleft superficially, or, in severe cases, it may be split down to the chin involving the mandible.

Philtral length is measured from the base of the nose (subnasion) to the superior aspect of the vermilion border of the lip in the midline (Fig. 2–33). Ideal measurement utilizes sliding calipers. However, a calibrated transparent ruler could be used.

## Mouth and palate

Variation in size of the mouth is well documented but mouth width is a particularly difficult soft tissue measurement to assess without the aid of a cooperative, relaxed patient. One measures from one cheilion (corner of the mouth) to the other cheilion (Fig. 2–34) using sliding calipers. A tape measure, or calibrated transparent ruler may be substituted.

Variation in lip size and shape is extensively seen and may or may not be associated with differences in philtral development. A well-formed, deeply grooved philtrum is generally associated with wide-spaced peaks to the vermillion border of the upper lip. Conversely, a poorly formed, flat philtrum is usually associated with a relatively thin, even surface to the vermillion border. A tented upper lip usually results from long-standing, bilateral facial weakness, such as that seen in congenital myotonic dystrophy.

Congenital pits or recesses of the lips are present in 2 to 3% of neonates. They are generally found on the lower lips where they may be bilateral or unilateral, showing a well-defined circular depression on the vermillion border. They represent the orifice of mucous tracts that extend into the substance of the lip.

Frenula are strands of tissue extending between the buccal and alveolar mucosae. Abnormal numbers of frenula may be associated with various craniofacial syndromes. An assessment of alveolar ridge thickness should be included in the evaluation of the mouth. Thickening may be congenital or acquired, for example, following prolonged anticonvulsant therapy.

Cleft palate, with or without cleft lip, occurs about once in every 2,500 births and is more common in females than males. A cleft may involve the uvula or may extend through the soft palate or all the way forward to the hard palate. The cleft may be overt or submucous. In severe cases associated with cleft

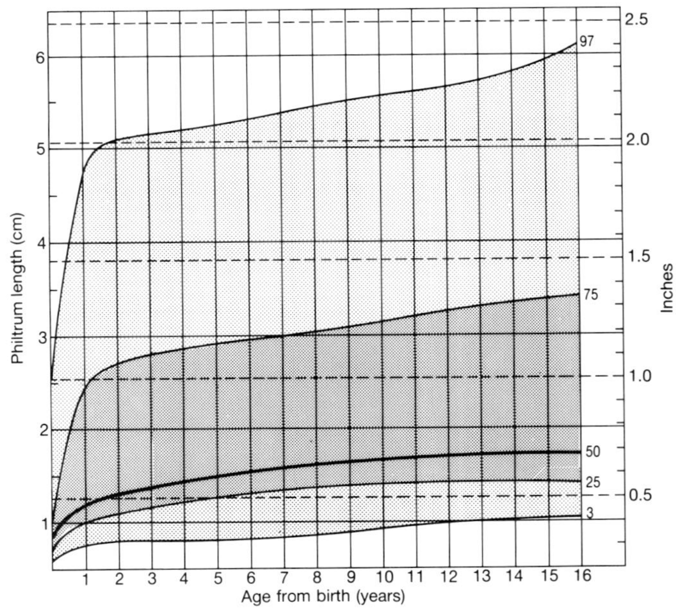


**Fig. 2–33.** Philtrum length, both sexes, birth to 16 years. (From Feingold and Bossert, Birth Defects 10:1–6, 1974[6] with permission.)

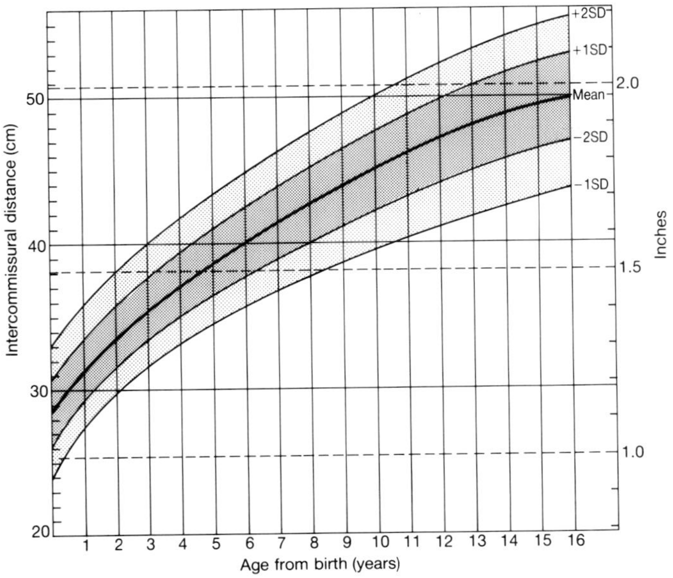


**Fig. 2–34.** Intercommissural distance, both sexes, birth to 16 years. (From Feingold and Bossert, Birth Defects 10:1–6, 1974,[6] and Farkas, 1981,[4] *Anthropometry of the Head and Face in Medicine,* Elsevier, New York, with permission.)

lip, the cleft of the palate extends through the alveolar process and lip on both sides. The majority of cases of cleft palate are associated with multifactorial inheritance. Others are part of single gene or chromosomal syndromes, especially Stickler syndrome. A few cases appear to be caused by teratogenic exposure, particularly to anticonvulsants and alcohol. Genetic factors are more important in cleft lip, with or without cleft palate, than in cleft palate alone.

The palate is often stated to be abnormally high when, in fact, no measurement has been carried out. Devices have been designed to directly measure palatal height, width, and length. In the "field" a rough estimate of palate height can be obtained by comparing it with height of the teeth. If the maximum height of the palate is greater than twice the height of the teeth, it can be considered abnormal. Unusually prominent lateral palatine ridges are a nonspecific feature of a variety of disorders in which there is either neuromuscular dysfunction or an anatomic defect which prevents or limits tongue thrust into the palatal vault. The lateral palatine ridges are normally more prominent during prenatal life and infancy. With increasing age, they become progressively flattened by the molding forces of the tongue and usually disappear by 5 years of age. Prominent lateral palatine ridges may be misinterpreted as a true narrow high-arched palate, which is a much less common anomaly.

Palate length may be assessed cephalometrically.[7] From a radiograph, the dimension from the anterior to the posterior nasal spine is measured, using sliding calipers. Soft tissue measurement of palate length is difficult and requires special instrumentation.[18] With this instrument, palate length is defined as the distance from the labial point of the incisive papilla to the midline of the junction of the hard and soft palates.[16] The majority of clinicians will not have access to such instrumentation.

The width of the palate is the distance between the maxillary first permanent molar on the right side and the maxillary first permanent molar on the left side at the lingual cervical line.[16] Palate width is again measured with a specific device.[18]

The height of the palate is measured by establishing the shortest distance between the midline of the junction of the hard and soft palates, and the plane established using the reference points noted in the evaluation of palate length and width.[16] This measurement point, the fovea palatinus, is not always the highest dimension of the palatal vault. Once again, a palatal measuring device is necessary.

## Maxilla

Unilateral maxillary absence is a rare condition resulting from the failure of development of one maxillary process. Absence of the premaxillary area is found in cyclopia when the frontonasal processes do not form. Subtle hypoplasia of the maxilla is best appreciated on X-rays, and is an important feature to be looked for in first-degree relatives of patients with Treacher Collins syndrome. Clinical evaluation of the maxilla is extremely subjective and is best performed in profile, while looking at prominence of maxilla in comparison to prominence of the supraorbital ridges, malar area, and mandible. No objective clinical measurements appear to be available.

To assess the size and prominence of the maxilla (effective midfacial length), one utilizes several cephalometric landmarks, measuring from the condylion of the mandible (the most posterosuperior point of the condylar outline) to point A (the deepest midline point on the maxilla between the anterior nasal spine and the prosthion, which is the inferior labial termination of the cortical plate just above the maxillary incisors).[11]

## Mandible

Agnathia, or absence of the mandible, is a developmental defect of the first branchial arch. The mandible may be missing on one side only, a condition sometimes associated with microtia, anotia, or unilateral congenital macrostomia. Micrognathia may be severe enough to lead to cleft palate in the Pierre Robin sequence. This can be an isolated anomaly or associated with other features as part of a syndrome diagnosis. Macrognathia or large jaw is otherwise termed *prognathism* and is best appreciated in profile. The shape of the jaw can vary markedly depending on the relative proportions of the ramus and body of the mandible. The jaw articulates with the skull at the temporomandibular joint. Restricted movement at that joint may produce limited mouth opening or trismus. The size and shape of the chin contribute to the overall facial shape. A wide chin will tend to produce a round or square face, while a narrow, pointed chin promotes the appearance of an inverted triangular face, secondary to the relative width of the forehead and cranial vault. Various measurements of the jaw can be made from radiographs. The main clinical measurement, for which a graph is provided, is mandibular width or bigonial distance.

The mandibular width, or bigonial distance, is measured from the most lateral aspect at the angle of the jaw (gonion) to the same point on the other side of the face, with spreading calipers (Fig. 2–35). Marked asymmetry of the mandible or malformation of the mandible may make it difficult to define the gonial points.

Two cephalometric measurements are also available. The effective length and prominence of the mandible can be ascertained if one measures from the condylion to the anatomic gnathion (determined by the intersection of the facial and

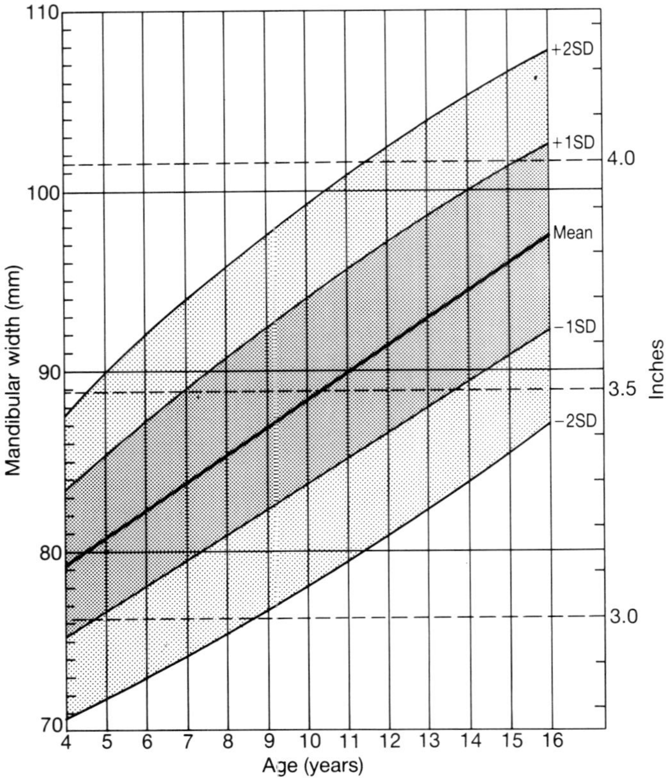


**Fig. 2–35.** Mandibular width, both sexes, 4 to 16 years. (From Farkas, *Anthropometry of the Head and Face in Medicine,* Elsevier, New York, 1981,[4] with permission.)

mandibular planes).[11] If one subtracts the effective midfacial length from the effective mandibular length, one has the maxillomandibular differential.[11]

## Neck

Most of the congenital malformations of the neck originate during transformation of the branchial apparatus into adult structures. Branchial cysts, sinuses, or fistulae may develop from part of the second branchial groove, the cervical sinus, or the second pharyngeal pouch, if there is failure of regression. The thyroglossal duct may persist, or remnants of it may give rise to thyroglossal duct cysts. These cysts, if infected, may form thyroglossal duct sinuses, which open in the middle of the neck, in contrast to the branchial sinuses, which open off center and close to the borders of the sternocleidomastoid muscle.

Torticollis usually is attributed to injury of the sternocleidomastoid muscle during delivery. However, prenatal onset of the anomaly cannot be ruled out. Torticollis additionally can be due to malformations of the cervical vertebrae. The presence of unequal muscle pull on the developing cranium, by torticollis, may lead to unequal growth of the skull with resultant plagiocephaly. A contralateral epicanthal fold is frequently seen.

In approximately one-third of cases, torticollis is associated with congenital hip dislocation. Both are thought to be caused by cramped circumstances in utero, for example, secondary to abnormal uterine anatomy, a uterine fibroid, or oligohydramnios.

Estimation of the length and width of the neck is very subjective and normal age-related charts are not available. The neck is generally short in the neonate and begins to elongate in the older child. The width of the neck obviously varies, increasing from a superior to an inferior aspect. A wide neck may be associated with skin folds or webs, or with prominence of the trapezius muscle. These latter anomalies may be related to prenatal onset of jugular lymphatic obstruction, which, in the newborn period, is correlated with excess nuchal skin, posteriorly rotated auricles, and upturned lobules.

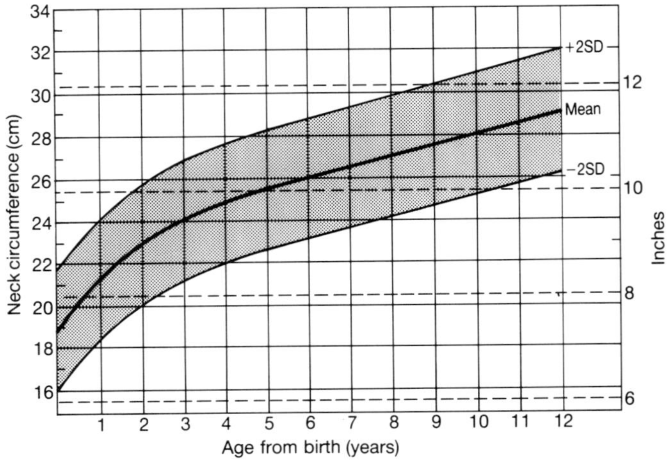


**Fig. 2–36.** Neck circumference, both sexes, birth to 12 years. (From Feingold and Bossert, Birth Defects 10:1–6, 1974,[6] with permission.)

Neck circumference can be quantified. The neck should be measured in a horizontal plane at the level of the most prominent portion of the thyroid cartilage (Fig. 2–36). A tape measure is the best tool for this dimension. In the presence of prominent folds of skin or webs at the side of the neck, the tape measure should carefully follow the surface of the skin to reflect circumference accurately.

### References


1. Caffey J: J. Caffey's Pediatric X-ray Diagnosis, 7th ed. Year Book Publishers, Chicago, 1978.
2. Currarino G, Silverman FN: Orbital hypotelorism, arhinencephaly, and trigonocephaly. Radiology 74:206–217, 1960.
3. Faix RG: Fontanelle size in black and white term newborn infants. J Pediatr 100:304–306, 1982.
4. Farkas LG: Anthropometry of the Head and Face in Medicine. Elsevier, New York, 1981.
5. Farkas LG, Munro IR: Anthropometric Facial Proportions in Medicine. Charles C. Thomas, Springfield, IL, 1987.
6. Feingold M, Bossert WH: Normal values for selected physical parameters: an aid to syndrome delineation. Birth Defects 10:1–6, 1974.
7. Garn SM, Smith BH, LaVelle M: Applications of pattern profile analysis to malformations of the head and face. Radiology 150:683–690, 1984.

7a. Goodman RM, Gorlin RJ: Atlas of the Face in Genetic Disorders, 2nd ed., CV Mosby Company, St Louis, 1977.

7b. Hall JG, Froster-Iskenius UG, Allanson JE: Handbook of Normal Physical Measurements. Oxford University Press, Oxford, 1989, pp 89–220.

8. Hansman CF: Growth of interorbital distance and skull thickness as observed in roentgenographic measurements. Radiology 86:87–96, 1966.
9. Iosub S, Fuchs M, Bingol N, Stone RK, Gromisch DS, Wasserman E: Palpebral fissure length in black and Hispanic children: correlation with head circumference. Pediatrics 75:318–320, 1985.

10. Laestadius ND, Aase JM, Smith DW: Normal inner canthal and outer orbital dimensions. J Pediatr 74:465–468, 1969.
11. McNamara JA, Jr: A method of cephalometric evaluation. Am J Orthod 86:449–469, 1984.
12. Nellhaus G: Head circumference form birth to eighteen years. Practical composite international and interracial graphs. Pediatrics 41:106–114, 1968.
13. Pashayan H, Pruzansky S, Putterman A: A family with belpharo-naso-facial malformations. Am J Dis Child, 125:389–393, 1973.
14. Popich GA, Smith DW: Fontanels: range of normal size. J Pediatr 80:749–752, 1972.
15. Pruzansky S: Clinical investigation of the experiments of nature. ASHA 8:62–94, 1973.
16. Redman RS: Measurement of normal and reportedly malformed palatal vaults II: normal juvenile measurements. J Dent Res 45:266, 1966.
17. Saksena SS, Walker GF, Bixler D, Yu P-L Clinical Atlas of Roentgenocephalometry in Norma Lateralis. Alan R Liss, New York, 1987.
18. Shapiro BL, Redman RS, Gorlin RJ: Measurement of normal and reportedly malformed palatal vaults I: normal adult measurements. J Dent Res 42:1039, 1963.
19. Tanner JM: Physical growth and development. In: Textbook of Pediatrics, JC Forfar, GC Arneil, eds. Churchill Livingstone, Edinburgh, 1978, pp 253–303.
20. Thomas IT, Gaitantzis YA, Frias JL: Palpebral fissure length from 29 weeks gestation to 14 years. J Pediatr 111:267–268, 1987.
21. Ward RE: Facial morphology as determined by anthropometry: keeping it simple. J Craniofac Genet Dev Biol 9:45–60, 1989.

# 3

# Epidemiology

MUIN J. KHOURY, RICHARD S. OLNEY, and J. DAVID ERICKSON

Epidemiology is concerned with patterns of disease occurrence in human populations and the factors that influence these patterns.[83,118] In the context of birth defects, and specifically otolaryngologic anomalies, epidemiology seeks

1) to characterize the distribution of these defects in human populations and evaluate geographic, temporal, social, and personal variations in risks (descriptive epidemiology);
2) to assess causes of defects including genetic, nutritional, infectious, drug-related, environmental, and other factors (analytic epidemiology); and
3) to provide a scientific basis for applying public health prevention and intervention strategies.[68,81]

Over the past decade, epidemiology has found increasing applications in the area of human reproduction, birth defects and genetic diseases.[64,68,74] Most epidemiologic studies of causes of adverse reproductive outcomes are observational, i.e., comparing pregnancy outcomes of women who have or do not have a certain attribute or exposure (cohort studies), or comparing past pregnancy exposures among mothers who delivered babies with or without birth defects (case–control studies). The observational nature of epidemiologic studies makes them particularly vulnerable to certain biases such as confounding, selection, and recall.[83] Nevertheless, a relatively new area in epidemiology is the field of randomized clinical trials where investigators evaluate the outcomes of pregnancies among women randomized to a certain preventive intervention and those to a placebo.[93] The most notable example here is the relatively recent documentation of a protective effect of periconceptional folic acid supplementation in reducing the risk of neural tube defects in pregnancies subsequent to an affected pregnancy,[100] and in the general population.[28] Randomized clinical trials are considered the gold standard of epidemiologic research and will find increasing applications in future studies that evaluate birth defects prevention strategies.

In this chapter, we review the epidemiology of selected otolaryngologic defects. We first give an overview of the available sources of data used to study the epidemiology of these defects. We next give an overview of otolaryngologic anomalies as a group, their overall frequency, and contribution to birth defects and infant morbidity and mortality. Because of the anatomic and pathogenetic heterogeneity of otolaryngologic anomalies, we review the epidemiology of five relatively common selected defects: microtia/anotia, choanal atresia, cleft lip and palate, esophageal atresia, and congenital deafness.

## Sources of data on the epidemiology of otolaryngologic anomalies

Much of the current information on the epidemiology of otolaryngologic anomalies comes from population-based birth defects surveillance systems and registries in North America, Europe, and other parts of the world.[61] These programs started as a result of the thalidomide tragedy and have continued to proliferate over the past 25 years.[58,65] In the United States, birth defects programs are available at the federal level and at the state level, as many states have passed legislation for reporting birth defects.[34,71,86] For example, the Metropolitan Atlanta Congenital Defects Program (MACDP) is a population-based birth defects system operated by the Centers for Disease Control (CDC) since 1967. The system ascertains all stillbirths and liveborn infants with major serious structural defects with onset in the first year of life among offspring of Atlanta residents.[34] While MACDP and other similar birth defects programs provide good quality data in ascertaining serious birth defects, the ascertainment of minor anomalies is less than complete. This is particularly pertinent to craniofacial features, some of which could be variably detected and recorded by clinicians and specialists. Another limitation of such programs is the lack of ascertainment of important developmental disabilities such as congenital deafness, which tends not to be related to structural or anatomic defects.

In addition, other sources of information on the epidemiology of otolaryngologic anomalies and their risk factors have come from special studies ranging from cross-sectional surveys, case–control studies based on hospitals and universities, cohort studies, and family studies.

## Public health impact of otolaryngologic anomalies

Serious structural birth defects are an important public health problem. About 3% of all infants are born with a major defect that is diagnosed within the first year of life. More infants have minor anomalies and developmental disabilities that are primarily nonstructural in origin (e.g., congenital deafness). Overall, birth defects are the leading cause of infant mortality in the United States, accounting for more than 20% of all infant deaths,[14] and are a major contributor to child hospitalizations and general morbidity.

To assess the overall relative importance of otolaryngologic anomalies within the spectrum of birth defects requires explicit inclusion criteria for what should be considered otolaryngologic defects. It is important to recognize that otolaryngologic anomalies include a variety of anatomic, embryologic, and pathogenetic disorders with different epidemiologic characteristics and causal pathways. Overall, if one considers this group of anomalies to include defects involving the ear, nose and sinuses, mouth, palate and pharynx, larynx, trachea and esophagus, as well as craniofacial and neck anomalies, then a substantial proportion of infants with serious birth defects have an otolaryngologic anomaly. For example, in the population-based data of about 25,000 infants with major birth defects ascertained in metropolitan Atlanta, we found that about 20% of all such infants have a defect in this group (CDC, unpublished data). Moreover, among infants with multiple congenital anomalies (defined as having two or more unrelated serious birth defects), about 62% have otolaryngologic defects. For those infants with multiple congenital anomalies of known cause (single gene, chromosomal, and teratogenic), the vast majority of such infants (84%) have an otolaryngologic defect.[107] The contribution of otolaryngologic anomalies is likely to be higher if one includes infants with congenital deafness and those with minor craniofacial anomalies not well ascertained in birth defects surveillance systems. Infants with otolaryngologic anomalies have an increased risk of early mortality. In Atlanta, for example, 3% of all such infants are stillbirths and an additional 10% die within the first year of life (10 times the general infant mortality rate in the population) (CDC, unpublished data). Undoubtedly, the impact of such anomalies on general morbidity could be even higher, although not easily quantifiable, as many such infants may require one or more corrective surgeries and long-term medical and nursing care.

Causes of otolaryngologic anomalies include single gene disorders, chromosomal defects, and known teratogenic agents such as alcohol, isotretinoin, and diphenylhydantoin. Nevertheless, the contribution of different causes to these defects will vary by the type of defect. In metropolitan Atlanta between 1989 and 1991, of 119 infants with multiple congenital anomalies involving otolaryngologic defects, most (51%) have an unknown cause, 25% have a chromosomal abnormality, 10% a known mendelian condition, 3% a teratogenic exposure, and 10% have a clinically known pattern of defects of unknown cause.[107]

**Table 3–1.** Epidemiologic characteristics of cleft lip with or without cleft palate (CL+/−P) and cleft palate (CP)

| Characteristics | Notes |
|---|---|
| Clinical presentation | 70% of cases with CL also have CP; 25% of cases with CL+/−P and 40% of cases with CP have additional defects |
| Prevalence | CL+/−P: 10 per 10,000 births; CP: 5 per 10,000 births |
| Geographic variation | CL+/−P: high rates (>15 per 10,000) in China, Japan, Denmark, Norway; CP: high rate (12 per 10,000) in Finland |
| Racial/ethnic differences | CL+/−P: in the U.S.: Asian descent and Native Americans > European descent > African Americans |
| Gender differences | CL+/−P: 60%–65% males: CP: 55% females |
| Temporal trends | Stable rates in most places |
| Maternal age | CP+/−P & CP: U-shaped maternal age distribution for multiple malformed cases in some studies |
| Birth weight | CL+/−P & CP: increased proportion with low birth weight among multiple malformed cases only |
| Twinning | CL+/−P monozygotic concordance 40%, dizygotic, 7%; CP monozygotic concordance 15%, dizygotic 6% |
| Familial patterns | Sibling recurrence: 3%–4%; many single gene syndromes |
| Causes/risk factors | Occasionally chromosomal (trisomy 13); occasionally single gene; smoking may increase risk; vitamin supplement use may decrease risk |

## Epidemiology of selected otolaryngologic anomalies

### Oral clefts

The epidemiologic characteristics of cleft lip and cleft palate are shown in Table 3–1. Oral clefts are among the most common of congenital anomalies, and numerous articles have been written on the epidemiology of these defects. The review article by Burdi[9] and the more recent review by Lettieri[82] are useful references for the reader wanting more details.

In embryological considerations, oral clefts are subdivided into two major categories: cleft of the upper lip (CL), with or without cleft palate (CL+/−P), and cleft palate (CP). CL+/−P derives from the so-called embryological *primary palate*, and CP derives from the *secondary palate*. Clefts of the primary palate involve the lip and the alveolar ridge anterior to the incisive foramen, while clefts of secondary palate involve the hard and soft palate, from the incisive foramen posterior to the uvula. Both types of clefts vary in severity, ranging from relatively minor clefts of the lip or clefts of the soft palate, to complete clefts of the lip and/or palate. CL can be unilateral or bilateral; when unilateral, the left side is more frequently affected than the right.[33] Infants with oral clefts often have additional defects[45,124] which could be components of recognizable phenotypes.[24,82] In some instances, a straightforward genetic pattern of occurrence can be discerned. Some are simple mendelian traits, while others reflect an underlying chromosomal aberration. However, patterns of relatively simple genesis are not apparent in the majority of cases. More complicated origins must therefore be postulated—probably as interactions between genetic susceptibilities and environmental influences.[41]

Numerous articles have presented data on the birth prevalence of oral clefts from various types of samples, from different geographical areas, times, and racial groups. In general, between 10 and 20 babies in each 10,000 births are affected by one or the other or both of these defects; atypical facial clefts, such as median cleft lip, are much less frequent. Data from the 25 International Clearinghouse for Birth Defects Monitoring Systems surveillance programs[61] for 1985–1988 show relatively wide variations in rates for CL+/−P, ranging from about 5 per 10,000 births in France, Italy, and Spain to 1.5 per 10,000 births in China, Japan, Norway, and Denmark. Data from these surveillance programs for CP show rates generally in the range of 4 to 6 per 10,000. Finland is the notable exception, with a rate of about 12 CP cases per 10,000 births.

It is well known that in the United States there are substantial racial variations in the rates of CL+/−P, while there are less variations for CP. Data from the CDC's Metropolitan Atlanta Congenital Defects Program[16] has shown the CL+/−P rate for whites to be at about 12 per 10,000 births, and for blacks at about 8 per 10,000; for CP the Atlanta rates have been about 6 and 5 per 10,000 births for whites and blacks, respectively. Persons of Asian heritage typically have high rates of CL+/−P, as do American Indians.[96,103,105,132]

Males have a higher rate of CL+/−P than females, while females are, less strikingly, at increased risk than males for

CP. The Atlanta rate for CL+/−P for males is 12 per 10,000 compared to 9 for females; for CP the rate for males is 5 per 10,000 and for females, 6 per 10,000 births. The differences for males and females are less pronounced among cases with other defects than among those who have isolated cleft defects.[37]

As for most types of defects, there are many causes of oral clefts. Some cases may be associated with chromosomal abnormalities (e.g., trisomy 13), and there are numerous defined malformation syndromes, many of them single gene disorders, that have CL+/−P or CP as a feature. The multifactorial model has been a popular theory used to explain the relatively low familial risks of oral clefts.[42] A particularly exciting finding is that a genetic variant at the transforming growth factor alpha locus may be associated with an increased risk for nonsyndromic CL+/−P,[3,18,56] although the association has not been consistently found.[54] In addition, no association could be found in eight families transmitting an apparently dominant form of CL+/−P.[138] Another potentially important finding is an association between nonsyndromic CL+/−P and a particular genetic variant at the retinoic acid receptor locus;[19] retinoic acid is a well-known and widely studied animal teratogen. A number of elegant statistical analyses of familial aggregation for CL+/−P have been done recently, some suggesting involvement of a major genetic locus contribution,[88] but these analyses have been found lacking by other observers.[99]

The risk of clefting is increased among the offspring of women with epilepsy; this risk is thought to be due to exposure to anti-epileptic drugs rather than to something directly associated with the epilepsy.[53] At least one study found an association between maternal benzodiazepine use and the occurrence of CL+/−P.[119] Maternal cigarette smoking has been found to be associated with CL+/−P and CP in some studies[38,73,123b] but not others.[141] In a small study of mothers of babies with CL+/−P, Niebyl et al.[104] could not demonstrate substantial differences from controls relative to a large number of serum chemistries. A study in New York found no association with exposure to 60 hertz electrical fields (electric blankets, heated water beds).[32] An exciting possibility is that the use of vitamin supplements might reduce the risk of recurrence of CL+/−P.[113,130]

## Microtia/anotia

The epidemiologic characteristics of microtia/anotia are summarized in Table 3–2. Most investigators consider microtia and anotia to be part of a continuum that includes even more extensive defects of the lateral face, such as hemifacial microsomia.[10] At the other end of the spectrum, the mildest forms of microtia (classified alternatively as grade or type I, or first degree) may often be described as cup ear or small ear and are variably ascertained by birth defect surveillance systems. In spite of these methodologic difficulties, reported rates of microtia are remarkably similar in many different countries, ranging between 1 and 3 per 10,000 births. With few exceptions, these rates have remained stable since early studies were done in the 1950s and 1960s[94] and since international surveillance began in the 1970s.[61] There also appears to be no seasonal variation in the occurrence of these defects.[13] Significantly higher rates (4–6 per 10,000) have been found in epidemiologic studies in Sichuan, Mexico, Ecuador, and six other countries in South America,[12,61] and in clinical studies among the Navajo Indians in New Mexico.[2]

**Table 3–2.** Epidemiologic characteristics of microtia/anotia

| Characteristics | Notes |
|---|---|
| Clinical presentation | Usually unilateral; 1/3 with multiple anomalies |
| Prevalence | 1–3 per 10,000 births |
| Geographic variation | Relatively high rates in Sichuan, Mexico, and South America (4–6 per 10,000 births) |
| Racial/ethnic differences | Not well studied; high rates among Native Americans in New Mexico (5.3 per 10,000 births) |
| Gender differences | M/F 2:1 |
| Temporal trends | Relatively stable rates since 1950s; no seasonal variation |
| Maternal age | No significant variation in rates by age |
| Birth weight/gestational age | Prematurity rate not increased; lower mean birth weights in some populations |
| Twinning | Rate of twinning not increased |
| Familial patterns | Multifactorial/threshold model usually applied (6%–8% of 1st degree relatives affected); single gene etiology in a minority of cases (usually autosomal dominant with incomplete penetrance) |
| Causes | Single genes, chromosomal abnormalities, or known teratogens (thalidomide, diabetes, isotretinoin) rarely implicated |

In a case–control study of microtia in South America,[12] there was no significant difference between affected and unaffected liveborn infants in maternal ages or gestational ages. Birth weights of infants with microtia were significantly lower in one of two populations studied, perhaps reflecting intrauterine growth retardation among those with multiple defects. The rate of twinning was not significantly higher among infants with microtia; indeed, even case reports of twins with microtia are rare.[102]

The male:female ratio among series of children with these defects is usually about 2:1, with a range of 1.2–2.4:1.[1,10,94] In most series and epidemiologic studies, 80%–90% of microtia/anotia cases are unilateral, usually with only the right side involved; the mandible is often hypoplastic and the external auditory meatus is usually atretic on the involved side, causing hearing impairment.[1,10,12,61,67] A minority (about one-third) of children with microtia/anotia have other types of defects or a recognized syndrome,[10,94] particularly involving the eye, cervical spine, and palate.[117]

Various degrees of microtia/anotia, usually with abnormal configurations of the pinnae, are features of several recognized patterns of multiple malformations.[1,63] A few of these phenotypes are well established and clearly inherited in a (dominant) mendelian fashion such as Treacher Collins syndrome. Nonsyndromic microtia with meatal atresia or anotia has also been described among several unrelated families, with both autosomal dominant and autosomal recessive inheritance suggested.[36,109,122] Extensive pedigree analyses have been performed in large clinical series of individuals affected with various degrees of microtia.[1,2,117] Results of these studies indicated empiric recurrence risks of 3%–4%. Such figures suggest that the multifactorial/threshold model of inheritance applies to most families with microtia, although autosomal dominant inheritance with incomplete penetrance undoubtedly applies in a few instances.[10]

Two classic teratogens have been associated with microtia/anotia (along with multiple defects): thalidomide and isotretinoin.[80,126] However, since the use of these drugs is now prohibited in pregnancy, they probably rarely cause these defects today. More common exposures in pregnancy that have been associated with microtia/anotia include diabetes[62] and maternal alcohol use,[10] although true microtia is not classically described among large series of infants with fetal alcohol syndrome[22] or diabetic embryopathy.[78] Case–control studies of microtia/anotia such as that done in South America[12] have failed to consistently identify any particular maternal exposures or illnesses that are significantly associated with these defects.

Aneuploidy is a well-known cause of ear malformations. However, true microtia occurs rarely in Down syndrome. The ears are more likely to be simply below the 5th percentile in size, square, and thickened. Small structural chromosomal abnormalities, for instance involving 22q,[121] are rarely reported among infants with microtia. The overall contribution of currently detectable cytogenetic abnormalities to the etiology of microtia/anotia is probably minimal, although this topic has not been well studied epidemiologically. Future research should help to pinpoint genetic polymorphisms that contribute to ear formation[10] and are likely to further elucidate the molecular basis of the epidemiologic heterogeneity of microtia/anotia.

### Choanal atresia

The epidemiologic characteristics of choanal atresia are summarized in Table 3–3. Congenital obstruction of the posterior nose is usually (90%–95%) bony in nature.[40,114,127] Complete bilateral atresia presents as severe respiratory distress immediately after birth, which may account for more frequent ascertainment of this type in some clinical series,[127] whereas most authors state that the unilateral type is more common.[40,87,101,114]

**Table 3–3.** Epidemiologic characteristics of choanal atresia

| Characteristics | Notes |
|---|---|
| Clinical presentation | 90%–95% bony; most unilateral; 1/2 with multiple anomalies |
| Prevalence | 1–2 per 10,000 births |
| Geographic variation | Not well studied; no statistical differences between Atlanta, California, and North African rates |
| Racial/ethnic differences | No differences between whites and blacks in California or Atlanta |
| Gender differences | M/F 0.5–0.8 |
| Maternal age | No significant variation in rates by age |
| Birth weight/gestational age | Lower mean birth weight due to increased rate of preterm delivery and growth retardation |
| Familial patterns | Familial cases < 10% in most series; recurrence risk for CHARGE < 1% |
| Causes | At least 9% chromosomal; occasionally single gene; few teratogens alleged but unconfirmed |

Most of the epidemiologic studies of this defect do not analyze clinical subtypes, nor do they stratify analyses according to whether the atresia is isolated or associated with other major or minor defects. Multiple defects do occur in at least half of all cases of choanal atresia,[87,101,114,127] with cardiovascular defects coinciding with as many as one-fourth of all cases of choanal atresia.[50] Choanal atresia is a frequent feature of four recognized multiple congenital anomaly phenotypes,[63] particularly the CHARGE (**c**oloboma, **h**eart defects, **a**tresia choanae, **r**etarded growth and development, **g**enital hypoplasia, and **e**ar anomalies or deafness) association,[84,112] for which this defect is often considered the cardinal feature.[51] Choanal atresia is occasionally seen in at least 10 other eponymic phenotypes;[63] of particular note is the DiGeorge sequence, many clinical features of which overlap with the CHARGE association.[23] Numerous case reports document other purported associations with major defects.[20,46,47a,49,75,106]

Birth prevalences of choanal atresia (1–2 per 10,000 live births) are similar among both whites and blacks in California and metropolitan Atlanta, two areas of the United States where birth defects surveillance is well established;[15] these prevalences differ little from less well-documented figures found in the clinical literature.[87,101,114] A hospital-based survey[98] in Benghazi, Libya (North Africa) found a higher birth prevalence of 3.2 per 10,000 births; however, this rate does not differ statistically from those in California and Atlanta because the birth population is relatively small.

A male:female ratio of 0.5 was reported in one early clinical series[40] and is widely quoted in reviews of choanal atresia,[52,87,101,114] whereas some series have found a more equal prevalence among males and females.[98,127] Population-based surveillance in Atlanta from 1968 to 1991 showed a male:female ratio of 0.8 (CDC, unpublished data). In the Atlanta population, no significant variation in choanal atresia rates is seen with varying maternal age. Rates of choanal atresia are significantly elevated among low birth-weight infants.[95] The relative risk for intrauterine growth retardation is high among Atlanta infants with choanal atresia,[72] and over one-third are premature (CDC, unpublished data). The combination of these factors, along with the high rate of associated defects, are undoubtedly responsible for the high mortality rate among infants with choanal atresia: one-fifth of all infants with choanal atresia in the Atlanta population died in the perinatal period.

Among infants born with choanal atresia in Atlanta from 1968 to 1991, 9% were found to have abnormal karyotypes, primarily trisomy 18 and 21. Another 17% were tested and no chromosome abnormalities were found. Since 1980, numerous small structural abnormalities such as chromosome deletions, duplications, and translocations have been reported in association with multiple congenital anomaly phenotypes, including choanal atresia, such as DiGeorge sequence and CHARGE association.[23,60,66,77,97,131] Cytogenetic evaluations in the 1960s and 70s may not have utilized the high resolution banding techniques necessary to ascertain such abnormalities, which are therefore probably underrepresented in the Atlanta data. However, even with current techniques, including molecular probes for chromosomal regions which appear to be specific for such phenotypes as the DiGeorge sequence, the proportion of children with chromosome abnormalities among those with choanal atresia and multiple congenital anomalies is not known.

The overall contribution of single gene defects to the etiology of choanal atresia is also poorly documented in the literature. The proportion of cases of choanal atresia that are inherited in a mendelian fashion has been estimated to be as high as 8%;[92] in one relatively large clinical series of 30 children who underwent surgical procedures, 3 (10%) were from the same family.[40] Familial choanal atresia associated with other defects, for example, spiky hair, athyrosis, and cleft palate,[4] is occasionally reported in the clinical literature. In these few cases, as well as those defects associated with established mendelian phenotypes such as ectrodactyly-ectodermal dysplasia-clefting (EEC) syndrome,[20] the defect appears to have been inherited in either an autosomal dominant or recessive fashion;[25] however, the recurrence risk for other types of choanal atresia is said to be either unknown (for isolated defects)[52] or less than 1% (for CHARGE with "nongenetic etiology").[39] On the other hand, McKusick[92] states that isolated choanal atresia is "probably a multifactorial trait." Reports of possible teratogens such as methimazole[49] and diazepam[51] are even less frequent and have not been confirmed by epidemiologic studies; the only agent that is strongly linked with choanal atresia is thalidomide.[126] In summary, familial patterns and causes of choanal atresia are quite heterogeneous, making skilled family history–taking, dysmorphological examination, and laboratory evaluation important prerequisites for accurate genetic counseling.

**Table 3–4.** Epidemiologic characteristics of esophageal atresia/tracheoesophageal fistula

| Characteristics | Notes |
|---|---|
| Clinical presentation | 85%–90% of cases have EA and distal TEF >50% of cases have multiple anomalies (VACTERL type) |
| Prevalence | 2–3 per 10,000 births |
| Geographic variation | Low rates in China (Sizchuan), 0.4 per 10,000 births; high rates in Finland, 4.1 per 10,000 births |
| Racial/ethnic differences | Not well studied; some studies show excess among whites compared to blacks |
| Gender differences | Slight excess in males in some studies (M/F of 1.1–1.4) |
| Temporal trends | Stable rates in most places; space–time clusters observed in some places |
| Maternal age | U-shaped maternal age distribution in some studies |
| Birth weight/gestational age | Lower mean birth weight due to increased rate of preterm delivery and growth retardation |
| Twinning | Increased rate of twinning in some studies (3 times) |
| Familial patterns | Sibling recurrence < 1%; rarely single gene etiology |
| Causes | Chromosomal < 5% (commonly trisomy 18 and 21); rarely single gene; multifactorial/threshold model may not fit well-observed data |

### Esophageal atresia/tracheoesophageal fistula (EA/TEF)

There is considerable anatomic and clinical variability in the presentation of EA/TEF. There are several subtypes of esophageal atresia according to the presence and location of TEF. Most cases (85–90%), however, have an esophageal atresia with a distal tracheoesophageal fistula.[31,61,139] Occasionally, TEF occurs in the absence of esophageal atresia (H-type). The epidemiologic characteristics of the less common anatomic subtypes of EA/TEF have been poorly described, however. In addition, about half of EA/TEF cases have other associated defects,[31,43,139] notably those that fall in the VACTERL (**v**ertebral anomalies, **a**nal atresia, **c**ardiac defects, **t**racheoesophageal fistula, **e**sophageal atresia, **r**enal anomalies, **l**imb defects) association and other midline defects spectrum.[69,70] As discussed below, these patterns of multiple congenital anomalies indicate underlying etiologic and pathogenetic heterogeneity. Unfortunately, much of the epidemiologic literature summarized below does not classify cases according to the presence or absence of other anomalies.

Information on the birth prevalence of EA/TEF has been obtained from birth defects surveillance systems worldwide (Table 3–4). The prevalence at birth has been recently summarized from 25 such programs and is of the order of 2 to 3 per 10,000 births.[61] In Atlanta, the rate of EA/TEF was 2.2 per 10,000 births between 1968 and 1980 (CDC, unpublished data). Recently, a population-based study of EA/TEF and other midline defects in the Maryland-Washington-northern Virginia area found that the rate of EA/TEF was 2.1 per 10,000 births between 1980 and 1987.[139] There has been little long term change in the rate of EA/TEF although space–time clusters have been observed in some parts of the world but not others.[43,76,79,110] There is little geographic variation in the rates of EA/TEF, although rates in China (Sichuan) have been consistently lower than in other parts of the world: 0.4 per 10,000 births.[61] On the other hand, rates in Finland, for example, have been consistently higher than in other places (4.1 per 10,000 births).[79]

There is little information on racial/ethnic variation in the rates of EA/TEF. In Atlanta for the period 1968–1990, rates were higher for whites compared to blacks (rates of 2.7 vs. 1.3 per 10,000 births, respectively; CDC, unpublished data). In Maryland-Washington-northern Virginia, there was a slight excess of EA/TEF among whites compared with other groups (predominantly blacks) (rates of 2.4 vs. 2.1 per 10,000 births, respectively).[139] In several studies, a slight male excess has been observed, with sex ratios (male:female) in the range of 1.1 to 1.4 (CDC, unpublished data.[31,43,47,79,139] No excess of EA/TEF among males was observed in data from British Columbia.[43]

Variations in rates of EA/TEF by maternal age and birth order have not been well characterized. In southwest England, David and O'Callaghan found evidence for a U-shaped maternal age effect, with excess of EA/TEF in children of mothers under age 20 years and over age 35 years.[31] A similar maternal age effect in isolated esophageal atresia has been observed in Hungary.[128] Yang et al. did not show maternal age effects in the Maryland-Washington-Virginia study.[139]

There is a reported association between EA/TEF and twinning. Several studies have shown a preponderance (up to three times) of twins among EA/TEF cases compared with the general population.[30,31,47] The excess twinning has not been observed in data from Hungary, however.[128]

Infants with EA/TEF tend to have a lower mean birth weight than normal infants.[79,128] This is related to a higher prevalence of both preterm delivery and intrauterine growth retardation (IUGR) in these infants.[31,128] In Atlanta, more than half the EA/TEF cases have IUGR (defined as birth weight under the 10th percentile for gestational age, race, and sex).[72]

There is considerable etiologic heterogeneity among cases of EA/TEF. Chromosomal abnormalities (most commonly trisomy 18 and 21) account for a small proportion of the cases (5%).[31,43] Also, EA/TEF is a variable feature of several single gene disorders and contiguous gene disorders.[59,91] No clear-cut teratogenic exposures have been documented in the etiology of EA/TEF, although maternal diabetes[31] and heavy alcohol ingestion[90] have been suggested as risk factors. However, in the majority of EA/TEF cases, the cause remains unknown. Sibling recurrence risks are generally low (under 1%).[91] For such cases, the multifactorial/threshold model of inheritance has been used as the basis for empiric risk estimates in genetic counseling.[17,137] However, Szendrey et al. have suggested that patterns of familial recurrence do not fit well with the expectations of the multifactorial model.[128] Also, some studies have suggested an increase in the risk of neural tube defects among siblings of infants with EA/TEF.[44] Based on a more recent synthesis of the literature, Little has concluded that the risk of neural tube defects in the pooled sibling data is not significantly higher than in the general population.[85]

The association between EA/TEF and other malformations notably cardiac, anorectal, and vertebral defects (part of the VACTERL spectrum), while most likely unrelated to a single cause or pathogenetic event, suggests underlying commonalities in developmental processes. These defects occur together much more than expected on the basis of chance alone, which may be due to multiple factors acting during the vulnerable period of blastogenesis.[108]

## Congenital Deafness

In contrast to the four otolaryngologic anomalies discussed above which tend to be serious birth defects that are relatively easily recognizable at birth, congenital deafness tends to be more variably ascertained during infancy and childhood and may or may not be associated with structural birth defects and genetic syndromes.[5] As a result, information on the epidemiology of congenital deafness tends to be more variable and inconsistent across studies and populations (Table 3–5). Some of the methodologic difficulties involved in describing and comparing congenital deafness in different populations include the following issues:

1. *Definition of deafness.* Studies have used a variety of definitions of deafness, ranging from mild to severe hearing impairment. For example, in a recent population-based study of developmental disabilities in metropolitan Atlanta, the authors defined hearing impairment as unaided, bilateral pure tone hearing loss that averaged 40 dB or worse in the better ear.[32a] In this study, moderate loss was defined as impairment from 40 to 70 dB, severe impairment from 71 to 90 and profound hearing impairment was defined as loss averaging more than 90 dB in the better ear. Many consider deafness to include severe to profound impairment (i.e. more than 90 dB loss in the better ear).[26,27] Nevertheless, in reviewing various surveys of childhood deafness, there is considerable variation in the cutoff used as an inclusion criterion (e.g., 25 dB, 35 dB, and 65 dB, as summarized by van Rijn and Cremers).[136] A study of childhood deafness in the European Community used 50 dB as a cutoff for case definition.[89] Such variation makes it difficult to compare population frequencies as well as causes of deafness in different studies.

2. *Age at onset and evaluation.* The ascertainment of congenital deafness is related to the early recognition and detection of the hearing impairment. While many infants with congenital deafness are recognized at birth or shortly thereafter, some may not be detected early. Often it is difficult to distinguish between congenital deafness and deafness that has an onset in the first few months of life.[11] Therefore, some of the variation in the epidemiologic studies of congenital deafness is related to the age of the study population. These studies range from newborn surveys[140] to the evaluation of children at different age-groups.[135]

3. *Methods of ascertainment.* Some variation in epidemiologic studies of congenital deafness is due to differences in case ascertainment which have varied from retrospective medical record reviews to systematic evaluation of hearing function in defined cohorts of infants and children.[32a,111] In addition, the types of populations studied include newborn surveys,[140] institutionalized patients,[129] children attending special schools,[29,57,123,136] and those that are referred to specialty centers.[6,35,111]

4. *Extent of diagnostic evaluation.* Finally, in describing and comparing causes of childhood deafness in different populations, one is faced with variations in the extent of clinical, audiological, genetic, and other medical work-up in different studies. Such work-up ranges from retrospective review of available records to extensive medical and genetic evaluations.[32a,111,135]

**Table 3–5.** Epidemiologic characteristics of congenital deafness

| Characteristics | Notes |
|---|---|
| Clinical presentation | Types are conductive, sensorineural, or both; onset at birth or early, variable degrees of severity; some cases associated with recognized syndromes |
| Prevalence | 0.8–2 per 1,000 births |
| Geographic variation | May be partly due to differences in case definition and ascertainment |
| Racial/ethnic differences | Unclear |
| Gender differences | Male excess, M/F ranging from 1.1 to 1.5 |
| Temporal trends | Decline in rubella-related deafness |
| Familial patterns | Depend on cause and mode of inheritance; empiric risk estimates are available (see text) |
| Causes | Considerable etiologic heterogeneity; 20%–55% of cases have genetic etiology (mostly autosomal recessive with several loci involved); 30%–50% cases have environmental etiology; 10%–40% have unknown cause |

Keeping these methodologic issues in mind, the prevalence of early childhood deafness has been reported mostly in the range of 0.8 to 2 per 1,000 births (Table 3–5). In the metropolitan Atlanta study,[32a] the prevalence of hearing impairment (40 dB or more) in 10–year-old children was 1.2 per 1,000. The rate of profound hearing impairment (90 dB) was 0.5 per 1,000. In a European Community study, the prevalence of hearing impairment (50 dB or more) among children born in 1969 was 0.8 per 1000.[89] In Hungary, the prevalence of profound deafness (>90 dB) among school-age children was 1 per 1,000.[29]

Deafness and congenital deafness in particular are worldwide problems.[55] Nevertheless, it is unclear to what extent the geographic variation in the frequency of congenital deafness may be due to differences in case definition and ascertainment or to different causal mechanisms. In the United States, Schein reported the lowest prevalence of childhood deafness in the northeast region and the highest in the north central region.[120] In an epidemiologic study of childhood deafness in Australia, Upfold and Isepy found among children born between 1949 and 1980 a rate of deafness by age 18 years of 2.6 per 1,000 births, with 41% of cases having severe or profound deafness.[134] Congenital rubella accounted for 11% of the cases overall. However, there has been a significant reduction in the rate of rubella-related deafness after 1976, which was accompanied by a reduction in the overall rate of severe and profound deafness.[133]

Most studies of childhood deafness have documented a slight excess among male infants compared with females. The male-to-female ratio ranges from 1.1 to 1.5. In the Atlanta study, the male-to-female ratio of the prevalence of hearing impairment at age 10 years was 1.2.[32a] In the European Community study of childhood deafness, the male-to-female ratio was also 1.2.[89]

There is considerable heterogeneity in the etiology of congenital deafness. Genetic factors play an important role, accounting for 20–55% of all cases.[5,26,27] Among cases with the inherited type, deafness is a component of numerous well-delineated mendelian or contiguous gene syndromes, involving craniofacial, dental, ocular, and other anomalies.[5,48] This syndromal type of deafness can account for up to 30% of inherited deafness.[5,115] Among the undifferentiated or nonsyndromal genetic deafness, autosomal recessive inheritance accounts for the majority of cases (60%–75%), followed by autosomal dominant inheritance (10%–30%) and X-linked deafness (1%–3%).[5,115] The more severe the deafness, the more likely the autosomal recessive etiology.[26,136] In single gene congenital deafness, it has been well documented that multiple loci are involved. In autosomal recessive deafness, the number of loci involved have been estimated to range from 5 to 45.[21,116] In a genetic analysis of autosomal recessive deafness in Israel, Brownstein et al. estimated that 8–9 loci were associated with deafness.[7] Genetic heterogeneity is also present for autosomal dominant and X-linked deafness and leads to complications in genetic counseling. To estimate recurrence risks, an accurate diagnosis, the mode of inheritance, the presence or absence of genetic heterogeneity, and the penetrance of each genotype are required. Unfortunately, many of these variables are often unknown and only empiric values for recurrence risks can be given.[125] Based on data from several studies, Smith found remarkable consistency in recurrence risks across studies. For example, the empiric recurrence after the birth of an affected infant whose parents have normal hearing is about 10%. The risk increases to 25% after the birth of more than one affected infant. The empiric risk of congenital deafness in offspring of one affected parent is 6% and increases to 40% after the birth of one affected infant. The empiric risk of congenital deafness in the offspring is 10% if both parents are affected and increases to more than 59% after the birth of one affected infant.[125] Advances in molecular genetics will improve the ability to map and sequence genes associated with congenital deafness, thereby refining estimates of familial risks.[8,115]

Acquired or environmental causes of childhood deafness have been found to account for 30%–50% of cases. Among prenatal factors are teratogenic drugs and infectious agents such as rubella, syphilis and cytomegalovirus. Acquired causes of deafness also include perinatal factors such as hypoxia and kernicterus, and postnatal factors such as otitis media and meningoencephalitis.[5,27] In the Atlanta study of the prevalence of childhood deafness among 10-year-olds, 32% of the cases had an environmental cause, primarily including meningitis, rubella, and ototoxic drugs.[32a]

## References


1. Aase JM: Microtia-clinical observations. Birth Defects 16:289–297, 1980.
2. Aase JM, Tegtmeier RE: Microtia in New Mexico: evidence for multifactorial causation. Birth Defects 13:113–116, 1977.
3. Ardinger HH, Buetow KH, Bell GI, Bardach J, VanDemark DR, Murray JC: Association of genetic variation of the transforming growth factor alpha gene with cleft lip and palate. Am J Hum Genet 45:348–353, 1989.
4. Bamforth JS, Hughes IA, Lazarus JH, Weaver CM, Harper PS: Congenital hypothyroidism, spiky hair, and cleft palate. J Med Genet 26:49–51, 1989.
5. Beighton P: Hereditary deafness. In: Principles and Practice of Medical Genetics Vol I, 2nd ed., AEH Emery, DL Rimoin, eds. Churchill Livingstone, Edinburgh, 1990, pp 733–748.
6. Ben Arab S, Bonaiti-Pellie C, Belkahia A: An epidemiological and genetic study of congenital profound deafness in Tunisia (governorate of Nabeul). J Med Genet 27:29–33, 1990.
7. Brownstein Z, Friedlander Y, Peritz E, Cohen T: Estimated number of loci for autosomal recessive severe nerve deafness within the Israeli Jewish population, with implications for genetic counselling. Am J Med Genet 41:306–312, 1991.
8. Brunner HG, Smeets B, Smeets D, Nelen M, Cremers CWRJ, Ropers HH: Molecular genetics of X-linked hearing impairment. Ann N Y Acad Sci 630:176–190, 1991.
9. Burdi AR: Cleft lip and palate research: an updated state of the art. Section I: epidemiology, etiology and pathogenesis of cleft lip and palate. Cleft Palate J 14:261–269, 1977.
10. Carey JC: External ear. In: Human Malformations and Related Anomalies, Vol II, RE Stevenson, JG Hall, RM Goodman, eds. Oxford University Press, New York, 1993, pp 193–198.
11. Carter CO: Genetics of severe congenital deafness. Dev Med Child Neurol 24:525–526, 1982.
12. Castilla EE, Orioli IM: Prevalence rates of microtia in South America. Int J Epidemiol 15:364–368, 1986.
13. Castilla EE, Orioli IM, Lugarinho R, Dutra GP, Lopez-Camelo JS, Campana HE, Spagnolo A, Mastroiacovo P: Monthly and seasonal variations in the frequency of congenital anomalies. Int J Epidemiol 19:399–404, 1990.
14. Centers for Disease Control and Prevention: Infant mortality—United States, 1990. MMWR 42:161–165, 1993.
15. Centers for Disease Control and Prevention. Surveillance for and comparison of birth defect prevalences in two geographic areas—United States, 1983–1988. In: CDC Surveillance Summaries, March 19, 1993. MMWR 42: (No. SS-1):1–8, 1993.
16. Centers for Disease Control and Prevention: Congenital malformations surveillance. Teratology 48:545–709, 1993.
17. Chen H, Goei GS, Hertzler JH: Family studies on congenital esophageal atresia with or without tracheoesophageal fistula. Birth Defects 15:117–144, 1979.
18. Chenevix-Trench G, Jones K, Green A, Martin N: Further evidence for an association between genetic variation in transforming growth factor alpha and cleft lip and palate. Am J Hum Genet 48:1012–1013, 1991.
19. Chenevix-Trench G, Jones K, Green AC, Duffy DL, Martin NG: Cleft lip with or without cleft palate: associations with transforming growth factor alpha and retinoic acid receptor loci. Am J Hum Genet 51:1377–1385, 1992.
20. Christodoulou J, McDougall PN, Sheffield LJ: Choanal atresia as a feature of ectrodactyly-ectodermal dysplasia-clefting (EEC) syndrome. J Med Genet 26:586–589, 1989.
21. Chung CS, Brown KS: Family studies of early childhood deafness ascertained through the Clarke School for the Deaf. Am J Hum Genet 22:630–644, 1970.
22. Clarren SK, Smith DW: The fetal alcohol syndrome. N Engl J Med 298:1063–1067, 1978.
23. Clementi M, Tenconi R, Turolla L, Silvan C, Bortotto L, Artifoni L:

Apparent CHARGE association and chromosome anomaly: chance or contiguous gene syndrome. Am J Med Genet 41:246–250, 1991.
24. Cohen MM Jr: Syndromes with cleft lip and cleft palate. Cleft Palate J 15:328, 1978.
25. Cohen MM Jr: The nose. In: Human Malformations and Related Anomalies, Vol II, RE Stevenson, JG Hall, RM Goodman, eds. Oxford University Press, New York, 1993, pp 327–328.
26. Cremers CWRJ, Marres HAM, van Rijn PM: Nonsyndromal profound genetic deafness in childhood. Ann N Y Acad Sci 630:191–196, 1991.
27. Cremers CWRJ, van Rijn PM: Acquired causes of deafness in childhood. Ann N Y Acad Sci 630: 197–202, 1991.
28. Czeizel AE, Dudás I: Prevention of the first occurrence of neural tube defects by periconceptional vitamin supplementation. N Engl J Med 327:1832–1835, 1992.
29. Czeizel A, Skirpeczky K, Mester E, Sankaranarayanan K: The load of genetic and partially genetic disease in man. IV. Severe visual handicaps and profound childhood deafness in Hungarian school-age children. Mutat Res 270:103–114, 1992.
30. David TJ, O'Callaghan SE: Twinning and oesophageal atresia. Arch Dis Child 49:660–662, 1974.
31. David TJ, O'Callaghan SE: Oesophageal atresia in the South West of England. J Med Genet 12:1–11, 1975.
32. Dlugosz L, Vena J, Byers T, Sever L, Bracken M, Marshall E: Congenital defects and electric bed heating in New York State: a register-based case-control study. Am J Epidemiol 135:1000–1011, 1992.
32a. Drews CD, Yeargin-Allsopp M, Murphy CC, Decouflé P: Hearing impairment among 10-year-old children: metropolitan Atlanta, 1985 through 1987. Am J Public Health 84:1164–1166, 1994.
33. Drillien CM, Ingram TTS, Wilkinson J: The Causes and Natural History of Cleft Lip and Palate. E & S Livingstone, Edinburgh and London, 1966.
34. Edmonds LD, Layde PM, James LM, Flynt JW, Erickson JD, Oakley GP Jr: Congenital malformations surveillance: two American systems. Int J Epidemiol 10:247–252, 1981.
35. Elango S, Chand RP, Purohit GN. Childhood deafness in Malaysia. Int J Pediat Otorhinolaryngol 24:11–17, 1992.
36. Ellwood LC, Winter ST, Dar H: Familial microtia with meatal atresia in two sibships. J Med Genet 5:289–291, 1968.
37. Emanuel I, Culver BH, Erickson JD, Guthrie B, Schuldberg D: The further epidemiological differentiation of cleft lip and palate: a population study of clefts in King County, Washington, 1956–1965. Teratology 7:271–281, 1973.
38. Ericson A, Kallen B, Westerholm P: Cigarette smoking as an etiologic factor in cleft lip and palate. Am J Obstet Gynecol 135:348–351, 1979.
39. Escobar LF, Weaver DD: CHARGE Association. In: Birth Defects Encyclopedia, ML Buyse, ed. Blackwell, Cambridge, 1990, pp 308–309.
40. Flake CG, Ferguson CF: Congenital choanal atresia in infants and older children. Ann Otol Rhinol Laryngol 73;458–473, 1964.
41. Fraser FC: The genetics of cleft lip and cleft palate. Am J Hum Genet 22:336–352, 1970.
42. Fraser FC: The William Allan Memorial Award Address: evolution of a palatable multifactorial threshold model. Am J Hum Genet 32:796–813, 1980.
43. Fraser C, Baird PA, Sadovnick AD: A comparison of incidence trends for esophageal atresia and tracheoesophageal fistula, and infectious disease. Teratology 36:363–369, 1987.
44. Fraser FC, Nussbaum E: Neural tube defects in sibs of children with tracheo-oesophageal dysraphism. Lancet ii: 807, 1980.
45. Fraser GR, Calnan JS: Cleft lip and palate: seasonal incidence, birth weight, birth rank, sex, site, associated malformations and parental age. Arch Dis Child 36:420–423, 1961.
46. Friedman N, Levitsky LL, Edidin DV, Weiss E: Choanal atresia and associated anomalies. J Pediatr 96:1123, 1980.
47. German JC, Mahour GH, Woolley MM: The twin with esophageal atresia. J Pediatr Surg 14:432–435, 1979.
47a. Glustein JZ, Weill M, Steinberg A: Anomalies of the nipple: an additional finding in CHARGE syndrome. Am J Med Genet 61:201, 1996.
48. Gorlin RJ, Cohen MM, Levin LS: Syndromes of the Head and Neck, 3rd ed. Oxford University Press, New York, 1990.
49. Greenberg F: Choanal atresia and athelia: methimazole teratogenicity or a new syndrome? Am J Med Genet 28:931–934, 1987.
50. Greenwood RD, Deddish RB: Cardiovascular malformations associated with choanal atresia. South Med J 70:195–196, 1977.
51. Hall BD: Choanal atresia and associated multiple anomalies. J Pediatr 95:395–398, 1979.
52. Hardcastle B: Nose, posterior atresia. In: Birth Defects Encyclopedia, ML Buyse, ed. Blackwell, Cambridge 1990, pp 1265–1266.
53. Hecht JT, Annegers JF, Kurland LT: Epilepsy and clefting disorders: lack of evidence of a familial association. Am J Med Genet 33:244–247, 1989.
54. Hecht JT, Wang Y, Blanton SH, Michels VV, Daiger SP: Cleft lip and palate: no evidence of linkage to transforming growth factor alpha. Am J Hum Genet 49:682–686, 1991.
55. Holborow C: Deafness as a world problem. Adv Otorhinolaryngol 29:174–182, 1983.
56. Holder SE, Vintiner GM, Farren B, Malcolm S, Winter RM: Confirmation of an association between RFLPs at the transforming growth factor-alpha locus and non-syndromic cleft lip and palate. J Med Genet 29:390–392, 1992.
57. Holten A, Parving A: Aetiology of hearing disorders in children at the schools for the deaf. Int J Pediatr Otorhinolaryngol 10:229–236, 1985.
58. Holtzman NA, Khoury MJ: Monitoring for congenital malformations. Annu Rev Public Health 7:237–266, 1986.
59. Hoyme HE: The upper gastrointestinal system. In: Human Malformations and Related Anomalies, Vol II, RE Stevenson, JG Hall, RM Goodman, eds. Oxford University Press, New York, 1993, pp 421–423.
60. Hurst JA, Meinecke P, Baraitser M: Balanced t(6;8) (6p8p;6q8q) and the CHARGE association. J Med Genet 28:54–55, 1991.
61. International Clearinghouse for Birth Defects Monitoring Systems: Congenital Malformations Worldwide. Elsevier, Amsterdam, 1991.
62. Johnson JP, Fineman RM: Branchial arch malformations in infants of diabetic mothers: two case reports and a review. Am J Med Genet 13:125–130, 1982.
63. Jones KL: Smith's Recognizable Patterns of Human Malformation, 5th ed. WB Saunders, Philadelphia, 1996.
64. Källén B: Epidemiology of Human Reproduction, CRC Press, Boca Raton, 1988.
65. Källén B, Hay S, Klinberg M: Birth defects monitoring systems: accomplishments and goals. In: Issues and Reviews in Teratology, Vol 2, H Kalter ed. Plenum Press, New York, 1984, pp 1–22.
66. Katafuchi Y, Fukuda T, Maruoka T, Tokunaga Y, Yamashita Y, Matsuishi T: Partial trisomy 6p with agenesis of the corpus callosum and choanal atresia. J Child Neurol 7:114–116, 1992.
67. Kaye CI, Rollnick BR, Hauck WW, Martin AO, Richtsmeier JT, Nagatoshi K: Microtia and associated anomalies: statistical analysis. Am J Med Genet 34:574–578, 1989.
68. Khoury MJ, Beaty TH, Cohen BH: Fundamentals of Genetic Epidemiology. Oxford University Press, New York, 1993.
69. Khoury MJ, Cordero JF, Greenberg F, James LM, Erickson JD: A population study of the VACTERL association: evidence for its etiologic heterogeneity. Pediatrics 71:815–820, 1983.
70. Khoury MJ, Cordero JF, Mulinare J, Opitz JM: Selected midline defect associations: a population study. Pediatrics 84:266–272, 1989.
71. Khoury MJ, Edmonds LD: Metropolitan Atlanta Congenital Defects Program: twenty-five years of birth defects surveillance at the Centers for Disease Control. In: Proceedings of the III ASM International Symposium on Birth Defects, P Mastroiacovo, ed. ICARO-ASM Press House, Rome, 1992, pp 1–7.
72. Khoury MJ, Erickson JD, Cordero JF, McCarthy BJ: Congenital malformations and intrauterine growth retardation: a population study. Pediatrics 82:83–90, 1988.
73. Khoury MJ, Gomez-Farias M, Mulinare J: Does maternal cigarette smoking during pregnancy cause cleft lip and palate in offspring? Am J Dis Child 143:333–337, 1989.
74. Kline J, Stein Z, Susser M: Conception to Birth: Epidemiology of Prenatal Development. Oxford University Press, New York, 1989.
75. Knowles JC, Brandt IK, Bull MJ: Kaufman syndrome (hydrometrocolpos, polydactyly, and congenital heart disease) with pituitary dysplasia, choanal atresia, and vertebral anomalies. Am J Med Genet 8:389–393, 1981.
76. Knox EG: Secular pattern of congenital oesophageal atresia. Br J Prev Soc Med 13:222–226, 1959.
77. Kousseff BG, Papenhausen P, Neu RL, Essig YP, Saraceno CA: Cleft palate and complex chromosome rearrangements. Clin Genet 42:135–142, 1992.
78. Kučera J: Rate and type of congenital anomalies among offspring of diabetic women. J Reprod Med 7:61–70, 1971.
79. Kyyronen P, Hemminki K: Gastro-intestinal atresias in Finland in 1970–79, indicating time-place clustering. J Epidemiol Community Health 42:257–265, 1988.
80. Lammer EJ, Chen DT, Hoar RM, Agnish ND, Benke PJ, Braun JT,

Curry CJ, Fernhoff PM, Grix AW, Lott IT, Richard JM, Sun SC: Retinoic acid embryopathy. N Engl J Med 313:837–841, 1985.
81. Leck I: The contribution of epidemiologic studies to understanding human malformations. In: Human Malformations and Related Anomalies, Vol I, RE Stevenson, JG Hall, RM Goodman, eds. Oxford University Press, New York, 1993, pp 65–93.
82. Lettieri J: Lips and oral cavity. In: Human Malformations and Related Anomalies, Vol II, RE Stevenson, JG Hall, RM Goodman, eds. Oxford University Press, New York, 1993, pp 367–381.
83. Lilienfeld AM, Lilienfeld DE: Foundations of Epidemiology, 2nd ed. Oxford University Press, New York, 1980.
84. Lin AE, Siebert JR, Graham JM Jr: Central nervous system malformations in the CHARGE association. Am J Med Genet 37:304–310, 1990.
85. Little J: Risks in siblings and other relatives. In: Epidemiology and Control of Neural Tube Defects, JM Elwood, J Little, JH Elwood, eds. Oxford Medical Publications, Oxford, 1992, pp 604–676.
86. Lynberg MC, Edmonds LD: Surveillance of birth defects. In: Public Health Surveillance, W Halperin, EL Baker Jr, RR Monson eds. Van Nostrand Reinhold, New York, 1992, pp 157–177.
87. Maniglia AJ, Goodwin WJ Jr: Congenital choanal atresia. Otolaryngol Clin North Am 14:167–173, 1981.
88. Marazita ML, Hu DN, Spence MA, Liu YE, Melnick M: Cleft lip with or without cleft palate in Shanghai, China: evidence for an autosomal major locus. Am J Hum Genet 51:648–653, 1992
89. Martin JAM: Aetiological factors relating to childhood deafness in the European Community. Audiology 21:149–158, 1982.
90. Martínez-Frías ML, Rodríguez-Pinilla E: Tracheoesophageal and anal atresia in prenatal children exposed to a high dose of alcohol. Am J Med Genet 40:128, 1991.
91. McKusick VA: Mendelian Inheritance in Man, 10th ed. The Johns Hopkins University Press, Baltimore, 1992, pp 1090–1091.
92. McKusick VA: Mendelian Inheritance in Man, 10th ed. The Johns Hopkins University Press, Baltimore, 1992, pp 1282–1283.
93. Meinert CL: Clinical Trials: Design, Conduct, Analysis. Oxford University Press, New York, 1986.
94. Melnick M, Myrianthopoulos N: External ear malformations: epidemiology, genetics and natural history. Birth Defects 15:1–140, 1979.
95. Mili F, Edmonds LD, Khoury MJ, McClearn AB: Prevalence of birth defects among low-birth-weight infants: a population study. Am J Dis Child 145:1313–1318, 1991.
96. Miller JR: The use of registries and vital statistics in the study of congenital malformations. In: International Conference on Congenital Malformations, 1963, International Medical Congress, ltd, ed., New York, 1964.
97. Milunsky JM, Wyandt HE, Milunsky A: Emerging phenotype of duplication (7p): a report of three cases and review of the literature. Am J Med Genet 33:364–368, 1989.
98. Mir NA, Grewal BS, Kishan J, Elzouki AY, Bhatia JN: Congenital choanal atresia in North African infants. Ann Trop Paediatr 6:141–144, 1986.
99. Mitchell LE, Risch N: Mode of inheritance of nonsyndromic cleft lip with or without cleft palate: a reanalysis. Am J Hum Genet 51:323–332, 1992.
100. [MRC] Medical Research Council Vitamin Study Research Group: Prevention of neural tube defects: results of the Medical Research Council Vitamin Study. Lancet 338:131–137, 1991.
101. Myer CM 3d, Cotton RT: Nasal obstruction in the pediatric patient. Pediatrics 72:766–77, 1983.
102. Neal GS, Hankins GD: Left microtia in one monozygotic twin. A case report. J Reprod Med 37:375–377, 1992.
103. Neel JV: A study of major congenital defects in Japanese infants. Am J Hum Genet 10:398–445, 1958.
104. Niebyl JR, Blake DA, Rocco LE, Baumgardner R, Mellits ED: Lack of maternal metabolic, endocrine and environmental influences in the etiology of cleft lip with or without cleft palate. Cleft Palate J 22:20–28, 1985.
105. Niswander JD, Adams MS: Oral clefts in the American Indian. Public Health Rep 82:807–812, 1967.
106. Oestreich AE: Choanal atresia with achondroplasia. J Pediatr 96:343–344, 1980.
107. Olney RS, Khoury MJ, Moore CA, Fernhoff PM, Cordero JF: Etiologic analysis of multiple congenital anomalies, Atlanta, 1990: comparison of a population-based registry with a genetic referral center. Teratology 45:454, 1992.
108. Opitz JM: Blastogenesis and the primary field in human development. In Blastogenesis: Normal and Abnormal, JM Opitz, ed. Wiley-Liss, New York, 1993.
109. Ørstavik KH, Medbø S, Mair IW: Right-sided microtia and conductive hearing loss with variable expressivity in three generations. Clin Genet 38:117–120, 1990.
110. Ozimek CD, Grimson RC, Aylsworth AS: An epidemiologic study of tracheoesophageal fistula and esophageal atresia in North Carolina. Teratology 25:53–59, 1982.
111. Pabla HS, McCormick B, Gibbin KP: Retrospective study of the prevalence of bilateral sensorineural deafness in childhood. Int J Pediatr Otorhinolaryngol 22:161–165, 1991.
112. Pagon RA, Graham JM Jr, Zonana J, Yong SL: Coloboma, congenital heart disease, and choanal atresia with multiple anomalies: CHARGE association. J Pediatr 99:223–227, 1981.
113. Peer LA, Gordon HW, Bernhard WG: Effect of vitamins on human teratology. Plast Reconstr Surg 34:358–362, 1964.
114. Qazi QH, Kanchanapoomi R, Beller E, Collins R: Inheritance of posterior choanal atresia. Am J Med Genet 13:413–416, 1982.
115. Reardon W: Genetic deafness. J Med Genet 29:521–526, 1992.
116. Reardon W, Pembrey M: The genetics of deafness. Arch Dis Child 65:1196–1197, 1990.
117. Rollnick BR, Kaye CI: Hemifacial microsomia and variants: pedigree data. Am J Med Genet 15:233–253, 1983.
118. Rothman KM: Modern Epidemiology. Little, Brown & Co., Boston, 1986.
119. Safra MJ, Oakley GP Jr: Association between cleft lip with or without cleft palate and prenatal exposure to diazepam. Lancet 2:478–480, 1975.
120. Schein JD: Childhood hearing loss: epidemiology and implications. Birth Defects 16:3–7, 1980.
121. Schinzel A, Schmid W, Fraccaro M, Tiepolo L, Zuffardi O, Opitz JM, Lindsten J, Zetterqvist P, Enell H, Baccichetti C, Tenconi R, Pagon RA: The "cat eye syndrome": dicentric small marker chromosome probably derived from a no.22 (tetrasomy 22pter to q11) associated with a characteristic phenotype. Report of 11 patients and delineation of the clinical picture. Hum Genet 57:148–158, 1981.
122. Schmid M, Schröder M, Langenbeck U: Familial microtia, meatal atresia, and conductive deafness in three siblings. Am J Med Genet 22:327–332, 1985.
123. Sellars S, Beighton P: Childhood deafness in southern Africa: an aetiological survey of 3,064 deaf children. J Laryngol Otol 97:885–889, 1983.
123a. Shaw GM, Lammer EJ, Wasserman CR, O'Malley CD, Tolarova MM: Risks of orofacial clefts in children born to women using multivitamins containing folic acid periconceptionally. Lancet 345:393–396, 1995.
123b. Shaw GM, Wasserman CR, Lammer EJ, O'Malley CD, Murray JC, Basart AM, Tolarova MM: Orofacial clefts, parental cigarette smoking, and transforming growth factor-alpha gene variants. Am J Hum Genet 58:551–561, 1996.
124. Shprintzen RJ, Siegel-Sadewitz VL, Amato J, Goldberg RB: Anomalies associated with cleft lip, cleft palate, or both. Am J Med Genet 20:585–595, 1985.
125. Smith SD: Recurrence risks. Ann N Y Acad Sci 630:203–211, 1991.
126. Smithells RW: Defects and disabilities of thalidomide children. Br Med J 1:269–272, 1973.
127. Stahl RS, Jurkiewicz MJ: Congenital posterior choanal atresia. Pediatrics 76:429–436, 1985.
128. Szendrey T, Danyi G, Czeizel A: Etiological study on isolated esophageal atresia. Hum Genet 70:51–58, 1985.
129. Tamayo ML, Bernal JE, Tamayo GE, Frias JL: Study of the etiology of deafness in an institutionalized population in Columbia. Am J Med Genet 44:405–408, 1992.
130. Tolarova M: Orofacial clefts in Czechoslovakia: incidence, genetics and prevention of cleft lip and palate over a 19-year period. Scand J Plast Reconstr Surg Hand Surg 21:19–25, 1987.
131. Tomkins DJ, Hunter AGW, Uchida IA, Roberts MH: Two children with deletion of the long arm of chromosome 4 with breakpoint at band q33. Clin Genet 22:348–355, 1982.
132. Tretsven V: Incidence of cleft lip and palate in Montana Indians. J Hear Speech 28:52–57, 1963.
133. Upfold LJ: Changes in the significance of maternal rubella as a factor in childhood deafness—1954 to 1982. Med J Aust 140:641–644, 1984.
134. Upfold LJ, Isepy J: Childhood deafness in Australia: incidence and maternal rubella, 1949–1980. Med J Aust 2:323–326, 1982.

135. van Rijn PM: Causes of Early Childhood Deafness. Thesis, University of Nijmegen, Nijmegen, The Netherlands, 1989.
136. van Rijn PM, Cremers CWRJ: Causes of childhood deafness at a dutch school for the hearing impaired. Ann Otol Rhinol Laryngol 100:903–908, 1991.
137. van Staey M, De Bie S, Matton MTh, De Roose J: Familial congenital esophageal atresia: personal case report and review of the literature. Hum Genet 66:260–266, 1984.
138. Vintiner GM, Holder SE, Winter RM, Malcolm S: No evidence of linkage between the transforming growth factor-alpha gene in families with apparently autosomal dominant inheritance of cleft lip and palate. J Med Genet 29:393–397, 1992.
139. Yang P, Khoury MJ, Stewart WF, Beaty TH, Chee E, Beatty JC, Diamond EL, Gordis L: Comparative epidemiology of selected midline congenital abnormalities. Genet Epidemiol 11:141–154, 1994.
140. Watkin PM, Baldwin M, McEnery G: Neonatal at risk screening and the identification of deafness. Arch Dis Child 66:1130–1135, 1991.
141. Werler MM, Lammer EJ, Rosenberg L, Mitchell AA: Maternal cigarette smoking during pregnancy in relation to oral clefts. Am J Epidemiol 132:926–932, 1990.

# 4

# Human Teratogens

EDWARD J. LAMMER and LEWIS B. HOLMES

## Principles

A wide variety of environmental agents may adversely affect the growth and development of the embryo or fetus. These include intrauterine infections, medications, occupational chemicals, physical agents, and maternal metabolic disturbances. The magnitude of risk posed by different teratogens and the phenotypes they induce, however, show remarkable variability. Because this book is intended for an otolaryngology audience, this chapter focuses on teratogen-induced craniofacial anomalies and hearing loss, and will not address the full range of adverse outcomes that may result from an environmental exposure, such as fetal death, neuropsychological dysfunction, etc. In addition, the environmental agents selected for inclusion in this chapter are primarily those for which epidemiologic studies have demonstrated teratogenic effects after exposure during the embryonic rather than the fetal period. Even when the discussion is limited to craniofacial anomalies as the outcome, however, the phenotypes induced by teratogenic agents still show marked variability, some of which may be explained by considering the following principles of teratology.[105,108,128]

### Dose-response effect

For most teratogenic agents, experimental studies show that there is a threshold dose below which identifiable malformations do not occur but at which more subtle effects, such as behavioral phenotypes[120] or biochemical changes, may be detectable. At even lower doses, the frequency of these subtle effects approaches that of the background population. Such relationships have proven difficult to demonstrate in humans. In general though, higher exposure translates into higher magnitude of risk for most human teratogens. Dose–reponse effects in humans are especially difficult to discern for medications that have a narrow therapeutic dose range (e.g., isotretinoin),[72] but they may be more discernible with other quantifiable exposures, such as cigarette smoking or alcohol intake.[88,125] Correlating measurements of maternal serum levels of medications chronically taken during pregnancy, such as anticonvulsants, with malformation outcomes has produced inconsistent results.[20,93] While use of such measurements has potential value for predicting differential risk, they are currently of unproven value in counseling and prevention.

### Timing of exposure

The stage(s) of embryonic or fetal development during which an exposure occurs sets limits on the potential range of adverse outcomes that it may cause. While an exposure may cause a malformation if it occurs before or during the active period of organogenesis of a structure, it cannot cause a malformation if the exposure occurs after an organ anlage has already formed (except anomalies resulting from a disruptive process).[18] Most major malformations, such as cleft palate or microtia, occur in the embryonic period of the first 60 days post-conception. A few craniofacial malformations, however, can occur much later in pregnancy (such as craniosynostosis or skull defects), and they, as well as neurosensory deficits such as hearing loss or speech problems, may result from exposure limited to the fetal period of development that begins at 60 days after conception. Congenital rubella syndrome demonstrates this phenomena very well. When rubella infection begins more than 55 days after conception, deafness and retinopathy frequently result, whereas the induction of cataracts and congenital heart defects is limited to infections that begin before that developmental stage.[115]

Many minor craniofacial anomalies can be induced during either the embryonic or fetal periods. For example, isotretinoin may cause epicanthus and auricular malformations after an exposure limited to the embryonic period. After fetal exposure, epicanthus may again result, but not major malformations of external ear morphogenesis; similarly craniosynostosis or speech problems may occur after embryonic or fetal isotretinoin exposure.[67,73] Another example of the effect of timing of exposure on outcomes concerns the association of early chorionic villus sampling (CVS) and the oromandibular limb hypogenesis syndrome. This malformation complex is thought to result from altered vascular regulation within the embryo and placenta, so the malformations are, in fact, disruptions of initially normal structures in the hindbrain, limb, and craniofacies. Most studies have found a correlation between CVS procedures and the malformation complex, while a few have not.[51] If the occurrence of the malformations is related primarily to placental injury that occurs only before, or at, certain susceptible times in development, as some studies suggest, then only epidemiologic research that incorporates timing of the event into the data analysis will be able to detect the adverse events.[87]

### Range of outcomes

The initial clinical delineation of the phenotypes caused by many teratogens has involved the recognition of a pattern of minor craniofacial anomalies rather than the observation that an agent increased the risk for individual major malformations. From cohort studies of several known human teratogens, it is apparent that the absolute risks of adverse outcomes other than major malformation are invariably higher;[2,52,56,79] these other adverse outcomes may include increased risks of perinatal mortality, premature delivery, pre- or postnatal growth deficiency, immune deficiencies, hormonal deficiencies, and central nervous system (CNS) dysfunction (sensory, motor, or psychological).[120] Nonmalformation adverse outcomes that are of particular relevance to otolaryngology and that have been associated with some human teratogens are sensorineural and conductive hearing loss and speech problems.

### Pathogenetic mechanisms

Most human teratogens induce a characteristic pattern of abnormalities that includes structural malformations, neuropsychological deficits, and pre- or postnatal growth retardation. If an agent causes major malformations, only rarely does it increase the risk of all malformations; rather, the occurrence of specific major malformations is more characteristic of most human teratogens.[43,50] These patterns reflect the limits on adverse outcomes that are determined by the specific pathogenetic mechanisms through which each environmental agent acts. For example, several teratogens probably act as ligands that can bind to cellular or nuclear receptors in embryonic tissues. The specificity of which organs become malformed may be determined by the tissue- and temporal-specific distribution of the matching receptors during the time that the teratogenic exposure occurs. Examples of such teratogens that induce specific patterns, probably through a receptor-mediated process, include diethystilbestrol and retinoic acid.[41,89] Some agents may exert a physiological effect on the fetus that is related to the pharmacologic effect intended to benefit the mother, as in the goitrogenic effects of maternal propylthiouracil on the fetus.[14] In other instances, an agent may induce a specific pattern of anomalies because it adversely affects one of the limited number of specific morphogenetic processes: cell division, cell differentiation, cell migration, epithelial–mesenchymal interactions, cell death, or extracellular matrix composition.

### Genetic variation and pharmacogenetics

Experimental studies using inbred strains of mice have unequivocally demonstrated the importance of genetic host factors in determining the presence and magnitude of teratogenic risks.[28,31] Unlike the experimental setting, humans are not exposed to agents under controlled conditions, nor do they share common genotypes. Teratogenic risks may be altered by genetic variation of (1) metabolic activation or conversion of xenobiotic medications; (2) immune response to infectious agents; (3) DNA or protein repair mechanisms; and (4) the extent of redundancy of genetic programs that control developmental processes. An example that demonstrates the potential importance of human pharmacogenetic variation is from a preliminary study which shows that lower epoxide hydrolase activity correlates with higher risk of the occurrence of features of the phenytoin embryopathy.[13,29] Genetic variation of alcohol metabolism may also play a role in determining some of the susceptibility to maternal alcohol use.[119] Variants of the alcohol dehydrogenases or acetaldehyde dehydrogenases are potential candidate genes.[25]

## Congenital infectious diseases

Few congenital infections cause malformations or neurological dysfunction that are likely to come to the attention of the otolaryngologist. The most likely setting in which children adversely affected by prenatal exposure to infectious agents would be seen by an otolaryngologist is for evaluation of hearing loss or speech problems. Sensorineural hearing loss is one of the cardinal features of congenital rubella infection; speech problems are also common.[35,37,104] Sensorineural hearing loss may also be a sequela of congenital cytomegalovirus or toxoplasma infections.[103] Neonatal chronic rhinitis is a well-known feature of congenital syphyllis infection.[36] Sensorineural hearing loss is an uncommon sequela of syphillis infection, however, and it is more likely to begin at a later age in this disorder, if it occurs.

## Ethanol

Although it is likely that alcohol embryopathy has existed since grain was first fermented into palatable beverages, its original recognition among offspring of French maternal alcoholics appeared only in 1968.[74] This was rapidly followed by Jones and co-workers' delineation of fetal alcohol syndrome (FAS), a constellation of minor craniofacial anomalies, growth deficiencies, and mental deficiency found among offspring of chronically alcoholic women.[54,56,57] Longitudinal follow-up of such severely affected children with FAS has revealed that the adult manifestations include short stature, microcephaly, subnormal intellectual function, and maladaptive adult behaviors.[17,109] FAS is probably one of the most common of the clinically diagnosed causes of mental retardation. Although its true incidence is unknown and is dependent on the diagnostic criteria used to define it, an estimate of 2 per 1,000 livebirths is frequently quoted.[1] This is almost certainly an underestimate of the total childhood morbidity attributable to excessive alcohol use during pregnancy.[1,54]

Cohort studies suggest that the pattern of defects that comprises FAS probably represents the more severe end of the spectrum of outcomes following alcohol exposure.[5] In a study employing facial photographs, Clarren and co-workers showed that experienced clinical geneticists accurately differentiated the faces of alcohol-exposed infants from those non-exposed only when the maternal use exceeded 4 ounces of absolute alcohol per day.[16] Women who drink less alcohol may be at increased risk for delivering infants who lack growth retardation but show some of the craniofacial features and/or motor and neuropsychological deficits. Studies have shown that less alcohol exposure may cause a much wider range of adverse effects, from attention deficits to slow reactive motor responses, and components of the FAS facial phenotype.[110] These abnormalities are frequently referred to as *fetal alcohol effects* (FAE) when they occur following significant maternal alcohol use but in the absence of the cardinal features of FAS: growth deficiency, characteristic facial phenotype, and neurological deficits.[5] Undoubtedly, FAE is much more common than FAS, among infants delivered of both alcoholic mothers and women who drink less during pregnancy. Assessing the magnitude of adverse effects potentially attributable to smaller amounts of maternal alcohol intake remains controversial. A committee of the American Academy of Pediatrics, however, recently recommended ". . . abstinence from alcohol for women who are pregnant or who are planning a pregnancy."[5]

### Clinical features

When a history of maternal excessive alcohol use is obtained, the diagnosis of FAS may be made based upon (1) prenatal and/or postnatal growth retardation; (2) a characteristic facial appearance; and (3) microcephaly, and/or motor or neuropsychological dysfunction (see Table 4–1).[5,54] Growth retardation is more commonly of prenatal than postnatal onset, and both length and weight are frequently affected. The characteristic facial features that have been observed include short palpebral fissures, short nose, long smooth philtrum, and thin vermillion of the upper lip (see Fig. 4–1); other craniofacial features are listed in Table 4–1. Microcephaly is probably as common as growth retardation, but even more frequent are motor and neuropsychological deficits. CNS abnormalities may be manifested as motor deficits (hypotonia and delayed development, clumsiness, and poor eye–hand coordination) and sensory organ malformation or dysfunction (sensorineural hearing loss, strabismus, ptosis, optic nerve hypoplasia, anterior chamber malformations).[54,109,110] Neuropsychological studies have found that full-scale intelligence testing scores are lower, with many children functioning in the mild or moderate range of mental retardation. Longitudinal studies, however, have reported significant maladaptive social function in adults with FAS even when their full-scale IQs are scored in the 70–85 range.[109] Learning disabilities, hyperactivity, attention deficit disorders, and impulsive behavior are included among the wide range of behavioral teratogenicity attributable to alcohol.

A variety of major malformations, including cardiac and renal defects, have been reported to occur with the above components of FAS. While major malformations have been reported as part of FAS in case series,[17,56] few case–control or prospective cohort studies have identified specific major malformations associated with maternal alcohol use, even at higher measures of exposure.[4,45,126] These malformations generally do not include major craniofacial defects. Epidemiologic studies of individual major craniofacial malformations, such as cleft lip or cleft palate, have not been associated with excess alcohol exposure.[5,126]

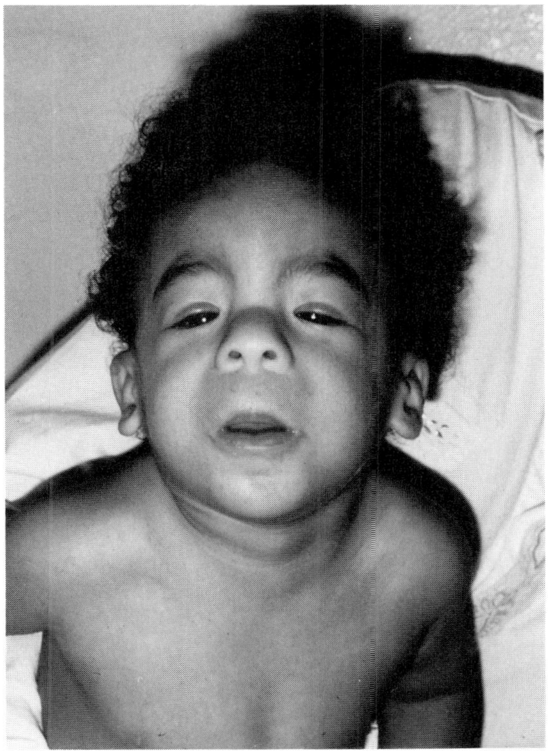

**Fig 4–1.** Fetal alcohol syndrome in a 15-month-old boy. Note ptosis, short palpebral fissures, upturned nares, and long, smooth philtrum. Courtesy of Dr. Kenneth Jones.

## Coumarin anticoagulants

Women requiring anticoagulant therapy during pregnancy face serious risks for themselves and for their fetuses. The increased maternal risks arise from maternal hemorrhages and the underlying diseases for which these women need treatment, such as deep vein thrombosis or the presence of artificial heart valves. Early in pregnancy, the maternal use of coumarin derivatives poses an increased risk of fetal demise and major malformations.[40,121] Later in pregnancy, anticoagulation may lead to fetal hemorrhages, possibly resulting in fetal or neonatal death.[40] Based on a cohort of 37 pregnancies, some features of coumarin embryopathy occured in about 30% of pregnancies in which it was used throughout the first trimester.[53] Because coumarin derivatives (warfarin, acenocoumarol, coumadin) are used for several months, it has been difficult to correlate abnormal outcomes with specific exposure intervals during pregnancy. A small clinical trial showed, however, that none of 23 children born to women who were switched from a coumarin derivative to heparin from before the 6th gestational week and remained on heparin until the 12th week, had features suggestive of coumarin embryopathy.[53] Of 12 women switched to heparin after the 7th week, 3 had children with anomalies. Other observations also support the idea that the risk of primary malformations (not disruptions) is largely limited to the interval between the sixth and ninth weeks of gestational age.[59] In another small cohort study of 20 pregnancies in which warfarin was used only in the second and third trimesters, an increase in perinatal mortality was found (9%), but liveborn infants were all normal.[15]

**Table 4–1.** Phenotypic features of fetal alcohol syndrome

| |
|---|
| *GROWTH RETARDATION* |
| Prenatal or postnatal onset |
| *CRANIOFACIAL* |
| Short palpebral fissures |
| Smooth, long philtrum with thin upper lip |
| Short upturned nose |
| Micrognathia |
| Maxillary hypoplasia |
| Orthodontic malocclusion |
| Excessive dental caries and/or enamel defects |
| *NEUROLOGICAL AND NEUROPSYCHOLOGICAL* |
| Microcephaly |
| Developmental delay and/or mental retardation |
| Speech problems |
| Sensorineural hearing loss |
| Hypotonia, poor coordination |
| Attention deficits, hyperactivity |
| Poor fine motor skills |
| Maladaptive adult behaviors |

### Clinical features

Prenatal growth deficiency and malformations of midfacial development and the central nervous system are the most characteristic abnormalities. The facial features are quite striking and resemble those of chondrodysplasia punctata. Midfacial hypoplasia may be severe with the nose very small and upturned, occasionally with notching of the nasal alae (Fig. 4–2). Among brain anomalies, characteristic findings include microcephaly, hydrocephaly, absence of the corpus callosum, and Dandy-Walker anomaly.[40,59] Eye development may also be affected: corneal opacities or cataracts, and optic nerve hypoplasia. Stippled epiphyses, or paravertebral calcific stippling, particularly in the lumbar-sacral area, are often found in the infant period, much as in chondrodysplasia punctata. This radiographic feature usually disappears in infancy, however, and is diagnostically helpful only during that time period.

A clue to the pathogenesis of this embryopathy was developed by Pauli and co-workers, who identified an identical pattern of malformation in a child who had congenital deficiency of multiple, vitamin K–dependent coagulation factors.[95] They hypothesized that, rather than the phenotype resulting from a primary pharmacologic effect of warfarin, the bone abnormalities were a consequence of warfarin's interference with vitamin K–dependent, post-translational carboxylation, which led to decreased carboxylation of proteins specifically involved in bone development. In addition, warfarin has been shown to inhibit the activity of a vitamin K reductase.[114]

## Anticonvulsants

The offspring of women whose seizure disorders are treated with anticonvulsants during pregnancy are at increased risk of developmental toxicity from the anticonvulsant medications. This toxicity may be manifested by growth retardation, minor anomalies, major malformation, or neuropsychological deficits. Most studies of the offspring of paternal epileptics, or of epileptic mothers who were off therapy during pregnancy, do not show an increased risk of malformation, which strongly suggests that the medications cause the developmental toxicity. Experimental studies also support the view that maternal antiepileptic drugs, and not the epilepsy itself, pose the risk to the embryo and fetus. Human and experimental studies have recently been comprehensively reviewed by Dansky and Finnell.[20,30] Many cohort studies have shown that polytherapy carries a higher risk for major malformations than monotherapy. The relationship is not so easily attributed to polytherapy alone, however, because mothers who require polytherapy are more likely to be taking higher doses of individual medications, and some human studies show a dose-related risk of birth defects. The risk for developmental toxicity probably differs for each anticonvulsant agent, but current data do not allow for many conclusions to be reached about the magnitude of risk of one anticonvulsant (or anticonvulsant combination) specifically compared to any other, especially concerning risks for major malformations. Nevertheless, the overall magnitude of risk of major malformation among offspring of women taking anticonvulsant medications appears to be two- to threefold higher than that of the general population.[30] In particular, cardiac and facial anomalies occur more frequently among offspring exposed to anticonvulsants in utero compared to children born to untreated mothers with epilepsy. A summary of 53 cohort studies showed a 1.3% absolute risk of cleft lip and a 0.2% risk of cleft palate among anticonvulsant-exposed offspring.[30] The absolute risk of a cardiac defect was 2%. Despite this summary data, however, not all cohort studies have found increased risks for these specific defects.

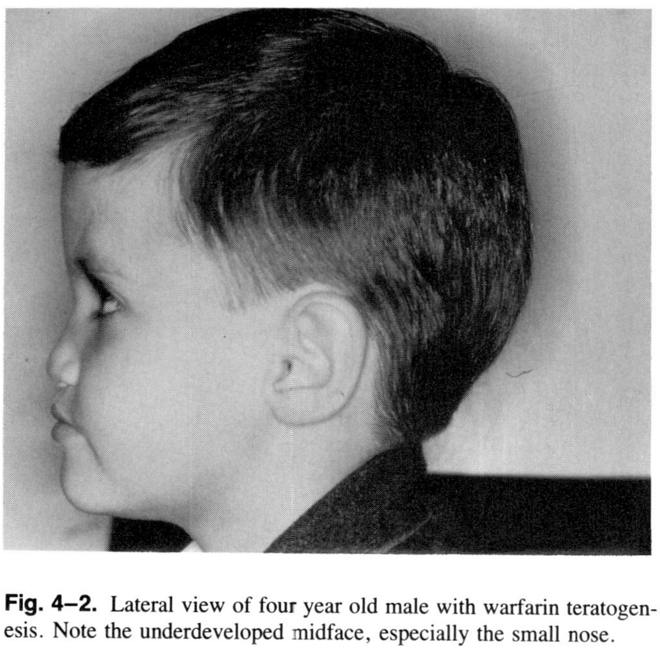

**Fig. 4–2.** Lateral view of four year old male with warfarin teratogenesis. Note the underdeveloped midface, especially the small nose.

### Clinical features

A distinctive facial phenotype was described in the initial reports of the fetal hydantoin (phenytoin) syndrome by Hanson and colleagues,[43,44] although some of the children in the initial report were exposed to additional anticonvulsants. Human studies over the past 20 years involving phenytoin and other anticonvulsants suggest that aspects of the anticonvulsant syndromes, especially their facial phenotypes, significantly overlap. An "anticonvulsant face" has been identified as a component of the teratogenic effects of monotherapy with all of the following anticonvulsants: phenytoin,[43,44] carbamazepine,[55] phenobarbital,[83,96] and valproic acid.[23] The features of the anticonvulsant face include (Fig. 4–3) broad and/or depressed nasal bridge, short nose with anteverted nostrils and a long philtrum, epicanthal folds, and maxillary hypoplasia. Among some anticonvulsant-exposed infants, the nasal bridge may be wide enough to be hyperteloric; much less commonly, infants have been reported with a decreased interorbital distance. Radiographs of older children who had been exposed to phenytoin in utero showed that those with the anticonvulsant face had a shortened anterior cranial base, small maxilla, and shortened nasal cartilage.[118] Prominence of the metopic suture has been specifically linked to valproic acid exposure, sometimes requiring surgical intervention.[23,39]

Several other notable noncraniofacial features have been associated with exposure to individual anticonvulsants. Among phenytoin-exposed children, microcephaly, growth retardation, and distal phalangeal and nail hypoplasia may occur.[83] Valproic acid use during pregnancy has an absolute risk of 1–2% for low open spina bifida, but anencephaly rarely occurs with this anticonvulsant exposure.[10,76,77,97] A more recent cohort study found a slightly higher risk of 5% for spina bifida.[93] The impact of valproic acid exposure in causing other major malformations or other adverse outcomes of pregnancy is less clear.[6] Carbamazepine's potential teratogenicity is also suspected but requires confirmation with additional cohort studies in which it is used as monotherapy. It appears to increase the risk of major malformation largely when taken in combination with other anticonvulsants.[55,129] Recent evidence has increasingly implicated

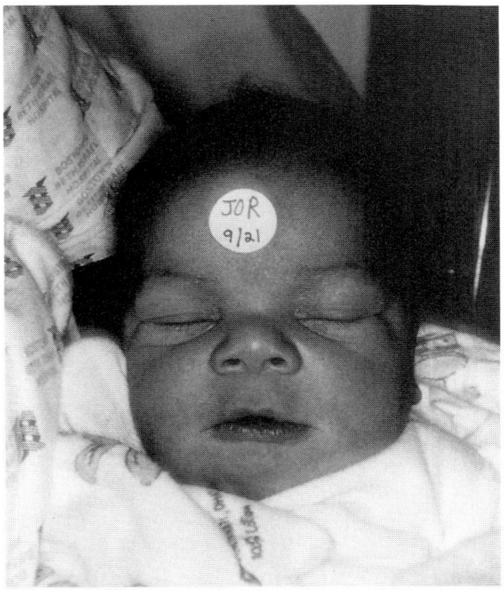


**Fig. 4–3.** The "anticonvulsant face" resulting from phenytoin exposure in this infant. Note epicanthal folds, broad nasal bridge, short nose with anteverted nares, and long philtrum.

carbamazepine monotherapy as a cause of spina bifida as well.[98]

Many issues remain unresolved concerning anticonvulsant teratogenicity: the relative risks posed by monotherapies versus polytherapy; the role of maternal seizures; the role of genetic differences in metabolism of anticonvulsants; and the underlying pathogenetic processes that lead to abnormal morphogenesis and histogenesis. Recent studies of the role of pharmacogenetics in fetal metabolism of phenytoin and the potential contribution of reactive epoxide (arene oxide) intermediates in inducing embryopathic effects suggest that lower fetal epoxide hydrolase activity is important in determining risk of malformation. In a preliminary prospective study of 19 phenytoin-exposed pregnancies, Buehler and co-workers found that each of 4 children who were born with features of the phenytoin embryopathy had low epoxide hydrolase activity, while the 15 normal outcomes had higher enzyme activities.[13,29] Such approaches may prove useful in predicting which fetuses are at higher risk of malformation if certain anticonvulsants are taken by a mother. Other laboratory research suggests that the teratogenicity of phenytoin and oxazolidinedione anticonvulsants may be influenced by the production of teratogenic intermediates (that are not arene oxide intermediates) produced by prostaglandin synthetase.[124]

## Retinoids

A number of retinoids are normally present in maternal serum during pregnancy, including retinol (vitamin A), retinyl esters, and retinoic acid (13-cis- and all-trans-). Within the embryo, these retinoids play important roles in the morphogenesis of many organs, including craniofacies, brain, heart, limbs, and axial skeleton.[11,12,27,81,86,89,94] This is primarily accomplished by retinoic acid and related compounds (9–cis-retinoic acid) acting as ligands that bind to nuclear receptors of the steroid-thyroid hormone receptor superfamily. The receptor complexes are transcription factors capable of activating major genetic programs involved in development.[11,48,75,84,85]

Maternal serum retinoids are derived from liver storage and diet, which contributes 7,000–8,000 International Units (IU) per day of vitamin A to a typical North American woman. Additional vitamin A intake may be derived from vitamin supplementation or therapy. The types of vitamin A supplements that women might take during pregnancy, exclusive of prenatal multivitamin preparations, include $\beta$-carotene, retinol, and retinyl esters. Ingestion of large amounts of $\beta$-carotene does not cause symptoms of hypervitaminosis A in humans, and there is no biological reason to suspect that it poses a risk for developmental toxicity.[116] The policy paper "Recommendations for vitamin A use during pregnancy" from the Teratology Society thoroughly reviews the small number of published case reports of malformations associated with daily intake of 25,000 IU or more of vitamin A.[112] In summary, epidemiologic studies of vitamin A exposure and malformation outcomes are few, but they suggest a small increased risk for malformations at doses that exceed by at least severalfold the dose of vitamin A present in most prenatal multivitamins.[91] Recent evidence that vitamin A supplementation at doses above 25,000 IU increases serum concentrations of a number of retinoids in humans, including teratogenic retinoic acid isomers, raises concern about the potential for vitamin A teratogenicity.[26] Supplementation of 8,000 IU should be considered the maximum amount of vitamin A per unit dosage prior to or during pregnancy. Ideally, a $\beta$-carotene source for vitamin A supplements should be recommended for women in their reproductive years, at least in those countries where vitamin A deficiency is rare.

Another way in which a pregnant woman might increase her serum levels of retinoids is from therapeutic ingestion of isotretinoin or etretinate. Isotretinoin (13–cis-retinoic acid) is taken orally at doses of 0.5–2 mg/kg in most countries for treating severe nodulocystic acne. It has an elimination half-life of 16–20 hours with chronic dosing; thus, maternal serum levels will remain elevated for several days after the last dose.[3] Unlike retinyl esters, isotretinoin is not stored in human adipose or hepatic tissues. Isotretinoin exposure in the first trimester poses an exceptionally high risk for major malformation (about 25% for pregnancies reaching 20 gestational weeks), comparable in its magnitude of risk to only thalidomide and congenital rubella infection among environmental developmental toxicants (Lammer, Hayes, and Holmes, personal communication).[69,113] Isotretinoin exposure during that period also significantly increases the risk of spontaneous abortion, premature delivery, and developmental disabilities (Lammer, Hayes, and Holmes, personal communication).[70]

Etretinate is an aromatic retinoid used mainly for the treatment of severe psoriasis and with varying success in other chronic dermatoses. Acitretin is the pharmacologically active compound that is derived from etretinate in the gut and liver; it is also available for therapy in some countries. The compounds are mainly distinguished by their pharmacokinetic differences. Etretinate accumulates in a deep peripheral compartment with an apparent mean human elimination half-life of 121 days. It has been detected in the serum of some patients more than 2 years after therapy ended.[22] In contrast, acitretin has a mean elimination half-life of 2–4 days after chronic dosing. Recent evidence, however, has suggested that, in some patients, acitretin is biotransformed into etretinate, which then distributes into a deep compartment and persists in serum.[3] The pharmacokinetic properties of these medications create an unusual situation where the teratogenic potential persists for periods of months (or years?) after therapy has ended. Unanswered questions remain about the magnitude of risk posed by etretinate use during pregnancy or before conception.

### Clinical features

Isotretinoin causes a specific phenotype characterized by malformations of the brain, heart and major arteries, craniofacies, and thymus (Table 4–2). [55] Of craniofacial malformations, facial asymmetry is most common, followed by abnormalities of external ear development. The auricular malformations can range from clinically insignificant pits and dimples on the posterior aspect of the lobule to anotia. The auricular malformations can take on many forms (Figs. 4–4 and 4–5), but are very similar to those found in thalidomide embryopathy; the parts of the external ear that are derived from the second branchial arch appear to be more susceptible than those derived from the first arch, and occasionally only a tragus and slit-like canal is present.[67] Middle ear bones are less frequently affected, and inner ear malformations are rare. The temporal bone is frequently malformed. Also as in thalidomide embryopathy, ear malformations are often accompanied by facial nerve paresis ipsilateral to the more severely affected ear. External ear malformations are usually bilateral, but the severity may not be comparable on both sides. Chronic otitis media is a common problem and may be exacerbated by the T-cell immunodeficiency that some children have. Ectopic thymus tissue has been noted in the lateral neck of several affected children at autopsy. Cleft palate has occured in a small number of affected children, but not cleft lip. Other less frequently occurring craniofacial anomalies include branchial cleft sinus and anomalous tracheal ring segmentation.

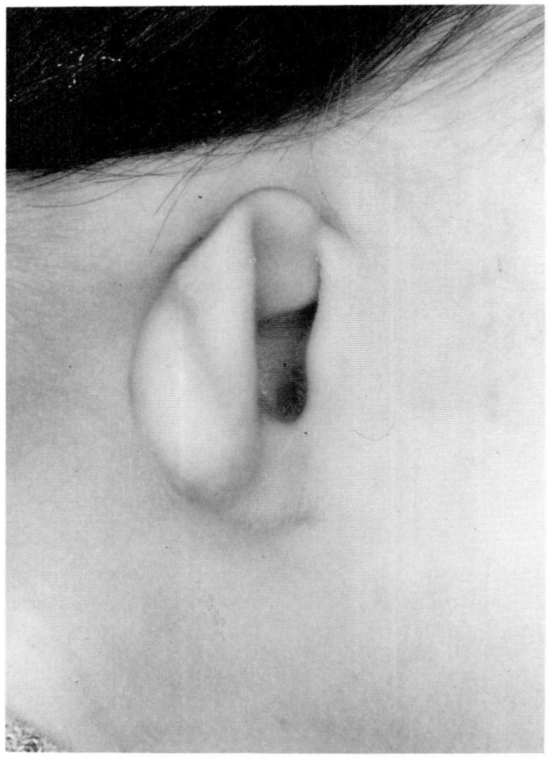

**Fig. 4–4.** Malformed external ear with slit-like ear canal associated with isotretinoin (13-cis-retinoic acid) teratogenesis. Note characteristic displacement of the lobule away from the cheek and the abnormal angle of the merger of the crus helicis and the superior helix.

**Table 4–2.** Phenotypic features of retinoic acid embryopathy

| |
|---|
| Spontaneous abortion |
| Premature delivery |
| *CRANIOFACIAL FEATURES* |
| Facial asymmetry |
| Microtia or external ear malformation |
| Stenotic external ear canals |
| Auricular pits and dimples |
| Epicanthal folds |
| Branchial cleft sinus |
| Malformed middle ear bones |
| Mottled teeth and excessive dental caries |
| Cardiac defects |
| Thymic deficiency |
| Mondini malformation |
| *NEUROLOGICAL AND NEUROPSYCHOLOGICAL* |
| Microcephaly |
| Developmental delay and/or mental retardation |
| Speech problems |
| Sensorineural and/or conductive hearing loss |
| Hypotonia, poor coordination |
| Attention deficits |
| Poor fine motor skills |
| Cranial nerve deficits II, III, VI, VIII, IX |

Isotretinoin-induced brain malformations include ventriculomegaly, hydrocephalus (Fig. 4–5), cranial nerve deficits, and specific malformations of the cerebellum and brainstem.[68] Cardiac defects caused by isotretinoin generally involve defects resulting from abnormal aorticopulmonary septation and aortic arch malformations.[71] Isotretinoin exposure can cause all of the features that are components of the DiGeorge anomaly, in varying combinations. Thymic deficiency usually, but not always, is limited to children with other severe malformations, especially cardiac defects.

Evidence of human etretinate teratogenicity is based solely upon case reports, but these are suggestive of at least some

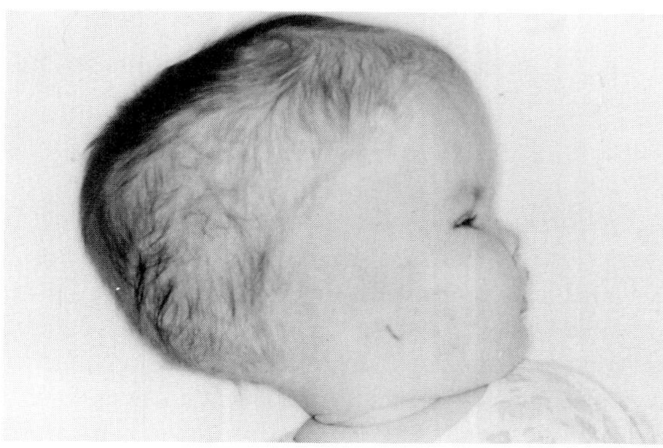

**Fig. 4–5.** 10 month old infant with isotretinoin teratogenesis showing severe congenital hydrocephalus (aqueductal stenosis) and a low-set, malformed external ear in which only the tragus developed, with a stenotic ear canal. This type of ear malformation has also been seen in thalidomide embryopathy.

causal associations. Malformed infants have been reported after preconceptional or postconceptional exposure to etretinate;[62,66] but there are no systematically conducted epidemiologic studies to confirm this.

The pathogenetic mechanisms through which isotretinoin induces these malformations are still poorly understood. There is evidence to support a role for retinoic acid in nearly every developmental process: cell migration, cell death, cell differentiation, and extracellular matrix composition.[49,60,90,107,111] Experimental studies suggest important roles for cellular retinoic acid binding proteins (CRABP-I) and nuclear receptors that bind all-trans- and 9-cis-retinoic acid (RARs and RXRs).[80,85,101] In experimental studies, mRNA and these proteins co-localize within many, but not all, of the apparently susceptible tissues during critical periods of embryogenesis.[24,38,80,82,100] How an excessively high concentration of retinoic acid within certain cells leads to malformation, however, is not understood.

## Other medications and environmental exposures

Tetracyclines taken after 20 weeks gestation may cause yellow-brown discoloration of teeth or occasionally, enamel defects or hypoplasia.[19] They do not appear to affect development of other craniofacial structures. Methotrexate use during pregnancy has been associated with a syndrome of growth deficiency, mental retardation, and effects on skull and craniofacial development.[123] Features include abnormal calvarial development with large sutures, misshapen skull, or craniosynostosis. The frequency of abnormal outcomes is not known. Recently, a new syndrome affecting offspring of women using angiotensin converting enzyme (ACE) inhibitors during the second and third trimesters of pregnancy was described. The phenotype includes enlarged kidneys, neonatal oliguria and renal failure, and skull hypoplasia.[9,63]

Thalidomide, although not available in North America except under special research protocols, deserves mention because of its historical importance in teratology.[122] External,[21,33,78] middle, and inner ear[58,64,99] malformations are major components of this embryopathy and are frequently accompanied by cranial nerve deficits including the facial, abducens, and oculomotor nerves. A few cases with narrow windows of exposure have allowed correlations between timing of exposure and ear malformations and have proven very valuable.[92] Dental anomalies and cleft lip also occur as part of this syndrome.[7,33]

Oromandibular-limb hypogenesis syndrome has been linked to chorionic villus sampling (CVS).[32,87] A recent National Institutes of Health (NIH) workshop concluded that its occurrence seems to correlate with CVS procedures done earlier than 7 weeks after conception, but that it might not be limited just to procedures done before that gestational age.[51] Tobacco smoking during pregnancy is one of the most frequent environmental exposures during pregnancy and its association with intrauterine growth retardation is clear.[102] Some case–control studies of oral clefts have found associations with maternal smoking, while others have not. Other cohort studies looking at overall major malformation rates among smokers have not found elevated rates.[61,106,117,125,127] Inhalation of toluene has been anecdotally linked to the occurrence of midfacial hypoplasia, short palpebral fissures, micrognathia, growth retardation, and abnormal neuropsychological development.[46,47]

## References


1. Abel EL, Sokol RJ: Incidence of fetal alcohol syndrome and economic impact of FAS-related anomalies. Drug Alcohol Depend 19:51–70, 1987.
2. Adams J, Lammer EJ: Relationship between dysmorphology and neuropsychological function in children exposed to isotretinoin "in utero". In: Functional Neuroteratology of Short-Term Exposure to Drugs, T Fujii, GJ Boer, eds. Teikyo University Press, Tokyo, 1991, pp 159–170.
3. Allen JG, Bloxham DP: The pharmacology and pharmacokinetics of the retinoids. Pharmacol Ther 40:1–27, 1989.
4. Alpert JJ, Zuckerman B: Alcohol use during pregnancy: what is the risk? Pediatr Rev 12:375–379, 1991.
5. American Academy of Pediatrics Committee on Substance Abuse and Committee on Children with Disabilities: Fetal alcohol syndrome and fetal alcohol effects. Pediatrics 91:1004–1006, 1993.
6. Ardinger HH, Atkin JF, Blackston RD, Elsas LJ, Clarren SK, Livingstone S, Flannery DB, Pellock JM, Harrod MJ, Lammer EJ, Majewski F, Schinzel A, Toriello HV, Hanson JW: Verification of the fetal valproate syndrome phenotype. Am J Med Genet 29:171–185, 1988.
7. Axrup K, d'Avignon M, Hellgren K, Henrikson C-O, Juhlin I-M, Larsson KS, Persson GG, Welander E: Children with thalidomide embryopathy: odontologic observations and aspects. Acta Odontol Scand 24:3–21, 1966.
8. Bantz EW: Valproic acid and congenital malformations. Clin Pediatr 23:352–353, 1984.
9. Barr M Jr, Cohen MM Jr.: ACE inhibitor fetopathy and hypocalvaria: the kidney-skull connection. Teratology 44:485–495, 1991.
10. Bertollini R, Källen B, Mastroiacovo P, Robert E: Anticonvulsant drugs in monotherapy: effect on the fetus. Eur J Epidemiol 3:164–171, 1987.
11. Boncinelli E, Simeone A, Acampora D, Mavilio F: HOX gene activation by retinoic acid. Trends Genet 7:329–334, 1991.
12. Bryant SV, Gardiner DM: Retinoic acid, local cell-cell interactions, and pattern formation in vertebrate limbs. Dev Biol 152:1–25, 1992.
13. Buehler BA, Delmont D, van Waes M, Finnell RH: Prenatal prediction of risk of the fetal hydantoin syndrome. N Engl J Med 322:1567–1572, 1990.
14. Cheron RG, Kaplan MM, Larsen PR, Selenkow HA, Crigler JF Jr.: Neonatal thyroid function after propylthiouracil therapy for maternal Graves' disease. N Engl J Med 304:525–528, 1981.
15. Chong MK, Harvey D, de Swiet M: Follow-up study of children whose mothers were treated with warfarin during pregnancy. Br J Obstet Gynaecol 91:1070–1073, 1984.
16. Clarren SK, Sampson PD, Larsen J, Donnell DJ, Barr HM, Bookstein FL, Martin DC, Streissguth AP: Facial effects of fetal alcohol exposure: assessment by photographs and morphometric analysis. Am J Med Genet 26:651–666, 1987.
17. Clarren SK, Smith DW: The fetal alcohol syndrome. N Engl J Med 298:1063–1067, 1978.
18. Cohen MM Jr: The Child with Multiple Birth Defects, Raven Press, New York, 1982.
19. Cohlan SQ: Tetracycline staining of teeth. Teratology 15:127–129, 1977.
20. Dansky LV, Finnell RH: Parental epilepsy, anticonvulsant drugs, and reproductive outcome: epidemiologic and experimental findings spanning three decades; 2: Human studies. Reprod Toxicol 5:301–335, 1991.
21. d'Avignon M, Barr B: Ear abnormalities and cranial nerve palsies in thalidomide children. Arch Otolaryngol 80:136–140 1964.
22. DiGiovanna JJ, Zech LA, Ruddel ME, Gantt G, Peck GL: Etretinate. Persistent serum levels after long-term therapy. Arch Dermatol 125:246–251, 1989.
23. DiLiberti JH, Farndon PA, Dennis NR, Curry CJ: The fetal valproate syndrome. Am J Med Genet 19:473–481, 1984.
24. Dollé P, Ruberte E, Leroy P, Morriss-Kay G, Chambon P: Retinoic acid receptors and cellular retinoid binding proteins. I. A systematic study of their differential pattern of transcription during mouse organogenesis. Development 110:1133–1151, 1990.
25. Duester G, Shean ML, McBride MS, Stewart MJ: Retinoic acid response element in the human alcohol dehydrogenase gene ADH3: implications for regulation of retinoic acid synthesis. Mol Cell Biol 11:1638–1646, 1991.
26. Eckhoff C, Nau H: Vitamin A supplementation increases levels of retinoic acid compounds in human plasma: possible implications for teratogenesis. Arch Toxicol 64:502–503, 1990.

27. Eichele G: Retinoids and vertebrate limb pattern formation. Trends Genet 5:246–251, 1989.
28. Finnell RH: Genetic differences in susceptibility to anticonvulsant drug-induced developmental defects. Pharmacol Toxicol 69:223–227, 1991.
29. Finnell RH, Buehler BA, Kerr BM, Ager PL, Levy RH: Clinical and experimental studies linking oxidative metabolism to phenytoin-induced teratogenesis. Neurology 42(Suppl 5):25–31, 1992.
30. Finnell RH, Dansky LV: Parental epilepsy, anticonvulsant drugs, and reproductive outcome: epidemiologic and experimental findings spanning three decades: 1. Animal studies. Reprod Toxicol 5:281–299, 1991.
31. Finnell RH, Shields HE, Taylor SM, Chernoff GF: Strain differences in phenobarbital-induced teratogenesis in mice. Teratology 35:177–185, 1987.
32. Firth HV, Boyd PA, Chamberlain P, MacKenzie IZ, Lindenbaum RH, Huson SM: Severe limb abnormalities after chorion villus sampling at 56–66 days' gestation. Lancet 337:762–763, 1991.
33. Fogh-Andersen P: Thalidomid und Lippen-Kiefer-Gaumen-Spalte. Dtsch Stomat 15:343–346, 1965.
34. German J, Kowal A, Ehlers KH: Trimethadione and human teratogenesis. Teratology 3:349–362, 1970.
35. Gray JE: Rubella in pregnancy; fetal pathology in the internal ear. Ann Otol Rhinol Laryngol 68:170–174, 1959.
36. Grossman J 3rd: Congenital syphilis. Teratology 16:217–219, 1977.
37. Gumpel SM, Hayes K, Dudgeon JA: Congenital perceptive deafness: role of intrauterine rubella. Br Med J 2:300–304, 1971.
38. Gustafson AL, Dencker L, Eriksson U: Non-overlapping expression of CRBPI and CRABPI during pattern formation of limbs and craniofacial structures in the early mouse embryo. Development 117:451–460, 1993.
39. Hall BD: Metopic suture fusion in fetal valproate syndrome (Abstract). Teratology 47:420, 1993.
40. Hall JG, Pauli RM, Wilson KM: Maternal and fetal sequelae of anticoagulation during pregnancy. Am J Med 68:122–140, 1980.
41. Haney AF: Structural and functional consequences of prenatal exposure to diethylstilbestrol in women. In: Banbury Report 26: Developmental Toxicology: Mechanisms and Risk, JA McLachlan, RM Pratt, CL Markert, eds. Cold Spring Harbor Laboratory, Cold Spring Harbor, 1987, pp 271–286.
42. Hanson JW: Teratogenic agents. In: Principles and Practice of Medical Genetics, Vol. 2, A Emery, D Rimoin, eds. Livingston, NY, 1992, pp 183–213.
43. Hanson JW, Myrianthopoulos NC, Harvey MA, Smith DW: Risks to the offspring of women treated with hydantoin anticonvulsants, with emphasis on fetal hydantoin syndrome. J Pediatr 89:662–668, 1976.
44. Hanson JW, Smith DW: The fetal hydantoin syndrome. J Pediatr 87:285–290, 1975.
45. Hanson JW, Streissguth AP, Smith DW: The effect of moderate alcohol consumption during pregnancy on fetal growth and morphogenesis. J Pediatr 92:457–460, 1978.
46. Hersh JH: Toluene embryopathy: two new cases. J Med Genet 26:333–337, 1989.
47. Hersh JH, Podruch PE, Rogers G, Weisskopf B: Toluene embryopathy. J Pediatr 106:922–927, 1985.
48. Heyman RA, Mangelsdorf DJ, Dyck JA, Stein RB, Eichele G, Evans RM, Thaller C: 9–cis retinoic acid is a high affinity ligand for the retinoid X receptor. Cell 68:397–406, 1992.
49. Holder N, Hill J: Retinoic acid modifies development of the midbrain-hindbrain border and affects cranial ganglion formation in zebrafish embryos. Development 113 1159–1170, 1991.
50. Holmes LB: Human teratogens: delineating the phenotypic effects, the period of greatest sensitivity, the dose-response relationship and mechanisms of action. In: Transplacental Effects on Fetal Health, DG Scarpelli, G Migaki, eds. Alan R. Liss, New York, 1988, pp 177–191.
51. Holmes LB: Report of National Institute of Child Health and Human Development workshop on chorionic villus sampling and limb and other defects, October 20, 1992. Teratology 48:7–13, 1993.
52. Holmes LB, Harvey EA, Hayes AM, Brown KS, Schoenfeld DA, Khoshbin S: The teratogenic effects of anticonvulsant monotherapy: phenobarbital (PB), carbamazepine (CBZ), and phenytoin (PHT) [Abstract]. Teratology 41:565, 1990.
53. Iturbe-Alessio I, Fonseca MC, Mutchinik O, Santos MA, Zajarias A, Salazar E: Risks of anticoagulant therapy in pregnant women with artificial heart valves. N Engl J Med 315:1390–1393, 1986.
54. Jones KL: Fetal alcohol syndrome. Pediatr Rev 8:122–126, 1986.
55. Jones KL, Lacro RV, Johnson KA, Adams J: Pattern of malformations in the children of women treated with carbamazepine during pregnancy. N Engl J Med 320:1661–1666, 1989.
56. Jones KL, Smith DW, Streissguth AP, Myrianthopoulos NC: Outcome in offspring of chronic alcoholic women. Lancet i:1076–1078, 1974.
57. Jones KL, Smith DW, Ulleland CN, Streissguth AP: Pattern of malformation in offspring of chronic alcoholic mothers. Lancet i:1267–1271, 1973.
58. Jorgensen MB, Kristensen HK, Buch NH: Thalidomide-induced aplasia of the inner ear. J Laryngol 78:1095–1101, 1964.
59. Kaplan LC: Congenital Dandy-Walker malformation associated with first trimester warfarin: a case report and literature review. Teratology 32:333–337, 1985.
60. Kessel M, Gruss P: Homeotic transformations of murine vertebrae and concomitant alteration of Hox codes induced by retinoic acid. Cell 67:89–104, 1991.
61. Khoury MJ, Weinstein A, Panny S, Holtzman NA, Lindsay PK, Farrel K, Eisenberg M: Maternal cigarette smoking and oral clefts: a population-based study. Am J Public Health 77:623–625, 1987.
62. Kietzmann H, Schwarze I, Grote W, Ravens U, Janig U, Harms D: Embryonale Fehlbildung bei Etretinat-Therapie der Mutter wegen Morbus Darier. Dtsch Med Wochensch 111:60–62, 1986.
63. Kreft-Jais C, Plouin PF, Tchobroutsky C, Boutray MJ: Angiotensin-converting enzyme inhibitors during pregnancy: a survey of 22 patients given captopril and nine given enalapril. Br J Obstet Gynaecol 95:420–422, 1988.
64. Kreipe U: Mißbildungen innerer Organe bei Thalidomidembryopathie. Ein Beitrag zur Bestimmung der sensiblen Phase bei Thalidomideinnahme in der Frühschwangerschaft. Arch Kinderheilk 176:33–61, 1967.
65. Lammer EJ: Developmental toxicity of synthetic retinoids in humans. In: Progress in Clinical and Biological Research Volume 281: Transplacental Effects on Fetal Health, DG Scarpelli, G Migaki, eds. Alan R. Liss, Inc., New York, 1988, pp 193–202.
66. Lammer EJ: Embryopathy in infant conceived one year after termination of maternal etretinate. Lancet ii:1080–1081, 1988.
67. Lammer EJ: Preliminary observations on isotretinoin-induced ear malformations and pattern formation of the external ear. J Craniofac Genet Dev Biol 11:292–295, 1991.
68. Lammer EJ, Armstrong DL: Malformations of hindbrain structures among humans exposed to isotretinoin (13–cis-retinoic acid) during early embryogenesis. In: Retinoids in Normal Development and Teratogenesis, G Morriss-Kay ed. Oxford University Press, Oxford, 1992, pp 281–295.
69. Lammer EJ, Chen DT, Hoar RM, Agnish ND, Benke PJ, Braun JT, Curry CJ, Fernhoff PM, Grix AW Jr, Lott IT, Richard JM, Sun SC: Retinoic acid embryopathy. N Engl J Med 313:837–841, 1985.
70. Lammer EJ, Hayes AM, Schunior A, Holmes LB: Unusually high risk for adverse outcomes of pregnancy following fetal isotretinoin exposure. Am J Hum Genet 43:A58, 1988.
71. Lammer EJ, Opitz JM: The DiGeorge anomaly as a developmental field defect. Am J Med Genet Suppl 2:113–127, 1986.
72. Lammer EJ, Schunior A, Hayes AM, Holmes LB: Isotretinoin dose and teratogenicity. Lancet ii:503–504, 1988.
73. Lammer EJ, Schunior A, Holmes LB: Retinoic acid fetopathy (Abstract). Proc Greenwood Genet Center 68, 1990.
74. Lemoine P, Rousseau HA, Borteyru JP: Les enfants de parents alcooliques. Anomalies observées à propos de 127 cas. Ouest Med 21:476–482, 1968.
75. Leroy P, Krust A, Kastner P, Mendelsohn C, Zelent A, Chambon P: Retinoic acid receptors. In: Retinoids in Normal Development and Teratogenesis, G Morriss-Kay, ed. Oxford University Press, New York, 1992, pp 7–26.
76. Lindhout D, Omtzigt JG, Cornel MC: Spectrum of neural-tube defects in 34 infants prenatally exposed to antiepileptic drugs. Neurology 42(Suppl 5):111–118, 1992.
77. Lindhout D, Schmidt D: In-utero exposure to valproate and neural tube defects. Lancet 1:1392–1393, 1986.
78. Livingstone G: Congenital ear abnormalities due to thalidomide. Proc R Soc Med 58:493–497, 1965.
79. MacGregor SN, Keith LG, Chasnoff IJ, Rosner MA, Chisum GM, Shaw P, Minogue JP: Cocaine use during pregnancy: adverse perinatal outcome. Am J Obstet Gynecol 157:686–690, 1987.
80. Maden M, Gale E, Horton C, Smith JC: Retinoid binding proteins in the developing vertebrate nervous system. In: Retinoids in Normal Development and Teratogenesis, G Morriss-Kay, ed. Oxford University Press, New York, 1992, pp 119–136.
81. Maden M, Holder N: The involvement of retinoic acid in the develop-

ment of the vertebrate central nervous system. Development Suppl 2:87–94, 1991.

82. Maden M, Hunt P, Eriksson U, Kuroiwa A, Krumlauf R, Summerbell D: Retinoic acid-binding protein, rhombomeres and the neural crest. Development 111:35–43, 1991.

83. Majewski F, Steger M, Richter B, Gill J, Rabe F: The teratogenicity of hydantoins and barbiturates in humans with considerations on the etiology of malformations and cerebral disturbances in the children of epileptic parents. Int J Biol Res Pregnancy 2:37–45, 1981.

84. Mangelsdorf DJ, Borgmeyer U, Heyman RA, Zhou JY, Ong ES, Oro AE, Kakizuka A, Evans RM: Characterization of three RXR genes that mediate the action of 9–cis retinoic acid. Genes Dev 6:329–344, 1992.

85. Mangelsdorf DJ, Evans RM: Vitamin A receptors: new insights on retinoid control of transcription. In: Retinoids in Normal Development and Teratogenesis, G Morriss-Kay, ed. Oxford University Press, New York, 1992, pp 27–50.

86. Marshall H, Nonchev S, Sham MH, Muchamore I, Lumsden A, Krumlauf R: Retinoic acid alters hindbrain Hox code and induces transformation of rhombomeres 2/3 into a 4/5 identity. Nature 360:737–741, 1992.

87. Mastroiacovo P, Botto LD, Cavalcanti DP, Lalatta F, Selicorni A, Tozzi AE, Baronciani D, Cigolotti AC, Giordono S, Petroni F, et al: Limb anomalies following chorionic villus sampling: a registry based case-control study. Am J Med Genet 44:856–864, 1992.

88. Mills JL, Graubard BI, Harley EE, Rhoads GG, Berendes HW: Maternal alcohol consumption and birth weight. How much drinking during pregnancy is safe? JAMA 252:1875–1879, 1984.

89. Morriss-Kay G: Retinoic acid and craniofacial development: molecules and morphogenesis. Bioessays 15:9–15, 1993.

90. Morriss-Kay G, Mahmood R: Morphogenesis-related changes in extracellular matrix induced by retinoic acid. In: Retinoids in Normal Development and Teratogenesis, G Morriss-Kay, ed. Oxford University Press, New York, 1992, pp 165–180.

91. Nau H, Chahoud I, Dencker L, Lammer EJ, Scott WJ Jr: Teratogenicity of vitamin A and retinoids. In: Vitamin A in Health and Disease: Basic Science and Clinical Aspects, R Blomhoff, ed. Marcel Dekker, New York, 1993.

92. Nowack E: Die sensible Phase bie der Thalidomide-Embryopathie. Humangenetik 1:516–536, 1965.

93. Omtzigt JG, Los FJ, Grobbee DE, Pijpers L, Jahoda MG, Brandenburg H, Stewart PA, Gaillard HL, Sachs ES, Wladimiroff JW, Lindhout D: The risk of spina bifida aperta after first-trimester exposure to valproate in a prenatal cohort. Neurology 42(Suppl 5):119–125, 1992.

94. Papalopulu N, Hunt P, Wilkinson D, Graham D, Krumlauf R: Hox-2 homeobox genes and retinoic acid: potential roles in patterning the vertebrate nervous system. In: Advances in Neural Regeneration Research. Wiley-Liss, New York, 1990, pp 291–307.

95. Pauli RM, Lian JB, Mosher DF, Suttie JW: Association of congenital deficiency of multiple vitamin K-dependent coagulation factors and the phenotype of the warfarin embryopathy: clues to the mechanism of teratogenicity of coumarin derivatives. Am J Hum Genet 41:566–583, 1987.

96. Rating D, Jäger-Roman E, Koch S, Diechl A, Hartmann H, Jacob S, Beck-Mannagetta G, Nau H, Helge H: Major malformations and minor anomalies in the offspring of epileptic parents: the role of antiepileptic drugs. In: Pharmacokinetics in Teratogenesis, H Nau, WJ Scott Jr, eds. CRC Press, Boca Raton, FL, 1987, pp 205–224.

97. Robert E, Löfkvist E, Maugiere F: Valproate and spina bifida. Lancet 2:1392, 1984.

98. Rosa FW: Spina bifida in infants of women treated with carbamazepine during pregnancy. N Engl J Med 324:674–677, 1991.

99. Rosendal T: Aplasia-hypoplasia of the otic labyrinth after thalidomide. Acta Radiol Diagn 3:225–236, 1965.

100. Ruberte E, Dolle P, Chambon P, Morriss-Kay G: Retinoic acid receptors and cellular retinoid binding proteins. II. Their differential pattern of transcription during early morphogenesis in mouse embryos. Development 111:45–60, 1991.

101. Ruberte E, Friederich V, Morriss-Kay G, Chambon P: Differential distribution patterns of CRABP1 and CRABP2 transcripts during mouse embryogenesis. Development 115:973–987, 1992.

102. Rush D, Cassano P: Relationship of cigarette smoking and social class to birth weight and perinatal mortality among all births in Britain, 5–11 April 1970. J Epidemiol Community Health 37:249–255, 1983.

103. Sever JL, Ellenberg JH, Ley AC, Madden DL, Fuccillo DA, Tzan NR, Edmonds DM: Toxoplasmosis: maternal and pediatric findings in 23,000 pregnancies. Pediatrics 82:181–192, 1988.

104. Sever JL, South MA, Shaver KA: Delayed manifestations of congenital rubella. Rev Infect Dis 7(Suppl 1):S164–S169, 1985.

105. Shepard TH: Detection of human teratogenic agents. J Pediatr 101:810–815, 1982.

106. Shiono PH, Klebanoff MA, Berendes HW: Congenital malformations and maternal smoking during pregnancy. Teratology 34:65–71, 1986.

107. Smith-Thomas L, Lott I, Bronner-Fraser M: Effects of isotretinoin on the behavior of neural crest cells in vitro. Dev Biol 123:276–281, 1987.

108. Stein Z, Kline J, Kharrazi M: What is a teratogen? Epidemiological criteria. In: Issues and Reviews in Teratology, Vol 2, H Kalter, ed. Plenum Press, New York, 1984, pp 23–65.

109. Streissguth AP, Aase JM, Clarren SK, Randels SP, LaDue RA, Smith DF: Fetal alcohol syndrome in adolescents and adults. JAMA 265:1961–1967, 1991.

110. Streissguth AP, Barr HM, Sampson PD, Parrish-Johnson JC, Kirchner GL, Martin DC: Attention, distraction, and reaction time at age 7 years and prenatal alcohol exposure. Neurobehav Toxicol Teratol 8:717–725, 1986.

111. Sulik KK, Cook CS, Webster WS: Teratogens and craniofacial malformations: relationships to cell death. Development 103 (Suppl):213–231, 1988.

112. Teratology Society: Recommendations for vitamin A use during pregnancy. Teratology 35:269–275, 1987.

113. Teratology Society: Recommendations for isotretinoin use in women of childbearing potential. Teratology 44:1–6, 1991.

114. Thijssen HH, Baars LG, Vervoort-Peters HT: Vitamin K 2,3–epoxide reductase: the basis for stereoselectivity of 4–hydroxycoumarin anticoagulant activity. Br J Pharmacol 95:675–682, 1988.

115. Ueda K, Nishida Y, Oshima K, Shepard TH: Congenital rubella syndrome: correlation of gestational age at time of maternal rubella with type of defect. J Pediatr 94:763–765, 1979.

116. Underwood BA: The Safe Use of Vitamin A by Women during the Reproductive Years: Report of the International Vitamin A Consultative Group. Nutrition Foundation, Washington, DC, 1984,

117. Van den Eeden SK, Karagas MR, Daling JR, Vaughan TL: A case-control study of maternal smoking and congenital malformations. Paediatr Perinat Epidemiol 4:147–155, 1990.

118. VanLang QN, Tassinari MS, Keith DA, Holmes LB: Effect of in utero exposure to anticonvulsants on craniofacial development and growth. J Craniofac Genet Dev Biol 4:115–133, 1984.

119. Véghelyi PV: Fetal abnormality and maternal ethanol metabolism. Lancet 2:53–54, 1983.

120. Vorhees CV: Principles of behavioral teratology. In: Handbook of Behavioral Teratology, EP Riley, CV Vorhees, eds. Plenum Press, New York, 1986, pp 23–48.

121. Warkany J: Warfarin embryopathy. Teratology 14:205–209, 1970.

122. Warkany J: Congenital Malformations: Notes and Comments, Yearbook Medical Publishers, San Diego, 1972.

123. Warkany J: Aminopterin and methotrexate: folic acid deficiency. Teratology 17:353–357, 1978.

124. Wells PG, Nagai MK, Greco GS: Inhibition of trimethadione and dimethadione teratogenicity by the cyclooxygenase inhibitor acetylsalicylic acid: a unifying hypothesis for the teratologic effects of hydantoin anticonvulsants and structurally related compounds. Toxicol Appl Pharmacol 97:406–414, 1989.

125. Werler MM, Lammer EJ, Rosenberg L, Mitchell AA: Maternal cigarette smoking during pregnancy in relation to oral clefts. Am J Epidemiol 132:926–932, 1990.

126. Werler MM, Lammer EJ, Rosenberg L, Mitchell AA: Maternal alcohol use in relation to selected birth defects. Am J Epidemiol 134:691–698, 1991.

127. Werler MM, Pober BR, Holmes LB: Smoking and pregnancy. In: Teratogen Update: Environmentally Induced Birth Defects, Sever JL, Brent RL (eds), AR Liss, Inc., New York, 1986, pp 131–139.

128. Wilson JG: Current status of teratology: general principles and mechanisms derived from animal studies, in Handbook of Teratology: General Principles and Etiology, Vol. 1, Wilson JG, Fraser FC (eds), Plenum Press, New York, 1977, pp 49–60.

129. Wladimiroff JW, Stewart PA, Reuss A, van Swaay E, Lindhout D, Sachs ES: The role of ultrasound in the early diagnosis of fetal structural defects following maternal anticonvulsant therapy. Ultrasound Med Biol 14:657–660, 1988.

# 5

# Prenatal Diagnosis

PATRICE EYDOUX and SAMIR KHALIFÉ

Otolaryngologic anomalies are common at birth. In about 20% of newborns with a major birth defect, there is an otolaryngologic anomaly (involving the face, nose, mouth, pharynx, larynx, esophagus, trachea, or neck). About 85% of infants with multisystem malformations have an otolaryngologic defect, not including deafness. These malformations are serious, and the perinatal and first year mortality rate is approximately 13%. Their etiology is often unknown (69%). However, 15% percent are known to be of chromosomal, 4% monogenic, 9% multifactorial, and 3% teratogenic causation.

The development of the head and neck is closely related to the development of the central nervous system.[64] A defect involving the central nervous system is likely to be accompanied by facial abnormalities ranging from minor anomalies, e.g., hypertelorism, to major malformations, e.g., cebocephaly. Conversely, facial anomalies often coexist with neurological abnormalities. Thus the prenatal detection of cranial or facial anomalies may help in the diagnosis of serious conditions with grave prognosis.

Prenatal diagnosis of genetic diseases may be offered when there is a high risk of a very serious condition, threatening fetal life or leading to major defects and/or mental retardation. Many of these anomalies are not amenable to treatment and if so wished by the parents, these pregnancies may be terminated.

The main diagnostic tool for prenatal diagnosis is ultrasonography, allowing both the visualization of the fetus and intrauterine sampling. Ultrasonographic examination is considered harmless and allows an almost complete prenatal examination of the fetal body. This examination is now routinely done during the second trimester of pregnancy and permits the detection of numerous fetal malformations, even in low-risk situations. However, it also leads to a high degree of anxiety in the patient whenever a structural anomaly is discovered.

Dramatic improvement of ultrasonographic examination during the past 10 years allows a detailed study of many of the structures in the head and neck. Prenatal discovery of any otolaryngologic anomaly should prompt a thorough search for another structural anomaly, especially of a neurological nature.

Intrauterine sampling is usually proposed whenever a significant structural anomaly is detected in the fetus. Amniocentesis, chorionic villus sampling (CVS), and fetal blood sampling are various possibilities allowing a fetal karyotype. DNA or biochemical testing may also be offered in specific situations. These invasive techniques carry a risk of fetal death and should be extensively discussed with the parents prior to any decision.

It is most important to detail fetal malformations as accurately as possible with repeated ultrasound examinations in order to assess the prognosis and decide the therapeutic action that should be taken.

## Methods in prenatal diagnosis

### Non-invasive procedures

#### Ultrasonography

Ultrasound is now the primary tool for prenatal diagnosis of malformations. Numerous malformations have been described prenatally, resulting in early diagnosis of serious fetal conditions. Ultrasound is also of great value as a guide for sampling techniques (amniocentesis, chorionic villi sampling, cordocentesis).

A detailed ultrasound view of the fetal face, using a transvaginal approach, can be achieved starting at 13–15 weeks gestation. Similar views can be obtained transabdominally only 3–4 weeks later. Examining the fetal face requires ingenuity, patience, and good luck on the part of the ultrasonographer. Familiarity with normal anatomy is essential. A systematic approach should include sagittal, axial, and coronal planes.

The sagittal plane allows the assessment of the fetal profile: forehead, nose, and jaw (Fig. 5–1). Parasagittal planes tangential to the calvarium allow the visualization of the ears. The axial plane identifies both orbits (Fig. 5–2), the anterior palate, and the tongue within the oral cavity. The coronal planes are the most important for evaluation of craniofacial anatomy, allowing the visualization of the orbits, eyelids, nose, and lips (Fig 5–3).[34,52]

The ears are amenable to examination by ultrasonography, but a detailed study does not yield good results before the third trimester. The helix, scaphoid fossa, triangular fossa, concha, antihelix, tragus, intertragic incisure, and lobule can be seen.[35] Occasionally, the basal turn of the cochlea or superior semicircular canal may be visualized within the petrous portion of the temporal bone.[33]

The section demonstrating the upper lip and nose is easily obtained. The tip of the nose, the alae nasi, and the columella are seen above the upper lip. The lower lip is also seen in the same plane. The intranasal portion of the upper airways between the concha is seen on transverse sections.[35]

Tooth buds of the incisors, canines, and the premolars are usually recognized. They start calcifying between the fourth and fifth month of gestation.[35]

The tongue, the epiglottis, and the vestibulum of the larynx can also be identified. The vocal cords are seen slightly below these.[2,35] The esophagus can also be visualized.[2]

Apart from the morphological examination, fetal movements can also be observed: swallowing, sucking, yawning, protrusion of the tongue, breathing, hiccups, and regurgitation.

Ultrasonography has thus become very accurate and allows a complete and systematic examination of the head and neck,

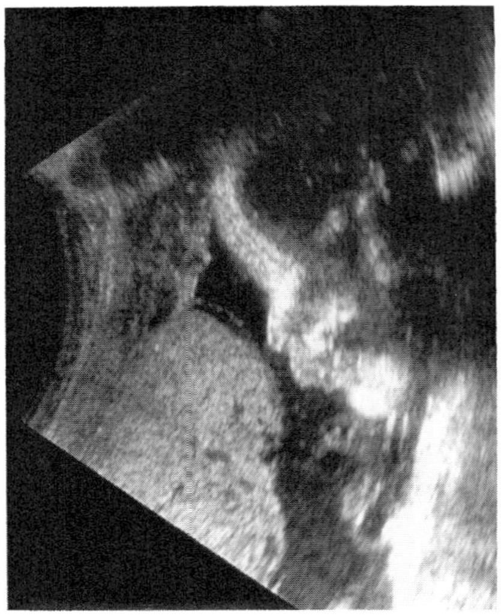

**Fig. 5–1.** Fetal profile, second trimester. Forehead, nose, chin, and upper and lower lip are clearly identified.

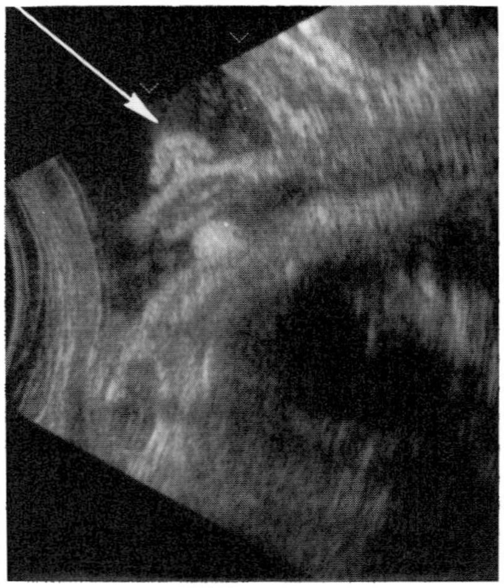

**Fig. 5–3.** Coronal plane, second trimester, showing the nose, mouth, and chin.

as well as of the entire fetal body. New improvements in this technology are expected, both in the definition of ultrasound and the computer treatment of the data obtained. Three-dimensional ultrasonography will potentially add a better morphometric evaluation of the fetal face, especially in the case of complex anomalies.[69]

It should be emphasized that ultrasonographic results are operator and equipment dependent. Patients should be referred to specialized centers for these examinations.

### Magnetic resonance imaging (MRI)

MRI may be performed without curarization during the third trimester. It is not commonly used in prenatal diagnosis, but numerous studies are being undertaken to assess its application to fetal examination. In some cases, it may provide additional information to that provided by ultrasonography.

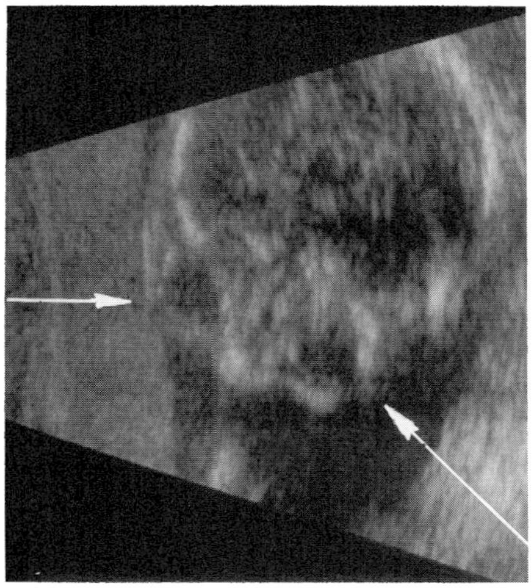

**Fig. 5–2.** Axial plane, second trimester showing the two orbits. Orbital diameters can be measured from this plane.

MRI allows the evaluation of the maturation of the surface of the fetal brain.[41] Anomalies such as megalencephaly,[49] hydrocephalus, agenesis of the corpus callosum, subarachnoidal nodules in tuberous sclerosis,[50] and intracranial teratoma[23,66] have been diagnosed using this method. MRI may also be useful for the diagnosis and evaluation of cervical teratoma.[53]

### Maternal blood sampling

*Triple screen.* Biochemical markers of chromosomal anomalies, primarily trisomy 21, have been assessed over the past few years. The *triple screen* is a combined test of three maternal serum parameters: human chorionic gonadotropin (hCG), alpha-fetoprotein (AFP), and unconjugated estriol ($UE_3$).[29] These parameters have been used extensively. If the entire population at risk were screened, about 5% of patients would be identified as "high risk." These patients would then be offered amniocentesis, yielding a detection rate of 60%–70% of trisomy 21. Ongoing studies involve newer parameters, such as human placental lactogen (HPL).[54] Of all these parameters, hCG seems to be the most discriminating, and the free beta fraction is now used for first trimester diagnosis. In addition to screening for chromosomal anomalies, AFP is useful in the diagnosis of neural tube defects and seems to be a good marker for unfavorable pregnancy outcome.

*Fetal cells in maternal circulation.* Fetal cells, e.g., trophoblasts, erythroblasts, macrophages, and granulocytes, are known to circulate in maternal blood. The kinetics of transplacental passage is under study, but it appears that a detectable number of cells is present in most women by 11 weeks of gestation, and that their number increases throughout pregnancy. Some of these cells, such as trophoblastic cells, remain permanently in the maternal circulation. Using sorting technology, such as a fluorescence activated cell sorter (FACS) with monoclonal antibodies which recognize specific cell lines, it is possible to increase the concentration of fetal cells in a sample of maternal blood. These cells may then be subject to genetic analysis, such as fluorescent in situ hybridization (FISH) or polymerase chain reaction (PCR).[26] This strategy is being tested as a method for screening chromosomal anomalies during the first trimester of pregnancy.

### Invasive procedures

In many cases, prenatal diagnosis involves laboratory testing of fetal or parafetal tissues (amniotic sac, placenta, umbilical cord). All of the following procedures are performed under ultrasound guidance. They all carry the risk, however small, of fetal death.

#### Amniocentesis

Amniocentesis is performed from 15 weeks gestation to term. Under ultrasonic guidance, using a 22 gauge needle, 20–30 cc of fluid is withdrawn transabdominally from the amniotic sac. It is possible to withdraw fluid from the amniotic sac even before 10 weeks of gestation, but the risk of such an early procedure is still unknown.

During the third trimester, amniocentesis may also be performed for amnioreduction or amnioinfusion in cases of polyhydramnios or oligohydramnios, respectively.

Genetic amniocentesis is performed primarily for karyotyping. Chromosomal studies are carried out by culturing the few viable cells present in the amniotic fluid. The success rate is approximately 99.4%.

The biochemical diagnosis of many inborn errors of metabolism is possible from the cultured cells or the analysis of the amniotic fluid supernatant. DNA from these cells may also be studied, although chorionic villus sampling is usually preferred for these analyses because the procedure can be performed earlier for those patients at high genetic risk (vide infra). Amniotic fluid can also be assayed under specific conditions for other fetal products, e.g., alphafetoprotein and acetylcholinesterase in neural tube defects, or bilirubin in defects of the digestive system.

Mid-trimester amniocentesis carries an estimated risk of fetal loss of 0.5% to 1.0%.[62,73]

#### Chorionic villi sampling (CVS)

Chorionic villi may be obtained by aspiration through a transabdominal needle or a transcervical catheter. The procedure is usually performed between 9 and 12 weeks gestation, but may also be performed transabdominally until late in the third trimester for chromosomal diagnosis.[44] Preliminary results can be obtained from a semidirect preparation of spontaneously dividing cells and final results from cultured cells. More tissue is obtained than with amniocentesis, allowing direct DNA or enzymatic analysis.

The success rate of CVS for chromosome analysis (97.8%) is slightly lower than that with amniocentesis. Also, given the relatively high rate of false-negative (1/1000) and false-positive (1%) chromosomal results, both direct and long-term cultures must be performed in order to analyze two different cell populations, thus increasing the workload of the cytogenetic laboratory. Some maternal tissue may also be present, especially after cell culture, and may be responsible for false negative results. The quality of chromosome analysis is lower than that achieved with amniocentesis.

According to published data, CVS carries an estimated rate of fetal loss of 0.6%[13] to 0.8%[51] in excess of second trimester amniocentesis. This difference is not considered to be statistically significant. Concern has been expressed regarding a possible association of oromandibular and limb hypoplasia with CVS. Recent data from the literature seem to acknowledge this potential danger in procedures performed before 10 weeks of gestation.[32,38]

#### Fetal blood sampling

Fetal blood sampling can be performed from approximately 18 weeks gestation to term. A 20 or 22 gauge heparinized needle is inserted into the umbilical cord, usually near its insertion into the placenta. The intrahepatic vein may also be used as a sampling site. Up to 3 ml of fetal blood is taken, depending upon gestational age.

Access to fetal blood allows for rapid cytogenetic results from fetal lymphocyte culture, the evaluation of fetal hematological or immunological abnormalities, the diagnosis of certain inborn errors of metabolism, the assessment of certain fetal infections, the evaluation of the fetal acid–base status, and the possible direct intravascular treatment of some of these conditions.

The risk of fetal loss from diagnostic fetal blood sampling is estimated at 1%–2%.[45]

#### Fetal biopsies

Biopsies of fetal skin, liver, muscle, lung, and kidney have been performed for different rare fetal disorders in which a diagnosis has not been possible using other techniques.[22,52]

#### Fetoscopy, Embryoscopy

The development of ultrasound technology in the early 1980s induced a rapid decline in the use of fetoscopy. The current development of endoscopy, using thin-gauge fiberoptic instruments, may soon allow early diagnosis of congenital anomalies with greater accuracy than ultrasound examination, earlier access to fetal circulation, and, owing to operative fetoscopic techniques, an improved prenatal management of some fetal conditions.[48]

#### Preimplantation diagnosis (PID)

Following in vitro fertilization (IVF), one or two cells may be sampled from the morula and studied with appropriate techniques. Genetic analysis of these few cells is currently under extensive study, the most promising methods being PCR and FISH. Only normal embryos are then reimplanted, avoiding the

**Table 5–1.** Invasive sampling for prenatal diagnosis

| Sampling | Age of pregnancy | Quantity | Duration of cell culture | Turnaround time | Quality of the karyotype | Risk of procedure |
|---|---|---|---|---|---|---|
| Amniocentesis | 14–39 weeks | 20–40 ml | 10–20 days | 15–30 days | excellent | 1/200 |
| Chorionic villus sampling | 10–39 weeks | 5–15 mg | 1–20 days | 2–20 days | middle | 1/100 |
| Fetal blood sampling | 20–39 weeks | 1–2 ml | 3 days | 7 days | excellent; high resolution | 2/100 |

need for termination of an ensuing genetically abnormal pregnancy. This approach would allow a very early diagnosis of chromosomal and mendelian conditions.[61]

The applications of PID will probably remain scarce, as IVF is needed as a first step. Moreover, at least for the foreseeable future, an invasive prenatal diagnostic procedure will remain necessary to rule out a false-negative result. Another drawback of PID is the occurrence of frequent mosaicism of chromosomal anomalies in early embryos. Nonetheless, some indications for this method remain of interest, e.g., patients who have previously undergone terminations of pregnancy because of affected fetuses, and patients undergoing IVF who are at risk for a genetic disease.[61]

## Fetal ultrasononography and anomalies of the ear, nose, and throat

Fetal ultrasound at 18–20 weeks is now part of routine antenatal practice. Many malformations may be identified at this gestational age, although it should be possible to detect at least some of them earlier.

### Hypertelorism

#### General considerations

*Hypertelorism* is defined as an increase greater than two standard deviation (SD) of the mean interorbital distance (orbital hypertelorism), or the interpupillary distance (ocular hypertelorism). Orbital and ocular hypertelorism usually coexist if there is no associated strabismus.

Isolated hypertelorism is very rare. It is usually a feature of a syndrome, e.g., Aarskog, DiGeorge, Noonan, and midfacial cleft syndromes. It may also be caused by chromosomal aberrations (monosomy 4p, monosomy 5p, monosomy X, monosomy 18p) or teratogenic factors.

#### Ultrasonography and prenatal diagnosis

Normograms for fetal ocular parameters exist, starting at the age of 11 weeks of intrauterine life. There are tables of gestational age–normative values for interocular distance, binocular distance, and ocular diameter.[34,39,52] Hypertelorism may be a serendipitous finding during fetal development, and must prompt a careful search for other fetal structural abnormalities. Its detection may also help in the diagnosis of a mendelian syndrome that has previously been diagnosed in an older sibling. As with other fetal anomalies, karyotyping should be offered. If a cardiac malformation is also present, the use of fluorescent in situ hybridization may be considered for the diagnosis of DiGeorge syndrome.

### Hypotelorism

#### General considerations

In hypotelorism the measurement of the interocular and interorbital distances is decreased. Cyclopia is the most severe form of hypotelorism, with complete fusion of the orbits.

This rare anomaly is usually part of the holoprosencephaly spectrum. Hypotelorism may also be associated with microcephaly or cleft palate. It is a feature of Williams syndrome and Langer-Giedion syndrome, which may be explored using DNA probes mapping to the regions of interest on chromosome 7 and chromosome 8, respectively. Other conditions associated with hypotelorism include Meckel syndrome, with its concomitant encephalocele, polydactyly and renal cysts, and Coffin-Siris syndrome, with its limb abnormalities. Both should be detected by ultrasound.

Chromosome aberrations are detected in 26% of cases of holoprosencephaly, in association with facial and extrafacial defects (trisomy 13 and 18, triploidies, structural aberrations).[42]

#### Ultrasonography and prenatal diagnosis

Detailed examination is necessary whenever hypotelorism is found on ultrasound examination. Attention should be focused on the brain to detect holoprosencephaly. Any associated intrauterine anomaly is an indication for fetal karyotyping.

### Anomalies of the nose

#### General considerations

Anomalies of the nose may be part of the holoprosencephaly spectrum, resulting from cleavage abnormalities of the prosencephalon. As isolated anomalies, they are often monogenic, but when associated with extrafacial malformations, an underlying chromosomal anomaly must be sought.[9]

#### Proboscis

The proboscis is a tube-like, blind appendage which has developed in place of or laterally to the nose. It is associated with arhinencephaly or other anomalies of the olfactory cortex and may be a feature of holoprosencephaly. It is very rare (<1/10,000) and may be associated with chromosomal abnormalities (trisomy 13, 18, triploidy, and structure anomalies). In utero ultrasound diagnosis is feasible and fetal karyotyping must be offered.

#### Arhinia

Arhinia is an extremely rare condition. The nose is absent and there is micrognathia and a high-arched palate. It may be isolated or associated with other malformations, including meningocele.

### Cleft lip and cleft palate

#### General considerations

Cleft lip and/or palate is common in newborns (1/700), accounting for 13% of all anomalies at birth.[27,51,61] In 25% of cases, only the lip is involved, in 25% the palate only, and in 50%, both lip and palate.

Cleft lip with or without cleft palate (cleft lip/palate), and isolated cleft palate are usually considered to be genetically separate groups.[24,25] Anticonvulsivant treatment during pregnancy,[25] including hydantoin, trimethadione, and valproate have been associated with these defects. Other causes include numerous single gene syndromes (e.g., oral-facial-digital [OFD], ectrodactyly-ectodermal dyplasia, cleft lip/palate [EEC], velo-cardio-facial [VCF] syndrome) and chromosomal anomalies (trisomy 13, 18, and 9, but also structural anomalies).[18,60] Association of cleft lip and/or cleft palate with other anomalies is frequent. The systems involved, with their relative frequencies, are the following: central nervous system anomalies (29%), microcephaly (25%), eye defects (15%), micrognathia (9%), skeletal anomalies (12%, including polydactyly) and cardiac defects (7%).

### Ultrasonography and prenatal diagnosis

Routine diagnosis of cleft lip and/or cleft palate is often made only as late as the third trimester of pregnancy. An accurate ultrasonographic diagnosis of complete cleft lip is possible after 16 weeks of gestation and of incomplete cleft lip sometimes only after 27 weeks.[8] Nonetheless, diagnosis of bilateral cleft lip as part of an EEC syndrome has been reported as early as 14 weeks, using a transvaginal probe.[11] Premaxillary protrusion is visible as a paranasal mass and is seen in most cases of bilateral cleft lip and palate.[12,46]

When such a defect is discovered, the family history may reveal multifactorial clefting or a mendelian syndrome. Associated malformations, growth retardation, or polyhydramnios should be carefully looked for, with detailed scanning not just of the face but also of the entire fetus. Fetal echocardiography should also be performed.

When concomitant malformations are present, chromosome anomalies, mainly trisomy 13 or 18, are detected in 40%–48% of cases.[43,56] When an isolated cleft lip or palate is found, fetal karyotyping is advisable in order to rule out a structural chromosomal rearrangement.

One of the possible causes of an association of cleft palate with a cardiac anomaly is velo-cardio-facial (VCF) syndrome, which may be diagnosed using in situ hybridization mapping to the region of interest (22q11).[20]

When a cleft lip or cleft palate is discovered at ultrasonic examination, the patient should be referred for genetic counseling. Family history and examination of the parents or siblings may give valuable information and, once the result of the karyotype is available, the prognosis of this anomaly will be more accurate. A consultation with a pediatric surgeon familiar with prenatal diagnosis should be scheduled to inform the patient of the possible difficulties related to cleft palate (feeding, breathing, and phonation), to evaluate the possibility of surgical treatment, to assess the prognosis after surgery, and to organize the management at delivery.

## Macroglossia

### General considerations

*True macroglossia* is defined as enlargement of the tongue, which is related to histological findings such as vascular malformations (hemangioma, lymphangioma), muscular enlargement (hemihypertrophy, Beckwith-Wiedemann syndrome [BWS]), anomalies resulting from a storage disease (Pompe disease, mucopolysaccharidosis types I, II, and VI, mannosidosis, I-cell disease), or tumors and cysts (neurofibromas, hamartomas).[68]

No abnormal histological findings are found in relative macroglossia, the main cause of which is Down syndrome.

### Ultrasonographic and prenatal diagnosis

Enlargement of the tongue may be demonstrated at ultrasonic examination by using a midsagittal view of the face. A karyotype should be performed in cases of relative macroglossia to rule out an aneuploidy, mainly trisomy 21. In one study, 13 fetuses with macroglossia were detected. Nine were found to have trisomy 21, and 2 had BWS. Macroglossia was found in 13% of fetuses with trisomy 21 (10% before 28 weeks, 20% after 28 weeks of gestation).[44]

Family history or other ultrasonographic findings may point to one of the conditions listed above that are associated with macroglossia. BWS may be suspected because of an abdominal wall defect,[72] visceromegaly,[67] or adrenal hemorrhagic macrocysts.[40] Probes mapping to the chromosomal region of interest for BWS (11p15) may facilitate the diagnosis. Prenatal diagnosis of BWS is of importance, as immediate management of possible neonatal hypoglycemia may prevent long-term intellectual impairment.

## Micrognathia

### General considerations

*Micrognathia* is defined as the reduction in the size of the mandible, resulting from hypoplasia of the ectomesenchyme in the first branchial arch. It may be difficult to distinguish from *retrognathia,* which refers to a posteriorly positioned mandible. *Agnathia,* or absence of the mandible, is a rare finding, and is usually associated with holoprosencephaly.

Micrognathia may be associated with ear anomalies. Although it may be a familial trait, it is usually part of a syndrome and is a common finding in chromosomal anomalies. Such a discovery should thus be followed by a detailed fetal ultrasonographic examination.

### Ultrasonography and prenatal diagnosis

Attempts have been made to determine normograms for measurements of the fetal mandible during pregnancy.[17,70] Only severe micrognathia may be detected with ultrasound. It is rarely an isolated finding and is often associated with fetal structural anomalies that may point towards one of the numerous syndromes listed in association with a small jaw.[21] Micrognathia is also a feature of chromosomal anomalies in association with multisystem defects; over 80% of fetuses with a trisomy 18 have micrognathia.[6] Even in these cases, it may be difficult to detect.[42] A high incidence of abnormal karyotypes in fetuses with an abnormal profile, of which most had micrognathia, has been reported. In the same series, skeletal dysplasias were also frequent.[65]

## Abnormal external ear

### General considerations

Although gross anomalies of the ear are detectable by ultrasonographic examination, they are rarely a reason for referral to prenatal diagnosis centers.

Microtia represents a spectrum ranging from a small auricle with an overall normal structure to total absence of the pinna (anotia). Auditory canal atresia and mandibular hypoplasia are often associated with microtia. Hearing loss depends upon the presence of middle ear malformations, the frequency of which is to a certain extent correlated with the degree of the external ear defect. Sensorineural hearing loss is also a frequent occurrence (present in 16% of individuals with microtia and/or hemifacial microsomia). Twenty to forty percent of children with microtia/anotia have an associated defect, including the oculo-auriculo-vertebral spectrum (OAV), or an associated renal malformation.[14]

### Ultrasonography, prenatal diagnosis

Normograms of fetal ear length have been established for the second and third trimester. This measurement can therefore be included as a criterion in the screening of aneuploidies during pregnancy and has given encouraging results.[3,37,59]

The sonographic discovery of an external ear malformation during pregnancy should prompt the search for other facial, neurological, spinal, or renal malformations. The question of invasive sampling for fetal karyotyping should be answered on an individual basis, taking into consideration the extent of the malformation, the presence of concomitant defects, and the gestational age.

## Hearing loss

Moderate to severe hearing loss is found in 1/1,000 to 1/2,000 infants. Recognized syndromes account for 10% of hearing loss in schools for the hearing impaired. Waardenburg, Pendred, and Usher syndromes are a few of the most common.[15]

Attempts at nonspecific prenatal diagnosis of hearing loss have been made, e.g., measuring the fetal heart response to acoustic stimulation during the second and third trimester; the results are promising but should be assessed further.[36] In addition, prenatal diagnosis of hearing loss may rely upon ultrasound examination if a syndrome is suspected or upon DNA studies if a genetic defect has already been identified in the family.

## Esophageal and tracheal malformations

### General considerations

Esophageal and tracheal malformations usually result from an anomaly of tracheoesophageal separation occurring at 3–5 weeks gestation. Esophageal atresia (EA) is a complete obstruction of the esophageal lumen; in esophageal stenosis, the lumen is only narrowed. A tracheoesophageal fistula (TEF) is associated with tracheal atresia (TA) in 96% of cases.[31] In a recent European collaborative study, a chromosomal anomaly (mostly trisomy 18 and 21) was found in 10% of neonates with EA/TEF. Of the remaining cases, 50% had multiple malformations.[19]

VACTERL association (**V**ertebral anomalies, **A**nal atresia, **C**ardiac malformation, TEF/EA, **R**enal and **L**imb malformations) is a frequent occurrence. EA/TEF may be a feature of DiGeorge syndrome, associated with hypertelorism, micrognathia, thymic aplasia, aortic arch anomalies, persistent truncus arteriosus, and other visceral abnormalities.

### Ultrasonography and prenatal diagnosis

Prenatal diagnosis is usually made during the third trimester, although one diagnosis of EA associated with duodenal stenosis has been reported as early as the first trimester.[63]

Polyhydramnios is a common feature of EA (30% of cases with TEF and 50% without TEF);[31] failure to visualize the stomach on successive examinations is also an indirect ultrasonographic sign. EA is diagnosed at ultrasonography when, in association with polyhydramnios, the stomach is not seen after repeated examinations. Bilirubin, gamma-glutamyltranspeptidase, and microvillar intestinal enzymes are normal in the amniotic fluid. Doppler studies of the amniotic fluid flow in the upper respiratory tract show potential for the evaluation of this malformation.

Trisomy 18 and other chromosome anomalies are frequent causes of EA. Therefore, when EA/TEF is suspected prenatally, fetal karyotyping should be proposed. In some instances, FISH studies with probes mapping to chromosome 22q11 may be useful for the diagnosis of a suspected DiGeorge syndrome.

Prenatal diagnosis of EA/TEF, with or without concomitant malformations, may be important to the neonate, as it facilitates the planning of optimal care in an appropriate unit. Consequently, once the ultrasonographic diagnosis is made, the patient should be referred for genetic counseling and to a pediatric surgeon.

## Nuchal edema and Hygroma

### General considerations

*Hygroma* is a fluid-filled cavity, present most often in the nuchal region, caused by failure or delay in jugular lymphaticovenous communication. Hygromas are usually bilateral and medially septated and may be multiloculated as well. They are often associated with malformations of the major lymph trunks. Generalized hydrops is present in 60%–90% of cases of fetal cystic hygroma.[1] In a retrospective study of 13 newborns with hygromas, 9 were detected prenatally at ultrasound examination, and 6 out of the 11 who were karyotyped had a monosomy X.[16]

### Ultrasonography and prenatal diagnosis

Examination of the neck is an important component of the first and the second trimester fetal ultrasound. Anomalies which may be detected include either hygroma or edema.

*Cervical hygroma* may easily be detected during the first or second trimester. A nuchal pouch is visualized, with one or more septa lobulating the cavity. The skull and spine are intact. Rarely, it may disappear in the course of successive examinations.

Prenatally, cystic hygroma is found in approximately 1% of fetuses when a transvaginal probe is used. It accounts for 1%–5% of malformations seen before 26 weeks gestation. It is frequently associated with other malformations. Cardiac defects are present in up to 92% of cases, and renal malformations are also frequent. Chromosome anomalies are a common cause of fetal cystic hygromas: between 50% and 75% of all cases are cytogenetically abnormal. The most common abnormality is monosomy X (40% to 80%), while the majority of the remainder are autosomal trisomies.

Hygromas may also be a feature of syndromes such as achondrogenesis type II, lethal multiple pterygium, or Noonan syndrome, or may be teratogenic in origin (fetal alcohol, trimethadione, aminopterin syndromes).

Cystic hygroma should be distinguished from nuchal edema and from unilateral cyst of the neck, the prognosis of which is good after postnatal surgery.

*Edema* of the posterior area of the neck is identified as a hypoechogenic area in this region. It is a frequent finding, and may be seen as early as 12–13 weeks of gestation. It may disappear completely or evolve into fetal hydrops.

Cervical edema may be seen during the second or third trimester. As with hygroma, it may be associated with chromosomal anomalies, but instead of monosomy X, autosomal trisomies including trisomy 21 are more common. Frequencies of 45% have been reported in trisomies in contrast to 0.06% in normal fetuses. This ultrasound finding, although nonspecific, may be considered as a marker for trisomy 21. Nuchal edema of 7 mm or more was reported to be associated with a high rate of chromosomal anomalies, mainly trisomy 21.[43] Chromosomally normal fetuses with nuchal edema may also have a very poor prognosis because of concomitant malformations or genetic conditions.[5,7]

During the first trimester of pregnancy, posterior cervical edema is referred to as *fetal nuchal translucency*. In a higher-risk population (i.e, with increased maternal age), the risk of chromosomal anomalies associated with a nuchal translucency of 3 mm or more was found to be increased more than tenfold. As in second trimester edema, the chromosomal defects are mainly autosomal trisomies. The incidence of this sign is around 4%, and the sensitivity of the test as a marker for trisomy 21 more than 75%.[43]

## Teratomas

Teratomas are usually benign tumors. They contain elements of all three germ layers which may be differentiated into cartilage, bone, nerves, muscle, and cavities surrounded by tissues of various origins.

The prognosis depends on the location and extension of the tumor. For example, the prognosis following surgical excision of a teratoma of the tongue is excellent,[28] whereas a cervical teratoma or an epignathus extending to the brain is almost always lethal.

### Ultrasonography and prenatal diagnosis

Ultrasonographic diagnosis of a teratoma is not uncommon. Cervical and oropharyngeal teratomas may occur during the second trimester and may cause polyhydramnios. Perinatal morbidity may be high, resulting from airway or esophageal obstruction or hemorrhage.[58] Malignant transformation of this tumor is extremely rare.[4]

Prenatal MRI may be useful. Delivery is performed by cesarean section to allow fetal intubation, while the fetomaternal circulation is maintained to avoid respiratory distress.[53] Prenatal diagnosis of this condition is critical, since a perinatal team may be organized, if needed, for rapid intubation and perinatal care of the newborn.[74]

## Goiters

### General considerations

An enlargement of the thyroid may be detected at fetal ultrasonography. It may be associated with either hyper- or hypothyroidism. Neonatal hyperthyroidism is rare and is secondary to maternal thyroid-stimulating antibodies, regardless whether the mother has clinically active Graves disease.

Hypothyroid goiters may be acquired (secondary to thyroid-stimulating hormone [TSH] receptor–blocking maternal antibodies, or iodide-containing drugs) or genetic, involving complete or incomplete block of the enzymes involved in thyroxin synthesis. These cases probably account for 10%–20% of non-endemic hypothyroid goiters at birth. Goiter is a feature of such genetic conditions as cystinosis, Johanson-Blizzard, Hansen-Larsen-Berg, Young-Fryns, Holmes, hypothyroidism–spiky hair–cleft palate syndromes, as well as hypohydrotic ectodermal dysplasia with hypothyroidism.[57]

### Ultrasonography and prenatal diagnosis

Normograms are available for the measurements of the transverse width and the circumference of the fetal thyroid at different gestational ages.[10]

A few cases of prenatal diagnosis of fetal thyroid anomalies resulting from maternal Graves disease have been reported.[30,71] In cases of maternal Graves disease or maternal iodide treatment, fetal thyroid enlargement should be looked for in order to monitor a possibly abnormal thyroid function.

Whenever an enlargement of the fetal thyroid is noted, the fetal phenotype should be studied: epiphyseal ossification should be assessed with ultrasound, and TSH and T4 levels may be measured from amniotic fluid or fetal blood samples. Maternal and fetal thyroid-stimulating and thyroid-inhibiting immunoglobulins should be assessed and maternal propylthiouracil treatment may be indicated. Fetal hypothyroidism resulting from maternal drug treatment should be evaluated as early as the second trimester of pregnancy, as neurological sequelae may occur even if a treatment is started at birth. Intra-amniotic injection of T4 can prevent fetal hypothyroidism and its ensuing perinatal complications.[47,55]

## Conclusion

Genetic counseling includes the diagnosis of genetic diseases, assessment of risk for individuals from populations or families at risk, provision of information to patients, and proposal of prenatal diagnostic and management options for the individuals at risk.

The consultation may take place in two different situations: either the parents have already been identified as being at risk for a genetic condition, or an unexpected fetal anomaly has been detected at fetal ultrasound examination.

1. In a minority of cases, the family is known to be at risk for a genetic disease. Prenatal diagnosis is easier in these cases; the disorder in question has already been identified and the prognosis is usually known. Appropriate testing is scheduled early during the pregnancy, and the risk, sensitivity, and specificity of the test as well as its possible results are explained to the patient. These tests may include an ultrasonographic examination, with or without CVS or amniocentesis for karyotyping, or DNA, biochemical, or any other specialized laboratory testing.
2. Usually fetal anomalies are serendipitous findings at ultrasonographic examination. The genetic diagnosis has not been previously made, and a detailed ultrasonography of the fetus by experienced operators becomes necessary. This investigation will detect any concomitant structural anomaly. The search for neurological abnormalities is of particular importance, as they are frequent and potentially serious. In most cases, it may be necessary to present the patient with options of laboratory testing which involve invasive procedures, including chromosomal analysis and other more specialized tests.

The management of these cases may be complicated because of late diagnosis and difficulty in reaching a clear-cut conclusion and in assessing the impact of the particular malformation on the future life of the child. Emphasis should be placed on the possibilities of early and effective surgical correction of relatively benign defects such as cleft lip. Consultation with a pediatric surgeon is imperative to provide the parents with complete information and to enable the surgeon to plan postnatal treatment beforehand. Referral to an appropriate tertiary health care center may be necessary. Fetal surgery still has very few indications in the area of otolaryngology.

### References


1. Allanson JE: Lymphatic circulation. In: Human Malformations and Related Anomalies, Vol II, RE Stevenson, JG Hall, RM Goodman, eds. Oxford University Press, New York, 1993, pp 271–305.
2. Avni EF, Rypens F, Milaire J: Fetal esophagus: normal sonographic appearance. J Ultrasound Med, 13:175–180, 1994.
3. Awwad JT, Azar GB, Karam KS, Nicolaides KH: Ear length: a potential sonographic marker of Down syndrome. Int J Gynaecol Obstet 44:233–238, 1994.
4. Baumann FR, Nerlich A: Metastasizing cervical teratoma of the fetus. Pediatr Pathol 13:21–27, 1993.
5. Benacerraf BR, Barss VA, Laboda LA: A sonographic sign for the detection in the second trimester of the fetus with Down's syndrome. Am J Obstet Gynecol 151:1078–1079, 1985.
6. Benacerraf BR, Frigoletto FD Jr, Greene MF: Abnormal facial features and extremities in human trisomy syndromes: prenatal US appearance. Radiology 159:243–246, 1986.
7. Benacerraf BR, Gelman R, Frigoletto FD Jr: Sonographic identification of second trimester fetuses with Down's syndrome. N Engl J Med, 317:1371–1376, 1987.
8. Benacerraf BR, Mulliken JB: Fetal cleft lip and palate: sonographic diagnosis and postnatal outcome. Plast Reconstr Surg 92:1045–1051, 1993.
9. Berry SM, Gosden C, Snijders RJ, Nicolaides KH: Fetal holoprosencephaly: associated malformations and chromosomal defects. Fetal Diagn Ther 5:92–99, 1990.
10. Bromley B, Frigoletto FD Jr, Cramer D, Osathanondh R, Benacerraf BR: The fetal thyroid: normal and abnormal sonographic measurements. J Ultrasound Med 11:25–28, 1992.
11. Bronshtein M, Gershoni-Baruch R: Prenatal transvaginal diagnosis of the ectrodactyly, ectodermal dysplasia, cleft palate (EEC) syndrome. Prenat Diagn 13:519–522, 1993.
12. Bronshtein M, Mashiah N, Blumenfeld I, Blumenfeld Z: Pseudoprognathism: an auxiliary ultrasonographic sign for transvaginal ultrasonographic diagnosis of cleft lip and palate in the early second trimester. Am J Obstet Gynecol 165:1314–1316, 1991.
13. Canadian Collaborative CVS-Amniocentesis Clinical Trial Group: Multicentre randomised clinical trial of chorionic villus sampling and amniocentesis. First report. Lancet 1:1–6, 1989.
14. Carey JC: External ear. In Human Malformations and Related Anomalies, Vol II, RE Stevenson, JG Hall, RM Goodman, eds. Oxford University Press, New York, 1993, pp 221–230.
15. Carey JC: Inner ear. In: Human Malformations and Related Anomalies, Vol II, RE Stevenson, JG Hall, RM Goodman, eds. Oxford University Press, New York, 1993, pp 231–235.
16. Carson HJ, Taxy JB: Role of the autopsy in congenital cystic hygroma. Pediatr Pathol 14:183–189, 1994.
17. Chitty LS, Campbell S, Altman DG: Measurement of the fetal mandible—feasibility and construction of a centile chart. Prenat Diagn 13:749–756, 1993.
18. Cohen MM Jr: Syndromes with cleft lip and cleft palate. Cleft Palate J 15:306–328, 1978.
19. Depaepe A, Dolk H, Lechat MF: The epidemiology of tracheo-oesophageal fistula and oesophageal atresia in Europe. EUROCAT Working Group. Arch Dis Child 68:743–748, 1993.
20. Driscoll DA, Salvin J, Sellinger B, Budarf ML, McDonald-McGinn DM, Zackai EH, Emanuel BS: Prevalence of 22q11 microdeletions in DiGeorge and velocardiofacial syndromes: implications for genetic counseling and prenatal diagnosis. J Med Genet 30:813–817, 1993.
21. Escobar LF: Facial bones. In: Human Malformations and Related Anomalies, Vol II, RE Stevenson, JG Hall, RM Goodman, eds. Oxford University Press, New York, 1993, pp 629–653.
22. Evans MI, Hoffman EP, Cadrin C, Johnson MP, Quintero RA, Golbus MS: Fetal muscle biopsy: collaborative experience with varied indications. Obstet Gynecol 84:913–917, 1994.
23. Ferreira J, Eviatar L, Schneider S, Grossman R: Prenatal diagnosis of intracranial teratoma. Prolonged survival after resection of a malignant teratoma diagnosed prenatally by ultrasound: a case report and literature review. Pediatr Neurosurg 19:84–88, 1993.
24. Fraser FC: The genetics of cleft lip and palate. Am J Hum Genet 22:336–352, 1970.
25. Fraser GR, Calnan JS: Cleft lip and palate: seasonal incidence, birth weight, birth rank, sex, site, associated malformations and parental age. Arch Dis Child 36:420–423, 1961.
26. Geifman-Holtzman O, Blatman RN, Bianchi DW: Prenatal genetic diagnosis by isolation and analysis of fetal cells circulating in maternal blood. Semin Perinatol 18:366–375, 1994.
27. Gorlin RJ, Cervenka J, Pruzanski S: Facial clefting and its syndromes. Birth Defects 7:3–49, 1971.
28. Gorlin RJ, Sedano HO: The tongue. In: Human Malformations and Related Anomalies, Vol II, RE Stevenson, JG Hall, RM Goodman, eds. Oxford University Press, New York, 1993, pp 397–414.
29. Haddow JE, Palomaki GE, Knight GJ, Williams J, Pulkkinen A, Canick JA, Saller DN Jr, Bowers GB: Prenatal screening for Down's syndrome with use of maternal serum markers. N Engl J Med 327:588–593, 1992.
30. Hatjis CG: Diagnosis and successful treatment of fetal goitrous hyperthyroidism caused by maternal Graves disease. Obstet Gynecol 81:837–839, 1993.
31. Hoyme HE: The upper gastrointestinal system. In: Human Malformations and Related Anomalies, Vol II, RE Stevenson, JG Hall, RM Goodman, eds. Oxford University Press, New York, 1993, pp 415–443.
32. Hsieh FJ, Shyu MK, Sheu BC, Lin SP, Chen CP, Huang FY: Limb defects after chorionic villus sampling. Obstet Gynecol 85:84–88, 1995.
33. Isaacson G, Mintz MC: Prenatal sonographic visualization of the inner ear. J Ultrasound Med 5:409–410, 1986.
34. Jeanty P, Romero R: Fetal ocular biometry. In: Obstetrical Ultrasound. McGraw-Hill, New York, 1984, pp 93–98.
35. Jeanty P, Romero R, Staudach A, Hobbins JC: Facial anatomy of the fetus. J Ultrasound Med 5:607–616, 1986.
36. Johansson B, Wedenberg E, Westin B: Fetal heart rate response to acoustic stimulation in relation to fetal development and hearing impairment. Acta Obstet Gynecol Scand 71:610–615, 1992.
37. Lettieri L, Rodis JF, Vintzileos AM, Feeney L, Ciarleglio L, Craffey A: Ear length in second-trimester aneuploid fetuses. Obstet Gynecol 81:57–60, 1993.
38. Mastroiacovo P, Botto LD, Cavalcanti DP, Lalatta F, Selicorni A, Tozzi AE, Baronciani D, Cigolotti AC, Giordano S, Petroni F, et al: Limb anomalies following chorionic villus sampling: a registry based case-control study. Am J Med Genet 44:856–864, 1992.
39. Mayden KL, Tortora M, Berkowitz RL, Bracken M, Hobbins JC: Orbital diameters: a new parameter for prenatal diagnosis and dating. Am J Obstet Gynecol 144:289–297, 1982.
40. McCauley RG, Beckwith JB, Elias ER, Faerber EN, Prewitt LH Jr, Berdon WE: Benign hemorrhagic adrenocortical macrocysts in Beckwith-Wiedemann syndrome. Am J Roentgenol 157:549–552, 1991.
41. Naidich TP, Grant JL, Altman N, Zimmerman RA, Birchansky SB, Braffman B, Daniel JL: The developing cerebral surface. Preliminary report on the patterns of sulcal and gyral maturation-anatomy, ultrasound, and magnetic resonance imaging. Neuroimaging Clin North Am 4:201–240, 1994.
42. Nicolaides KH, Salvesen DR, Snijders RJ, Gosden CM: Fetal facial defects: associated malformations and chromosomal abnormalities. Fetal Diagn Ther 8:1–9, 1993.
43. Nicolaides K, Shawwa M, Brizot M, Snijders R: Ultrasonographically detectable markers of fetal chromosomal defects. Ultrasound Obstet Gynecol 3:56–69, 1993.
44. Nicolaides KH, Soothill PW, Rodeck CH, Warren RC, Gosden CM: Why confine chorionic villus (placental) biopsy to the first trimester? Lancet 1:543–544, 1986.
45. Nicolini U, Rodeck CH: Fetal blood and tissue sampling. In: Prenatal Diagnosis and Screening, DJH Brock, CH Rodeck, MA Ferguson-Smith, eds. Churchill Livingstone, Edinburgh, 1992, pp 39–51.
46. Nyberg DA, Hegge FN, Kramer D, Mahony BS, Kropp RJ: Premaxillary protrusion: a sonographic clue to bilateral cleft lip and palate. J Ultrasound Med 12:331–335, 1993.
47. Perelman AH, Johnson RL, Clemons RD, Finberg HJ, Clewell WH, Trujillo L: Intrauterine diagnosis and treatment of fetal goitrous hypothyroidism. J Clin Endocrinol Metab 3:618–621, 1990.

48. Quintero RA, Puder KS, Cotton DB: Embryoscopy and fetoscopy. Obstet Gynecol Clin North Am 20:563–581, 1993.
49. Ramirez M, Wilkins I, Kramer L, Slopis J, Taylor SR: Prenatal diagnosis of unilateral megalencephaly by real-time ultrasonography. Am J Obstet Gynecol 170:1384–1385, 1994.
50. Revel MP, Pons JC, Lelaidier C, Fournet P, Vial M, Musset D, Labrune M, Frydman R: Magnetic resonance imaging of the fetus: a study of 20 cases performed without curarization. Prenat Diagn 13:775–799, 1993.
51. Rhoads GG, Jackson LG, Schlesselman SE, de la Cruz FF, Desnick RJ, Golbus MS, Ledbetter DH, Lubs HA, Mahoney MJ, Pergament E, et al: The safety and efficacy of chorionic villus sampling for early prenatal diagnosis of cytogenetic abnormalities. N Engl J Med 320:609–617, 1989.
52. Romero R, Pilu G, Jeanty P, Ghidini A, Hobbins JC: Prenatal Diagnosis of Congenital Anomalies. Appleton and Lange, Norwalk, 1988, pp 81–112.
53. Rothschild MA, Catalano P, Urken M, Brandwein M, Som P, Norton K, Biller HF: Evaluation and management of congenital cervical teratoma. Case report and review. Arch Otolaryngol Head Neck Surg 120:444–448, 1994.
54. Ryall RG, Staples AJ, Robertson EF, Pollard AC: Improved performance in a prenatal screening programme for Down's syndrome incorporating serum-free hCG subunit analyses. Prenat Diagn 12:251–261, 1992.
55. Sagot P, David A, Yvinec M, Pousset P, Papon V, Mouzard A, Boog G: Intrauterine treatment of thyroid goiters. Fetal Diagn Ther 6:28–33, 1991.
56. Saltzman DH, Benacerraf BR, Frigoletto FD: Diagnosis and management of fetal facial clefts. Am J Obstet Gynecol 155:377–379, 1986.
57. Schimke RN: The endocrine glands. In: Human Malformations and Related Anomalies, Vol II, RE Stevenson, JG Hall, RM Goodman, eds. Oxford University Press, New York, 1993, pp 1017–1030.
58. Sherer DM, Woods JR Jr, Abramowicz JS, Dipreta JA, Metlay LA, Jaffe R: Prenatal sonographic assessment of early, rapidly growing fetal cervical teratoma. Prenat Diagn 13:1079–1084, 1993.
59. Shimizu T, Salvador L, Allanson J, Hughes-Benzie R, Nimrod C: Ultrasonic measurements of fetal ear. Obstet Gynecol 80:381–384, 1992.
60. Shprintzen RJ, Siegel-Sadewitz VL, Amato J, Goldberg RB: Anomalies associated with cleft lip, cleft palate, or both. Am J Med Genet, 20:585–595, 1985.
61. Simpson JL, Carson SA, Buster JE, Elias S: Future horizons in prenatal genetic diagnosis: preimplantation diagnosis and noninvasive screening. In: Human Prenatal Diagnosis, 2nd ed, K Filkins, JF Russo, eds. Marcel Dekker, New York, 1990, pp 547–577.
62. Tabor A, Philip J, Madsen M, Bang J, Obel EB, Norgaard-Pedersen B: Randomised controlled trial of genetic amniocentesis in 4606 low-risk women. Lancet 1:1287–1292, 1986.
63. Tsukerman GL, Krapiva GA, Kirillova IA: First-trimester diagnosis of duodenal stenosis associated with oesophageal atresia. Prenat Diagn 13:371–376, 1993.
64. Tuchmann-Duplessis H, Haegel P: Illustrated Human Embryology, Vol 2. Springer–Verlag, New York, 1972.
65. Turner GM, Twining P: The facial profile in the diagnosis of fetal abnormalities. Clin Radiol 47:389–395, 1993.
66. Ulreich S, Hanieh A, Furness ME: Positive outcome of fetal intracranial teratoma. J Ultrasound Med 12:163–165, 1993.
67. Viljoen DL, Jaquire Z, Woods DL: Prenatal diagnosis in autosomal dominant Beckwith-Wiedemann syndrome. Prenat Diagn 11:167–75, 1991.
68. Vogel JE, Mulliken JB, Kaban LB: Macroglossia: a review of the condition and a new classification. Plast Reconstr Surg 78:715–23, 1986.
69. Warkin KL, Baer LH, Mathur S, Jones R, El-Hakim S, Diouf I, Nuwayhid B, Khalifé S: Three-dimensional reconstruction and enhancement of arbitrarily oriented and positioned 2D medical ultrasonic images. IEEE Trans Electr Comput Eng 1188–1195, 1993.
70. Watson WJ, Katz VL: Sonographic measurement of the fetal mandible: standards for normal pregnancy. J Perinat 10:226–228, 1993.
71. Wenstrom KD, Weiner CP, Williamson RA, Grant SS: Prenatal diagnosis of fetal hyperthyroidism using funipuncture. Obstet Gynecol 76:513–517, 1990.
72. Whisson CC, Whyte A, Ziesing P: Beckwith-Wiedemann syndrome: antenatal diagnosis. Australas Radiol 38:130–131, 1994.
73. Working party on amniocentesis: An assessment of the hazards of amniocentesis. Br J Obstet Gyneacol 85(Supp 2):1–14, 1978.
74. Zerella JT, Finberg FJ: Obstruction of the neonatal airway from teratomas. Surg Gynecol Obstet 170:126–131, 1990.

# II

# THE EAR

# 6

# Developmental Biology of the Ear

MALCOLM C. JOHNSTON

The embryological origins of the tissues involved in the formation of the ear are now quite well known. Some progress has been made recently in understanding the nature of developmental interactions, including a number of studies utilizing transgenic mice. Besides presenting data about the normal genetic and molecular mechanisms involved in the formation of the different parts of the ear, this chapter will also discuss the alterations (molecular and histological) that occur in certain types of anomalies of the ear. Development of the pharynx is particularly relevant to development of the external and middle ear and is presented in detail in Chapter 12.

## Normal development

### The initiation of ear development

The ear develops from two initially independent components illustrated in Figure 6–1. The outer and middle ear develop from the first and second pharyngeal (branchial, visceral) arches, and the inner ear from the otic placode and underlying mesenchyme. As will be discussed in detail later, the origin of the mesenchyme is also entirely different. On a histological basis, developmental biologists distinguish between two types of embryonic tissues at these stages: loosely arranged mesenchyme and compactly arranged epithelia. The mesenchyme interacting with the otic palcodes is of mesodermal origin, while the mesenchyme involved in external and middle ear formation (and the rest of the face and anterior neck) arises from neural crest cells.[28,29,35,37,47,62,71] Crest cells migrate from the margins (folds or "crests") of the neural plate (or tube) and consequently are of ectodermal origin. The difference in origin of the mesenchymes is important for both normal and abnormal development.

### Development of the external ear

There is still some disagreement as to the exact contributions of the mesenchymes of the mandibular and hyoid arches to the external ear (Fig. 6–2).[67,77] The auricular hillocks appear to represent growth centers, the nature of which is unknown. It is generally agreed that most of the pinna arises from the hyoid arch. Hillocks are found in species such as fish which do not have pinna.[66]

Virtually no direct information is available concerning the interactions involved in external ear development. In contrast, information concerning the development of other facial growth centers, such as the facial prominences, is accumulating rapidly and some of this information is probably applicable to external ear development. For example, regional growth of the auricular hillocks is probably dependent on extensive epithelial–mesenchymal interactions. Presumably, a number of growth factors are involved, such as the fibroblast growth factors (FGFs) that support facial prominence mesenchyme in culture in the absence of epithelia.[59] One would also expect that auricular cartilage formation involves epithelial mesenchymal interactions, as do other cartilages and bone of neural crest origin.

### Development of the middle ear

The middle ear also develops from the first and second visceral arches. The epithelial lining of the middle ear is derived from the endoderm of the first pharyngeal pouch. In the mesenchyme surrounding the pouch, groups of cells condense to form the primordia of the middle ear cartilages (Figs. 6–3, 6–4). These condensations are continuous with those of the first (Meckel's) and second (Reicher's) arch cartilages (Fig. 6–4). The malleus and incus develop from first arch mesenchyme, while the stapes develops primarily from second arch mesenchyme. As these primordia are forming, the pouch (tubotympanic recess) epithelium invades the mesenchymes surrounding them, eventually enveloping the cartilages completely. The major process of the malleus remains connected to the ear drum and the foot plate of the stapes connected to the inner ear at the oval window (Figs. 6–3, 6–4). In postnatal life, this epithelium also invades the mastoid process, providing the lining for the mastoid air cells. Also in postnatal life, the middle ear cartilages undergo endochondral ossification to form the middle ear ossicles.

The skeletal and connective tissues of the middle ear are derived almost entirely from neural crest mesenchyme. As noted earlier, these cells migrate from the folds of the ectodermal neural plate (tube), and Figure 6–5 A shows these cells approaching the completion of their migrations. The foot plate of stapes is largely of mesodermal origin, as is the rest of the otic capsule, of which the foot plate appears to be an early component (Fig. 6–3C). The only middle ear connective tissue components not of neural crest, but mesodermal, origin are the endothelial linings of the blood vessels.[52] The myoblasts of the tensor tympani are also of mesodermal origin, migrating from somite-like structures[49] (Fig. 6–5A) to the core of the mandibular (first) arch and then to the middle ear (see Chapter 12, Figs. 12–5 and 12–11). Myoblasts of the stapedius are of similar origin but from the second arch.

There have been major advances in our understanding of the molecular mechanisms controlling head segmentation that are highly relevant to understanding the mechanisms of both normal and abnormal ear development (Figs. 6–5, 6–6). The segmental pattern appears to be under the control of homeobox genes which are derived from the same genes that regulate seg-

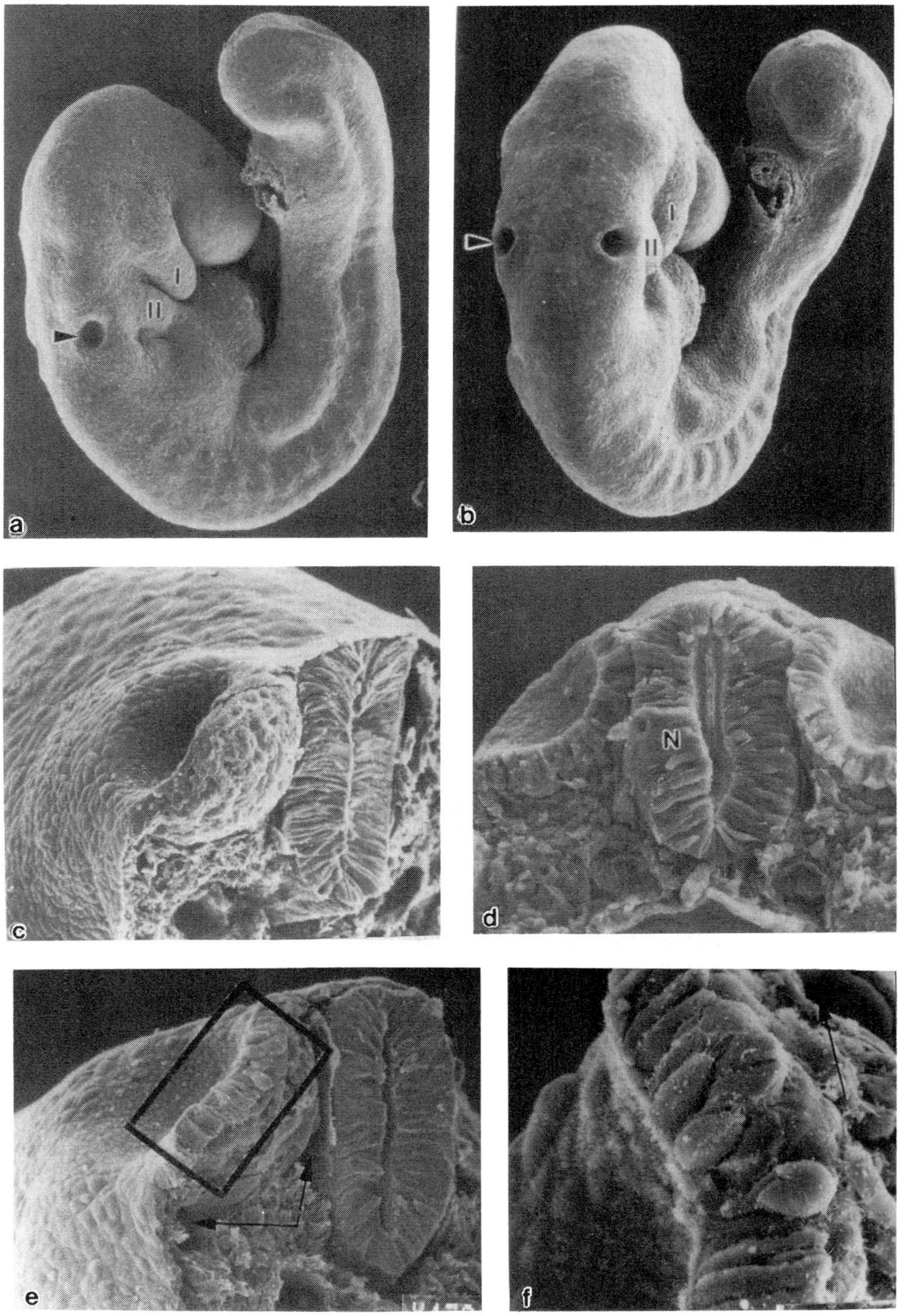


**Fig. 6–1.** Scanning electron micrographs of otocyst development in the mouse embryo. The position of the invaginating otic placode (arrowheads) and its relation to the first (I) and second (II) pharyngeal arches is illustrated in a and b. The sectioned embryos in c and d illustrate the close relationship of the invaginating placode to the neural tube (N), while the cellular arrangement of the placodal pseudostratified epithelium is illustrated in e and f. (From Sulik, Embryology of the ear. In *Hereditary Hearing Loss and Its Syndromes*, RJ Gorlin et al., eds., Oxford University Press, New York, 1995, pp. 22–42,[67] with permission.)

mentation in the Drosophila (fruit fly). Genes that regulate the activity of other genes contain a *box* that is responsible for that portion of the protein derived from it that binds to DNA and permits the alteration of expression of associated genes. The designation *Hox* is now reserved for those genes derived from the original *Drosophila* segmentation genes.[55,61] In mammals, the *Hox* genes have been duplicated as intact sets on four different chromosomes with the same head-to-tail organization on each chromosome (Fig. 6–6).

In mamalian and avian embryos, *Hox* gene activity (as measured by in situ hybridization for specific mRNAs) forms an overlapping cascade, first in the neuromeres and then in the neural crest cells derived from them (Fig. 6–6). This activity has been best documented for hindbrain rhombomeres 2 through 7 and the crest cells derived from them. Although there is considerable other homeobox gene activity in more rostral brain and neural crest, its relation to the *Hox* genes is unclear. This portion of the head forms the midbrain, forebrain, and face, which have been progressively added in higher vertebrates; the organizational plan is somewhat different.[33,51,52,81]

The overlapping cascade of *Hox* gene activity seems to be responsible for the specification of hindbrain rhombomeres (Fig. 6–6) and their derivatives. This pattern is established very early in development, as shown by experimental substitutions of one prospective rhombomere for another.[25] In *Hox-A1* (Hox 1.6, Fig. 6–6) knockouts,[6,41] (replacement of normal genes with non-functional genes) the development of rhombomeres 4 and 5 is severely disrupted, with rhombomere 5 apparently eliminated. Elements such as the motor neurons for the facial (hyoid arch) and abducens nerves are either missing[41] or abnormal.[6] The *Int-2* gene, which directs the formation of FGF3 and may be involved in the induction of the otic placode, is abnormal, as is the development of the otocyst (see below). Similar deficiencies in rhombomeres can be induced by retinoic acid administration.[44,45]

The axial (rostral-caudal) patterning of crest cells has been studied by Noden[47,48,50–52,55] by transplanting crest cells from one position in the neural folds to another. Trunk neural crest cells, transplanted to the head in place of the mandibular arch crest, migrated normally into the mandibular arch and formed neural elements (e.g., portions of the trigeminal ganglion) but were unable to form skeletal elements in response to the inductive influences of first arch epithelia. Mandibular arch, or more rostral maxillary and frontonasal, crest cells respond to the inductive influences of hyoid arch epithelia when used to replace hyoid arch crest cells. However, they form mandibular skeletal elements (e.g., Meckel's cartilage) rather than hyoid arch skeletal elements (e.g., the main portion of the columella which is equivalent to the mammalian stapes).

The molecular basis for Noden's results has been clarified through the use of transgenic mice in which the *Hox* gene *Hox-A2* (Fig. 6–6) was "knocked out."[20,60] In both studies, the mandibular arch pattern was repeated in the hyoid arch, including duplicate malleus and incus cartilages, a result very similar to Noden's. The interpretation of these results was that the normal addition of Hox-A2 expression in hyoid crest cells changes their response to the inductive effects of hyoid arch epithelia so that hyoid arch skeletal elements are made rather than mandibular arch skeletal elements. If this interpretation is correct, then the further addition of *Hox* gene expression, e.g., of *Hox-B4* (Fig. 6–6) in the third (glossopharyngeal) arch crest could convert the response of these cells to third arch epithelia. Thus they would form third arch skeletal elements rather than hyoid (second) arch skeletal elements.

Although there is very considerable information on the inter-

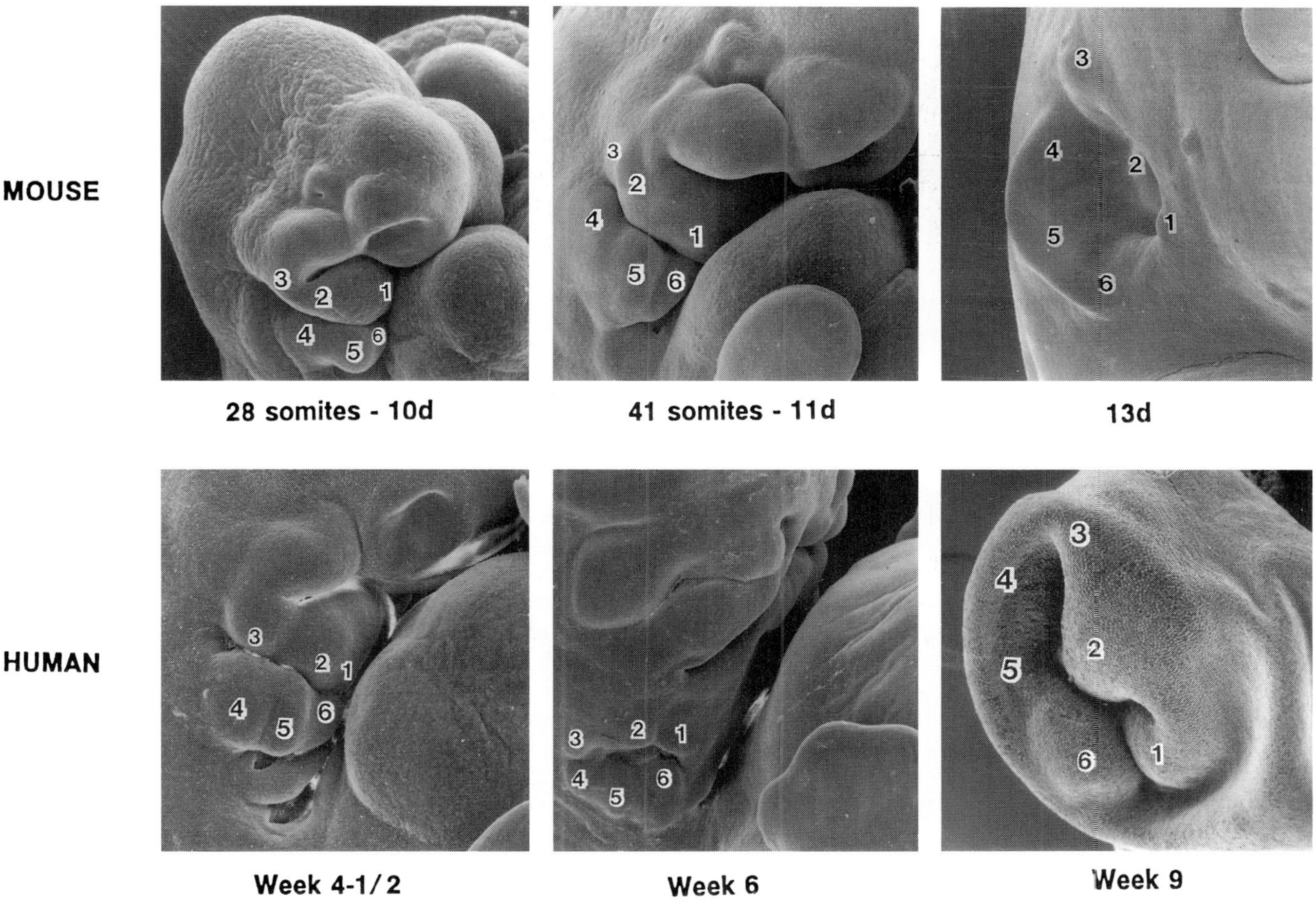


**Fig. 6–2.** Scanning electron micrographs of the developing external ear in mouse and human embryos. The numbering of the hillocks and portions of the ear derived from them in somewhat arbitrary and definitive numbering will require marking studies. (From Jarvis et al., Otolaryngol Head Neck Surg 102:391–401,[27] with permission.)

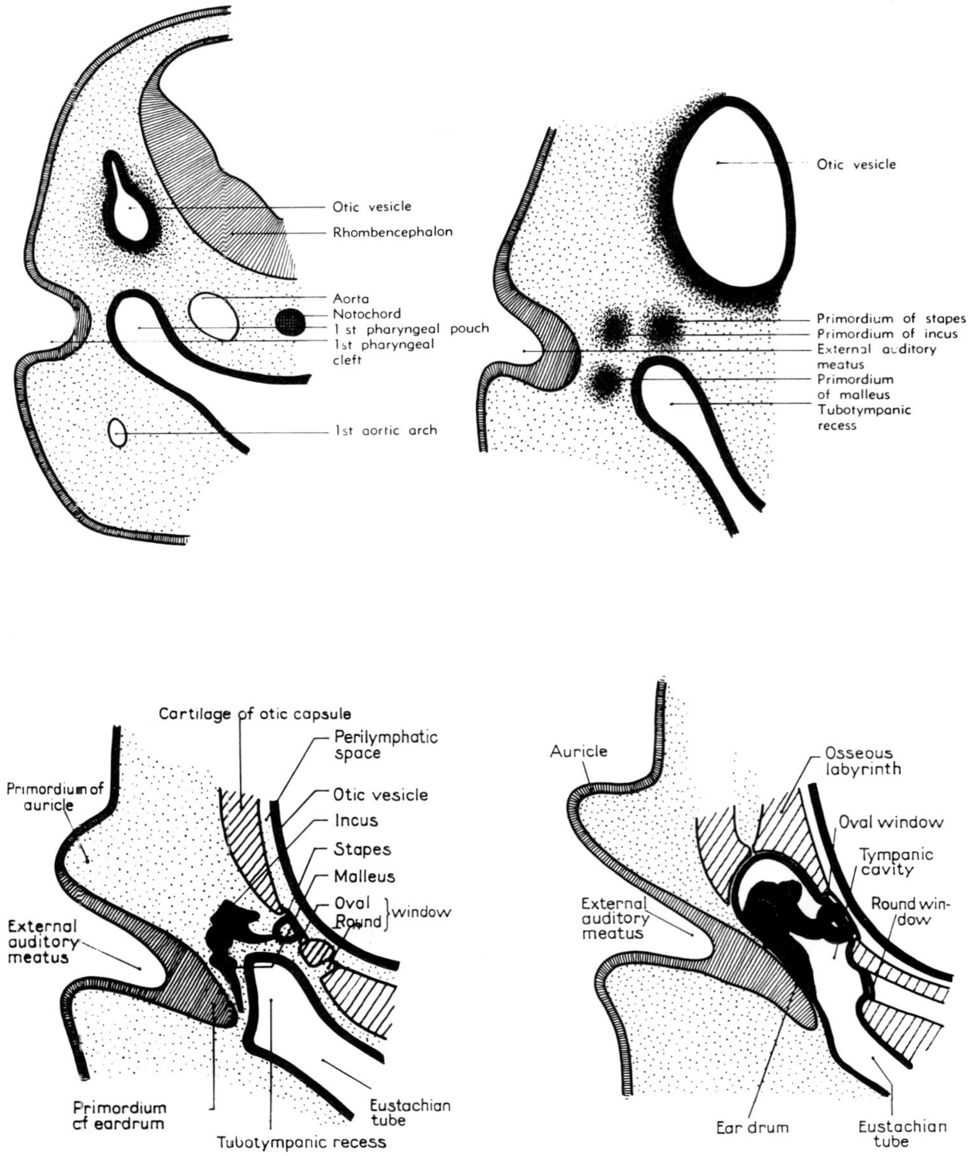


**Fig. 6–3.** Schematic diagram depicting development of the middle ear. The only mesenchyme involved in ear development that is not of neural crest origin is the capsule (denser stipple) around the otocyst and at least part of the foot plate of the stapes. For details, see text. (From Tuchmann-Duplessis, *Illustrated Human Embryology,* Springer-Verlag, New York, 1975,[75] with permission.)

actions of crest cells with the local environment with respect to cartilage and bone in general (particularly their interactions with various epithelia) and with respect to tooth development, there is little specific information on the middle ear bones, the tympanic ring, and the Eustachian tube cartilage. The possible involvement of retinoic acid will be considered later under *Abnormal development.*

### Development of the inner ear

The otic placode develops with its dorsal half in close apposition to the neural tube (Fig. 6–1). Toward the end of its invagination, and as it separates from the surface, it becomes completely surrounded by mesodermal mesencyme which condenses to form the otic capsule and other connnective tissues involved in inner ear development (Fig. 6–3). Through complex extensions, foldings, fusions, and epithelial breakdown, the semicircular ducts (and other vestibular structures) as well as the cochlea and endolymphatic sac are formed (Fig. 6–7).

The vestibulo-cochlear (acoustico-vestibular) ganglion initially develops fused with the facial nerve ganglion (Fig. 6–7A).[4,31,54] The three components gradually separate. The neuroblasts of the vestibular and cochlear (acoustic) ganglia are derived almost entirely from the otocyst epithelium (Fig. 6–8), in contrast to other cranial sensory ganglia in which both neural crest and ganglionic placodes make extensive contributions to the neuroblast populations. As in all cranial ganglia, supporting Schwann and satellite cells are exclusively of neural crest origin (Fig. 6–8), apparently arising via the facial nerve ganglion.[13,31,54]

The key sensory element in the ear is the hair cell, a structure which is basically similar to that of the lateral line organs (flow detectors) on the external surfaces of aquatic vertebrates.

The "hairs" are stereocilia which are embedded in a gelatinous matrix. The simplest receptor structure is found in the ampullae of the semicircular ducts where the stereocilia and matrix form paddle-shaped structures that detect fluid motion resulting from head movements (Fig. 6–9). Surface mineralized otoconia (gravity detectors) are added in the maculae (Fig. 6–10) of the utricle and saccule. The most complex structures are the hair cells' arrangements in the cochlea (Fig. 6–11).

Details of hair cell structures are presented in Figure 6–10. They are interspersed among support cells. They become innervated both by sensory axons extending from neuroblasts in the ganglia and by motor axons (involved in modulating hair cell responses) extending from the neural tube.

Development and structure of the exquisitely complex cochlear receptors are presented in Figure 6–11. Here the gelatinous matrix, in which the stereocilia of the inner and outer hair cells are found, is in the tectorial membrane (Fig. 6–11e, f). Changing arrangements of the stereocilia (Fig. 6–11g, h) at different positions along the cochlea are apparently related to the detection of fluid vibrations of different wave lengths.

While it has been known for many years that the hindbrain has a major inductive effect on the epithelium that gives rise to the otic placode (Fig. 6–1; for reviews see Lim and Ryan,[38a] van de Water,[76] van de Water and Represa,[78] and Sulik[67]), there has been little information on the nature of the interaction. An apparent breakthrough was the observation that inactivation of FGF3 formation by antisense (complimentary) DNA to FGF mRNA in cultures of neural tube and surface ectoderm prevented induction of the otic placode and otocyst formation.[58] *Int-2* (sometimes called *Wnt-2*), the gene regulating FGF3 formation, is active in rhombomeres 4 and 5 at the appropriate time in development.[40] However, when *Int-2* was knocked out in transgenic mice, the otocyst formed normally.[40] Later development of the inner ear, particularly the endolymphatic duct, was abnormal, which, the authors concluded, resulted in the cystic development of the cochlea. The endolymphatic duct is normally involved in fluid removal and its experimental extirpation leads to cystic development of the cochlea. The authors of the knockout study[40] concluded that FGF3 is required for endolymphatic duct development. There are some problems with this interpretation. As the authors point out, there were severe deficiencies in the acoustic-vestibular ganglion at a stage prior to the normal initiation of endolymphatic duct formation. Also, the otocysts appear to be very thin walled at even earlier stages in the knockout mice. It seems possible that the otic placode is only partially induced, with problems related to formation of

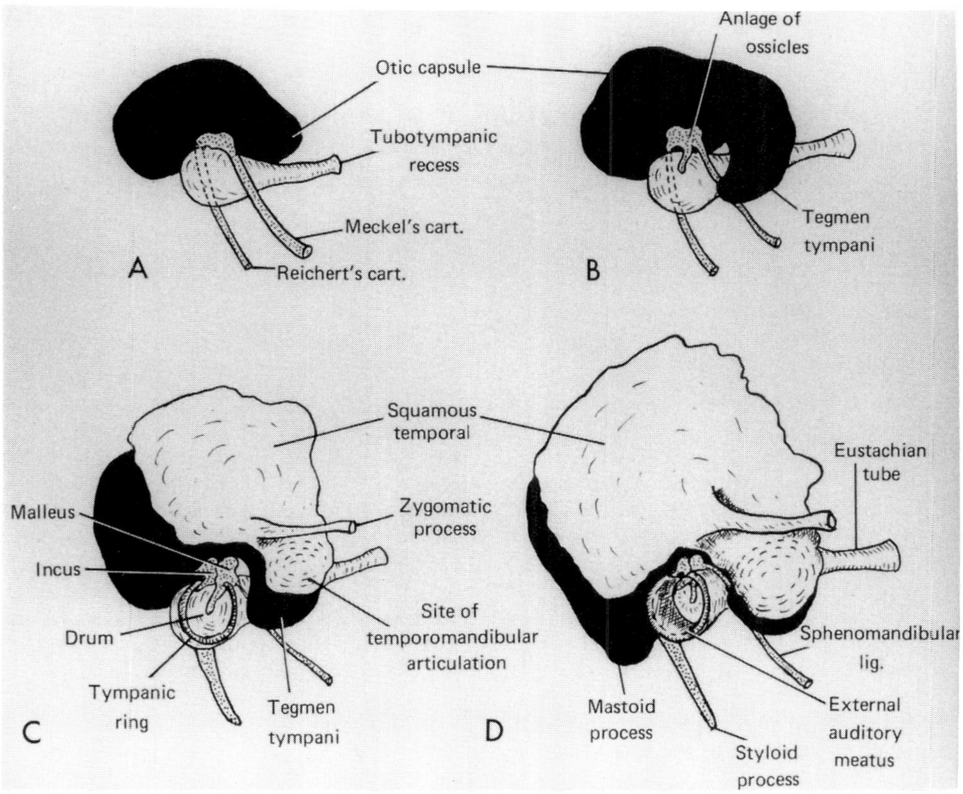


**Fig. 6–4.** Three-dimensional depiction of developing components of the middle (stippled and hatched areas) and internal (black area) ear. (From Anson and Davies, Embryology of the ear. In: *Otolaryngology*, MM Paparella, DA Shumrick, eds., WB Saunders, Philadelphia, 1980, pp. 3–25,[3] with permission). The anlage of Meckel's (first arch) and Reichert's (second arch) cartilages are connected as they wrap around the tubotympanic recess (A). The early anlage of the middle ear ossicles, which develop as part of the above connections, are depicted in B, and the derived malleus and incus in C. Most of the stapes forms from the proximal portion of Reichert's cartilage and is hidden by the tubotympanic recess in C. The attachment of the major process of the malleus to the ear drum, which form at the end of the tubotympanic recess (see also Fig. 6–3) and the tympanic ring at the periphery of the drum, is also illustrated. The proximal portion of Meckel's and Reichert's cartilages become, respectively, the sphenomandibular ligament and styloid process (D). Early formation of the external auditory meatus is also depicted in D.

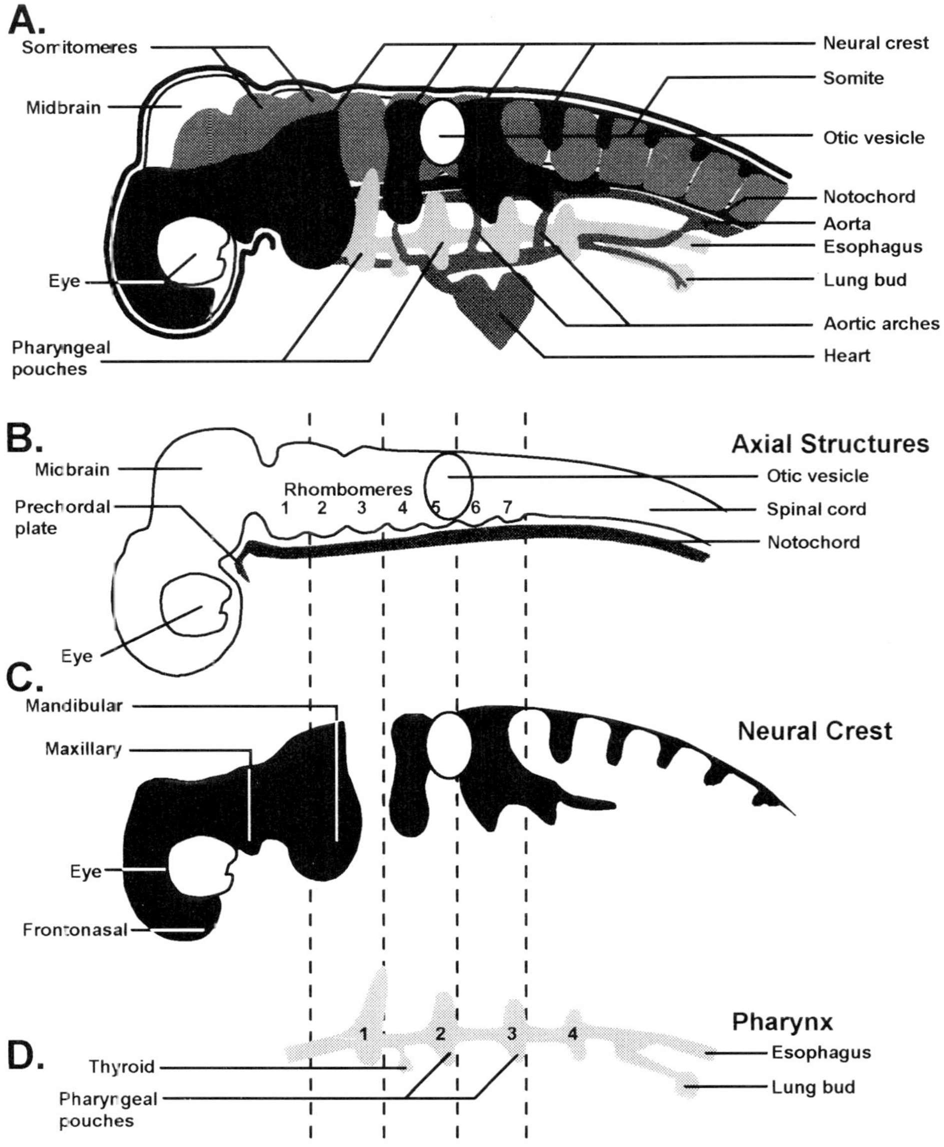


**Fig. 6–5.** Schematic diagrams depicting the segmental origins of different cell populations giving rise to the head and neck. In B–D the different components have been separated ("exploded"), with vertical lines showing the segmental relationships. The initial segmental control may lie in the notochord and its rostral (anterior) extension, the prechordal plate, but by the stages of development illustrated, segmental control lies principally in the rhombomeres (hindbrain neuromeres, B, and the segmented pharynx, D). The neural crest (C) is derived from the neuromeres (e.g., second or hyoid arch crest from rhombomere 4) and migrates into the immediately ventral pharyngeal (branchial, visceral) arches. The otic vesicle (otocyst) develops from the otic placode which is induced by rhombomeres 5 and 6. It becomes surrounded by underlying mesoderm. The external and middle ear epithelia develop from the endoderm of the first pharyngeal pouch and from the epithelia of the first and second arches, while the mesenchyme is derived from the neural crest. As can be seen in the upper diagram, these structures are initially located rostral (anterior) to the developing otocyst. Only later do they come into register with the otocyst as the more rapid growth of the brain carries the more dorsal tissues, including the otocyst, forward (rostrally) relative to the more ventral pharyngeal arches and heart. Almost all other skeletal and connective tissues in the face and anterior neck are derived from the neural crest. Skeletal and connective tissues in other portions of the head and neck are derived from mesoderm, as are all the myoblasts of "voluntary" muscles (e.g., tensor tympani) and the endothelial lining of blood vessels. (Diagrams modified from Noden, Brain Behav Evol 38:190–255, 1991,[51] with permission.)

ganglion and endolymphatic duct arising secondarily. Failure of closure of the otocyst in the Represa et al. study[58] could be related to further developmental inhibition related to organ culture.

Although little is known about the molecular aspects of other tissue interactions, some interdependencies have been established. Explant studies and analysis of other epithelial–mesenchymal interactions suggest that most of the morphogenetic control of development of the endolymphatic duct, semicircular vestibular canals, and the cochlea (Fig. 6–7) lies in the mesenchyme rather than the epithelia. Explantation studies show that the very complex sensory receptors (Figs. 6–10, 6–11) do not depend on innervation for their development but that they regulate their own innervation,[76] perhaps by growth factors such as nerve growth factor (NGF).

Little direct information on the development of the stria vascularis (Fig. 6–11d, e) is available, but studies of mouse mutants (see below) with combined pigmentary and inner ear defects (e.g., Deol,[14–17] Steel and Barkway[65]) are helpful. Melanoblasts (presumably of crest origin) are normally found between the marginal layer of cells which abuts the fluid-filled scala media and a subjacent layer of basal cells. All three cell types interdigitate with each other. A rich plexus of vessels is also found interspersed between all three cell types. The melanoblasts are absent in the mutants (or have failed to make melanosomes),[14–16,65] and eventually, the other two cell types become deficient.[65] The low negative charge of the ear fluids fails to materialize.[65]

## Abnormal development

Discussion here will be largely limited to those abnormalities whose pathogenesis is relatively well understood and where these abnormalities shed some light on the mechanisms of normal ear development. A number of abnormalities fit these criteria particularly well.

### Defects of otic placode induction

While these defects have been fairly extensively studied in mice,[6,7,18,39] there are few such cases in humans. The gene for one such mouse mutant, Kreisler,[8] results in abnormalities of

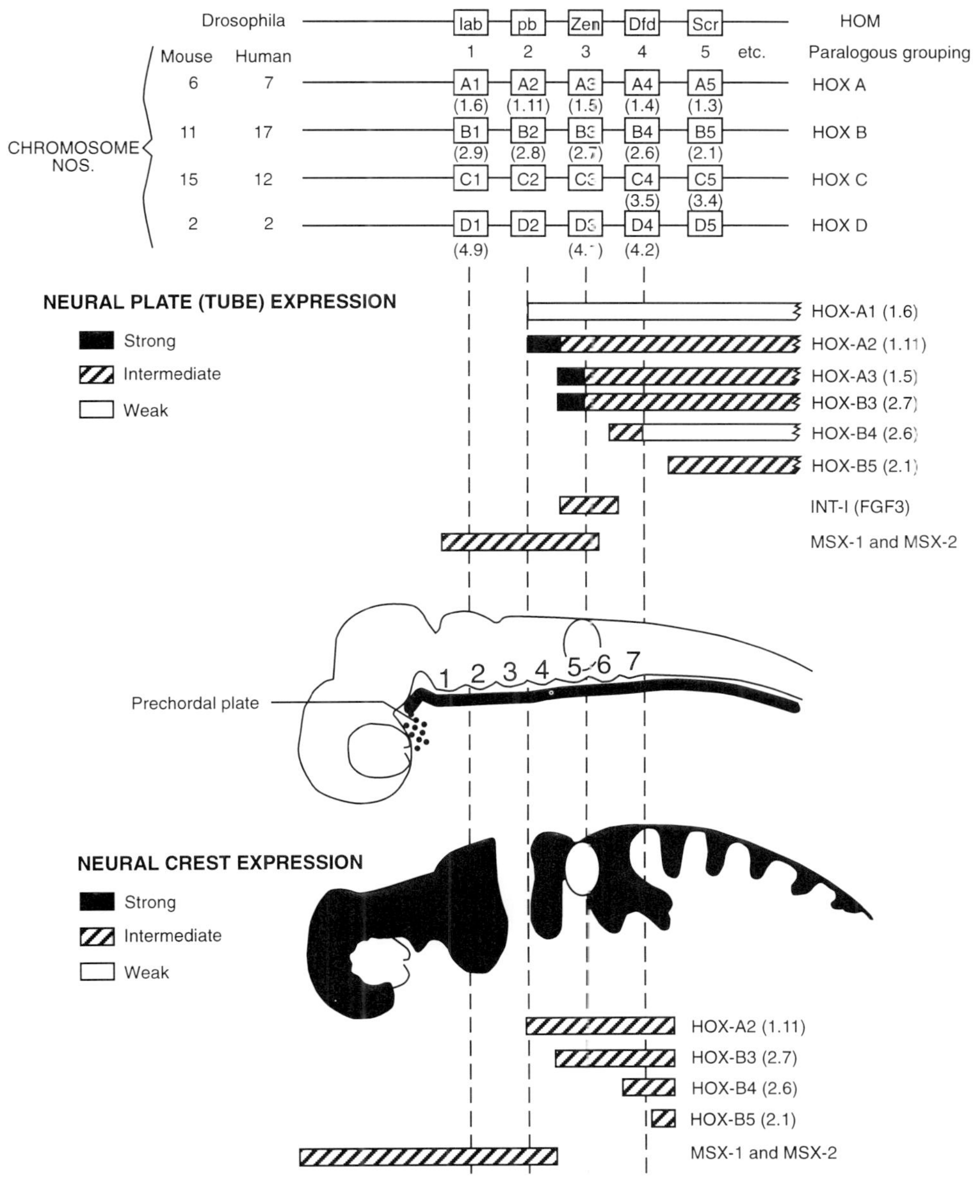


**Fig 6–6.** Homeobox gene expression in the neural tube and neural crest. The *HOM* genes of *Drosophila* (fruit fly), which are involved in the axial development of the embryo, have been replicated (as *Hox* genes) on four different chromosomes of the human and the mouse, where they have similar functions. The older numbering system used for mice is given in parentheses (see Scott, 1992).[61] The *Hox* genes are expressed in all species studied as an overlapping cascade, with new gene expression added segmentally (1–7) in a rostral-to-caudal fashion, as illustrated for the neural plate (tube) and neural crest. These additions modify the inductive responses of crest cells in different pharyngeal arches (see text). The expression of other homeobox genes not in the HOM/Hox series, such as *Msx-1*, *Msx-2* and *Int-1*, are also illustrated. (Diagram modified from Noden, Brain Behav Evol 38:190–225, 1991,[51] with permission.)

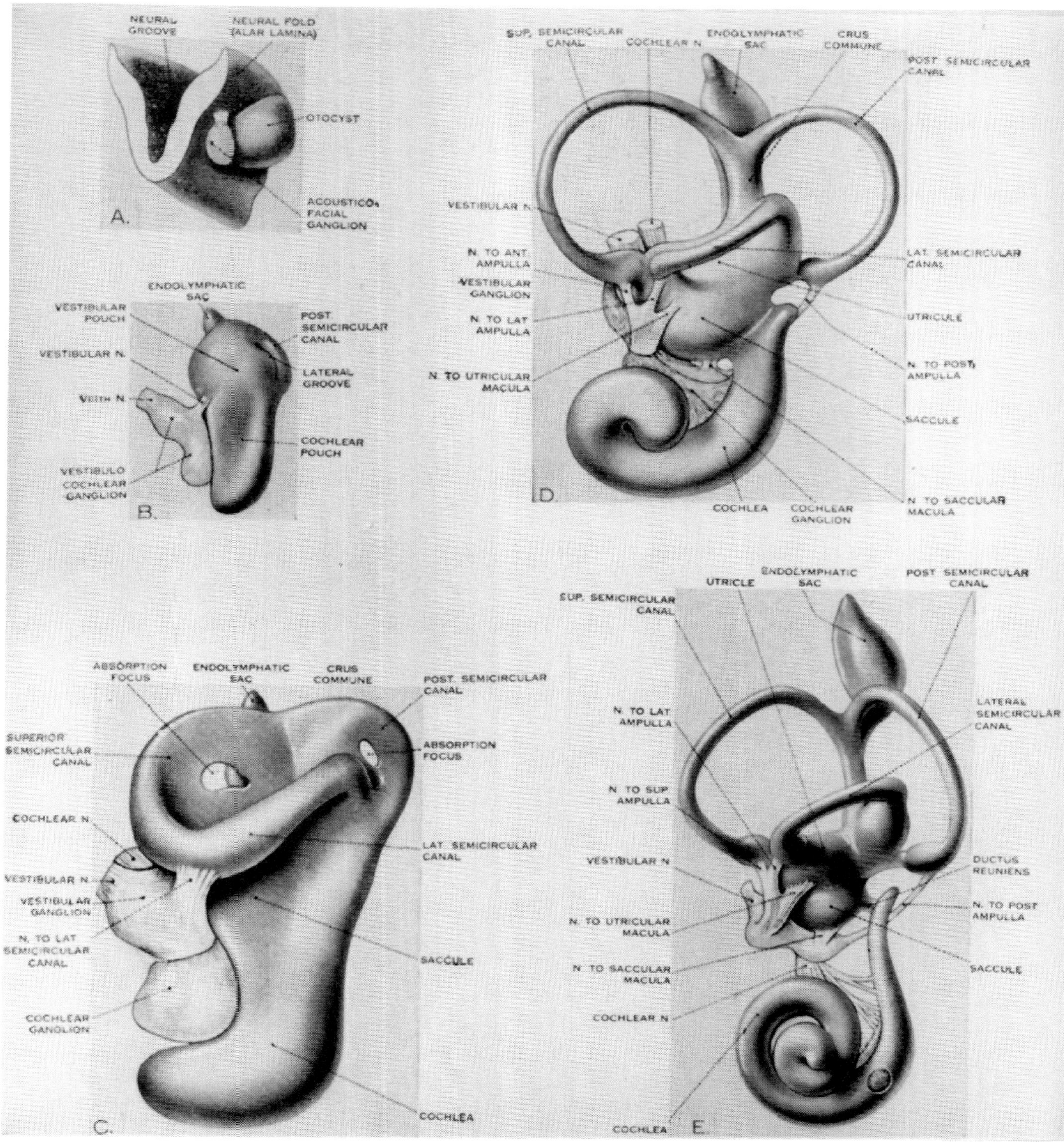

**Fig. 6–7.** Progressive development of the otic epithelium (A–E) which, through complex interactions with the associated mesoderm, forms the semicircular canals of the vestibular apparatus, the endolymphatic duct or sac (which is apparently involved in fluid removal), and the cochlea. The developing acoustic-vestibular ganglion is also illustrated. (From Hamilton and Mossman, *Human Embryology,* Macmillan, London, 1976,[26] with permission.)

rhombomere differentiation with secondary effects on otic placode induction.

### Defects in hair cell development

The gene products of two well-known mouse mutations for inner ear deafness (*shaker*[21]; *waltzer*[1]) have been shown to be unconventional myosins that appear to be responsible for the integrity of hair cells. Their names suggest that these mutants were intially identified because of vestibular problems. Deol and Green[17] showed many years ago that the *waltzer* organ of Corti develops normally to postnatal day 8, indicating that initial differentiation is normal and that failure of stereocilia development leads to degeneration of hair cells and subsequently degeneration of supporting cells.

### Pigmentation and ear defects

While such combinations of defects account for only a limited percentage of hearing defects (perhaps 10%),[5,64] and an even smaller percentage of vestibular problems, they are of very considerable interest from a developmental point of view. The most studied human combination of this nature is in the Waardenburg syndrome, where there is hypopigmentation of the skin and iris, a moderate incidence of hearing defects, and occasionally, neural tube defects (NTDs) and cleft lip with or without cleft palate.[21a] It now appears that type I Waardenburg syndrome (with telecanthus) results from a defect in one of the

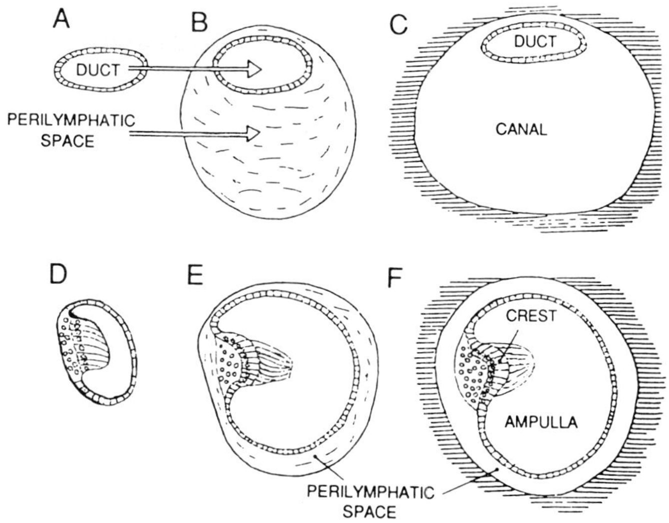


**Fig. 6–9.** Sketches illustrating development of ampulla of the semicircular duct. The ducts develop as outpunchings from the otocyst and become converted to ducts (canals) as illustrated in Figure 6–7B–D. A portion of the duct epithelium thickens to form a paddle-like crest, the hair cells of which form stereo cilia that are embedded in a gelatinous matrix to further extend this "paddle" into the lumen of the ampulla. Fluid movement in the ducts caused by head rotations bends the paddle and the hair cell response is transmitted to nerve fibers innervating them. The detailed structure is the same as that of the macula illustrated in Figure 6–10, except for the otoconia. (From O'Rahilly and Müller, Development of the human ear. In *Diseases of the Nose, Throat, Ear, Head and Neck,* JJ Ballenger, JB Snow, eds., Lea and Febiger, Philadelphia, 1996, pp. 829–837,[55a] with permission.)

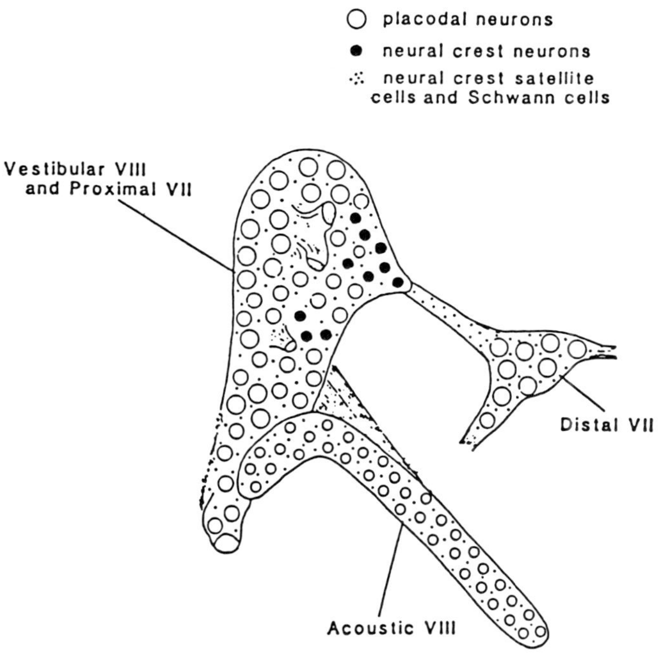


**Fig. 6–8.** Cell-making studies in avian embryos show that almost all neurons in the vestibular and acoustic ganglia are derived from the otocyst as "placodal" neurons. In contrast, all the supporting satellite and Schwann cells are derived from neural crest cells, apparently from the VIIth nerve ganglion to which the acoustic-vestibular (vestibulocochlear) ganglion is initially attached. (From Noden and van de Water, The developing ear: tissue origins and interactions. In *The Biology of Change in Otolaryngology,* RJ Ruben, TR van de Water, eds., Elsevier, Amsterdam, 1986, pp. 15–46,[54] with permission.)

*Pax* homeobox genes (*PAX-3*).[72] The mouse homologue is Splotch. *Pax-3* genes are expressed in the dorsal half of the neural tube and appear to affect numerous aspects of the development of crest cells derived from it, as well as those of cells in a number of other areas.[24] *Pax-3* appears to affect many aspects of neural crest development. In Splotch mouse embryos, abnormalities of the neural folds lead to problems of neural tube closure defects (NTDs) as well as crest cell migration.[42] There are also ganglionic and pigmentation defects. The phenotype of the Dancer mouse is somewhat similar to that of Waardenburg syndrome (it also has vestibular involvement), but only pathogenetic studies[15,16,74] have been conducted.

### Regeneration of the sensory epithelia

This phenomenon is of considerable interest because it increases the possibility of repair after environmental damage. Regeneration of hair cells occurs normally in lower vertebrates[9–12,19,63] and may occur spontaneously in vestibular hair cells in guinea pigs and humans.[19,79] Regeneration can apparently be induced in mice with the growth factor TGF$\alpha$[5] and further potentiated by retinoic acid (RA).[36,63]

### Otofacial syndromes

The retinoic acid syndrome (RAS, Fig. 6–12, Table 6–1) has stimulated considerable interest in the pathogenesis of a number of otofacial malformations as well as the role of RA in normal craniofacial development. RAS frequently has severe defects of

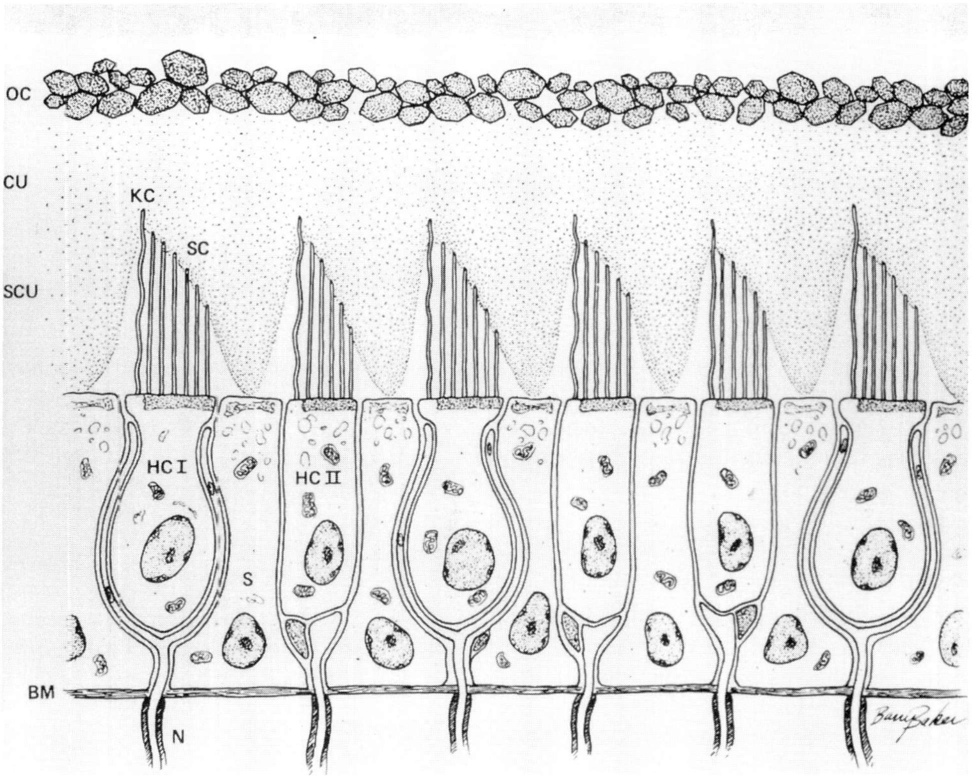


**Fig. 6–10.** Detailed structure of the macula which develops in the floor of the utricle and saccule of Figure 6–7. The mineralized otoconia (OC) develop on the surface of the gelatinous matrix (stipple) in which the stereocilia (KC and SC) of the hair cells (HCI and HCII) are embedded. Endings from the nerve fibers (N), which extend through the basement membrane (BM), surround the hair cells. Supporting cells (S) are interposed between the hair cells. The "heavy" otoconia permit the maculae to sense orientation of the head related to gravity. (Diagram from Austin, The ear: anatomy and embryology. In *Diseases of the Nose, Throat, Ear, Head and Neck,* JJ Ballenger, JB Snow, eds., Lea and Febiger, Philadelphia, 1996, pp. 838–857,[4] with permission.)

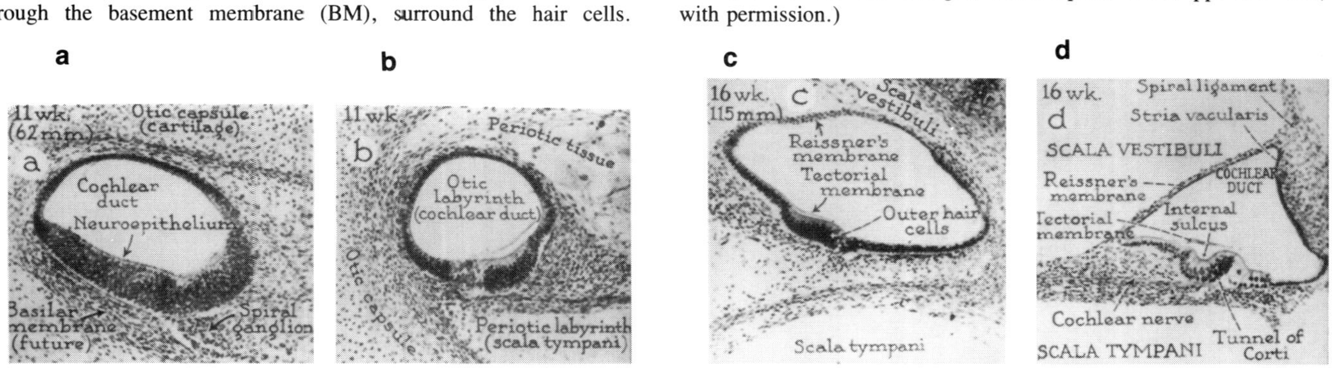


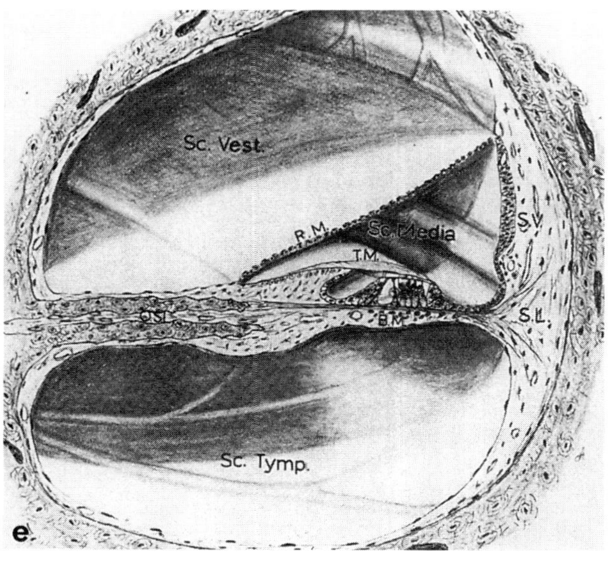


**Fig. 6–11.** The same basic cellular configuration as in Figure 6–10 is used by hair cells of the much more complex cochlea. These hair cells sense vibrations in the cochlear fluid transmitted from the ear drum, by the middle ear ossicles, to the oval window at the base of the cochlea. a, b, and c, d illustrate development at 11 and 16 weeks, respectively. Reissner's membrane separates the cochlear duct cavity (future scala media) from the scala vestibuli, a connective tissue-lined, fluid-filled space. e and f are cross-sectional sketches of the mature cochlea showing the relations of the above-mentioned cavities to a second connective tissue cavity, the scala tympani, which is separated from the scala media by the basilar membrane (BM). The function of the pigmented stria vascularis (SV) is poorly understood, but it is known to play a key role in a number of pigmentation (auditory/vestibular) abnormalities; see text). The stereocilia of the inner (ihc) and outer (ohc) hair cells are embedded in the gelatinous matrix of the tectorial membrane (TM). BC = border cells; CC = cells of Clau-

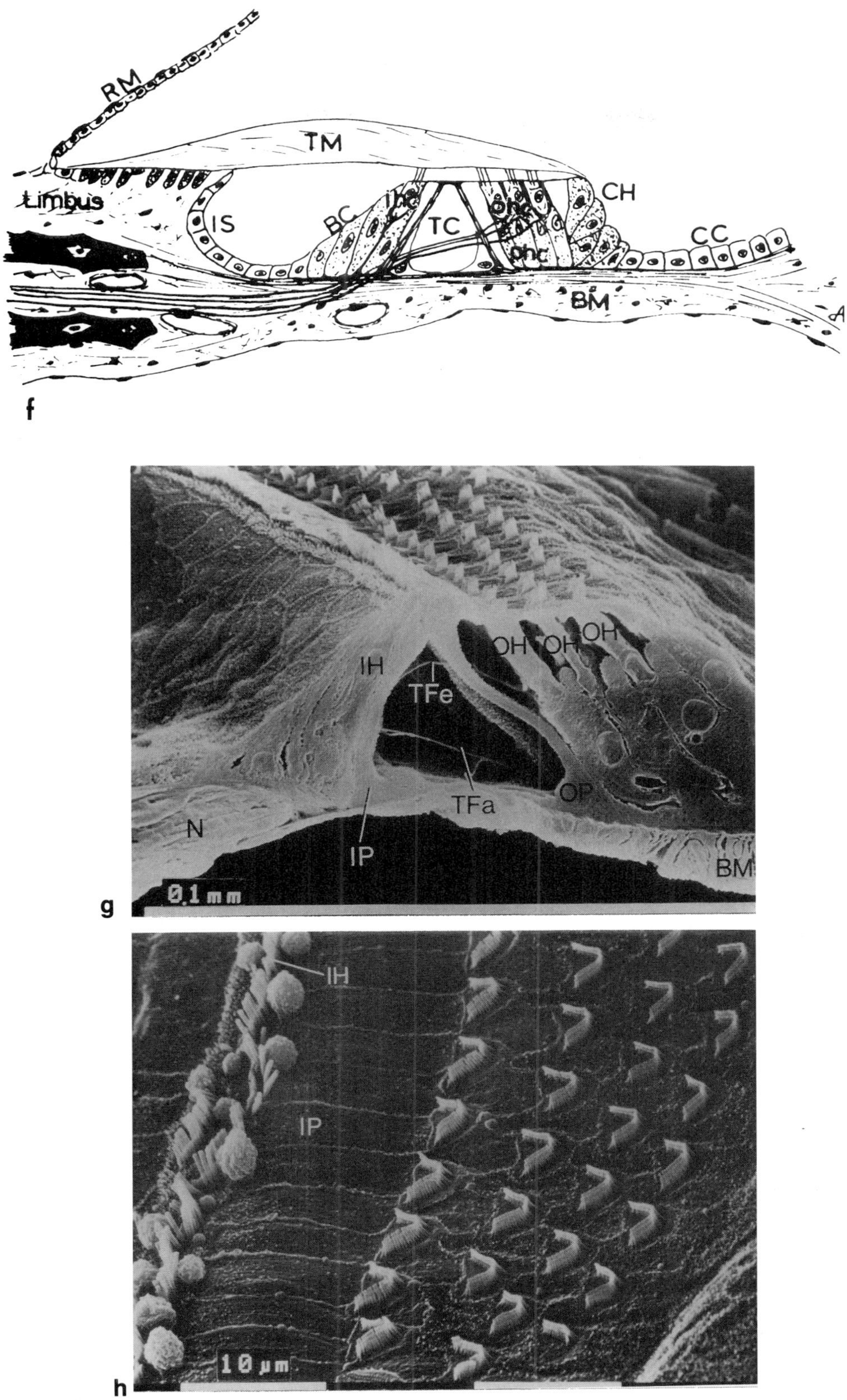


dius; CH = cells of Hansen; IS = inner sulcus; RM = Reissner's membrane; SL = spiral ligament; TC = tunnel of Corti. g and h are scanning electron micrographs of the inner (IH) and outer (OH) hair cells (tectorial membrane removed) of a mouse embryo. The higher-power SEM in h is of the same specimen (slightly different orientation) showing the exquisite arrangements of the stereocilia of the inner and outer hair cells. BM = basement membrane; IP = inner pillar cells; N = myelinated nerve fibers; OP = outer pillar cells; TFa = tunnel fibers (afferent); TFe = tunnel fibers (efferent). (a–d from Anson and Davies, Embryology of the ear. In: *Otolaryngology,* MM Paparella, DA Shumrick, eds., WB Saunders, Philadelphia, 1980, pp. 3–25,[3] with permission; e and f from Austin, The ear: anatomy and embryology. In: *Diseases of the Nose, Throat, Ear, Head and Neck,* JJ Ballenger, JB Snow, eds. Lea & Febiger, Philadelphia, 1996, pp. 838–857, with permission; g and h from Lim and Anniko, Acta Otolaryngol 422(Suppl):1–69, 1985,[38] with permission.)

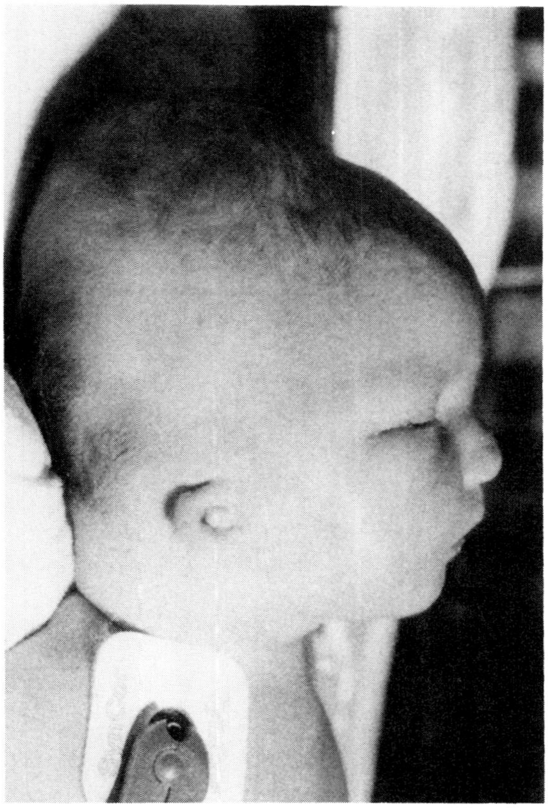

**Fig. 6–12.** Infant showing the retinoic acid syndrome (RAS). (Courtesy of Paul M. Fernhoff).

the external and middle ear, as well as of the cerebellum, pharyngeal glands, and cardiovascular systems.[34] It results from the inadvertent use of the drug Accutane®, a stereoisomer of RA which is used successfully in the treatment of severe cystic acne.

The pathogenesis of RAS has been extensively studied in experimental animals (Fig. 6–13).[22,30,46,57,59,68,80,82] Sorting out the pathogenesis was greatly enhanced by the studies of Kirby and co-workers.[32] They,[32] and others,[53] have shown that much of the mesenchyme of the conotruncal septum of the developing heart is derived from 3rd and 4th arch neural crest. Normally, the septum splits with the two halves of the conotruncus, forming the proximal portions of the arch of the aorta and pulmonary artery. Kirby and co-workers[32] also showed that extirpation of these crest cells prior to migration resulted in cardiovascular malformations of the conotruncal outflow tract type, the same as the malformations associated with RAS and other otofacial malformations. It appears that the ear and cerebellar malformations in RAS can be largely accounted for by excessive death of cells in the dorsal portions of rhombomeres 3 and 4 (Fig. 6–5), including cells which normally give rise to the hyoid (second) arch crest and the affected portions of the cerebellum. There is normally a certain amount of cell death (apoptosis) in the dorsal neural tube, which appears to be largely limited to the neural folds of rhombomere 3, and may be involved in eliminating the crest cells that would normally fill the gap between the mandibular and hyoid crest (Fig. 6–5).[23] Graham et al.[23] have provided convincing evidence that this cell death is controlled by the homeobox gene *Msx-2* and that the activity of the gene is expanded by RA to include a higher percentage of cells in a larger area of the neural tube. Although deficits in first arch crest cells can be compensated for by regulation of more anterior crest cells, the isolated location of hyoid crest (Fig. 6–5A, C) apparently inhibits such

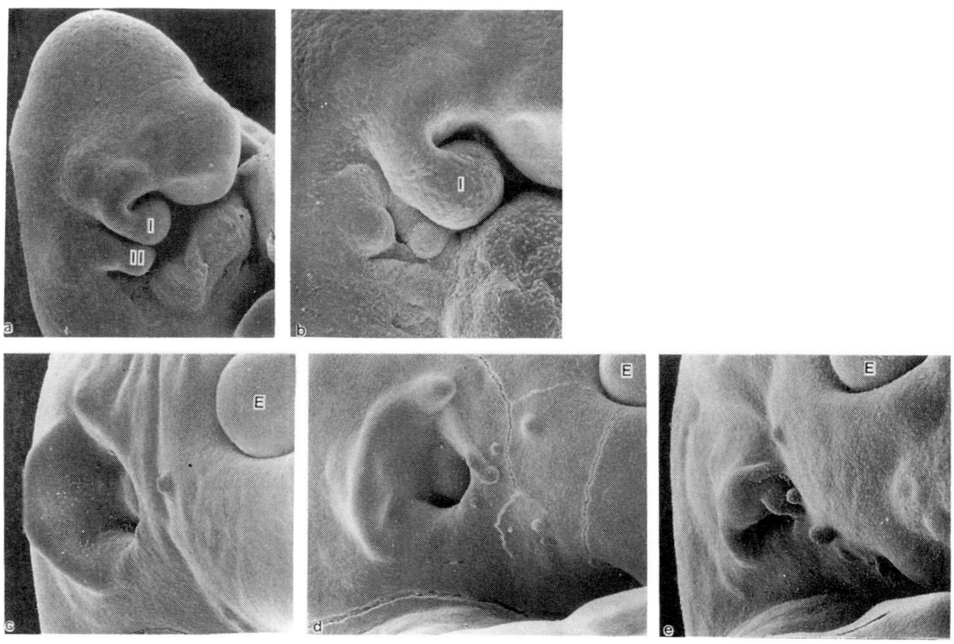


**Fig. 6–13.** RAS in the mouse. The normal hyoid arch (II) in (a) is almost obliterated in the embryo from an RA-treated mother (b). The ear tags in the affected fetuses (d,e) are frequently observed in the common human malformation. I: 1$^{st}$ brachial arch; II: 2$^{nd}$ branchial arch; E: eye. (From Sulik, Embryology of the ear. In: *Hereditary Hearing Loss and Its Syndromes,* RJ Gorlin et al, eds. Oxford University Press, New York, 1995, pp. 22–42,[67] with permission.)

**Table 6–1.** Comparison of three syndromes (with apparent primary cranial neural crest involvement) and the Treacher Collins syndrome (in which there appears to be primary ganglionic placodal cell death and secondary localized crest cell involvement) (From Johnston and Bronsky[30])

| Syndromes | Developmental abnormalities | | | | | | Etiology | Possible Pathogenesis |
|---|---|---|---|---|---|---|---|---|
| | Ear | Facial bones | Cardiovascular | Pharyngeal glands | Facial clefts (variable incidence) | Other associated malformations (variable incidence) | | |
| Retinoic acid syndrome (Fig. 6–12) | Primarily middle and external ear | Mandibular and other deficiencies | Conotruncal defects | Thymus, etc. deficient or absent | Cleft palate (8%) | Brain (particularly cerebellum) | 13-cis-retinoic acid (isotretinoin, Accutane®) | Cranial neural crest; kills 2nd arch crest before migration along with other neural plate cells—retards migration? other cell populations in some cases |
| Di George syndrome | External and middle ear | Variable maxillary and mandibular deficiencies | Conotruncal defects | Thymus, etc. deficient or absent | Cleft lip and/or palate (10%) | Brain | Heterogeneous; frequently associated with chromosome 22, sometimes with ethanol | Cranial neural crest; ethanol kills before and during migration |
| Hemifacial microsomias (Fig. 6–14) | Primarily middle and external ear | Usually asymmetrical deficiencies of mandible, squamous temporal, and other bones | Conotruncal defects | No reported abnormalities | Cleft lip and/or palate (7%–22%) | Eye, brain (in severe cases), vertebrae in oculo-auriculo-vertebral variant | Heterogeneous; many multifactorial | Cranial neural crest; selective death of 2nd arch crest retards migrations; sometimes other cell populations affected |
| Treacher Collins syndrome | External, middle, and particularly inner ear | Symmetrical deficiencies or absence of zygoma, underdevelopment of posterior maxilla and mandible | No increase in CV malformations | No reported abnormalities | Cleft palate (35%) | Rarely with limb defects, e.g., Nager syndrome | Dominant gene | Ganglionic placodal cell death with secondary crest cell involvement |

compensation, thereby accounting for the virtual absence of hyoid arch in an animal model (Fig. 6–13a and b).

Explanation of the other RAS malformations is not so simple. The peak incidence for conotruncal and pharyngeal gland abnormalities in experimental RAS is associated with the administration of the drug well after the 3rd and 4th arch crest cells have left the neural folds.[80] RA also appears to have effects on migrating crest cells,[43,57,73,80] and the crest cells migrating to the conotruncus have particularly long migration paths.

The DiGeorge sequence (Table 6–1), which is sometimes associated with maternal ethanol consumption,[2] is similar to RAS except that the effects on the ear are much less severe and there are few, if any, cerebellar defects. In an ethanol-induced animal model for the DiGeorge sequence, it was found that the malformations were associated with excessive cell death of premigratory and migrating crest cells.[69] The principal effects of ethanol on cells appears to be the labilization of membranes.[6a] The major involvement of membranes in migrating cells may make them particularly sensitive.

The possibility of crest cell involvement in hemifacial microsomia (Fig. 6–14, Table 6–1), which also has conotruncal defects but not pharyngeal gland defects, has been thoroughly discussed by Johnston and Bronsky.[30] Treacher Collins syndrome is also included in Table 6–1 as an example of an otofacial malformation where crest cell involvement appears to be sec-

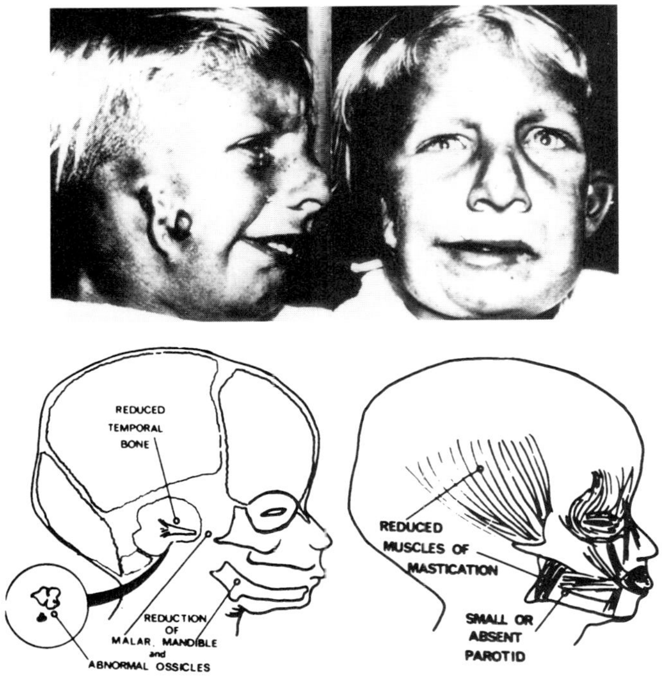


**Fig. 6–14.** Features and diagrams of hemifacial microsomia. (From Poswillo, Oral Surg 35:302–328, 1973,[56] with permission.)

ondary to excessive death of placodal cells contributing to the formation of cranial sensory ganglia (Fig. 12–4, Chapter 12).[70] Excessive death of otic placodal cells contributing to the formation of the acoustic ganglion (Fig. 6–8) may account for the increased incidence of neural deafness in Treacher Collins syndrome.

## References


1. Abraham KB, Hasson T, Steel KP, Kingsley DM, Russell LB, Mooseker MS, Kopland NG, Jenkins NA: The mouse *Snell's waltzer* deafness gene encodes an unconventional myosin required for the structural integrity of inner ear hair cells. Nat Genet 11:369–375, 1995.
2. Ammann AJ, Wara DW, Cowan MJ, Barrett DJ, Stiehm ER: The DiGeorge syndrome and the fetal alcohol syndrome. Am J Dis Child 136:906–908, 1982.
3. Anson BJ, Davies J: Embryology of the ear. In: Otolaryngology, MM Paparella, DA Shumrick, eds. WB Saunders, Philadelphia, 1980, pp. 3–25.
4. Austin DF: The ear: anatomy and embryology. In: Diseases of the Nose, Throat, Ear, Head and Neck, JJ Ballenger, JB Snow, eds. Lea & Febiger, Philadelphia, 1996, pp 838–857.
5. Beighton P, Ramesar R, Winship I, Viljoen D, Greenberg J, Young K, Curis D, Sellars S: Hearing impairment and pigmentary disturbance. Ann NY Acad Sci 630:152–166, 1991.
6. Carpenter EM, Goddard JM, Chisaka O, Manley NR, Capecchi MR: Loss of Hox-A1 (Hox-1.6) function results in the reorganization of the murine hindbrain. Development 118:1063–1075, 1993.

6a. Chin JH, Goldstein DA, Parsons LM: Fluidity and lipid composition of mouse biomembranes during adaptation to ethanol. Alcoholism Clin Exp Res 3:47–49, 1979.

7. Chisaka O, Musci, TS, Capecchi MR: Developmental defects of the ear, cranial nerves and hindbrain resulting from targeted disruption of the mouse homeobox gene Hox-1.6. Nature 355:516–520, 1992.
8. Cordes SP, Barsh GS: The mouse segmentation gene kr encodes a novel basic domain-leucine zipper transcription factor. Cell 79:1025–1034, 1994.
9. Corwin JT: Perpetual production of hair cells and maturational changes in hair cell ultrastructure accompany postembryonic growth in an amphibian ear. Proc Natl Acad Sci USA 82:3911–3915, 1985.
10. Corwin JT, Cotanche DE: Regeneration of sensory hair cells after acoustic trauma. Science 240:1772–1774, 1988.
11. Cotanche DA: Regeneration of hair cell stereociliary bundles in the chick cochlea following severe acoustic trauma. Hear Res 30:181–195. 1987.
12. Cotanche DA, Lee KH, Stone JS, Picard DA: Hair cell regeneration in the bird cochlea following noise damage or ototoxic drug damage. Anat Embryol 189:1–18, 1994.
13. D'Amico-Martel A, Noden DM: Contributions of placodal and neural crest cells to avian cranial peripheral ganglia. Am J Anat 166:445–468,1983.
14. Deol MS: Influence of the neural tube on the differentiation of the inner ear in the mammalian embryo. Nature 209:219–220, 1966.
15. Deol MS: The relationship between abnormalities of pigmentation and development of the inner ear. Proc R Soc London B Biol Sci 175:201–217, 1970.
16. Deol MS: Genetic malformation of the inner ear in the mouse and man. Birth Defects 16:243–261, 1980.
17. Deol MS, Green MC: Snell's waltzer, a new mutation affecting behaviour and inner ear of the mouse. Genet Res 8:339–345, 1966.
18. Dollé P, Lufkin T, Krumlauf R, Mark M, Duboule D, Chambon P: Local alterations of Krox-20 and Hox gene expression in the hindbrain suggest lack of rhombomeres 4 and 5 in homozygote null Hoxa-1 (Hox-1.6) mutant embryos. Proc Natl Acad Sci USA 90:7666–7670, 1993.
19. Forge A, Li L, Corwin JT, Nevill G: Ultrastructural evidence for hair cell regeneration in the mammalian inner ear. Science 259:1616–1619, 1993.
20. Gendron-Maguire M, Mallo M, Zhang M, Gridley T: Hoxa-2 mutant mice exhibit homeotic transformation of skeletal elements derived from cranial neural crest. Cell 75:1317–1331, 1993.
21. Gibson F, Walsh J, Mburu P, Varela A, Brown KA, Antonio M, Beisel KW, Steel KP, Brown SD: A type VII myosin encoded by the mouse deafness gene shaker-1. Nature 374:62–64, 1995.

21a. Gorlin RJ, Cohen MM Jr, Levin LS: Syndromes of the Head and Neck, 3rd ed. Oxford University Press, New York, 1990, p 977.

22. Goulding EH, Pratt RM: Isotretinoin teratogenicity in mouse whole embryo culture. J Craniofac Genet Dev Biol 6:99–112, 1986.
23. Graham A, Heyman I, Lumsden A: Even-numbered rhombomeres control the apoptotic elimination of neural crest cells from odd-numbered rhombomeres in the chick hindbrain. Development 119:233–245, 1993.
24. Gruss P, Walther C: Pax in development. Cell 69:719–722, 1992.
25. Guthrie S, Muchamore I, Kuroiwa A, Marshall H, Krumlauf R, Lumsden A: Neuroectodermal autonomy of Hox-2.9 expression revealed by rhombomere transposition. Nature 356:157–159, 1992.
26. Hamilton WJ, Mossman HW: Human Embryology, Macmillan Press, London, 1976.
27. Jarvis BL, Johnston MC, Sulik KK: Congenital malformations of the external, middle and inner ear produced by isotretinoin exposure in mouse embryos. Otolaryngol Head Neck Surg 102:391–401, 1990.
28. Johnston MC: A radioautographic study of the migration and fate of cranial neural crest cells in the chick embryo. Anat Rec 156:143–156, 1966.
29. Johnston MC, Bhakdinaronk A, Reid YC: An expanded role for the neural crest in oral and pharyngeal development. In: Oral Sensation and Perception, JF Bosma, ed. U.S. Govt Printing Office, Washington D.C., 1974, pp 37–52.
30. Johnston MC, Bronsky PT: Prenatal craniofacial development: new insights on normal and abnormal mechanisms. Crit Rev Oral Biol Med 4:25–79, 1995.
31. Johnston MC, Hazelton RB: Embryonic origins of facial structures related to oral sensory and motor function. In: Oral Sensory Perception, JF Bosma, ed. Charles C Thomas, Springfield, 1972, pp 96–97.
32. Kirby ML, Gale TF, Stewart DE: Neural crest cells contribute to normal aorticopulmonary septation. Science 220:1059–1061, 1983.
33. Krumlauf R: Hox genes and pattern formation in the branchial region of the verebrate head. Trends Genet 9:106–112, 1993.
34. Lammer EJ, Chen DT, Hoar RM, Agnish DN, Benke PJ, Braun JT, Curry CJ, Fernhoff PM, Grix AW Jr, Lott IT, et al: Retinoic acid embryopathy. N Engl J Med 313:837–841, 1985.
35. LeDouarin N: The Neural Crest. Cambridge University Press, Cambridge, 1983.
36. Lefebvre PP, Malgrange B, Staecker H, Moonen G, van de Water TR:

Retinoic acid stimulates regeneration of mammalian auditory hair cells. Science 260:692–695, 1993.
37. LeLievre C: Role des cellules mésectodermiques issues des crêtes neurales céphaliques dans la formation des arcs branchiaux et du squelette viscéral. J Embryol Exp Morphol 31:453–477, 1974.
38. Lim D, Anniko M: Developmental morphology of the mouse inner ear: a scanning electron microscopic observation. Acta Otolaryngol 422 (Suppl):1–69, 1985.
38a. Lim D, Ryan AF: Molecular biology of the ear. In: Diseases of the Nose, Throat, Ear, Head and Neck, JJ Ballenger, JB Snow (eds.), Lea A. Febiger, Philadelphia, 1996, pp 858– 873.
39. Lufkin T, Dierich A, LeMeur M, Mark M, Chambon P: Disruption of the Hox 1.6 homeobox gene results in defects in a region corresponding to its rostral domain of expression. Cell 66:1105–1119, 1991.
40. Mansour SL, Goddard JM, Capecchi MR: Mice homozygous for a targeted disruption of the proto-oncogene *int*-2 have developmental defects in the tail and inner ear. Development 117:13–28, 1993.
41. Mark M, Lufkin T, Vonesch J-L, Ruberte E, Olivo J-C, Dollé P, Gorry P, Lumsden A, Chambon P: Two rhombomeres are altered in Hoxa-1 mutant mice. Development 119:319–338, 1993.
42. Moase CE, Trasler DG: Splotch locus mouse mutants: models for neural tube defects and Waardenburg syndrome type I in humans. J Med Genet 29:145–151, 1992.
43. Morriss GM, Thorogood PV: An approach to cranial neural crest cell migration and differentiation in mammalian embryos. In: Development in Mammals, MH Johnson, ed. North Holland, Amsterdam, 1978, pp 363–412.
44. Morriss-Kay G: Retinoic acid and craniofacial development: molecules and morphogenesis. Bioessays 15:9–15, 1993.
45. Morriss-Kay GM, Murphy P, Hill RE, Davidson DR: Effects of retinoic acid excess on expression of Hox-2.9 and Krox-20 and on morphological segmentation in the hindbrain of mouse embryos. EMBO J 10:2985–2995, 1991.
46. Nau H, Chahoud I, Dencker L, Lammer EJ, Scott WJ: Teratogenicity of vitamin A and retinoids. In: Vitamin A in Health and Disease, R Blomhoff, ed. Marcel Dekker, New York, 1994, pp 615–664.
47. Noden DM: An analysis of migratory behavior of avian cephalic neural crest cells. Dev Biol 42:106–130, 1975.
48. Noden DM: The role of the neural crest in patterning of avian cranial skeletal, connective, and muscle tissues. Dev Biol 96:144–165, 1983.
49. Noden DM: The embryonic origins of avian cephalic and cervical muscles and associated connective tissues. Am J Anat 186:257–276, 1983.
50. Noden DM: Interactions and fates of avian craniofacial mesenchyme. Development 103(Suppl):121–140, 1988.
51. Noden DM: Vertebrate craniofacial development: the relation between ontogenetic process and morphological outcome. Brain Behav Evol 38:190–225, 1991.
52. Noden DM: Cell movements and control of patterned tissue assembly during craniofacial development. J Craniofac Genet Dev Biol 11:192–213, 1991.
53. Noden DM, Poelmann RE, Gittenberger-de Groot AC: Cell origins and tissue boundaries during outflow tract development. Trends Cardiovasc Med 5: 69–75, 1995.
54. Noden DM, van de Water TR: The developing ear: tissue origins and interactions. In: The Biology of Change in Otolaryngology, RJ Ruben, TR van de Water, eds. Elsevier/North-Holland, Amsterdam, 1986, pp 15–46.
55. Noden DM, van de Water TR: Genetic analyses of mammalian ear development. Trends Neurosci 14:235–237, 1992.
55a. O'Rahilly R, Müller F: Development of the human ear. In: Diseases of the Nose, Throat, Ear, Head and Neck, JJ Ballenger, JB Snow (eds), Lea & Febiger, Philadelphia, 1996, pp 829– 837.
56. Poswillo D: The pathogenesis of the first and second branchial arch syndrome. Oral Surg 35:302–328, 1973.
57. Pratt RM, Goulding EH, Abbott BD: Retinoic acid inhibits migration of cranial neural crest cells in the cultured mouse embryos. J Craniofac Genet Dev Biol 7:205–217, 1987.
58. Represa J, Leon Y, Miner C, Giraldez F: The int-2 proto-oncogene is responsible for induction of the inner ear. Nature 353:561–563, 1991.
59. Richman JM: The role of retinoids in normal and abnormal embryonic craniofacial morphogenesis. Crit Rev Oral Biol Med 4:93–109, 1992.
60. Rijli FM, Mark M, Lakkaraju S, Dierich A, Dollé P, Chambon P: A homeotic transformation is generated in the rostral branchial region of the head by disruption of Hoxa-2, which acts as a selector gene. Cell 75:1333–1349, 1993.
61. Scott MP: Vertebrate homeobox gene nomenclature. Cell 71:551–553, 1992.
62. Serbedzija GN, Bronner-Fraser M, Fraser SE: Vital dye analysis of cranial neural crest cell migration in the mouse embryo. Development 116:297–307, 1992.
63. Staecker H, Lefebvre P, Malgrange B, Moonen G, van de Water TR: Response to letters from Chardin S and Romand R on Regeneration and mammalian auditory hair cells. Science 267:707–711, 1995.
64. Steel KP: Similarities between mice and humans with hereditary deafness. Ann NY Acad Sci 630:68–79, 1991.
65. Steel KP, Barkway C: Another role for melanocytes: their importance for normal stria vascularis development in the mammalian inner ear. Development 107:453–463, 1989.
66. Streeter GL: Development of the auricle in the human embryo. Contrib Embryol Carnegie Inst 14:111–138, 1922.
67. Sulik KK: Embryology of the ear. In: Hereditary Hearing Loss and Its Syndromes, RJ Gorlin, HV Toriello, MM Cohen, eds. Oxford University Press, New York, 1995, pp 22–42.
68. Sulik KK, Cook CS, Webster WS: Teratogens and craniofacial malformations: relationships to cell death. Development 103(Suppl): 213–231, 1988.
69. Sulik KK, Johnston MC, Daft PA, Russell WE, Dehart DB: Fetal alcohol syndrome and DiGeorge anomaly: critical ethanol exposure periods for craniofacial malformations as illustrated in an animal model. Am J Med Genet (Suppl)2:97–112, 1986.
70. Sulik KK, Johnston MC, Smiley SJ, Speight HS, Jarvis BE: Mandibulofacial dysostosis (Treacher Collins syndrome): a new proposal for its pathogenesis. Am J Med Genet 27:359–372, 1987.
71. Tan SS, Morriss-Kay G: The development and distribution of cranial neural crest in the rat embryo. Cell Tissue Res 240:403–416, 1985.
72. Tassabehji M, Read AP, Newton VE, Patton M, Gruss P, Harris R, Strachan T: Mutations in the PAX3 gene causing Waardenburg syndrome type 1 and type 2. Nat Genet 3:26–30, 1993.
73. Thorogood P, Smith L, Nicol A, McGinty R, Garrod D: Effects of vitamin A on the behaviour of migratory neural crest cells in vitro. J Cell Sci 57:331–350, 1982.
74. Trasler DG: Differences in the face shape of mouse embryos with and without the gene Dancer predisposing to cleft lip. Teratology 2:271, 1969.
75. Tuchmann-Duplessis H: Illustrated Human Embryology. Springer-Verlag, New York, 1975.
76. van de Water TR: Tissue interactions and cell differentiation: neurone-sensory cell interaction during otic development. Development 103(Suppl):185–193, 1988.
77. van de Water TR, Noden DM, Maderson PFA: Embryology of the ear: outer, middle, and inner. In: Otologic Medicine and Surgery, Vol I, PW Albert, RJ Ruben, eds. Churchill Livingstone, New York, 1988.
78. van de Water TR, Represa J: Tissue interactions and growth factors that control development of the inner ear. Neural tube-otic anlage interaction. Ann NY Acad Sci 630:116–128, 1991.
79. Warchol ME, Lambert PR, Goldstein BJ, Forge A, Corwin JT: Regenerative proliferation in inner ear sensory epithelia from adult guinea pigs and humans. Science 259:1619–1622, 1993.
80. Webster WS, Johnston MC, Lammer EJ, Sulik KK: Isotretinoin embryopathy and the cranial neural crest: an in vivo and in vitro study. J Craniofac Genet Dev Biol 6:211–222, 1986.
81. Wilkinson DG: Molecular mechanisms of segmental patterning in the vertebrate hindbrain and neural crest. Bioessays 15:499–505, 1993.
82. Willhite CC, Hill RM, Irving DW: Isotretinoin-induced craniofacial malformations in humans and hamsters. J Craniofac Genet Dev Biol (Suppl)2:193–209, 1986.

# 7

# Prelingual Deafness: Diagnosis and Treatment

PATRICK E. BROOKHOUSER

Congenital or early-onset sensorineural hearing loss (SNHL), which is educationally significant, should be identified by 1 year of age to permit early intervention aimed at promoting age-appropriate linguistic development. Past public health initiatives have included public awareness campaigns, hearing risk factor questionnaires for new parents and newborn nursery personnel, and an array of infant screening modalities. Beginning in the early 1980s, efforts of the Joint Committee on Infant Hearing (1982)[25] were directed toward promulgating specific risk factors (e.g., congenital and neonatal infections, ear deformities, etc.) to identify neonates and older infants at risk for hearing impairment who could be targeted for hearing screening. This risk indicator list was augmented in the Committee's 1990[36] statement to include factors which become manifest after the neonatal period. A major deficiency of early identification programs targeted at only high-risk infants has been such programs' propensity to miss up to 50% of children who subsequently present with an SNHL during elementary school.

Heightened interest in the concept of universal newborn screening for hearing has followed the development of simplified, but reliable, screening technologies such as evoked otoacoustic emission (EOAE) testing and automated auditory brainstem response (ABR) systems.[26] A recently issued NIH Consensus Statement on early identification of childhood hearing loss (1993)[18] recommends that all infants admitted to a neonatal intensive care unit should be screened and that universal hearing screening should be carried out for all other infants within the first 3 months of life. Techniques based on evoked otoacoustic emissions were recommended for the initial screening of all babies with EOAE failures being rescreened with ABR. Infants who fail an ABR screening would be referred for comprehensive audiologic evaluation.

The 1994 Statement of the Joint Committee on Infant Hearing[27] also addressed sensorineural hearing loss that has onset after 3 months of age. The statement includes an expanded list of "indicators associated with sensorineural and/or conductive hearing loss" for use with neonates in environments where universal screening capability is not available and for use with all infants who require rescreening or periodic monitoring of hearing. Indicators identifying neonates at risk for SNHL include family history of hereditary childhood sensorineural hearing loss; prenatally acquired infections such as cytomegalovirus, rubella, syphilis, herpes, and toxoplasmosis; craniofacial anomalies, particularly those involving abnormalities of the pinna and ear canal; birth weight less than 1,500 grams (3.3 lbs.); serum hyperbilirubinemia sufficient to prompt exchange transfusion; ototoxic medications (e.g., aminoglycosides) in multiple courses or in combination with loop diuretics; bacterial meningitis; Apgar scores of 0–4 at 1 minute or 0–6 at 5 minutes; the use of mechanical ventilation for periods exceeding 4 days; and syndromic findings known to be associated with SNHL.

With children (29 days–2 years), parent or caregiver concern regarding developmental delay of hearing, speech, and/or language should raise a red flag and prompt hearing assessment. In addition to the infectious processes, ototoxic medications, and syndromic features listed for neonates, indicators for infants also include head trauma accompanied by unconsciousness or skull fracture, and recurrent otitis media or otitis media with effusion persisting for at least 3 months.

Children (29 days–3 years) who should have periodic monitoring of hearing are those with a family history of hereditary hearing loss; a history of in utero infections, such as cytomegalovirus, rubella, toxoplasmosis and syphilis; neurofibromatosis type II and neurodegenerative disorders; and persistent pulmonary hypertension. Conductive hearing loss is associated with recurrent or persistent otitis media with effusion, eustachian tube anomalies or dysfunction, and certain neurodegenerative disorders.

## Patterns of sensorineural hearing loss etiology

Congenital defects can be produced by a continuum of abnormal events involving numerical or structural alterations of chromosomes, defects within the structure of individual genes, a breakdown in normal genetic regulation, or disturbances of genetic and environmental interactions during prenatal development. Complex inheritance patterns result from such factors as variable penetrance and segregation of multiple single gene traits interacting with one another. Congenital defects can also be traced to the action of environmental teratogens, such as physical factors (e.g., hyperthermia, and radiation); intrauterine infections (cytomegalovirus [CMV], herpes simplex virus [HSV], human immunodeficiency virus [HIV], and toxoplasma); maternal metabolic disturbances such as diabetes and hypothyroidism; maternal intake of alcohol and/or illicit drugs (cocaine), maternal contact with industrial chemicals (solvents, pesticides, maternal cigarette smoking, pharmacologic agents), synthetic retinoids (e.g., isotretinoin), and chemotherapeutic agents (Developmental Biology, Genetics and Teratology Branch Report, 1994).[17]

Epidemiologic studies have typically attributed 50% of childhood hearing impairment to genetic factors and 20%–25% to prenatal, perinatal, or postnatal environmental causes, while the etiology of the remaining 25%–30% of cases remains uncertain. Childhood hearing loss may be congenital or delayed in onset, variable in severity and audiometric configuration, progressive or nonprogressive, unilateral or bilateral, and syndromic (involving other identifiable physical characteristics) or nonsyndromic. (Appendix B of section 2 and last chapter). Syndromic deafness may be categorized according to other involved organ systems: craniofacial/cervical, skeletal, integumentary, ocular, neurological, renal, cardiovascular, or metabolic. Nonsyndromic genetic hearing disorders (i.e., isolated hearing loss) are described in terms of audiological characteristics, age of onset, presence or absence of progression, associated vestibular deficit, if any, and mode of inheritance. Dominant inheritance accounts for approximately 18%–20% of genetic hearing loss in surveys of schools for the deaf, while recessive inheritance is implicated in about 80% of cases, half of which entail recognizable syndromes. Sex-linked genetic inheritance is involved in only 1%–2% of all hereditary losses but may be responsible for about 6% of nonsyndromic profound hearing impairment in males. Some genetic hearing disorders appear to result from multifactorial inheritance whereby a combination of genetic factors interact with environmental influences.

Public health initiatives aimed at preventive intervention are changing the mix of etiologies operative in each successive age cohort of children with SNHL. Effective immunization programs against mumps, measles, and rubella have all but eradicated these once formidable SNHL etiologies. Administration of a recently developed *H. influenza* type B conjugate vaccine early in the first year of life can achieve a 90% reduction in the incidence of invasive *H. influenza* disease, including meningitis, among infants and children. Conjugate vaccines against meningococcal, *E. coli,* and pneumococcal disease are presently being evaluated in clinical trials and efforts are underway to develop a subunit conjugate vaccine against cytomegalovirus. New diagnostic techniques utilizing polymerase chain reaction (PCR) methodologies should achieve rapid and precise detection of congenital infectious agents, such as CMV and toxoplasma, beginning during the prenatal period. Mitochondrial inheritance has been invoked to explain enhanced familial susceptibility to ototoxic drugs and chemicals pointing toward pre-exposure identification of at-risk individuals. As historical nongenetic causes of SNHL respond to prevention or therapeutic initiatives, genetic etiologies should receive even greater consideration in the differential diagnosis of SNHL in children.

## Evaluation of children with hearing loss

Evaluation, treatment, and (re)habilitation of children with educationally significant hearing loss requires the efforts of a multidisciplinary team of professionals prepared to respond to the needs of the patient and immediate family. Parents are particularly in need of the information necessary to make informed choices regarding the complex array of medical, audiologic, and educational options involved in their child's care and education. A typical team might include: an otolaryngologist with special expertise in pediatrics; audiologists competent in both behavioral and electrophysiologic techniques; an aural rehabilitation specialist to determine amplification needs; a pediatric vestibular specialist; a pediatrician with knowledge of dysmorphology; a geneticist or genetic counselor; a pediatric ophthalmologist able to perform electroretinography; a psychologist skilled in both cognitive and behavioral evaluation; specialists in early childhood intervention and deaf education; and, finally, a speech/language pathologist to evaluate oral motor function and language development. Specialists in pediatric neurology and neuroradiology should be available for consultation on a regular basis.

A comprehensive case history should address prenatal, perinatal, and postnatal factors known to be associated with hearing loss. A review of medical records of the pregnancy, birth, and immediate postnatal period may be necessary to identify evidence of fetal anoxia or distress (e.g., Apgar scores), bilirubin levels or transfusions, sepsis, potentially ototoxic medications, and prolonged ventilatory assistance. Any history of trauma (physical or noise) and serious early childhood infection (including otomastoiditis) should be sought. Diagnostic points of interest in the family history include consanguineous relationships involving parents, grandparents, or earlier ancestors, early-onset hearing loss or use of hearing aids, use of sign language or admission to a state school or institution for the deaf, and suspected mental retardation (often confused with deafness in past decades). A history of multiple miscarriages and stillbirths could indicate a genetic disorder.

The patient's family history and the physical examination of the patient should both be reviewed for evidence of organ system anomalies and disorders associated with genetic hearing loss. Clinically significant information and findings include the following: holes, pits, or skin tags in or near the ear (branchio-oto-renal [BOR] syndrome); external ear deformity (e.g., microtia), auricular displacement, or stenosis/atresia of the external ear canal (bilateral Treacher Collins syndrome; unilateral Goldenhar complex); white forelock (Waardenburg syndrome), café-au-lait spots and peripheral neurofibromas (von Recklinghausen syndrome); cervical cysts or fistulae (BOR); previous middle ear or mastoid surgery (middle ear anomalies, otosclerosis); intracranial tumor affecting hearing or balance (e.g., neurofibromatosis); motor milestone delay, spatial disorientation in the dark, difficulty with unipedal balancing or objective evidence of vestibular deficit (e.g., Usher type I syndrome); early-onset myopia requiring corrective lenses, retinal detachment and cataracts (Stickler syndrome); congenital blindness or microphthalmia (Norrie syndrome); night blindness and retinitis pigmentosa (Usher syndrome 1 and 2); widely spaced eyes (dystopia canthorum) and heterochromia iridis (Waardenburg); lid abnormalities—coloboma and downslanting palpebral fissures (Treacher Collins syndrome); blue sclerae (osteogenesis imperfecta); optic atrophy (e.g., Cockayne syndrome); recurrent long bone fractures (osteogenesis imperfecta); abnormal fingers or toes, including web-type deformity or abnormal nails (oto-palato-digital); vertebral deformities (Wildervanck or Goldenhar syndrome); early arthritis, joint enlargement or hyperextensibility (Stickler syndrome); short stature, webbed neck and/or shield chest deformity (Turner syndrome); cleft lip or palate, as well as micrognathia (Stickler syndrome or Robin sequence); facial asymmetry (Goldenhar syndrome); lip pits or mounds (Van der Woude syndrome); nasal or facial deformities (Treacher Collins syndrome); renal anomalies or disorders, including a history of dialysis or renal transplant (BOR or Alport syndrome); euthyroid goiter apparent during first decade (Pendred syndrome); and childhood syncopal or fainting episode, or family history of sudden unexplained childhood death (Jervell and Lange-Nielsen syndrome). Ophthalmologic evaluation is essential to document visual acuity and produce findings such as retinitis pigmentosa (electroretinography).

In cases of uncertain etiology, selected laboratory studies could include a complete blood count with differential; sickle cell prep, if appropriate; routine blood chemistries expanded to include lipids, blood sugar, creatinine, blood urea nitrogen (BUN), and thyroid function tests; and urinalysis extended to renal ultrasound if evidence of kidney disease (e.g., hematuria or "red diaper") is present. Because congenital toxoplasmosis and syphilis are potentially treatable, specific serological and microbiological tests (e.g., fluorescent treponemal antibody absorption [FTA-Abs]) should be carried out if indicated. If the mother did not receive rubella vaccine before pregnancy, rubella serology or viral isolation may also be in order. Congenital cytomegalovirus infection can be confirmed by viral isolation obtained within the first few weeks of life, but perinatally or postnatally acquired infection can cloud the diagnosis, as viral shedding can begin within 8–10 weeks. Sensorineural hearing loss has been found in patients with immune mediated systemic disorders, such as Cogan syndrome (nonsyphilitic interstitial keratitis with hearing loss and vestibular dysfunction); polyarteritis nodosa; systemic lupus erythematosus; relapsing polychondritis; Behçet syndrome; and giant-cell arteritis. The role of autoimmunity in the etiology of SNHL in children is presently unclear and the cost-effectiveness of studies aimed at detecting such disease processes must be considered on a case-by-case basis.

Studies of children and adolescents with severe to profound SNHL revealed vestibular deficits in 20% or more cases.[9] Young children may not tolerate standard electronystagmography (ENG) procedures utilizing caloric irrigation, and technical modifications may be necessary to assess vestibular function. Computerized rotational testing is particularly useful for longitudinal assessment of vestibular function in children receiving potentially vestibulotoxic medications. Progressive and fluctuating SNHL should alert the clinician to a possible perilymphatic fistula (PLF). A history of mechanical stress factors such as head/ear trauma[33] or exertional activity (e.g., gymnastics) would reinforce this diagnostic possibility. A monitored fistula test may be helpful in confirming the diagnosis if positive, but a negative result is inconclusive, based on reported series.

Temporal bone imaging may identify middle ear anomalies in children with conductive or mixed losses, as well as inner ear or internal auditory canal anomalies or lesions in cases of SNHL. The relatively low yield and high cost of such studies make their uniform application questionable. Fluctuation or progression of an SNHL or consideration of cochlear implant candidacy would be indications for more aggressive use of temporal bone imaging.

### Detection and measurement of hearing loss

The pediatric audiologic team is charged with characterizing the type of hearing loss (i.e., conductive, sensorineural, or mixed); the degree of loss (i.e., mild, moderate, severe, profound, or anacusic); the audiometric configuration and symmetry; and, with serial assessment, the stability or progression of the loss. The team should be acquainted with and competent in utilization of selected components of the available techniques for detecting and measuring hearing loss.

### Otoacoustic emissions

A sensitive acoustic probe placed in the external auditory canal can detect faint acoustic energy, called *otoacoustic emissions* (OAE),[28] emanating from the inner ear itself. Outer hair cells appear to play a critical role in generating OAEs. In 30%–50% of normal ears, spontaneous otoacoustic emissions (SOAE) occur continuously in the absence of external stimulation, whereas evoked emissions (EOAE) occur with variable latency following an eliciting auditory stimulus in about 98% of normal hearing ears. Infants, children, and young adults are more likely to exhibit SOAEs than persons over 50 years of age. Spontaneous emissions are also more common in normal-hearing females than comparable males (52% vs. 30%) for reasons as yet unclear.

Transiently evoked otoacoustic emissions (TEOAE) are elicited by brief acoustic stimuli, such as clicks or tone bursts, after latencies of several milliseconds in 98% of normal hearing ears,[22] but are usually absent if hearing loss exceeds 30 dB HL. Both ears of the same individual tend to exhibit TEOAEs with similar characteristics, but TEOAEs cannot generally be detected if hearing loss is 35 dB or worse at 0.5, 1, 2, and 4 kHz and 40 dB or worse at 1 kHz.[22] Detection of TEOAEs is possible in ears with isolated retrocochlear hearing loss. Presentation of two stimuli of different frequencies will elicit distortion product otoacoustic emissions (DPOAE), comprised of frequencies distinct from the stimuli, in about 90% of normal hearing ears. The most robust DPOAE is the so-called cubic difference tone, calculated as 2F1 − F2, where F1 and F2 represent the frequencies of the two stimuli. Aspirin intake and hypoxia/anoxia can temporarily reduce or abolish SOAEs in humans but have a less dramatic, although measurable, suppressant effect on TEOAEs. In most ears with significant middle ear dysfunction, which can disrupt the transmission of OAEs, emissions would not be recordable.

Evoked otoacoustic emission measurement holds promise as a rapid and sensitive technique for infant hearing screening. Current EOAE methods can be useful in identifying the presence of high-frequency hearing loss, but do not as yet provide reliable information about hearing over a wide range of other frequencies. A screening procedure utilizing DPOAEs at 4,000 Hz can correctly identify at least 90% of ears with hearing impairment with a false alarm rate of 5%, and results are comparable at 8,000 Hz. At decreasing test frequencies, the false alarm rate increased to 15% at 2,000 Hz, 25%–60% at 1,000 Hz, and 50% at 500 Hz. At 4,000 Hz, DPOAEs or TEOAEs could identify hearing loss with about the same degree of accuracy.[22]

### Electrocochleography and auditory brainstem response

Techniques for measurement of responses from the cochlea and eighth nerve, including the summating potential (SP), cochlear microphonic (CM), and whole-nerve action potential (AP), comprise electrocochleography. Sensory cell responses within the cochlea are reflected in the CM and SP, the so-called AC and DC responses, respectively. The complex, additive combination of discharges from neurons within the auditory nerve generate the whole-nerve action potential. High quality electrocochleographic recording necessitates transtympanic promontory electrode placement, making the procedure unsuitable for mass hearing screening.

The auditory brainstem response procedure[24] employs a large number of short-duration stimuli, broadband clicks, or tone bursts, which generate electric activity detected by surface electrodes and analyzed by using computer signal averaging techniques. In most clinical situations, auditory thresholds obtained with broadband click stimuli correlate best with pure-tone behavioral thresholds in the 2,000 to 4,000 Hz region and not with thresholds at 1,000 Hz or lower. As a result, click-evoked ABR measures will fail to detect low-frequency hearing loss, especially when high-frequency hearing is normal (i.e., a rising audiometric configuration). Because most educationally significant sensorineural hearing losses involve at least these higher-frequency regions, the value of click-evoked ABR testing as a screening procedure is undiminished. Evoked potential measurements are not as inherently sensitive as behavioral audiologic techniques for definitive determination of audiologic thresholds. Children who have no click-evoked auditory brainstem responses at the upper limits of the equipment (100 dB HLn; peak sound pressure 130–136 dB) may still have measurable thresholds utilizing behavioral techniques. In one study,[10] the probability of observing either an unaided or aided behavioral response decreased as frequency increased (Fig. 7–1). Among the ears with no measurable ABR, 58% had thresholds of 100 dB hearing level (HL) or better at 250 Hz while only 12% had them at 4,000 Hz. Seventy percent of all ears had unaided speech awareness thresholds (SATs) of 100 dB or better and 45% of the ears had SATs of 50 dB or less. Click-evoked ABR accurately detected severe to profound hearing loss, permitting early (re)habilitative intervention, but it failed to distinguish between severe and profound degrees of impairment. Absence of a click-evoked ABR does not necessarily mean that the ear is anacusic, even for high frequencies. Tone burst–evoked ABRs tend to be less sensitive than behavioral thresholds by 10 to 30 dB. While EOAEs simply cannot be elicited in the presence of a 25–30 dB hearing loss, ABR thresholds, if present, do provide useful information about the degree of hearing loss, thus facilitating early intervention.

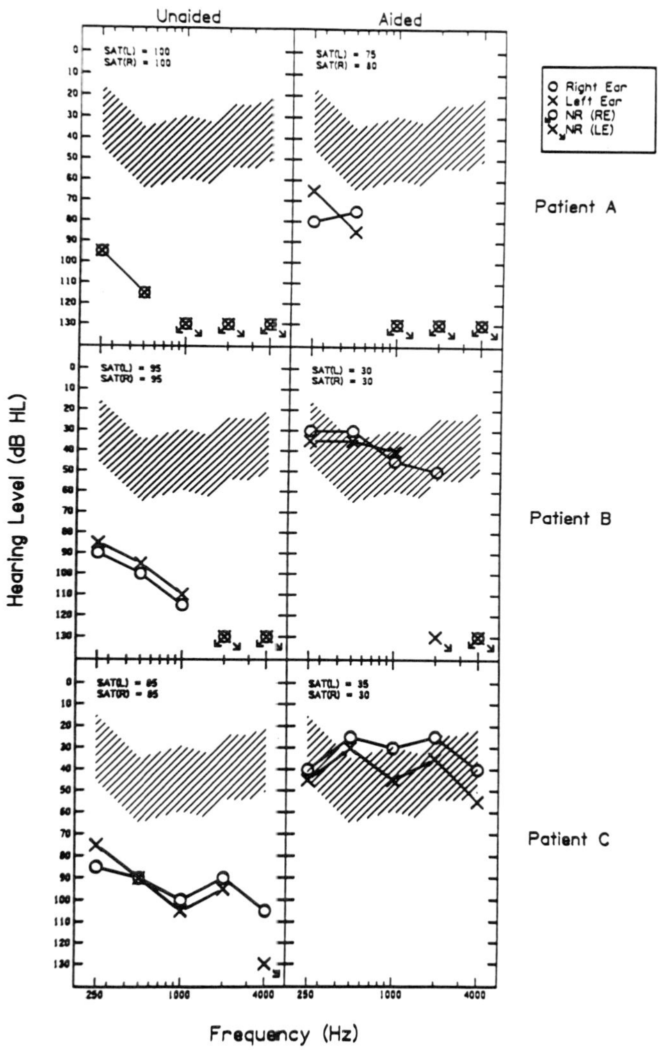


**Fig. 7–1.** Examples of unaided and aided behavioral audiograms in three children who had no click-evolved auditory brainstem responses (ABRs) at 100 dB HLn bilaterally. Speech awareness thresholds (SATs) are given in the left corner of each panel. The shaded portion in each panel represents the long-term speech spectrum converted to hearing level, including a 30 dB range that is typical speech. (Reprinted with permission from Brookhouser et al., Laryngoscope 100:803–810, 1990.[10])

## Behavioral audiologic evaluation

Evaluation of a child with suspected hearing loss is often limited as much by the clinical limitations of the examiner as the response capabilities of the child. The continued use of gross screening measures (e.g., hand-clapping, noise makers, and loud speech) to assess hearing sensitivity as a substitute for formal audiologic techniques cannot be justified. A pediatric audiologic test battery should include a comprehensive case history, acoustic emmitance measures, pure-tone thresholds, speech awareness and reception thresholds, electrophysiologic measures (if indicated), and auditory discrimination testing, utilizing speech or nonspeech signals.

Behavioral observation audiometry (BOA), which does not require conditioned or voluntary behavior, may be employed with infants under 6 months of age. The minimal sound intensity at which behavioral changes are observed (e.g., Moro response, alerting, scanning, aural-palpebral reflex, cessation of activity, increase in activity, flexion or extension of limbs, grimacing, change in sucking, or change in breathing pattern) in response to a variety of stimuli is determined. Because relatively high sound intensity levels are required to elicit an unconditioned response, only severe and profound losses can be ruled out by this technique. Rapid habituation may also occur. In visual reinforcement audiometry (VRA), visual stimuli (e.g., flashing lights, toys) serve to reinforce a child's correct head-turn response toward an auditory stimulus. Because a conditioned bond is established, habituation is slower to emerge and useful threshold information can be obtained with infants as young as 5 months (developmental age). If sound-field threshold information is obtained, it is primarily reflective of auditory acuity in the better hearing ear and unilateral losses may be missed. Ear-specific data may often be elicited even with infants utilizing small insert earphones rather than the circumaural style. Conditioned play audiometry (CPA) pairs an auditory stimulus and some play activity (e.g., putting rings on a peg, marbles in a container, or pegs in a peg board) as a reinforcer. Positive verbal encouragement from the examiner helps encourage continued participation by toddlers and preschoolers. Retarded, hyperactive, and other difficult-to-test youngsters often respond best to tangible reinforcement operant conditioning audiometry (TROCA), which employs tangible reward tokens (e.g., stickers, edible morsels, etc.). A hierarchy of materials, ranging from open-set vocabulary word lists to closed-set response tasks using pictures or objects, should be available to assess auditory discrimination in children. For children with extremely limited discrimination abilities, simple syllable recognition tests or nonspeech measures (e.g., environmental sounds, sound effects recognition) may be applicable. Accurate monitoring of threshold stability is facilitated by obtaining the maximum amount of information at each audiologic visit.

## Unilateral hearing loss

Unilateral sensorineural hearing loss (USNHL) in children has traditionally been regarded as developmentally innocuous if appropriate compensatory strategies, such as preferential classroom seating, are implemented early and consistently. Reports in the last decade,[4,11] however, suggest that early onset, severe USNHL may be associated with significant deficits in auditory and psycholinguistic skills and school performance. Otherwise normal children with USNHL appear to have a higher likelihood of experiencing academic difficulty and manifesting school behavior problems than comparable children with normal binaural hearing (Fig. 7–2).

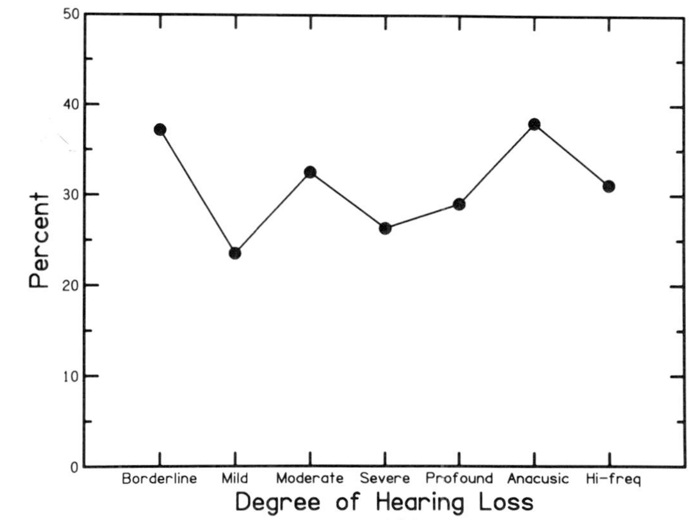


**Fig. 7–2.** Percentage of reporting school problems. (Reprinted with permission from Brookhouser et al., Laryngoscope 101:1264–1272, 1991.[11])

## Coexisting middle ear disease

### Conventional amplification

If an educationally significant hearing loss is not medically remediable, a loaner hearing aid should be fitted promptly. Over- or underamplification in young patients can be avoided by ear canal probe tube techniques for determining the intensity of sound being delivered at the level of the child's tympanic membrane. Assessing the benefit from conventional amplification is a dynamic, longitudinal process during which the interplay of multiple variables (e.g., type of aid, volume settings, auditory responsiveness, otitis media history, parental cooperation, aural rehabilitation program, and additional handicaps) must be determined. As the child wears the hearing aid and attends to soft acoustic stimuli, reliable, aided threshold information begins to emerge. Young children with sudden losses, such as postmeningitic impairments, are particularly challenging patients who require longer trial periods than older children and adults to determine the degree of aided benefit. These considerations are important for rehabilitative decisions, such as the possibility of cochlear implant candidacy.

Accurate determination of the severity and configuration of an SNHL, a requisite for fitting appropriate amplification, can be hampered by coexisting middle ear disease. A longitudinal study of preschool youngsters with bilateral sensorineural hearing losses[13] revealed that a coexisting effusion produced an average mean shift in pure-tone air conduction thresholds, as follows: thresholds were 25.0 dB at 250 Hz, 28.5 dB at 500 Hz, 29.5 dB at 1000 Hz, 24.5 dB at 2,000 Hz, and 27.5 dB at 4,000 Hz. Nine out of 10 demonstrated more than a 20 dB threshold shift at 500 Hz, 79% at 1,000 Hz, and 67% at 2,000 Hz; keep in mind that a downward shift of 20 dB could move the child's hearing loss from one category to another (e.g., moderate to severe) (Fig. 7–3, 7–4). When applying this criterion across frequencies, 67%–90% of ears shifted downward at least one category of hearing loss severity and 20% of affected ears by 40 dB or more (i.e., two hearing loss categories). Only vibrotactile responses could be obtained in 59 ears in the presence of effusion, while only 8 ears in an effusion-free condition were classified as anacusic.

Because delivery of stimuli in excess of 60–70 dB HL through a standard bone conduction vibrator will result in significant signal distortion, it is not feasible to measure residual sensorineural acuity in patients with severe to profound SNHL. Evaluation of a young child with suspected SNHL must include otologic examination, including pneumatic otoscopy, pure-tone audiometry (air and bone conduction), speech measures, and acoustic immitance testing. Electrophysiologic measures (e.g., ABR) should be obtained in infants and other difficult-to-test children. Coexisting middle ear effusions must be eliminated medically or surgically to avoid diagnostic errors and inappropriate conclusions regarding expected benefit from conventional amplification and (re)habilitative recommendations.

### Neonatal intensive care

Admission criteria for a neonatal intensive care unit (NICU) may include anoxia/hypoxia, sepsis, hyperbilirubinemia, low birth weight, dysmaturity, and orofacial anomalies, all of which are high-risk indicators for SNHL. Premature infants (birth weight less than 2,500 g) exhibit a 20-fold increase in the incidence of SNHL as compared with full-term, normal controls. As a consequence, NICU admission serves as a reliable identifier for infants needing auditory screening and follow-up.

## Selected nongenetic sensorineural hearing loss etiologies

### Viral labyrinthitis: an overview

Diverse mechanisms are involved in the replication and spread of viral infections in humans.[44] While initial replication occurs within a cell's nucleus, eventual lysis of infected cells disperses large quantities of free virus throughout the blood and lymphatic systems. Specific viruses have a predilection for invading particular cell types, such as neurons, lymphocytes, or myocardial cells. The multifaceted defense mounted by the host in response to viral invasion ranges from formation of nonspecific and viral-specific antibodies to production of specific cytotoxic lymphocytes and nonspecific immune-response mediators,

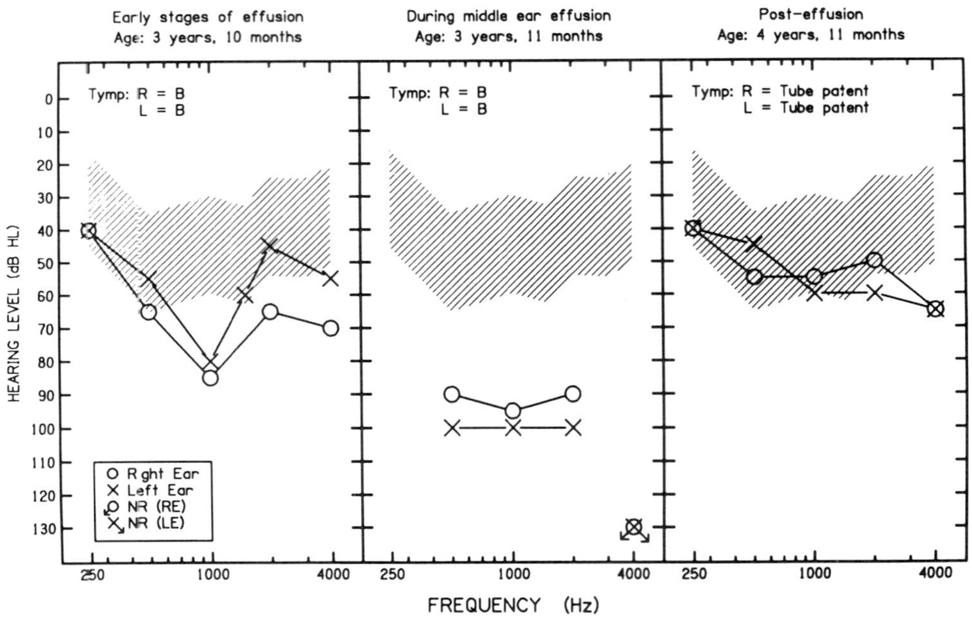


**Fig. 7–3.** Effect of a middle ear effusion on a patient with moderate sensorineural hearing loss (SNHL). (Reprinted with permission from Brookhouser et al., Laryngoscope 103:371–378, 1993.[13])

including the complement system, interferons, and lymphokines. If the virus is not eliminated, fulminant infection may ensue or alternatively, a chronic or latent (i.e., nonactive) infection may persist. Experimental evidence suggests that the body's immunologic response may actually enhance the pathogenic effect of the infection, necessitating strategies for downward modulation of the host–immune response. Molecular techniques including DNA/RNA hybridization and the polymerase chain reaction (PCR) permit detection of extremely limited quantities of viral material and determination of viral loci during latent infection.

Cytomegalovirus (CMV), rubella, mumps, and rubeola (measles) have been shown to infect the human labyrinth. In animal models, each virus demonstrates a trophism for specific cells within the inner ear. Mumps virus infects non-neuroepithelial cells found in Reissner's membrane, the stria vascularis, Hensen- and Claudius-type supporting cells, and the utricular and saccular walls. A neurotropic mumps strain has been shown to infect the spiral and vestibular ganglion neurons while sparing hair cells. Mumps-associated deafness has its onset toward the end of the first week of parotitis, gaining entry into the inner ear either during initial viremia or through direct

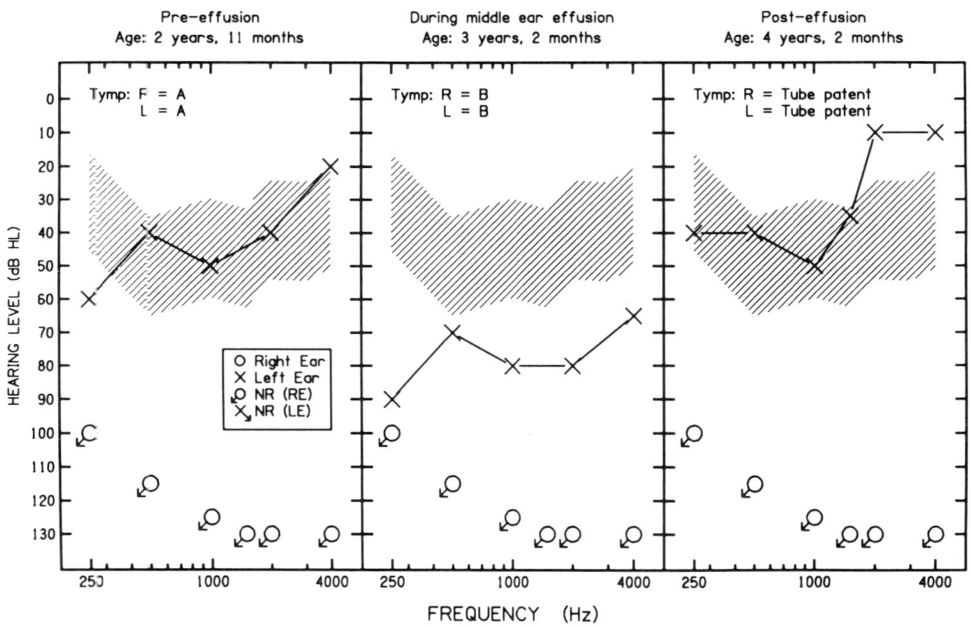


**Fig. 7–4.** Effect of middle ear effusion on audiogram of patient with asymmetrical bilateral SNHL. (Reprinted with permission from Brookhouser et al., Laryngoscope 103:371–378, 1993.[13])

spread from infected cerebrospinal fluid. Neuroepithelial structures of the cochlea, utricle, saccule, and semicircular canals, as well as spiral and vestibular ganglion cells are most likely to harbor rubeola virus. Temporal bone histopathology in such cases generally reveals sensory and neural degeneration in cochlear and vestibular organs, thickened tectorial membrane, stria vascularis atrophy, and saccular/utricular collapse. Human cytomegalovirus is most often found in endolymphatic cells and evidence indicates that the virus can persist in the inner ear, leading to delayed-onset hearing loss after years of quiescence. Human temporal bone sections in patients with CMV infection reveal classic CMV inclusions in both the cochlear and vestibular endolymphatic ducts. Neurosensory structural damage resulting from host–immune response may be as important as viral cytopathology resulting from CMV labyrinthitis.

### Anoxia/hypoxia

Placental insufficiency, umbilical cord compression, or neonatal seizures may be associated with hypoxia/anoxia during the perinatal period, as well as enhanced risk of SNHL. Objective clinical evidence of oxygen deprivation and fetal distress includes neonatal acidosis, meconium staining, primary apnea (e.g., low Apgar score at 1 and 5 minutes), resuscitation at birth, or prolonged ventilatory assistance. While the precise pathophysiologic mechanism leading to SNHL is uncertain, 20% of neonates with chronic hypoxemia secondary to persistent fetal circulation have SNHL, 75% of the losses being moderate to severe and 25%, profound.

### Hyperbilirubinemia

Neonates with elevated serum bilirubin and kernicterus have increased risk for SNHL. Decreased conjugation of bilirubin, impaired serum albumin binding, or increased unconjugated bilirubin production can produce serum levels sufficient to permit passage through the blood-brain barrier, leading to bilirubin deposition in the basal ganglia, including the ventrocochlear nucleus. Some authors suggest that "bili lights" and exchange transfusions should be employed more aggressively, while recent follow-up studies from a very large collaborative perinatal project denigrate the risk of transient neonatal hyperbilirubinemia.[35]

### Congenital cytomegalovirus infection

As much as 20%–30% of congenital deafness in the U.S.A. may be caused by congenital infection with cytomegalovirus, a member of the herpes family. Congenital CMV infection rates range from 0.5% to 1.2% of live births, making it the most common type of intrauterine infection. Additionally, 4%–10% of infants acquire CMV perinatally or postnatally as a result of cervical virus shedding, virus in breast milk, and blood transfusions. Only 10% of approximately 40,000 infants born annually with congenital CMV infection in the U.S.A. are symptomatic, and 90% of these babies suffer severe CNS sequelae, including mental retardation, severe to profound hearing loss, language or learning disorders, vision problems, and cerebral palsy by 2 years of age. These infants, who acquire cytomegalic inclusion disease (CID), typically suffer damage of both the central nervous system and the reticuloendothelial system, with hepatosplenomegaly, petechiae, and jaundice being common presenting findings. They are also prone to microcephaly, intrauterine growth retardation, and prematurity, and experience an overall mortality rate as high as 30%. Severe to profound sensorineural hearing impairment and such ocular abnormalities as chorioretinitis with optic atrophy can be documented in 25–30% of cases. More moderate sequelae occur in about 15% of asymptomatic children, although low birth weight is associated with a higher rate of congenital infection, as well as below normal head size in full-term CMV-infected infants.

The prognosis for the 90% of congenital CMV infants who are asymptomatic is much better than for symptomatic neonates, with only 10%–15% of asymptomatic infants developing significant sensorineural hearing loss, ranging from mild to profound. Fetal infection early in gestation generally results in greater involvement, with sensorineural hearing loss being the most common irreversible sequela of congenital CMV infection—30%–50% incidence in symptomatic and 10%–15% in asymptomatic infants. The SNHL is bilateral in about 50% of cases, varying in magnitude from 50–100 dB. Nearly 25% of SNHL associated with congenital CMV infection either develops or increases in severity after the first year of life.

The CMV can be transmitted in utero during either primary maternal infection or infection resulting from the reactivation of latent virus in immune women. The probability of a harmful congenital CMV infection is nine times greater among women who suffer the primary-type infection. Infants born to mothers who suffered primary CMV infection during pregnancy are at highest risk to suffer symptomatic involvement, with a transplacental transmission rate in the 25%–40% range. Pregnant women under 20 years of age from lower socioeconomic (SES) groups are particularly at risk of having symptomatic CMV babies. Expectant mothers from higher SES groups are at increased risk for seroconversion if their other infants and toddlers attend typical day care centers, where CMV seropositivity has been documented in 9%–70% of attendees, of which 50% may be shedding virus. It has been postulated that 20%–40% of congenital CMV may be day care–related.

Because as many as 95% of primary CMV cases and essentially all recurrent infections are asymptomatic, maternal seroconversion is usually necessary to document infection during pregnancy. Documentation of congenital cytomegalovirus infection necessitates isolation of the virus from infected neonates in the first few weeks of life because infants infected through perinatal or postnatal exposure generally begin to excrete virus between 3 and 12 weeks of age. Time-consuming techniques for viral isolation from urine samples may soon give way to PCR-based methods for neonatal saliva screening as early as the second day of life.[2]

### Congenital rubella infection

The sequelae of congenital rubella infection were described by Australian clinicians in the early 1940s,[14] but isolation of the rubella myxovirus in 1962 paved the way for serological and viral isolation techniques for confirming prenatal and congenital infection. An expanded rubella syndrome was described, including deafness, eye defects, congenital heart defects, microcephaly, mental and/or motor retardation, newborn hepatosplenomegaly, thrombocytopenia, radiolucencies in long bones, interstitial pneumonitis, encephalitis, and low birth weight. Among laboratory-documented cases of maternal rubella in one study population,[6] 49% were clinically apparent, while 51% were subclinical. The greatest fetal involvement resulted from first-trimester maternal infection, but deafness, microcephaly, cataracts, and mental or motor retardation were present in offspring of mothers with laboratory-confirmed second-trimester infection. Hearing loss was the most common deficit among all infants with congenital rubella infection and was the only disability in 22% of cases. Among offspring of mothers with subclinical infection, about 30% of babies had SNHL, which ranged in severity and was not always symmetrical. The most frequently observed audiometric pattern was a "cookie-bite" type audiogram with greatest loss in the mid-frequencies between 500 and 2,000 Hz. Progressive decrease in auditory acuity was documented by serial audiograms in approximately 25% of cases.

### Measles and mumps

Widespread measles and mumps immunization has decreased the incidence of these diseases in the U.S. by 90% to 95%. Prior studies revealed a common otologic sequela associated with mumps infection to be unilateral profound SNHL, often anacusis, in the absence of vertigo or vestibular impairment. Temporal bones histopathology in cases of mumps- or measles-associated deafness implicates two distinct pathogenetic mechanisms. Absent meningoencephalitis, the virus appears to access the inner ear via the striae vascularis during viremia. If meningoencephalitis occurs in conjunction with measles and mumps, histopathologic changes are similar to those noted in meningogenic bacterial labyrinthitis. The viral inflammatory process appears to extend directly along the nerves and vessels in the internal auditory canal into the inner ear.

### Congenital toxoplasmosis

The protozoan *Toxoplasma gondii* can infect a number of warm-blooded species, including humans, and members of the cat family serve as natural reservoirs for the infection, excreting oocyst-containing sporozoites in their feces. Because cats are initially infected through carnivorism, the typical house-dwelling domestic cat poses minimal risk. A recently developed antitoxoplasma vaccine for kittens has proven 84% effective at preventing oocyst excretion in animals challenged with *Toxoplasma*.[21] Humans may acquire the infection through ingestion of *Toxoplasma* cysts in undercooked meat or oocysts in food contaminated with cat feces by transplacental transmission to a developing fetus or as a transplant recipient receiving an infected donor organ. Heating to a minimum temperature of 70°C for 10 minutes or more will render *Toxoplasma*-contaminated food safe for human consumption. In some cultural groups (e.g., French) relatively undercooked meat is consumed routinely and *Toxoplasma* seroprevalence among childbearing women in France approaches 85%. In the U.S., seronegativity among women of childbearing age approaches 85%–90%, placing the vast majority at risk for primary toxoplasma infection during pregnancy. Primary infection in immunocompetent individuals may be subclinical or minimally symptomatic with fatigue, muscle spasms, and lymphadenopathy in about 10%–20% of cases. Immunosuppression through pharmacological agents or diseases, especially AIDS, permits reactivation of latent infection with diffuse organ system involvement, including life-threatening *Toxoplasma* encephalitis. Untreated mothers with primary infection run an overall 50% risk of transplacental transmission of the organism, increasing to 90% if infection occurs in the third trimester.[38] Of the estimated 3,000 infants born in the U.S. annually with congenital toxoplasmosis, approximately 5%–10% manifest severe involvement at birth. Left untreated, congenital infection can lead to serious sequelae in adolescence or early adulthood, such as sight-threatening bilateral chorioretinitis caused by intraocular cyst rupture. Hearing loss occurs in about 25% of these untreated congenital infections, with educationally significant bilateral SNHL in about 10%–15%.

Laboratory confirmation of toxoplasmosis is achieved by identifying antibodies in serum, plasma, cerebrospinal fluid, or intraocular fluid. The traditional methylene blue dye test (DT) of Sabin and Feldman[46] has recently been supplemented by an indirect fluorescent antibody test (IFA), an enzyme immunoassay (EIA), and an enzyme-linked immunosorbent assay (ELISA). Congenital toxoplasmosis is confirmed by documenting an acute maternal infection during pregnancy, coupled with detection of infection in the fetus prenatally or in the neonate. The *Toxoplasma* organism may be recovered from amniotic fluid or fetal blood and *Toxoplasma*-specific IgM antibodies can be detected in fetal serum. Cerebral calcification in the developing fetus can also be identified by ultrasonography. Diagnostic sensitivity may be enhanced by using PCR techniques which can detect even a single organism, targeting a *Toxoplasma*-specific rDNA repetitive gene. Postnatal computed tomography (CT) head scans may also reveal characteristic cerebral calcifications. Suspected cases of maternal toxoplasma infection should be treated with spiramycin until a definitive diagnosis is achieved. Confirmation of fetal involvement dictates pyrimethamine/sulfonamide combination therapy during the remainder of the pregnancy to limit fetal damage. Infected neonates should receive a pyrimethamine/sulfadiazine combination alternating with spiramycin therapy for at least 1 year.[16] Evidence crediting this treatment strategy with preventing early emergence of sensory deficits such as SNHL has been forthcoming in recent reports.

### Congenital syphilis

Transplacental passage of the *Treponema pallidum* organism after the fourth month of gestation may infect the developing fetus, leading to sequelae including the classic signs of congenital syphilitic infection: hearing loss (SNHL), interstitial keratitis, Hutchinson's teeth (notched incisors), and nasal septal perforation. Prevalence estimates for hearing loss range from 3% to 38%, with 37% of these cases presenting prior to the child's tenth birthday. In some instances, the infection may remain clinically inapparent until much later. Various degrees of hearing loss have been described in children with otosyphilis, a common pattern being a bilateral flat configuration which may be sudden in onset. Characteristic findings may also include particular impairment of speech discrimination, severe loudness recruitment, a positive fistula test (Hennebert's sign), and disequilibrium in the presence of loud sounds (Tullio's phenomenon).

Since its introduction, the fluorescent treponema antibody absorption test (FTA-Abs) has demonstrated a high degree of specificity with minimal false positivity during all stages of syphilis. The microhemagluttination assay for T-pallidum (MHA-TP) and the treponema pallidum inhibition test (TPI) are highly specific but costly alternatives for confirming the diagnosis in equivocal cases. The observation that treponema-specific tests may remain positive following an adequate treatment regimen has led to the development of a Western blot assay to detect treponema antibody isotypes.[5] While IgM and

IgG antibodies are detectable during active infection, only those of IgG type persist following successful treatment. Parenteral penicillin at adequate dosage levels to overcome the blood-CSF (cerebrospinal fluid) and blood-perilymph barriers remains the recommended treatment in nonpenicillin-allergic patients. The most recent treatment guidelines from public health agencies should be consulted regarding recommended treatment regimens for penicillin-allergic patients. Supplemental systemic corticosteroids are effective in stabilizing or improving auditory acuity, particularly speech discrimination, in approximately 50% of otosyphilitics.

### Herpes simplex encephalitis

About 25%–30% of herpes simplex encephalitis (HSE) occurs in children, and primary genital infection during pregnancy with herpes simplex type I or II may be responsible for spontaneous abortion, premature labor, CNS damage, or intrauterine growth retardation (Developmental Biology, Genetics and Teratology Branch Report, 1994).[17] The infection may spread to the developing fetus through either transplacental transmission or by ascending from infected genitalia. Approximately 1 of 2,000 newborns acquire HSV infection perinatally, with fatality rates approaching 10% and another 60% suffering severe CNS sequelae. Neonatal infection may be limited to mucocutaneous areas or may present as a disseminated infection with about a 25%–30% incidence of meningoencephalitis. Focal meningoencephalitis is detectable by electroencephalography and brain imaging studies (e.g., CT scan and MRI). Brain biopsy, which is positive in about 30%–35% of cases, remains the most reliable diagnostic method. Treatment recommendations include Acyclovir administration over a 10 to 14–day course. Sensorineural hearing loss associated with HSE has been postulated to involve central nervous system mechanisms.

### Bacterial meningitis

Effective antimicrobial agents have reduced the mortality rate for childhood bacterial meningitis from over 90% to 2%–3% for patients older than 1 month of age. *Escherichia coli* and group-B and beta-hemolytic streptococci are most often implicated in neonatal infections, whereas *Haemophilus influenzae, Neisseria meningitidis* and *Streptococcus pneumoniae* have traditionally been the most common pathogens in children 6–9 months of age. These latter three organisms are encapsulated bacteria which colonize the respiratory tract, causing both bacteremia and invasive disease. Historically, prevention strategies have included hyperimmune globulins for passive immunization during epidemic periods, treatment of high-risk patients or contacts with prophylactic antibiotics, and finally, active immunization.[31] The bacterial capsular component in *H. influenza B* (HIB) which elicits a host–immune response is a polysaccharide, a heteropolymer of ribosyribitol phosphate (i.e., PRP). In the most effective conjugated HIB vaccine, a protein carrier is covalently linked with the PRP component to elicit a long-lasting T-cell–based immune response, even in young patients, and the vaccine has been licensed for use with infants exceeding 2 months of age. In geographic areas where aggressive immunization programs among infants have been implemented, the incidence of invasive *H. influenza* disease has decreased by 90% or more.

*Neisseria meningitidis* accounts for about 20% of meningitis cases reported annually to the Centers for Disease Control and Prevention's National Bacterial Meningitis Reporting System.[40] Infants in the first year of life have the greatest susceptibility while mortality across all ages is about 10%. Meningococcal serotypes B (50%) and C (20%) account for most meningococcal meningitis in the United States and a recently developed polyvalent protein conjugate vaccine can evoke antibodies against both Groups B and C meningococcus and E. Coli K1. Clinical trials of the vaccine must precede final recommendations regarding general administration to infants and children.

*Streptococcus pneumoniae* has been responsible for about 13% of U.S. meningitis cases, an incidence of 1.2% to 2.8% per 100,000 annually. Children younger than 2 years of age have greater susceptibility and the mortality rate across all age-groups (26%) is the highest observed of the three leading pathogens. Serotypes 4, 6, 14, 18, 19, and 23 most commonly affect children in the United States. A conjugate vaccine which links pneumococcal polysaccharide with tetanus toxoid and provides increased immunogenicity in children ages 2 to 5 years has recently been developed. Unfortunately, each serotype must be conjugated individually, limiting the number that can be included in a single vaccine.

Bacterial meningitis is responsible for both immediate (e.g., seizures in 28%–40% of cases) and long-term sequelae. Twelve months following discharge from the hospital, 57% of pneumoncoccal meningitis survivors and 14.5% of those with *H. influenza* meningitis have at least one detectable handicap, such as SNHL, seizure disorders, motor abnormalities (cerebral palsy, hemiparesis, diplegia, quadriplegia, etc.), hydrocephalus, vestibular deficits, speech/language disorders, attention deficit disorder, visual impairment, and learning disabilities. Approximately 15%–20% of survivors suffer SNHL, most of which is permanent and bilateral severe to profound loss. In one series of 64 cases,[8] 38% had bilateral asymmetric SNHL while 11% exhibited unilateral losses. The hearing loss associated with meningitis has its onset early in the clinical course. Although otitis media with direct spread through labyrinthine windows may serve as a means of ingress into the inner ear, a more likely route is penetration of bacteria and bacterial toxins via the cochlear aqueduct or internal auditory canal contents, resulting in perineuritis or neuritis of the cochleovestibular nerve and/or suppurative labyrinthitis. Serous or toxic labyrinthitis, thrombophlebitis, or embolization of labyrinthine vessels and hypoxia/anoxia of the eighth nerve and central auditory pathways may also be important pathophysiologically.[34] A meningitis victim exhibiting a normal ABR after the first few days of inpatient antibiotic therapy is unlikely to develop SNHL later. In some patients, an initially abnormal ABR, probably attributable to serous labyrinthitis, may revert to normal by discharge or shortly thereafter, suggesting a resolving serous labyrinthitis. Rarely, meningitis survivors with documented mild to moderate SNHL at hospital discharge can experience some improvement over time, while more severe losses, in some children, have fluctuated for as long as a year post-hospital discharge. Well-documented late progression of post-meningitic SNHL after years of stability has been reported in a few cases. Postmeningitic sensory and neurologic sequelae may result from direct bacterial action on affected tissue and/or host inflammatory response. Tissue damage in experimental models during initial antibiotic therapy has been attributed to the inflammatory response evoked by bacterial disintegration products. Down-modulation of host inflammatory response with corticosteroids (e.g., dexamethasone) has led to a decrease in indices of meningeal inflammation at 24 hours and fewer neurologic sequelae in dexamethasone-treated patients compared to placebo controls.[39] Extensive clinical studies are underway to assess the effectiveness of this regimen in decreasing the incidence of postmeningitic hearing loss.

### Ototoxic drugs and chemicals

The Aminoglycoside class of bactericidal antibiotics, which includes streptomycin, neomycin, kanamycin, gentamicin, tobramycin, sisomycin, amikacin, lividomycin and netilmicin, can accumulate in the serum of treated patients with compromised renal status. These medications can cause nephrotoxicity, which can be reversible, and ototoxicity, which is irreversible in most cases. Streptomycin and gentamicin are primarily vestibulotoxic, while amikacin, kanamycin and neomycin are generally considered to be cochleotoxic. The toxic actions of these medications, mediated through a metabolite rather than the drug per se, can initially cause outer hair cell degeneration followed by inner hair cell damage commencing at the basal coil of the cochlea and proceeding apically. Reversible in some instances, aminoglycoside ototoxicity can also progress after cessation of therapy. Synergism between aminoglycosides and loop diuretics depends on the order of administration of the medications. If the aminoglycoside is administered following a loop diuretic, the synergism is minimized, whereas the converse order of administration produces significant synergistic effect. Permeability alterations during the administration of an aminoglycoside appears to enhance the loop diuretic's toxicity. Transplacental passage of aminoglycosides has been documented in pregnant women treated with streptomycin for tuberculosis, the blood levels in the fetus and amniotic fluid reaching approximately 50% of maternal blood levels. Because fetal susceptibility to ototoxicity is somewhat less than the mother's, overall risk of severe prenatal cochlear or vestibular damage appears to be slight.

Relative risks of ototoxicity among the aminoglycosides are as follows: gentamicin in 5% to 8.6% of cases; amikacin in 7.5% to 13.9%, tobramycin in 6.1%, and netilmicin in 2.4% of cases.[32] Because parenteral neomycin and kanamycin are highly toxic, they are restricted to topical use. Kanamycin and amikacin show greater cochleotoxicity than either gentamicin or tobramycin. Gentamicin is twice as likely to be vestibulotoxic as cochleotoxic, and the cochlear effects are reversible in about 50% of cases over a 1–week to 6–month period. Premature infants appear to be more sensitive than full-term infants to the ototoxic effects of aminoglycosides, particularly if they have a complicated perinatal course and prolonged high-dose aminoglycoside treatment. Reported incidence figures range from 0% to 36%, depending upon age, the patient population, dose duration, and specific aminoglycoside antibiotic employed. One study of infants receiving kanamycin and gentamicin during the perinatal period reported a 7% incidence of SNHL, together with delayed head and posture control in 18.6% of patients.[19] In contrast, Finitzo-Hieber et al.[20] observed only some transient auditory impairment which resolved following cessation of treatment among neonates, gestational age 27–42 weeks, who received amikacin and netilimicin in therapeutic doses. Recent evidence supports a role for mitochondrial inheritance of a predisposition toward aminoglycoside toxicity.

Ototoxic effects have been documented for the loop diuretics ethacrynic acid and furosemide, which are used to treat bronchopulmonary dysplasia. Furosemide crosses the placenta so readily that levels in the fetus may exceed maternal levels after multiple doses. Sensorineural hearing loss, which is generally reversible, has been associated with higher doses, longer duration of treatment, and concurrent aminoglycoside therapy. A prolonged drug effect has been observed in low birth weight, premature infants and standard dosage regimens may yield potentially toxic plasma levels. Ethacrynic acid inhibits the potassium pump and the adenylate cyclase system in the stria vascularis and may have a direct effect on the outer hair cells and stereocilia. While furosemide effects are rapid in onset and quickly reversible, ethacrynic acid exerts a more gradual effect on hearing, with a prolonged recovery period. Organic acid pretreatment ameliorates furosemide effects but not those produced by ethacrynic acid.

Synthetic retinoids, such as isotretinoin (Accutane),[30] administered to a mother during embryonic development can result in either spontaneous abortion or severe malformations of the central nervous, cardiovascular and respiratory systems, as well as cleft lip, cleft palate, and defects of the external ears, with or without ear canal agenesis.

Relatively high doses of the macrolide antibiotic erythromycin can be associated with SNHL, which is reversible in most cases and characteristically affects the speech frequencies.[29] While the ototoxic mechanism is unclear, observed auditory brainstem response changes suggest a central nervous system site of lesion. Erythromycin ototoxicity appears to be dose related with greater severity in patients with impaired hepatic or renal function.

### Chemotherapeutic agents

Cisplatin (cisplatinum) is a divalent platinum compound, with side effects that include a dose-limiting, high-frequency sensorineural hearing loss, peripheral neuropathy, and dose-related, cumulative renal insufficiency with tubular necrosis and interstitial nephritis. Tinnitus, which is often reversible, is present in about 7% of cases. The severity of associated SNHL depends upon the mode of drug administration, tumor site, patient's age, renal function, prior cranial irradiation, temporally related noise exposure, concurrently administered aminoglycosides and diuretics, the cumulative dose and, finally, the total dose per treatment.[42] Susceptibility to toxic effects varies among individuals, and severe hearing deterioration has been observed after a single dose. About 62% (range 11%–97%) of cisplatin-treated patients experience some ototoxicity, with bilateral SNHL occurring in most instances, although asymmetric and isolated high-frequency impairment (i.e., 4,000 and 8,000 Hz) can occur as early as 3 to 4 days after the initial dose. It appears that cisplatin ototoxicity is more severe in the pediatric population, ranging from 84% to 100%, and may be enhanced by concurrent or pretreatment cranial irradiation. High-frequency losses (40 dB or greater at 1,000 Hz and above) have been documented in nearly 50% of children receiving a standard dose of cisplatin (60 to 100 milligrams/$m^2$ per course). Losses in nearly one-third of affected children are of sufficient severity to require amplification. If a specific cisplatin dosage is spread over 6 months rather than the typical 1– or 3–month protocols, observed ototoxicity is decreased and unilateral impairment is more common with low-dose regimens. Careful audiologic monitoring at 6,000 and 8,000 Hz may provide early evidence of ototoxicity.

## Recurrent otitis media and mastoid disease

Some longitudinal studies of children with middle ear and mastoid disease suggest a higher risk of developing sensorineural loss. Animal studies of experimental otitis media confirm that round window membrane permeability permits diffusion of toxins and potentially ototoxic topical medications into the inner ear. Similar pathogenic mechanisms have been postulated in humans, but widespread clinical experience with otic drops containing potentially ototoxic drugs and chemicals in patients with nonintact tympanic membranes (e.g., perforation or patent tympanostomy tubes) without apparent sequelae confounds the issue. A protective role has been suggested for middle ear mucosal edema and granulation tissue which generally accompany otitis media.

## Ear and temporal bone trauma

Ear and temporal bone trauma can result from both penetrating and blunt injuries to the ear and skull, with or without accompanying fracture. Closed head trauma, without fracture, can damage delicate intralabyrinthine structures, resulting in tinnitus, vertigo, and SNHL, typically involving the high frequencies. Perilymphatic fistulae can also be sequalae of hearing trauma. One retrospective study of children admitted to the hospital following head trauma revealed a 7% incidence of temporal bone fracture while 13% had SNHL.[33] Among a study population of 324 children and adolescents with unilateral SNHL, 10.8% of the losses were attributed to head trauma, 35% of which occurred prior to age eight.[11]

## Perilymphatic fistula

A perilymphatic fistula (PLF) results from discontinuity in the bony/membranous enclosure which normally surrounds the perilymphatic spaces to prevent leakage of perilymph. Associated conditions and precipitating events related to PLF formation are ear surgery (stapes or chronic ear procedures), head/ear trauma, noise trauma, barotrauma, significant physical exertion, cranial or inner ear anomalies, and ossicular/middle ear deformities, particularly involving the stapes or round window. Perilymphatic fistula has been suggested as a contributing etiology for sudden, fluctuating and progressive SNHL in children by a number of authors.[23,37,43] Pathophysiologically, accumulation of air in the labyrinthine spaces may play a more important role in producing characteristic signs and symptoms than actual leakage of perilymph.

Signs and symptoms of a PLF may include aural fullness; sudden, fluctuating, and/or progressive SNHL; fluctuating speech discrimination scores; tinnitus (i.e., roaring); and balance disturbances (unsteadiness rather than true vertigo). Symptoms may be exacerbated by nose blowing, straining, valsalva maneuver, eustachian tube dysfunction, or physical exertion. Fistula tests utilizing pneumatic otoscopy or tympanometry, with or without concurrent posture platform testing, are helpful if results are positive but not exclusionary if negative. Without the benefit of pathognomonic symptoms or a reliable noninvasive technique for confirming the diagnosis of PLF, the clinician may be prompted to undertake direct inspection of the middle ear either surgically or endoscopically through a myringotomy incision, either through a tympanotomy approach or a myringotomy (e.g., with otologic endoscopes) as the definitive approach to diagnosis. Beta-2 transferrin has been advocated as a marker unique to perilymph and cerebrospinal fluid which could distinguish perliymph from other fluids present in the middle ear at surgery, such as mucus or local anesthetic solution. Clinical trials of alternative detection methods are presently underway.[3,7,41,45] The availability of sensitive and specific diagnostic tools will permit an accurate assessment of the prevalence of PLF among children with sudden, fluctuating, and/or progressive SNHL.

## Noise-induced hearing loss

Exposure to sounds of sufficient intensity and duration can result in temporary or permanent hearing loss, often accompanied by tinnitus which could impair speech discrimination enough to have an impact on performance in the classroom. A 1990 National Institutes of Health (NIH) Consensus Statement on Noise and Hearing Loss[15] addressing potentially harmful noise sources at home, on the farm, and in recreational environments places increasing numbers of unsuspecting people at risk for noise-induced hearing loss (NIHL).

Short-duration and very high sound intensity levels, 132–170 dB(A) are characteristic of impulse noises, such as gunfire or firecrackers. Infants exposed to these may sustain permanent hearing loss.[1,12]

## References


1. Axelsson A: Noise exposure in adolescents and young adults [Abstract]. NIH Consensus Development Conference on Noise and Hearing Loss, Office of Medical Applications of Research, National Institutes of Health, Bethesda, MD, January 1990, pp 22–24 and 77–82.
2. Balcarek KB, Warren W, Smith RJ, Lyon MD, Pass RF: Neonatal screening for congenital cytomegalovirus infection by detection of virus in saliva. J Infect Dis 167:1433–1436, 1993.
3. Bassiouny M, Hirsch BE, Kelly RH, Kamerer DB, Cass SP: Beta 2 transferrin application in otology. Am J Otol 13:552–555, 1992.
4. Bess FH, Klee T, Culbertson JL: Identification, assessment and management of children with unilateral sensorineual hearing loss. Ear Hear 7:43–51, 1986.
5. Birdsall HH, Baughn RE, Jenkins HA: The diagnostic dilemma of otosyphilis. A new western blot assay. Arch Otolaryngol Head Neck Surg 116:617–621, 1990.
6. Bordley JE, Brookhouser PE, Hardy J, Hardy WG: Prenatal rubella. Acta Otolaryngol 66:1–9, 1968.
7. Brookhouser, PE: Perilymphatic fistula in children. In: Common Problems in Pediatric Otolaryngology, GB Healy, ed. Year Book Medical Publishers, Chicago, 1990, pp 138–147.
8. Brookhouser PE, Auslander MC, Meskan ME: The pattern and stability of postmeningitic hearing loss in children. Laryngoscope 98:940–948, 1988.
9. Brookhouser PE, Cyr DG, Beauchaine K: Vestibular findings in the deaf and hard of hearing. Otolaryngol Head Neck Surg 90:773–777, 1982.
10. Brookhouser PE, Gorga MP, Kelly WJ: Auditory brainstem response results as predictors of behavioral auditory thresholds in severe and profound hearing impairment. Laryngoscope 100:803–810, 1990.
11. Brookhouser PE, Worthington DW, Kelly WJ: Unilateral hearing loss in children. Laryngoscope 101:1264–1272, 1991.
12. Brookhouser PE, Worthington DW, Kelly WJ: Noise-induced hearing loss in children. Laryngoscope 102:645–655, 1992.
13. Brookhouser PE, Worthington DW, Kelly WJ: Middle ear disease in young children with sensorineural hearing loss. Laryngoscope 103:371–378, 1993.
14. Carruthers DB: Congenital deaf-mutism as a sequela of a rubella-like maternal infection during pregnancy. Med J Aust 1:315–320, 1945.
15. Clark WW: Noise exposure and hearing loss from leisure activities

[Abstract]. NIH Consensus Development Conference on Noise and Hearing Loss, 22–24, Office of Medical Applications of Research, National Institutes of Health, Bethesda, MD, January 1990, pp. 55–58.
16. Daffos F, Forestier F, Capella-Pavlovsky M, Thulliez P, Aufrant C, Valenti D, Cox WL: Prenatal management of 746 pregnancies at risk for congenital toxoplasmosis. N Engl J Med 318:271–275, 1988.
17. Developmental Biology, Genetics and Teratology Branch Report to the National Advisory Child Health and Human Develpment Council. January, 1994. Bethesda, MD.
18. Early identification of hearing impairment in infants and young children. NIH Consens Statement 11:1–24, 1993.
19. Eviatar L, Eviatar A: Development of head control and vestibular responses in infants treated with aminoglycosides. Dev Med Child Neurol 24:372–379, 1982.
20. Finitzo-Hieber T, McCracken GH Jr, Brown KC: Prospective controlled evaluation of auditory function in neonates given netilmicin or amikacin. J Pediatr 106:129–136, 1985.
21. Frenkel JK, Pfefferkorn ER, Smith DD, Fishback JL: Prospective vaccine prepared from a new mutant of Toxoplasma gondii for use in cats. Am J Vet Res 52:759–63, 1991.
22. Gorga MP, Neely ST, Bergman B, Beauchaine KL, Kaminski JK, Peters J, Jesteadt W: Otoacoustic emissions from normal-hearing and hearing-impaired subjects: distortion product respones. J Acoust Soc Am 93:2050–2060, 1993.
23. Grundfast KM, Bluestone CD: Sudden or fluctuating hearing loss and vertigo in children due to perilymph fistula. Ann Otol Rhinol Laryngol 87:761–771, 1978.
24. Jewett DL, Williston JS: Auditory evoked far fields averaged from the scalp of humans. Brain 94:681–696, 1971.
25. Joint Committee on Infant Hearing: 1982 position statement. ASHA 24: 1017–1018, 1982
26. Joint Committee on Infant Hearing: 1990 position statement. ASHA 33:3–6, 1991.
27. Joint Committee on Infant Hearing: 1994 position statement. ASHA 36:38–41, 1994.
28. Kemp DT: Stimulated acoustic emissions from within the human auditory system. J Acoust Soc Am 64:1386–1391, 1978.
29. Kroboth PD, McNeil MA, Kreeger A, Dominguez J, Rault R: Hearing loss and erythromycin pharmacokinetics in a patient receiving hemodialysis. Arch Inter Med 143:1263–1265, 1983.
30. Lammer EJ, Chen DT, Hoar RM, Agnish ND, Benke PJ, Braun JT, Curry CJ, Fernhoff PM, Grix AW Jr, Lott IT, et al: Retinoic acid embryopathy. N Engl J Med 313:837–841, 1985.
31. Lieberman JM, Greenberg DP, Ward JI: Prevention of bacterial meningitis—vaccines and chemoprophylaxis. Infect Dis Clin North Am 4:703–729, 1990.
32. Matz GJ: Aminoglycoside cochlear ototoxicity. Otolaryngol Clin North Am 26:705–712, 1993.
33. McGuirt WF Jr, Stool SE: Temporal bone fractures in children: a review with emphasis on long-term sequelae. Clin Pediatr 31:12–18, 1992.
34. Nadol JB Jr: Hearing loss. N Engl J Med 329:1092–1102, 1993.
35. Newman TB, Klebanoff MA: Neonatal hyperbilirubinemia and long-term outcome: another look at the collaborative perinatal project. Pediatrics 92:651–657, 1993.
36. Noise and hearing loss. NIH Consensus Statement 8:3–20, 1990.
37. Parnes LS, McCabe BF: Perilymph fistula: an important cause of deafness and dizziness in children. Pediatrics 80:524–528, 1987.
38. Remington JS: The tragedy of toxoplasmosis. Pediatr Infect Dis J 9:762–763, 1990.
39. Schaad UB, Lips U, Gnehm HE, Blumberg A, Heinzer I, Wedgwood J: Dexamethasone therapy for bacterial meningitis in children. Swiss Meningitis Study Group. Lancet 342:457–461, 1993.
40. Schlech WF 3rd, Ward JI, Band JD, Hightower A, Fraser DW, Broome CV: Bacterial meningitis in the United States, 1978 through 1981. The National Bacterial Meningitis Surveillance Study. JAMA 253:1749–1754, 1985.
41. Skedros DG, Cass SP, Hirsch BE, Kelly RH: Sources of error in the use of beta-2 transferrin analysis for diagnosing perilymphatic and cerebral spinal fluid leaks. Otolaryngol Head Neck Surg 109:861–864, 1993.
42. Strauss M, Towfighi J, Lord S, Lipton A, Harvey HA, Brown B: Cisplatinum ototoxicity: clinical experience and temporal bone histopathology. Laryngoscope 93:1544–1549, 1983.
43. Supance JS, Bluestone CD: Perilymph fistulas in infants and children. Otolaryngol Head Neck Surg 91:663–671, 1983.
44. Tinghitella TJ: Pathogenesis of viral infections: the role of the immune response. Am J Otolaryngol 11:309–312, 1990.
45. Weber PC, Kelly RH, Bluestone CD, Bassiouny M: Beta 2–transferrin confirms perilymphatic fistula in children. Otolaryngol Head Neck Surg 110:381–386, 1994.
46. Wilson M, McAuley JB: Laboratory diagnosis of toxoplasmosis. Clin Laborat Med 11:923–939, 1991.

# 8

# Congenital Anomalies of the Pinna: Surgical Management

KANT Y.K. LIN and THOMAS J. GAMPPER

The surgical correction of congenital anomalies of the pinna has evolved from techniques first developed for the correction and reconstruction of traumatic auricular injuries. The Susruta Samhita, an ancient Indian textbook of medicine believed to have been written around 900 B.C., describes a partial reconstruction of an earlobe injury using a cheek flap.[4] Tagliacozzi (1597) described transferring a flap from the arm of a monk to reconstruct his defective auricle.[25] Dieffenbach (1845) reconstructed an ear that had been partially severed following a sword injury, by fashioning a flap of skin from the mastoid region.[13] Pierce (1930) and Gillies (1937) were the first to demonstrate successful auricular reconstruction using cartilage grafts to provide the rigid framework of the ear.[24,54] Since then, various types and combinations of homografts, heterografts, and prosthetic materials have been used in seeking the ideal reconstructive framework. With demonstrably poor long-term outcomes using alloplastic materials it has now become generally accepted that native cartilage offers the best hope for a stable long-term result.[11,12,22,38,58,62] In a series of landmark papers on total ear reconstruction using autologous costal cartilage grafts, Tanzer (1959), initiated the modern period of ear reconstruction.[67,68] Brent (1992) reviewed his own personal experience for the past 20 years of over 600 ear reconstructions with excellent results.[6]

## External anatomy of the ear

Details of the external anatomy of the ear are dictated by a highly complex and intricate cartilaginous framework, which in turn is enclosed by a thin and extremely pliable cutaneous cover. Topographic landmarks are illustrated in Figure 8–1. Overall size, position, and orientation of the ear on the side of the head are as important in auricular reconstruction as are the fine intrinsic details of the framework. Typically, the auricle or pinna lies between horizontal lines drawn from the superior orbital rim and the nasal spine.[2] The distance from the lateral orbital rim to the root of the helix is equal to the vertical height of the ear.[18] The framework protrudes a variable distance from the mastoid bone—depending on which portion of the outer helical rim is measured, 20–22mm at the top, 16–18mm in the midportion, and 10–12mm in the lower third, with an angle of protrusion ranging from 21 to 25 degrees.[1,3]

The longitudinal or vertical axis of the ear is posteriorly inclined at an average angle of 25 degrees, with a standard deviation of 6 degrees.[18] Contrary to earlier beliefs, the angle between the long axis of the ear and the bridge of the nose is not parallel, but in fact, varies on the average by roughly 15 degrees.[60]

There are six intrinsic and three extrinsic muscles of the ear, but all are vestigial in nature. The sensory nerve supply to the ear has its main source from the great auricular nerve (C2,C3), which lies in the plane just beneath the platysma and superficial to the external jugular vein. The nerve courses from behind the posterior border of the sternocleidomastoid muscle and ascends superiorly toward the auricle, where it provides sensation to the inferior portion of the ear. The superior surface is supplied by the lesser occipital nerve and the auriculotemporal nerve, which also serves to supply the entire tympanic membrane. The concha and external auditory canal are innervated by Arnold's nerve, an auricular branch of the vagus.

A rich vascular arterial network surrounds the ear and is comprised of branches from the posterior auricular artery, which arises from the external carotid, and the superficial temporal. Venous outflow is through auricular veins emptying into the external jugular, superficial temporal, and posterior facial veins. Draining lymphatic basins are divided with the cranial surface and external auditory canal emptying into the mastoid and infra-auricular lymph nodes, and the concha and meatus into the pre- and infra-auricular nodes.

When performing surgery on the infant or child, it is important to be aware of the unusual course of the facial nerve as it exits the stylomastoid foramen, to avoid inadvertent transection. Because of the lack of early pneumatization of the mastoid, the nerve lies in a much higher and more horizontal position than in the adult. It is only with the development of the mastoid air cells that the nerve is pushed inferiorly and deep to the mastoid process where it becomes more protected and less prone to iatrogenic injury.

## Etiology

### Genetic considerations

A review of the literature reveals strong evidence for hereditary transmission of congenital anomalies of the pinna. Preauricular pits, fistulae, appendages, cupping deformities, and deafness have been reported to exhibit both autosomal dominant and recessive inheritance patterns.[47,73] In a review of over several hundred patients with ear deformities, Rogers demonstrated that morphologic, anatomic, and genetic interrelationships exist between microtia and constricted and protruding ears. He hypothesized that these entities represented different points on a continuum, and that variable expression of a defective gene was responsible for the different morphologic manifestations.[55] In another study of 96 families with 171 microtia patients, the authors excluded chromosomal aberration as the sole cause of the deformity and instead concluded that the etiology must be multifactorial, with a 5.7% risk of recurrence.[64]

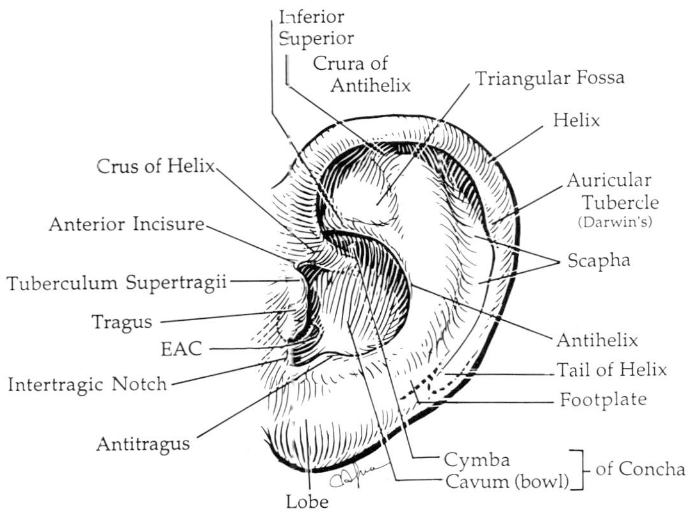


**Fig. 8–1** Important surface anatomical landmarks of the lateral surface of the pinna.

### Environmental considerations

In utero obliteration of the stapedial artery,[44] intrauterine infection with rubella, and exposure to specific teratogenic drugs such as thalidomide during the first trimester of pregnancy have all been implicated as possible causal factors in the occurrence of deafness and deformities of the pinna.[5]

## Classification

Congenital anomalies of the pinna are generally classified into three groups: (1) microtia; (2) constricted ears; and (3) prominent ears. Within each group, various sub-classifications have been developed, which will be discussed along with each individual anomaly.

### Microtia

#### General considerations

*Microtia* refers to a spectrum of congenital auricular size and shape deformities varying from the complete absence of ear tissue to a near normal but small ear with an atretic canal. Because of the wide range of variations encountered, microtia represents one of the greatest challenges to the reconstructive surgeon. Complete absence of the ear, or anotia, is extremely rare and is thought to result from the complete failure of development of the helix through a lack of mesenchymal proliferation.[45] The most common variant of microtia is a vertically oriented, sausage-like remnant with varying amounts of skin and cartilage.[5] The overall incidence of microtia varies with the extent of the deformity and between ethnic groups, with the more significant deformities occuring in 1:7,000 to 1:8,000 births in the Western world[27,32] and becoming as frequent as 1:4,000 births in Japan.[64] Ogino found that more males were affected than females by a ratio of 2:1,[51] and Tanzer found an even greater sex disparity in his series with a ratio of 3:1.[70] Dupertuis and Musgrave noted that the right side was affected twice as often as the left and that there was bilateral involvment in 10% of cases.[14]

Microtia can occur both as a sporadic, isolated event and as an inherited condition. It has been noted to be associated with several craniofacial syndromes. A review of Tanzer's series demonstrated that 50% of his patients with microtia had overt evidence of the first and second branchial arch syndrome.[70] Gorlin has grouped the wide variety of anomalies seen with branchial arch deformities under a broad classification term, the *oculo-auriculo-vertebral* (OAV) spectrum, which encompasses such diverse syndromes as Goldenhar's, hemifacial microsomia, unilateral mandibulofacial dysostosis, and acrofacial dysostosis.[26] Some authors have suggested that unilateral microtia or an ear abnormality such as an accessory tag, is the mandatory feature within this spectrum.[56]

Controversy exists as to whether there is a correlation between the severity of the external ear defect and the degree of middle ear deformity. Schuknecht found no correlation[59], yet all of Tanzer's patients had some deformity of the ear canal, middle ear, or both.[70] It is known that the external ear is formed at an earlier embryologic stage than the middle ear, and depending upon the timing of the disrupting event, it could theoretically be possible to have a normal outer ear associated with an abnormal middle ear. On the other hand, it is unlikely to have microtia with a normal middle ear. This is borne out with clinical observations.[8] Cole and Jahrsdoerfer recommend that these patients require the services of both a plastic surgeon and an otologist, to maximize efforts in achieving both a cosmetic and functionally successful reconstruction.[8] All of these patients require a thorough physical examination, conventional audiologic response testing, an auditory brain stem response (ABR) to differentiate conductive loss from sensorineural hearing loss, and a high resolution computed tomography (CT) scan of the temporal bone. A detailed discussion of surgery for atresia is beyond the scope of this chapter.

#### Classification

Several broad classification systems have been proposed encompassing the full spectrum of external pinna deformities ranging from anotia and microtia to prominent ears.[55,69] A classification system involving only variants of microtia was proposed by Marx (Table 8–1, Fig. 8–2a–c) and is most commonly used today.[40]

#### Surgical timing

The "foundation" of auricular reconstruction is the cartilage framework, most frequently obtained as a free graft from costal cartilage. Others have advocated the use of alloplastic materials such as silastic, but follow-up has revealed poor long-term results with materials other than autogenous cartilage.[11,12,22,38,58,62] With this in mind, critical considerations in the timing of ear reconstruction are (1) the rate at which costal cartilage develops; (2)correspondence between the size of the fabricated framework and the contralateral normal growing ear;

**Table 8–1.** Clinical classification of microtia[40]

| | |
|---|---|
| I. | Auricle is small; different structures of each part of ear are recognizable. |
| II. | Ear is smaller than normal; auricular remnant retains some structural resemblance to a helix in its configuration. |
| III. | Auricular configuration absent; only a narrow remnant or irregular ridge of tissue is present. |

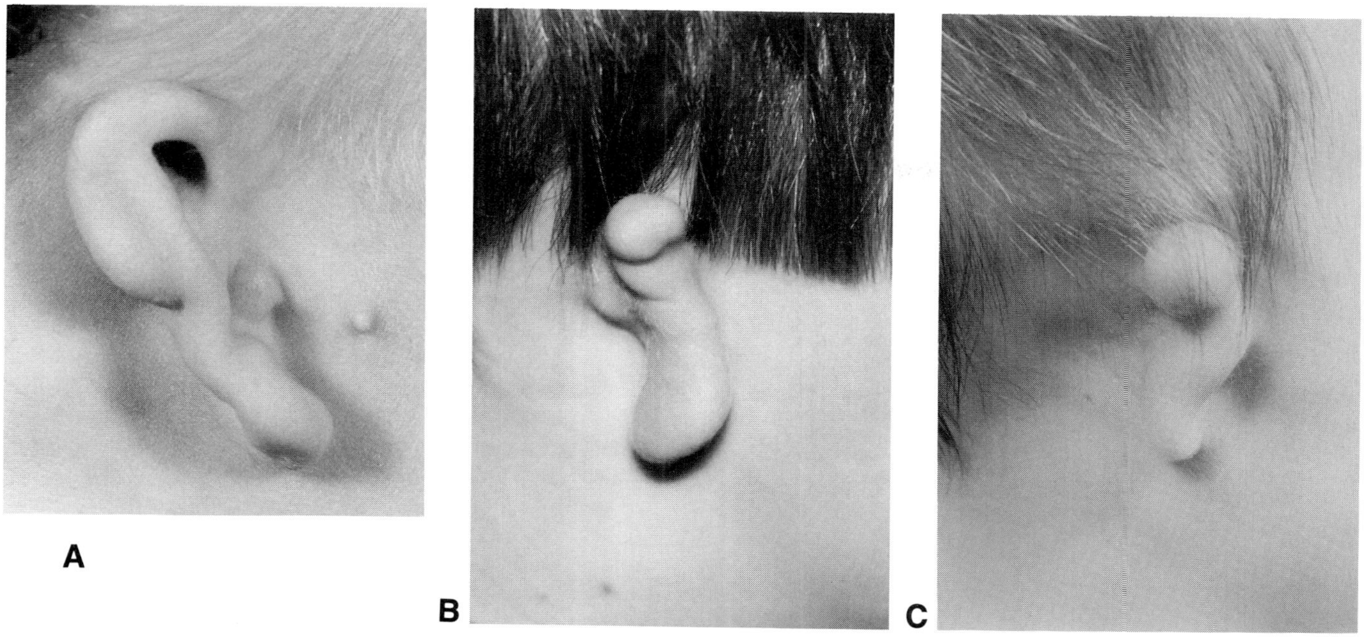

**Fig. 8–2.** Marx's classification scheme for microtia. A: Class 1 deformity; B: class 2 deformity; C: class 3 deformity.

and (3) risk to the child of exposure to psychological trauma.[39] Studies have shown that body image relating to the face develops between 4 and 5 years of age.[36] Brent states that in his series of over 400 patients with microtia, psychological disturbances "rarely began before age 7 years."[5] There is general consensus that the reconstruction should be undertaken prior to this age and usually prior to introduction of the child to his peers at school, i.e, at age 5 to 6 years.[5,21,52,57] Farkas has shown that by age 6, the normal ear will have grown to within 6 to 7 mm of its full vertical height,[18] which would allow for a reasonable reconstruction at that age with proper symmetry. Although the normal ear will continue to grow, studies have now shown that the reconstructed framework can itself grow with time and can even outgrow the opposite normal ear.[6,70] There is some difference of opinion whether overcorrection of the fabricated framework is necessary, or whether a one-to-one match in size is all that is necessary.[71] Finally, by the age of 5, most children will have enough costal cartilage from consecutive ribs to construct a full auricular framework.[6,57]

### Surgical sequence

Many different surgical protocols have been described,[6,7,21,50,70] but in essence, involve four separate events: (1) framework harvest, construction, and implanatation; (2) framework elevation; (3) lobule construction and rotation; and (4) tragal construction and conchal refinement. These different protocols involve various combinations of the separate events into two or three surgical procedures to accomplish the full reconstruction. The otologist will typically undertake middle ear reconstruction only after the final work has been completed on the pinna.

We will briefly outline the protocol used in the plastic surgery clinics at the University of Virginia.

*First stage.* As previously discussed, the location and orientation of the ear with respect to facial planes, and symmetry with the contralateral ear, are paramount. In unilateral microtia, the normal ear's outline is traced onto a piece of clear roentgenographic film along with its position relative to the patient's nose, lateral canthus, and eyebrow. The film is then sterilized, and when reversed, can be used intraoperatively as a template to locate the proper site for the framework. In bilateral microtia, knowledge of proper ear positioning with respect to other fixed landmarks of the head, and careful attention to creating symmetry, will guide the reconstruction.

An appreciation of the finest details in any fabricated framework will be lost if it is covered by a thick and nonpliant skin covering. The best skin available for coverage, in terms of pliability, thinness, color and texture match, and elasticity is usually that which surrounds the ear remnant. Preliminary procedures which would cause the formation of scar tissue in this skin should be avoided. The first stage in our protocol entails harvesting the costal cartilage, framework fabrication, and implantation into a virginal subcutaneous pocket at the desired new ear position. Careful dissection of the pocket is crucial to the success of the entire reconstruction and is carried out just beneath the subdermal plexus. Often, the roots of the hair follicles in the postauricular region will be visible during the skin elevation. The pocket should be widely undermined, extending at least 2 cm beyond the margins of the framework in the superior, inferior, and posterior directions. Meticulous hemostasis should be sought.

The cartilage can be harvested simultaneously by a second surgical team. The framework is created from the synchondrosis at the sternal junction of the sixth and seventh ribs. The helical rim is created from a separate piece of cartilage usually harvested from the first free-floating rib (Fig. 8–3). Brent emphasizes two aspects of the harvest: (1) the rib cartilage should be harvested from the contralateral chest wall in order to take advantage of the natural curve in the cartilage to match the ear contour, and (2) the dissection should take place in the extraperichondrial plane in order to obtain an unmarred specimen.[6] The framework is then fabricated at a separate side table while the chest wound is closed.

Sculpturing the framework requires artistic skill and an

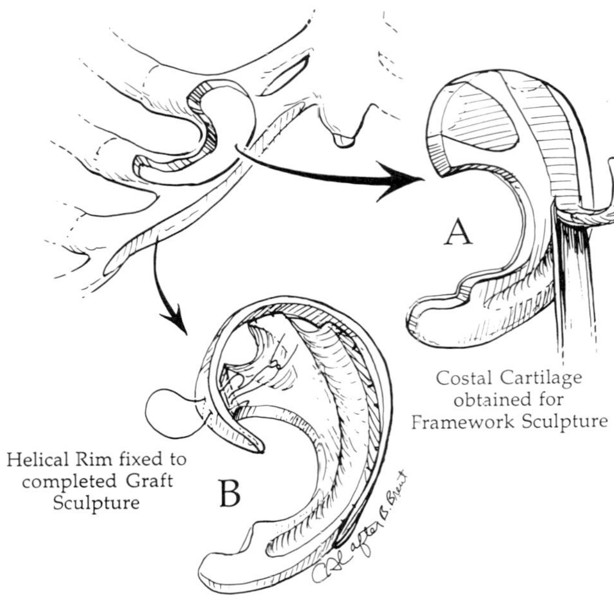


**Fig. 8–3.** Method of costal cartilage harvest for framework reconstruction.

appreciation for proportions which can only be developed through practice. Novices may need to practice carving (a raw potato is ideal for this) before the actual surgery in order to gain an appreciation of the delicacy required for this part of the procedure. Only hand-held instruments should be used, a rounded wood-chisel being the ideal tool, to create the intricate sulci and prominences of the pinna. Power-driven tools should be avoided as they generate heat, which could destroy the chondrocytes. After appropriate shaping, the separate helical rim is attached to the rest of the framework with clear nylon sutures (Fig. 8–4) An important aspect of the sculpturing is the final height or lateral projection of the framework. Brent emphasizes maximizing this projection by affixing the terminal helix on top of the main cartilage block along its posterior border.[6] Because of the degree of projection he is able to achieve, Brent does not usually need a second procedure to elevate the framework from the side of the head. We have found this to be more problematic, as increased projection can cause the already thin periauricular skin flaps to become ischemic. We choose instead to elevate the framework at a second stage by inserting an additional cartilage wedge behind the main framework, while simultaneously recreating the postauricular sulcus.

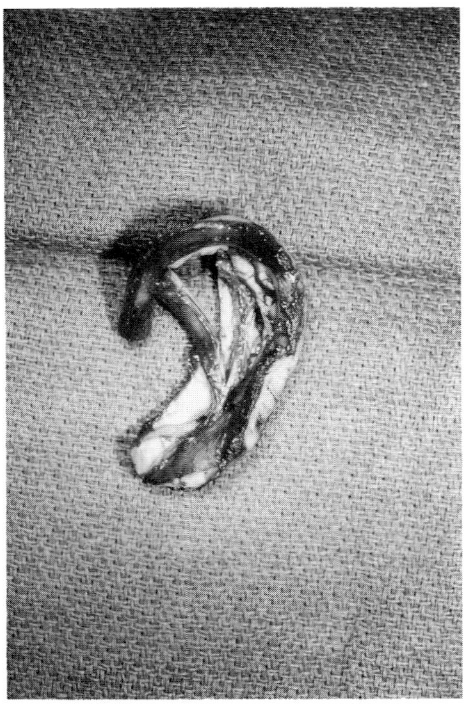

**Fig. 8–4.** A left ear framework sculptured from costal cartilage.

Once the cartilage is adequately shaped, it is inserted into the subcutaneous pocket. Tanzer's principle of an anterior incision followed by centrifugal skin relaxation is utilized, which allows for the use of more hairless skin cover and preserves the circulation to the helical border by avoiding any incisions in that region.[67] Once the correct position has been achieved, the underside of the framework is anchored to the temporoparietal fascia with a long-lasting absorbable suture to prevent displacement. A mini-flap silicone catheter drain is always used to allow for close coaptation of the skin to the cartilage framework postoperatively. Bolster sutures are avoided to prevent ischemia of the skin flap. A special donut-type dressing is fabricated before the patient is awakened from anesthesia. Thick wads of cotton are used to create a circumferential pad, so that the ear sits isolated within the "donut hole." The entire head, along with the cotton pad, is then wrapped with gauze wraps and adhesive tape, while the hole in the pad is left open (Fig. 8–5) A generous coating of topical antibiotic salve is then applied to the ear and incision line, and the hole is covered with $4 \times 4$ gauze sponges to create a window flap. Frequent inspection postoperatively can be achieved by removing the $4 \times 4$ sponges without having to remove the entire head dressing. Postoperative chest roentgenogram and intravenous antibiotics until the drain is removed are part of the postoperative routine. We believe in maintaining the suction drain for at least 4 days to allow full coaptation and to prevent seroma formation, regardless of earlier cessation of drainage. Following drain removal, the entire head dressing is removed, and a custom-fitted ear guard is fashioned and secured with velcro straps. The patients wear their guard continuously for 2 weeks and then only at night for another 2 weeks. Activity restrictions apply for 4 to 6 weeks.

*Second stage*. Goals to be accomplished in this stage include: (1) lobule transposition, and (2) framework elevation. Even in the most severe cases of microtia, there is almost always a lobule remnant found. If present, it is typically sausage-shaped and oriented vertically, rather than horizontally. Transposition is achieved through a z-plasty of unequal flaps, with the lobule being based on a narrow inferior pedicle.[70] If the lobule is totally absent, Converse described a method of elevating a lobule-shaped flap at the desired position from the skin inferior to the framework, designed one-third oversize, and covering the posterior surface with a full-thickness skin graft.[9]

Framework elevation is begun with an incision parallel to the posterior border of the ear immediately behind the helical rim. The dissection is carried out posteriorly in the subdermal plane to create a thin flap of hair bearing skin. It is of paramount importance to preserve the underlying temporoparietal fascia in this dissection. An anteriorly based fascial banner flap is then

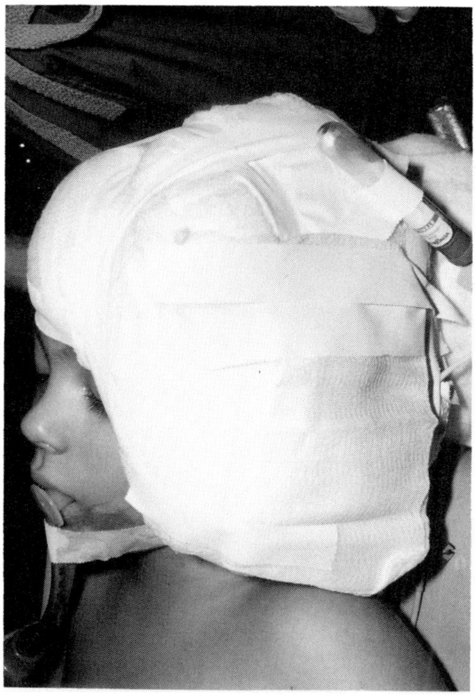

**Fig. 8–5.** Postoperative head dressing used to protect the reconstructed ear. There is a window on the side covered with a gauze sponge that allows easy access and viewing of the new ear. A vacuum test tube connected to a mini-flap drain is used for drainage.

raised in a posterior-to-anterior direction off the deep temporal fascia, the length of which approximates the anticipated vertical height of the framework. The length should be such that it would allow for this flap to be folded onto itself to cover the posterior and undersurface of the framework once it is elevated. After this fascial flap has been raised, the undersurface of the framework is exposed and elevated from the side of the head. A wedge of cartilage (usually an extra piece of costal cartilage harvested at the first stage and stored or "banked" as an extension of the inferior framework) is then wedged and secured with nonabsorbable, clear sutures behind the framework to maintain the newly elevated position. The fascial banner flap is then folded back onto itself to cover all of the exposed posterior framework cartilage, thus providing a vascularized bed to support a skin graft. A full-thickness skin graft harvested from the groin is then bolstered onto the fascial flap to complete the procedure. Similar postoperative methods are used in the second stage, including suction drainage and full head dressings (Fig. 8–6a–f).

*Third stage.* Goals of this stage include (1) tragal construction, and (2) conchal bowl excavation. Kirkham has described a method where a U-shaped, anteriorly based skin flap is raised at the proposed tragal site.[34] This skin flap is then folded back onto itself and secured with mattress sutures to create the new tragus. A full-thickness skin graft is placed onto the hollowed-out donor site which recreates the posterior wall of the conchal bowl. Brent accomplishes both goals in a single procedure, by inserting an arched composite chondrocutaneous graft, harvested from the anterolateral conchal surface of the normal ear, through a J-shaped incision in the conchal region.[5] Excess soft tissue beneath the tragal flap is excised to deepen the conchal bowl.

### Complications

With what is perhaps the world's largest experience, Brent recently reviewed his complications in 606 patients who have undergone microtia repair[6] and found that the most common complications related to the cartilage harvest was pneumothorax and atelectasis. Pneumothoraces resulted from violation of the pleura which allowed air to enter the thoracic cavity, and was not due to lung parenchymal injury. This can be readily treated with catheter aspiration of the air and closure of the pleural lining. Atelectasis was usually secondary to postoperative splinting from pain and is preventable with adequate analgesia and aggressive pulmonary toilet. The total complication rate for the newly reconstructed ear in his series was 1.6%, with 0.5% infection, 0.3% hematoma, and 0.8% skin loss with cartilage exposure. Brent felt that his complications occured early in his experience and decreased as his technique improved, and that most were preventable. Fukuda reported on his series of 500 reconstructions and noted a 4% infection rate, a 2% incidence of keloid formation, and a nearly 10% incidence of exposure of the wire used to connect the parts of the auricular framework.[21] Tanzer also mentions a significant incidence of wire exposure in his series,[70] which has lead to his abandonment of this material and instead to using nonabsorbable clear nylon sutures as utilized at the University of Virginia.

### Tissue expansion

Expansion of insufficient glabrous skin to provide coverage of auricular frameworks has been described in the repair of microtia.[3,53] In theory, this technique has the advantage over conventional treatments in providing donor skin that is virtually the same color, texture, and sensation as the recipient site, as well as being hairless, and in obviating the need for additional skin harvest and grafting. The total number of stages in the reconstruction, however, may be increased, as well as requiring more outpatient visits as the expansion takes place. Tanino and Miyasaka have reviewed their 10–year experience in 35 patients where tissue expansion was used.[66] Using a rectangular Radovan type expander, with a total expansion time of 3 months, their reconstruction consisted of 4 separate stages. Removal of the expander capsule is advocated to obtain the most extensible skin possible. A special silicone rubber splint is constructed and placed over the expanded skin after the framework has been inserted in an effort to retain internal details of the framework. In an average follow-up time of 8.7 years of their 35 patients, they had 14 with excellent, 12 with good, and 8 with poor contour. One patient's reconstruction was totally lost due to framework infection. Due to the high rate of expander exposure (14%), partial flap necrosis leading to cartilage framework exposure (11%), and poor ear contour (23%) in their series, the authors conclude that this technique is still under investigation.

### Osseointegrated implants

With advancements in rubber technology, it is now possible to construct an auricular prosthesis so life-like as to be indistinguishable, both in appearance and in texture, from the real ear. The idea of using external prostheses has been long considered and attempted in cases of severe or complete microtia, but success has been limited by problems of prosthesis retention. Tjellström has described his group's attempts over

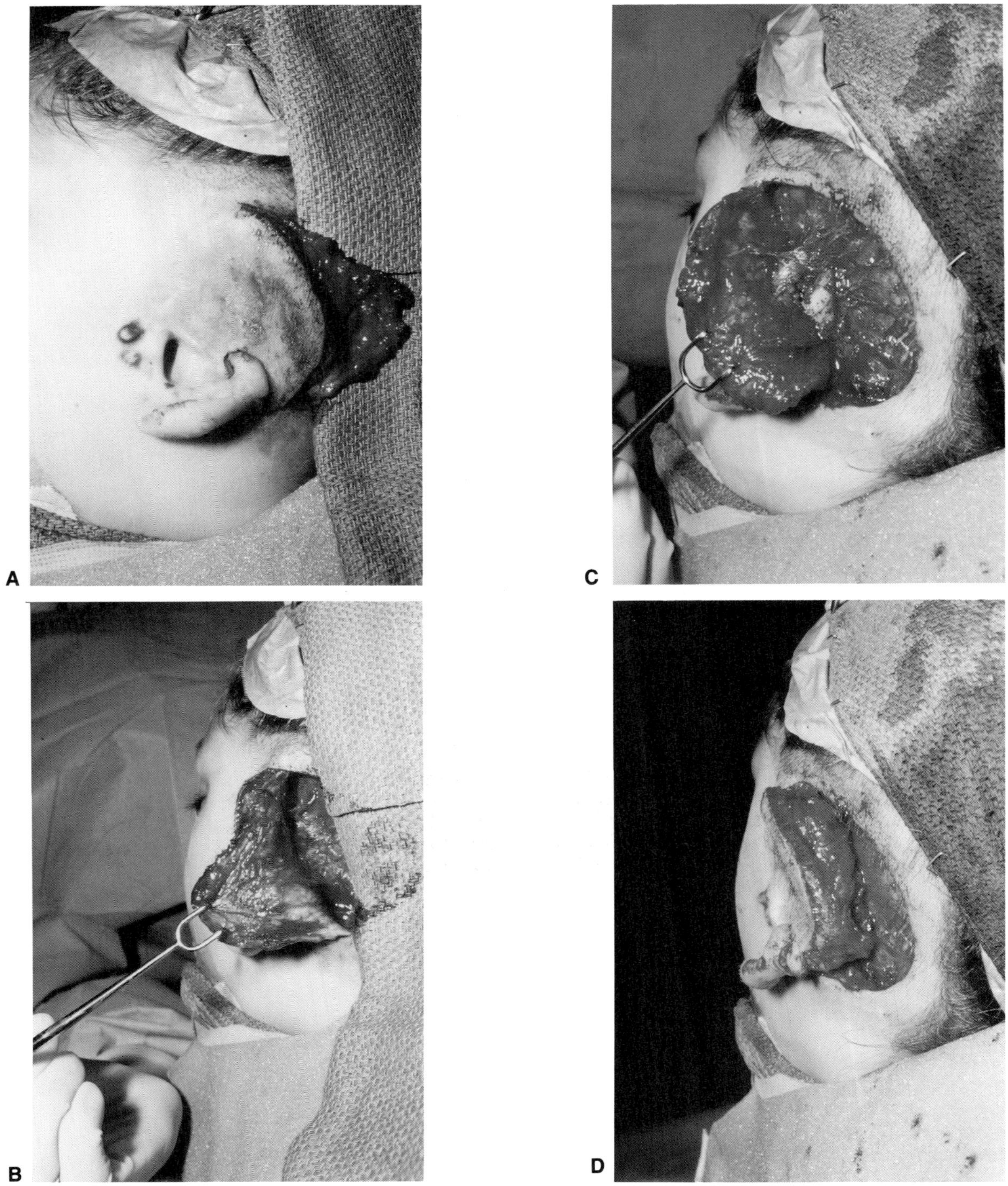

**Fig. 8–6.** Second stage ear reconstruction. A,B: Dissection of anterior-based superficial temporal fascia fan flap. C: Placement of additional cartilaginous wedge (center) behind framework for additional projection. D: Folding the fascial flap onto itself to cover the cartilage wedge. E: Placement of split thickness skin graft to create new postauricular sulcus. F: Bolster in place to stent postauricular skin graft.

the past 10 years in using osseointegrated implants as a method to secure the prosthesis, with impressive results.[72] Of 94 treated patients, only 2 were not using their implants at long-term follow-up. Autogenous tissue should always be the preferred method of reconstruction for best results in terms of growth and long-term durability. However, in certain selected cases, particularly in post-traumatic adult patients who may not tolerate multiple staged procedures, prosthetic implants may provide a reasonable alternative in total ear reconstruction.

## The constricted ear

Tanzer coined the term *constricted ear* to describe one where the rim of the ear had been tightened "as if by a purse string."[69] Other descriptive terms used to describe this group

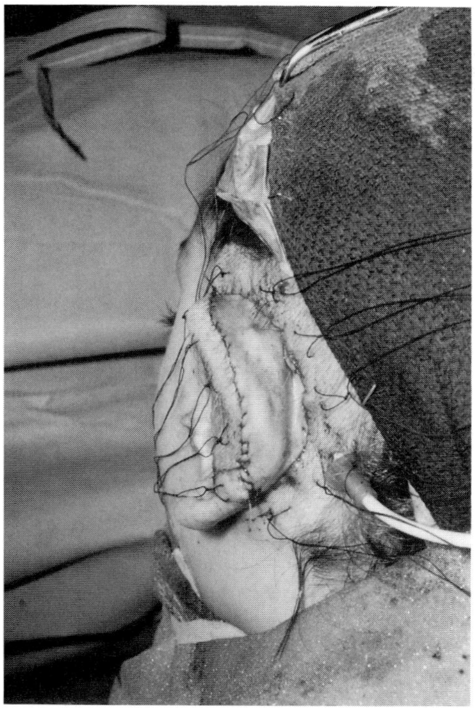

E

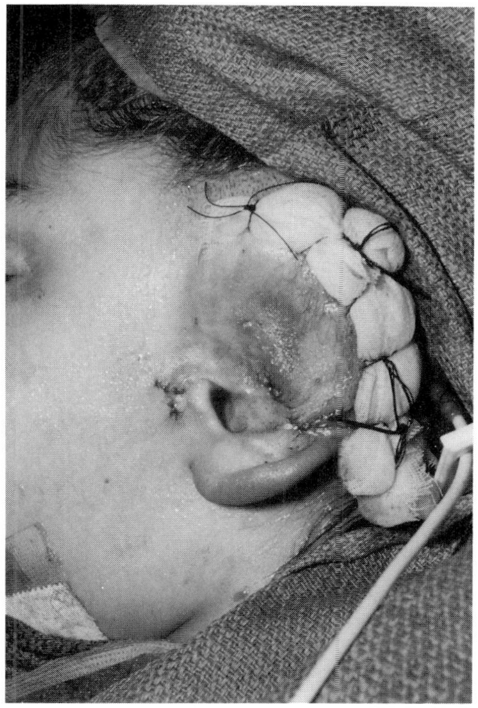

F

of ear deformities include the *lop* and the *cup* ear. This is a clinical entity seen relatively infrequently, with repeated surveys suggesting that its incidence is 3 to 5 percent in a general clinic population, and approaching 10 to 15 percent in the black population.[10] According to Cosman, four aspects of their appearance emerge as fundamental to the viewer's perception of the defect: (1) lidding, (2) protrusion, (3) decreased ear size, and (4) low ear position.[10]

The lop ear is one where the major deformity is an acute downward angling of the auricular cartilage, most commonly at the level of Darwin's tubercle, which involves the helix and often the scapha.[10] This may be due to a folding of the cartilage, or due to a true tissue deficiency. Often, there is an associated malformation of the superior crus of the antihelix. (Fig. 8–7a)

The cup ear is typically more of a deformed protruding ear, seen with an extremely deep, cup-shaped conchal bowl, along with a deficiency in both the helical margin and the antihelical crura.[10] This folded-over configuration is often referred to as a *hooding* of the helical rim. (Fig. 8–7b)

Tanzer classified constricted ears into three groups and two subgroups, representing a range of severity in the constricted portion, but primarily based on the type of surgical correction needed (Table 8–2).[69] In practical terms, however, the key to the surgical correction is whether the repair can be done by simply reshaping the existing tissue, or whether additional tissue needs to be brought in to make up for a true tissue deficiency.[10]

The surgical approach is based on comparing the difference in ear size between the normal and the abnormal, and in clearly defining the anatomic defect. If lidding is the major problem, and there is no protrusion and a height difference greater than 1 cm, Cosman suggests direct excision of the overhanging helical curl.[10] With a height difference between 1 and 1.5 cm, a banner flap using the cartilage lid is used. With lidding, protrusion, and a height difference of 1–1.5cm, height expansion and protrusion correction can both be accomplished through Cosman's technique.[10] With severe scaphal compression (height difference of 1.5–2 cm), additional skin and cartilage must be added, and Kislov's technique is the method of choice.[35]

Recently, Matsuo et al. have described the nonsurgical correction for congenital auricular deformities.[41,42] When applied in the early neonatal period, within the first 6 weeks of life, by using a dental compound as an external mold they have successfully and permanently altered the shape of the auricle in such conditions as lop ear, Stahl's ear, the protruding ear, and in cryptotia. This technique is not applicable with hypoplastic ears.

### Cryptotia

This condition is more commonly seen among Asians (1:400), and is believed to arise due to an intrinsic deformity of the antihelix, whereby an abnormal folding secondary to abnormalities in the intrinsic transverse and oblique ear muscles causes impingement of the upper pole of the auricle onto the temporal region.[5] This results in a gradual invagination of the ear into the temporal scalp. The right side is more commonly involved than the left, but in 40% of cases, it is bilateral. Hirose et al. have proposed a classification system based on the type of antihelical deformity and the state of the intrinsic auricular musculature.[30] Nonsurgical treatment with splinting has been successfully performed when the child is less than 6 months old, but beyond that age, surgical division of the muscle, combined with either a local flap or skin graft for the retroauricular sulcus, is required.

### The prominent ear

#### Morphology

This condition is characterized by a protruding appearance of the pinna with excessive distance between the helical rim and

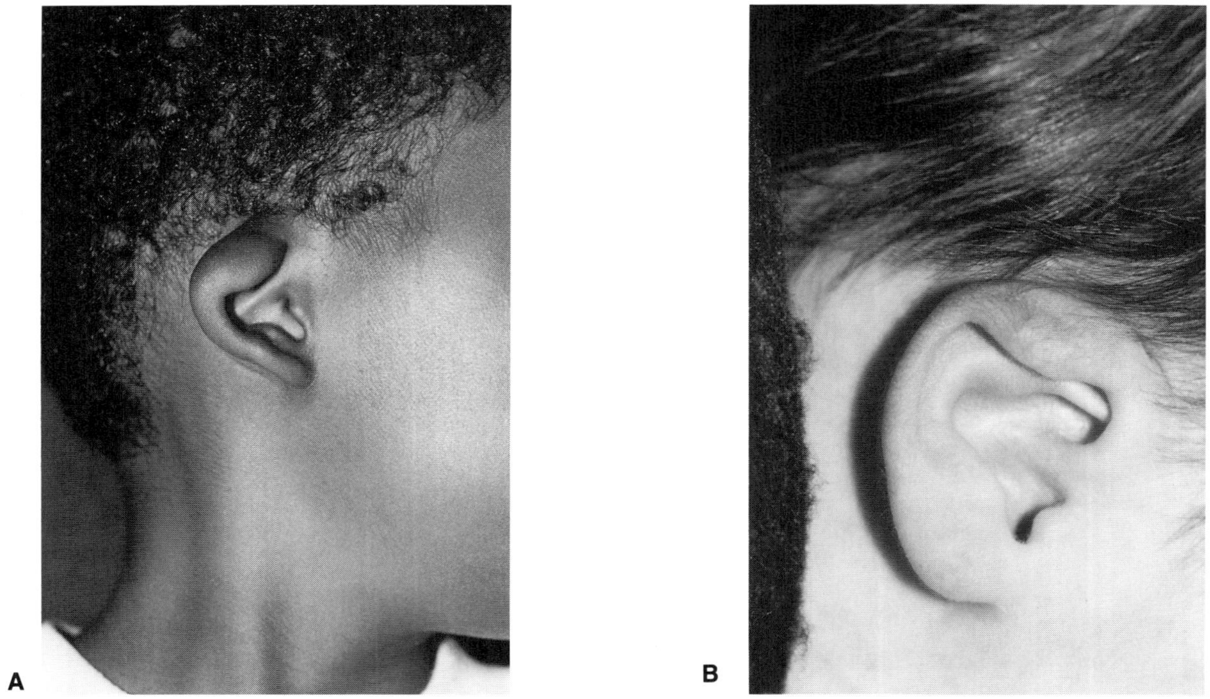

Fig. 8–7. A: Lop ear deformity; B: cup ear deformity.

the mastoid. It is thought to arise from an embryonic arrest in development of the infolding of the auricular cartilage, particularly from a failure of formation of the antihelical fold and/or crura.[31] The typical appearance is one with a greatly widened (greater than 90 degrees) concho-scaphal angle, and/or a very deep conchal bowl. This is usually seen bilaterally, and tends to run in families, suggesting an inherited transmission.[16]

### Surgical goals

The goals of surgical repair of this condition are clearly outlined by McDowell.[43] These include: (1) all traces of protrusion in the upper third of the ear should be corrected; (2) from the front view, the helix of both ears should be seen beyond the antihelix (at least down to the mid-ear); (3) the helix should have a smooth and regular line throughout; (4) the postauricular sulcus should not be markedly decreased or distorted; (5) the ear should not be placed too close to the head, particularly in boys; and (6) the distance of the two ears from the lateral border to the head should match fairly closely, to within 3 mm at any given point.

### Operative management

These goals are attainable through a variety of surgical methods. The technique chosen must specifically address that portion of the ear considered abnormal. If the protrusion centers about the upper pole of the ear, due to lack of an antihelical fold, then a new antihelix must be formed. If the middle portion is too prominent, then a conchal bowl recession must be considered, either by cartilage excision or through suture fixation. If the lower lobule is abnormal, it should then either be resected or retropositioned.

*Creation of antihelix.* Lack of an antihelical fold is perhaps the most common cause of a prominent ear. Many varying methods have been described that address this problem, but they all have in common either directly suturing the cartilage,

**Table 8–2.** Clinical classification of constricted ears[69]

| |
|---|
| I. Involvement of helix only |
| II. Involvement of helix and scapha |
| A. No supplemental skin needed at auricular margin |
| B. Supplemental skin needed at auricular margin |
| III. Extreme cupping deformity |

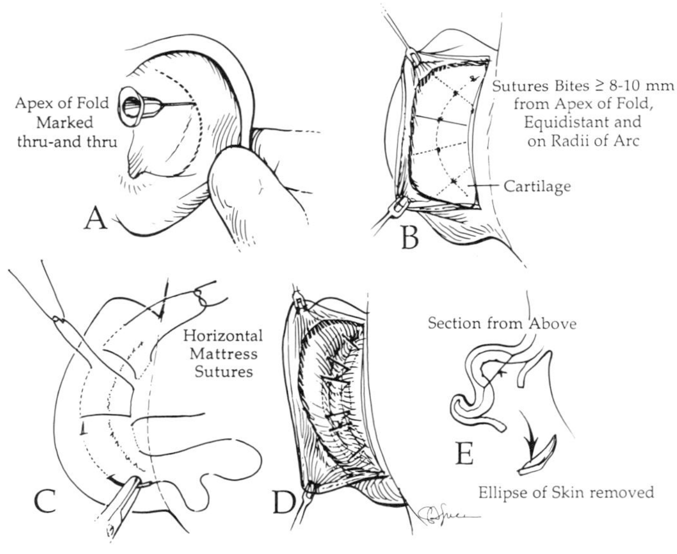


**Fig. 8–8.** The Mustarde otoplasty technique. A: Marking the new antihelical fold with ink and needle. B: Careful placement of horizontal mattress sutures. C,D: Creation of new antihelical fold. E: Cross-sectional view of auricular cartilage, and excision of skin ellipse from postauricular sulcus.

E

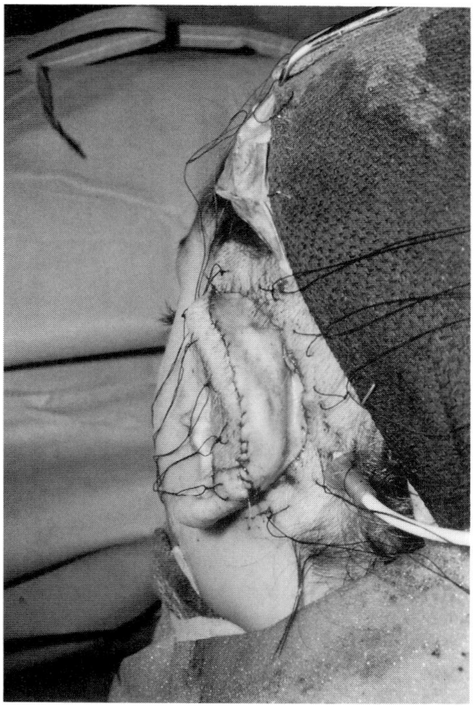

F

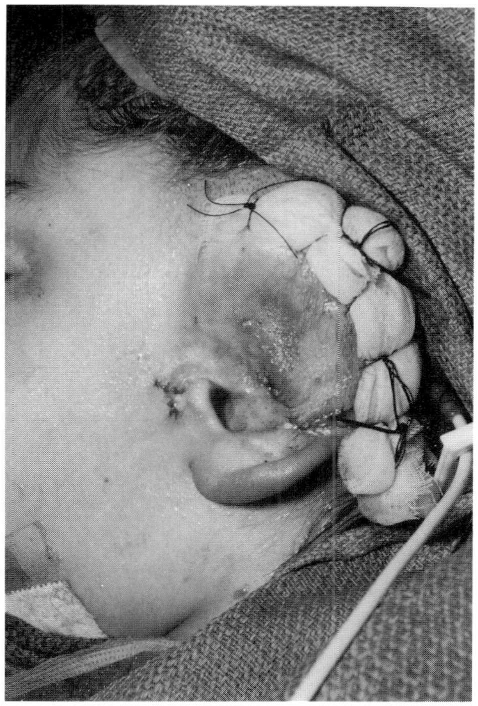

of ear deformities include the *lop* and the *cup* ear. This is a clinical entity seen relatively infrequently, with repeated surveys suggesting that its incidence is 3 to 5 percent in a general clinic population, and approaching 10 to 15 percent in the black population.[10] According to Cosman, four aspects of their appearance emerge as fundamental to the viewer's perception of the defect: (1) lidding, (2) protrusion, (3) decreased ear size, and (4) low ear position.[10]

The lop ear is one where the major deformity is an acute downward angling of the auricular cartilage, most commonly at the level of Darwin's tubercle, which involves the helix and often the scapha.[10] This may be due to a folding of the cartilage, or due to a true tissue deficiency. Often, there is an associated malformation of the superior crus of the antihelix. (Fig. 8–7a)

The cup ear is typically more of a deformed protruding ear, seen with an extremely deep, cup-shaped conchal bowl, along with a deficiency in both the helical margin and the antihelical crura.[10] This folded-over configuration is often referred to as a *hooding* of the helical rim. (Fig. 8–7b)

Tanzer classified constricted ears into three groups and two subgroups, representing a range of severity in the constricted portion, but primarily based on the type of surgical correction needed (Table 8–2).[69] In practical terms, however, the key to the surgical correction is whether the repair can be done by simply reshaping the existing tissue, or whether additional tissue needs to be brought in to make up for a true tissue deficiency.[10]

The surgical approach is based on comparing the difference in ear size between the normal and the abnormal, and in clearly defining the anatomic defect. If lidding is the major problem, and there is no protrusion and a height difference greater than 1 cm, Cosman suggests direct excision of the overhanging helical curl.[10] With a height difference between 1 and 1.5 cm, a banner flap using the cartilage lid is used. With lidding, protrusion, and a height difference of 1–1.5cm, height expansion and protrusion correction can both be accomplished through Cosman's technique.[10] With severe scaphal compression (height difference of 1.5–2 cm), additional skin and cartilage must be added, and Kislov's technique is the method of choice.[35]

Recently, Matsuo et al. have described the nonsurgical correction for congenital auricular deformities.[41,42] When applied in the early neonatal period, within the first 6 weeks of life, by using a dental compound as an external mold they have successfully and permanently altered the shape of the auricle in such conditions as lop ear, Stahl's ear, the protruding ear, and in cryptotia. This technique is not applicable with hypoplastic ears.

### Cryptotia

This condition is more commonly seen among Asians (1:400), and is believed to arise due to an intrinsic deformity of the antihelix, whereby an abnormal folding secondary to abnormalities in the intrinsic transverse and oblique ear muscles causes impingement of the upper pole of the auricle onto the temporal region.[5] This results in a gradual invagination of the ear into the temporal scalp. The right side is more commonly involved than the left, but in 40% of cases, it is bilateral. Hirose et al. have proposed a classification system based on the type of antihelical deformity and the state of the intrinsic auricular musculature.[30] Nonsurgical treatment with splinting has been successfully performed when the child is less than 6 months old, but beyond that age, surgical division of the muscle, combined with either a local flap or skin graft for the retroauricular sulcus, is required.

### The prominent ear

#### Morphology

This condition is characterized by a protruding appearance of the pinna with excessive distance between the helical rim and

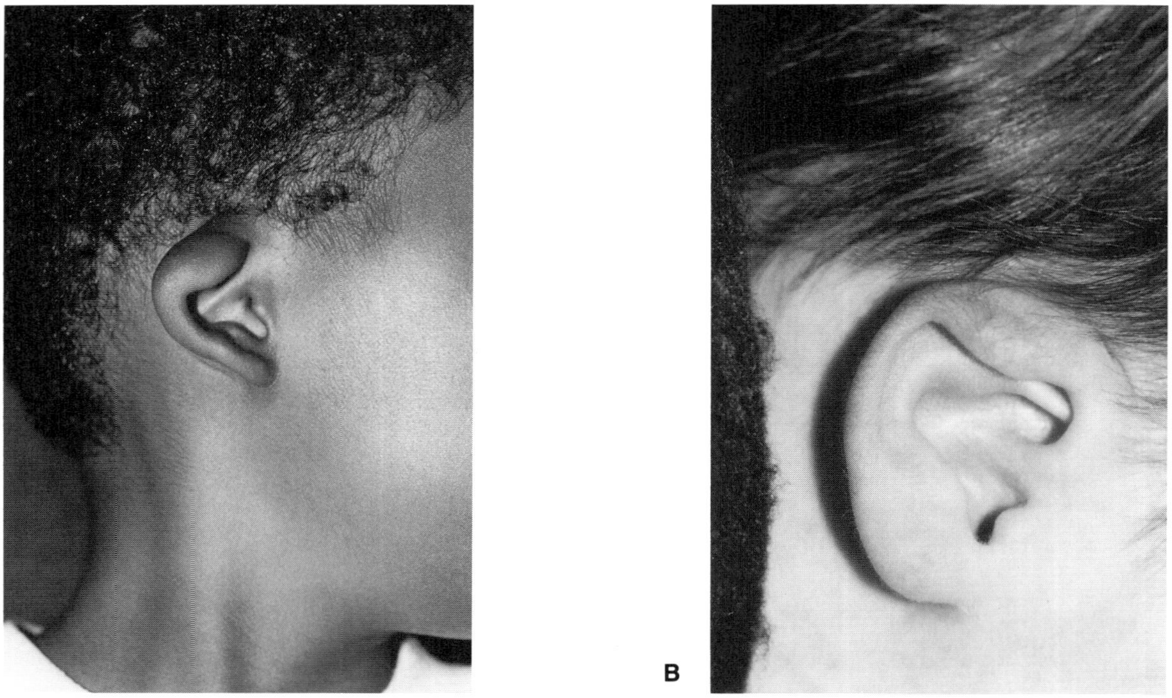


**Fig. 8–7.** A: Lop ear deformity; B: cup ear deformity.

the mastoid. It is thought to arise from an embryonic arrest in development of the infolding of the auricular cartilage, particularly from a failure of formation of the antihelical fold and/or crura.[31] The typical appearance is one with a greatly widened (greater than 90 degrees) concho-scaphal angle, and/or a very deep conchal bowl. This is usually seen bilaterally, and tends to run in families, suggesting an inherited transmission.[16]

### Surgical goals

The goals of surgical repair of this condition are clearly outlined by McDowell.[43] These include: (1) all traces of protrusion in the upper third of the ear should be corrected; (2) from the front view, the helix of both ears should be seen beyond the antihelix (at least down to the mid-ear); (3) the helix should have a smooth and regular line throughout; (4) the postauricular sulcus should not be markedly decreased or distorted; (5) the ear should not be placed too close to the head, particularly in boys; and (6) the distance of the two ears from the lateral border to the head should match fairly closely, to within 3 mm at any given point.

### Operative management

These goals are attainable through a variety of surgical methods. The technique chosen must specifically address that portion of the ear considered abnormal. If the protrusion centers about the upper pole of the ear, due to lack of an antihelical fold, then a new antihelix must be formed. If the middle portion is too prominent, then a conchal bowl recession must be considered, either by cartilage excision or through suture fixation. If the lower lobule is abnormal, it should then either be resected or retropositioned.

*Creation of antihelix.* Lack of an antihelical fold is perhaps the most common cause of a prominent ear. Many varying methods have been described that address this problem, but they all have in common either directly suturing the cartilage,

**Table 8–2.** Clinical classification of constricted ears[69]

- I. Involvement of helix only
- II. Involvement of helix and scapha
  - A. No supplemental skin needed at auricular margin
  - B. Supplemental skin needed at auricular margin
- III. Extreme cupping deformity

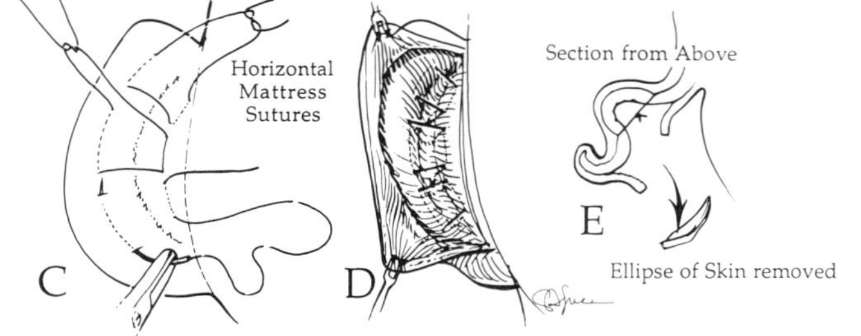


**Fig. 8–8.** The Mustarde otoplasty technique. A: Marking the new antihelical fold with ink and needle. B: Careful placement of horizontal mattress sutures. C,D: Creation of new antihelical fold. E: Cross-sectional view of auricular cartilage, and excision of skin ellipse from postauricular sulcus.

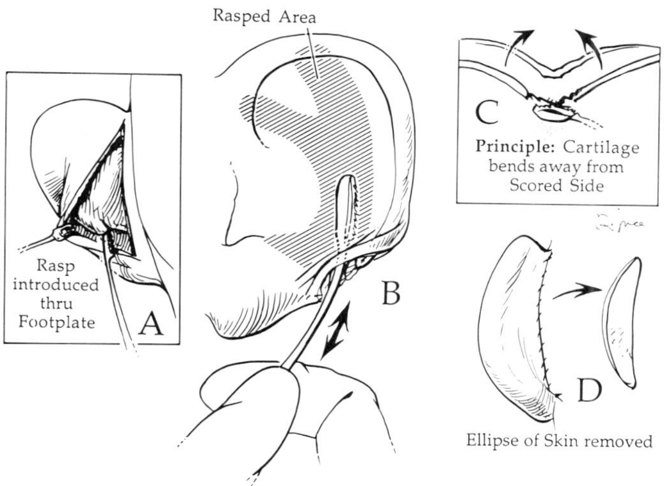


**Fig. 8–9.** The Stenstrom otoplasty technique. A: Dissection of the posterior aspect of the auricular framework to expose the foot plate of the helix. B: Placement of the otoabrader onto the anterior surface of the cartilage and area of abrasion (cross-hatched area). C: Cartilage will bend away from abraded surface. D: Completion of procedure with excision of skin ellipse from postauricular sulcus.

as described by Mustarde,[49] or scoring the cartilage, as described by Stenstrom.[63]

Luckett originally described the lack of an antihelical fold as the cause of a prominent ear, and attempted to restore the fold by excising a crescent of medial skin and cartilage.[37] His technique, however, resulted in an abruptly sharp and very noticeable step-off at the antihelical fold, which was considered aesthetically undesirable. Mustarde advocated molding the antihelix without directly cutting the cartilage, thereby creating a smoother fold.[49] The fold would be held in place by a row of nonabsorbable mattress sutures placed on the cranial cartilaginous surface in a full-thickness manner, through cartilage and perichondrium. The summit of the proposed fold is first carefully marked in ink on the anterior skin surface, and the mattress sutures are placed so that each bite of the lower sutures lies 8 to 10 mm from the summit of the fold. An ellipse of skin is excised from the posterior surface of the ear before the sutures are tightened. Next, the sutures are drawn together, tightening the intervening cartilage but only sufficiently to produce the desired gentle fold, without creating a sharp angle. The procedure is completed with direct closure of the postauricular skin. (Fig. 8–8)

Stenstrom's technique of scoring the cartilage was based on his observations while preparing cadaveric specimens of cartilage sections that had been scratched, curled strongly and uniformly toward their intact side.[63] He felt that it was natural to exploit this phenomenon in the correction of prominent ears by simply abrading the anterior surface of the cartilage instead of the posterior surface. Gibson and Davis studied this bending tendency and concluded that it was "due to differences in tension between the outermost layers of cartilage and the inner zone."[23] Stenstrom believes, however, that it is the perichondrium that is responsible and that disruption of the perichondrium on the anterior surface of the ear cartilage leads to contraction of the intact perichondrium on the posterior side. More recently, attention has been focused on the osmotic hydrostatic pressure within the internal cartilage, aptly termed the *swelling pressure*.[20] This pressure is thought to be generated by the interlocking of protein polysaccharide complexes within the cartilage and their binding of large amounts of water. Although normally held in check by the intact perichondrium, when the perichondrium is disrupted on one side, the internal cartilage will tend to extrude outward through the disruption, causing the surface to warp toward the side of the intact perichondrium.[19,20]

The Stenstrom technique involves making a postauricular incision, exposing the tail of the helix and adjacent cartilage, dissecting forward to elevate the skin from the anterior surface of the ear, and placing scratches over the entire anterior cartilage surface with special intensity over the antihelix, the anterior and posterior crura, and the posterior conchal wall. Once the cartilage has been weakened to an appropriate consistency, the ear is brought into the precise position desired by excision of a carefully calculated amount of postauricular skin, followed by closure of the cut skin edges (Fig. 8–9).[63]

Other modifications incorporate variations of these two basic philosophies and in various combinations, in order to avoid the disadvantages of using either technique in isolation (Fig. 8–10a, b).[15,33] Both Mustarde and Stenstrom have reviewed their extensive experiences over time. Review of Mustarde's results with 600 ears operated on over a 20–year period revealed only 10 patients whose ears relapsed so significantly after surgery that they required reoperation. Others have not found the Must-

A

B

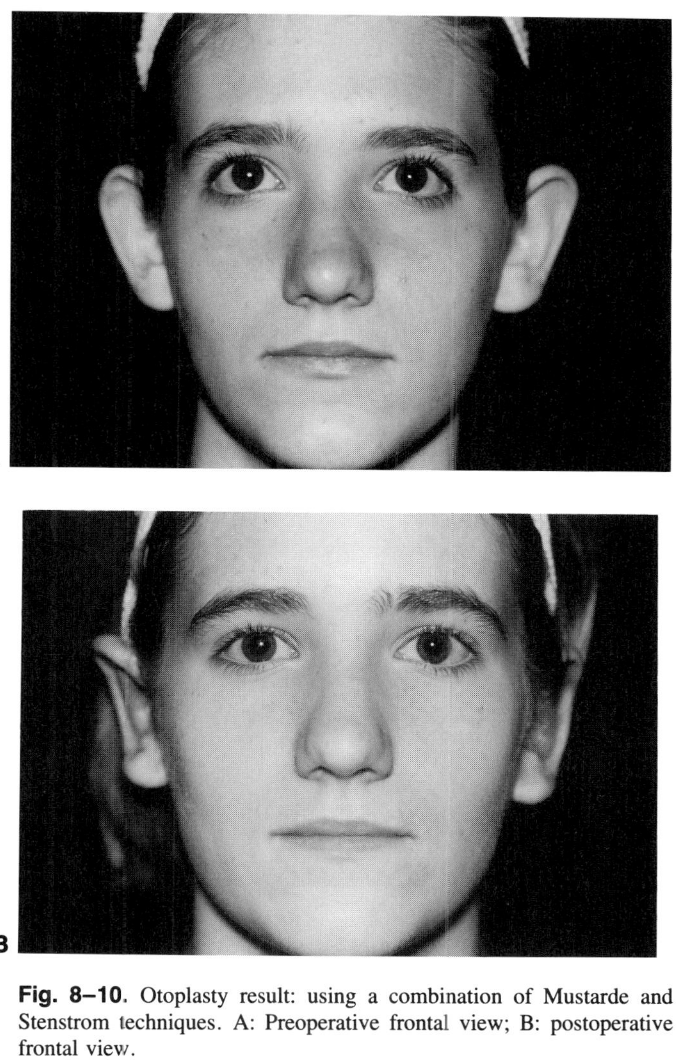

**Fig. 8–10.** Otoplasty result: using a combination of Mustarde and Stenstrom techniques. A: Preoperative frontal view; B: postoperative frontal view.

arde technique to be so reliable, with a large number of relatively minor complications and a high rate of partial recurrence of the deformity.[16,46,65] One hundred sixty-seven patients with Stenstrom otoplasties were surveyed over a period of 11 years, and it was found that only 7% were unsatisfied upon follow-up, and fully 82% were considered to have a good result based on symmetry, setting, and the roundedness of the superior helical crus on physician assessment.[28] Tan compared the two methods retrospectively over a 4–year period on 146 patients, where 45 were repaired with the Mustarde technique and 101 had anterior scoring. He found that 24% of the Mustarde group required reoperation, compared to 9.9% of the Stenstrom group ($P < 0.05$), but that the reoperation was required not for cosmetic dissatisfaction, but for minor complications specific to the Mustarde technique, such as sutures causing sinus tracts and wound infections.[65]

*Reduction of excessive conchal height.* Most described techniques involve partial or circumferential excision of the conchal wall and/or creation of a conchal flap, followed by tacking of the concha to the mastoid periosteum, thereby achieving a reduction in the depth of the postauricular sulcus.[17,29,48,61]

## Nonsurgical management

Matsuo et al. have described effective nonoperative correction of the protruding ear by affixing the posterior helical rim to the posterior retroauricular region using surgical tape, reinforced by a tubular elastic net bandage cut like a headband or earmuffs.[41] He found that if the treatments were started earlier, the total length of treatment was shorter to achieve a more lasting effect. The ideal age to begin treatment was less than 6 months old, and if started later, surgery would probably be more effective in correcting the deformity.

### References

1. Adamson JE, Horton CE, Crawford HH: The growth pattern of the external ear. Plast Reconstr Surg 36:466–470, 1965.
2. Allison GR: Anatomy of the external ear. Clin Plast Surg 5:419–422, 1978.
3. Bauer BS: Reconstruction of the microtic ear. J Pediatr Surg 19:440–445, 1984.
4. Bhishagratna KKL: An English Translation of the Susruta Samhita. Wilkens Press, Calcutta, 1907.
5. Brent B: Reconstruction of the auricle. In: Plastic Surgery, JG McCarthy, ed. WB Saunders, Philadelphia, 1990, pp 2094–2152.
6. Brent B: Auricular repair with autogenous rib cartilage grafts: two decades of experience with 600 cases. Plast Reconstr Surg 90:355–374, 1992.
7. Broadbent TR, Woolf RM: A bilateral approach to the middle ear. In: Symposium on Reconstruction of the Auricle, RC Tanzer, MT Edgerton, eds. CV Mosby, St. Louis, 1974, pp 168–173.
8. Cole RR, Jahrsdoerfer RA: Congenital aural atresia. Clin Plast Surg 17:367–371, 1990.
9. Converse JM: Construction of the auricle in congenital microtia. Plast Reconstr Surg 32:425–433, 1963.
10. Cosman B: The constricted ear. Clin Plast Surg 5:389–400, 1978.
11. Cronin TD, Greenberg RL, Brauer RO: Follow-up study of silastic frame for reconstruction of external ear. Plast Reconstr Surg 42:522–529, 1968.
12. Curtin JW, Bader KF: Improved techniques for the successful silicone reconstruction of the external ear. Plast Reconstr Surg 44:372–377, 1969.
13. Dieffenbach JE: Die Operative Chirurgie. FA Brockhaus, Leipzig, 1845.
14. Dupertuis SM, Musgrave RH: Experiences with the reconstruction of the congenitally deformed ear. Plast Reconstr Surg 23:361–373, 1959.
15. Elliot RA Jr: Otoplasty: a combined approach. Clin Plast Surg 17:373–381, 1990.
16. Elliot RA Jr: Complications in the treatment of prominent ears. Clin Plast Surg 5:479–490, 1978.
17. Ely ET: An operation for prominent auricles. Arch Otolaryn 10:97, 1881.
18. Farkas LG: Anthropometry of normal and anomalous ears. Clin Plast Surg 5:401–412, 1978.
19. Fry H: Cartilage and cartilage grafts: the basic properties of the tissue and the components responsible for them. Plast Reconstr Surg 40:526–539, 1967.
20. Fry HJ: Interlocked stresses in human nasal septal cartilage. Br J Plast Surg 19:276–278, 1966.
21. Fukuda O: Long-term evaluation of modified Tanzer ear reconstruction. Clin Plast Surg 17:241–249, 1990.
22. Gibson T, Davis WB: The fate of preserved bovine cartilage implants in man. Br J Plast Surg 6:4–25, 1953.
23. Gibson T, Davis WB: The distortion of autogenous cartilage grafts: its cause and prevention. Br J Plast Surg 10:257–274, 1958.
24. Gillies HD: Reconstruction of the external ear with special reference to the use of maternal ear cartilage as the supporting structure. Rev Chir Struct 7:169–179, 1937.
25. Gnudi MT, Webster JP. The Life and Times of Gaspare Tagliacozzi (1545–1590). Herbert Reichner, New York, 1950.
26. Gorlin RJ, Cohen MM Jr, Levin S: Syndromes of the Head and Neck, 3rd ed. Oxford University Press, New York, 1990, pp 641–649.
27. Grabb WC: The first and second branchial arch syndrome. Plast Reconstr Surg 36:485–508, 1965.
28. Hefter J: The Stenstrom otoplasty. Clin Plast Surg 5:465–470, 1978.
29. Hinderer UT, del Rio JL, Fregenal FJ: Macrotia. Aesth Plast Surg 11:81–85, 1987.
30. Hirose T, Tomono T, Matsuo K, Katohda S, Takahashi N, Iwasawa M, Satoh R: Cryptotia: our classification and treatment. Br J Plast Surg 38:352–360, 1985.
31. Jaffe BF: Deformities of the external ear associated with middle ear, inner ear, or distant malformations. Clin Plast Surg 5:413–418, 1978.
32. Kaseff LG: Investigation of congenital malformations of the ear with tomography. Plast Reconstr Surg 39:282–286, 1967.
33. Kaye BL: A simplified method for correcting the prominent ear. Plast Reconstr Surg 40:44–48, 1967.
34. Kirkham HL Jr: The use of preserved cartilage in ear reconstuction. Ann Surg 111:896–902, 1940.
35. Kislov R: Surgical correction of the cupped ear. Plast Reconstr Surg 48:121–125, 1971.
36. Knorr NJ, Edgerton MT, Barbarie M: Psychological factors in the reconstruction of the ear. In: Symposium on Reconstruction of the Auricle, RC Tanzer, MT Edgerton, eds. CV Mosby, St. Louis, 1974, p 187.
37. Luckett WH: A new operation for prominent ears based on the anatomy of the deformity. Surg Gynecol Obstet 10:635–637, 1910.
38. Lynch JB, Pousti A, Doyle JE, Lewis S: Our experiences with silastic ear implants. Plast Reconstr Surg 49:283–285, 1972.
39. MacGregor FC: Ear deformities: social and psychological implications. Clin Plast Surg 5:347–350, 1978.
40. Marx H: Die Missbildungen des Ohres. In: Handbuch der Morphologie der Missbildungen des Menschen und der Tiere, E Schwalbe, G Fischer, eds. Springer-Verlag, Jena Austria, 1911, p 565.
41. Matsuo K, Hayashi R, Kiyono M, Hirose T, Netsu Y: Nonsurgical correction of congenital auricular deformities. Clin Plast Surg 17:383–395, 1990.
42. Matsuo K, Hirose T, Tomono T, Iwasawa M, Katohda S, Takahashi N, Koh B: Nonsurgical correction of congenital auricular deformities in the early neonate: a preliminary report. Plast Reconstr Surg 73:38–51, 1984.
43. McDowell AJ: Goals in otoplasty for protruding ears. Plast Reconstr Surg 41:17–27, 1968.
44. McKenzie J, Craig J: Mandibulo-facial dysostosis (Treacher Collins syndrome). Arch Dis Child 30:391–395, 1955.
45. Melnick M, Myrianthopoulos NC, Paul NW: External ear malformations: epidemiology, genetics and natural history. Birth Defects 15:1–140, 1979.
46. Minderjahn A, Huttl WR, Hildmann H: Mustarde's otoplasty- evaluation of correlation between clinical and statistical findings. J Maxillofacial Surg 8:241–250, 1980.
47. Minkowitz S, Minkowitz F: Congenital aural sinuses. Surg Gynecol Obstet 118:801–806, 1964.

48. Morestin MH: De la reposition et du plissement cosmetiques du pavillon de l'oreille. Rev Orthopedie 14:289–303, 1903.
49. Mustarde JC: Correction of prominent ears using buried mattress sutures. Clin Plast Surg 5:459–464, 1978.
50. Nager GT: Congenital aural atresia: anatomy and surgical management. Birth Defects 7:33–51, 1971.
51. Ogino Y: Reconstruction of the external ear. Trans Third Inter Congr Plast Surg. Excerpta Medica, Amsterdam, 1964, p 461.
52. Ohmori S: Reconstruction of microtia using the Silastic frame. Clin Plast Surg 5:379–387, 1978.
53. O'Neal RM, Rohrich RJ, Izenberg PH: Skin expansion as an adjunct to reconstruction of the external ear. Br J Plast Surg 37:517–519, 1984.
54. Pierce GW: Reconstruction of the external ear. Surg Gynecol Obstet 50:601–605, 1930.
55. Rogers BO: Microtic, lop, cup and protruding ears: four directly inheritable deformities. Plast Reconstr Surg 41: 208–231, 1968.
56. Rollnick BR, Kaye CI: Hemifacial microsomia and variants: pedigree data. Am J Med Genet 15:233–253, 1983.
57. Rueckert F, Brown FE, Tanzer RC: Overview of experience of Tanzer's group with microtia. Clin Plast Surg 17:223–240, 1990.
58. Schofield AL: A preliminary report on the use of preserved homogenous cartilage implants. Br J Plast Surg 6:26–31, 1953.
59. Schukneckt HF: Reconstructive procedure for congenital aural atresia. Arch Otolaryngol 101:170–172, 1975.
60. Skiles MS, Randall P: The aesthetics of ear placement: an experimental study. Plast Reconstr Surg 72:133–138, 1983.
61. Spira M, Stal S: The conchal flap: an adjunct in otoplasty. Ann Plast Surg 11:291–298, 1983.
62. Steffensen WH: Comments on reconstruction of the external ear. Plast Reconstr Surg 16:194–200, 1955.
63. Stenstrom SJ, Heftner J: The Stenstrom otoplasty. Clin Plast Surg 5:465–470, 1978.
64. Takahashi H, Maeda K: Survey of familial occurrence in 171 microtia cases. Jpn J Plast Reconstr Surg 25:310–319, 1982.
65. Tan KH: Long-term survey of prominent ear surgery: a comparison of two methods. Br J Plast Surg 39:270–273, 1986.
66. Tanino R, Miyasaka M: Reconstruction of microtia using tissue expander. Clin Plast Surg 17:339–353, 1990.
67. Tanzer RC: Total reconstuction of the external ear. Plast Reconstr Surg 23:1–15, 1959.
68. Tanzer RC: An analysis of ear reconstruction. Plast Reconstr Surg 31:16–30, 1963.
69. Tanzer RC: The constricted (cup and lop) ear. Plast Reconstr Surg 55:406–415, 1975.
70. Tanzer RC: Microtia. Clin Plast Surg 5:317–336, 1978.
71. Tanzer RC: Microtia: a long-term follow-up of 44 reconstructed auricles. Plast Reconstr Surg 61:161–166, 1978.
72. Tjellström A: Osseointegrated implants for replacement of absent or defective ears. Clin Plast Surg 17:355–366, 1990.
73. Wildervanck LS. Hereditary malformations of the ear in three generations. Marginal pits, pre-auricular appendages, malformations of the auricle and conductive deafness. Acta Otolaryngol 54:553–560, 1962.

# 9

# Congenital Anomalies of the External Auditory Canal and the Middle Ear: Surgical Management

MELVIN D. SCHLOSS

Congenital malformations of the external auditory canal and the middle ear are associated with hearing loss, facial nerve abnormalities, and occasionally, recurrent meningitis. The goal of surgical intervention is to correct the hearing loss and to prevent further sequelae such as meningitis.

The incidence and prevalence of malformations of the pinna, external auditory canal, and middle ear cavity have been reported by different investigators and are summarized in Table 9–1.[16] The total number of external ear malformations has been reported to be from 2.41 to 88.4 per 10,000 births.[16] The data in Table 9–1 are those obtained from the National Institute of Neurological Diseases, Communicative Disorders and Stroke Collaborative Perinatal Project.[16] There are no prospective data on the incidence of middle ear malformations with or without malformations of the pinna or external auditory canal.[16,17] This type of malformation usually may be syndromic or nonsyndromic.[17] In a small group of children, the diagnosis of congenital malformation of the middle ear may be made later in life. These are children who have less than severe types of hearing losses and may not have obvious malformations of the pinna. The effects of hearing loss secondary to malformations of the external auditory canal and middle ear are well documented. Children with one hearing-impaired ear have more educational difficulties than similar children with binaural hearing.[5,22]

## Interventions for hearing loss

The ultimate goal of all interventions for hearing loss is to produce the best possible hearing with the smallest risk. There are basically two effective interventions available.[21] The first is use of amplification in the form of a hearing aid, and the second is some type of operative reconstruction of the external ear and sound-conducting mechanism. A third promising intervention is the use of a bone-conducting implantable hearing device.[26,27] At present, there are two different systems commercially available: (1) the Nobel Pharma Auditory System HC 200 percutaneous bone-anchored device developed by Tjellström,[26] and (2) the transcutaneous Xomed Audiant Bone Conductor developed by Hough.[11,12]

A hearing aid will usually give better hearing acuity than a surgical intervention (Fig. 9–1).[21,22] The hearing aid will be able to correct the conductive loss and may be able to compensate for some of the sensorineural hearing loss, if present. It does not expose the patient to perioperative morbidity since no operation is involved. The hearing aid, however, has several disadvantages, the most significant being the lack of acceptance by many patients and their families. Other disadvantages are the need for batteries, the tendency of children to lose their hearing aids, and interference with such sports as swimming. With the advent of bone conduction implants, the surgeon and patient have been provided with an alternative to actual surgical correction of the atretic external auditory canal and abnormalities of the middle ear.[26,27]

The efficacy of surgical intervention for hearing loss in a selected group of surgical interventions for malformations is given in Table 9–2.[3,13,14,15,18,25] The authors have analyzed the postoperative air conduction values for a combination of 500, 1,000 and 2,000 Hz and/or reported a speech reception threshold. The results in this table are short-term for a select population.

Approximately one-third (32%) of the ears reported in Table 9–2 had hearing above 20 dB and 70% were better than 30 dB.[3,13–15,18,25] Significant hearing impairment was defined as worse than 40 dB and was found in about 30% of the patients. The overall efficacy of the reported operative results is that 30% of the patients have average hearing and 70% have hearing worse than 21 dB, thus requiring some other form of hearing therapy.

The associated morbidity of the operative procedures are also important to understand. Surgery in these cases resulted in approximately 5 out of 100 patients having further hearing loss.[21] It is also important to consider the possibility of facial nerve dysfunction and postoperative infection in the cavities created in the ears with atresia.[21]

The results of hearing aids providing improvement in the hearing in patients with congenital anomalies of the external auditory canal and middle ear should be quite good. Most ears can be corrected to at least the bone conduction level and many are overcorrected (Fig. 9–1).[21,22] Lack of acceptance of a hearing aid is relatively common. If the hearing aid is introduced early in life, the patient may be more likely to accept the aid throughout childhood, adolescence, and adulthood.[5] There are other problems associated with hearing aids, such as otitis externa and allergic reaction to the hearing aid mold. Most of the time, these conditions can be managed rather easily, but in some cases this curtails the possibility of using a hearing aid.

**Table 9–1.** Findings in 600 children with malformations of pinna and external ear

| Malformation | Number | Rate per 10,000 |
|---|---|---|
| Preauricular sinus | 446 | 83.74 |
| Preauricular tags | 91 | 17.09 |
| Microtia | 16 | 3.00 |
| Other malformed pinna | 61 | 11.45 |

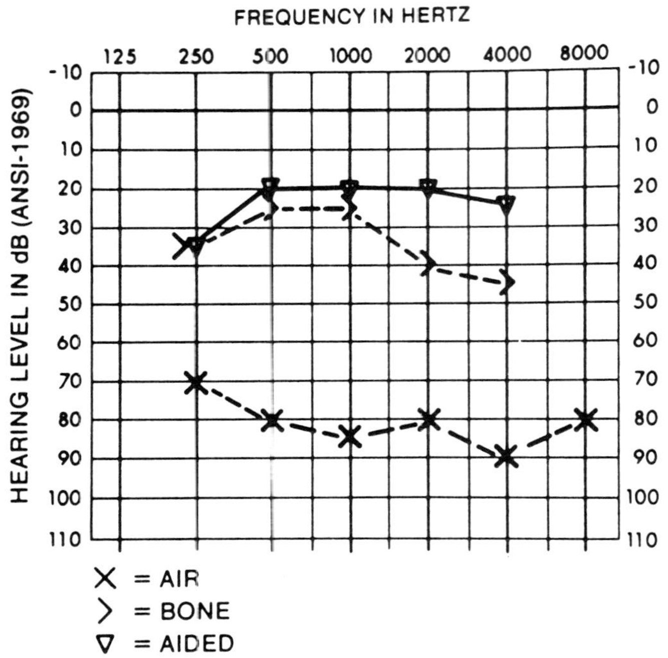


Audiogram shows for the left ear the efficacy of a hearing aid in the care of a child with bilateral malformations of the middle ear. The hearing threshold with the aid is better than the bone conduction threshold.

**Fig. 9–1.**

There are a number of patients with congenital anomalies of the external auditory canal and middle ear that are unable to wear a hearing aid at ear level or a conventional bone conduction aid. The bone-anchored hearing device has been developed for just this type of patient.[9,26,27] In both the percutaneous and transcutaneous device, an external sound processor, which may be either a body or an ear-level processor, converts sound energy into electromagnetic vibrations that are transmitted either transcutaneously or percutaneously to an internally implanted fixture. Vibrations then simultaneously stimulate both inner ears, providing the patient with nearly distortion-free sound at normal intensity levels.[26,27]

When deciding the treatment plan for a child with congenital malformations, the outcome of surgery, hearing aid, or implantable device must be considered. The advice given to parents of children with malformations must reflect all information available.[2,5,6,21,22,24] Initially, children should be prescribed a proper hearing aid. Operative procedures for the improvement of hearing should not be undertaken until the child's hearing can be accurately and precisely determined.[1,24] Proper radiographic imaging must be performed preoperatively so that the maximal information is available. This involves computed tomography (CT) or magnetic resonance imaging (MRI). The child must also be able to cooperate with postoperative care.[21] The side that is operated on is always the worse-hearing ear.[2,3,7] A hearing aid must be prescribed without any consideration of surgical intervention if the malformation is in the only hearing ear.[2,22] It must be decided and calculated whether the operation will achieve hearing of a level better than 20 dB pure-tone average of 500, 1,000 and 2,000 Hz.[21]

## External auditory canal stenosis and atresia

Congenital stenosis and atresia of the external auditory canal are usually associated with other malformations of the tympanic membrane, middle ear cavity, and ossicular chain (Table 9–3).[7] These anomalies or malformations are frequently associated with malformations of the inner ear. They are also commonly associated with other malformations of the head and neck and can be associated with systemic abnormalities.[7,10]

The most common malformation of the external auditory canal is its narrowing. In some cases, the stenosis is more medial than lateral.[16,17] These ears may or may not have a normal tympanic membrane with annulus associated with them.[16,17] A rare malformation is the double external auditory canal.[21] This has been considered a branchial cleft fistula or sinus. External canal stenosis and atresia creates three problems for the patient. The first is hearing loss, the second is an area associated with a disease process, such as infection or cholesteatoma, and the third is the lack of a canal in which a hearing aid may be fitted. The operative procedure contemplated should take into consideration the care of these problems.

There have been many operative procedures for creating an external auditory canal and at the same time exploring congenital malformations of the middle ear cavity.[1,3,4,7,8,13–15,18–20] They are as follows:

1. *Zuhlke's incision.*[19] The incision and transposition of the flap are illustrated in Figure 9–2. These flaps cover most of the meatus with transposition or rotation flaps, and any remaining defect on the meatal roof is covered with a split-thickness skin graft.

2. *Lange's incision.*[19] This incision utilizes the Z-plasty. The base of the flap lies opposite to that in Zuhlke's technique (Fig. 9–3). The roof and inferior wall of the meatus are lined with this flap. A split-thickness skin graft is used to cover the anterior and posterior meatal walls.

**Table 9–2.** Results of operative interventions for congenital malformations of the middle ear

| | Postoperative hearing dB[a] | | | | | | |
|---|---|---|---|---|---|---|---|
| Study | 0–10 | 11–20 | 21–30 | 31–40 | 41–50 | 51–60 | >61 |
| Sooy 1960[24a] | 2 | 1 | 0 | 2 | 0 | 0 | 0 |
| Crabtree 1968[2a] | 0 | 5 | 6 | 5 | 4 | 1 | 3 |
| Steele 1969[25] | 8 | 10 | 8 | 3 | 6 | 6 | 1 |
| Jahrsdoerfer 1978[13] | 0 | 4 | 6 | 3 | 2 | 1 | 4 |
| Morimitsu et al. 1980[18] | 0 | 6 | 2 | 3 | 0 | 1 | 1 |
| Total | 10 | 26 | 22 | 16 | 12 | 9 | 9 |
| % n/104 | 9.6 | 25.0 | 21.2 | 15.4 | 11.5 | 8.7 | 8.7 |

[a]Given as either pure-tone air average of 500, 1,000, 2,000 Hz and/or air conduction speech reception threshold.

**Table 9–3.** Classification of congenital meatal atresia

| Type I | Type II | Type III | Type IV |
|---|---|---|---|
| Normal or slightly deformed pinna | Pinna deformed either minimally or grossly | Gross deformity of pinna | Almost normal pinna |
| External auditory meatus present in at least the inner third | No external auditory meatus | No external auditory meatus | Almost normal external auditory meatus but normal curves exaggerated |
| Tympanic membrane always present but may be deformed or ossified | No tympanic membrane | No tympanic membrane | Tympanic membrane normal |
| Malleus, incus, and stapes all present and distinct but may be slightly deformed | Only head of malleus present and may be fused with incus; long process of incus may be present, represented by a strand of tissue going to capitulum of stapes, or absent; stapes usually present and normal or slightly deformed | Ossicles not present, or unrecognizable | Normal malleus; incus grossly deformed; stapes grossly deformed or absent |
| Middle ear cleft, mastoid process, and Eustachian tubes and cushion normal | Middle ear cleft, mastoid process, and Eustachian tubes and cushion almost normal | No middle ear cleft or only a few cells present; mastoid process densely sclerotic or Eustachian cushion deformed | Middle ear cleft, mastoid process, and Eustachian tubes and cushion normal |

Types III and IV are usually found in association with the Treacher Collins syndrome. There may be overlap between the different types. For example, it is not uncommon for type I cases to show stapedial malformations.

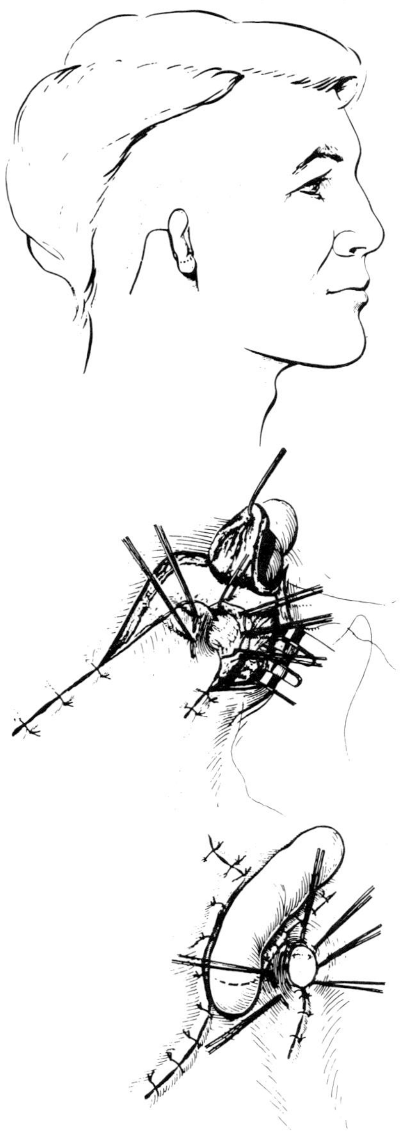

Fig. 9–2.

3. *Crabtree's incision.*[3] This technique combines postauricular access with a preauricular flap for anterior meatal wall coverage. Figure 9–4a shows the anterior incision which includes the rudimentary tragus in the base of the flap. Elevation of this flap is shown in Figures 9–4b and 4c. A sickle-shaped piece of skin is excised from the postauricular area (Fig. 9–4d). Figure 9–4e shows the stage after the postauricular excision of skin and the undermining of the auricular rudiment. The connective tissue beneath the auricular rudiment is excised and later used for obliteration of the mastoid cavity. Figure 9–4f is a cross section at the completion of the procedure. The anterior wall of the meatus is covered by the preauricular flap (1). The sickle-shaped piece of skin from the postauricular area is designed to cover the remaining meatus (2). The mastoid cavity is partially obliterated with the connective tissue previously removed (3). A free cartilage graft replaces the posterior part of the tympanic annulus (4). A transposed incus lies on the mobile stapedial head and is covered with fascia (5). The edges of the fascial graft are overlapped with the meatal skin.

4. *Marquet's incision.*[19] This technique is ideal for later reconstruc-

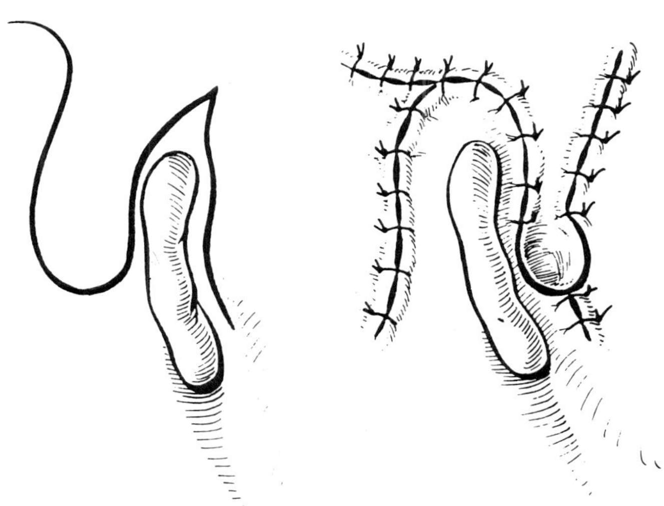

Fig. 9–3.

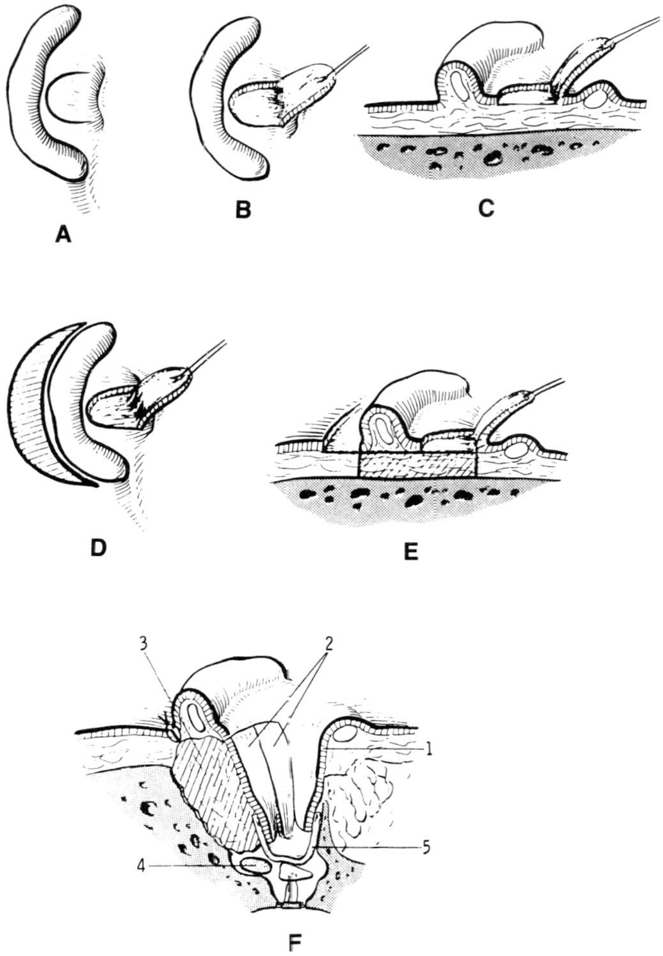


Fig. 9–4.

tion of the auricle. Figure 9–5a demonstrates the incision posterior to the hairline. A flap with a wide base on the cheek is elevated (Fig. 9–5b). This flap includes the rudiment of the auricle. A second incision is made anteriorly to the rudiment of the auricle (Fig. 9–5c). This allows the auricle to be transported posteriorly. The mastoid is now exposed and a new meatus is formed. Figure 9–5d show the new meatus formed. Figure 9–5e and f show the new meatus at completion of the procedure.

The many techniques described have all attempted to minimize a restenosis, which is a very common complication.

The surgeon must understand that the facial nerve may be in an abnormal location. It can be lateral to the usual course of the nerve and also may consist of one or more branches. A facial nerve stimulator should be used throughout the procedure. The facial nerve or a branch of the facial nerve may be small when compared to the normal facial nerve. The patient should be draped so that the surgeon can see the face during the procedure. The patient should not be paralyzed during anesthesia, so that facial movement can be observed.

The most cautious technique is to enter the middle ear cleft via the mastoid antrum. This approach is the safest, as it permits adequate visualization of the facial nerve canal, the labyrinth, and the ossicles. The surgeon must be continually cognisant of abnormalities in the course of the facial nerve. After the middle ear cavity is defined, the external auditory canal can be formed. The external auditory canal can only be extended ventrally to the dorsal portion of temporal mandibular joint. The joint space should not be entered. The dorsal limit of the canal may involve a number of structures, including an abnormal coursing facial nerve, the sigmoid sinus, or the posterior cranial fossa. Usually more space can be committed dorsally than ventrally to form a new external auditory canal. A cavity similar to a modified radical mastoid is created without necessarily defining the sinodural angle or posterior fossa. The middle ear and tympanic membrane are reconstructed before completion of the external auditory canal. The lining of the new external auditory canal is fashioned after completion of the reconstruction of the middle ear and tympanic membrane. Numerous techniques have been used to obtain an open canal. Currently, the most popular technique is with the use of a split-thickness skin graft. It is important when harvesting the skin graft that enough skin is taken to easily cover all exposed bone. The split-thickness skin graft must be taken from a non–hair-bearing area such as the medial aspect of the upper arm. The split-thickness skin graft after placement into the cavity is usually sutured into position. The newly created ear canal is then stented with packing. Numerous packing techniques have been described: silk, gauze, strips filled with antibiotic-soaked sponges or cottonballs provide adequate stenting. The antibiotic used must not be ototoxic. The packing is kept in place from 1 to 2 weeks and then is removed in an outpatient setting, either with or without anaesthesia. It is very important to examine the patient frequently, along with cleansing of the external auditory canal and the use of antibiotic-steroid drops, until healing is complete.

## The Middle Ear

The computed tomography (CT) scan may delineate ossicular malformations.[10] Any or all of the ossicles may be affected in the middle ear cavity. This is consistent with the embryologic development of these structures. The most commonly encountered malformations with a normal or near normal external canal and tympanic membrane are fixation of the head of the malleus, fusion of the malleoincudal joint, fixation of the long process of the incus, absence of the long process of the incus, lack of crura of the stapes, fixation of the footplate, absence of the oval window, and absence of the round window.[10,11,23]

Abnormalities of the facial nerve are relatively common when dealing with middle ear malformations. It has been reported that up to 24% of these cases demonstrate abnormalities of the facial nerve. Other malformations that the surgeon may encounter are vascular malformations or malpositions, encephalocele, and congenital tumors.

Surgical correction of ossicular malformations has been attempted by various means, including the use of homografts, synthetic materials, fenestration procedures, allografts, and autografts.

It is not uncommon for massive inner ear fluid leaks in congenitally malformed ears.[8] The otologic surgeon must be aware of this possibility preoperatively and know how to handle a perilymph leak if it is encountered. There should be mimimal manipulation of the oval window in patients with congenital middle ear malformations as there is an enhanced risk of further hearing loss from manipulation of the footplate.

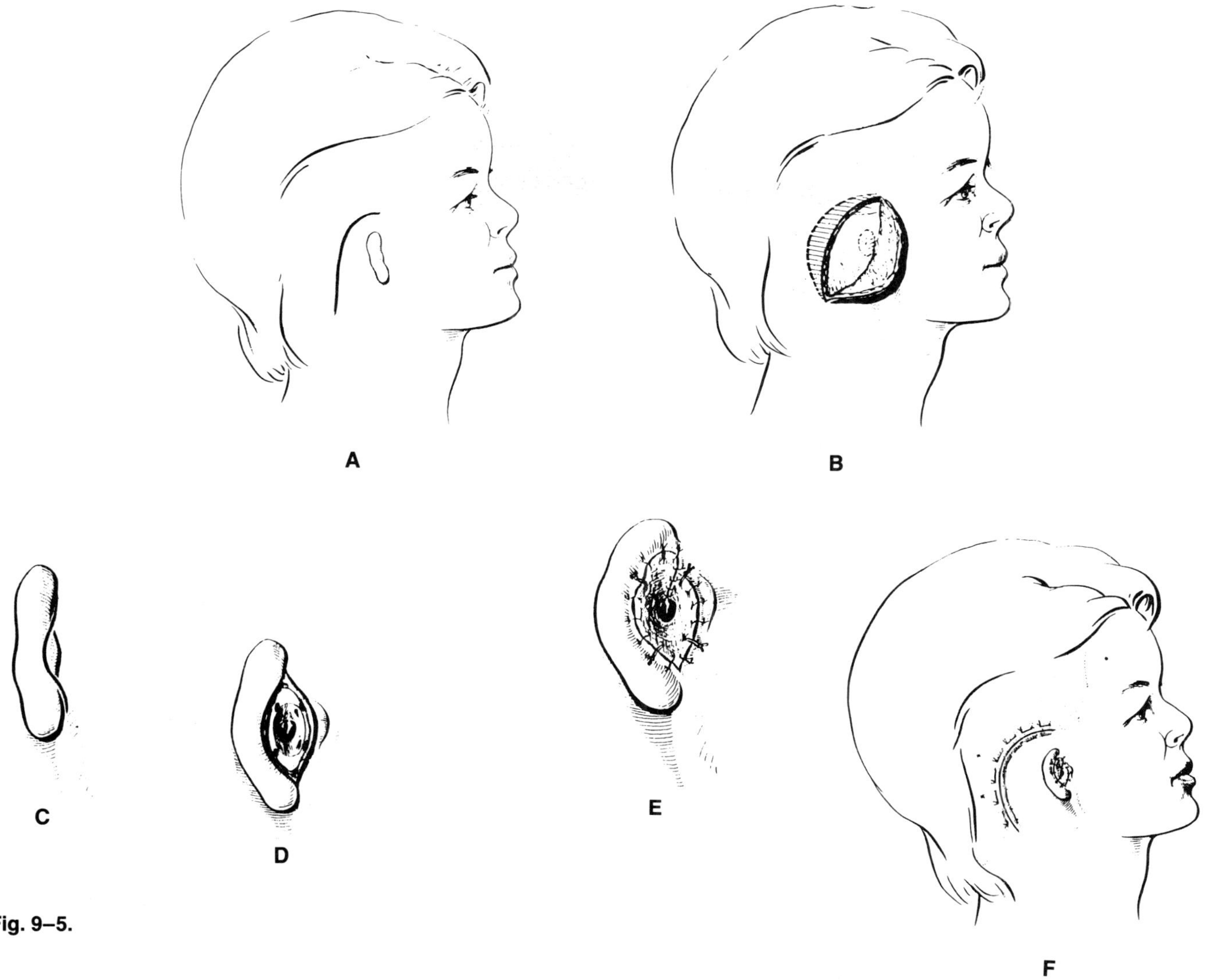


Fig. 9–5.

## References


1. Bellucci RJ: Congenital auricular malformations: Indications, contraindications, and timing of middle ear surgery. Ann Otol Rhinol Laryngol 81:659–663, 1972.
2. Bess FH, Tharpe AM: Unilateral hearing impairment in children. Pediatrics 74:206–216, 1984.

2a. Crabtree JA: Tympanoplastic techniques in congenital atresia. *Arch Otolaryngol* 88:63–70, 1968.

3. Crabtree JA: Atresia of the external auditory canal. In: Otolaryngology—Head and Neck Surgery. CW Cummings, JM Frederickson, LA Harker, CJ Krause, DE Schuller, eds. CV Mosby, St Louis, 1988, pp. 2952–2961.
4. De la Cruz A, Linthicum FH, Luxford WM: Congenital atresia of the external auditory canal. Laryngoscope 95:421–427, 1985.
5. Downs M: Amplifications in the habilitation of the young deaf child. In: Early Management of Hearing Loss. FT Mencher, SE Gerber, eds. Grune & Stratton, Orlando, 1980, p 199.
6. Dunham ME, Friedman HI: Audiologic management of bilateral external auditory canal atresia with the bone conducting implantable device. Cleft Palate J 27:369–373, 1990.
7. Gill NW: Surgery of meatal atresia. In: Operative Surgery, 4th ed, JC Ballantyne, A Morrison, eds. Butterworths, London, 1986, p 16.
8. Glasscock ME III: The stapes gusher. Arch Otorhinolaryngol 98:82–91, 1973.
9. Håkansson B, Lidén G, Tjellström A, Ringdahl A, Jacobsson M, Carlsson P, Erlandson BE: Ten years of experience with the Swedish bone-anchored hearing system. Ann Otol Rhinol Laryngol Suppl 151:1–16, 1990.
10. Herman HK, Kimmelman CP: Congenital anomalies limited to the middle ear. Otolaryngol Head Neck Surg 106:285–287, 1991.
11. Hough JVD: Malformations and anatomical variations seen in the middle ear during the operation for mobilization of the stapes. Laryngoscope 68:1337–1379, 1958.
12. Hough JVD, McGee M, Himelick T, Vernon T: The surgical technique for implantation of the temporal bone stimulator (Audiant ABC). Am J Otol 7:315–321, 1986.
13. Jahrsdoerfer RA: Congenital atresia of the ear. Laryngoscope 88 (Suppl 13):1–48, 1978.
14. Jahrsdoerfer RA: The facial nerve in congenital middle ear malformations. Laryngoscope 91:1217–1225, 1981.
15. Jahrsdoerfer RA, Yeakley JW, Hall JW III, Robbins KT, Gray LC: High-resolution CT scanning and auditory brain stem response in congenital aural atresia: patient selection and surgical correlation. Otolaryngol Head Neck Surg 93:292–298, 1985.
16. Melnick M: The etiology of external ear malformations and its relation to abnormalities of the middle ear, inner ear, and other organ systems. Birth Defects 16:303–331, 1980.
17. Melnick M, Myrianthopoulos NC, Paul NW: External ear malformations: epidemiology, genetics, and natural history. Birth Defects 15:1–140, 1979.
18. Morimitsu T, Matsumoto I, Takahashi M, Komune S: Vestibular fenestration and stapedioplasty in congenital stapes and vestibular window abnormality. Arch Otorhinolaryngol 226:27–33, 1980.
19. Mundrich K: Operations for congenital anomalies of the ear. In: Head & Neck Surgery—Ear, Vol 3, HH Naumann, ed. WB Saunders, Philadelphia, 1982, pp 395–398.
20. Ombrédanne M: Chirurgie des surdités congénitales par malfor-

mations ossiculaires. Acta Otorhinolaryngol Belg 25:837–869, 1971.

21. Ruben RJ: Management and therapy of congenital malformations of the external and middle ears. In: Otologic Medicine and Surgery, PW Alberti, RJ Ruben, eds. Churchill Livingstone, New York, 1989, pp 1135–1151.
22. Rubin M: Hearing aids for infants. In: Early Management of Hearing Loss, GT Mencher, SE Gerber, eds. Grune & Stratton, Orlando, 1980, p 183.
23. Sakashita T, Sando I, Kanerer D: Congenital anomalies of the external and middle ear. In: Pediatric Otolaryngology, 3rd ed CD Bluestone, SE Stool, MA Kenna eds. WB Saunders, Philadelphia, 1996, pp 333–370.
24. Schuknecht HF: Reconstructive procedures for congenital aural atresia. Arch Otolaryngol 101:170–172, 1975.

24a. Sooy FA: The management of middle ear lesions simulating otosclerosis. Ann Otol Rhinol Laryngol 69:540–558, 1960.

25. Steele BC: Congenital fixation of the stapes footplate. Acta Otolaryngol Suppl 245:1–20, 1969.
26. Tjellström A, Rosenhall U, Lindström J, Hallén O, Albrektsson T, Brånemark PI: Five-year experience with skin-penetrating bone-anchored implants in the temporal bone. Acta Otolaryngol Stockh 95:568–575, 1983.
27. Wade PS, Halik JJ, Chasin M: Bone conduction implants: transcutaneous vs percutaneous. Otolaryngol Head and Neck Surg 106:68–74, 1992.

# Appendix A

## Syndromes and Conditions Associated with Congenital Anomalies of the Ear

TED L. TEWFIK, AHMAD S. TEEBI, and VAZKEN M. DER KALOUSTIAN

| Syndrome or condition | MIM No. and POSSUM No.[a] | Inheritance[b] | Ear, nose, and throat manifestations | Other manifestations |
|---|---|---|---|---|
| PREDOMINANTLY ABNORMAL EAR STRUCTURES | | | | |
| Ablepharon and macrostomia[83] | **200110** 3910 | AR | Microtia, low-set dysplastic ears, abnormal ear size, abnormal tragus, coloboma of nostrils, large mouth, microdontia, high-arched palate, webbed neck | Decreased body hair, dry skin and loose skin, long palpebral fissures, absent eyelids, cryptophthalmos, ectropion, ambiguous genitalia, small penis |
| Acrocraniofacial dysostosis, Kaplan type[92] | **201050** 4407 | AR | Preauricular tags/pits, low-set malformed ears, atresia of the external auditory canal, choanal atresia, deafness, cleft palate, short neck | Microcephaly, sutural synostosis, large fontanelles, myopia, ptosis, short phalanges, ulnar deviation of fingers, coxa valga, short great toe, mental retardation |
| Acrofacial dysostosis, Arens-Goodman type[7] | 4950 | AR | Low-set ears, atresia of the external auditory canal, small nose, depressed nasal bridge, down-turned mouth angles, microstomia, micrognathia, short neck | Intrauterine growth retardation (IUGR), hypertelorism, blepharophimosis, abnormal metacarpals, syndactyly of fingers, camptodactyly, abnormal dermatoglyphics, dislocated hip, talipes valgus *or* varus, ureteric anomalies |
| Acrofacial dysostosis, cleft lip/palate, triphalangeal thumb[150] | **154400** 3610 | AR | Microtia, atresia of the external auditory canal, high nasal bridge, cleft palate, midface hypoplasia, conductive deafness | Frontal bossing, hypertelorism, deep-set eyes, hypoplastic radius, single palmar creases, abnormal palmar dermatoglyphics, hypoplastic thumbs |
| Acrofacial dysostosis, facial cleft, tetramelic limb defects[69,95] | 4609 | | Low-set ears, abnormal tragus and antitragus, abnormal helix, atresia of the external auditory canal, abnormal middle ear, depressed premaxillary region, lateral facial cleft, macrostomia | Short limbs, club hand, missing fingers, severe limb reduction, abnormal long bones, syndactyly, coloboma of eyelids, hydrocephalus, heart defect (?spectrum of Nager syndrome) |
| Alopecia, anosmia, deafness[89] | **147770** 3595 | AD | Microtia, atresia of the external auditory canal, deafness, cleft hard palate, anosmia, facial paralysis, micrognathia | Decreased sweating, sparse scalp hair, atrophic testes, delayed puberty, coarctation of the aorta, hydrocephalus, mental retardation |
| Antley-Bixler syndrome (multisynostotic osteodysgenesis with fractures)[22,44] | ***207410** 3570 | AR | Preauricular tags, atresia of the external canal, abnormal antihelix, low-set ears, microtia or anotia, midface hypoplasia, small nose, choanal atresia/stenosis, depressed nasal bridge, long philtrum | Craniosynostosis, brachycephaly, hydrocephalus, flat supraorbital ridges, prominent eyes, scoliosis, vaginal abnormalities, large hands, camptodactyly, radiohumeral synostosis, femoral bowing-fractures, flexion deformity of toes, rocker-bottom feet |
| Anus-hand-ear syndrome (Townes-Brocks syndrome)[23,68,72] | ***107480** 3026 | AD | Folded-down ear, microtia, preauricular tags, conductive deafness, asymmetry of the jaw | Short stature, syndactyly of fingers, preaxial polydactyly, triphalangeal or hypoplastic thumb, hypoplastic kidney, ureteric and urethral anomalies, imperforate malplaced anus |

**Appendix A** Syndromes and Conditions Associated with Congenital Anomalies of the Ear (*Continued*)

| Syndrome or condition | MIM No. and POSSUM No.[a] | Inheritance[b] | Ear, nose, and throat manifestations | Other manifestations |
|---|---|---|---|---|
| Beals auriculo-osteo-dysplasia[91] | ***109000** 3035 | AD | Abnormal ear pinna, short neck | Short stature, winged scapula, hypoplastic or absent metacarpals, abnormal shoulder, dislocation of the radioulnar joints, dislocated hip |
| Beals contractural arachnodactyly[16,104] | ***121050** 3027 | AD | Low-set and "crumpled" ears, prominent antihelix, abnormal antitragus, high- arched palate, micrognathia | Long and thin limbs, subluxated lens, myopia, thoracolumbar kyphosis, scoliosis, pectus carinatum, large hand with long fingers, camptodactyly, overlapping toes, coarctation of the aorta, defect in fibrillin 2(FBN2), chromosome 5q23–q31 |
| Beckwith-Wiedemann syndrome[2] | ***130650** 3036 | AD | Posterior helical indentations and Irving linear ear lobe creases, enlarged tongue | Omphalocele, gigantism, hypoglycemia in the neonatal period, hemihypertrophy, predisposition to Wilms tumor/embryonic tumors |
| Branchio-oto-renal (BOR) syndrome (Melnick-Fraser syndrome)[53] | ***113650** 3133 | AD | Preauricular pits, hearing loss, branchial fistulas or cysts, anomalous pinna, malformed middle or inner ear | Renal dysplasia, lacrimal duct stenosis/aplasia |
| Branchio-oto-ureteral syndrome (BOU syndrome, Fraser-Aymé-Halal syndrome)[52] | ***113650** 3588 | AD | Preauricular tags/pits, microtia, deafness | Single palmar creases, ureteric abnormalities; probably the same as branchio-oto-renal syndrome |
| C syndrome (see Opitz trigonocephaly syndrome) | | | | |
| Cat-eye syndrome (Chromosome 22, partial trisomy 22)[111] | **#115470** 3267 | | Preauricular appendages or fistulae, depressed nose, micrognathia, cleft palate | Colobomatous anomalies of the eye, anal atresia, mental retardation; chromosomal region 22pter-q11 |
| CHARGE association (**C**oloboma, **H**eart defect, **A**tresia choanae, **R**etardation, **G**rowth deficiency/ **G**enital hypoplasia in males, **E**ar anomalies)[117,126] | **214800** 3480 | Sporadic ?AR form | Prominent ears, folded-down ear, absent helix, abnormal size of earlobes, deafness, micrognathia, midface hypoplasia, short neck, dysphagia | Short stature, ptosis, microphthalmos, coloboma of iris, retinal coloboma, omphalocele, cryptorchidism, small penis, delayed skeletal maturation, cyanotic heart disease, syndactyly of fingers, hypoplastic kidney, hypothyroidism, pituitary defects, hypocalcemia |
| Chromosome 6, partial del 6p[102,132] | 4051 | | Hypoplastic antihelix, microtia, posteriorly angulated ears, broad and depressed nasal bridge, cleft palate, nystagmus, short neck | Short stature, marble skin, abnormal scalp hair, microcephaly, plagiocephaly, large fontanelle, hypertelorism, prominent eyes, epicanthic folds, microphthalmos, hyperopia, scoliosis, umbilical hernia, syndactyly of fingers, spasticity, mental retardation |
| Chromosome 11, partial del 11q[189] | 3087 | | Microtia, low-set and malformed ears, down-turned mouth angles, short nose, broad nasal bridge, micrognathia, short neck | Short stature, hypertelorism, ptosis, coloboma of iris, small penis, ectopic testes, brachydactyly, clinodactyly of 5th finger, aortic stenosis, moderate to profound psychomotor retardation, cerebellar hypoplasia |
| Chromosome 18, i18p (tetrasomy 18p)[194] | 3702 | | Microtia, low-set ears, preauricular tags, cleft palate, large nose, microstomia, long face | Growth retardation, microcephaly, acrocephaly, downslanting palpebral fissures, epicanthic folds, scoliosis, small penis, diffuse osteoporosis, radioulnar synostosis, large hands, arachnodactyly, camptodactyly, coxa valga, moderate to severe mental retardation, ataxia, hypotonia |

| Syndrome or condition | MIM No. and POSSUM No.[a] | Inheritance[b] | Ear, nose, and throat manifestations | Other manifestations |
|---|---|---|---|---|
| Chromosome 22, partial trisomy 22 (see cat-eye syndrome) | | | | |
| Chromosome 49 XXXXY[84] | 3111 | | Abnormal helix, hypoplastic antihelix, macrostomia, anteverted nostrils, broad nasal bridge, flat nose | Short stature, microcephaly, prognathism, severe visual loss, scoliosis, small penis, cryptorchidism, delayed skeletal maturation, restriction of joint mobility, radioulnar synostosis, camptodactyly of 5th finger, mental retardation |
| Cleft lip/palate, ectrodactyly[152] | | | Thickened helix, hypoplastic antihelix, cleft palate, lateral cleft lip, nystagmus | Ectrodactyly, syndactyly of fingers, hypoplasia of corpus callosum, hypotonia, cryptorchidism, diabetes insipidus |
| Coffin-Siris syndrome[51,147] | **135900** 3151 | AR | Preauricular tags, cleft palate, short philtrum, thick lips, macrostomia, bulbous nasal tip, broad nasal bridge, flat face | Short stature, increased body hair, hypoplastic or absent fifth fingernails, hypoplasia of toenails, bushy eyebrows, ptosis, scoliosis, small penis, hypermobile joints and hypotonia, mental retardation |
| Deafness, conductive, malformed ears, facial palsy[161] | **124490** 4430 | AD | Microtia, abnormal helix, preauricular tags, atresia of the external auditory canal, abnormal middle ear, conductive deafness, facial palsy | Overlaps with the spectrum of branchio-oto-renal syndrome and facio-auriculo-vertebral spectrum |
| Deafness, conductive, malformed external ears (Mengel-Konigsmark syndrome)[100] | ***221300** 3449 | AR | Microtia, thickened helix, folded-down ear, low-set ears, malformation of the ossicles in the middle ear, narrow and high palate | Cryptorchidism, small penis, mental retardation |
| Deafness, conductive, micrognathia[159] | 4604 | AD | Abnormal size of ear lobe, cup-shaped ears, abnormal middle ear, conductive deafness, facial palsy, open bite, micrognathia | |
| Deafness, conductive, microtia, meatal atresia[165] | ***251800** 4324 | AD AR | Atresia of the external auditory canal, preauricular tags, low-set ears, microtia, immobile soft palate | |
| Deafness, myoclonic seizures, cleft palate[142] | 3869 | | Microtia, preauricular pits/sinuses, posteriorly angulated low-set ears, thickened helix, sensorineural deafness, small nose, microstomia | IUGR/short stature, coarse hair, narrow forehead, broad cheeks, prominent eyes, hypoplastic/absent nipples, inguinal hernia, short phalanges, brachydactyly, pes cavus, mental retardation, seizures, EEG abnormalities |
| De Barsy syndrome[93] | ***219150** 3680 | AR | Large and dysplastic ears, absent helix, anteverted nostrils, webbed neck, microstomia, nystagmus, prematurely-aged face | Failure to thrive/short stature, dry, thin excessive skin with wrinkling, microcephaly, hypertelorism, cataract, corneal clouding, thin lips |
| Diastrophic dysplasia[187] | | | Cauliflower ears with calcified cartilage, cleft palate, micrognathia | Short stature, short limbs, talipes, hitch-hiker thumb, contractures, kyphoscoliosis, respiratory difficulties |
| Facial dysmorphism, right-sided aortic arch, mental retardation (Strong syndrome)[167] | **107500** 3448 | AD | Long ears, large beaked nose, abnormal columella, deviated nasal septum, prognathism, asymmetry of the face, microstomia | Microcephaly, broad forehead, dental caries, right-sided aortic arch, mental retardation |
| Facio-auriculo-radial dysplasia (Harding-Hall-Baraitser syndrome)[77] | 3544 | AD | Microtia, abnormal middle ear, conductive deafness, small nose, long philtrum, midface hypoplasia | Multiple vertebral anomalies, joint dislocations, hypoplastic radius, club hand, missing fingers, camptodactyly, short thumb |

**Appendix A** Syndromes and Conditions Associated with Congenital Anomalies of the Ear (*Continued*)

| Syndrome or condition | MIM No. and POSSUM No.[a] | Inheritance[b] | Ear, nose, and throat manifestations | Other manifestations |
|---|---|---|---|---|
| Facio-auriculo-vertebral dysplasia (Oculo-auriculo-vertebral dysplasia *or* Goldenhar syndrome)[30,154] | 3339 | ?AR (usually sporadic) | Preauricular pits *or* tags, epibulbar dermoids, microtia or anotia, low-set ears, abnormal middle ear, deafness, macrostomia midfacial hypoplasia, facial asymmetry, laryngeal anomaly | IUGR, microcephaly, coloboma of eyelids, cataract, retinal coloboma, micropthalmos, visual loss, oligodontia, abnormal rib number, talipes varus/valgus, vertebral/rib defects, dysplastic kidney, hydrocephalus, mental retardation |
| Focal dermal hypoplasia (Goltz-Gorlin syndrome)[172] | ***305600** 3204 | XLD | Low-set simple ears, abnormal antihelix, cleft lip/palate, bulbous nasal tip, coloboma/hypoplasia of nostrils, nystagmus, hypoplasia, asymmetry of the face, sensorineural and conductive hearing loss, nasal and perioral papillomata | Short stature, sparse and thin scalp hair, microcephaly, microphthalmos, coloboma of iris/optic nerve, paresis of ocular muscles, hypoplastic clavicles, hernias, small penis, syndactyly, preaxial polydactyly of fingers/toes, missing fingers/toes or part of a limb, asymmetric areas of pigmentation, variable skin changes with atrophy and subcutaneous collection of fat, osteopathia striata |
| Freeman-Sheldon syndrome (see Whistling face syndrome) | | | | |
| Goldenhar (see Facio-auriculo-vertebral dysplasia) | | | | |
| Goltz-Gorlin syndrome (see Focal dermal hypoplasia) | | | | |
| GOMBO syndrome (multiple congenital anomalies, mental retardation, Verloes-Lambotte type) (*G*rowth retardation, *O*cular abnormalities, *M*icrocephaly, *B*rachydactyly, *O*ligophrenia)[183] | **233270** 4939 | AR | Prominent antihelix, abnormal tragus, neurosensory deafness, prominent nose, abnormal columella, prognathism, dental anomalies | Failure to thrive, decreased body hair, excessive skin wrinking (premature aging), small nails, microcephaly, flat occiput, ptosis, atrophic testes, brachydactyly, irregular length of fingers, diaphragmatic hernia, moderate to severe mental retardation |
| Hemifacial microsomia, radial ray defects[118] | **141400** 4346 | AD | Preauricular tags/pits, microtia, atresia of the external auditory canal, conductive deafness, facial asymmetry | Short limbs, radial ray defects, scoliosis, carpal fusion, preaxial polydactyly, triphalangeal thumb, overlapping toes, malplaced anus |
| Hemimegalencephaly or diffuse enlargement of one hemisphere[151,179] | 4691 | | Atresia of the external auditory canal, abnormal antitragus, depressed nasal bridge, flat face | Asymmetry of the body, decreased skin pigmentation, macrocephaly, frontal bossing, hypertelorism, cardiac tumors, atrophy of cerebral cortex, mental retardation, seizures, ataxia (may be isolated or a part of tuberous sclerosis or in association with hypomelanosis of Ito) |
| Hennekam syndrome (lymphangiectasia, mental retardation, distinctive facies)[57] | ***235510** 4750 | AR | Microtia, thickened helix, atresia of the external auditory canal, conductive deafness, bulbous tip of nose with flat nasal bridge, microstomia, short philtrum, delayed eruption of teeth | Growth retardation, sparse scalp hair, prominent metopic suture, hypertelorism, downward slant of palpebral fissures, epicanthic folds, puffy eyelids, pectus excavatum, scoliosis, cryptorchidism, syndactyly of fingers, ureteric abnormalities, intestinal lymphangiectasia, lymphedema, mental retardation |
| Hittner syndrome (colobomatous microphthalmia, heart defects, deafness, mental retardation)[81] | 4193 | AD | Atresia of the external auditory canal, posteriorly angulated low-set ears, facial palsy, conductive deafness | Microphthalmia, eye colobomas, cyanotic heart defect, mental retardation (may be a part of CHARGE association) |

| Syndrome or condition | MIM No. and POSSUM No.[a] | Inheritance[b] | Ear, nose, and throat manifestations | Other manifestations |
|---|---|---|---|---|
| Holoprosencephaly (arrhinencephaly)[29,78] | ***236100** 3460 | (Heterogeneous) AD AR sporadic | Preauricular pits/tags, flattened nose, depressed nasal bridge, small nostrils/single nostril, abnormal nasal septum, midline cleft lip and palate, midline central incisor | Microcephaly, hypotelorism, cyclopia, coloboma of iris, corneal opacities, small penis, hypoplasia of corpus callosum, mental retardation, pituitary defect, stillbirth or neonatal death |
| Hypertelorism, microtia, clefting syndrome (Bixler syndrome)[69] | ***239800** 3259 | AR | Atresia of the external auditory canal, abnormal size of ear lobe, middle ear anomalies, conductive deafness, cleft palate, bifid nose, microstomia | Short stature, microcephaly, telecanthus/hypertelorism, cardiovascular anomalies, ureteric abnormalities, horseshoe kidney, mental retardation |
| Hypothalamic-hamartoblastoma syndrome (Pallister-Hall syndrome)[42,47] | **146510** 3259 | Unknown ?AD | Prominent and low-set ears, ear cartilage deficiency, glossoptosis, cleft palate, flat face, micrognathia, laryngeal cleft | IUGR, macrocephaly, prominent occiput, abnormal sella turcica, hypothalamic hamartomas, agenesis of corpus callosum, hypopituitarism, scoliosis, small penis, multiple vertebral anomalies, cryptorchidism, postaxial polydactyly, short limbs, syndactyly, heart defect, imperforate anus |
| Keutel syndrome (Pulmonary stenosis, brachydactyly, deafness, cartilage defect)[56] | ***245150** 3675 | AR | Calcified ear cartilage, cup-shaped ears, deafness, flattened nose, short philtrum, abnormal columella, small nostrils, midface hypoplasia, laryngeal/tracheal abnormality | Small nails, hypertelorism, carpal fusion, brachytelephalangy, soft tarsal fusion, syndactyly, cardiac conduction defects, mental retardation, short stature |
| Lambotte syndrome[184] | **245552** 4785 | AR | Large ears, atresia of the external auditory canal, beaked nose, flat face, microstomia | IUGR, microcephaly, hypertelorism, brachydactyly, preaxial polydactyly of feet, heart defect, severe neurological impairment, death in infancy or childhood |
| Madokoro-Ohdo syndrome[110] | 4286 | AR | Preauricular tags, cleft palate, microstomia, high nasal bridge, abnormal cry, dysphagia, micrognathia | Short stature, severe microcephaly, downward slant of palpebral fissures, blepharophimosis, simian creases, clinodactyly of 5th finger, heart defect, mental retardation |
| Mandibulofacial dysostosis, Toriello type[176] | **301950** 4291 | XLR | Low-set protruding ears, preauricular tags, high-arched palate, broad nasal bridge, deafness, facial asymmetry, webbed neck | Microcephaly, triangular asymmetric face, ptosis, cryptorchidism, heart defect, mental retardation |
| Marshall-Smith syndrome (accelerated skeletal maturation, short stature, unusual face)[25,41] | 3316 | Sporadic | Ear cartilage deficiency, choanal atresia *or* stenosis, flat face, abnormal cry, low nasal bridge, upturned nose, micrognathia, laryngomalacia | Failure to thrive, tall stature, high forehead, prominent eyes, blue sclera, myopia, broad phalanges, mental retardation, hypotonia, death in infancy? |
| Melnick-Fraser syndrome (see branchio-oto-renal [BOR] syndrome) | | | | |
| Mental retardation, cataracts, calcified pinnae, muscle wasting (Primrose syndrome)[144] | 3868 | | Calcified ear pinnae, pointed ears, short philtrum, prognathism, midface hypoplasia | Mental retardation, congenital cataracts, thoracolumbar kyphosis, abnormal vertebrae, hypogonadism, muscle wasting, contractures of long joints, cystic metaphyseal changes, seizures |
| Michels syndrome (cleft lip/palate, deafness, eye abnormalities)[33] | **257920** 3984 | AR | Preauricular tags, high-arched palate, sensorineural/conductive deafness, nystagmus, cleft lip/palate | Failure to thrive, facial asymmetry, hypertelorism, corneal opacities, blepharophimosis, epicanthus inversus, ptosis, severe visual loss, contracture of large joints, radioulnar synostosis, brachydactyly, mild mental retardation, seizures |

**Appendix A** Syndromes and Conditions Associated with Congenital Anomalies of the Ear (*Continued*)

| Syndrome or condition | **MIM No.** and POSSUM No.[a] | Inheritance[b] | Ear, nose, and throat manifestations | Other manifestations |
|---|---|---|---|---|
| Nager acrofacial dysostosis (Mandibulofacial dysostosis, limb anomalies)[35,63] | **154400** 3141 | Sporadic ?heterogeneous AD AR | Microtia, atresia of the external auditory canal, low-set ears, cleft hard palate, high nasal bridge, midface hypoplasia, lateral facial cleft, conductive deafness | Short stature, coloboma of eyelids, hypoplastic nipples, heart defect, restriction of joint mobility, syndactyly of fingers, missing fingers, radial ray defects and usually normal lower limbs |
| Nance-Sweeny syndrome (chondrodystrophy, sensorineural deafness)[64] | ***215150** 3062 | AR | Rigid ear cartilage, abnormal location or orientation of ears, cleft palate, long philtrum, depressed nasal bridge, small nose with anteverted nostrils, sensorineural deafness, prognathism | Short stature, thick skin, frontal bossing, high forehead, hyperopia, kyphosis, platyspondyly, epiphyseal abnormality, restriction of joint mobility, brachydactyly, hypoplastic thumb |
| Opitz-trigonocephaly syndrome, C syndrome[143] | ***211750** 3048 | AR | Ear cartilage deficiency, low-set posteriorly angulated ears, high-arched palate, oral synechiae, long philtrum, small nose, broad nasal bridge, short neck | Short stature, short limbs, microcephaly, trigonocephaly, prominent metopic sutures, upward slant of palpebral fissures, epicanthic folds, Brushfield spots, squint, omphalocele, hypogonadism, multiple joint contractures, syndactyly, talipes varus/valgus, complex heart defect, lung anomalies, mental retardation, hypotonia |
| Oto-onycho-peroneal syndrome[138] | **259780** 3582 | AR | Abnormal helix, low-set ears, small ear lobe, midface hypoplasia | Hypoplastic nails, camptodactyly, restriction of joint mobility, webbing of lower limb joints, hypoplastic fibula/tibia, irregular shape of toes |
| Paes-Alves syndrome[130] | 4955 | ?AR | Preauricular tags, low-set ears, atresia of the external auditory canal, mixed deafness, abnormal columella, broad nasal tip, dysphagia, speech defect | Short stature, hyperkeratosis, nevi, microcephaly, hypertelorism, short palpebral fissures, puffy eyelids, pseudopapilledema, oligodontia, pectus excavatum, brachydactyly, pes cavus, syndactyly, seizures |
| Pallister-Hall syndrome (see Hypothalamic-hamartoblastoma syndrome) | | | | |
| Peters anomaly, short limb dwarfism[96] | ***261540** 4483 | AR | Atresia of the external auditory canal, low-set ears, high-arched cleft palate, abnormal columella, depressed nasal bridge, anteverted nostrils, abnormal cry | Failure to thrive, short limbs, flat occiput, blepharophimosis, microcornea, glaucoma, cataract, hypospadias, heart defect, delayed skeletal maturation, mental retardation |
| Pfeiffer syndrome (acro-cephalo-syndactyly type 5)[66] | ***101600** 3008 | AD | Abnormal middle ear, conductive deafness, small nose, depressed nasal bridge, dental malocclusion, tracheal abnormality | Coronal craniosynostosis, abnormal skull shape, hypertelorism, downward slant of palpebral fissures, broad great toes, soft tissue syndactyly |
| Pfeiffer-Palm-Teller (PPT) syndrome[139] | **261560** 3879 | ?AR | Cup-shaped ears, high-arched narrow palate, high-pitched voice | Short stature, short limbs, thick skin, short palpebral fissures, epicanthic folds, coloboma of eyelids, small hands, cone-shaped epiphyses, coarctation of aorta, mitral valve prolapse, spasticity, progressive joint stiffness |
| Pseudoisotretinoin syndrome[94] | **243440** 4475 | ?AR | Atresia of the external auditory canals, microtia, folded-down ears, micrognathia, facial palsy | Death in infancy, prominent occiput, hypertelorism, interrupted aortic arch (no history of drug exposure) |

| Syndrome or condition | MIM No. and POSSUM No.[a] | Inheritance[b] | Ear, nose, and throat manifestations | Other manifestations |
|---|---|---|---|---|
| Pseudoprogeria syndrome (pseudoprogeria-Hallermann-Streiff)[75] | **200130** 3867 | ?AR | Microtia, prominent ears, small beaked nose, high nasal bridge, abnormal nasal septum, webbed neck | Microcephaly, absent or decreased eyebrows and eyelashes, glaucoma, cataract, optic nerve anomalies, kyphosis, diffuse osteoporosis, contracture of large joints, hip abnormalities, seizures, spasticity, mental retardation, short stature |
| Rüdiger syndrome (mental retardation, coarse face, limb hypoplasia, stenotic urethra)[70] | **268650** 3148 | AR | Coarse facies, ear cartilage deficiency, small nose, depressed nasal bridge, anteverted nostrils, cleft palate, macrostomia, long philtrum, abnormal cry | Distal limb hypoplasia, ureteral stenosis, hypertelorism, inguinal hernia, camptodactyly, small hands and feet, mental retardation |
| Seaver-Cassidy syndrome[160] | 4934 | ?AD | Low-set posteriorly angulated ears, linear indentation of ear lobes, thin lips, high and broad nasal bridge, large mouth, prognathism | Hypertelorism, downward slant of palpebral fissures, ptosis, umbilical hernia, hyperextensible joints, shawl scrotum, borderline mental retardation |
| Simpson-Golabi-Behmel syndrome (Golabi-Rosen syndrome)[99,127] | ***312870** 3325 | XLR | Coarse facies, preauricular tags, prominent ears, macrostomia, macroglossia, high nasal bridge, anteverted nostrils, hypoplasia of the midface, submucous cleft palate | Overgrowth, microcephaly, tall stature, lax skin, upward slant of palpebral fissures, retinal coloboma, visual loss, squint, pectus excavatum, kyphoscoliosis multiple vertebral segmentation defects, cardiac arrhythmias, cryptorchidism, abnormal palmar dermatoglyphics, overlapping toes, syndactyly, mental retardation, seizures, hypotonia |
| Split hand, split foot, mandibulofacial dysostosis (Patterson-Stevenson syndrome)[50] | ***183700** 3880 | AD | Atresia of the external auditory canal, folded ear, abnormal ear lobule, cleft palate, conductive, deafness, coloboma of nostrils, micrognathia | Ectrodactyly, cleft hand, short or absent phalanges, syndactyly of fingers |
| Symphalangism-brachydactyly syndrome *or* WL syndrome[86] | ***186500** 3402 | AD | Hypoplastic antihelix conductive deafness, broad nasal bridge, long nose, short philtrum, thin lips | Multiple fusions involving midphalangeal joints and elbows, short stature, small hands, irregular shape of fingers, abnormal palmar dermatoglyphics, short feet, overlapping toes |
| Teebi hypertelorism syndrome (brachycephalo-fronto-nasal dysplasia)[164,171] | ***145420** | AD | Ear cartilage deficiency, prominent ears, high-arched palate, midface hypoplasia, short nose, broad and depressed nasal bridge, bulbous nasal tip, thin lips, long philtrum deeply grooved philtrum | Flat occiput, frontal bossing, pronounced hypertelorism, ptosis, squint, webbed fingers, small hands, umbilical hernia, clinodactyly of 5th finger, normal intelligence |
| Townes-Brocks syndrome (see Anus-hand-ear syndrome) | | | | |
| Uropathy, distal obstructive, polydactyly[73] | 4532 | | Low-set ears, ear cartilage deficiency, micrognathia, beaked nose | Stillbirth, oligohydramnios, cryptochidism, syndactyly of fingers, postaxial polydactyly, ureteric, bladder and urethral anomalies |
| VACTERL association with hydrocephalus[87] | 4843 | Sporadic | Microtia, atresia of the external auditory canal, low-set ears, micrognathia, tracheoesophageal fistula | CNS defects, macrocephaly, hypertelorism, vertebral defects, heart defect, hypoplastic radius, hypoplastic kidneys, ureteric/urethral anomalies, anal stenosis, mental retardation |
| Whistling face syndrome[34,48] | **193700** 3156 | AD AR | Ear cartilage deficiency, puckered appearance of the mouth | Ulnar deviation of hands, possible hypertonicity at birth, with vomiting in infancy, normal intelligence |

**Appendix A** Syndromes and Conditions Associated with Congenital Anomalies of the Ear (*Continued*)

| Syndrome or condition | **MIM No.** and POSSUM No.[a] | Inheritance[b] | Ear, nose, and throat manifestations | Other manifestations |
|---|---|---|---|---|
| Wildervanck syndrome (cervico-oculo-acoustic syndrome)[166] | **314600** 3059 | ? | Preauricular tags, atresia of external auditory canal, low-set ears, abnormal middle and inner ear, sensorineural deafness, cleft palate, short webbed neck | Klippel-Feil anomaly, Duane retraction syndrome, cerebellar and brain stem atrophy, short stature, mental retardation |
| PREDOMINANTLY ABNORMAL EAR POSITION | | | | |
| Acrofacial dysostosis, Palomeque type[133] | 4789 | | Microtia, posteriorly angulated ears, cleft palate, macrostomia, broad nasal bridge, oblique facial cleft, midfacial hypoplasia | Short stature, microcephaly, backward sloping forehead, prominent supraorbital ridges, coloboma of iris, radio-ulnar synostosis, clinodactyly of 5th finger, short thumbs, talipes, syndactyly |
| Amyoplasia with mandibulofacial dysostosis[115] | 4234 | | Microtia, low-set ears, micrognathia | Poor muscle build, muscular atrophy, downward slant of palpebral fissures, scoliosis, camptodactyly, talipes |
| Baller-Gerold syndrome (craniosynoaplasia syndrome)[67,182] | ***218600** 3165 | AR | Microtia, low-set ears, cleft palate, high nasal bridge, micrognathia | Short stature, acrocephaly, sutural synostosis, hypoplastic radius, absent phalanges, carpal fusion, horseshoe kidney, imperforate or malplaced anus, hydrocephalus, premature centromere separation as in Roberts syndrome |
| Carnevale-Bonvino syndrome[24] | **265050** 4946 | AR | Low-set ears, abnormal helix, abnormal size of earlobe, depressed nasal bridge, narrow palate | Short stature, blepharophimosis, ptosis, open bite, lumbar lordosis, ectopic testes, dislocated hip, mild mental retardation, brisk reflexes |
| Catel-Manzke syndrome (Pierre Robin sequence and symmetric hyperphalangy of index finger)[18,38] | **302380** 3557 | ?XL | Low-set and posteriorly angulated ears, prominent antihelix, abnormal size of earlobes, cleft soft palate, short neck, micrognathia | Hypertelorism, short stature, abnormal metacarpals, irregular shape of fingers, abnormal palmar dermatoglyphics, short feet, cyanotic heart disease, mild mental retardation |
| Chromosome 3, del 3p (p25–pter)[116,121] | 3520 | | Low-set ears, high-arched palate, thick lips, small nostrils, high nasal bridge, beaked nose, structural asymmetry of the face | Pre- and postnatal growth retardation, epicanthic folds, ptosis, visual loss, scoliosis, umbilical hernia, small penis, delayed skeletal maturation, abnormal urinary tract, polydactyly of toes, abnormal gait, mental retardation |
| Chromosome 5, partial del 5p (Cri du chat syndrome)[103,129] | 3073 | | Preauricular tags, posteriorly angulated ears, depressed nasal bridge, prominent supraorbital ridges, round face, laryngeal anomaly, abnormal (cat) cry, large frontal sinuses (in adults) | Short stature, premature graying of hair in adults, broad cheeks, hypertelorism, heart defect, scoliosis, hypospadias, small hands, partial syndactyly, moderate to severe mental retardation, hypotonia |
| Chromosome 5, partial dup 5q[113] | 4671 | | Low-set ears, deafness, downturned mouth, microstomia, broad depressed nasal bridge, depressed premaxillary region, dysphagia, speech defect | Failure to thrive, fine hair, microcephaly, hypertelorism, umbilical hernia, arachnodactyly, clinodactyly of 5th finger, moderate to severe mental retardation |
| Chromosome 9, partial del 9p[20] | 3081 | | Microtia, low-set and posteriorly angulated ears, depressed nasal bridge, small nose, midface hypoplasia, short neck, micrognathia | Hypoplastic nails, hypertelorism, upward slant of palpebral fissures, bushy eyebrows, umbilical hernia, polydactyly, abnormal external female genitalia, seizures, hypotonia, mental retardation |
| Chromosome 12, del 12p13[15] | 4775 | | Low-set and posteriorly angulated ears, protruding tongue, cleft lip, deeply grooved philtrum, large nose | Microcephaly, hypoplastic left heart, hypoplastic kidneys, abnormal liver |

| Syndrome or condition | MIM No. and POSSUM No.[a] | Inheritance[b] | Ear, nose, and throat manifestations | Other manifestations |
|---|---|---|---|---|
| Costello syndrome[37] | ***218040** 3475 | AR | Low-set ears, abnormal size of ear lobe, short neck, coarse face, variable onset of nasal and perioral papillomata | Short stature, thick redundant skin, fuzzy hair, macrocephaly, epicanthic folds, tooth discoloration, abnormal palmar/plantar creases, mild to moderate mental retardation, happy personality |
| Crane-Heise syndrome[32] | 3407 | AR | Low-set and posteriorly angulated ears, absent helix, cleft lip/palate, micrognathia, anteverted nostrils, short neck | Macrocephaly, hypertelorism, small scapula, absence of cervical vertebrae and clavicles, small penis, syndactyly of fingers, single palmar creases, agenesis of corpus callosum, lethal |
| Craniosynoaplasia syndrome (see Baller-Gerold syndrome) | | | | |
| Craniosynostosis, arachnodactyly, abdominal hernias (Shprintzen-Goldberg syndrome)[27,193] | **182212** 3669 | ?AD | Low-set and posteriorly angulated ears, soft ears with cartilage deficiency, "pseudocleft" of the palate, micrognathia, midface hypoplasia | Sutural synostosis, hypertelorism, downward slant of palpebral fissures, pectus carinatum/excavatum, scoliosis, omphalocele, hernia, large hands, camptodactyly, arachnodactyly, mitral valve prolapse, Hirschsprung disease, mental retardation, hypotonia |
| Craniosynostosis, Fontaine type[49] | 4133 | | Low-set ears, microtia, depressed nasal bridge, anteverted nostrils | Sparse or absent scalp hair, phalangeal hypoplasia with small or no nails, acrocephaly, sutural synostosis, flat supraorbital ridges, hypospadias and genital anomalies, syndactyly of fingers, brain and cardiac anomalies |
| Dwarfism, (intrauterine), ataxia, diabetes[9] | **210740** 3772 | AR | Low-set ears, abnormal antihelix, abnormal ear lobe size, large beaked nose, abnormal columella, flared nostrils, micrognathia, long face | Short stature, deep-set eyes, cryptorchidism, hypogonadism, small hand, clinodactyly of 5th fingers, short foot, mental retardation, ataxia, insulin resistant diabetes, goiter |
| Facio-auricular syndrome, Simosa type[162] | 4638 | AD | Low-set posteriorly angulated ears, abnormal tragus, large nose, coloboma of nostrils, downturned mouth angles, midface hypoplasia, abnormal cry and voice | High forehead, high-arched eyebrow, blepharophimosis, kyphosis, scoliosis, inguinal hernia, cryptorchidism, normal intelligence |
| Fetal valproate syndrome[31,39] | 3650 | | Microtia, low-set ears, short nose with anteverted nostrils, long and flat philtrum, nystagmus, midfacial hypoplasia, microstomia | Narrow forehead, hypoplastic nails, sutural synostosis, flat supraorbital ridges, squint, hypospadias, radial ray defects, cardiovascular anomalies, duodenal atresia, neural tube defect, mental retardation |
| FG syndrome (Opitz-Kaveggia syndrome)[128] | ***305450** 3566 | XLR | Microtia, posteriorly angulated and low-set ears, high-arched palate, thick lips, micrognathia, long face, trismus, sensorineural deafness | Short stature, abnormal scalp hair, macrocephaly, hypertelorism, prominent supraorbital ridges, deep-set eyes, pectus excavatum, lordosis, inguinal hernia, syndactyly of fingers, talipes valgus/varus, heart defect, imperforate stenotic/malplaced anus, hydrocephalus, hypoplasia of corpus callosum, mental retardation, hypotonia, chronic constipation |
| Fibrochondrogenesis[11] | ***228520** 3642 | AR | Microtia, posteriorly-angulated ears, cleft palate, flattened and hypoplastic nose, anteverted nostrils, absent nasal cartilage, microstomia, short neck | Short stature, rhizomelic limb shortness, broad forehead, prominent eyes, pectus excavatum, anomalies of vertebral bodies, camptodactyly, clinodactyly of 5th fingers, cerebral cortex atrophy, lethal |

**Appendix A** Syndromes and Conditions Associated with Congenital Anomalies of the Ear (*Continued*)

| Syndrome or condition | **MIM No.** and POSSUM No.[a] | Inheritance[b] | Ear, nose, and throat manifestations | Other manifestations |
|---|---|---|---|---|
| Herrmann-Opitz acrocephalosyndactyly syndrome (craniosyndactyly, brachysyndactyly, absent toes)[65] | 3440 | | Microtia, low-set ears, midfacial hypoplasia, high-arched narrow palate, micrognathia | Short stature, hypertelorism, squint, restricted joint movement, brachydactyly, missing toes, craniosynostosis, mental retardation |
| Herrmann-Opitz arthrogryposis syndrome[79] | 3252 | AD | Posteriorly-angulated large ears, cleft palate, abnormal facies, abnormal sinuses | Short stature, joint contractures, delayed fusion of sutures, ectropion, bell-shaped chest, scoliosis, anomalies of vertebrae, short limbs, camptodactyly |
| Idaho 2 syndrome[27,28] | 3169 | | Microtia, posteriorly-angulated low-set ears, preauricular tags, beaked and short nose, micrognathia, microglossia often associated with bifid epiglottis or laryngeal cleft | Sagittal craniosynostosis, dolichocephaly, antimongoloid slant of palpebral fissures, mental retardation, sloping shoulders/winged scapulae, long chest, cubitus valgus, marfanoid habitus |
| MacDermot-Winter syndrome[109] | **247990** 4947 | AR | Large posteriorly-angulated ears, narrow nasal bridge, small nose, round face, abnormal cry, dysphagia | IUGR, short stature, microcephaly, puffy eyelids, hypoplastic genitalia, camptodactyly, seizures, moderate to severe mental retardation, hypotonia, early death |
| Multiple congenital anomalies, Thakker-Donnai type[173] | **227255** 4904 | AR | Large posteriorly-angulated ears, downturned mouth angle, broad nasal bridge, short neck, microstomia | Failure to thrive, macrocephaly, hypertelorism, broad nasal tip, abnormal rib number, vertebral segmentation defects, heart defect, hypoplasia of corpus callosum, imperforate anus/anal stenosis (resembles Lambotte syndrome) |
| Multiple pterygium syndrome[114,148] | ***265000** 3472 | AR | Low-set ears, conductive deafness, abnormal middle ear, cleft palate, glossoptosis, micrognathia, expressionless face, short webbed neck | Short stature, hypertelorism, epicanthic folds, ptosis, pterygia of neck, axilla, elbows, knees with joint contractures, syndactyly, camptodactyly, lumbar lordosis, vertebral defects, dislocated hip, rocker-bottom foot, abnormal external genitalia |
| Mulvihill-Smith syndrome[12] | **176690** 4573 | | Low-set ears, abnormal size of ear lobe, high nasal bridge, microstomia, abnormal sinuses, open bite, abnormal cry, disproportionately small face | Growth retardation, pigmented nevi, premature aging, short stature, sparse hair, microcephaly, myopia, oligodontia, hepatomegaly, mental retardation, diabetes mellitus |
| Nevo syndrome[123] | 3848 | AR | Low-set ears, high-arched palate, general enlargement of the jaw, abnormal voice | Tall stature, cerebral gigantism, frontal bossing, generalized edema, flexion contracture of feet, kyphoscoliosis, advanced bone age, coxa vara, single palmar creases, mental retardation, (one family) |
| Noonan-like syndrome with slow hair growth[13] | 4342 | | Low-set posteriorly-angulated ears, small nose, broad nasal bridge, anteverted nostrils, thin lips, deeply grooved philtrum, mixed deafness, dysphagia | Short stature, shield chest, heart defects, sparse scalp hair, hypertelorism, pectus excavatum, delayed skeletal maturation, brachydactyly, cryptorchidism, mental retardation |
| Potter sequence (bilateral renal agenesis and oligohydramnios sequence)[10,192] | ***191830** 3368 | Sporadic AD | Low-set ears, cleft palate, flattened nose, micrognathia, webbed neck | Microcephaly, hypertelorism, epicanthic folds, ambiguous genitalia, hypoplastic lower limbs, dysplastic kidneys, bladder anomalies, imperforate anus (urinary tract abnormalities may be isolated or part of multiple congenital anomalies) |

| Syndrome or condition | MIM No. and POSSUM No.[a] | Inheritance[b] | Ear, nose, and throat manifestations | Other manifestations |
|---|---|---|---|---|
| Progeroid, congenital syndrome, Petty-Wiedemann type[137] | 4882 | | Posteriorly angulated and low-set ears, prominent mandible and lower lip | Pre- and postnatal growth retardation, diminished subcutaneous fat, wrinkled skin, aged appearance from birth, sparse hair, hypoplastic distal phalanges, umbilical hernia, normal mental development |
| Seckel syndrome (microcephalic primordial dwarfism type 1)[21,90] | ***210600** 3387 | AR | Microtia, low-set ears, abnormal size of ear lobule, high palate, large beaked nose, high nasal bridge, prominent midface, oligodontia, micrognathia | Severe growth retardation, joint dislocations, increased body hair, narrow forehead, microcephaly, squint, abnormal rib number, single palmar creases, talipes varus/valgus, dysplastic kidney, irregular shape of fingers, moderate to severe mental retardation (pancytopenia and chromosomal instability in 2 cases) |
| Seckel-like with short limbs (microcephalic primordial dwarfism type II *or* osteodysplastic primordial dwarfism type 2)[185,191] | ***210720** 3345 | AR | Microtia, low-set ears, high-arched and narrow palate, prominent nose, micrognathia, short neck | Growth retardation, receding forehead, upward slanting of palpebral fissures, abnormal pelvis, hypospadias, atrophic testes, small hand, brachydactyly, short limbs with abnormal tibia/fibula, moderate to severe mental retardation |
| Short stature, deafness, neutrophil dysfunction, dysmorphism (Thong-Douglas-Ferrante syndrome)[174] | 4334 | | Microtia, low-set ears, sensorineural deafness, high-arched narrow palate, micrognathia | Short stature, hypertelorism, coronal synostosis, malplaced anus, diffuse osteoporosis, abnormal neutrophil chemotaxis, osteosarcoma (2 siblings) |
| X-linked mental retardation, alpha-thalassemia[60] | ***301040** 4919 | XLR | Microtia, low-set ears, macroglossia, midface hypoplasia, broad nasal bridge, small nose | Severe mental retardation, hemoglobin H, telecanthus, squint, scoliosis, multiple vertebral anomalies, genital anomalies, hypotonia/spasticity, severe mental retardation |
| Yunis-Varon syndrome (Cleidocranial dysostosis, micrognathia, digital anomalies)[195] | ***216340** 3485 | AR | Low-set or posteriorly angulated or cup-shaped ears, abnormal tragus, abnormal size of ear lobe, micrognathia, short midface, webbed neck | Absent thumb, absent distal phalanges, absent clavicles, growth deficiency, small nails, delayed fusion of sutures, poorly ossified calvarium, upward slanting of palpebral fissures, prominent eyes, microphthalmos, abnormal pelvis, brachydactyly, coxa valga, rocker-bottom foot, hypotonia |
| PREDOMINANTLY ABNORMAL EAR SIZE | | | | |
| Acardia[19,120] | 4406 | | Anotia or microtia | Microphthalmos, abnormal genitalia, short limbs, syndactyly of fingers, talipes varus/valgus, missing toes, malsegmentation defects of lungs |
| Acrocephalospondylosyndactyly, Wells type[190] | 4772 | | Large ears, thin lips, down-turned mouth, small nostrils, beaked nose, midfacial hypoplasia | Abnormal distribution of scalp hair,sutural synostosis, hypertelorism, prominent eyes, inguinal hernia, radioulnar dislocation, syndactyly of fingers, block thoracic vertebrae, widely open neural arches and fan-shaped thoracic cage |
| Acrofacial dysostosis, Rodriguez type[136,153] | **201170** 4804 | AR | Microtia, small external auditory canal, cleft palate, high nasal bridge, marked micrognathia | IUGR, short limbs, abnormal rib number, hypoplastic ulna, missing fingers, pulmonic atresia, hydrocephalus, agenesis of corpus callosum, lethal |

**Appendix A** Syndromes and Conditions Associated with Congenital Anomalies of the Ear (*Continued*)

| Syndrome or condition | MIM No. and POSSUM No.[a] | Inheritance[b] | Ear, nose, and throat manifestations | Other manifestations |
|---|---|---|---|---|
| Allan-Herndon syndrome[158] | ***309600** 4784 | XLR | Long ears, expressionless face | Abnormal gait/ataxia, narrow forehead, camptodactyly, muscle weakness |
| Anotia, facial weakness, congenital heart defect[135] | 4556 | | Anotia, atresia of the external canal, facial palsy, preauricular tags | Congenital heart disease, ptosis, scoliosis |
| Beare-Stevenson type cutis gyratum (cutis gyratum—acanthosis nigricans)[163] | 3831 | | Abnormal size pinna, cleft palate, micrognathia, small nose, depressed nasal bridge, abnormal facial skin folds | Thick skin, acanthosis nigricans, flat occiput, large fontanelles, prominent eyes, abnormal palmar dermatoglyphics, pyloric stenosis, hypoglycemia, hepatomegaly, mental retardation |
| Blepharoptosis, ectopia lentis, myopia[62] | **110150** 3903 | AD | Long ears | Discolored nails, ptosis, dislocated lens, retinal pigmentary changes, visual loss |
| Börjeson-Forssman-Lehmann syndrome (mental retardation, microcephaly, epilepsy, hypogonadism)[180] | ***301900** 3502 | XLR | Long and large low-set ears, round and coarse facies, nystagmus, depressed nasal bridge, short neck, speech defect | Generalized obesity, thick skin, microcephaly, broad cheeks, deep-set eyes, retinal detachment, optic nerve abnormality, visual loss, scoliosis, small hands/brachydactyly, mental retardation, seizures, hypotonia, diabetes mellitus, pituitary defects, hypogonadism |
| Brachydactyly, microtia[175] | **123560** 4547 | AD | Microtia, abnormal sinuses | Excessive freckling, hypoplastic nails, epiphyseal abnormality, brachydactyly, abnormal palmar dermatoglyphics, short and broad feet, scrotal abnormality |
| CAMFAK syndrome (Cockayne syndrome type 2)[169] | **212540** 4758 | AR | Long and large ears, small face | Failure to thrive, microcephaly, scoliosis, camptodactyly, dislocated hip, cerebral cortex atrophy, mental retardation, absent reflexes |
| Chromosome 1, dup 1 (p21.2–p32)[119] | 4701 | | Long and large ears, anteverted nostrils, long philtrum, lateral cleft lip, micrognathia | Failure to thrive, microcephaly, inguinal hernia, squint, cryptorchidism, clinodactyly of 5th fingers, single palmar creases, mental retardation |
| Chromosome 3, partial del 3 (p12–p14)[80] | 3687 | | Abnormal size of ear lobe, microtia, low-set ears, broad nasal bridge | Acrocephaly, narrow and high forehead, flat supraorbital ridges, epicanthic folds, short sternum, pectus carinatum, camptodactyly, overlapping fingers, single palmar creases, bifid great toe, mental retardation |
| Chromosome 4, partial del 4p (Wolf-Hirschhorn syndrome)[146] | 3069 | | Microtia, preauricular tags, cleft palate, short philtrum, hypertelorism, broad nasal bridge, prominent glabella, beaked nose, nystagmus, round face, down-turned mouth angles, trismus | Pre- and postnatal growth retardation, microcephaly, frontal bossing, poorly ossified calvarium, high-arched eyebrow, ptosis, ectropion, epicanthic folds, microphthalmos, cataract, scoliosis, congenital heart disease, severe psychomotor retardation |
| Chromosome 4, partial del 4q[45] | 3072 | | Microtia, cup-shaped ears, cleft palate, cleft lip, anteverted nostrils, flattened nose, micrognathia | Short stature, microcephaly, hypertelorism, micrognathia, hypospadias, contracture of large joints, clinodactyly of 5th finger, nail defects, urinary tract defects, moderate to severe mental retardation |

| Syndrome or condition | **MIM No.** and POSSUM No.[a] | Inheritance[b] | Ear, nose, and throat manifestations | Other manifestations |
|---|---|---|---|---|
| Chromosome 8, partial dup 8q[122] | 3120 | | Microtia, cup-shaped ears, posteriorly angulated ears, cleft palate, thin lips, down-turned mouth angles, depressed nasal bridge, anteverted nostrils, short webbed neck, long face, micrognathia | Failure to thrive, increased body hair, high forehead, small penis, hypospadias, cryptorchidism, clinodactyly of 5th fingers, syndactyly, wide space between 1st and 2nd toes, dysplastic kidneys, abnormal gall bladder, mental retardation |
| Chromosome 12, partial dup 12p[170] | 3088 | | Microtia, cleft palate, long philtrum, drooping lower lip, anteverted nostrils, small nose, depressed nasal bridge, midfacial hypoplasia | Short stature, acrocephaly, flat occiput, hypertelorism, microphthalmos, aniridia, severe visual loss, short sternum, small hand/brachydactyly, syndactyly, imperforate anus, mental retardation, hypotonia |
| Chromosome 22, trisomy 22[5,168] | 3703 | | Preauricular tags/sinuses, large posteriorly angulated, low-set and abnormally-shaped ears, flat nose, macrostomia, cleft palate, micrognathia, short neck | Stillbirth or neonatal death, small for gestational age, microcephaly, coloboma of iris, hypotonia, mental retardation |
| Cohen-Lockwood-Wyborney syndrome (mental retardation, blepharophimosis, ptosis, syndactyly)[54] | 3966 | | Hypoplastic antihelix, microtia, low-set cup-shaped ears, macrostomia, broad nasal tip, hypoplasia of midface, abnormal voice | Short stature, broad forehead, blepharophimosis, asymmetry of the chest, inguinal hernia, syndactyly of fingers, dislocated hip, overlapping toes, mental retardation |
| Coxoauricular syndrome (short stature, ear malformations and hip dislocation)[40] | **122780**<br>3522 | AD | Microtia, atresia of the external auditory canal, abnormal middle ear, conductive hearing loss | Lumbar lordosis, delayed ossification of pubic bones, abnormal femur, dislocated hip |
| Cutis laxa, osteoporosis, growth/mental retardation[134] | 4013 | AR | Long and large ears, significantly abnormal facies | Short stature, sagging cheeks, downward slant of palpebral fissures, medial flare of eyebrows, dental caries, diffuse osteoporosis, delayed skeletal maturation, hypermobile joints, mental retardation, lethal arterial dissection |
| Cutis laxa, skeletal defects, ambiguous genitalia[101] | 4582 | | Long and large ears, webbed neck, high-arched palate, micrognathia, glossoptosis | Failure to thrive, macrocephaly, poorly ossified calvarium, hypertelorism, umbilical hernia, hypospadias, small penis, short digits, enamel hypoplasia, mental retardation |
| Deafness, cleft palate, colobomata, radial synostosis (Abruzzo-Erickson syndrome)[1] | **214800**<br>4057 | ?AR<br>?XLR | Large anteverted ears, deafness, cleft palate, midface hypoplasia, flat face, micrognathia | Short stature, coloboma of iris, retinal coloboma, hypospadias, cryptorchidism, clinodactyly of fingers, radial synostosis, atrial septal defect; distinguished from CHARGE association |
| Deafness, nephritis, anorectal malformation[108] | **107100**<br>4141 | AD | Large ears, preauricular tags, sensorineural deafness | Sacral dimple, renal failure, imperforate or malplaced anus (possible anus-hand-ear syndrome without limb anomalies) |
| Dermatoleuko-dystrophy[112] | **221790**<br>3922 | AR | Large ears, large nose, expressionless aged face, dysphagia | Hyperkeratosis, ichthyosis, excessive skin wrinkling, optic nerve atrophy, large hand, large foot, cerebral cortex atrophy, mental retardation, seizures (progressive neurological deterioration with death in infancy) |
| Dermotrichic syndrome[140] | 3850 | | Large ears | Short stature, decreased sweating, ichthyosis, sparse scalp hair, frontal bossing, clubbing of toes, anemia, mental retardation |

**Appendix A** Syndromes and Conditions Associated with Congenital Anomalies of the Ear (*Continued*)

| Syndrome or condition | MIM No. and POSSUM No.[a] | Inheritance[b] | Ear, nose, and throat manifestations | Other manifestations |
|---|---|---|---|---|
| Dubowitz syndrome type 2[88] | 4800 | | Large ears, high-arched palate, thick lips, large nose, abnormal cry, micrognathia | Eczema, pigmented nevi, microcephaly, sutural synostosis, short palpebral fissures, ptosis, squint, atrophic testes, syndactyly of fingers, clinodactyly of 5th fingers, imperforate anus, mental retardation (seen in an isolated Russian population) |
| Ear lobes thickened, deafness, incudostapedial defects (Escher-Hirt syndrome)[43] | ***128980** 3444 | AD | Abnormal size of ear lobe, abnormal middle ear, conductive deafness | |
| Facio-cardio-renal syndrome (Eastman-Bixler syndrome)[124] | **227280** 3500 | AR | Microtia, long and pointed ears, high and broad nasal bridge, micrognathia, long face, cleft lip and palate | Abnormal posture, small nails, corneal opacities, camptodactyly, mitral valve stenosis, ectopic *or* horseshoe kidney, cryptorchidism, vertebral anomalies, moderate to severe mental retardation |
| Gingival fibromatosis, hepatosplenomegaly, other anomalies (Zimmermann-Laband syndrome)[71] | ***135500** 3433 | AD | Coarse face, large and long ears, macroglossia, protruding lips, gingival fibromatosis, large nose, flared nostrils | Increased body hair, small nails, abnormal phalanges, hepatosplenomegaly, mental retardation |
| Greig cephalopolysyndactyly (Hootnick-Holmes syndrome *or* Frontodigital syndrome)[141,156,186] | **#175700** 3489 | AD | Abnormal size of ear lobe, broad nasal bridge | Macrocephaly, scaphocephaly, flat occiput, broad forehead, hypertelorism, oligondontia, abnormal metacarpals, polydactyly, camptodactyly, syndactyly, hypoplasia of corpus callosum (distinguished from acrocallosal syndrome) |
| Growth retardation, intrauterine, mandibular/malar hypoplasia[46] | 4198 | | Microtia, low-set ears, marked hypoplasia of the facial bones, micrognathia | Pre- and postnatal growth retardation, microcephaly, hypoplastic nipples, delayed skeletal maturation, camptodactyly, overlapping fingers, hypoplastic nails |
| Holoprosencephaly, hypokinesia[82] | **306990** 4666 | XLR | Abnormal or absent helix, long ears | Decreased fetal movements, microcephaly, short ribs, hypospadias, hypoplastic lungs, agenesis of kidney, joint contractures, stillbirth or neonatal death |
| Holzgreve-Wagner-Rehder syndrome[105] | 4694 | | Large and low-set folded ears, micrognathia, cleft palate | Renal agenesis, hypoplastic lungs, postaxial polydactyly, talipes, valgus/varus, cardiac and intestinal defects, hypoplasia of corpus callosum, stillbirth or neonatal death |
| Kabuki make-up syndrome (Niikawa-Kuroki syndrome)[74,125] | **147920** 2355 | AD | Large cup-shaped ears, preauricular pits, open bite, cleft palate, abnormal nasal septum, bulbous nasal tip, beaked nose, micrognathia | Short stature, long palpebral fissures, everted lateral third of lower lid, epicanthic folds, blue sclera, paresis of the ocular muscles, discoloration of teeth, scoliosis, prominent finger pads, cone-shaped epiphyses, mental retardation, hypotonia |
| Killian-Teschler-Nicola syndrome (Pallister mosaic syndrome)[61,145,157] | 3800 | | Large low-set ears, thickened helix, short neck, cleft palate, down-turned mouth, speech defect | Dry skin, sparse hair, irregular skin pigmentation, accessory nipples, puffy eyelids, inguinal hernia, imperforate anus, caudal appendage, severe mental retardation, seizures, hypotonia, chromosome 12p tetrasomy mosaic |

| Syndrome or condition | MIM No. and POSSUM No.[a] | Inheritance[b] | Ear, nose, and throat manifestations | Other manifestations |
|---|---|---|---|---|
| Lin-Gettig syndrome[106] | **218649** 4783 | | Microtia, low-set ears, small nose, hypoplastic nostrils, long philtrum, abnormal columella, midfacial hypoplasia, small face | Macrocephaly, craniosynostosis, ptosis, agenesis of corpus callosum, joint contractures, urogenital anomalies, mental retardation |
| Low birth weight syndrome, Kogut-Sensenbrenner type[97] | 4295 | | Microtia, large nose, high nasal bridge, hearing loss, dysphagia, micrognathia | Microcephaly, short stature, scoliosis, diffuse osteoporosis, dislocated radial heads, brachydactyly, aminoaciduria, borderline mental retardation |
| Microtia, absent patella, short stature, (Meier-Gorlin syndrome, includes Hurst-Winter-Baraitser syndrome)[17,26,85] | **224690** 4906 4408 | AR | Bilateral microtia, atresia of external auditory canal, high-arched palate, microstomia, distinctive triangular face | Short stature, microcephaly, thin skin, absent patellae, delayed skeletal maturation, radioulnar dislocation, clinodactyly of 5th finger, mild mental retardation to normal intelligence |
| Nance-Horan syndrome (Oculo-dental syndrome, X-linked)[188] | ***302350** 3464 | XLR | Large, anteverted and pointed ears, nystagmus, multiple dental anomalies | Microphthalmos, congenital cataracts, microcorneas, short metacarpals |
| Oculo-palato-cerebral dwarfism[55] | **257910** 3993 | AR | Long and large ears, cleft palate | Microcephaly, mental retardation, spasticity, short stature, smooth doughy skin, microphthalmos, corneal opacity, scoliosis, small hands and feet |
| Pallister mosaic syndrome (see Killian-Teschler-Nicola syndrome) | | | | |
| Patterson pseudoleprechaunism syndrome[36] | **169170** 3494 | ?AD | Large ears, thick lips, large nose, bulbous nasal tip, significantly abnormal facies | Growth retardation, increased body hair, lack of subcutaneous tissue, loose skin, abnormal rib number, kyphoscoliosis, platyspondyly, large penis, abnormal metaphyses and epiphyses, symphalangism, talipes varus/valgus, diabetes mellitus, adrenal malfunction, mental retardation |
| Postaxial acrofacial dysostosis syndrome (Genee-Wiedemann syndrome or Miller syndrome)[14] | ***263750** 3487 | AR | Microtia, cleft palate, cleft lip, micrognathia | Short limbs, hypertelorism, downward slant of palpebral fissures, ectropion, pectus excavatum, ulnar ray defect with missing fingers, hypoplastic thumb, mental retardation |
| Schilbach-Rott syndrome[155] | **164220** 4630 | AD | Abnormal size of ear lobe, conductive deafness, submucous cleft palate | Hypotelorism, upward slant of palpebral fissures, hypospadias |
| Shprintzen syndrome (see velo-cardio-facial syndrome) | | | | |
| Tel-Hashomer camptodactyly (camptodactyly, muscular hypoplasia, skeletal dysplasia)[131,177] | ***211960** 3051 | AR | Microtia, high-arched palate, large nose, broad nasal bridge, facial asymmetry, microsomia | Short stature, abnormal palmar creases, hypertelorism, scoliosis, humeroradial fusion, camptodactyly, syndactyly of fingers, tapered fingers, talipes valgus/varus, muscular hypoplasia |
| Tetra-amelia with multiple malformations (X-linked tetra-amelia syndrome)[58] | **301090** 3715 | XLR | Anotia/microtia, abnormal mouth, absent nasal cartilage, anosmia, facial cleft, abnormal mouth, abnormal neck | Multiple limb deficiences, absent pelvic bones, anal atresia, vertebral anomalies, rib anomalies, hypoplastic nipples, cardiovascular defects, bladder abnormalities, hypoplasia of corpus callosum, hydrocephalus, distinguished from Roberts syndrome |

**Appendix A** Syndromes and Conditions Associated with Congenital Anomalies of the Ear (*Continued*)

| Syndrome or condition | MIM No. and POSSUM No.[a] | Inheritance[b] | Ear, nose, and throat manifestations | Other manifestations |
|---|---|---|---|---|
| Thrombocytopenia, absent radius, van Haeringen type[181] | 4348 | ? | Microtia, cleft palate, micrognathia, short neck, tracheal anomalies | Intermittent thrombocytopenia, short stature, short limbs, absent radius/ulna, microcephaly, narrow shoulder, duodenal atresia, bow legs, chromosome breaks with Xrays |
| Trichorhinophalangeal syndrome type I[76] | ***190350** 3415 | AD AR | Prominent (cup-shaped) and large ears, large nose, high nasal bridge, bulbous nasal tip, small nostrils, abnormal columella, thin lips, long philtrum, micrognathia, long face | Sparse hair, short metacarpals/metatarsals, coned epiphyses, dysplastic nails, decreased eyebrows, winged scapula, pectus carinatum, small hand, clinodactyly of 5th finger, kyphoscoliosis |
| Velo-cardio-facial syndrome (Shprintzen syndrome)[107] | **#192430** 3132 | AD | Microtia, thickened helix, conductive deafness, cleft palate (often submucous), long midface, high nasal bridge, nasal speech, laryngeal anomaly | Short stature, microcephaly, scoliosis, thymic hypoplasia, cardiovascular defects, ocular abnormalities, mental retardation, deletion of 22q |
| Vitamin A embryopathy (retinoic acid embryopathy)[3] | 3624 | Teratogenicity | Anotia/microtia, low-set ears, beaked nose, protruding lips, cleft palate, depressed nasal bridge | Hydrocephalus, CNS defects, thymic aplasia/hypoplasia, cardiovascular anomalies, hypoplastic fibula/ulna, abnormal palmar creases, hypotonia, early death? |
| Walker-Warburg syndrome (HARD-E syndrome; *H*ydrocephalus, *A*gyria, *R*etinal *D*ysplasia, *E*ncephalocele)[59] | ***236670** 3656 | AR | Microtia, cleft palate, atresia of the external auditory canal, abnormal cry | Macrocephaly, hydrocephalus, cataract, megalocornea, transilluminable iris, retinal coloboma/detachment, contracture of large joints, encephalocele, Dandy-Walker malformation, agenesis of corpus callosum, mental retardation |
| Weaver syndrome (Camptodactyly, overgrowth, unusual facies)[4,6,98,149] | 3429 | | Low-set large ears, long philtrum, abnormal voice and cry, dysphagia | Large at birth, advanced skeletal maturation, feeding problems in infancy, macrocephaly, hypertelorism, metaphyseal abnormality, camptodactyly, terminal clubbing of fingers, bifid/broad thumb, mental retardation |
| X-linked mental retardation, macrocephaly, short stature, coarse face (Atkin-Flaitz-Patil syndrome)[8] | ***309530** 3724 | AD XLR | Coarse facies, large ears, high-arched palate, thick lips, broad nasal bridge, anteverted nostrils | Frontal bossing, high forehead, prominent supraorbital ridges, epicanthic folds, kyphosis, macrotestes, small hand, genu recurvatum, seizures, ataxia, mental retardation, short stature |
| X-linked mental retardation, Tranebjaerg type[178] | **309480** 4522 | XLR | Long ears, high-arched palate, hypotonic face, macrostomia, thick lips, prognathism | Hyperkeratosis, psoriasis, hypertelorism, scoliosis, large penis, single palmar creases, ataxias, hypotonia, mental retardation, seizures |

[a]MIM, *M*endelian *I*nheritance in *M*an. A Catalog of Human Genes and Genetic Disorders, by Victor A. McKusick, 11th ed, The Johns Hopkins University Press, Baltimore, 1994; POSSUM, *P*ictures *O*f *S*tandard *S*yndromes and *U*ndiagnosed *M*alformations, by Agnes Bankier et al., Murdoch Institute, Royal Children's Hospital, Victoria, Australia.
[b]AD, autosomal dominant; AR, autosomal recessive; XLR, X-linked recessive; XLD, X-linked dominant.
*confirmed gene and inheritance.
#phenotype that can be caused by mutation in any of 2 or more genes.

## References


1. Abruzzo MA, Erickson RP: Re-evaluation of new X-linked syndrome for evidence of CHARGE syndrome or association Am J Med Genet 34:397–400, 1989.
2. Aleck KA, Hadro TA: Dominant inheritance of Wiedemann-Beckwith syndrome: further evidence for transmission of "unstable premutation" through carrier women. Am J Med Genet 33:155–160, 1989.
3. Alles AJ, Sulik KK: Retinoic-acid-induced limb-reduction defects: perturbation of zones of programmed cell death as a pathogenetic mechanism. Teratology 40:163–171, 1989.
4. Amir N, Gross-Kieselstein E, Hirsch HJ, Lax E, Silverberg-Shalev R: Weaver-Smith syndrome. A case study with long-term follow-up. Am J Dis Child 138:1113–1117, 1984.
5. Antle CM, Pantzar JT, White VA: The ocular pathology of trisomy 22: a report of two cases and review. J Pediatr Ophthalmol Strabismus 27:310–314, 1990.
6. Ardinger HH, Hansen JW, Harrod MJE, Cohen MM Jr, Tibbles JAR, Welch JP, Young-Wee T, Sommer A, Goldberg R, Shprintzen RJ, Sidoti EJ, Leichtman LG, Hoyme HE: Further delineation of the Weaver syndrome. J Pediatr 108:228–235, 1986.
7. Arens R, Reichman B, Katznelson MB, Goodman RM: New form of postaxial acrofacial dysostosis? Am J Med Genet 41:438–443, 1991.
8. Atkin JF, Flaitz K, Patil S, Smith W: A new X-linked mental retardation syndrome. Am J Med Genet 21:697–705, 1985.
9. Bangstad HJ, Beck-Nielsen H, Hother-Nielsen O,Nystad R, Trygstad O, Pedersen O, Aagenaes O: Primordial birdheaded nanism associated with progressive ataxia, early onset insulin resistant diabetes, goiter and primary gonadal insufficiency. A new syndrome. Acta Paediatr Scand 78:488–493, 1989.
10. Bankier A, de Campo M, Newell R, Rogers JG, Danks DM: A pedigree study of perinatally lethal renal disease. J Med Genet 22:104–111, 1985.
11. Bankier A, Fortune D, Duke J, Sillence DO: Fibrochondrogenesis in male twins at 24 weeks gestation. Am J Med Genet 38:95–98, 1991.
12. Baraitser M, Insley J, Winter RM: A recognisable short stature syndrome with premature aging and pigmented naevi. J Med Genet 25:53–56, 1988.
13. Baraitser M, Patton MA: A Noonan-like short stature syndrome with sparse hair. J Med Genet 23:161–164, 1986.
14. Barbuti D, Orazi C, Reale A, Paradisi C: Postaxial acrofacial dysostosis or Miller syndrome. A case report. Eur J Pediatr 148:445–446, 1989.
15. Baroncini A, Avellini C, Neri C, Forabosco A: Distal 12p deletion in a stillborn infant. Am J Med Genet 36:358–360, 1990.
16. Bawle E, Quigg MH: Ectopia lentis and aortic root dilatation in congenital contractural arachnodactyly. Am J Med Genet 42:19–21, 1992.
17. Boles RG, Teebi AS, Schwartz D, Harper JF: Further delineation of the ear, patella, short stature syndrome (Meier-Gorlin syndrome). Clin Dysmorphol 3:207–214, 1994.
18. Brude E: Pierre Robin sequence and hyperphalangy—a genetic entity (Catel-Manzke syndrome). Eur J Pediatr 142:222–223, 1984.
19. Buntinx IM, Bourgeois N, Buytaert PM, Dumon JE: Acardiac amorphous twin with prune belly sequence in the co-twin. Am J Med Genet 39:453–457, 1991.
20. Burton BK, Pettenati MJ, Block SM, Bensen J, Roach ES: Nonketotic hyperglycinemia in a patient with the 9p- syndrome. Am J Med Genet 32:504–505, 1989.
21. Butler MG, Hall BD, Maclean RN, Lozzio CB: Do some patients with Seckel syndrome have hematological problems and/or chromosome breakage? Am J Med Genet 27:645–649, 1987.
22. Butler MG, Hassell S, Feingold M, Tunnessen WW Jr: Picture of the month. Antley-Bixler syndrome. Am J Dis Child 145:701–702, 1991.
23. Cameron TH, Lachiewicz AM, Aylsworth AS: Townes-Brocks syndrome in two mentally retarded youngsters. Am J Med Genet 41:1–4, 1991.
24. Carnevale F, Krajewska G, Fischetto R, Greco MG, Bonvino A: Ptosis of eyelids, strabismus, diastasis recti, hip defect, cryptorchidism, and developmental delay in two sibs. Am J Med Genet 33:186–189, 1989.
25. Charon A, Gillerot Y, Van Maldergem L, Van Schaftingen MH, de Bont B, Koulischer L: The Marshall-Smith syndrome. Eur J Pediatr 150:54–55, 1990.
26. Cohen B, Temple IK, Symons JC, Hall CM, Shaw DG, Bhamra M, Jackson AM, Pembrey ME: Microtia and short stature: a new syndrome. J Med Genet 28:786–790, 1991.
27. Cohen MM Jr: Craniosynostosis and syndromes with craniosynostosis: incidence, genetics, penetrance, variability, and new syndrome updating. Birth Defects 15:13–63, 1979.
28. Cohen MM Jr: Craniosynostosis update 1987. Am J Med Genet (Suppl.) 4:99–148, 1988.
29. Cohen MM Jr: Perspectives on holoprosencephaly: part I. Epidemiology, genetics and syndromology. Teratology 40:211–235, 1989.
30. Cohen MM Jr, Rollnick BR, Kaye CI: Oculoauriculovertebral spectrum: an updated critique. Cleft Palate J 26:276–286, 1989.
31. Coulter DL: Carnitine, valproate, and toxicity. J Child Neurol 6:7–14, 1991.
32. Crane JP, Heise RL: New syndrome in three affected siblings. Pediatrics 68:235–237, 1981.
33. Cunniff C, Jones KL: Craniosynostosis and lid anomalies: report of a girl with Michels syndrome. Am J Med Genet 37:28–30, 1990.
34. Dallapiccola B, Giannotti A, Lembo A, Sagui L: Autosomal recessive form of whistling face syndrome in sibs. Am J Med Genet 33:542–544, 1989.
35. Danziger I, Brodsky L, Perry R, Nusbaum S, Bernat J, Robinson L: Nager's acrofacial dysostosis. Case report and review of the literature. J Pediatr Otorhinolaryngol 20:225–240, 1990.
36. David TJ, Webb BW, Gordon IR: The Patterson syndrome, leprechaunism, and pseudoleprechaunism. J Med Genet 18:294–298, 1981.
37. Der Kaloustian VM, Moroz B, McIntosh N, Watters AK, Blaichman S: Costello syndrome. Am J Med Genet 41:69–73, 1991.
38. Dignan PS, Martin LW, Zenni EJ Jr: Pierre Robin anomaly with an accessory metacarpal of the index fingers. The Catel-Manzke syndrome. Clin Genet 29:168–173, 1986.
39. DiLiberti JH, Farndon PA, Dennis NR, Curry CJ: The fetal valproate syndrome. Am J Med Genet 19:473–481, 1984.
40. Duca D, Paña I, Ciovirnache M, Simionesu L, Ispas I, Maximilian C: A previously unreported, dominantly inherited syndrome of shortness of stature, ear malformations, and hip dislocation: the coxoauricular syndrome—autosomal or X-linked male-lethal. Am J Med Genet 8:173–180, 1981.
41. Eich GF, Silver MM, Weksberg R, Daneman A, Costa T: Marshall-Smith syndrome: new radiographic, clinical and pathological observations. Radiology 181:183–188, 1986.
42. Encha-Razavi F, Larroche JC, Roume J, Migne G, Delezoide AL, Gonzales M, Mulliez N: Congenital hypothalamic hamartoma syndrome: nosological discussion and minimun diagnostic criteria of a possibly familial form. Am J Med Genet 42:44–50, 1992.
43. Escher F, Hirt H: Dominant hereditary conductive deafness through lack of incus-stapes junction. Acta Otolaryngol 65:25–32, 1968.
44. Escobar LF, Bixler D, Sadove M, Bull MJ: Antley-Bixler syndrome from a prognostic perspective: report of a case and review of the literature. Am J Med Genet 29:829–836, 1988.
45. Fagan K, Gill A: A new interstitial deletion of 4q (q21.1::q22.1) J Med Genet 26:644–647, 1989.
46. Fernhoff PM, Blackston RD, Oakley GP: Intrauterine growth retardation, abnormal facial appearance. Syndr Identif 6:10–11, 1980.
47. Finnigan DP, Clarren SK, Haas JE: Extending the Pallister-Hall syndrome to include other central nervous system malformations. Am J Med Genet 40:395–400, 1991.
48. Fitzsimmons JS, Zaldua V, Chrispin AR: Genetic heterogeneity in the Freeman-Sheldon syndrome: two adults with probable autosomal recessive inheritance. J Med Genet 21:364–368, 1984.
49. Fontaine G, Farriaux JP, Blanckaert D, Lefebvre C: Un nouveau syndrome polymalformatif complexe. J Genet Hum 25:109–119, 1977.
50. Fontaine G, Farriaux JP, Delattre P, Gidlecki Z, Poupard B, Durieux G, Piquet JJ: Une observation familiale du syndrome ectrodactylie et dysostose mandibulo-faciale. J Genet Hum 22:289–307, 1974.
51. Franceschini P, Cirillo Silengo M, Bianco R, Biagioli M, Guala A, Lopez Bell G: The Coffin-Siris syndrome in two siblings. Pediatr Radiol 16:330–333, 1986.
52. Fraser FC, Aymé S, Halal F, Sproule J: Autosomal dominant duplication of the renal collecting system, hearing loss, and external ear anomalies: a new syndrome? Am J Med Genet 14:473–478, 1983.
53. Fraser FC, Sproule JR, Halal F: Frequency of the branchio-oto-renal (BOR) syndrome in children with profound hearing loss. Am J Med Genet 7:341–349, 1980.
54. Friedman JM: Cohen-Lockwood-Wyborney syndrome: delineation of a clinically recognized entity. Proc Greenwood Genet Center 7:178, 1988.
55. Frydman M, Kauschansky A, Leshem I, Savir H: Oculo-palato-cerebral dwarfism: a new syndrome. Clin Genet 27:414–419, 1985.
56. Fryns JP, van Fleteren A, Mattelaer P, van de Berghe H: Calcification of cartilages, brachytelephalangy and peripheral pulmonary stenosis.

Confirmation of the Keutel syndrome. Eur J Pediatr 142:201–203, 1984.
57. Gabrielli O, Catassi C, Carlucci A, Coppa GV, Giorgi P: Intestinal lymphangiectasia, lymphedema, mental retardation, and typical face: confirmation of the Hennekam syndrome. Am J Med Genet 40:244–247, 1991.
58. Gershoni-Baruch R, Drugan A, Bronshtein M, Zimmer EZ : Roberts syndrome or "X-linked amelia"? Am J Med Genet 37:569–572, 1990.
59. Gershoni-Baruch R, Mandel H, Miller B, Sujov P, Braun J: Walker-Warburg syndrome with microtia and absent auditory canals. Am J Med Genet 37:87–91, 1990.
60. Gibbons RJ, Wilkie AO, Weatherall DJ, Higgs DR: A newly defined X-linked mental retardation syndrome associated with alpha thalassaemia. J Med Genet 28:729–733, 1991.
61. Gilgenkrantz S, Droulle P, Schweitzer M, Foliguet B, Chadefaux B, Lombard M, Chery M, Prieur M: Mosaic tetrasomy 12p. Clin Genet 28:495–502, 1985.
62. Gillum WN, Anderson RL: Dominantly inherited blepharoptosis, high myopia, and ectopia lentis. Arch Ophthal 100:282–284, 1982.
63. Goldstein DJ, Mirkin LD: Nager acrofacial dysostosis: evidence for apparent heterogeneity. Am J Med Genet 30:741–746, 1988.
64. Gorlin RJ, Cohen MM Jr, Levin LS: Syndromes of the Head and Neck, 3rd ed. Oxford University Press, New York, 1990, p 213.
65. Gorlin RJ, Cohen MM Jr, Levin LS: Syndromes of the Head and Neck, 3rd ed. Oxford University Press, New York, 1990, p 550.
66. Gorlin RJ, Cohen MM Jr, Levin LS: Syndromes of the Head and Neck, 3rd ed. Oxford University Press, New York, 1990, pp 526–527.
67. Gorlin RJ, Cohen MM Jr, Levin LS: Syndromes of the Head and Neck, 3rd ed. Oxford University Press, New York, 1990, pp 535–536.
68. Gorlin RJ, Cohen MM Jr, Levin LS: Syndromes of the Head and Neck, 3rd ed. Oxford University Press, New York, 1990, pp 661–662.
69. Gorlin RJ, Cohen MM Jr, Levin LS: Syndromes of the Head and Neck, 3rd ed. Oxford University Press, New York, 1990, p 663.
70. Gorlin RJ, Cohen MM Jr, Levin LS: Syndromes of the Head and Neck, 3rd ed. Oxford University Press, New York, 1990, p 771.
71. Gorlin RJ, Cohen MM Jr, Levin LS: Syndromes of the Head and Neck, 3rd ed. Oxford University Press, New York, 1990, pp 851–852.
72. Gorlin RJ, Toriello HV, Cohen MM Jr: Hereditary Hearing Loss and Its Syndromes. Oxford University Press, New York, 1995, pp 73–75.
73. Halal F: Distal obstructive uropathy with polydactyly: a new syndrome? Am J Med Genet 24:753–757, 1986.
74. Halal F, Gledhill R, Dudkiewicz A: Autosomal dominant inheritance of the Kabuki make-up (Niikawa-Kuroki) syndrome. Am J Med Genet 33:376–381, 1989.
75. Hall BD, Berg BO, Rudolph RS, Epstein CJ: Pseudoprogeria-Hallermann-Streiff (PHS) syndrome. Birth Defects 10:137–146, 1974.
76. Hamers A, Jongbloet P, Peeters G, Fryns JP, Geraedts J: Severe mental retardation in a patient with tricho-rhino-phalangeal syndrome type I and 8q deletion. Eur J Pediatr 149:618–620, 1990.
77. Harding AE, Hall CM, Baraitser M: Autosomal dominant asymmetrical radial dysplasia, dysmorphic facies, and conductive hearing loss (facioauriculoradial dysplasia). J Med Genet 19:110–115, 1982.
78. Hennekam RCM, Van Noort G, de la Fuente FA, Norbruis OF: Agenesis of the nasal septal cartilage: another sign in autosomal dominant holoprosencephaly [letter]. Am J Med Genet 39:121–122, 1991.
79. Herrmann J, Opitz JM: The VSR syndrome. Studies of malformation syndromes of man XXXII. Birth Defects 10:227–239, 1974.
80. Hertz JM, Coerdt W, Hahnemann N, Schwartz M: Interstitial deletion of the short arm of chromosome 3. Fetal pathology and exclusion of the gene for beta-galactosidase-1 (GLB-1) from 3(p11→p14.2). Hum Genet 79:389–391, 1988.
81. Hittner HM, Hirsch NJ, Kreh GM, Rudolf AJ: Colobomatous microphthalmia, heart disease, hearing loss, and mental retardation—a syndrome. J Pediatr Ophthalmol Strabismus 16:122–128, 1979.
82. Hockey A, Crowhurst J, Cullity G: Microcephaly, holoprosencephaly, hypokinesia—second report of a new syndrome. Prenat Diagn 8:683–686, 1988.
83. Hornblass A, Reifler DM: Ablepharon macrostomia syndrome. Am J Ophthalmol 99:552–556, 1985.
84. Huang TH, Greenberg F, Ledbetter DH: Determination of the origin of nondisjunction in a 49,XXXXY male using hypervariable dinucleotide repeat sequences. Hum Genet 86:619–620, 1991.
85. Hurst JA, Winter RM, Baraitser M: Distinctive syndrome of short stature, craniosynostosis, skeletal changes and malformed ears. Am J Med Genet 29:107–115, 1988.
86. Hurvitz SA, Goodman RM, Hertz M, Katznelson MB-M, Sack Y: The facio-audio-symphalangism syndrome: report of a case and review of the literature. Clin Genet 28:61–68, 1985.
87. Iafolla AK, McConkie-Rosell S, Chen YT: VATER and hydrocephalus: distinct syndrome? Am J Med Genet 38:46–51, 1991.
88. Ilyina HG Lurie IW: Dubowitz syndrome: Possible evidence for a clinical subtype. Am J Med Genet 35:561–565, 1990.
89. Johnston K, Golabi M, Hall B, Ito M, Grix A: Alopecia-anosmia-deafness-hypogonadism syndrome revisited: report of a new case. Am J Med Genet 26:925–927, 1987.
90. Jones KL: Smith's Recognizable Patterns of Human Malformation, 5th ed. WB Saunders, Philadelphia, 1996, p 108–109.
91. Jones KL: Smith's Recognizable Patterns of Human Malformation, 5th ed. WB Saunders, Philadelphia, 1996, p 476–477.
92. Kaplan P, Plauchu H, Fitch N, Jéquier S : A new acro-cranio-facial dysostosis syndrome in sisters. Am J Med Genet 29:95–106, 1988.
93. Karnes PS, Shamban AT, Olsen DR, Fazio MJ, Falk RE: De Barsy syndrome: report of a case, literature review, and elastin gene expression studies of the skin. Am J Med Genet 42:29–34, 1992.
94. Kawashima H, Ohno I, Ueno Y, Nakaya S, Kato E, Taniguchi N: Syndrome of microtia and aortic arch anomalies resembling isotretinoin embryopathy. J Pediatr 111:738–740, 1987.
95. Kawira EL, Weaver DD, Bender HA: Acrofacial dysostosis with severe facial clefting and limb reduction. Am J Med Genet 17:641–647, 1984.
96. Kivlin JD, Fineman RM, Crandall AS, Olson RJ: Peters' anomaly as a consequence of genetic and nongenetic syndromes. Arch Ophthalmol 104:61–64, 1986.
97. Kogut MD, Sensenbrenner J: Low birthweight syndrome in two brothers. Birth Defects 11:450–452, 1975.
98. Kondo I, Mori Y, Kuwajima K: Weaver syndrome in two Japanese children. Am J Med Genet 41:221–224, 1991.
99. Konig R, Fuchs S, Kern C, Langenbeck U: Simpson-Golabi-Behmel syndrome with severe cardiac arrhythmias. Am J Med Genet 38:244–247, 1991.
100. Konigsmark BW, Gorlin RJ: Genetic and Metabolic Deafness, WB Saunders, Philadelphia, 1976, pp 65–68.
101. Koppe R, Kaplan P, Hunter A, McMurray B: Ambiguous genitalia associated with skeletal abnormalities, cutis laxa, craniostenosis, psychomotor retardation, and facial abnormalities (SCARF syndrome). Am J Med Genet 34:305–312, 1989.
102. Kormann-Bortolotto MH, Farah LMS, Soares D, Corbani M, Müller R, Adell ACA: Terminal deletion 6p23: a case report. Am J Med Genet 37:475–477, 1990.
103. Kushnick T, Rao KW, Lamb AN: Familial 5p- syndrome. Clin Genet 26:472–476, 1984.
104. Lee B, Godfrey M, Vitale E, Hori H, Mattei M-G, Sarfarazi M, Tsipouras P, Ramirez F, Hollister DW: Linkage of Marfan syndrome and a phenotypically related disorder to two different fibrillin genes. Nature 352:330–334, 1991.
105. Legius E, Moerman P, Fryns JP, Vandenberghe K, Eggermont E: Holzgreve-Wagner-Rehder syndrome. Potter sequence associated with persistent buccopharyngeal membrane. A second observation. Am J Med Genet 31:269–272, 1988.
106. Lin AE, Gettig E: Craniosynostosis, agenesis of the corpus callosum, severe mental retardation, distinctive facies, camptodactyly, and hypogonadism. Am J Med Genet 35:582–585, 1990.
107. Lipson AH, Yuille D, Angel M, Thompson PG, Vandervoord JG, Beckenham EJ: Velocardiofacial (Shprintzen) syndrome: an important syndrome for the dysmorphologist to recognize. J Med Genet 28:596–604, 1991.
108. Lowe J, Kohn G, Cohen O, Mogilner M, Schiller M: Dominant anorectal malformation, nephritis and nerve-deafness: a possible new entity? Clin Genet 24:191–193, 1983.
109. MacDermot KD, Winter RM: Two brothers with facial anomalies, microcephaly, hypoplastic genitalia and a failure of psychomotor development. Am J Med Genet 32:60–62, 1989.
110. Madokoro H, Ohdo S, Sonoda T, Ohba K, Hayakawa K: Association of severe microcephaly, short palpebral fissures, micrognathia, growth retardation and early death: a new syndrome. Acta Paediatr Jpn 29:186–188, 1987.
111. Magenis RE, Sheehy RR, Brown MG, McDermid HE, White BN, Zonana J, Weleber R: Parental origin of the extra chromosome in the cat eye syndrome: evidence from heteromorphism and in situ hybridization analysis. Am J Med Genet 29:9–19, 1988.

112. Matsuyama H, Watanabe I, Mihm MC, Richardson EP Jr: Dermatoleukodystrophy with neuroaxonal spheroids. Arch Neurol 35:329–336, 1978.
113. McGillivray BC, Bassett AS, Langlois S, Pantzar T, Wood S: Familial 5q11.2→q13.3 segmental duplication cosegregating with multiple anomalies, including schizophrenia. Am J Med Genet 35:10–13, 1990.
114. McKeown CM, Harris R: An autosomal dominant multiple pterygium syndrome. J Med Genet 25:96–103, 1988.
115. Meier VZ, Rothschild M: Ein Fall von Arthrogryposis multiplex congenita kombiniert mit Dysostosis mandibulofacialis (Franceschetti-Syndrom). Helv Pediatr Acta 2:213–216, 1959.
116. Meinecke P: Terminal deletion of chromosome 3p in adults: a fourth observation [letter]. Am J Med Genet 36:519–520, 1990.
117. Meinecke P, Polke A, Schmiegelow P: Limb anomalies in the CHARGE association. J Med Genet 26:202–203, 1989.
118. Moeschler J, Clarren SK: Familial occurrence of hemifacial microsomia with radial limb defects. Am J Med Genet 12:371–375, 1982.
119. Mohammed FM, Farag TI, Gunawardana SS, al-Digashim DD, al-Awadi SA, al-Othman SA, Sundareshan TS: Direct duplication of chromosome 1, dir dup (1) (p21.2→p32) in a Bedouin boy with multiple congenital anomalies. Am J Med Genet 32:353–355, 1989.
120. Moore CA, Buehler BA, McManus BM, Harmon JP, Mirkin LD, Goldstein DJ: Acephalus-acardia in twins with aneuploidy. Am J Med Genet (Suppl.) 3:139–143, 1987.
121. Narahara K, Kikkawa K, Murakami M, Hiramoto K, Namba H, Tsuji K, Yokoyama Y, Kimoto H: Loss of the 3p25.3 band is critical in the manifestation of del (3p) syndrome: karyotype-phenotype correlation in cases with deficiency of the distal portion of the short arm of chromosome 3. Am J Med Genet 35:269–273, 1990.
122. Naritomi K, Hirayama K: Partial trisomy of distal 8q derived from mother with mosaic 8q23.3→24.13 deletion and relatively mild expression of trichorhinophalangeal syndrome I. Hum Genet 82:199–201, 1989.
123. Nevo S, Zeltzer M, Benderly A, Levy J: Evidence for autosomal recessive inheritance in cerebral gigantism. J Med Genet 11:158–165, 1974.
124. Nevin NC, Hill AE, Carson DJ: Facio-cardio-renal (Eastman-Bixler) syndrome. Am J Med Genet 40:31–33, 1991.
125. Niikawa N, Kuroki Y, Kajii T, Matsuura N, Ishikiriyama S, Tonoki H, Ishikawa N, Yamada Y, Fujita M, Umemoto H, et al.: Kabuki make-up (Niikawa-Kuroki) syndrome: a study of 62 patients. Am J Med Genet 31:565–589, 1988.
126. Oley CA, Baraitser M, Grant DB: A reappraisal of the CHARGE association. J Med Genet 25:147–156, 1988.
127. Opitz JM, Herrmann J, Gilbert EF, Matalon R: Simpson-Golabi-Behmel syndrome: follow-up of the Michigan family. Am J Med Genet 30:301–308, 1988.
128. Opitz JM, Richieri-da Costa A, Aase JM, Benke PJ: FG syndrome update 1988: note of 5 new patients and bibliography. Am J Med Genet 30:309–328, 1988.
129. Overhauser J, McMahon J, Oberlender S, Carlin ME, Niebuhr E, Wasmuth JJ, Lee-Chen J: Parental origin of chromosome 5 deletions in the cri-du-chat syndrome. Am J Med Genet 37:83–86, 1990.
130. Paes-Alves AF, Azevêdo ES, Sousa MGF, Almeida-Melo N, Oliveira-Filho OJ: Autosomal recessive malformation syndrome with minor manifestation in the heterozygotes: a preliminary report of a possible new syndrome. Am J Med Genet 41:141–152, 1991.
131. Pagnan NAB, Gollop TR, Lederman H: The Tel Hashomer camptodactyly syndrome: report of a new case and review of the literature. Am J Med Genet 29:411–417, 1988.
132. Palmer CG, Bader P, Slovak ML, Comings DE, Pettenati MJ: Partial deletion of chromosome 6p:a delineation of the syndrome. Am J Med Genet 39:155–160, 1991.
133. Palomeque A, Pastor X, Ballesta F: Nager anomaly with severe facial involvement, microcephaly, and mental retardation. Am J Med Genet 36:356–357, 1990.
134. Patton MA, Tolmie J, Ruthnum P, Bamforth S, Baraitser M, Pembrey M: Congenital cutis laxa with retardation of growth and development. J Med Genet 24:556–561, 1987.
135. Pearl W: Syndrome of anotia, facial paralysis and congenital heart disease. J Pediatr 105:441–442, 1984.
136. Petit P, Moerman P, Fryns JP: Acrofacial dysostosis syndrome type Rodriguez: a new lethal MCA syndrome. Am J Med Genet 42:343–345, 1992.
137. Petty EM, Laxova R, Wiedemann HR: Previously unrecognized congenital progeroid disorder. Am J Med Genet 35:383–387, 1990.
138. Pfeiffer RA: The oto-onycho-peroneal syndrome. A probably new genetic entity. Eur J Pediatr 138:317–320, 1982.
139. Pfeiffer RA, Palm D, Teller W: A syndrome of short stature, amimic facies, enamel hypoplasia, slowly progressive stiffness of the joints and high-pitched voice in two siblings. J Pediatr 91:955–957, 1977.
140. Pinheiro M, Freire-Maia N: Atrichias and hypotrichoses: a brief review with description of a recessive atrichia in two brothers. Hum Hered 35:53–55, 1985.
141. Pliskin ME, Haber B, Kornbrot A, Madani F, Lally ET: The occurrence of a fibro-osseous lesion and multiple dental anomalies in a patient with the Greig cephalopolysyndactyly syndrome. Oral Surg Oral Med Oral Pathol 66:475–479, 1988.
142. Preus M, Cooper AR, O'Leary E: Sensorineural hearing loss, small facial features, submucous cleft palate and myoclonic seizures. J Clin Dysmorphol 2:30–31, 1984.
143. Preus M, Vekemans M, Kaplan P: Diagnosis of chromosome 3 duplication q23→qter, deletion p25→pter in a patient with the C (trigonocephaly) syndrome. Am J Med Genet 23:935–943, 1986.
144. Primrose DA: A slowly progressive degenerative condition characterized by mental deficiency, wasting of limb musculature and bone abnormalities, including ossification of the pinnae. J Ment Defic Res 26:101–106, 1982.
145. Quarrell OW, Hamill MA, Hughes HE: Pallister-Killian mosaic syndrome with emphasis on the adult phenotype. Am J Med Genet 31:841–844, 1988.
146. Quarrell OW, Snell RG, Curtis MA, Roberts SH, Harper PS, Shaw DJ: Paternal origin of the chromosomal deletion resulting in Wolf-Hirschhorn syndrome. J Med Genet 28:256–259, 1991.
147. Rabe P, Haverkamp F, Emons D, Rosskamp R, Zerres K, Passarge E: Syndrome of developmental retardation, facial and skeletal anomalies and hyperphosphatasia in two sisters: nosology and genetics of the Coffin-Siris syndrome. Am J Med Genet 41:350–354, 1991.
148. Ramer JC, Ladda RL, Demuth WW: Multiple pterygium syndrome. An overview. Am J Dis Child 142:794–798, 1988.
149. Ramos-Arroyo MA, Weaver DD, Banks ER: Weaver syndrome: a case without early overgrowth and review of the literature. Pediatrics 88:1106–1110, 1991.
150. Richieri-Costa A, Gollop TR, Colletto GM: Syndrome of acrofacial dysostosis, cleft lip/palate and triphalangeal thumb in a Brazilian family. J Med Genet 14:225–229, 1983.
151. Robain O, Floquet C, Heldt N, Rozenberg F: Hemimegalencephaly: a clinicopathological study of four cases. Neuropathol Appl Neurobiol 14:125–135, 1988.
152. Rodini ES, Freitas JAS, Richieri-Costa A: Ectrodactyly, cleft lip/palate syndrome. Am J Med Genet 38:539–541, 1991.
153. Rodriguez JI, Palacios J, Urioste M: New acrofacial dysostosis syndrome in 3 sibs. Am J Med Genet 35:484–489, 1990.
154. Rollnick BR, Kaye CI, Nagatoshi K, Martin AO: Oculoauriculovertebral dysplasia and variants: phenotypic characteristics of 294 patients. Am J Med Genet 26:361–375, 1987.
155. Schilbach U, Rott HD: Ocular hypotelorism, submucosal cleft palate, and hypospadias: a new autosomal dominant syndrome. Am J Med Genet 31:863–870, 1988.
156. Schinzel A: Microdeletion syndromes, balanced translocations, and gene mapping. J Med Genet 25:454–462, 1988.
157. Schinzel A: tetrasomy 12p (Pallister-Killian syndrome). J Med Genet 28:122–125, 1991.
158. Schwartz CE, Ulmer J, Brown A, Pancoast I, Goodman HO, Stevenson RE: Allan-Herndon syndrome II. Linkage to DNA markers in Xq21. Am J Hum Genet 47:454–458, 1990.
159. Schweitzer VG, Kemink JL, Graham MD: Conductive hearing loss, middle ear ossicular anomalies, malformed thickened lop auricles, and micrognathia. A rare autosomal dominant congenital syndrome. Am J Otol 5:387–391, 1984.
160. Seaver LH, Cassidy SB: New syndrome: mother and son with hypertelorism, downslanting palpebral fissures, malar hypoplasia and apparently low-set ears associated with joint and scrotal anomalies. Am J Med Genet 41:405–409, 1991.
161. Sellars S, Beighton P: Autosomal dominant inheritance of conductive deafness due to stapedial anomalies, external ear malformations and congenital facial palsy. Clin Genet 23:376–379, 1983.
162. Simosa V, Penchaszadeh VB, Bustos T: A new syndrome with distinct facial and auricular malformations and dominant inheritance. Am J Med Genet 32:184–186, 1980.
163. Stevenson RE, Ferlauto GJ, Taylor HA: Cutis gyratum and acanthosis nigricans associated with other anomalies: a distinctive syndrome. J Pediatr 92:950–952, 1978.

164. Stratton RF: Teebi hypertelorism syndrome (brachycephalofrontonasal dysplasia) in a U.S. family. Am J Med Genet 39:78–80, 1991.
165. Strisciuglio P, Ballabio A, Parenti G: Microtia with meatal atresia and conductive deafness: mild and severe manifestations within the same sibship. J Med Genet 23:459–460, 1986.
166. Strisciuglio P, Raia V, Di Meo A, Rinaldi E, Andria G: Wildervanck's syndrome with bilateral subluxation of lens and facial paralysis. J Med Genet 20:72–73, 1983.
167. Strong WB: Familial syndrome of right-sided aortic arch, mental deficiency, and facial dysmorphism. J Pediatr 73:882–888, 1968.
168. Sundareshan TS, Naguib KK, Al-Awadi SA, Redha MA, Hamoud MS: Apparently nonmosaic trisomy 22:clinical report and review. Am J Med Genet 36:7–10, 1990.
169. Talwar D, Smith SA: CAMFAK syndrome: a demyelinating inherited disease similar to Cockayne syndrome. Am J Med Genet 34:194–198, 1989.
170. Tayel S, McCorquodale MM, Rutherford T, Kurczynski TW, Abdel-Aziz AM, el-Gabaldy F, Sharaf EA: A case of de novo trisomy 12p syndrome. Clin Genet 35:382–386, 1989.
171. Teebi AS: New autosomal dominant syndrome resembling craniofrontonasal dysplasia. Am J Med Genet 28:581–591, 1987.
172. Temple IK, MacDowall P, Baraitser M, Atherton DJ: Focal dermal hypoplasia (Goltz syndrome). J Med Genet 27:180–187, 1990.
173. Thakker Y, Donnai D: A new recessive syndrome of unusual facies and multiple structural abnormalities. J Med Genet 28:633–635, 1991.
174. Thong YH, Simpson DA: The syndrome of abnormal neutrophil chemotaxis, unusual facies, proportionate small stature and sensorineural deafness-mutism (letter). Acta Paediatr Scand 70:575, 1981.
175. Tonoki H, Ohura T, Niikawa N: Cryptomicrotia and short, stubby fingers with excess fingertip arch patterns in a mother and son. Am J Med Genet 29:857–862, 1988.
176. Toriello HV, Higgins JV, Abrahamson J, Waterman DF, Moore WD: X-linked syndrome of branchial arch and other defects. Am J Med Genet 21:137–142, 1985.
177. Toriello HV, Higgins JV, Malvitz T, Waterman DF: Two siblings with Tel Hashomer camptodactyly and mitral valve prolapse. Am J Med Genet 36:398–403, 1990.
178. Tranebjaerg L, Svejgaard A, Lykkesfeldt G: X-linked mental retardation associated with psoriasis: a new syndrome? Am J Med Genet 30:263–273, 1988.
179. Trounce JQ, Rutter N, Mellor DH: Hemimegalencephaly: diagnosis and treatment. Dev Med Child Neurol 33:261–266, 1991.
180. Turner G, Gedeon A, Mulley J, Sutherland G, Rae J, Power K, Arthur I: Börjeson-Forssman-Lehmann syndrome: clinical manifestations and gene localization to Xq26–27. Am J Med Genet 34:463–469, 1989.
181. Van Haeringen A, Veenstra F, Maaswinkel-Mooij PD, van de Kamp JJ: Intermittent thrombocytopenia and absent radii: report of a patient with additional unusual manifestations. Am J Med Genet 34:202–206, 1989.
182. Van Maldergem L, Verloes A, Lejeune L, Gillerot Y: The Baller-Gerold syndrome. J Med Genet 29:266–268, 1992.
183. Verloes A, Delfortrie J, Lambotte C: GOMBO syndrome of growth retardation, ocular abnormalities, microcephaly, brachydactyly, and oligophrenia: a possible "new" recessively inherited MCA/MR syndrome. Am J Med Genet 32:15–18, 1989.
184. Verloes A, Dodinval P, Beco L, Bonnivert J, Lambotte C: Lambotte syndrome: microcephaly, holoprosencephaly, intrauterine growth retardation, facial anomalies and early lethality—a new sublethal multiple congenital anomaly/mental retardation syndrome in four sibs. Am J Med Genet 37:119–123, 1990.
185. Verloes A, Lambrechts L, Senterre J, Lambotte C: Microcephalic osteodysplastic dwarfism (type II-like) in siblings. Clin Genet 32:88–94, 1987.
186. Wagner K, Kroisel PM, Rosenkranz W: Molecular and cytogenetic analysis in two patients with microdeletions of 7p and Greig syndrome: hemizygosity for PGAM2 and TCRG genes. Genomics 8:487–491, 1990.
187. Walker BA, Scott CI Jr, Hall JG, Murdoch JL, McKusick VA: Diastrophic dwarfism. Medicine 51:41–60, 1972.
188. Walpole IR, Hockey A, Nicoll A: The Nance-Horan syndrome. J Med Genet 27:632–634, 1990.
189. Wardinsky TD, Weinberger E, Pagon RA, Clarren SK, Thuline HC: Partial deletion of the long arm of chromosome 11 [del (11)(q23.3→qter)] with abnormal white matter. Am J Med Genet 35:60–63, 1990.
190. Wells TR, Falk RE, Senac MO, Vachon L: Acrocephalospondylosyndactyly-a possible new syndrome: analysis of the vertebral and intervertebral components. Pediatr Pathol 10:117–131, 1990.
191. Willems PJ, Rouwe C, Smit GP: A new case of the osteodysplastic primordial dwarfism type II. Am J Med Genet 26:819–824, 1987.
192. Wilson RD, Baird PA: Renal agenesis in British Columbia. Am J Med Genet 21:153–169, 1985.
193. Yomo A, Taira T, Kondo I: Goldberg-Shprintzen syndrome: Hirschprung disease, hypotonia, and ptosis in sibs. Am J Med Genet 41:188–191, 1991.
194. Yoshihara S, Iinuma K, Nihei K, Naito H : Case report of tetrasomy 18p in a girl. Acta Paediatr Jpn 30:635–637, 1988.
195. Yunis E, Varon H: Cleidocranial dysostosis, severe micrognathism, bilateral absence of thumbs and first metatarsal bone, and distal aphalangia: a new genetic syndrome. Am J Dis Child 134:649–653, 1980.

# Appendix B

## Syndromes and Conditions Associated with Genetic Deafness

TED L. TEWFIK, AHMAD S. TEEBI, and VAZKEN M. DER KALOUSTIAN

Heredity is a very important cause of significant hearing impairment in humans. Well over half of all cases of childhood deafness have a genetic etiology. Most of these (70%) are not associated with other anomalies or syndromes. Severe inherited childhood nonsyndromic deafness has an incidence of 1 per 2,000 births. It represents the most common inherited sensory disorder. The inheritance of nonsyndromic deafness is mainly autosomal recessive (over 75%), while autosomal dominant (12%–24%), X-linked (1%–3%), and mitochondrial patterns of inheritance are also noted.[50,225]

Non-syndromic recessive deafness (NSRD) is genetically heterogeneous. A rough estimate of autosomal recessive loci contributing to sensorineural deafness was considered to be 13.[227a] To date, 11 autosomal recessive loci have been mapped, along with 11 autosomal dominant, 4 X-linked and 2 mitochondrial loci (See Appendix B-1.)

When deafness is associated with syndromes, it is hard to separate them into different categories. The most useful classification we have found is presented in the book *Hereditary Hearing Loss and Its Syndromes* by Gorlin et al.,[151a] and we have followed it in the preparation of our tables.

**Appendix B-1** Location of DFN Loci Causing Non-Syndromic Deafness in Humans*

DOMINANT

| Locus name | Location | Most important reference |
|---|---|---|
| DFNA1 | 5q31 | Leon *et al.*, 1992[247a] |
| DFNA2 | 1p32 | Coucke *et al.*, 1994[76a] |
| DFNA3 | 13q12 | Chaib *et al.*, 1994[62a]<br>Guilford *et al.*, 1995[160c] |
| DFNA4 | 19q13 | Chen *et al.*, 1995[66a] |
| DFNA5 | 7p15 | Van Camp *et al.*, 1995[419a] |
| DFNA6 | 4p16.3 | Lesperance *et al.*, 1995[248a] |
| DFNA7 | 1q21–q23 | Fagerheim *et al.*, 1996[113a] |
| DFNA8 | 15q15–q21 | Kirschhofer *et al.*, 1995[226a] |
| DFNA9 | 14q12–q13 | Manolis *et al.*, 1996[258a] |
| DFNA10 | 6q22–q23 | O'Neill *et al.*, 1996[296a] |
| DFNA11 | 11q13.5 | Tamagawa *et al.*, 1996[393a] |

RECESSIVE

| Locus name | Location | Most important reference |
|---|---|---|
| DFNB1 | 13q12 | Guilford *et al.*, 1994 and 1995[b,c] |
| DFNB2 | 11q13.5 | Guilford *et al.*, 1994[160a] |
| DFNB3 | 17p11.2–q12 | Friedman *et al.*, 1995[126a] |
| DFNB4 | 7q31 | Baldwin *et al.*, 1995[19a] |
| DFNB5 | 14q12 | Fukushima *et al.*, 1995[130a] |
| DFNB6 | 3p14–p21 | Fukushima *et al.*, 1995[130b] |
| DFNB7 | 9q13–q21 | Jain *et al.*, 1995[201a] |
| DFNB8 | 21q22 | Veske *et al.*, 1996[421] |
| DFNB9 | 2p22–p23 | Chaib *et al.*, 1996[62b] |
| DFNB10 | 21q22.3 | Bonné-Tamir *et al.*, 1996[41a] |
| DFNB11 | reserved | |
| DFNB12 | 10q21–q22 | Chaib *et al.*, 1996[62c] |

X-LINKED

| Locus name | Location | Most important reference |
|---|---|---|
| DFN1** | Xq22 | Tranebjaerg *et al.*, 1995[405a] |
| DFN2 | ? | OMIM 304500 |
| DFN3 | Xq21.1 | De Kok *et al.*, 1995[94a]<br>Dahl *et al.*, 1995[88a] |
| DFN4 | Xp21.2 | Lalwani *et al.*, 1994[243a] |
| DFN5 | reserved | |
| DFN6 | Xp22 | del Castillo *et al.*, 1996[94b] |

**Non-syndromic X-linked deafness of DFN1 locus was shown to be associated with blindness, dystonia, fractures and mental deficiency. Therefore, it was reclassified as syndromic (Mohr-Tranebjaerg syndrome)

MITOCHONDRIAL

| Locus name | Mutation | Most important reference |
|---|---|---|
| 12Sr RNA | A1555G | Prezant *et al.*, 1993[319] |
| tRNA-Ser(UCN) | T7445C | Reid *et al.*, 1994[330a] |

*Modified from Smith and Van Camp, Hereditary Deafness Newsletter, June 1996, with permission. This table, with additional information on the gene and screening markers, is continuously updated. It is available on line at http://alt-www.uia.ac.be/u/dnalab/hhh.html and is maintained by Drs. Richard Smith and Guy Van Camp.

**Appendix B-2** Genetic hearing loss with no associated abnormalities

| Condition or syndrome | Mode of inheritance[a] | MIM No. POSSUM No.[b] | Type of deafness[c] | Ear, nose, and throat manifestations | Other manifestations |
|---|---|---|---|---|---|
| Congenital moderate sensorineural hearing loss[229] | AR | | SND | Hearing loss noted in childhood. No progression. Normal vestibular function | Two sibs in each of three sibships |
| Congenital retrocochlear hearing loss[39] | AR | | SND | Mild (30–40 dB) loss at 250–500 Hz, 60–90 db loss from 1,000 to 4,000 Hz. Improvement at 8,000 Hz. | Two pairs of sibs |
| Congenital sensorineural hearing loss[326,341] | XLR | | SND | Normal vestibular function | Mental deficiency in some cases |
| Deafness, congenital, dominant, severe, sensorineural[146] | | | | | |
| Deafness, congenital, severe to profound[266,382] | AR | ***220700**<br>***220800** | SND<br>SND | | |
| Deafness, low-frequency hearing loss, mixed conductive and sensorineural type[302] | AD | **124910** | SND<br>CD | | |
| Deafness, midfrequency, neural[235] | AD | ***124700** | SND | Affected frequencies 500–4,000 Hz | |
| Deafness, progressive, low-frequency (Konigsmark syndrome; Monge hearing loss, DFNA 1)[234] | AD | ***124900** | SND | Hearing is normal above 2,000 cycles | |
| Deafness, sensorineural, early onset[267] | AR | **221600** | SND | Progressive severe loss of hearing in later childhood | |
| Deafness, unilateral[112] | AD | **125000** | SND | | |
| Deafness with stapes fixation (Perilymphatic gusher-deafness syndrome DFN3)[17,80,283] | XLR | ***304400** | SND<br>CD | Vestibular disturbance, fixed footplate of stapes; at operation, profuse drainage of perilymph and cerebrospinal fluid indicating abnormal patency of cochlear duct | |
| Hereditary Ménière syndrome[37,215] | AD<br>AR | | SND | Episodic vertigo | 15% inherited, 85% sporadic. Severe unilateral headache |
| High-frequency sensorineural hearing loss[430] | XLR | | SND | Nonprogressive | |
| Konigsmark syndrome (see Deafness, progressive, low frequency) | | | | | |
| Moderate sensorineural hearing loss[309] | XLR | | SND | Onset at adolescence, slowly progressive, moderate hearing loss. Normal vestibular function | |
| Otosclerosis[145] | Probably multifactorial | | CD or mixed | Gradual onset of hearing loss in early decades of life. Usually normal vestibular function | |
| Progressive high-frequency sensorineural hearing loss[257] | AR | | SND | Normal vestibular function | Three reports of four families |
| Progressive mixed hearing loss[113] | AD | | SND<br>CD | Starting around 3–5 years of age | |
| Progressive sensorineural hearing loss[41,54] | AD | | SND | Begins in childhood with high tone loss. Middle and lower frequencies involved with increased age. Abrupt bilateral symmetrical loss above 2,000 Hz | |
| Sensorineural hearing loss[319,320] | Mitochondrial | | SND | Severe to profound, progressive, involving all frequencies | Both antibiotic-induced and non-syndromic deafness |

**Appendix B–3** Genetic hearing loss associated with external ear abnormalities

| Condition or syndrome | Mode of inheritance[a] | MIM NO. POSSUM No.[b] | Type of deafness[c] | Ear, nose, and throat manifestations | Other manifestations |
|---|---|---|---|---|---|
| Acro-cranio-facial dysostosis, Kaplan type[218] | AR | **201050** 4407 | SND and CD | Malformation of auricles with narrow external auditory canals, preauricular pits. Hearing loss is nonprogressive, moderately severe | Short stature, developmental delay |
| Aural atresia, microtia, conductive hearing loss[296] | AD | | CD | Microtia, aural atresia (unilateral or bilateral) | |
| Aural atresia, microtia, conductive hearing loss[79] | AR | | CD | Microtia, meatal atresia (unilateral or bilateral) | |
| Aural atresia, vertical talus (Rasmussen syndrome)[323] | AD | | CD | Atresia of lateral auditory canals with normal pinnae | Bilateral clubfeet with vertical talus |
| Aural atresia, mental retardation, multiple congenital anomalies, conductive hearing loss (Cooper-Jabs syndrome)[73] | AR | | CD or mixed | Bilateral auricular deformities, atresia of external auditory meatus | Short stature, developmental delay, ventricular septal defect, anterior placement of anus |
| Aural atresia, microtia, aortic arch anomalies, conductive hearing loss[219] | AR XLR | | CD | Malformation of auricles | Aortic arch anomalies |
| Aural atresia, microtia, unusual facies, pseudopapilledema[300] | AR | | Mixed | Aural atresia, microtia | Pseudopapilledema, microcephaly, multiple pigmented nevi and café-au-lait spots |
| Aural atresia, microtia, skin mastocytosis, short stature, conductive hearing loss[180] | AR | | CD or mixed | | Short stature, hyperpigmentation of skin of trunk and extremities |
| Aural atresia, conductive hearing loss (Hefter-Ganz syndrome)[339] | AD | | CD | Meatal atresia | |
| Bixler syndrome (see Hypertelorism, microtia, clefting syndrome) | | | | | |
| BOR syndrome (see Branchio-oto-renal syndrome) | | | | | |
| Branchio-oculo-facial (BOF) syndrome[130] | AD | ***113620** | CD | Pseudocleft of upper lip, cleft lip/palate, obstruction of the nasolacrimal duct, malformed pinnae | |
| Branchio-oto-renal syndrome (Melnick-Fraser syndrome or BOR syndrome)[155] | AD | ***113650** 2224 | SND CD | Facial palsy, abnormal ear shape and size, preauricular tags or pits, abnormal middle ear, branchial cleft sinus or fistula | Renal aplasia or hypoplasia, ureteric abnormalities, defects of the nasolacrimal duct |
| CHARGE association[2] | Sporadic or AD (occasional) or AR or XLR (rare) | 3480 | SND or mixed | Abnormalities of external ear, choanal atresia | Colobomatous microphthalmia, congenital conotruncal heart defects, retarded growth and development, genital hypoplasia |
| Coxoauricular syndrome[101] | AD | **122780** 3522 | CD | Microtia | Short stature, hip dislocation |
| Cupped pinnae, microcephaly, mental retardation, sensorineural hearing loss[220] | | | | | |
| Deafness, anal anomalies, triphalangeal thumb (see Townes-Brocks syndrome) | | | | | |
| Deafness, conductive, with microtia, and meatal atresia[298,387] | AR AD | ***251800** 4324 | CD | Low-set ears, microtia | |
| Deafness, ear malformations, mental retardation[59] | AR | ***221300** | SND CD | Malformed, low-set ears | Mental retardation, hypogonadism |

**Appendix B-3** Genetic hearing loss associated with external ear abnormalities (*Continued*)

| Condition or syndrome | Mode of inheritance[a] | **MIM No.** POSSUM No.[b] | Type of deafness[c] | Ear, nose, and throat manifestations | Other manifestations |
|---|---|---|---|---|---|
| Deafness, ear pits[124] | AD | ***125100** | SND | Mild to severe deafness, branchial pits or fistulas, preauricular pits or appendages | |
| DiGeorge sequence[156,429] | Sporadic | ***188400** 3186 | CD | Micrognathia; low-set, small, posteriorly-angulated ears; short philtrum, cleft palate or bifid uvula, choanal atresia | Hypoplasia or aplasia of parathyroid glands and thymus, interrupted aortic arch or truncus arteriosus. Chromosome 22q deletion |
| Dysmorphic pinnae, facial palsy, and stapedial anomalies[361] | AD | 4430 | | Abnormal pinnae, with absence of upper half; narrow external auditory canals; pre- or postauricular sinuses; stapedial anomalies with severe hearing loss | Unilateral or bilateral facial palsy. |
| Dysmorphic pinnae and conductive hearing loss[258] | AR | | CD | Low-set ears, malformed pinnae | Mental retardation in 50%, hypogonadism in males. Two sibships in single Mennonite kindred |
| Facio-auriculo-vertebral dysplasia (Oculo-auriculo-vertebral dysplasia, Goldenhar syndrome, Hemifacial microsomia)[72,161,344] | AD AR | **164210** **257700** 3339 | SND CD | Facial palsy, asymmetry of the face, midfacial hypoplasia, micrognathia, macrostomia, cleft lip, cleft palate, notched tongue, low-set ears, preauricular tags, laryngeal anomalies | Microcephaly, coloboma of eyelids, lateral facial cleft, epibulbar dermoids, glaucoma, cataract, vision loss, abnormal rib number, multiple vertebral anomalies, talipes deformities, uterine abnormality, coarctation of the aorta, hypoplastic lungs, dysplastic kidneys, mental retardation |
| Franceschetti-Klein syndrome (see Treacher Collins syndrome) | | | | | |
| Goldenhar syndrome (see Facio-auriculo-vertebral dysplasia) | | | | | |
| Hemifacial microsomia (see Facio-auriculo-vertebral dysplasia) | | | | | |
| Hypertelorism, microtia, clefting syndrome (Bixler syndrome)[148] | AR | ***239800** 3259 | CD | Micrognathia, cleft nose, small mouth, cleft palate, microtia, abnormal middle ear | Microcephaly, short stature, horseshoe kidney, mental retardation |
| Lacrimo-auriculo-dento-digital) syndrome (Levy-Hollister syndrome) (LADD)[238,397] | AD | ***149730** 3546 | SND | Low-set ears, microtia, hypoplasia of antihelix, dysplasia of pinna | Contractures of large joints, defects of lacrimal system, hypodontia, syndactyly of fingers, polydactyly, clinodactyly of 5th finger, hypoplastic thumb, hypoplastic kidneys |
| Levy-Hollister syndrome (see Lacrimo-auriculo-dento-digital syndrome) | | | | | |
| Lop ears, deafness, incudo-stapedial defects (Escher-Hirt syndrome)[110] | AD | ***128980** 3444 | CD | Abnormal earlobe size, abnormal middle ear, deafness is congenital and nonprogressive. Malformation of the incudostapedial junction | |
| Mandibulofacial dysostosis (see Treacher Collins syndrome) | | | | | |
| Melnick-Fraser syndrome (see Branchio-oto-renal syndrome) | | | | | |

| Condition or syndrome | Mode of inheritance[a] | MIM No. POSSUM No.[b] | Type of deafness[c] | Ear, nose, and throat manifestations | Other manifestations |
|---|---|---|---|---|---|
| Miller syndrome (Genée-Wiedemann syndrome)[294] | Probable AR | ***263750** 3487 | CD | Micrognathia, cleft palate, cupped and simple ears | Malar hypoplasia, ectropion, long philtrum, postaxial limb anomalies |
| Nager acrofacial dysostosis syndrome[42,66] | Mostly sporadic, some AD or AR | ***154400** 3143 | CD | Malformations of external ear | Abnormalities of radial ray (thumb or radius hypoplasia or aplasia), downward slanting palpebral fissures, zygomatic hypoplasia, retromicrognathia |
| Oculo-auriculo-vertebral dysplasia (see Facio-auriculo-vertebral dysplasia) | | | | | |
| Oto-facio-cervical syndrome[114] | AD | **166780** 3998 | CD | Prominent auricles with deep conchae, preauricular pits | Lateral cervical fistulas, characteristic radiographic abnormalities |
| Townes-Brocks syndrome (Deafness, imperforate anus, hypoplastic thumbs)[115,405] | AD | ***107480** 3026 | SND | Hypoplastic and malformed ears, preauricular tags | Imperforate anus, prominent perineal raphe, rectoperineal fistula, triphalangeal thumbs or supernumerary thumbs, other anomalies of fingers, corneal anomalies |
| Treacher Collins syndrome (Mandibulofacial dysostosis, Franceschetti-Klein syndrome)[209,390,406] | AD | ***154500** 3282 | CD | Midfacial hypoplasia, micrognathia, high nasal bridge, choanal stenosis, macrostomia, cleft palate, low-set ears, malformed ears with meatal atresia, microtia | Coloboma of eyelids, defect of lacrimal system, anophthalmos, microphthalmos, coloboma of iris, visual loss, mild mental retardation. Localized to chromosome 5q32–q33.1 |
| Wilms tumor, auditory canal stenosis, conductive hearing loss[355] | ? AD | | CD | | |

**Appendix B–4** Genetic hearing loss associated with eye disorders

| Condition or syndrome | Mode of inheritance[a] | MIM No. POSSUM No.[b] | Type of deafness[c] | Ear, nose, and throat manifestations | Other manifestations |
|---|---|---|---|---|---|
| Abruzzo-Erickson syndrome[2] | XLR | 4057 | SND | Cleft palate | Coloboma of iris, choroid and retina, short stature, radial synostosis, hypospadias |
| Albinism, ocular, with late-onset sensorineural deafness[437] | XLR | **300650** | SND | Deafness moderately severe by late middle age in the XLR form | Reduced visual acuity, photophobia, translucent irides, strabismus, hypermetropia, albinoid fundus with foveal hypoplasia |
| Alström syndrome[140] | AR | ***203800** 3020 | SND Deafness by 1st decade | Nystagmus | Acanthosis nigricans, glaucoma, cataract, optic nerve anomaly, photophobia, visual loss, hypogonadism, hypertelorism, diabetes mellitus |
| Aniridia and sensorineural hearing loss[77] | AD | | SND | | |
| Arthropathy, rash, chronic meningitis, eye lesions and mental retardation or Prieur-Griscelli syndrome[321] | | 3550 | SND | | Urticaria, macrocephaly, large fontanelle, optic nerve atrophy, symmetrical large joint arthritis, mental retardation, chronic meningitis, cerebral cortex atrophy, seizures |
| Atrophia bulborum hereditaria (see Norrie disease) | | | | | |
| Berk-Tabatznik syndrome[174] | ? | 3894 | SND | | Congenital optic atrophy, cervical kyphosis, spastic quadriparesis, short stature |

**Appendix B-4** Genetic hearing loss associated with eye disorders (*Continued*)

| Condition or syndrome | Mode of inheritance[a] | **MIM No.** POSSUM No.[b] | Type of deafness[c] | Ear, nose, and throat manifestations | Other manifestations |
|---|---|---|---|---|---|
| Cataracts and progressive sensorineural hearing loss[160] | AD | | SND | | Cataracts |
| Choroideremia, obesity, congenital deafness[270] | XL | **303110** 4173 | SND or mixed | | |
| Congenital cataracts, hypercholesterolemia, spasticity of lower limbs, sensorineural hearing loss[292] | AD or XLR | | SND | | |
| Congenital total color blindness, cataracts, hyperinsulinism[168] | AR | | SND | | Retinal pigmentation, mild mental retardation |
| Corneal anesthesia, retinal abnormalities, mental retardation, unusual facies[322] | AD | 4237 | SND | | Absence of retinal pigment epithelium |
| Corneal dystrophy, sensorineural deafness (Harboyan syndrome)[170] | AR | **217400** 3153 | SND | | Corneal clouding, loss of vision is progressive |
| Cryptophthalmos multiple congenital anomalies syndrome (Fraser syndrome)[46,131] | AR | ***219000** 3179 | CD | Asymmetry of the face, high nasal bridge, coloboma of nostrils, choanal atresia, low-set ears, atresia of external auditory canal, abnormal middle ear, cleft lip + palate, laryngeal abnormalities | Hypertelorism, cryptophthalmos (not obligatory), anal atresia, hypospadias, abnormally placed nipples, ambiguous genitalia, thymic aplasia, mental retardation |
| Deafness, keratoconus, blue sclera, spondylolisthesis[158] | AR | 4523 | CD | Nystagmus | Corneal opacities, severe vision loss, scoliosis |
| Deafness, optic atrophy, progressive (Gernet syndrome)[233] | AD | **125250** 3196 | SND | Profound hearing loss of 60 to over 90 db, may be present from early childhood on | Vision loss is slowly progressive, optic atrophy |
| Deafness, myopia, cataract, saddle nose (Marshall syndrome)[286] | AD | ***154780** 3200 | SND | Midface hypoplasia, depressed nasal bridge, anteverted nostrils, cleft palate | Short stature, frontal bossing, cataract, glaucoma, myopia, vision loss, platyspondyly, abnormal phalanges, intracranial calcification |
| Deafness, myopia, intellectual impairment[105] | AR | **221200** | SND Cochlear | | Intellectual impairment, severe myopia |
| Edwards syndrome (Pigmentary retinopathy, labyrinthine deafnesss)[43] | AR | 4584 | SND | Nystagmus, progressive hearing loss | Pigmentary retinopathy, progressive blindness, photophobia, diabetes mellitus, mental retardation |
| Ehlers-Danlos syndrome type VI[159] | AR | **225400** 3406 | Mixed | | Keratoconus, blue sclerae, loose ligaments |
| Familial band keratopathy, abnormal calcium metabolism[165] | AD | | Type? | Hearing loss | |
| Fraser syndrome (see Cryptophthalmos, MCA syndrome) | | | | | |
| Holmes-Schepens syndrome[193] | AR | | SND | Profound deafness | Myopia, choroidal atrophy, cataract, retinal detachement, hypertelorism, albuminuria |
| Iris dysplasia, hypertelorism, mental retardation, deafness (De Hauwere syndrome)[94] | AD | **147590** 3938 | SND | | Short stature, flat occiput, hypertelorism, strabismus, dislocated hips, hydrocephalus, mental retardation |
| Jensen syndrome[204] | XLR | **311150** 3468 | SND | | Optic atrophy, dementia |
| Jéquier-Deonna[205] syndrome | AR | | SND | | Optic atrophy, polyneuropathy |
| Marshall syndrome (see Deafness, myopia cataract, saddle nose) | | | | | |

| Condition or syndrome | Mode of inheritance[a] | **MIM No.** POSSUM No.[b] | Type of deafness[c] | Ear, nose, and throat manifestations | Other manifestations |
|---|---|---|---|---|---|
| Michels syndrome[271] | AR | **257920** 3984 | CD | Dysmorphic pinnae Cleft lip/palate | Blepharophimosis, ptosis, mental retardation |
| Mohr-Mageroy syndrome (Mohr-Tranebjaerg syndrome) (DFN1)[275,405b] | XLR | | SND | | Blindness, spastic paraplegia, dystonia, mental retardation, fractures |
| Myopia, hypertelorism, agenesis of corpus callosum, diaphragmatic hernia, exomphalos[99] | AR | | SND | | Developmental delay |
| Norrie disease (atrophia bulborum hereditaria)[370] | XLR | ***310600** 3336 | SND | | Deep-set eyes, cataract, corneal opacities, pseudoglioma of the retina, vision loss, hypogonadism, mental retardation |
| OHAHA syndrome (**O**phthalmoplegia, **H**ypotonia, **A**taxia, **H**ypoacusis)[217] | AR | | SND | Marked vestibular dysfunction | |
| Ohdo syndrome[295] | AR | **249620** 3875 | CD | Dysmorphic pinnae | Blepharophimosis, ptosis, mental retardation, congenital heart disease |
| Ophthalmoplegia, radial ray hypoplasia, thrombocytopenia, mixed hearing loss (IVIC syndrome)[350] | AD | ***147750** 3849 | Mixed | | |
| Refsum disease (phytanic acid oxidase deficiency, heredopathia atactica polyneuritiformis)[317,381] | AR | ***266500** 3463 | SND | Anosmia, nystagmus | Hyperkeratosis, ichthyosis, corneal opacities, retinitis pigmentosa, small hands, pes cavus, flexion deformity of toes, ataxia, multiple epiphyseal dysplasia, muscle weakness, absent reflexes, defective phytanic acid degradation |
| Refsum disease, infantile form[338] | AR | ***266510** 4516 | SND | Nystagmus, high-arched palate, low-set ears | Wasted build, short stature, optic nerve abnormalities, retinitis pigmentosa, cryptorchidism, single palmar creases, malabsorption, hepatic fibrosis, clotting disorder, seizure, ataxia, EEG abnormality, hyperlipidemia, peroxisomal disorder |
| Retinitis pigmentosa, congenital deafness (see Usher syndrome) | | | | | |
| Retinitis pigmentosa inversa, hypogonadism, deafness, (Hersh syndrome)[331] | AR | **268010** 4014 | SND | | Macular pigmentary abnormalities, retinal vascular changes, night blindness, visual loss, hypogonadism |
| Retinitis pigmentosa, nystagmus, hemiplegic migraine[444] | AD | | SND | Nystagmus | |
| Retinitis pigmentosa, vitiligo, sensorineural hearing loss[95] | | 4696 | SND | | |
| Rod-cone dystrophy, renal dysfunction, sensorineural hearing loss[32] | AR | 5328 | SND | | |
| Total color blindness, liver degeneration, endocrine dysfunction[168] | AR | | SND | | Sterility, hypothyroidism, diabetes mellitus |
| Usher syndrome (retinitis pigmentosa, congenital deafness)[81,366,427a] | AR | ***276901** 3421 | SND | Anosmia, abnormal inner ear, speech defect | Retinitis pigmentosa, night blindness, visual loss, cataract, ataxia |
| Wolfram syndrome (see Diabetes insipidus, optic atrophy, deafness—DIDMOAD, Appendix B-8) | | | | | |

**Appendix B–5** Genetic hearing loss associated with musculoskeletal disorders

| Condition or syndrome | Mode of inheritance[a] | MIM No. POSSUM No.[b] | Type of deafness[c] | Ear, nose, and throat manifestations | Other manifestations |
|---|---|---|---|---|---|
| Achondroplasia[33,118,177] | AD | ***100800** 3006 | CD | Significantly abnormal facies, midfacial hypoplasia, prognathism, small nose, depressed nasal bridge | Short stature, short limbs, macrocephaly, flat occiput, frontal bossing, small ribs, abnormal vertebral bodies, abnormal acetabulum, restriction of joint mobility, Mutation in FGFR3 |
| Acrocephalosyndactyly type I (see Apert syndrome) | | | | | |
| Acrocephalosyndactyly type III (Saethre-Chotzen syndrome)[287,438] | AD | ***101400** 3009 | | Mild deafness, facial asymmetry, deviated nasal septum | Craniosynostosis, brachydactyly, syndactyly, ptosis of eyelids. Mapped at 7p21 |
| Acrocephalosyndactyly type V (Pfeiffer syndrome)[78,301] | AD | ***101600** 3008 | | Mild deafness | Craniosynostosis and malformations of the thumb and great toe. Mutations in FGFR1 and FGFR2 |
| Acrofacial dysostosis, Kelly type[222] | ?AR | | | Maxillary and mandibular hypoplasia; bilateral, high-frequency hearing loss | Short stature, mild mental retardation, hypospadias, cryptorchidism, symphalangism of thumbs and distal interphalangeal joints |
| Acrofacial dysostosis, Reynolds type[333] | AD | | Mixed | Mild mandibulofacial dysostosis, high-arched palate, mild congenital, mixed hearing loss | |
| Albers-Schönberg disease (see Osteopetrosis, infantile) | | | | | |
| Apert syndrome (acrocephalosyndactyly type I)[71,301,305] | AD | ***101200** 3007 | CD | Congenital stapes fixation, wide cochlear aqueduct, flat face, midface hypoplasia, beaked nose, choanal atresia, cleft palate, low-set ears | Hemivertebrae, humeroradial anomalies, carpal fusion, tarsal fusion, small hands, syndactyly, coronal synostosis. Mutations in FGFR2 |
| Auralcephalosyndactyly[242] | AD | **109050** 4494 | CD | Ears shaped like question marks | Craniosynostosis, cutaneous syndactyly of fourth and fifth toes |
| Aural-digital-anal syndrome[362] | AD | | SND | | Bifid and/or triphalangeal thumbs and imperforate or anteriorly placed anus, coronal synostosis |
| Brachydactyly A1, dwarfism, ptosis, microcephaly, mental retardation[409] | ? | | Mixed | | Persistent iridopupillary membranes and myopia |
| Brachydactyly, broad first digits, hyperopia[399] | AD | | CD | Conductive hearing loss of 50–60 dB | |
| Brachydactyly, Char type, and congenital profound sensorineural hearing loss[64] | ? | | SND | | |
| Campomelic dysplasia[56,195,243,288,353] | AR | ***211970** 3049 | CD | | Relatively frequent sex reversal, frequent lethality, bent femora and tibiae |
| Camurati-Engelmann disease (progressive diaphyseal dysplasia)[376,443] | AD | ***131300** 3206 | CD | Mandibular hyperostosis, facial palsy | Progressive symmetrical diaphyseal sclerosis, fusiform enlargement of long bones with sclerosis of the skull bone, scoliosis, muscle weakness, abnormal gait |

| Condition or syndrome | Mode of inheritance[a] | **MIM No.** POSSUM No.[b] | Type of deafness[c] | Ear, nose, and throat manifestations | Other manifestations |
|---|---|---|---|---|---|
| Carpal and tarsal abnormalities, cleft palate, oligodontia[151] | AR | | CD | | Dorsiflexion of halluces, talonavicular and talocalcaneal fusion |
| Carraro syndrome[62] | ?AR | | Type? | Congenital profound hearing loss | Shortened tibiae |
| Chondrodysplasia, Khaldi type[224] | AR | | SND | | Osteochondrodysplasia, retinitis pigmentosa |
| Chondrodysplasia, Nance-Sweeney type[284] | ?AR | 3062 | Mixed | | Hypoplastic nasal bones, shortened long bones with bowing of tibiae |
| Chondrodysplasia, Temtamy type[398] | AR | | ? | Severe congenital hearing loss | Bone fractures, short stature, leukoderma |
| Cleidocranial dysplasia[100,132,203] | AD | ***119600**<br>3146 | CD | Small face, abnormal facies, cleft soft palate, delayed eruption of teeth, dental cysts | Short stature, flat occiput, frontal bossing, wormian bones, hypoplastic clavicles, scoliosis, small scapulae, delayed ossificaiton of pubic bones. Mapped on 6p21 |
| Coarse facies, skeletal dysplasia[324] | AR | | Mixed | Broad nose, prognathism | Mental retardation; two male and female siblings |
| Cranial hyperostosis[258] | AD | **144755** | Mixed | Broad nasal bridge | Large head circumference, elevated alkaline phosphatase |
| Craniodiaphyseal dysplasia[53] | ? | | Mixed | | Enlargement and sclerosis of cranial and facial bones, ribs, and clavicles; cylinderization of long bones, blindness |
| Craniometaphyseal dysplasia[61,375] | AD<br>AR | ***123000**<br>***218400**<br>3162 | CD | Facial palsy, short nose, broad nasal bridge, choanal atresia or stenosis | Hypertelorism, prominent supraorbital ridges, hyperostotic clavicle, scoliosis, diffuse osteosclerosis, metaphyseal and/or diaphyseal abnormalities |
| Crouzon craniofacial dysostosis[211,239,301] | AD | ***123500**<br>3158 | CD | Midface hypoplasia, sometimes with lateral cleft lip, cleft hard palate, macroglossia, beaked nose and a small jaw | Sutural synostosis, proptosis of the eyes secondary to shallow orbits, optic atrophy, hypoplasia of corpus callosum, usually of normal intelligence. Many mutations in *FGFR2* gene and one in *FGFR3* (associated with acanthosis nigricans) |
| Deafness, peripheral pulmonary stenosis, brachytelephalangy (see Keutel syndrome) | | | | | |
| Deafness, congenital, with split hands and feet[126] | AR | **220600** | SND<br>CD | Asymmetric face, choanal atresia or stenosis, dysplastic ears, high palate, irregular and crowded teeth, micrognathia, webbed neck | Microcephaly, mental retardation, short stature, split hands and/or feet, absent nails |
| Diastrophic dysplasia[141,163,175] | AR | ***222600**<br>3185 | CD | Cauliflower ears due to calcified cartilage, micrognathia, cleft palate, abnormal middle ears, atresia of the external auditory canal, laryngeal abnormalities, abnormal cry | Short stature, atlantoaxial instability, thoracolumbar kyphosis, scoliosis, abnormalities of epiphysis, diaphysis and/or metaphysis, bowed limbs carpal fusion symphalangism, claw hands, dislocated hips |

**Appendix B-5** Genetic hearing loss associated with musculoskeletal disorders (*Continued*)

| Condition or syndrome | Mode of inheritance[a] | MIM No. POSSUM No.[b] | Type of deafness[c] | Ear, nose, and throat manifestations | Other manifestations |
|---|---|---|---|---|---|
| Dwarfism, metatropic, type II (see Kniest dysplasia) | | | | | |
| Dyschondrosteosis (Madelung's deformity, Leri-Weil disease)[92] | AD | ***127300** 3190 | CD | | Deformity of distal radius and ulna and proximal carpal bones, mesomelic dwarfism |
| Dysosteosclerosis[69] | AR | ***224300** 3728 | CD | Otosclerosis | Short stature, bent tubular bones, macular atrophy of skin |
| Dysplasia of capital femoral epiphyses, severe myopia[313] | AD | | SND | Abrupt high-tone loss above 3,000 to 4,000 Hz | |
| Ectrodactyly, Ectodermal dysplasia, Clefting syndrome (EEC syndrome)[343,423] | AD | ***129900** 3211 | | Midfacial hypoplasia, trismus, flat nose, choanal stenosis, microtia, cleft lip, cleft palate | Thin skin, abnormal skin pigmentation, corneal clouding, photophobia, hypoplastic or absent nipples, cryptorchidism, ectrodactyly, syndactyly, cleft hand, vaginal abnormality |
| Facioauriculoradial dysplasia[171] | AD | **171480** 3544 | CD | Variable abnormalities of external ear, midface hypoplasia, long philtrum, bulbous nose | Variable abnormalities of radius |
| Facioscapulohumeral muscular dystrophy and sensorineural hearing loss[251] | AD | ***158900** | SND | | Weakness in face and shoulder girdle, retinal telangiectasia |
| Familial expansile osteolysis[24] | AD | | CD or mixed | Hearing loss evident before age of 10 years | Bone pain, with disordered trabecular ("fishnet") pattern, premature loss of teeth |
| Fibrodysplasia ossificans progressiva[31] | AD | ***135100** 3233 | CD SND | | Ectopic calcification with restriction of movement, malformation of hallux and reduction of digits, baldness |
| Frontometaphyseal dysplasia[202] | XLR | ***305620** 3236 | Mixed or CD | | Marked supraorbital ridges, wasting of arm and leg muscles |
| Fryns craniosynostosis syndrome[129] | AD | | SND | Sensorineural hearing loss of 35–45 dB in low and middle frequencies | Craniosynostosis affecting coronal and metopic sutures |
| Gorlin-Chaudhry-Moss syndrome[199] | AR | **233500** 3173 | CD | | Craniosynostosis, midface hypoplasia, hypertrichosis, anomalies of the eyes, teeth, heart, and external genitalia |
| Grebe-like chondrodysplasia[395] | ? | ***200700** 3755 | Mixed | | Short humeri, short deformed forearms and lower legs |
| Hajdu-Cheney syndrome[416] | AD | ***102500** 3013 | CD SND | | Dissolution of terminal phalanges, dolichocephaly with occipital prominence, short stature, premature loss of teeth |
| Hersh craniosynostosis syndrome[183a] | AR | | SND | Flat nasal bridge, broad nasal tip, micrognathia | Hypertelorism, sparse, curly hair |
| Horizontal gaze palsy, scoliosis[335] | AR | | SND | | Short neck |
| Humero-radio-ulnar synostosis[364] | ?AR | 3123 | SND | | |

| Condition or syndrome | Mode of inheritance[a] | MIM No. POSSUM No.[b] | Type of deafness[c] | Ear, nose, and throat manifestations | Other manifestations |
|---|---|---|---|---|---|
| Hyperostosis corticalis generalisata (Van Buchem disease, Endosteal hyperostosis)[415] | AR | **239100** 3256 | SND | Facial palsy, mandibular hyperostosis | Macrocephaly, frontal bossing, abnormal vision, cortical hyperostosis |
| Hyperphosphatasemia[373] | AR | ***239000** 5325 | Mixed | | Fever, bone pain and swelling, enlargement of the calvaria, pseudoxanthoma elasticum, elevated serum alkaline and acid phosphatase |
| Joint fusion, mitral insufficiency, and conductive hearing loss[123] | AD | **157800** 3303 | CD | 30–70 dB conductive hearing loss; fixation of the footplate of the stapes | Short stature, freckles, fused vertebrae |
| Keipert syndrome (see Naso-digito-acoustic syndrome) | | | | | |
| Keutel syndrome[75,223] | AR | ***245150** | SND | Calcification and/or ossification of the cartilage in the external ears, nose, larynx, trachea, and ribs | Multiple peripheral pulmonary stenoses, short terminal phalanges |
| Klippel-Feil deformity, absent vagina, deafness[19] | | **148860** 4329 | CD | Abnormal middle ear, webbed neck | Short stature, multiple vertebral anomalies, hypoplastic kidneys, absent vagina |
| Klippel-Feil syndrome[27,150,214] | AD AR | ***148900** | CD SND | Nystagmus, cleft palate, short neck | Optic nerve atrophy, squint, winged scapulae, scoliosis, Sprengel anomaly, mild mental retardation, hemiparesis |
| Kniest dysplasia (Metatropic dwarfism type II)[264,336,378,434] | AD | **#156550** | CD | Abnormal facies, depressed nasal bridge, lateral cleft lip, cleft palate | Micrognathia, glaucoma, atlantoaxial instability, lumbar lordosis, wedging of vertebral bodies, scoliosis, abnormal pelvic bones, umbilical hernia, inguinal hernia, accessory phalanges, dislocated hips |
| Larsen syndrome[254] | AD | ***150250** 3275 | CD SND Mixed | Hearing loss is rare | Flat facies, joint hyperextensibility with multiple joint dislocations |
| Lenz-Majewski syndrome[340] | | **151050** 3045 | SND | | Macrocephaly, loose skin, prominent veins, progressive sclerosis of the skull, mental retardation |
| Maxillofacial dysostosis, X-linked[404] | XLR | ***155000** 3921 | Mixed | Malar hypoplasia, outstanding pinnae | Microcephaly, mental retardation, downward slanting palpebral fissures, cryptorchidism |
| Mental and somatic retardation, short and clubbed digits, EEG abnormalities[312] | ?AR | | Mixed | Short broad nose | |
| Metaphyseal dysostosis, mental retardation, conductive deafness[337] | AR | **250420** 3194 | CD | Hearing difficulty first noticed in adolescence; recurrent middle ear infections | Short limb dwarfism, very short fingers suggesting peripheral dysostosis; coxa vara, scoliosis, lumbar lordosis |
| Metaphyseal dysplasia, retinal pigmentary changes[248] | ?AR | | SND | Profound hearing loss | |
| Multiple epiphyseal dysplasia, myopia[255] | AD | **132450** 3871 | CD | Small nose | Wide femoral necks, coxa valga, retinal thinning, crenated cataract |

**Appendix B-5** Genetic hearing loss associated with musculoskeletal disorders (*Continued*)

| Condition or syndrome | Mode of inheritance[a] | **MIM No.** POSSUM No.[b] | Type of deafness[c] | Ear, nose, and throat manifestations | Other manifestations |
|---|---|---|---|---|---|
| Myotonic dystrophy[198] | AD | ***160900** 3193 | SND | | Weakness and wasting of the face and distal muscles first, proximal muscles later; myotonia, cataracts, cardiac conduction defects, mental reatardation, retinal degeneration |
| Naso-digito-acoustic syndrome (Keipert syndrome)[142] | AR | **255980** 3047 | SND | Short nasal septum, flared nostrils, large mouth, everted lips, high and narrow palate | Macrocephaly, ptosis, paresis of ocular muscles, accessory phalanges, clinodactyly of fifth finger, short great toes, mental retardation |
| Oculodentoosseous dysplasia[303] | AD | **257850** | CD | | Thin nose with hypoplastic alae, microcornea, enamel hypoplasia, comptodactyly and frequent syndactyly of fourth and fifth fingers |
| OSMED, megepiphyseal dysplasia (**O**to-**S**pondylo-**ME**gepiphyseal **D**ysplasia)[137] | AR | ***215150** 3630 | SND | Low nasal bridge, hypoplastic midface, cleft palate | Short stature, large epiphyses, myopia |
| Osteogenesis imperfecta, types I, III, and IV[260,432] | AD | **#166200** 3349 | CD | Abormal middle ear | Short limbs, thin skin, macrocephaly, wormian bones, blue sclera, scoliosis, diffuse osteoporosis, multiple fractures, renal stones |
| Osteopathia striata[236] | AD | ***166500** 4249 | Mixed | Cleft palate in 50% of cases | Enlarged head circumference, combed radiographic appearance of bones, mild mental retardation in 30% of cases |
| Osteopetrosis, infantile (Albers-Schönberg disease, marble bone disease)[374,424] | AR | ***259700** 3374 | CD | Square face, mandibular sclerosis, abnormal sinuses | Macrocephaly, frontal bossing, ptosis, optic nerve atrophy, diffuse osteosclerosis, metaphyseal abnormality, mutiple fractures, hepatosplenomegaly, thrombocytopenia, hypotonia, hypocalcemia |
| Otopalatodigital syndrome type I (Taybi syndrome)[36,210,363] | XLD | ***311300** 3352 | CD | Small nose, broad nasal bridge, cleft palate, low-set ears, abnormal middle ear | Short stature, frontal bossing, small nails, prominent supraorbital ridges, dental caries, pectus deformity, carpal fusion, irregularity of length of fingers, hypoplastic thumbs, dislocated hips, syndactyly, mental retardation. Locus at Xq28 |
| Otopalatodigital syndrome type II[293,308,446] | XLD | **304120** 3352 | CD | Small nose, depressed nasal bridge, long philtrum, low-set ears | Distinguished from type I by facies and skeletal changes: long, curved clavicles; bowed legs, osteosclerosis, joint dislocation |
| Paget-like bone disorders[3] | AD | | Mixed or CD | | Paget-like changes in the bones of the extremities, elevated alkaline phosphatase |
| Pfeiffer syndrome (see Acrocephalosyndactyly type V) | | | | | |

| Condition or syndrome | Mode of inheritance[a] | MIM No. POSSUM No.[b] | Type of deafness[c] | Ear, nose, and throat manifestations | Other manifestations |
|---|---|---|---|---|---|
| Progressive diaphyseal dysplasia (see Camurati-Engelmann disease) | | | | | |
| Proximal symphalangism, deafness[106] | AD | ***185800** 4065 | CD | Abnormal middle ear | Carpal fusion, symphalangism, tarsal fusion |
| Saethre-Chotzen syndrome (see Acrocephalosyndactyly type III) | | | | | |
| Scapuloperoneal syndrome[11] | AD | | SND | | Weakness in the shoulder girdle and peroneal muscles |
| Sclerosteosis (cortical hyperostosis with syndactyly)[30] | AR | ***269500** 3386 | CD | Flat face, facial palsy, prognathism, asymmetry of the jaw, nystagmus, abnormal middle ear, depressed nasal bridge | Tall stature, small nails, sclerotic calvarium, abnormal sella turcica, optic nerve anomalies, visual loss, syndactyly of fingers, hydrocephalus |
| Skeletal malformations, ptosis of eyelids[201] | AR | | CD | Pinched nose | |
| Sorsby syndrome[403] | | **120400** 3282 | Mixed | Severe hearing loss | Brachydactyly B, macular colobomas |
| Spondylocarpotarsal coalition syndrome with or without unilateral unsegmented bar[433] | AR | ***272460** 4490 | SND or Mixed | Variable cleft palate | Scoliosis, cervical vertebral fusion |
| Spondyloepiphyseal dysplasia congenita[377] | AD | **#183900** 3394 | SND | Cleft palate in 15%-20%, moderately severe sensorineural hearing loss in 30% of cases | Short stature, short neck, bell-shaped chest, myopia |
| Spondyloepiphyseal dysplasia, myopia, deafness, MacDermot type[255] | AD | **184000** 4479 | SND | Triangular face, short neck | Short stature, proximal femoral epiphyseal dysplasia, blue slcera, myopia, retinal detachment, scoliosis, delayed skeletal maturation, dislocated hips |
| Stickler syndrome (Hereditary progressive arthroophthalmopathy)[4,34,372,396] | AD | **#108300** 3030 | SND | Flat, round face, micrognathia, small nose, anteverted nostrils, cleft palate, glossoptosis | Glaucoma, cataract, retinal detachement, myopia, scoliosis, restriction of joint mobility, arachnodactyly, large hands, hypotonia, pectus carinatum. Mutation in nonhelical 3′ end of type II procollagen gene *(COL2A1)* |
| Symphalangism-brachydactyly syndrome (Herrmann type)[183,190] | AD | ***186500** 3402 | CD | Deafness probably due to anomalies of the ossicles | Synostosis of elbow joints, fingers, wrist and foot with short middle phalanges and metacarpals |
| Symphalangism, proximal (Cushing symphalangism)[84,315] | AD | ***185800** | CD | Stapes ankylosis | |
| Taybi syndrome (see Oto-palatodigital syndrome, type I) | | | | | |
| Trichorhinophalangeal syndrome type II[253] | | ***150230** 3416 | Mixed | Bulbous nose, protruding ears | Clinodactyly, cone-shaped epiphyses, sparse, fine hair |

**Appendix B–6** Genetic hearing loss associated with renal disorders

| Condition or syndrome | Mode of inheritance[a] | MIM No. POSSUM No.[b] | Type of deafness[c] | Ear, nose, and throat manifestations | Other manifestations |
|---|---|---|---|---|---|
| Adolescent or young adult renal tubular acidosis and slowly progressive sensorineural hearing loss[422] | AR | ***267300** 4553 | SND | | |
| Alport syndrome[45,120,184,227,247] | AD AR XLR | ***104200 *153640 203780 #301050 *303630** 4509 | SND | Progressive, high-tone deafness; decreased responses to caloric stimulation | Cataract, keratoconus, macular degeneration, renal failure, abnormal esophagus |
| Barakat syndrome[22] | AR | **256340** | SND | | Steroid-resistant nephrosis with progressive renal failure, hypoparathyroidism |
| BOR syndrome (see Branchio-oto-renal syndrome) | | | | | |
| Deafness, hyperprolinuria, ichthyosis[153] | AD | ***239500** 3198 | SND | | Ichthyosis, renal tubular defect, hyperprolinemia, renal stones, proline oxidase deficiency |
| Deafness, renal tubular acidosis[8] | AR | ***267300** 4553 | SND | Speech defect | Short stature, splayed rib ends, metaphyseal abnormalities, renal tubular defects, hypercalcemia |
| Epstein syndrome (see Macrothrombocytopathy, nephritis and deafness)[109] | | | | | |
| Facio-oculo- acoustico-renal syndrome (FOAR syndrome)[299] | AR | **227290** 3338 | SND | Broad and depressed nasal bridge, high-arched palate | Macrocephaly, frontal bossing, coloboma of iris, retinal detachment, myopia, severe vision loss, tooth discoloration, epiphyseal abnormality, urinary tract defects |
| Fechtner syndrome[134] | AD | ***153640** 4598 | SND | | Nephropathy in males, giant platelets with thrombocytopenia, leukocyte inclusions |
| Fitzsimmons syndrome[119] | AD | **270710** 3596 | SND | | Mesangial IgA nephropathy, spastic paraplegia, mental retardation |
| Lemieux-Neemeh syndrome[136] | AD | | SND | | Nephrotic syndrome, neuropathy |
| Macrothrombocytopathy-nephritis and deafness (Epstein syndrome)[109] | AD | **153650** 3864 | SND | Moderate to severe, high-frequency sensorineural hearing loss | Thrombocytopenia with giant platelets, nephritis (mixed glomerulonephritis and interstitial nephritis) |
| Membranous glomerulonephritis and sensorineural hearing loss[269] | ?AR | | SND | | |
| Nephritis, hyperparathyroidism[103] | AR | | SND | | Progressive nephropathy |
| Nephritis, myopathy, corneal crystals[13] | ? | | CD | | Albuminuria |
| Renal anomalies, prune belly, pulmonic stenosis, mental retardation[251] | XL | | SND | | Lack of abdominal muscles, renal anomalies, mild mental retardation |
| Renal disease, digital anomalies[47] | XLR AR | | CD | Bifurcation of the uvula | Shortened bulbous thumbs and halluces, ureteral constriction and duplication of the renal pelvis |
| Renal failure, cataracts, recurrent infections[368] | AR | | CD | | Cataracts, early renal failure, chronic diarrhea |

| Condition or syndrome | Mode of inheritance[a] | MIM No. POSSUM No.[b] | Type of deafness[c] | Ear, nose, and throat manifestations | Other manifestations |
|---|---|---|---|---|---|
| Renal failure, severe hypertension, abnormal steroidogenesis, hypogenitalism[166] | AR | | SND | | Progressive renal failure |
| Renal, genital, and middle ear anomalies (Winter syndrome)[226] | AR | **267400** 3376 | CD | Micrognathia, beaked nose, low-set ears, abnormal middle ear | Oligohydramnios, uterine abnormality, clinodactyly of fifth finger, hypoplastic kidneys, mental retardation |
| Renal rickets, retinitis pigmentosa[152] | AR | | SND | | Relentless progression of visual handicap |
| Urticaria, deafness, amyloidosis, nephritis (Muckle-Wells syndrome)[63,279] | AD | | SND | Deafness noted in 85% of cases, usually appears in childhood or adolescence | Limb and joint pains, 35% develop nephrotic syndrome |

**Appendix B–7** Genetic hearing loss associated with nervous system disorders

| Condition or syndrome | Mode of inheritance[a] | MIM No. POSSUM No.[b] | Type of deafness[c] | Ear, nose, and throat manifestations | Other manifestations |
|---|---|---|---|---|---|
| Ataxia, deafness and cardiomyopathy (Jeune-Tommasi syndrome)[206] | AR | ***208750** | SND | Nystagmus, progressive deafness | Ataxia, mental deficiency, numerous freckles or lentigines, enlarged heart, heart block |
| Ataxia-deafness-retardation syndrome (Berman syndrome)[228] | AR | **208850** 4251 | SND | Nystagmus, high palate, speech defect | Ataxia, mental retardation, paresis of ocular muscles, pes cavus, flexion deformities of toes |
| Begeer syndrome[29] | AR | 4851 | SND | | Cataracts, mental retardation, ataxia, motor and sensory neuropathy |
| Boltshauser syndrome[40] | AD | | SND | Vocal cord paralysis | Mild motor neuropathy |
| Borud syndrome[44] | Mitochondrial | | SND | | Ataxia, cardiomyopathy, mitochondrial myopathy, pigmentary retinopathy |
| Brown-Vialetto-Van Leare syndrome[391] | AD | ***211530** 4748 | SND | | Pontobulbar paralysis |
| Charcot-Marie-Tooth disease and deafness[76,86,310,349] | AD AR | ***118300** **214370** 4384 | SND | Micrognathia, narrow palate, short neck, laryngeal abnormality | Pectus carinatum, umbilical hernia, camptodactyly, pes cavus, ataxia, hypotonia, abnormal gait |
| Chorea and sensorineural hearing loss[89] | AR | | SND | | Childhood onset, nonprogressive chorea, mild hypotonia |
| Cockayne syndrome type I[12,181,304] | AR | ***216400** 3149 | SND | Aged facies, small nose, nystagmus | Sun sensitivity resulting in bullae and desquamation of skin, death in infancy or childhood, short stature, thin skin, cataract, defect of the laryngeal system, thoracolumbar kyphosis, hypogonadism, contracture of large joints, hepatomegaly, mental retardation, chromosomal breakage on exposure of cells to UV light |
| Congenital neuroaxonal dystrophy with peripheral gangrene[196] | ?AR | | SND | | Dysmorphism, congenital hypotonia, mental retardation, blindness, distal gangrene, ichthyosis |
| Coppeto-Lessell syndrome[74] | AR | | SND | | Dystonia with blepharospasm, pigmentary retinopathy, dementia |
| Cruse syndrome[85] | AD | | SND | Trigeminal neuralgia | Motor and sensory neuropathy |
| Cutler syndrome[88] | ?AR ?Mitochondrial | | SND | | Ataxia, amyotrophy, bone marrow hypoplasia, nephropathy, goiter |

**Appendix B-7** Genetic hearing loss associated with nervous system disorders (*Continued*)

| Condition or syndrome | Mode of inheritance[a] | MIM No. POSSUM No.[b] | Type of deafness[c] | Ear, nose, and throat manifestations | Other manifestations |
|---|---|---|---|---|---|
| Deafness, hyperuricemia, ataxia[345] | XLR | ***311850** 4266 | SND | Nystagmus, speech defect | Cardiac conduction defect, hypertension, renal failure, muscle weakness |
| Deafness, optic atrophy, neuropathy (Rosenberg-Chutorian syndrome)[346] | XLR | **311070** 3196 | SND | Slowly progressive hearing loss | Mid-life optic atrophy with vision loss, distal muscular atrophy resembling Charcot-Marie-Tooth disease |
| Deafness, diabetes, myoclonus, nephropathy (Herrmann syndrome)[182] | AD | **172500** | SND | Progressive deafness, horizontal nystagmus | Diabetes mellitus, nephropathy, photomyoclonic seizures |
| Deafness, sensorineural, with peripheral neuropathy and arterial disease (Campbell-Clifton syndrome)[58,307] | AD | **124950** 4038 | SND | Mild saddle nose | Skin rash, peripheral arterial disease leading to gangrene, elevation of cerebrospinal fluid protein, papilledema, contracted retinal arteries |
| Dobyns syndrome[98] | AR | | SND | | Ataxia, optic atrophy |
| Dyck syndrome[102] | AR XLR | | SND | | Motor and sensory neuropathy, adrenocortical insufficiency, hepatosplenomegaly, optic atrophy |
| Dystonia, deafness syndrome[359] | XLR | **305050** | SND | Pathological changes are mainly neuronal loss and gliosis in the basal ganglia | Severe dysarthria, striking deterioration of handwriting, occasional bizarre positioning of ears and neck |
| Flynn-Aird syndrome[122] | AD | ***136300** 3437 | SND | | Ataxia, cataracts, motor and sensory neuropathy, myopia, pigmentary retinopathy, kyphoscoliosis, skin atrophy |
| Friedreich's ataxia[55,116a,167,392] | AR | ***229300** 3797 | SND | Nystagmus, speech defect | Optic nerve anomalies, scoliosis, pes cavus, cardiac conduction defects, heart failure, late-onset diabetes mellitus |
| Geminiani syndrome[133] | AR or XLR | | SND | | Ataxia, localized amyotrophy of hands, spastic paraparesis, hypogonadism, short stature |
| Golabi-Ito-Hall syndrome[139] | XL | 3590 | SND | | Unusual facies, microcephaly, mental retardation |
| Gordon syndrome[144] | AR or XL | | SND | | Spastic quadriparesis, mental retardation, dementia, optic atrophy, pigmentary retinopathy |
| Groll-Hirschowitz syndrome[316] | AR | **221400** 3731 | SND | Normal vestibular functions | Disturbances of cardiac rhythm, small bowel diverticulitis |
| Gustavson syndrome[162] | XLR | ***309555** 5234 | SND | | Microcephaly, severe mental retardation, optic atrophy, spasticity, seizures, restricted movement of large joints |
| Hagemoser syndrome[164] | AD | | SND | | Motor and sensory neuropathy, optic atrophy |
| Hallgren syndrome[38] | AR | | SND | | Ataxia, mild motor and sensory neuropathy, pigmentary retinopathy |
| Hers-Opitz syndrome (N syndrome)[121] | XLR | | | Hearing loss suspected | Mental retardation, multiple congenital anomalies, spastic quadriplegia, visual loss, susceptibility to neoplasia, increased chromosomal breakage |
| Hicks syndrome[194] | AD | | SND | | Sensory and autonomic neuropathy, dementia |
| Holoprosencephaly, myelomeningocele, abducens paralysis[70] | AR | | SND | | |

| Condition or syndrome | Mode of inheritance[a] | MIM No. POSSUM No.[b] | Type of deafness[c] | Ear, nose, and throat manifestations | Other manifestations |
|---|---|---|---|---|---|
| Iwashita syndrome[200] | AR | | SND | | Optic atrophy, hereditary motor and sensory neuropathy type II |
| Kearns-Sayre syndrome (Ophthalmoplegia, retinitis pigmentosa, cardiomyopathy)[245,282,420] | Mitochondrial | **#530000** 3747 | CD SND | Abnormal facies, facial palsy, speech defect, abnormal cry | Optic nerve abnormality, peripheral pigmentary retinal changes, kyphosis, scoliosis, ataxia, diabetes mellitus |
| Latham-Munro syndrome[246] | AR | | SND | | Myoclonic epilepsy, dementia |
| Lichtenstein-Knorr syndrome[386] | AR | | SND | | Ataxia, scoliosis |
| May-White syndrome[413] | AD | | SND | | Ataxia, myoclonic and other seizures |
| MELAS (**M**itochondrial **E**ncephalopathy, **L**actic **A**cidosis, **S**troke-like episodes)[419] | Mitochondrial | ***590050** 4935 | SND | | Mitochondrial myopathy with ragged-red fibers, headache, vomiting, hemiparesis, cortical blindness |
| MERRF (**M**yoclonic **E**pilepsy, **R**agged-**R**ed **F**ibers)[367] | Mitochondrial | **#545000** | SND | | Myoclonic epilepsy, mitochondrial myopathy with ragged-red fibers, ataxia, dementia |
| MNGIE syndrome (**M**yo-**n**euro-**g**astrointestinal **e**ncephalopathy)[23] | Mitochondrial | **#550900** | | | Mitochondrial myopathy with ragged-red fibers, ptosis, and ophthalmoplegia, motor and sensory neuropathy |
| Möbius syndrome (congenital facial diplegia)[241,256] | AD AR | **157900** 3217 | SND | Expressionless face, micrognathia, glossoptosis | Ptosis, short stature, small hands, brachydactyly, syndactyly, talipes, muscle weakness, mental retardation |
| Muller-Zeman syndrome[116] | AR | | SND | | Developmental delay, hypotonia, spastic quadriplegia, ataxia, dementia, optic atrophy |
| Muscle wasting of hands, congenital sensorineural deafness (Stewart Bergstrom syndrome)[383] | AR | **108200** 3486 | SND | | Congenital flexion contractures and atrophy of thenar, hypothenar and interosseous muscles |
| Nathalie syndrome (Oto-oculo-musculo-skeletal syndrome)[83] | AR | **255990** 3351 | SND | Deafness in early childhood | Cataract, muscular atrophy, EKG abnormalities |
| Neurofibromatosis 2 (central neurofibromatosis)[172,197,244] | AD | ***101000** 4258 | SND | Neurofibromas, acoustic neuromas | Corneal clouding, cataract, intracranial calcification, café-au-lait patches |
| Oculopalatocerebral dwarfism[127] | AR | | CD | Cleft palate | Microcephaly, mental retardation, spastic diplegia or quadriplegia, microphthalmia, asthma |
| Ophthalmoplegia, retinitis pigmentosa, cardiomyopathy (see Kearns-Sayre syndrome) | | | | | |
| Opjordsmoen-Nyberg-Hansen syndrome[297] | AD | | SND | | Spastic paraplagia, syndactyly |
| Optic atrophy, ophthalmoplegia, ptosis, deafness, myopathy (Treft-Sanborn syndrome)[407] | AD | **165490** 4360 | SND | Speech defect | Ptosis, optic nerve atrophy, abnormal electroretinogram, muscle weakness, absent relfexes, EMG abnormality |
| Pauli syndrome[307] | AD | | SND | | Pigmentary retinopathy, motor and sensory neuropathy |
| POLIP syndrome (**P**olyneuropathy, **O**phthalmoplegia, **L**eukoencephalopathy, **I**ntestinal **P**seudo-obstruction)[369] | Mitochondrial | **#550900** 4821 | SND | Chronic intestinal pseudo-obstruction | |
| Reardon syndrome[327] | AR or XLR | | SND | Onset of hearing loss at 2–3 years | Ataxia, global delay |

**Appendix B-7** Genetic hearing loss associated with nervous system disorders (*Continued*)

| Condition or syndrome | Mode of inheritance[a] | **MIM No.** POSSUM No.[b] | Type of deafness[c] | Ear, nose, and throat manifestations | Other manifestations |
|---|---|---|---|---|---|
| Renier syndrome[332] | XL | | SND | | Mental retardation, microcephaly, epilepsy, spastic paraplegia |
| Richards-Rundle syndrome (ataxia, hypogonadism, mental retardation, sensorineural deafness)[125,334] | AR | ***245100** 4549 | SND | Nystagmus, narrow palate, speech defect | Slowly progressive ataxia, premature, graying of hair, paresis of ocular muscles, hypogonadism, abnormal female genitalia, seizures, mental retardation, ketoaciduria |
| Robinson syndrome[342] | AD | ***124480** 3581 | SND | | Sensory ataxia, thoracolumbar scoliosis |
| Schimke-Horton syndrome[354] | XLR | **312840** 3706 | SND | "Pinched" nasal bridge | Congenital hypotonia, choreoathetosis, spastic quadriplegia, mental retardation, postnasal microcephaly and growth deficiency |
| Schmidley syndrome[357] | XLR | | SND | | Ataxia, dysphagia and choking, early hypotonia and later spasticity and areflexia, mental retardation, seizures, optic atrophy |
| Seitelberger disease[360] | AR | | SND | | Dysmorphism, congenital hypotonia, mental retardation, blindness, distal gangrene, ichthyosis |
| Strömgren syndrome[388] | AD | | SND | | Posterior polar cataracts, intrabulbar hemorrhage, late-onset ataxia, dementia, loss of vestibular function |
| Sylvester syndrome[392] | ?AD | | SND | | Ataxia, spasticity and amyotrophy, optic atrophy |
| Weaver-Williams syndrome[428] | AR | 4046 | Type? | Cleft palate | Brother and sister with microcephaly, mental retardation, skeletal abnormalities |
| Wells-Jankovic syndrome[431] | XLR | | SND | | Spastic paraplegia, cataracts, mild pigmentary retinopathy, hypogonadism |
| X-linked mental retardation, short stature, deafness, microgenitalism (Juberg-Marsidi mental retardation)[215a,263] | XLR | ***309590** 3584 | Abnormal hearing | Depressed nasal bridge, thickened helix, preauricular pits | Small for gestational age, short stature, microcephaly, small penis, hypospadias, camptodactyly, seizures, hypotonia |

**Appendix B–8** Genetic hearing loss associated with endocrine and metabolic disorders

| Condition or syndrome | Mode of inheritance[a] | **MIM No.** POSSUM No.[b] | Type of deafness[c] | Ear, nose, and throat manifestations | Other manifestations |
|---|---|---|---|---|---|
| Adrenoleuko dystrophy[291] | XLR | ***300100** | SND | | Progressive neurologic deterioration, with blindness; peroxisomal disease |
| Amyloidosis IV, Iowa type[414] | AD | ***107680** | SND | | Chronic progressive sensorimotor neuropathy, cataracts, duodenal ulcer, amyloid nephropathy, elevated spinal fluid protein |
| Amyloidosis VII (oculoleptomeningeal amyloidosis)[411] | AD | ***105210** | SND | Diminished vestibular function | Hemiplegic migraine, polyneuropathy, seizures, dementia, vision loss |
| Aspartylglucosaminuria[277] | AR | ***208400** 4607 | CD or SND | | Coarse facies, mild dysostosis multiplex, mental retardation |

| Condition or syndrome | Mode of inheritance[a] | MIM No. POSSUM No.[b] | Type of deafness[c] | Ear, nose, and throat manifestations | Other manifestations |
|---|---|---|---|---|---|
| Biotinidase deficiency (Multiple carboxylase deficiency)[440] | AR | ***253260** 5333 | | Hearing loss in 15–50% of cases | Rash, conjunctivitis, alopecia, seizures, ataxia, hyperammonemia, organic aciduria |
| Canavan disease (N-acetylaspartic aciduria)[262] | AR | ***271900** 4810 | SND | | Macrocephaly, seizures, optic atrophy, severe progressive psychomotor retardation, early death |
| Chanarin-Dorfman syndrome[435] | AR | ***275630** 4111 | SND | | Cataracts, ichthyosis, mild myopathy, cytoplasmic droplets in many cell types |
| Congenital absence of thyroid and sensorineural hearing loss[93] | | | SND | | |
| Congenital adrenal hypoplasia, gonadotrophin deficiency, and progressive high-frequency, sensorineural hearing loss[448] | XLR | ***300200** 4626 | SND | | |
| Cretinism, endemic (fetal iodine deficiency syndrome)[185] | ?AR | **228355** | SND | Deafness from fetal iodine deficiency | Mental deficiency, sometimes neuromuscular disorders, diplegia, squint |
| Deafness, diabetes mellitus, mitochondrial DNA deletion[20] | Mitochondrial | | | ? | Premature deafness, 10.4 kb mitochondrial DNA deletion, stroke |
| Deafness, goiter, stippled epiphyses (Refetoff syndrome)[329,330,393] | AR | **#274300** 4093 | SND | Midfacial hypoplasia, high nasal bridge, abnormal cry, deaf-mutism | Pectus carinatum, winged scapula, epiphyseal abnormality, goiter, end-organ unresponsiveness to thyroid hormone, hypothyroidism |
| Deafness-hypogonadism[281] | XLR | **304350** | SND CD | Congenital mixed deafness beginning in the 2d decade and progressing to severe deafness | Primary hypogonadism, and antisocial behavior in males |
| **D**iabetes **I**nsipidus, **D**iabetes **M**ellitus, **O**ptic **A**trophy, **D**eafness (DIDMOAD syndrome or Wolfram syndrome)[240] | AR | ***222300** 3516 | SND | Nystagmus, hearing loss is variable and slowly progressive | Diabetes insipidus, diabetes mellitus, optic atrophy, hydronephrosis, hydroureters |
| Diabetes mellitus, thiamine-dependent megaloblastic anemia, sensorineural hearing loss (α-keto-glutarate, dehydrogenase deficiency)[1] | AR | ***249270** | SND | | Variable heart anomalies |
| Fabry disease (α-galactosidase A deficiency)[276] | XLR | ***301500** 3023 | SND | High-tone sensorineural deafness | Cutaneous angiokeratoma, paresthesia, cataracts |
| Familial hypophosphatemic rickets[347] | XLD | ***307800** 3263 | SND or mixed | | Vitamin D–resistant rickets |
| Glucosylceramide-β-glucosidase deficiency[412] | ?AR | | SND | | Hydrocephalus, corneal opacities, valvular heart disease, calcification of aorta |
| Hunter syndrome (Mucopolysaccharidosis II [MPS II][65,285] | XLR | ***309900** 3309 | CD | Coarse facies, webbed neck, macroglossia | Increased body hair, macrocephaly, abnormal sella turcica, papilledema, retinal anomalies, diffuse osteoporosis, restriction of joint mobility, hepatosplenomegaly, herniae, claw hand. Distinguished from Hurler syndrome by clear cornea and usually milder or no mental retardation |
| Hurler syndrome (mucopolysaccharidosis IH [MPS IH][285,427] | AR | ***252800** 3308 | CD | Depressed nasal bridge, winged alae nasi, macroglossia, airway obstruction | Increased body hair, macrocephaly, abnormal sella turcica, coarse facies, corneal |

**Appendix B-8** Genetic hearing loss associated with endocrine and metabolic disorders (*Continued*)

| Condition or syndrome | Mode of inheritance[a] | MIM No. POSSUM No.[b] | Type of deafness[c] | Ear, nose, and throat manifestations | Other manifestations |
|---|---|---|---|---|---|
| | | | | | clouding, gibbus, retinal pigmentary changes, umbilical hernia, abnormal metacarpals, coxa valga, dislocated hips, cardiac valve abnormalities, hepatosplenomegaly, mental retardation |
| Insulin-resistant diabetes mellitus and progressive sensorineural hearing loss[417] | Mitochondrial | **#520000** | SND | Severe to profound, progressive, involving all frequencies | Inheritance only through mother |
| Johanson-Blizzard syndrome[135] | AR | ***243800** | SND | Notched or hypoplastic alae nasi, delayed tooth eruption and development, widely spaced small teeth | Scalp defects, microcephaly, short stature, heart defects, hypothyroidism, mental retardation, failure to thrive, pancreatic exocrine insufficiency |
| Juberg-Marsidi syndrome (see X-linked mental retardation, short stature, deafness, microgenitalism) | | | | | |
| Kallmann syndrome[92] | AD<br>AR<br>XL | ***308700**<br>4216 | SND or mixed | Anosmia, occasionally cleft lip or palate | Hypogonadism |
| Krabbe disease (galactosylceramide $\beta$-galactosidase deficiency, globoid cell leukodystrophy)[5] | AR | ***245200** | | Profound deafness in late phase of disorder | Psychomotor retardation, seizures, onset between 3 and 8 months |
| Mannosidosis $\alpha$-D[290,401] | AR | ***248500**<br>4458<br>***248510** | SND | Macroglossia, large ears, short neck | Coarse facies, hypertelorism, cataract, corneal opacities, delayed skeletal maturation, hepatosplenomegaly, recurrent respiratory infections, liver storage disease, hypotonia, diabetes, mild dysostosis multiplex |
| Methylglutaconic aciduria[68] | AR or XLR | ***250950** | SND | Deafness in at least 20% of cases | Choreoathetosis, dementia, seizures, optic atrophy, acidosis |
| Mucopolysaccharidosis IH (see Hurler syndrome) | | | | | |
| Mucopolysaccharidosis II (see Hunter syndrome) | | | | | |
| Mucosulfatidosis (Multiple sulfatase deficiency)[371] | AR | ***272200** | | Involvement of the retrocochlear auditory system | Ichthyosis, dysostosis multiplex, coarse facies, psychomotor retardation |
| Neonatal adrenoleukodystrophy[221] | AR | **#202370**<br>4188 | SND | | Progressive mental deficiency and dementia |
| Niemann-Pick type C[314] | | ***257220**<br>3334 | | | Hepatosplenomegaly, progressive neurologic deterioration |
| Pendred syndrome (goiter with deafness)[207,216] | AR | ***274600**<br>3910 | SND | | Thyroid enlargement, hypothyroidism, thyroid hormone organification defect |
| Peroxisomal disorders[49] | | | SND | All have sensorineural hearing loss (adult-type Refsum syndrome, acatalasia, Zellweger syndrome, infantile-type Refsum syndrome, Leber congenital amaurosis, chondrodysplasia punctata, rhizomelic type) | |
| Perrault syndrome (Gonadal dysgenesis, deafness)[289] | AR | ***233400**<br>3764 | SND | Nystagmus, microstomia, high-vaulted palate | Retrognathia, blue sclera, myopia, squint, scoliosis, streak gonads, delayed skeletal maturation, cubitus valgus, talipes, ataxia, pituitary defect |

| Condition or syndrome | Mode of inheritance[a] | MIM No. POSSUM No.[b] | Type of deafness[c] | Ear, nose, and throat manifestations | Other manifestations |
|---|---|---|---|---|---|
| Refetoff syndrome (see Deafness, goiter, stippled epiphyses) | | | | | |
| Rosenberg syndrome[28] | XL | **311070** 3196 | SND | Abnormal vestibular function | Ataxia, gout, hyperuricemia |
| Salivary gland insensitivity to aldosterone and sensorineural hearing loss[410] | AR or XLR | | SND or mixed | | |
| Seip-Berardinelli syndrome[149] | AR | ***269700** 3439 | CD | | Progressive lipodystrophy, hyperlipemia, acanthosis nigricans, insulin-resistant diabetes mellitus |
| Sialidosis (neuraminidase deficiency)[445] | AR | ***256550** 3305 | CD or mixed | | Dysostosis multiplex, ataxia, myoclonus, mental retardation, cherry-red spots of the retina |
| Tay-Sachs disease (infantile $Gm_2$ gangliosidosis)[111] | AR | ***272800** 3244 | SND | | Progressive psychomotor retardation, seizures, blindness, death usually before age of 3 years |
| Van Gemund syndrome[418] | AR or XLR | | SND | Congenital profound hearing loss | Prenatal dwarfism, elevated serum levels of immunoreactive growth hormone, mental retardation |
| Winkelmann syndrome[436] | AR | | SND | Hearing loss appears at 6–8 years of age and progresses rapidly to complete deafness | Somatic and sexual infantilism due to deficiency of growth hormone and gonadotropins, normal intelligence |
| Yumita syndrome[447] | AR | | SND | | Hypoparathyroidism; association with HLA-A9,A11 |

**Appendix B–9** Genetic hearing loss associated with chromosomal disorders

| Condition or syndrome | Mode of inheritance[a] | MIM No. POSSUM No.[b] | Type of deafness[c] | Ear, nose, and throat manifestations | Other manifestations |
|---|---|---|---|---|---|
| Cat-eye syndrome[265] | | 3267 | | Frequent hearing loss involving the middle ear, preauricular fistula, hypertelorism, atretic or absent external ear canals | Presence of an extra chromosome derived from a rearranged chromosome #22 and with a karyotype of inv dup (22) (pter→q11). Mental development mildly or moderately impaired. Striking feature is coloboma of iris, choroid and retina. Renal (50%) and cardiac (35%) anomalies |
| Chromosome 13, trisomy 13 (Patau syndrome)[237,358] | | 3090 | SND CD | Abnormal helices and low-set ears, cleft lip/palate, absent philtrum, micrognathia | Holoprosencephaly, microcephaly, microphthalmos, polydactyly, cardiac defect, severe mental retardation |
| Chromosome 18, trisomy 18 (Edwards syndrome)[237,261,358] | | 3094 | SND CD | Malformed auricles, low-set ears, microsomia, narrow palate, micrognathia | Growth deficiency, prominent occiput, clenched hands, short sternum, heart defect, severe mental retardation |
| Chromosme 18, del(18q) syndrome[273] | | | CD | Very narrow or atretic external ear canals, cleft palate | |
| Chromosome 21, trisomy 21 (Down's syndrome)[52] | | 3100 | Mild | Folded or small ears, small nose, flat nasal bridge, hypoplasia of frontal sinuses, short neck, redundant nuchal skin | Brachycephaly, upward slant of the eyes, epicanthic folds, Brushfield spots on iris, short broad hands, single palmar creases, cardiac defect, hypotonia, mental retardation |
| Chromosome X monosomy, 45X (Turner syndrome)[400] | | 3104 | SND | Down-turned mouth angles, high-arched palate, short/webbed neck | Short stature, pigmented nevi, streak gonads, primary or early secondary amenorrhea, conge- |

**Appendix B-9** Genetic hearing loss associated with chromosomal disorders (*Continued*)

| Condition or syndrome | Mode of inheritance[a] | MIM No. POSSUM No.[b] | Type of deafness[c] | Ear, nose, and throat manifestations | Other manifestations |
|---|---|---|---|---|---|
| | | | | | nital lymphedema (may be transient), delayed skeletal maturation, cubitus valgus, coarctation of the aorta, aortic valve problems, usually normal intelligence |
| Edwards syndrome (see Chromosome 18, trisomy 18) | | | | | |
| Klinefelter syndrome (47,XXY or 48,XXYY or 48,XXXY or 49,XXXXY)[9] | | 3107 | SND | Dips in the middle frequencies and high stapedius reflex threshold | Infertility, below average intelligence, gynecomastia (50%), female habitus |
| Smith-Magenis syndrome[157] | | **#182290** 4368 | CD | Misshapen and posteriorly angulated external ears, prominent chin, broad nasal bridge, cleft palate, delayed speech | Deletion of 17p [del(17p11.2)]. Growth and mental retardation, frontal bossing, synophrys |
| Turner syndrome (see Chromosome 45X) | | | | | |
| Unbalanced 11/22 translocation[356] | | | CD SND | Broad and flat nose, receding mandible, abnormal auricles, cleft palate (50%) | rcp (11;22)(q23;q11) is the most frequent non-Robertsonian balanced rearrangement in humans. Male genital hypoplasia with micropenis and cryptorchidism, heart defects (50%), anal atresia |

**Appendix B–10** Genetic hearing loss associated with integumentary disorders

| Condition or syndrome | Mode of inheritance[a] | MIM No. POSSUM No.[b] | Type of deafness[c] | Ear, nose, and throat manifestations | Other manifestations |
|---|---|---|---|---|---|
| Albinism, cutaneous, with deafness[365,450] | XLR | ***300700** 4629 | SND | | |
| Albinism, ocular, with sensorineural deafness[249] | AD | **103470** | SND | Nystagmus and deafness accompanied by vestibular hypofunction | |
| Albinism, oculocutaneous, with deafness (Tietz-Smith syndrome)[328] | AD | **103500** | SND | | Hypopigmentation and not true albinism |
| Albinism, oculocutaneous, with deafness, autosomal recessive type[449] | AR | | SND | | Albinism of entire body with optic fundi and irides |
| BADS syndrome (**B**lack locks, oculocutaneous **A**lbinism, **D**eafness **S**yndrome)[439] | AR | | SND | | White skin with brown macules, white hair with black locks |
| Björnstad syndrome[82] | ?AR | **262000** 3038 | SND | | Congenital pili torti |
| Buschke-Ollendorf syndrome[389] | AD | ***166700** 4673 | CD | | Elastic connective tissue nevi, osteopoikilosis |
| CHIME syndrome (**C**oloboma, **H**eart defect, **I**chthyosis, **Me**ntal retardation, **E**ar)[451] | ?AR | **280000** 3605 | CD | Cleft palate | Congenital ichthyosiform dermatosis, mental retardation, seizures, retinal colobomas |
| Congenital spiny hyperkeratosis, universal alopecia, congenital sensorineural hearing loss[48] | ? | | SND | | Hypohidrosis, obstruction of lacrimal punctae |
| Crandall syndrome (see Pili torti and nerve deafness) | | | | | |
| Davenport syndrome[91] | AD | | SND | | Hypopigmentation of skin, hair, and eyes, joint contractures, psoriasiform lesions, abnormal chemotaxis |

| Condition or syndrome | Mode of inheritance[a] | MIM No. POSSUM No.[b] | Type of deafness[c] | Ear, nose, and throat manifestations | Other manifestations |
|---|---|---|---|---|---|
| Deafness, atopic dermatitis[232] | AR | **221700** | SND | | Atopic dermatitis or late-onset and atypical distribution (ulnar aspects of forearms and antecubital fossae) |
| Deafness, congenital, with keratopachydermia and constrictions of fingers and toes (Vohwinkel-Nockemann syndrome)[6] | AD | ***124500** | SND | | Hyperkeratosis of palms and soles, epidermal thickening over knuckles, mental retardation |
| Deafness, knuckle pads, leukonychia (Schwann syndrome, Bart-Pumphrey syndrome)[25] | AR (semidominant) | ***149200** 4267 | SND CD | Hearing loss from infancy on with poor speech development | Hyperkeratosis, dysplastic nails, eczema, thickened skin over interphalangeal joints, gene carriers with white nails |
| Deafness, onychodystrophy (Robinson-Miller-Bensimon syndrome)[143] | AD ?AR | ***124480** 3581 | SND | | Small nails, grooved nails, teeth with crown-shaped coniform anomaly, abnormal phalanges, syndactyly of fingers, polydactyly |
| **D**eafness, **O**nycho-**O**steodystrophy, **R**etardation, **S**eizures (DOORS syndrome)[60,306] | AR | ***220500** 3733 | SND | Short, broad nose, large nostrils | Triphalangeal thumb, abnormal dermatoglyphics, hypoplastic nails, seizures and EEG abnormalities, elevated levels of plasma and urinary 2-oxyglutarate, mental retardation |
| Deafness, vitiligo, achalasia[231] | AR | ***221350** 3855 | SND | Tracheoesophageal fistula, achalasia | Short stature, vitiligo, muscle wasting, peripheral neuropathy |
| Desmons syndrome[96] | AR | | SND | | Ichthyosiform erythroderma of palms and soles, short stature |
| DOORS syndrome (see **D**eafness, **O**nycho-**O**steodystrophy, **R**etardation, **S**eizures) | | | | | |
| Goodman-Moghadam syndrome[274] | AD | | SND | | Onychodystrophy of fingernails and toenails, triphalangeal thumbs |
| Helweg-Larsen and Ludvigsen syndrome[179] | AD | | SND | Hearing loss in middle age | Congenital anhidrosis |
| Hypopigmentation, muscle wasting, achalasia, congenital sensorineural hearing loss[348] | AR | | SND | | Short stature |
| Johnson-McMillin syndrome[208] | AD | **147770** 3595 | CD | Variable malformation of the external ear, anosmia | Alopecia, hypogonadotropic hypogonadism, excessive dental caries, mental retardation, congenital heart disease |
| KID syndrome (**K**eratitis, **I**chthyosis, **D**eafness)[278] | ? | **148210** 3933 | SND | | Heterogeneous; peripheral neuropathy, frequent cutaneous squamous-cell carcinoma |
| LEOPARD syndrome (**L**entigines, **E**KG abnormalities, **O**cular hypertelorism, **P**ulmonic stenosis, **A**bnormalities of genitalia, **R**etardation of growth, and **D**eafness)[147,212] | AD | **151100** 3277 | SND | Prognathism, prominent pinnae, short neck | Short stature, pigmented nevi, delayed eruption of teeth, pectus deformity, hypospadias, small penis, cardiomyopathy, cardiac conduction defect, hypoplastic kidneys, mild mental retardation |
| Olmsted syndrome[15] | | 4802 | SND | Hearing loss at higher frequencies | Palmar and plantar hyperkeratosis, hyperhidrosis, nail dystrophy, hypotrichosis or alopecia |
| Piebald trait, neurological impairment (Telfer-Sugar-Saeher Mulcahy syndrome)[230,379,380,442] | AD | **172850** 4597 | SND | | Decreased skin pigmentation, patchy hair pigmentation, white forelock, mental retardation, abnormal gait |

**Appendix B-10** Genetic hearing loss associated with integumentary disorders (*Continued*)

| Condition or syndrome | Mode of inheritance[a] | **MIM No.** POSSUM No.[b] | Type of deafness[c] | Ear, nose, and throat manifestations | Other manifestations |
|---|---|---|---|---|---|
| Pili torti and nerve deafness (Crandall syndrome)[82] | AR | **262000** 3038 | SND | | Dry brittle hair, decreased eyebrows and eyelashes, delayed skeletal maturation, small penis, hypogonadism |
| Scanty hair, camptodactyly, and neurosensory hearing loss[272] | AR | | SND | | |
| Shepard-Elliot-Mulvihill syndrome[280] | ? | | SND | | Premature aging, growth retardation, nevi or lentigines, genital anomalies, mental retardation |
| Symmetrical lipomatosis with hearing loss[108] | AD | | SND | Variable expression of deafness | Stiff skin, peptic ulcer, renal stones |
| Tsakalakos ectodermal dysplasia[408] | ?AD | | SND | | Amastia with or without athelia, sparse hair, numerous skin tags in a mother and daughter |
| Waardenburg syndrome type I[14,18,214,394] | AD | ***193500** 3426 | SND | Broad, high nasal bridge; dystopia canthorum, prognathism, small nostrils, cleft palate/lip in some cases | Decreased skin pigmentation, white forelock, white eyelashes, retinal albinism, heterochromia irides, contractures of large joints, cyanotic heart disease, syndactyly of fingers. Mapped on chromosome 2q.A *PAX3* gene |
| Waardenburg syndrome type II[214,394] | AD | **193510** 4100 | SND | Broad high nasal bridge without dystopia canthorum, striking vestibular disturbances | Similar to type I with more frequent pigmentary disorders (this type of deafness is much more common than in type I) |
| Woodhouse-Sakati syndrome[441] | AR | ***241080** 3612 | SND | | Mental retardation, alopecia, diabetes mellitus, hypogonadism, ECG abnormalities |
| Woolf syndrome[442] | ?AR or XLR | | SND | Normal vestibular responses | Depigmentation of head and arms |
| Yemenite-type hypopigmentation, blindness, sensorineural hearing loss[425] | AR | | SND | Infantile onset of hearing loss | Hypopigmentation with areas of hyperpigmentation, microcornea and colobomata. Reported in a Yemenite brother and sister |
| Ziprkowsi-Margolis syndrome[259] | XLR | | SND | Depressed vestibular responses | Pigmentary changes of the skin (hypopigmentation and hyperpigmentation) |

**Appendix B–11** Genetic hearing loss associated with oral and dental disorders

| Condition or syndrome | Mode of inheritance[a] | **MIM No.** POSSUM No.[b] | Type of deafness[c] | Ear, nose, and throat manifestations | Other manifestations |
|---|---|---|---|---|---|
| Enamel hypoplasia, leukonychia, sensorineural hearing loss[178] | AR | | SND | | Minor nail anomalies |
| Gingival fibromatosis and sensorineural hearing loss (Jones syndrome)[173] | AD | ***135550** | SND | | |
| Oligodontia and congenital sensorineural hearing loss[138] | AR | | SND | | |
| Otodental syndrome[67] | AD | ***166750** 3350 | SND | Dental changes with globoid posterior teeth and taurodontism | |

**Appendix B–12** Hearing loss associated with miscellaneous disorders

| Condition or syndrome | Mode of inheritance[a] | **MIM No.** POSSUM No.[b] | Type of deafness[c] | Ear, nose, and throat manifestations | Other manifestations |
|---|---|---|---|---|---|
| Branchial arch defects[7] | AR | 3623 | SND | Preauricular pits, rudimentary retroauricular tubercles, dysphagia | Central hypoventilation, mental retardation, hypotonia |
| Burn syndrome[57] | AR | | SND | Anomalies of the external ear, bilateral choanal atresia | Cardiac defects, characteristic facies |
| Cleft lip and palate, sacral lipomas, misplaced supernumerary digits, sensorineural hearing loss[252] | AR or XLR | | SND | | |
| Coffin-Lowry syndrome[191] | XL | ***303600** 3150 | SND | | Characteristic facies, short stature, scoliosis, variable mental retardation |
| De Lange syndrome[104] | ? | **122470** 3183 | SND | Small nose, anteverted nostrils | Characteristic facies, severe mental retardation, synophrys, micromelia |
| Deafness, myoclonic seizures, cleft palate[318] | | 3869 | SND | Small nose, depressed nasal bridge, subcutaneous cleft palate, preauricular tags, microtia | Coarse hair, broad cheeks, prominent eyes, cryptorchidism, inguinal hernia, small hand, clinodactyly of fifth finger, abnormal skin creases, hypotonia, seizures and EEG abnormalities |
| Deafness, Pfaendler type[311] | AR | **221000** | SND | Congenital deafness | Present in eastern Switzerland; mental deficiency and hypogonadism may be associated; semilethal effect of the gene is possible |
| Deafness,progressive, high-tone, neural[188] | AD | ***124800** | SND | Hearing loss divided into 4 types, depending on audiogram | Talipes equinovarus, syndactyly, nail dystrophy, mild antimongoloid slant of the eyes, frontal upsweep of hair, absence of testes, mild mental retardation |
| Deafness, skeletal dysplasia, lip granuloma (Fountain syndrome)[128] | AR | **229120** 4162 | SND | Coarse facies, granulomatous swelling of cheeks and gingivae, prognathism, thick lips, abnormal inner ear, speech defect | Erythroderma, microdontia, dental caries, scoliosis, kyphosis, short phalanges, brachydactyly, short foot, spina bifida, hypotonia, mental retardation |
| Duane anomaly, deafness, radial ray defects (see Okihiro syndrome) | | | | | |
| Fanconi pancytopenia[16,169] | AR | ***227650** 3234 | CD | Hearing loss in 5%–15% of cases. Auricles malformed in 5%. External auditory meatus may be atretic and ossicles fused or malformed | Small stature, patchy melanotic hyperpigmentation of skin, hypoplastic or aplastic thumbs or radii |
| Fetal alcohol syndrome[154,250,385] | | 3218 | SND | Abnormal facies, midfacial hypoplasia, micrognathia, short nose, smooth and underdeveloped philtrum, thin lips, cleft palate, short neck | Failure to thrive, microcephaly, increased body hair, microphthalmos, myopia, fusion of ribs, delayed skeletal maturation, radioulnar synostosis, nail hypoplasia, camptodactyly, single palmar creases, congenital heart disease, neural tube defect, ataxia |
| Fetal aminoglycoside ototoxicity[189,319] | Mitochondrial | | SND | Vestibular disturbance | Occurs in offspring with maternal systemic exposure to streptomycin, kanamycn, gentamycin, tobramycin, amikacin, or other aminoglycosides |

**Appendix B-12** Hearing loss associated with miscellaneous disorders (*Continued*)

| Condition or syndrome | Mode of inheritance[a] | **MIM No.** POSSUM No.[b] | Type of deafness[c] | Ear, nose, and throat manifestations | Other manifestations |
|---|---|---|---|---|---|
| Fetal cytomegalovirus syndrome[35] | | 3220 | SND | | Small for gestational age, microcephaly, optic nerve anomalies, vision loss, inguinal hernia, hepatomegaly, thrombocytopenia, hydrocephalus, Dandy-Walker malformation, mental retardation, soft tissue calcification |
| Fetal rubella syndrome[90,213] | | 3222 | SND | | Small for gestational age, microcephaly, microphthalmos, glaucoma, cataract, corneal opacities, peripheral retinal changes, squint, delayed eruption of teeth, hypospadias, hypoplastic right heart, mental retardation, diabetes mellitus, pituitary defect |
| Fetal thalidomide syndrome[51] | | 3224 | | Abnormal hearing | Short stature, short limbs, abnormal long bones, missing toes, ureteric anomalies, renal failure, duodenal atresia |
| FG syndrome[402] | XL | ***305450** 3566 | SND | Hearing loss in 35% of patients | Relative microcephaly, soft sparse scalp hair, enlarged corneae, fetal finger and toe pads |
| Finucane syndrome[1[illegible]7] | ? | | SND | | Unusual facies, mental retardation, hypopigmented areas of skin |
| Fountain syndrome (see Deafness, skeletal dysplasia, lip granuloma) | | | | | |
| Glomus tympanicum (nonchromaffin paragangliomas, chemodectomas, familial glomus tumors) and hearing loss)[186] | AD | | SND, CD or mixed | | |
| Hypoplastic thumbs, coloboma of choroid, cataracts, developmental delay, sensorineural hearing loss[426] | AR | | SND | | |
| Jervell and Lange-Nielsen syndrome (cardioauditory syndrome)[87,187] | AR | ***220400** 3660 | SND | | Prolonged Q-T intervals, episodes of loss of consciousness or fainting, may die of arrhythmia if not treated |
| Kabuki make-up syndrome[352] | AD | **147920** | CD | Severe ossicular malformations | Mental retardation, postnatal dwarfism, long palpebral fissures, eversion of lateral third of lower lid, broad and depressed nasal tip, prominent finger and toe pads |
| Limb-oto-cardiac syndrome (Phocomelia, ectrodactyly, deafness, sinus arrhythmia)[384] | AD | **171480** 3280 | CD | Abnormal middle ear (absent incus and stapes) | Absent radius, sinus arrhythmia, abnormal humerus, missing fingers |
| Lymphedema of the lower limbs, hematologic abnormalities, sensorineural hearing loss[107] | AD | | SND | | |
| Okihiro syndrome (Duane anomaly, deafness, radial ray defects)[176] | AD | ***126800** 3713 | SND CD | Asymmetry of the face, microtia, atresia of the external auditory canal, speech defect | Multiple vertebral anomalies, hypoplastic radius, paresis of the ocular muscles, short thumb |

| Condition or syndrome | Mode of inheritance[a] | MIM No. POSSUM No.[b] | Type of deafness[c] | Ear, nose, and throat manifestations | Other manifestations |
|---|---|---|---|---|---|
| Orofaciodigital syndrome, type 2 (Mohr syndrome, OFD type II)[10,21,325] | AR | ***252100** 3348 | CD | Midfacial hypoplasia, micrognathia, broad nasal bridge, cleft lip/palate, notched tongue, oral synechiae, abnormal middle ear | Short stature, oligodontia, pectus excavatum, brachydactyly, syndactyly, clinodactyly of the fingers, metatarsal abnormalities, Dandy-Walker malformation, cerebral cortex atrophy, hypotonia |
| Unusual facies, microcephaly, joint laxity, conductive hearing loss[26] | ?AR | | CD | | |

[a]AD, autosomal dominant; AR, autosomal recessive; XLD, X-linked recessive; XLD, X-linked dominant.

[b]MIM, *M*endelian *I*nheritance in *M*an. A catalog of human genes and genetic disorders, by Victor A. McKusick, 11th ed, The Johns Hopkins University Press, Baltimore, 1994; POSSUM, *P*ictures *O*f *S*tandard *S*yndromes and *U*ndiagnosed *M*alformations, by Agnes Bankier et al., Murdoch Institute, Royal Children's Hospital, Victoria, Australia.

*confirmed gene and inheritance.

#phenotye that can be caused by mutation in any of 2 or more genes.

[c]CD, conductive deafness; SND, sensorineural deafness.

## References


1. Abboud MR, Alexander D, Najjar SS: Diabetes mellitus, thiamine-dependent megaloblastic anemia, and sensorineural deafness associated with deficient α-ketoglutarate dehydrogenase deficiency. J Pediatr 107:537–541, 1985.
2. Abruzzo MA, Erickson RP: Re-evaluation of new X-linked syndrome for evidence of CHARGE syndrome or association. Am J Med Genet 34:397–400, 1989.
3. Adams DA, Gormley PK, Kerr AG, Smyth GD, Osterberg P, Sloan J: Otological manifestations of a new familial polyostotic bone disorder. J Laryngol Otol 105:80–84, 1991.
4. Ahmad NN, Dimascio J, Knowlton RG, Tasman WS: Stickler syndrome—a mutation in the nonhelical 3′ end of type II procollagen gene. Arch Ophthalmol 113:1454–1457, 1995.
5. Aicardi J: The inherited leukodystrophies. J Inherit Metab Dis 16:733–743, 1993.
6. Aksu F, Mietens C: Keratopachydermie mit Schnurfurchen an Fingern und Zehen und Innenohrschwerhörigkeit. Paediatr Prax 23:303–310, 1980.
7. Aksu F, von Stockhausen HB, Wiebicke W, Froster-Iskenius U, Schwinger E, Schultz-Coulon HJ: Hereditary branchial arch defects in a Turkish family. Eur J Pediatr 142:232–233, 1984.
8. Anai T, Yamamoto J, Matsuda I, Taniguchi N, Kondo T, Nagai B: Siblings with renal tubular acidosis and nerve deafness. The first family in Japan. Hum Genet 66:282–285, 1984.
9. Anderson H, Lindsten J, Wedenberg E: Hearing defects in males with sex chromosome anomalies. Acta Otolaryngol 72:55–58, 1971.
10. Annerin G, Gustavson K-H, Jòzwiak S, Kjartansson S, Strömberg B: Abnormalities of the cerebellum in oro-facio-digital syndrome II (Mohr syndrome). Clin Genet **38:**69–73, 1990.
11. Ansher M, Smith LD, Ringel SP: Autosomal dominant scapuloperoneal syndrome with sensorineural hearing loss. Otolaryngol Head Neck Surg 100:242–244, 1989.
12. Arlett CF: Human DNA repair defects. J Inher Metab Dis 9 (Suppl 1):69–84, 1986.
13. Arnold RW, Stickler GB, Bourne WM, Mellinger JF: Corneal crystals, myopathy and nephropathy: a new syndrome. J Pediatr Ophthalmol Strabismus 24:151–155, 1987.
14. Asher JH Jr, Morell R, Friedman TB: Waardenburg syndrome (WS): The analysis of a single family with a WS1 mutation showing linkage to RFLP markers on human chromosome 2q. Am J Hum Genet 48: 43–52, 1991.
15. Atherton DJ, Sutton C, Jones BM: Mutilating palmoplantar keratoderma with periorificial keratotic plaques (Olmsted's syndrome). Br J Dermatol 122:245–252, 1990.
16. Auerbach AD, Sagi M, Adler B: Fanconi anemia: prenatal diagnosis in 30 fetuses at risk. Pediatrics 76:794–800, 1985.
17. Bach I, Brunner HG, Beighton P, Ruvalcaba RH, Reardon W, Pembrey ME, van der Velde-Visser SD, Bruns GA, Cremers CW, Cremers FP, et al: Microdeletions in patients with gusher-associated X-linked mixed deafness (DFN3). Am J Hum Genet 50:38–44, 1992.
18. Badner JA, Sieber WK, Garver KL, Chakravarti A: A genetic study of Hirschprung disease. Am J Hum Genet 46:568–580, 1990.
19. Baird PA, Lowry RB: Absent vagina and the Klippel-Feil anomaly. Am J Obst Gynec 118:290–291, 1974.

19a. Baldwin CT, Weiss S, Farrer LA, De Stefano AL, Adair R, Franklyn B, Kidd KK, Korostishevsky M, Bonné-Tamir B: Linkage of congenital, recessive deafness (DFNB4) to chromosome 7q31 and evidence for genetic heterogeneity in the Middle Eastern Druze population. Hum Mol Genet 4:1637–1642, 1995.

20. Ballinger SW, Shoffner JM, Hedaya EV, Trounce I, Polak MA, Koontz DA, Wallace DC: Maternally transmitted diabetes and deafness associated with a 10.4 Kb mitochondrial DNA deletion. Nat Genet 1:11–15, 1992.
21. Baraitser M: The orofaciodigital (OFD) syndromes. J Med Genet 23:116–119, 1986.
22. Barakat AY, D'Albora JB, Martin MM, Jose PA: Familial nephrosis, nerve deafness, and hypoparathyroidism. J Pediatr 91:61–64, 1977.
23. Bardosi A, Creutzfeldt W, Di Mauro S, Felgenhauer K, Friede RL, Goebel HH, Kohlschutter A, Mayer G, Rahlf G, Servidei S, et al: Myo-, neuro-, gastrointestinal encephalopathy (MNGIE syndrome) due to partial deficiency of cytochrome c oxidase: a new mitochondrial multisystem disorder. Acta Neuropathol 74:248–258, 1987.
24. Barr RJ, Hughes AE, Mollan RA, Nevin NC: Idiopathic multicentric osteolysis: report of two new cases and a review of the literature. Am J Med Genet 32:556, 1989.
25. Bart RS, Pumphrey RE: Knuckle pads, leukonychia and deafness—a dominantly inherited syndrome. N Engl J Med 276:202–207, 1967.
26. Bartsocas CS, Papamikalis T, Goumas P, Antonakopoulos C, Verygakis M: A new syndrome of multiple congenital anomalies, partial deafness, and mental subnormality. 5th Int Conf Birth Defects, Montreal, 21–27, 1977.
27. Bavinck JN, Weaver DD: Subclavian artery supply disruption sequence: hypothesis of a vascular etiology for Poland, Klippel-Feil, and Möbius anomalies. Am J Med Genet 23:903–918, 1986.
28. Becker MA, Puig JG, Mateos FA, Jimenez ML, Kim M, Simmonds HA: Inherited superactivity of phosphoribosylpyrophosphate synthetase: association of uric acid overproduction and sensorineural deafness. Am J Med 85:383–390, 1988.
29. Begeer JH, Scholte FA, van Essen AJ: Two sisters with mental retardation, cataract, ataxia, progressive hearing loss, and polyneuropathy. J Med Genet 28:884–885, 1991.
30. Beighton P: Sclerosteosis. J Med Genet 25:200–203, 1988.
31. Beighton P: Fibrodysplasia ossificans progressiva. In: McKusick's Heritable Disorders of Connective Tissue, 5th ed. P Beighton, ed. CV Mosby, St Louis, 1993, pp 501–518.
32. Beighton P, Bartmann L, Bingham G, Sellars S: Rod-cone dystrophy, sensorineural deafness, and renal dysfunction: An autosomal recessive syndromic entity? Am J Med Genet 47:832–836, 1993.
33. Bellus GA, McIntosh I, Smith EA, Aylsworth AS, Kaitila I, Horton

WA, Greenhaw GA, Hecht JT, Francomano CA: A recurrent mutation in the tyrosine kinase domain of fibroblast growth factor receptor 3 causes hypochondroplasia. Nat Genet 10:357–359, 1995.
34. Bennett JT, McMurray SW: Stickler syndrome. J Pediatr Orthop 10:760–763, 1990.
35. Beuhler BA, Shinefield HR: Fetal cytomegalovirus syndrome. In: Birth Defects Encyclopedia, ML Buyse, ed. Blackwell Scientific Publications, Cambridge, 1990, pp 691–692.
36. Biancala V, Le Marec B, Odent S, van den Hurk JA, Hanauer A: Oto-palato-digital syndrome type I: further evidence for assignment of the locus to Xq28. Hum Genet 88:228–230, 1991.
37. Birgerson L, Gustavson KH, Stahle J: Familial Ménière's disease: a genetic investigation. Am J Otol 8:323–326, 1987.
38. Bitoun P, Bandini D, Rigaudiere F: A hereditary syndrome with retinopathy and ataxia or deafness in two consanguineous brothers. Ophthalmol Paediatr Genet 12:149–152, 1991.
39. Blegvad B, Hvidegaard T: Hereditary dysfunction of the brainstem auditory pathways as a major cause of speech retardation. Scand Audiol 12:179–187, 1983.
40. Boltshauer E, Lang W, Spillmann T, Hof E: Hereditary distal muscular atrophy with vocal cord paralysis and sensorineural hearing loss: a dominant form of spinal muscular atrophy? J Med Genet 26:105–108, 1989.
41. Bonfils P, Avan P, Londero A, Narcy P, Trotoux J: Progressive hereditary deafness with predominant inner hair cell loss. Am J Otol 12:203–206, 1991.
41a. Bonné-Tamir B, De Stefano AL, Briggs CE, Adair R, Franklyn B, Weiss S, Korostishevsky M, Frydman M, Baldwin CT, Farrer LA: Linkage of congenital recessive deafness (gene DFNB10) to chromosome 21q22·3. Am J Hum Genet 58:1254–1259, 1996.
42. Bonthron DT, Macgregor DF, Barr DG: Nager acrofacial dysostosis—minor manifestations support dominant inheritance. Clin Genet 43:127–131, 1993.
43. Boor R, Herwig J, Schrezenmeir J, Pontz BF, Schonberger W: Familial insulin resistant diabetes associated with acanthosis nigricans, polycystic ovaries, hypogonadism, pigmentary retinopathy, labyrinthine deafness, and mental retardation. Am J Med Genet 45:649–653, 1993.
44. Borud O, Torbergsen T, Mathiesen E: Increased lactate in cerebrospinal fluid from 7 siblings in a family with mitochondrial myopathy and cerebellar ataxia. J Inher Metab Dis 10:400, 1987.
45. Boye E, Flinter F, Zhou J, Tryggvason K, Bobrow M, Harris A: Detection of 12 novel mutations in the collagenous domain of the COL4A5 gene in Alport syndrome patients. Hum Mutat 5:197–204, 1995.
46. Boyd PA, Keeling JW, Lindenbaum RH: Fraser syndrome (cryptophthalmos-syndactyly syndrome): a review of eleven cases with postmortem findings. Am J Med Genet 31:159–168, 1988.
47. Braun FC Jr, Bayer JF: Familial nephrosis associated with deafness and congenital urinary tract anomalies in siblings. J Pediatr 60:33–41, 1962.
48. Britton H, Lustig J, Thompson BJ, Meyer S, Esterly NB: Keratosis follicularis spinulosa decalvans. Arch Dermatol 114:761–764, 1978.
49. Brown FR 3d, Voigt R, Singh AK, Singh I: Peroxisomal disorders: neurodevelopmental and biochemical aspects. Am J Dis Child 147:617–626, 1993.
50. Brown KA, Janjua AH, Karbani G, Parry G, Noble A, Crockford G, Bishop DT, Newton VE, Marham AF, Mueller RF: Linkage studies of non-syndromic recessive deafness (NSRD) in a family orignating from the Mirpur region of Pakistan maps DFNB1 centromeric to D13S175. Hum Mol Genet 5:169–173, 1996.
51. Brown MA, Farrell C, Newton P, Child RP: Thalidomide, pregnancy and renal failure. Med J Aust 152:148–149, 1990.
52. Brown PM, Lewis GT, Parker AJ, Maw AR: The skull base and nasopharynx in Down's syndrome in relation to hearing impairment. Clin Otolaryngol 14:241–246, 1989.
53. Brueton LA, Winter RM: Craniodiaphyseal dysplasia. J Med Genet 27:701–706, 1990.
54. Bu XK, Ying MD, Guo HB, Cao Z: Audiologic investigation of autosomal dominant hereditary sensory hearing loss in a family of 507 members in 6 generations. Ann NY Acad Sci 630:310–312, 1991.
55. Bundey S: Genetics and Neurology. Churchill Livingstone, Edinburgh, 1985, pp 226–227.
56. Burgoyne P, Schafer AJ, Graves JAM: The role of SOX9 in autosomal sex reversal and campomelic dysplasia—discussion. Phil Trans R Soc Lond B Biol Sci 350:277–278, 1995.
57. Burn J, McKeown C, Wagget J, Bray R, Goodship J: New dysmorphic syndrome with choanal atresia in siblings. Clin Dysmorphol 1:137–144, 1992.
58. Campbell AMG, Clifton F: Adult toxoplasmosis in one family. Brain 73:281–290, 1950.
59. Cantú JM, Ruenes R, García-Cruz D: Autosomal recessive sensorineural-conductive deafness, mental retardation, and pinna anomalies. Hum Genet 40:231–234, 1978.
60. Cantwell RJ: Congenital sensory neural deafness associated with onycho-osteodystrophy and mental retardation (D.O.O.R. syndrome). Hum Genet 26:261–265, 1975.
61. Carnevale A, Grether P, del Castillo V, Takenaga R, Orzechowski A: Autosomal dominant craniometaphyseal dysplasia. Clinical variability. Clin Genet 23:17–22, 1983.
62. Carraro A: Assenza congenita della tibia e sordomutismo nel quattro fratelli. Chir Organi Mov 16:429–438, 1931.
62a. Chaib H, Lina-Granade G, Guilford P, Plauchu H, Levilliers J, Morgon A, Petit C: A gene responsible for a dominant form of neurosensory non-syndromic deafness maps to the NSRD1 recessive deafness gene interval. Hum Mol Genet 3:2219–2222, 1994.
62b. Chaib H, Place C, Salem N, Chardenoux S, Vincent C, Weissenbach J, El-Zir E, Loiselet J, Petit C: A gene responsible for a sensorineural nonsyndromic recessive deafness maps to chromosome 2p22–23. Hum Mol Genet 5:155–158, 1996.
62c. Chaib H, Place C, Salem N, Dode D, Chardenoux S, Weissenbach J, El-Zir E, Loiselet J, Petit C: Mapping of DFNB12, a gene for non-syndromal autosomal recessive deafness, to chromosome 10q21–22. Hum Mol Genet 5:1061–1064, 1996.
63. Champion RH: Muckle-Wells syndrome (urticaria, amyloidosis and deafness). Br J Dermatol 121 (Suppl 34):75, 1989.
64. Char F: An unusual form of brachydactyly associated with deafness. Birth Defects 13:228, 1977.
65. Chase DS, Morris AH, Ballabio A, Pepper S, Giannelli F, Adinolfi M: Genetics of Hunter syndrome: carrier detection, new mutations, segregation and linkage analysis. Ann Hum Genet 50:349–360, 1986.
66. Chemke J, Mogilner BM, Ben-Itzhak I, Zurkowski L, Ophir D: Autosomal recessive inheritance of Nager acrofacial dysostosis. J Med Genet 25:230–232, 1988.
66a. Chen AH, Ni L, Fukushima K, Marietta J, O'Neill M, Coucke P, Willems P, Smith RJ: Linkage of a gene for dominant non-syndromic deafness to chromosome 19. Hum Mol Genet 4:1073–1076, 1995.
67. Chen RJ, Chen HS, Lin LM, Lin CC, Jorgenson RJ: "Otodental" dysplasia. Oral Surg Oral Med Oral Pathol 66:353–358, 1988.
68. Chitayat D, Chemke J, Gibson KM, Mamer OA, Kronick JB, McGill JJ, Rosenblatt B, Sweetman L: 3-Methylglutaconic aciduria: a marker for as yet unspecified disorders and the relevance of prenatal deafness in a new type (type 4). J Inherit Metab Dis 15:204–212, 1992.
69. Chitayat D, Silver K, Azouz EM: Skeletal dysplasia, intracerebral calcifications, optic atrophy, hearing impairment, and mental retardation: nosology of dysosteosclerosis. Am J Med Genet 43:517–523, 1992.
70. Cohen MM Jr: Perspectives on holoprosencephaly: Part I. Epidemiology, genetics, and syndromology. Teratology 40:211–235, 1989.
71. Cohen MM Jr, Kreiborg S: The central nervous system in the Apert syndrome. Am J Med Genet 35:36–45, 1990.
72. Cohen MM Jr, Rollnick BR, Kaye CI: Oculoauriculovertebral spectrum: an updated critique. Cleft Palate J 26:276–286, 1989.
73. Cooper LF, Jabs EW: Aural atresia associated with multiple congenital anomalies and mental retardation: a new syndrome. J Pediatr 110:747–750, 1987.
74. Coppeto JR, Lessell S: A familial syndrome of dystonia, blepharospasm, and pigmentary retinopathy. Neurology 40:1359–1363, 1990.
75. Cormode EJ, Dawson M, Lowry RB: Keutel syndrome: clinical report and literature review. Am J Med Genet 24:289–294, 1986.
76. Cornell J, Sellars S, Beighton P: Autosomal recessive inheritance of Charcot-Marie-Tooth disease associated with sensorineural deafness. Clin Genet 25:163–165, 1984.
76a. Coucke P, Van Camp G, Djoyodiharjo B, Smith SD, Frants RR, Padberg GW, Darby JK, Huizing EH, Cremers CW, Kimberling WJ et al.: Linkage of autosomal dominant hearing loss to the short arm of chromosome 1 in two families. N Engl J Med 331:425–431, 1994.
77. Courteney-Harris RG, Mills RP: Aniridia and deafness: An inherited disorder. J Laryngol Otol 104:419–420, 1990.
78. Cremers CWRJ: Hearing loss in Pfeiffer's syndrome. Int J Pediatr Otorhinolaryngol 3:343–353, 1981.
79. Cremers CWRJ: Meatal atresia and hearing loss. Autosomal dominant and autosomal recessive inheritance. Int J Pediatr Otorhinolaryngol 8:211–213, 1985.
80. Cremers CW: Audiologic features of the X-linked progressive mixed

deafness syndrome with perilymphatic gusher during stapes gusher. Am J Otol 6:243–246, 1985.
81. Cremers CW, Delleman WJ: Usher's syndrome, temporal bone pathology. Int J Pediatr Otorhinolaryngol 16:23–30, 1988.
82. Cremers CWRJ, Geerts SJ: Sensorineural hearing loss and pili torti. Ann Otol Rhinol Laryngol 88:100–104, 1979.
83. Cremers CW, Ter Haar BG, Van Rens TJ: The Nathalie syndrome. A new hereditary syndrome. Clin Genet 8:330–340, 1975.
84. Cremers C, Theunissen E, Kuijpers W: Proximal symphalangia and stapes ankylosis. Arch Otolaryng 111:765–767, 1985.
85. Cruse RP, Conomy JP, Wilbourn AJ, Hanson MR: Hereditary hypertrophic neuropathy combining features of tic douloureux, Charcot-Marie-Tooth disease, and deafness. Cleve Clin Q 44:107–111, 1977.
86. Cudrey C, Chevillard C, Le Paslier D, Vignal A, Passage E, Fontes M: Assignment of microsatellite sequences to the region duplicated in CMT1A (17p12): a useful tool for diagnosis. J Med Genet 32:231–233, 1995.
87. Cusimano F, Martines E, Rizzo C: The Jervell and Lange-Nielsen syndrome. Int J Pediatr Otolaryngol 22:49–58, 1991.
88. Cutler EA, Bass J, Romshe CA, Hamoudi AB, Boesel CP, Bachman D, Kontras SB, Sotos JF: A familial thyrocerebral-renal syndrome: a newly recognized disorder. Birth Defects 14:265–274, 1978.
88a. Dahl N, Laporte J, Hu L, Biancalana V, LePaslier D, Cohen D, Piussan C, Mandel J-L: Deletion mapping of X-linked mixed deafness (DFN 3) identifies a 265–525 kb region centromeric of DX526. Am J Hum Genet 56:993–998, 1995.
89. Damasio H, Antunes L, Damasio AR: Familial nonprogressive involuntary movements of childhood. Ann Neurol 1:602–603, 1977.
90. Das BD, Lakhani P, Kurtz JB, Hunter N, Watson BE, Cartaright KA, Caul EO, Roome AP: Congenital rubella after previous maternal immunity. Arch Dis Child 65:545–546, 1990.
91. Davenport SL, Donlan MA, Dolan CR, Ochs HD: Dominant hearing loss, white hair, contractures, hyperkeratotic papillomata, and depressed chemotaxis. Birth Defects 15:227–237, 1979.
92. Dawe C, Wynne-Davies R, Fulford GE: Clinical variaton in dyschondrosteosis: a report on 13 individuals in 8 families. J Bone Joint Surg 64:377–381, 1982.
93. Debruyne F, Vanderschueren-Lodeweyckx M, Bastijns P: Hearing in congenital hypothyroidism. Audiology 22:404–409, 1983.
94. De Hauwere RC, Leroy JG, Adriaenssens K, Van Heule R: Iris dysplasia, orbital hypertelorism and psychomotor retardation: a dominantly inherited developmental syndrome. J Pediatr 82:679–681, 1973.
94a. de Kok YJ, van der Maarel SM, Bitner-Glindzicz M, Huber I, Monaco AP, Malcolm S, Pembrey ME, Ropers HH, Cremers FP: Association between X-linked mixed deafness and mutations in the POU domain gene POU3F4. Science 267:685–688, 1995.
94b. del Castillo I, Villamar M, Sarduy M, Romero L, Herraiz C, Hernández FJ, Rodríguez M, Borrás I, Montero Á, Bellón J, Tapia MC, Moreno F: A novel locus for non-syndromic sensorineural deafness *(DFN6)* maps to chromosome Xp22. Hum Mol Genet 5:1383–1387, 1996.
95. Dereymaeker AM, Fryns JP, Ars J, Andresescu J, van den Berghe H: Retinitis pigmentosa, hearing loss and vitiligo: report of two patients. Clin Genet 35:387–389, 1989.
96. Desmons F, Bar J, Chevillard Y: Erythrodermie ichthyosiforme congenitale sèche, surdimutité, hépatomégalie, de transmission récessive autosomique. Bull Soc Fr Dermatol Syph 78:585–591, 1971.
97. Dignan PS, Martin LW, Zenni EJ Jr: Pierre Robin anomaly with an accessory metacarpal of the index fingers. The Catel-Manzke syndrome. Clin Genet 29:168–173, 1986.
98. Dobyns WB: Genetic hearing loss associated with nervous system disorders. In: Hereditary Hearing Loss and Its Syndromes, RJ Gorlin, HV Toriello, MM Cohen Jr, eds. Oxford University Press, New York, 1995, pp 257–317.
99. Donnai D, Barrow M: Diaphragmatic hernia, exomphalos, absent corpus callosum, hypertelorism, myopia and sensorineural deafness—a newly recognized autosomal recessive disorder? Am J Med Genet 47:679–682, 1993.
100. Dore DD, MacEwen GD, Boulos MI: Cleidocranial dysostosis and syringomyelia. Review of the literature and case report. Clin Orthop 214:229–234, 1987.
101. Duca D, Pana I, Ciovirnache M, Simionesu L, Ispas I, Maximilian C: A previously unreported, dominantly inherited syndrome of shortness of stature, ear malformations, and hip dislocation: the oxauricular syndrome—autosomal or X-linked male lethal. Am J Med Genet 8:173–180, 1981.
102. Dyck PJ, Yao JK, Knickerbocker DE, Holman RT, Gomez MR, Hayles AB, Lambert EH: Multisystem neuronal degeneration, hepatosplenomegaly, and adrenocortical deficiency associated with reduced tissue arachidonic acid. Neurology 31:925–934, 1981.
103. Edwards BD, Patton MA, Dilly SA, Eastwood JB: A new syndrome of autosomal recessive nephropathy, deafness and hyperparathyroidism. J Med Genet 26:289–293, 1989.
104. Egelund EP: Congenital hearing loss in patients with Cornelia de Lange syndrome. J Laryngol Otol 101:1276–1279, 1987.
105. Eldridge R, Berlin CI, Money JW, McKusick VA: Cochlear deafness, myopia, and intellectual impairment in an Amish family. A new syndrome of hereditary deafness. Arch Otolaryngol 88:49–54, 1968.
106. Elkington SG, Huntsman RG: The Talbot fingers: a study in symphalangism. Br Med J 1:407–411, 1967.
107. Emberger JM, Navarro M, Dejean M, Izarn P: Surdi-mutité, lymphoedème des membres inférieurs et anomalies hématologiques (leukose aigue, cytopénies) à transmission autosomique dominante. J Genet Hum 27:237–245, 1979.
108. Enzi G, Angelini C, Negrin P, Armani M, Pierobon S, Fedele D: Sensory, motor and autonomic neuropathy in patients with multiple symmetric lipomatosis. Medicine 64:388–392, 1986.
109. Epstein CJ, Sahud MA, Piel CF, Goodman JR, Bernfield MR, Kushner JH, Ablin AR: Hereditary macrothrombocytopathia, nephritis and deafness. Am J Med 52:299–310, 1972.
110. Escher F, Hirt H: Dominant hereditary conductive deafness through lack of incus-stapes junction. Acta Otolaryngol 65:25–32, 1968.
111. Evans PR: Tay-Sachs disease: a centenary. Arch Dis Child 62:1056–1059, 1987.
112. Everberg G: Unilateral anacusis. Clinical, radiological and genetic investigations. Acta Otolaryngol 158 (Suppl):366–374, 1960.
113. Everberg G, Jensen J: Labyrinthine malformations and radiological aspects. Acta Otolaryngol 82:238–241, 1976.
113a. Fagerheim T, Nilssen O, Raeymaekers P, Brox V, Moum T, Elverland HH, Teig E, Omland HH, Fostad GK, Tranebjaerg L: Identification of a new locus for autosomal dominant non-syndromic hearing impairment (DFNA7) in a large Norwegian family. Hum Mol Genet 5:1187–1191, 1996.
114. Fára M, Chlupackova V, Hrivnakova J: Dismorphia oto-faciocervicalis familiaris. Acta Chir Plast 9:255–268, 1967.
115. Ferraz FG, Nunes L, Ferraz ME, Sousa JP, Santos M, Carvatho C, Maroteaux P: Townes-Brocks syndrome: report of a case and review of the literature. Ann Genet 32:120–123, 1989.
116. Ferrer I: Dégénérescence systématisée optico-cochléo-dentelée. J Neurol 234:416–420, 1987.
116a. Filla A, De Michele G, Cavalcanti F, Pianese L, Monticelli A, Campanella G, Cocozza S: The relationship between trinucleotide (GAA) repeat length and clinical features in Friedreich ataxia. Am J Hum Genet 59:554–560, 1996.
117. Finucane B, Kurtz MD, Scott CI JR: New mental retardation syndrome with deafness, distinctive facies, and skeletal anomalies. Am J Med Genet 43:844–847, 1992.
118. Fitzsimmons JS: Familial recurrence of achondroplasia. Am J Med Genet 22:609–613, 1985.
119. Fitzsimmons JS, Watson AR, Mellor D, Guilbert PR: Familial spastic paraplegia, bilateral sensorineural deafness, and intellectual retardation associated with a progressive nephropathy. J Med Genet 25:168–172, 1988.
120. Flinter FA, Cameron JS, Chantler C, Houston I, Bobrow M: Genetics of classic Alport's syndrome. Lancet 2:1005–1007, 1988.
121. Floy KM, Hess RO, Meisner LF: DNA polymerase alpha defect in the N syndrome. Am J Med Genet 35:301–305, 1990.
122. Flynn P, Aird RB: A neuroectodermal syndrome of dominant inheritance. J Neurol Sci 2:161–182, 1965.
123. Forney WR, Robinson SJ, Pascoe DJ: Congenital heart disease, deafness, and skeletal malformations: a new syndrome? J Pediatr 68:14–26, 1966.
124. Fourman P, Fourman J: Hereditary deafness in family with earpits (fistula auris congenita). Br Med J 2:1354–1356, 1955.
125. Franceschi M, Parmigiani F, Zamproni P, Cairoli G, Canal N: Richards-Rundle syndrome, cochleovestibular dysfunction and neurofibromatosis in a family. J Neurol 231:11–13, 1984.
126. Fraser GR: The Cause of Profound Deafness in Childhood. The Johns Hopkins University Press, Baltimore, 1976, p 70.
126a. Friedman TB, Liang Y, Weber JL, Hinnant JT, Barber TD, Winata S, Arhya IN, Asher Jr JH: A gene for congenital, recessive deafness

DFNB3 maps to the pericentromeric region of chromosome 17. Nat Genet 9:86–91, 1995.

127. Frydman M, Kauschansky A, Leshem I, Savir H: Oculo-palato-cerebral syndrome: a new syndrome. Clin Genet 27:414–419, 1985.

128. Fryns JP, Dereymaeker A, Hoefnagels M, Van den Berghe H: Mental retardation, deafness, skeletal abnormalities, and coarse face with full lips: confirmation of the Fountain syndrome. Am J Med Genet 26:551–555, 1987.

129. Fryns JP, Vogels A, van den Berghe H: Craniosynostosis and low middle frequency perceptive deafness in mother and son. A distinct entity? Genet Couns 1:63–66, 1990.

130. Fujimoto A, Lipson M, Lacro RV, Shinno NW, Boelter WD, Jones KL, Wilson MG: New autosomal dominant branchio-oculo-facial syndrome. Am J Med Genet 27:943–951, 1987.

130a. Fukushima K, Ramesh A, Srisailapathy CR, Ni L, Chen A, O'Neill M, Van Camp G, Coucke P, Smith SD, Kenyon JB et al.: Consanguineous nuclear families used to identify a new locus for recessive non-syndromic hearing loss on 14q. Hum Mol Genet 4:1643–1648, 1995.

130b. Fukushima K, Ramesh A, Srisailapathy CR, Ni L, Waynes S, O'Neill ME, Van Camp G, Coucke P, Jain P, Wilcox ER et al.: An autosomal recessive nonsyndromic form of sensorineural hearing loss maps to 3p-DFNB6. Genome Res 5:305–308, 1995.

131. Gattuso J, Patton MA, Baraitser M: The clinical spectrum of the Fraser syndrome: report of three new cases and review. J Med Genet 24:549–555, 1987.

132. Gelb BD, Cooper E, Shevell M, Desnick RJ: Genetic mapping of the cleidocranial dysplasia (CCD) locus on chromosome band 6p21 to include a microdeletion. Am J Med Genet 58:200–205, 1995.

133. Geminiani F: Spinocerebellar ataxia associated with localized amyotrophy of the hands, sensorineural deafness and spastic paraparesis in two brothers. J Neurogenet 3:125–133, 1986.

134. Gershoni-Baruch R, Baruch Y, Viener A, Lichtig C: Fechtner syndrome: clinical and genetic aspects. Am J Med Genet 31:357–367, 1988.

135. Gershoni-Baruch R, Lerner A, Braun J, Katzir Y, Iancu TC, Benderly A: Johansson-Blizzard syndrome: clinical spectrum and further deliniation of the syndrome. Am J Med Genet 35:546–551, 1990.

136. Gherardi R, Belghiti-Deprez D, Hirbec G, Bouche P, Weil B, Lagrue G: Focal glomerulosclerosis associated with Charcot-Marie-Tooth disease. Nephron 40:357–361, 1985.

137. Giedion A, Brandner M, Lecannellier J, Muhar U, Prader A, Sulzer J, Zweymuller E: Oto-spondylo-megaepiphyseal dysplasia (OSMED). Helv Paediatr Acta 37:361–380, 1982.

138. Glass L, Gorlin RJ: Congenital profound sensorineural deafness and oligodontia. A new syndrome. Arch Otolaryngol 105:621–622, 1979.

139. Golabi M, Ito M, Hall BD: A new X-linked multiple congenital anomalies/mental retardation syndrome. Am J Med Genet 17:367–374, 1984.

140. Goldstein JL, Fialkow PJ: The Alström syndrome. Report of 3 cases with further delination of the clinical, pathophysiological, and genetic aspects of the disorder. Medicine 52:53–71, 1973.

141. Gollop TR, Eigier A: Prenatal ultrasound diagnosis of diastrophic dysplasia at 16 weeks. Am J Med Genet 27:321–324, 1987.

142. Goodman RM, Gorlin RJ: Atlas of the Face in Genetic Disorders, CV Mosby, St Louis, 1977, p 228.

143. Goodman RM, Lockareff S, Gwinup G: Hereditary congenital deafness with onychodystrophy. Arch Otolaryngol 90:474–477, 1969.

144. Gordon AM, Capute AJ, Konigsmark BW: Progressive quadriparesis, mental retardation, retinitis pigmentosa, and hearing loss: Report of two sibs. Johns Hopkins Med J 138:142–145, 1976.

145. Gordon MA: The genetics of otosclerosis. A review. Am J Otol 10:426–438, 1989.

146. Gorlin RJ: Genetic hearing loss with no associated abnormalities. In Hereditary Hearing Loss and Its Syndromes, RJ Gorlin, HV Toriello, MM Cohen Jr, eds. Oxford University Press, New York, 1995, pp 43–44.

147. Gorlin RJ, Cohen MM Jr, Levin LS: Syndromes of the Head and Neck, 3rd ed. Oxford University Press, New York, 1990, pp 461–463.

148. Gorlin RJ, Cohen MM Jr, Levin LS: Syndromes of the Head and Neck, 3rd ed. Oxford University Press, New York, 1990, p 663.

149. Gorlin RJ, Cohen MM Jr, Levin LS: Syndromes of the Head and Neck, 3rd ed. Oxford University Press, New York, 1990, pp 824–827.

150. Gorlin RJ, Cohen MM Jr, Levin LS: Syndromes of the Head and Neck, 3rd ed. Oxford University Press, New York, 1990, pp 886–889.

151. Gorlin RJ, Schlorf RA, Paparella MM: Cleft palate, stapes fixation, and oligodontia: A new autosomal recessively inherited syndrome. Birth Defects 7:87–88, 1971.

151a. Gorlin RJ, Toriello HV, Cohen MM Jr (eds): Hereditary Hearing Loss and Its Syndromes, Oxford University Press, New York, 1995.

152. Gorlin RJ, Wester DC, Carey JC: Genetic hearing loss associated with renal disorders. In: Hereditary Hearing Loss and Its Syndromes, RJ Gorlin, HV Toriello, MM Cohen Jr, eds. Oxford University Press, New York, 1995, pp 234–256.

153. Goyer RA, Reynolds J Jr, Burke J, Burkholder P: Hereditary renal disease with neurosensory hearing loss, proteinuria, and ichthyosis. Am J Med Sci 256:166–179, 1968.

154. Graham JM Jr, Hanson JW, Darby BL, Barr HM, Streissguth AP: Independent dysmorphology evaluations at birth and 4 years of age for children exposed to varying amounts of alcohol in utero. Pediatrics 81:772–778, 1988.

155. Greenberg CR, Trevenen CL, Evans JA: The BOR syndrome and renal agenesis-prenatal diagnosis and further clinical delineation. Prenat Diagn 8:103–108, 1988.

156. Greenberg F: Di George syndrome: an historical review of clinical and cytogenetic features. J Med Genet 30:803–806, 1993.

157. Greenberg F, Guzzetta V, Montes de Oca-Luna R, Magenis RE, Smith AC, Richter SF, Kondo I, Dobyns WB, Patel PI, Lupski JR: Molecular analysis of the Smith-Magenis syndrome: a possible contiguous-gene syndrome associated with del (17)(p11.2). Am J Hum Genet 49:1207–1218, 1991.

158. Greenfield G, Romano A, Stein R, Goodman RM: Blue sclerae and keratoconus: key features of a distinct heritable disorder of connective tissue. Clin Genet 4:8–16, 1973.

159. Greenfield G, Stein R, Romano A, Goodman RM: Blue sclerae and keratoconus: key features of a distinct heritable disorder of connective tissue. Clin Genet 4:8–16, 1973.

160. Guala A, Germinetti V, Sebastiani F, Silengo MC: A syndrome of progressive sensorineural deafness as an autosomal dominant trait. Clin Genet 49:293–295, 1992.

160a. Guilford P, Ayadi H, Blanchard S, Chaib H, Le Paslier D, Weissenbach J, Drira M, Petit C: A human gene responsible for neurosensory, non-syndromic recessive deafness is a candidate homologue of the mouse sh-1 gene. Hum Mol Genet 3:989–993, 1994.

160b. Guilford P, Ben Arab S, Blanchard S, Levilliers J, Weissenbach J, Belkahia A, Petit C: A non-syndrome form of neurosensory region of chromosome 13q. Nat Genet 6: 24–28, 1994.

160c. Guilford P, Dodé C, Crozet F, Blanchard S, Chaïb H, Levilliers J, Levi-Acobas F, Weil D, Weissenbach J, Cohen D, et al: A YAC contig and an EST map in the pericentromeric region of chromosome 13 surrounding the loci for neurosensory nonsyndromic deafness (DFNB1 and DFNA3) and limb-girdle muscular dystrophy type 2C(LGMD2C). Genomics 29:163–169, 1995.

161. Gustavson EE, Chen H: Goldenhar syndrome, anterior encephalocele, and aqueductal stenosis following fetal primidone exposure. Teratology 32:13–17, 1985.

162. Gustavson KH, Anneren G, Malmgren H, Dahl N, Ljunggren CG, Backman H: New X-linked syndrome with severe mental retardation, severely impaired vision, severe hearing defect, epileptic seizures, spasticity, restricted joint mobility, and early death. Am J Med Genet 45:654–658, 1993.

163. Gustavson KH, Holmgren G, Jagell S, Jorulf M: Lethal and nonlethal diastrophic dysplasia. A study of 14 Swedish cases. Clin Genet 28:321–334, 1985.

164. Hagemoser K, Weinstein J, Bresnick G, Nellis R, Kirkpatrick S, Pauli RM: Optic atrophy, hearing loss, and peripheral neuropathy. Am J Med Genet 33:61–65, 1989.

165. Hallerman W, Doering P: Primäre bandförmigen Hornhautdegeneration, Schwerhörigkeit und gestörter Calciumumsatz—ein hereditäre Symptomenkomplex. Berl Dtsch Ophthalmol Ges 65:285–288, 1963.

166. Hamet P, Kuchel O, Nowaczynski W, Ortega JM, Sasaki C, Genest J: Hypertension with adrenal, genital, renal defects, and deafness. Arch Int Med 131:563–569, 1973.

167. Hanauer A, Chery M, Fujita R, Driesel AJ, Gilgenkrantz S, Mandel JL: The Friedreich ataxia gene is assigned to chromosome 9q13-q21 by mapping of tightly linked markers and shows linkage disequilibrium with DgS15. Am J Hum Genet 46:133–137, 1990.

168. Hansen E, Larsen IF, Berg K: A familial syndrome of progressive cone dystrophy, degenerative liver disease, endocrine dysfunction, and hearing deficit. I. Ophthalmological studies. Acta Ophthalmol 54:129–144, 1976.
169. Harada T, Sando I, Stool SE, Myers EN: Temporal bone histopathologic features in Fanconi's anemia syndrome. Arch Otolaryngol 106:275–279, 1980.
170. Harboyan G, Mamo J, Der Kaloustian VM, Karam FA: Congenital corneal dystrophy, progressive sensorineural deafness in a family. Arch Ophthal 85:27–32, 1971.
171. Harding AE, Hall CM, Baraitser M: Autosomal dominant asymmetric radial dysplasia, dysmorphic facies, and conductive hearing loss (facioauriculoradial dysplasia). J Med Genet 19:110–115, 1982.
172. Harsh GR 4th, MacCollin M, McKenna MJ, Nadol JB, Ojemann R, Short MP: Molecular genetic screening for children at risk of neurofibromatosis 2. Arch Otolaryngol Head Neck Surg 121:590–591, 1995.
173. Hartsfield JK Jr, Bixler D, Hazen RH: Gingival fibromatosis with sensorineural hearing loss: an autosomal dominant trait. Am J Med Genet 22:623–627, 1985.
174. Hartwell EA, Robinson LK, Robinson LH, Aceves J: Congenital optic atrophy and brachytelephalangy. The Berk-Tabatznik syndrome. Am J Med Genet 29:383–389, 1988.
175. Hastbacka J, de la Chapelle A, Mahtani MM, Clines G, Reeve-Daly MP, Daly M, Hamilton BA, Kusumi K, Trivedi B, Weaver A, et al: The diastrophic dysplasia gene encodes a sulfate transporter: positional cloning by fine-structure linkage disequilibrium mapping. Cell 78:1073–1087, 1994.
176. Hayes A, Costa T, Polomeno RC: The Okihiro syndrome of Duane anomaly, radial ray abnormalities, and deafness. Am J Med Genet 22:273–280, 1985.
177. Hecht JT, Butler IJ: Neurologic morbidity associated with achondroplasia. J Child Neurol 5:84–97, 1990.
178. Heimler A, Fox JE, Hershey JE, Crespi P: Sensorineural hearing loss, enamel hypoplasia and nail abnormalities in sibs. Am J Med Genet 39:192–195, 1991.
179. Helweg-Larsen HF, Ludvigsen K: Congenital familial anhidrosis and neurolabyrinthitis. Arch Dermatol Venereol 26:489–505, 1946.
180. Hennekam RCM, Beemer FA: Skin mastocytosis, hearing loss with mental retardation. Clin Dysmorphol 1:85–88, 1992.
181. Henning KA, Li L, Iyer N, McDaniel LD, Reagan MS, Legerski R, Schultz RA, Stefanini M, Lehmann AR, Mayne LV, et al: The Cockayne syndrome group A gene encodes a WD repeat protein that interacts with CSB protein and a subunit of RNA polymerase II TFIIH. Cell 82:555–564, 1995.
182. Herrmann C Jr, Aguilar MJ, Sacks OW: Hereditary photomyoclonus associated with diabetes mellitus, deafness, nephropathy, and cerebral dysfunction. Neurology 14:212–221, 1964.
183. Herrmann J: Symphalangism and brachydactyly syndrome: report of the WL symphalangism-brachydactyly syndrome: review of literature and classification. Birth Defects 10:23–53, 1974.
183a. Hersh JH, Martinez SA, Cohen MM Jr, Weisskopf B: Craniosynostosis, sensorineural hearing loss and craniofacial abnormalities in siblings. Proc Greenwood Genet Ctr 5:186, 1986.
184. Hertz JM, Heiskari N, Zhou J, Jensen UB, Tryggvason K: A nonsense mutation in the COL4A5 collagen gene in a family with X-linked juvenile Alport syndrome. Kidney Int 47:327–332, 1995.
185. Hetzel BS: Progress in the prevention and control of iodine-deficiency disorders. Lancet II:266, 1987.
186. Heutink P, van der Mey AG, Sandkuijl LA, van Gils AP, Bardoel A, Breedveld GJ, van Vliet M, van Ommen GJ, Cornelisse CJ, Oostra BA, et al: A gene subject to genomic imprinting and responsible for hereditary paragangliomas maps to chromosome 11q23-qter. Hum Mol Genet 1:7–10, 1992.
187. Hiejima K, Suzuki F, Satake S, Ishihara K: Electrophysiologic studies of Jervell, Lange-Nielsen syndrome. Chest 79:446–448, 1981.
188. Higashi K: Heterogeneity of dominant high-frequency sensorineural deafness. Clin Genet 33:424–428, 1988.
189. Higashi K: Unique inheritance of streptomycin-induced deafness. Clin Genet 35:433–436, 1989.
190. Higashi K, Inoue S: Conductive deafness, symphalangism, and facial abnormalities: the WL syndrome in a Japanese family. Am J Med Genet 16:105–109, 1983.
191. Higashi K, Matsuki C: Coffin-Lowry syndrome with sensorineural deafness and labyrinthine anomaly. J Laryngol Otol 108:147–148, 1994.
192. Hill J, Elliott C, Colquhoun I: Audiological vestibular and radiological abnormalities in Kallmann's syndrome. J Lanryngol Otol 106:530–534, 1992.
193. Holmes LB, Schepens CL: Syndromes of facial anomalies, telecanthus, and deafness. J Pediatr 81:552–555, 1972.
194. Horoupian DS: Hereditary sensory neuropathy with deafness: A familial multisystem atrophy. Neurology 39:244–248, 1989.
195. Houston CS, Opitz JM, Spranger JW, Macpherson RI, Reed MH, Gilbert EF, Herrmann J, Schinzel A: The campomelic syndrome: a review, report of 17 cases and follow-up on the currently 17-year-old boy first reported by Maroteaux in 1971. Am J Med Genet 15:3–28, 1983.
196. Hunter AG, Jimenez CL, Carpenter BF, MacDonald I: Neuroaxonal dystrophy presenting with neonatal dysmorphic features, early onset of peripheral gangrene, and a rapidly lethal course. Am J Med Genet 28:171–180, 1987.
197. Huson SM: Recent developments in the diagnosis and management of neurofibromatosis. Arch Dis Child 64:745–749, 1989.
198. Huygen PL, Verhagen WI, Noten JF: Auditory abnormalities, including "precocious presbyacusis," in myotonic dystrophy. Audiology 33:73–84, 1994.
199. Ippel PF, Gorlin RJ, Lenz W, van Doorne JM, Bijlsma JB: Craniofacial dysostosis, hypertrichosis, genital hypoplasia, ocular, dental, and digital defects. Confirmation of the Gorlin-Chaudhry-Moss syndrome. Am J Med Genet 44:518–522, 1992.
200. Iwashita H, Inoue N, Araki S, Kuroiwa Y: Optic atrophy, neural deafness, and distal neurogenic amyotrophy. Arch Neurol 22:357–364, 1970.
201. Jackson LG, Barr MA: Conductive deafness with ptosis and skeletal malformations in sibs: a probably autosomal recessive disorder. Birth Defects 14:199–204, 1978.
201a. Jain PK, Fukushima K, Deshmukh D, Arabandi R, Thomas E, Kumar S, Lalwani AK, Ploplis B, Skarka H, Srisailapathy CRS, Wayne S, Zbar RIS, Verma IC, Smith RJH, Wilcox ER: A human recessive neurosensory nonsyndromic hearing impairment locus is a potential homologue of the murine deafness (dn) locus. Hum Mol Genet 4:2391–2394, 1995.
202. Jend-Rossmann I, Jend HH, Ringe JD, Gundlach KK: Frontometaphyseal dysplasia: symptoms and possible mode of inheritance. J Oral Maxillofac Surg 42:743–748, 1984.
203. Jensen BL: Somatic development in cleidocranial dysplasia. Am J Med Genet 35:69–74, 1990.
204. Jensen PKA: Nerve deafness, optic nerve atrophy, and dementia: A new X-linked recessive syndrome? Am J Med Genet 9:55–60, 1981.
205. Jéquier M, Deonna T: A propos de dégénérescences neurosensorielles, surdité, atrophie optique et ataxie sensitive progressives chez deux soeurs. Schweiz Arch Neurol Neurochir Psychiatr 112:219–227, 1973.
206. Jeune M, Tommasi M, Freycon F, Nivelon J: Syndrome familial associant ataxie, surdité et oligophrénie; sclérose myocardique d'évolution fatale chez l'un des enfants. Pédiatrie 28:884–885, 1991.
207. Johnsen T, Larsen C, Friis J, Hougaard-Jensen F: Pendred's syndrome. Acoustic, vestibular and radiological findings in 17 unrelated patients. J Laryngol Otol 101:1187–1192, 1987.
208. Johnson VP, McMillin JM, Aceto T Jr, Bruins G: A newly recognized neuroectodermal syndrome of familial alopecia, anosmia, deafness and hypogonadism. Am J Med Genet 15:497–506, 1983.
209. Jones KL: Smith's Recognizable Patterns of Human Malformation, 5th ed. WB Saunders, Philadelphia, 1996, pp 250–251.
210. Jones KL: Smith's Recognizable Patterns of Human Malformation, 5th ed. WB Saunders, Philadelphia, 1996, pp 270–271.
211. Jones KL: Smith's Recognizable Patterns of Human Malformation, 5th ed. WB Saunders, Philadelphia, 1996, pp 420–421.
212. Jones KL: Smith's Recognizable Patterns of Human Malformation, 5th ed. WB Saunders, Philadelphia, 1996, pp 530–531.
213. Jones KL: Smith's Recognizable Patterns of Human Malformation, 5th ed. WB Saunders, Philadelphia, 1996, pp 574–575.
214. Jones KL: Smith's Recognizable Patterns of Human Malformation, 5th ed. Saunders, Philadelphia, 1996, pp 618–619.
215. Joutel A, Bousser MG, Biousse V, Labauge P, Chabriat H, Nibbio A, Maciazek J, Meyer B, Bach MA, Weissenbach J, et al: A gene for familial hemiplegic migraine maps to chromosome 19. Nat Genet 5:40–45, 1993.
215a. Juberg RC, Marsidi I: A new form of X-linked mental retardation with growth retardation, deafness and microgenitalism. Am J Hum Genet 32:714–722, 1980.

216. Kabakkaya Y, Bakan E, Yigitoglu MR, Gokce G, Dogan M: Pendred's syndrome. Ann Oto Rhino Laryngol 102:285–288, 1993.
217. Kallio AK, Jauhiainen T: A new syndrome of ophthalmoplegia, hypoacusis, ataxia, and athetosis (OHAHA). Adv Audiol 3:84–90, 1985.
218. Kaplan P, Plauchu H, Fitch N, Jequier S: A new acro-cranio-facial dysostosis syndrome in sisters. Am J Med Genet 29:95–106, 1988.
219. Kawashima H, Ohno I, Ueno Y, Nakaya S, Kato E, Taniguchi N: Syndrome of microtia and aortic arch anomalies resembling isotretinoin embryopathy. J Pediatr 111:738–740, 1987.
220. Kawashima H, Tsuji N: Syndrome of microcephaly, deafness/malformed ears, mental retardation, and peculiar facies in a mother and son. Clin Genet 31:303–307, 1987.
221. Kelley RI, Datta NS, Dobyns WB, Hajra AK, Moser AB, Noetzel MJ, Zackai EH, Moser HW: Neonatal adrenoleukodystrophy: new cases, biochemical studies, and differentiation from Zellweger and related peroxisomal polydystrophy syndromes. Am J Med Genet 23:869–901, 1989.
222. Kelly TE, Cooke RJ, Kester RW: Acrofacial dysostosis with growth and mental retardation, one with simultaneous Hermansky-Pudlak syndrome. Birth Defects 13:45–52, 1977.
223. Keutel J, Jorgensen G, Gabriel P: Ein neues autosomal-rezessiv vererbbares Syndrome. Multiple periphere Pulmonalstenosen, Brachytelephalangie, Innenohrschwerhorigkeit, Knorpelverknocherungen bzw.-verkalkungen. Dtsch Med Wochenschr 96:1676–1681, 1971.
224. Khaldi F, Bennaceur B, Gharbi HA: Nanisme ostéochondrodysplastique familial, associé à une surdité et une hérédo-dégénérescence tapéto-rétinienne. Arch Fr Pediatr 46:429–432, 1989.
225. Kimberling WJ: Current program in finding genes involved in hearing impairment. Adv Genet Deafness 1:1–4, 1995.
226. King LA, Sanchez-Ramos L, Talledo OE, Reindollar RH: Syndrome of genital, renal, and middle ear anomalies: a third family and report of a pregnancy. Obstet Gynecol 69:491–493, 1987.
226a. Kirshhofer K, Hoover DM, Kenyon JB, Franz P, Weipolthammer K, Wachtler F, Kimberling WJ: Localisation of a gene responsible for an autosomal dominant non-syndromic sensorineural hearing loss to chromosome 15. The Molecular Biology of Hearing and Deafness, Bethesda, USA, October 6–8, 1995.
227. Knebelmann B, Forestier L, Drouot L, Quinones S, Chuet C, Benessy F, Saus J, Antignac C: Splice-mediated insertion of an Alu sequence in the COL4A3 mRNA causing autosomal recessive Alport syndrome. Hum Mol Genet 4:675–679, 1995.
227a. Koehn D, Morgan K, Fraser FC: Recurrence risks for near relatives of children with sensori-neural deafness. Genet Counsel 38:127–132, 1990.
228. Koletzko S, Koletzko B, Lamprecht A, Lenard HG: Ataxia-deafness-retardation syndrome in 3 sisters. Neuropediatrics 18:18–21, 1987.
229. Konigsmark BW: Congenital nonprogressive moderate neural hearing loss. Birth Defects 7:140, 1971.
230. Konigsmark BW, Gorlin RJ: Genetic and Metabolic Deafness. WB Saunders, Philadelphia, 1976, p 244.
231. Konigsmark BW, Gorlin RJ: Genetic and Metabolic Deafness. WB Saunders, Philadelphia, 1976, p 246.
232. Konigsmark BW, Hollander MB, Berlin CI: Familial neural hearing loss and atopic dermatitis. JAMA 204:953–957, 1968.
233. Konigsmark BW, Knox DL, Hussels IE, Moses H: Dominant congenital deafness and progressive optic nerve atrophy. Arch Ophthalmol 91:99–103, 1974.
234. Konigsmark BW, Mengel MC, Berlin CI: Familial low frequency hearing loss. Laryngoscope 81:759–771, 1971.
235. Konigsmark BW, Salman S, Haskins H, Mengel M: Dominant mid-frequency hearing loss. Ann Otol Rhinol Laryngol 79:42–53, 1970.
236. Kornreich L, Grunebaum M, Ziv N, Shuper A, Mimouni M: Osteopathia striata, cranial sclerosis with cleft palate and facial nerve palsy. Eur J Pediatr 147:101–103, 1988.
237. Kos AO, Schuknecht HF, Singer JD: Temporal bone studies in 13–15 and 18 trisomy syndromes. Arch Otolaryngol 83:439–445, 1966.
238. Kreutz JM, Hoyme HE: Levy-Hollister syndrome. Pediatrics 82:96–99, 1988.
239. Kreiborg S, Cohen MM Jr: Germinal mosaicism in Crouzon syndrome. Hum Genet 84:487–488, 1990.
240. Kumaki S, Mori H, Suzuki H: DIDMOAD syndrome (Wolfram syndrome) in four male siblings. Acta Paediatr Jpn 29:856–861, 1987.
241. Kumar D: Möbius syndrome. J Med Genet 27:122–126, 1990.
242. Kurczynski TW, Casperson SM: Auralcephalosyndactyly: a new hereditary craniosynostosis syndrome. J Med Genet 25:491–493, 1988.
243. Kwok C, Weller PA, Guioli S, Foster JW, Mansour S, Zuffardi O, Punnett HH, Dominguez-Steglich MA, Brook JD, Young ID, Goodfellow PN, Schafer AJ: Mutations in *SOX9*, the gene responsible for campomelic dysplasia and autosomal sex reversal. Am J Hum Genet 57:1028–1036, 1995.
243a. Lalwani AK, Brister JR, Fex J, Grundfast KM, Pikus AT, Ploplis B, San Agustin T, Skarka H, Wilcox ER: A new nonsyndromic X-linked sensorineural hearing impairment linked to Xp21.2. Am J Hum Genet 55:685–694, 1994.
244. Landau K, Dossetor FM, Hoyt WF, Muci-Mendosa R: Retinal hamartoma in neurofibromatosis 2. Arch Ophthalmol 108:328–329, 1990.
245. Larsson NG, Holme E, Kristiansson B, Oldfors A, Tulinius M: Progressive increase of the mutated mitochondrial DNA fraction in Kearns-Sayre syndrome. Pediatr Res 28:131–136, 1990.
246. Latham AD, Munro TA: Familial myoclonus epilepsy associated with deaf-mutism in a family showing other psychological abnormalities. Ann Eugenics 8:166–175, 1937.
247. Legius E, Proesmans W, Van Damme B, Geboes K, Lerut T, Eggermont E: Muscular hypertrophy of the oesophagus and "Alport-like" glomerular lesions in a boy. Eur J Pediatr 149:623–627, 1990.
247a. Leon PE, Raventos H, Lynch E, Morrow J, King MC: The gene for an inherited form of deafness maps to chromosome 5q31. Proc Natl Acad Sci USA 89:5181–5184, 1992.
248. LeMerrer M, Maroteaux P: Unknown syndrome. Presented at First Mtg Bone Dysplasia Soc, June, 1993, Chicago, Illinois.
248a. Lesperance MM, Hall JW, Bess FH, Fukushima K, Jain PK, Ploplis B, San Agustin TB, Skarka H, Smith RJH, Wills M, Wilcox E: A gene for autosomal dominant nonsyndromic hereditary hearing impairment maps to 4p16.3. Hum Mol Genet 4:1967–1972, 1995.
249. Lewis RA: Ocular albinism and deafness [Abstract]. Am J Hum Genet 30:57A, 1978.
250. Little BB, Snell LM, Rosenfeld CR, Gilstrap LC 3d, Gant NF: Failure to recognize fetal alcohol syndrome in newborn infants. Am J Dis Child 144:1142–1146, 1990.
251. Lockhart JL, Reeve HR, Bredael JJ, Krueger RP: Siblings with prune belly syndrome and associated pulmonic stenosis, mental retardation, and deafness. Urology 14:140–142, 1979.
252. Lowry RB, Yong SL: Cleft lip and palate, sensorineural deafness, and sacral lipoma in two brothers: a possible example of the disorganization mutant. J Med Genet 28:135–137, 1991.
253. Lüdecke H-J, Johnson C, Wagner MJ, Wells DE, Turleau C, Tommerup N, Latos-Bielenska A, Sandig KR, Meinecke P, Zabel B, et al: Molecular definition of the shortest region of deletion overlap in the Langer-Giedion syndrome. Am J Hum Genet 49:1197–1206, 1991.
254. Maack RW, Muntz HR: Ossicular abnormality in Larsen's syndrome. Am J Otolaryngol 12:51–53, 1991.
255. MacDermot KD, Roth SC, Hall C, Winter RM: Epiphyseal dysplasia of femoral head, mild vertebral abnormality, myopia and sensorineural deafness: report of a pedigree with autosomal dominant inheritance. J Med Genet 24:602–608, 1987.
256. MacDermot KD, Winter RM, Taylor D, Baraitser M: Oculofacialbulbar palsy in mother and son: review of 26 reports of familial transmission within the 'Möbius spectrum of defects'. J Med Genet 28:18–26, 1991.
257. Madell JR, Sculerati N: Noncongenital hereditary hearing loss in children. Arch Otolaryngol Head Neck Surg 117:332–338, 1991.
258. Manni JJ, Scaf JJ, Huygen PL, Crysberg JR, Verhagen WI: Hyperostosis cranialis interna. A new hereditary syndrome with cranial nerve entrapment. N Engl J Med 332:450–454, 1990.
258a. Manolis EN, Yandavi N, Nadol JB, Eavey RD, McKenna M, Rosenbaum S, Khetarpal U, Halpin C, Merchant SN, Duyk GM, MacRae C, Seidman CE, Seidman JG: A gene for non-syndromic autosomal dominant progressive postlingual sensorineural hearing loss maps to chromosome 14q12–13. Hum Mol Genet 5:1047–1050, 1996.
259. Margolis E: A new hereditary syndrome-linked deaf-mutism associated with total albinism. Acta Genet 12:12–19, 1962.
260. Marini JC: Osteogenesis imperfecta: comprehensive management. Adv Pediatr 35:391–426, 1988.
261. Marion RW, Chitayat D, Hutcheon RG, Neidich JA, Zackai EH, Singer LP, Warman M: Trisomy 18 score: a rapid, reliable diagnostic test for trisomy 18. J Pediatr 113:45–48, 1988.
262. Matalon R, Michals K, Sebesta D, Deanching M, Gashkoff P, Casanova J: Aspartoacylase deficiency and N-acetylaspartic aciduria in patients with Canavan disease. Am J Med Genet 29:463–471, 1988.

263. Mattei JF, Collignon P, Aymé S, Giraud F: X-linked mental retardation, growth retardation, deafness and microgenitalism. A second familial report. Clin Genet 23:70–74, 1983.
264. Mawn LA, O'Brien JE, Hedges TR 3d: Congenital glaucoma and skeletal dysplasia. J Pediatr Ophtalmol Strabismus 27:322–324, 1990.
265. McDermid HE, Duncan AM, Brasch KR, Holden JJ, Magenis E, Sheehy R, Burn J, Kardon N, Noel B, Schinzel A, et al: Characterization of the supernumerary chromosome in cat eye syndrome. Science 232:646–648, 1986.
266. McKusick VA: Mendelian Inheritance in Man, 11th ed. Johns Hopkins University Press, Baltimore, 1994, pp 1756–1757.
267. Mengel MC, Konigsmark BW, Berlin CI, McKusick VA: Recessive early-onset neural deafness. Acta Otolaryngol 64:313–326, 1967.
268. Mengel MC, Konigsmark BW, Berlin CI, McKusick VA: Conductive hearing loss and malformed low-set ears as a possible recessive syndrome. J Med Genet 6:14–21, 1969.
269. Meroni M, Volpi A, Usberti M, Battini G, Tarelli LT, Giordano F, Sessa A: Two brothers with idiopathic membranous nephropathy and familial sensorineural deafness. Am J Kidney Dis 15:269–272, 1990.
270. Merry DE, Lesko JG, Sosnoski DM, Lewis RA, Lubinsky M, Trask B, van den Engh G, Collins FS, Nussbaum RL: Choroideremia and deafness with stapes fixation: a contiguous gene deletion syndrome in Xq21. Am J Hum Genet 45:530–540, 1989.
271. Michels VV, Hittner HM, Beaudet AL: A clefting syndrome with anterior chamber defect and lid anomalies. J Pediatr 93:444–446, 1978.
272. Mikaelian DO, Der Kaloustian VM, Shahin NA, Barsoumian VM: Congenital ectodermal dysplasia with hearing loss. Arch Otolaryngol 92:85–89, 1970.
273. Miller G, Mowrey PN, Hopper KD, Frankel CA, Ladda RL: Neurologic manifestations in 18q- syndrome. Am J Med Genet 37:128–132, 1990.
274. Moghadam H, Statten P: Herediatry sensorineural hearing loss associated with onychodystrophy and digital malformation. Can Med Assoc J 107:310–312, 1972.
275. Mohr J, Mageroy K: Sex-linked deafness of a possibly new type. Acta Genet 10:54–62, 1960.
276. Morgan SH, Rudge P, Smith SJ, Bronstein AM, Kendall BE, Holly E, Young EP, Crawford MD, Bannister R: The neurological complications of Anderson-Fabry disease ($\alpha$-galactosidase A deficiency)—investigation of symptomatic and presymptomatic patients. Q J Med 75:491–504, 1990.
277. Morris C, Heisterkamp N, Groffen J, Williams JC, Mononen I: Chromosomal localization of the human glycoasparaginase gene to 4q32-q33. Hum Genet 88:295–297, 1992.
278. Morris MR, Namon A, Shaw GY, Panje WR, Mhoon EE: The keratitis, ichthyosis and deafness syndrome. Otolaryngol Head Neck Surg 104:526–528, 1991.
279. Muckle T, Wells MV: Urticaria, deafness and amyloidosis: a new heredo-familial syndrome. Q J Med 31:235–248, 1962.
280. Mulvihill JJ, Smith DW: Another disorder with shortness of stature and premature aging. Birth Defects 11:368–371, 1975.
281. Myhre SA, Ruvalcaba RH, Kelley VC: Congenital deafness and hypogonadism. A new X-linked recessive disorder. Clin Genet 22:299–307, 1982.
282. Nakase H, Moraes CT, Rizzuto R, Lombes A, Di Mauro S, Schon EA: Transcription and translation of deleted mitochondrial genomes in Kearns-Sayre syndrome: implication for pathogenesis. Am J Hum Genet 46:418–427, 1990.
283. Nance WE, Setleff R, McLeod AC, Sweeney A, Cooper MC, McConnell FE: X-linked mixed deafness with congenital fixation of the stapedial footplate and perilymphatic gusher. Birth Defects VII (4):64–69, 1971.
284. Nance WE, Sweeney AA: A recessively inherited chondrodystrophy. Birth Defects 6:25–27, 1970.
285. Neufeld EF, Muenzer J: The mucopolysaccharidoses. In: The Metabolic and Molecular Bases of Inherited Disease, 7th ed. CR Scriver, AL Beaudet, WS Sly, D Valle, eds. McGraw Hill, New York, 1995, pp 2465–2494.
286. Nguyen J, Philip N, Arnaud JP, Sibille G, Tisne C, James F: Syndrome de Marshall. Arch Fr Pediatr 45:49–51, 1988.
287. Niemann-Seyde SC, Eber SW, Zoll B: Saethre-Chotzen syndrome (ACS III) in four generations. Clin Genet 40:271–276, 1991.
288. Ninomiya S, Isomura M, Narahara K, Seino Y, Nakamura Y: Isolation of a testis-specific cDNA on chromosome 17q from a region adjacent to the breakpoint of T(12–17) observed in a patient with acampomelic campomelic dysplasia and sex reversal. Hum Mol Genet 5:69–72, 1996.
289. Nishi Y, Hamamoto K, Kajiyama M, Kawamura I: The Perrault syndrome: clinical report and review. Am J Med Genet 31:623–629, 1988.
290. Noll RB, Netzloff ML, Kulkarni R: Long-term follow-up of biochemical and cognitive functioning in patients with mannosidosis. Arch Neurol 46:507–509, 1989.
291. Notarangelo LD, Parolini O, Baiguini G, Buzi F, Paterlini C, Perini A, Rimoldi M, Tiberti S, Uziel G, Notarangelo L, et al: Carrier detection in X-linked adrenoleukodystrophy by determination of very long chain fatty acid levels and by linkage analysis. Eur J Pediatr 151:761–763, 1992.
292. Nucci P, Mets MB: Cataract, hearing loss, and hypercholesterolemia. Acta Ophthalmol 68:739–742, 1990.
293. Ogata T, Matsuo N, Nishimura G, Hajikano H: Oto-palato-digital syndrome, type II: evidence for defective intramembranous ossification. Am J Med Genet 36:226–231, 1990.
294. Ogilvy-Stuart AL, Parsons AC: Miller syndrome (postaxial acrofacial dysostosis): further evidence for autosomal recessive inheritance and expansion of the phenotype. J Med Genet 28:695–700, 1991.
295. Ohdo S, Madokoro H, Sonoda T, Hayakawa K: Mental retardation associated with congenital heart disease, blepharophimosis, blepharoptosis, and hypoplastic teeth. J Med Genet 23:242–244, 1986.
296. Oliveira CA, Pinheiro LC, Gomes MR: External and middle ear malformations: autosomal dominant genetic transmission. Ann Otol Rhinol Laryngol 98:772–776, 1989.
296a. O-Neill ME, Marietta J, Nishimura D, Wayne S, Van Camp G, Van Laer L, Negrini C, Wilcox ER, Chen A, Fukushima K, Ni L, Sheffield V, Smith RJH: A gene for autosomal dominant late-onset progressive non-syndromic hearing loss maps to chromosome 6–DFNA10. Hum Mol Genet 5:853–856, 1996.
297. Opjordsmoen S, Nyberg-Hansen R: Hereditary spastic paraplegia with neurogenic bladder disturbances and syndactylia. Acta Neurol Scand 61:35–41, 1980.
298. Örstavik KH, Medbo S, Mair IWS: Right-sided microtia and conductive hearing loss with variable expressivity in three generations. Clin Genet 38:117–120, 1990.
299. Ozer FL: A possible "new" syndrome with eye and renal abnormalities. Birth Defects X(4):168, 1974.
300. Paes-Alves AF, Azevêdo ES, Sousa MDGF, Almeida-Melo N, Oliveira-Filho OJ: Autosomal recessive malformation syndrome with minor manifestation in the heterozygotes: a preliminary report of a possible new syndrome. Am J Med Genet 41:141–152, 1991.
301. Park W-J, Bellus GA, Jabs EW: Mutations in fibroblast growth factor receptors: phenotypic consequences during eukaryotic development. Am J Hum Genet 57:748–754, 1995.
302. Parving A: Inherited low-frequency hearing loss: a new mixed conductive/sensorineural entity? Scand Audiol 13:47–56, 1984.
303. Patton MA: Oculodentoosseous syndrome. J Med Genet 22:386–389, 1985.
304. Patton MA, Giannelli F, Francis AJ, Baraitser M, Harding B, Williams AJ: Early onset Cockayne's syndrome: case reports with neuropathological and fibroblast studies. J Med Genet 26:154–159, 1989.
305. Patton MA, Goodship J, Hayward R, Lansdown R: Intellectual development in Apert's syndrome: a long term follow up of 29 patients. J Med Genet 25:164–167, 1988.
306. Patton MA, Krywawych S, Winter RM, Brenton DP, Baraitser M: DOOR syndrome (deafness, onycho-osteodystrophy, and mental retardation): elevated plasma and urinary 2-oxoglutarate in three unrelated patients. Am J Med Genet 26:207–215, 1987.
307. Pauli RM: Sensorineural deafness and peripheral neuropathy. Clin Genet 26:383–384, 1984.
308. Pazzaglia UE, Beluffi G: Oto-palato-digital syndrome in four generations of a large family. Clin Genet 30:338–344, 1986.
309. Pelletier LP, Tanguay RB: X-linked recessive inheritance of sensorineural hearing loss expressed during adolescence. Am J Hum Genet 27:609–613, 1975.
310. Pericak-Vance MA, Barker DF, Bergoffen JA, Chance P, Cochrane S, Dahl N, Exler MC, Fain PR, Fairweather ND, Fischbek K, et al: Consortium fine localization of X-linked Charcot-Marie-Tooth disease (CMTX1): additional support that connexin 32 is the defect in CMTX1. Hum Hered 45:121–128, 1995.
311. Pfaendler U: Une forme semilétale de la surdimutité récessive dans différentes populations de la Suisse orientale. Bull Acad Suisse Sci Med 16:255–277, 1960.

312. Pfeiffer RA: Mixed hearing loss, mental deficiency, growth retardation, short clubbed digits and EEG abnormalities in monozygous female twins. Am J Med Genet 27:639–644, 1987.
313. Pfeiffer RA, Junemann G, Polster J, Bauer H: Epiphyseal dysplasia of the femoral head, severe myopia, and perceptive hearing loss in three brothers. Clin Genet 4:141–144, 1973.
314. Pikus A: Audiologic profile in Niemann-Pick C. Ann NY Acad Sci 630:313–314, 1991.
315. Polymeropoulos MH, Poush J, Rubenstein JR, Francomano CA: Localization of the gene (SYM1) for proximal symphalangism to human chromosome 17q21-q22. Genomics 27:225–229, 1995.
316. Potasman I, Stermer E, Levy N, Dar H, Bassan H: The Groll-Hirschowitz syndrome. Clin Genet 28:76–79, 1985.
317. Poulos A, Pollard AC, Mitchell JD, Wise G, Mortimer G: Patterns of Refsum's disease. Phytanic acid oxidase deficiency. Arch Dis Child 59:222–229, 1984.
318. Preus M, Cooper AR, O'Leary E: Sensorineural hearing loss, small facial features, submucous cleft palate, and myoclonic seizures. J Clin Dysmorphol 2:30–31, 1984.
319. Prezant TR, Agapian JV, Bohlman MC, Bu X, Ozlas S, Qiu WQ, Arnos KS, Cortopassi GA, Jaber L, Rotter JI, et al: Mitochondrial ribosomal RNA mutation associated with both antibiotic-induced and nonsyndromic deafness. Nature Genet 4:289–294, 1993.
320. Prezant TR, Shohat M, Jaber L, Pressman S, Fischel-Ghodsian N: Biochemical characterization of a pedigree with mitochondrially inherited deafness. Am J Med Genet 44:465–472, 1992.
321. Prieur AM, Griscelli C: Arthropathy with rash, chronic meningitis, eye lesions, and mental retardation. J Pediatr 99:79–83, 1981.
322. Ramos-Arroyo MA, Clark GG, Saksena SS, Hodes ME: Congenital corneal anesthesia with retinal abnormalities, deafness, unusual facies, persistent patent ductus arteriosus, and mental retardation: a new syndrome? Am J Med Genet 26:345–354, 1987.
323. Rasmussen N, Johnsen NJ, Thomsen J: Inherited congenital bilateral atresia of the external auditory canal, congenital bilateral vertical talus and increased interocular distance. Acta Otolaryngol 88:296–302, 1979.
324. Reardon W, Hall CM, Dillon MJ, Baraitser M: Sibs with mental retardation, supraorbital sclerosis, and metaphyseal dysplasia: frontometaphyseal dysplasia, craniometaphyseal dysplasia, or a new syndrome? J Med Genet 28:622–626, 1991.
325. Reardon W, Harbord MG, Hall-Craggs MA, Kendall B, Brett EM, Baraitser M: Central nervous system malformations in Mohr's syndrome. J Med Genet 26: 659–663, 1989.
326. Reardon W, Roberts S, Phelps PD, Thomas NS, Beck L, Issac R, Hughes HE: Phenotypic evidence for a common pathogenesis in X-linked deafness pedigrees and Xq13–21 deletion related deafness. Am J Med Genet 44:513–517, 1992.
327. Reardon W, Wilson J, Cavanagh N, Baraitser M: A new form of familial ataxia, deafness, and mental retardation. J Med Genet 30:694–695, 1993.
328. Reed WB, Stone VM, Boder E, Ziprkowski L: Pigmentary disorders in association with congenital deafness. Arch Dermatol 95:176–186, 1967.
329. Refetoff S: Syndromes of thyroid hormone resistance. Am J Physiol 243:E88-E98, 1982.
330. Refetoff S, DeWind LT, DeGroot LJ: Familial syndrome combining deaf-mutism, stippled epiphyses, goitre and abnormally high PBI: possible target organ refractoriness to thyroid hormone. J Clin Endocrinol 27:279–294, 1967.
330a. Reid FM, Vernham GA, Jacobs HT: A novel mitochondrial point mutation in a maternal pedigree with sensorineural deafness. Hum Mutation 3:243–247, 1994.
331. Reinstein NM, Chalfin AI: Inverse retinitis pigmentosa, deafness and hypogenitalism. Am J Ophthalmol 72:332–341, 1971.
332. Renier WO, Gabreels FJ, Jasper HH, Hustinx TW, Geelen JA, van Haelst UJ: An X-linked syndrome with microcephaly, severe mental retardation, spasticity, epilepsy and deafness. J Ment Def Res 26:27–40, 1982.
333. Reynolds JF, Webb MJ, Opitz JM: A new autosomal dominant acrofacial dysostosis syndrome. Am J Med Genet (Suppl) 2:143–150, 1986.
334. Richards BW, Rundle AT: A familial hormonal disorder associated with mental deficiency, deaf mutism and ataxia. J Ment Def Res 3:33–55, 1959.
335. Riley E, Swift M: Congenital horizontal gaze palsy and kyphoscoliosis in two brothers. J Med Genet 16:314–316, 1979.
336. Rimoin DL: The Chondrodystrophies. Adv Hum Genet 5:1–118, 1975.
337. Rimoin DL, McAlister WH: Metaphyseal dysostosis, conductive hearing loss, and mental retardation: a recessively inherited syndrome. Birth Defects VII(4):116–122, 1971.
338. Robertson EF, Poulos A, Sharp P, Manson J, Wise G, Jaunzems A, Carter R: Treatment of infantile phytanic acid storage disease: clinical, biochemical and ultrastructural findings in two children treated for 2 years. Eur J Pediatr 147:133–142, 1988.
339. Robinow M, Jahrsdoerfer RA: Autosomal dominant atresia of the auditory canal and conductive deafness. Am J Med Genet 4:89–94, 1979.
340. Robinow M, Johanson AJ, Smith TH: The Lenz-Majewski hyperostotic dwarfism: a syndrome of multiple congenital anomalies, mental retardation, and progressive skeletal sclerosis. J Pediatr 91:417–421, 1977.
341. Robinson D, Lamont M, Curtis G, Shield DC, Phelps P: A family with X-linked deafness showing linkage to the proximal Xq region of the X chromosome. Hum Genet 90:316–318, 1992.
342. Robinson GC, Jan JE, Miller JR: A new variety of hereditary sensory neuropathy. Hum Genet 35:153–161, 1977.
343. Rodini ESO, Nardi A, Guion-Almeida ML, Richieri-Costa A: Ectodermal dysplasia, ectrodactyly, clefting, anophthalmia/microphthalmia, and genitourinary anomalies: nosology of Goltz-Gorlin syndrome versus EEC syndrome. Am J Med Genet 42:276–280, 1992.
344. Rollnick BR, Kaye CI, Nagatoshi K, Hauck W, Martin AO: Oculoauriculovertebral dysplasia and variants: phenotypic characteristics of 294 patients. Am J Med Genet 26:361–375, 1987.
345. Rosenberg AL, Bergstrom L, Troost BT, Bartholomew BA: Hyperuricemia and neurological deficits. A familial study. N Engl J Med 282:992–997, 1970.
346. Rosenberg RN, Chutorian A: Familial opticoacoustic nerve degeneration and polyneuropathy. Neurology 17:827–832, 1967.
347. Rowe PS, Read AP, Mountford R, Benham F, Kruse TA, Camerino G, Davies KE, O'Riordan JL: Three DNA markers for hypophosphataemic rickets. Hum Genet 89:539–542, 1992.
348. Rozycki DL, Ruben RJ, Rapin I, Spiro AJ: Autosomal recessive hearing loss associated with short stature, vitiligo, muscle wasitng, and achalasia. Arch Otolaryngol 93:194–197, 1971.
349. Ruiz C, Rivas F, Ramirez-Casillas G, Vazquez-Santana R, Mendoza-Chalita B, Feria-Velasco A, Tapia-Arizmendi G, Cantú JM: A distinct congential motor and sensory neuropathy (neuronal type) with dysmorphic features in a father and two sons. A variant of Charcot-Marie-Tooth disease. Clin Genet 31:109–113, 1987.
350. Sammito V, Motta D, Capodieci G, Sanfilippo S, Neri G: IVIC syndrome: report of a second family. Am J Med Genet 29:875–881, 1988.
351. Sasfarazi M, Wijmenga C, Upadhyaya M, Weiffenbach B, Hyser C, Mathews K, Murray J, Gilbert J, Pericak-Vance M, Lunt P, et al: Regional mapping of facioscapulohumeral muscular dystrophy gene on 4q35: combined analysis of an international consortium. Am J Hum Genet 51:396–403, 1992.
352. Say B, McCutcheon L, Todd C, Hough JVD: Kabuki make-up syndrome and hearing impairment. Clin Dysmorphol 2:68–70, 1993.
353. Schafer AJ, Dominguezsteglich MA, Guioli S, Kwok C, Weller PA, Stevanovic M, Weissenbach J, Mansour S, Young ID, Goodfellow PN, Brook JD, Foster JW: The role of SOX9 in autosomal sex reversal and campomelic dysplasia. Phil Trans R Soc Lond B Biol Sci 350:271–277, 1995.
354. Schimke RN, Horton WA, Collins DL, Therou L: A new X-linked syndrome comprising progressive basal ganglion dysfunction, mental and growth retardation, external ophthalmoplegia, postnatal microcephaly and deafness. Am J Med Genet 17:323–332, 1984.
355. Schimmenti LA, Cich JA, Gorlin RJ, Berry SA: Autosmal dominant inheritance of Wilms' tumor and branchial cleft anomalies. A new syndrome. Am J Hum Genet (Suppl) 53:A503, 1993.
356. Schinzel A, Schmid W, Auf der Maur P, Moser H, Degenhardt KH, Geisler M, Grubisic A: Incomplete trisomy 22. I. Familial 11/22 translocation with 3:1 meiotic disjunction. Delineation of common clinical picture and report of nine new cases from six families. Hum Genet 56:249–261, 1981.
357. Schmidley JW, Levinsohn MW, Manetto V: Infantile X-linked ataxia and deafness: A new clinicopathologic entity? Neurology 37:1344–1349, 1987.
358. Schuknecht H: Mondini dysplasia, a clinical and pathological study. Ann Otol Rhinol Laryngol 89:3–23, 1980.

359. Scribanu N, Kennedy C: Familial syndrome with dystonia, neural deafness, and possible intellectual impairment: clinical course and pathological findings. Adv Neurol 14:235–243, 1976.

360. Seitelberger F: Infantile neuroaxonal dystrophy. In: Handbook of Clinical Neurology, Vol 42, Neurogenetics Directory, Part I, GW Bruyn, NC Myrianthopoulos, eds. North Holland Publishing, Amsterdam, 1981, pp 229–230.

361. Sellars S, Beighton P: Autosomal dominant inheritance of conductive deafness due to stapedial anomalies, external ear malformations and congenital facial palsy. Clin Genet 23:376–379, 1983.

362. Sheffield LJ, Rice JC, Simpson DA, Delaney S: Auro-digital-anal syndrome. Pathology 13:175–176, 1980.

363. Shi SR: Temporal bone findings in a case of otopalatodigital syndrome. Arch Otolaryngol 111:119–121, 1985.

364. Shih LY, Schmerler S, Kushnick T, Marquis J: Deafness associated with humero-radio-ulnar synostosis. A new syndrome? March of Dimes Birth Defects Conference, June 24–27, Chicago, 1979, p 211.

365. Shiloh Y, Litvak G, Ziv Y, Lehner T, Sandkuyl L, Hildesheimer M, Buchris V, Cremers FPM, Szabo P, White BN, Holden JJA, Ott J: Genetic mapping of X-linked albinism-deafness syndrome (ADFN) to Xq26.3-q27.1. Am J Hum Genet 47:20–27, 1990.

366. Shinkawa H, Nadol JB Jr: Histopathology of the inner ear in Usher's syndrome as observed by light and electron microscopy. Ann Otol Rhinol Laryngol 95:313–318, 1986.

367. Shoffner JM, Lott MT, Lezza AM, Seibel P, Ballinger SW, Wallace DC: Myoclonic epilepsy and ragged-red fiber disease (MERRF) is associated with a mitochondrial DNA $tRNA^{Lys}$ mutation. Cell 61:931–937, 1990.

368. Siegler RL, Brewer ED, Carey JC: New syndrome involving visual, auditory, respiratory, gastrointestinal, and renal systems. Am J Med Genet 44:461–464, 1992.

369. Simon LT, Horoupian DA, Dorfman LJ, Marks M, Herrick MK, Wasserstein P, Smith ME: Polyneuropathy, ophthalmoplegia, leukoencephalopathy, and intestinal pseudo-obstruction: POLIP syndrome. Ann Neurol 28:349–360, 1990.

370. Sims KB, Ozelius L, Corey T, Rinehart WB, Liberfarb R, Haines J, Chen WJ, Norio R, Sankila E, de la Chapelle A, Murphy DL, Gusella J, Breakfield XO: Norrie disease gene is distinct from the monoamine oxidase genes. Am J Hum Genet 45:424–434, 1989.

371. Soong BW, Casamassima AC, Fink JK, Constantopoulos G, Horwitz AL: Multiple sulfatase deficiency. Neurology 28:1273–1275, 1988.

372. Spallone A: Stickler's syndrome: a study of 12 families. Br J Ophthalnol 71:504–509, 1987.

373. Spindler A, Berman A, Mautalen C, Ubios J, Santini AE: Chronic idiopathic hyperphosphatasia: Report of a case treated with pamidronate and a review of the literature. J Rheumatol 19:642–645, 1992.

374. Spranger JW, Langer LO, Wiedemann HR: Bone Dysplasias. WB Saunders, Philadelphia, 1974, p 284.

375. Spranger JW, Langer LO, Wiedemann HR: Bone Dysplasias. WB Saunders, Philadelphia, 1974, pp 313–315.

376. Spranger JW, Langer LO, Wiedemann HR: Bone Dysplasias. WB Saunders, Philadelphia, 1974, p 340.

377. Spranger JW, Maroteaux P: Genetic heterogeneity of spondyloepiphyseal dysplasia congenita? Am J Med Genet 14:601–602, 1983.

378. Spranger J, Menger H, Mundlos S, Winterpacht A, Zabel B: Kniest dysplasia is caused by dominant collagen II (COL2A1) mutations: parental somatic mosaicism manifesting as Stickler phenotype and mild spondyloepiphyseal dysplasia. Pediatr Radiol 24:431–435, 1994.

379. Spritz RA, Droetto S, Fukushima Y: Deletion of the KIT and PDGFRA genes in a patient with piebaldism. Am J Med Genet 44:492–495, 1992.

380. Spritz RA, Giebel LB, Holmes SA: Dominant negative and loss of function mutations of the c-kit (mast stem cell growth factor receptor) proto-oncogenes in human piebaldism. Am J Hum Genet 50:261–269, 1992.

381. Steinberg D: Refsum Disease. In: The Metabolic and Molecular Bases of Inherited Disease, 7th ed. CR Scriver, AL Beaudet, WS Sly, D Valle, eds. McGraw-Hill, New York, 1995, pp 2351–2370.

382. Stevenson AC, Cheeseman EA: Hereditary deaf mutism, with particular reference to Nothern Ireland. Ann Hum Genet 20:177–231, 1956.

383. Stewart J, Bergstrom L: Familial hand abnormality and sensori-neural deafness: new syndrome. J Pediatr 78:102–110, 1971.

384. Stoll C, Levy JM, Francfort JJ, Roos R, Rohmer A: L'association phocomélie-ectrodactylie. Arch Fr Pediatr 31:669–680, 1974.

385. Streissguth AP, Clarren SK, Jones KL: Natural history of the fetal alcohol syndrome: a 10 year follow-up of eleven patients. Lancet 2:85–91, 1985.

386. Striano S, Barbieri F, Meo R, Bilo L, Cirillo S: Hearing loss associated with progressive ataxia (Lichtenstein-Knorr disease?). Report of a sporadic case with peculiar neuroradiological findings. Acta Neurol 11:351–359, 1989.

387. Strisciuglio P, Ballabio A, Parenti G: Microtia with meatal atresia and conductive deafness: mild and severe manifestations within the same sibship. J Med Genet 23:459–460, 1986.

388. Strömgren E: Heredopathia ophthalmo-oto-encephalica. In: Handbook of Clinical Neurology, Vol 42, Neurogenetics Directory, PJ Vinken et al, eds. North Holland Publishing, Amsterdam, 1981, pp 150–152.

389. Strosberg J, Adler RG: Otosclerosis associated with osteopoikilosis. JAMA 246:2030–2031, 1982.

390. Sulik KK, Johnston MC, Smiley SJ, Speight HS, Jarvis BE: Mandibulofacial dysostosis (Treacher Collins syndrome): a new proposal for its pathogenesis. Am J Med Genet 27:359–372, 1987.

391. Summers BA, Swash M, Schwartz MS, Ingram DA: Juvenile-onset bulbospinal muscular atrophy with deafness: Vialetto-Van Laere syndrome or Madras-type motor neuron disease. J Neurol 234:440–442, 1987.

392. Sylvester PE: Some unusual findings in a family with Friedreich's ataxia. Arch Dis Child 33:217–221, 1958.

393. Takeda K, Balzano S, Sakurai A, DeGroot LJ, Refetoff S: Screening of nineteen unrelated families with generalized resistance to thyroid hormone for known point mutations in the thyroid hormone receptor $\beta$-gene and the detection of a new mutation. J Clin Invest 87:486–502, 1991.

393a. Tamagawa Y, Kitamura K, Ishida T, Tanaka H, Tsuji S, Nishizawa M: A gene for a dominant form of non-syndromic sensorineural deafness (dfna11) maps within the region containing the DFNB2 recessive deafness gene. Hum Mol Genet 5:849–852, 1996.

394. Tassabehji M, Newton VE, Liu X-Z Brady A, Donnai D, Krajewski-Walasek M, Murday V, Normal A, Obersztyn E, Reardon W, Rice JC, Trembath R, Wieacker P, Whiteford M, Winter R, Read AP: The mutational spectrum in Waardenburg syndrome. Hum Mol Genet 4:2131–2137, 1995.

395. Teebi AS, Al-Awadi SA, Opitz JM, Spranger J: Severe short-limb dwarfism resembling Grebe chondrodysplasia. Hum Genet 74:386–390, 1986.

396. Temple IK: Stickler's syndrome. J Med Genet 26:119–126, 1989.

397. Temtamy S, McKusick V: The Genetics of Hand Malformations. Alan R Liss, 1978, pp 98–101.

398. Temtamy SA, Meligy RE, Osman NM, Meguid MS, Salem S: A "new" bone dysplasia with autosomal recessive inheritance. Birth Defects 10:165–170, 1974.

399. Teunissën E, Cremers CWRJ: An autosomal dominant inherited syndrome with congenital stapes fixation. Laryngoscope 100:380–384, 1990.

400. Therman E, Susman B: The similarity of phenotypic effects caused by Xp and Xq deletions in the female: a hypothesis. Hum Genet 85:175–183, 1990.

401. Thomas GH, Beaudet AL: Disorders of glycoprotein degradation and structure: $\alpha$-mannosidosis, $\beta$-mannosidosis, fucosidosis, sialidosis, aspartylglucosaminuria, and carbohydrate-deficient glycoprotein syndrome. In: The Metabolic and Molecular Bases of Inherited Disease, 7th ed, CR Scriver, AL Beaudet, WS Sly, D Valle, eds. McGraw-Hill, New York, 1995, pp 2509–2528.

402. Thompson E, Baraitser M: FG syndrome. J Med Genet 24:139–143, 1987.

403. Thompson EM, Baraitser M: Sorsby syndrome. A report on further genetics of the original family. J Med Genet 25:313–321, 1988.

404. Toriello HV, Higgins JV, Abrahamson J, Waterman DF, Moore WD: X-linked syndrome of branchial arch and other defects. Am J Med Genet 21:137–142, 1985.

405. Townes PL, Brocks ER: Hereditary syndrome of imperforate anus with hand, foot, and ear anomalies. J Pediatr 81:321–326, 1972.

405a. Tranebjaerg L, Schwartz C, Eriksen H, Andreasson S, Ponjavic V, Dahl A, Stevenson RE, May M, Arena F, Barker D, Elverland HH, Lubs H: A new X-linked recessive deafness syndrome with blindness, dystonia, fractures, and mental deficiency is linked to Xq22. J Med Genet 32:257–263, 1995.

406. Treacher Collins Syndrome Collaborative Groups: Positional cloning of a gene involved in the pathogenesis of Treacher Collins syndrome. Nat Genet 12:130–136, 1996.
407. Treft RL, Sanborn GE, Carey J, Swartz M, Crisp D, Wester DC, Creel D: Dominant optic atrophy, deafness, ptosis, ophthalmoplegia, dystaxia, and myopathy. A new syndrome. Ophthalmology 91:908–915, 1984.
408. Tsakalakos N, Jordaan FH, Taljaard JJ, Hough SF: A previously undescribed ectodermal dysplasia of the tricho-odonto-onychial subgroup in a family. Arch Dermatol 122:1047–1053, 1986.
409. Tsukahara M, Azuno Y, Kajii T: Type A1 brachydactyly, dwarfism, ptosis, mixed hearing loss, microcephaly, and mental retardation. Am J Med Genet 33:7–9, 1989.
410. Tungland OP, Savage MO, Bellman SC: A new syndrome: hearing loss and familial salivary gland insensitivity to aldosterone in two brothers. J Laryngol Otol 104:956–958, 1990.
411. Uitti RJ, Donat JR, Rozdilsky B, Schneider RJ, Koeppen AH: Familial oculoleptomeningeal amyloidosis: report of a new family with unusual features. Arch Neurol 45:1118–1122, 1988.
412. Uyama E, Takahashi K, Owada M, Okamura R, Naito M, Tsuji S, Kawasaki S, Araki S: Hydrocephalus, corneal opacities, deafness, valvular heart disease, deformed toes, and leptomeningeal fibrous thickening in adult sibship: a new syndrome associated with glucose cerebrosidase deficiency and a mosaic population of storage cells. Acta Neurol Scand 86:407–420, 1992.
413. Vaamonde J, Muruzabal J, Tunon T, Perez N, Artieda J, Rodriguez M, Obeso JA: Abnormal muscle and skin mitochondria in family with myoclonus, ataxia, and deafness (May-White syndrome). J Neurosurg Psychiatry 55:128–132, 1992.
414. Van Allen MW, Frohlich JA, Davis JR: Inherited predisposition to generalized amyloidosis: clinical and pathological study of a family with neuropathy, nephropathy, and peptic ulcer. Neurology 19:10–25, 1968.
415. Van Buchem FSP, Hadders HN, Hansen JF, Woldring MG: Hyperostosis corticalis generalisata: report of seven cases. Am J Med 33:387–397, 1962.
416. Van den Houten BR, Ten Kate LP, Gerding JC: The Hajdu-Cheney syndrome: a review of the literature and report of 3 cases. Int J Oral Surg 14:113–125, 1985.
417. Van den Ouweland JM, Lemkes HH, Ruitenbeek W, Sandkuijl LA, de Vijlder MF, Struyvenberg PA, van de Kamp JJ, Maassen JA: Mutation in mitochondrial $tRNA^{Leu(UUR)}$ gene in a large pedigree with maternally transmitted type II diabetes mellitus and deafness. Nat Genet 1:368–371, 1992.
418. Van Gemund JJ, Laurent de Angulo MS, van Gelderen HH: Familial prenatal dwarfism and elevated serum-immunoreactive growth hormone levels and end-organ unresponsiveness. Maandschr Kindergeneeskunde 37:372–382, 1969.
419. Van Hellenberg Hubar JL, Gabreels FJ, Ruitenbeek W, Sengers RC, Renier WO, Thijssen HO, ter Laak HJ: MELAS sydrome: report of two patients and comparison with data of 24 patients derived form the literature. Neuropediatrics 22:10–14, 1991.
419a. Van Camp G, Coucke P, Balemans W, Van Velzen D, Van der Bilt C, Smith RJH, Fukushima K, Padberg G, Frants RR, Van de Heyning P, Smith SD, Huizing EH, Willems PJ: Localization of a locus for non-syndromic hearing loss (DFNA5) to chromosome 7p. Hum Mol Genet 4:2159–2163, 1995.
420. Vazquez-Acevedo M, Coria R, Gonzalez-Astiazaran A, Medina-Crespo V, Ridaura-Sanz C, Gonzalez-Halphen D: Characterization of a 5025 base pair mitochondrial DNA deletion in Kearns-Sayre syndrome. Biochim Biophys Acta 1271:363–368, 1995.
421. Veske A, Oehlmann R, Younus F, Mohyuddin A, Müller-Myhsok B, Mehdi SQ, Gal A: Autosomal recessive non-syndromic deafness locus (DFNB 8) maps on chromosome 21q22 in a large consanguineous kindred from Pakistan. Hum Mol Genet 5:165–168, 1996.
422. Walker WG, Ozer FL, Whelton A: Syndrome of perceptive deafness and renal tubular acidosis. Birth Defects 10:163, 1974.
423. Wallis CE: Ectrodactyly (split hand/split foot) and ectodermal dysplasia with normal lip and palate in a four-generation kindred. Clin Genet 34:252–257, 1988.
424. Walpole IR, Nicoll A, Goldblatt J: Autosomal dominant osteopetrosis type II with "malignant" presentation. Further support for heterogeneity? Clin Genet 38:257–263, 1990.
425. Warburg M, Tommerup N, Vestermark S, Parving A, Weismann K, Russell B, Thomsen HK: The Yemenite deaf-blind hypopigmentation syndrome. Ophthalmic Paediatr Genet 11:201–207, 1990.
426. Ward JR, Saad de Owens C, Sierra IA: Upper limb defect associated with developmental delay, unilaterally poorly developed antihelix, hearing deficit, and bilateral choroid coloboma: A new syndrome. J Med Genet 29:589–591, 1992.
427. Watts RW, Spellacy E, Adams JH: Neuropathological and clinical correlations in Hurler disease. J Inherit Metab Dis 9:261–272, 1986.
427a. Wayne S, Der Kaloustian VM, Schloss M, Polomeno R, Scott DA, Sheffield VC, Smith RJH: Localization of the Usher Syndrome type ID gene (USH ID) to chromosome 10. Hum Mol Genet 5:1689–1692, 1996.
428. Weaver DD, Williams CPS: A syndrome of microcephaly, mental retardation, unusual facies, cleft palate and weight deficiency. Birth Defects 13:69–84, 1977.
429. Weinberg AG, Wright CG: Stapedial hypoplasia in partial Di George syndrome. Am J Dis Child 132:815–816, 1978.
430. Wellesley D, Goldblatt J: A new form of X-linked high frequency sensorineural deafness. Clin Genet 41:79–81, 1992.
431. Wells CR, Jankovic J: Familial spastic paraparesis and deafness: a new X-linked neurodegenerative disorder. Arch Neurol 43:943–946, 1986.
432. Wenstrup RJ, Willing MC, Starman BJ, Byers PH: Distinct biochemical phenotypes predict clinical severity in nonlethal variants of osteogenesis imperfecta. Am J Hum Genet 46:975–982, 1990.
433. Wiles CR, Taylor TF, Sillence DO: Congenital synspondylism. Am J Med Genet 42:288–295, 1992.
434. Wilkin DJ, Bogaert R, Lachman RS, Rimoin DL, Eyre DR, Cohn DH: A single amino acid substitution (G103D) in the type II collagen triple helix produces Kniest hysplasia. Hum Mol Genet 3:1999–2003, 1994.
435. Williams ML, Monger DJ, Rutherford SL, Hincenbergs M, Rehfeld SJ, Grunfeld C: Neutral lipid storage disease with ichthyosis: lipid content and metabolism of fibroblasts. J Inherit Metab Dis 11:131–143, 1988.
436. Winkelmann W, Solbach HG, Wiegelmann W, Bethge H, Pfeiffer RA: Hypothalamo-hypophysärer Minderwichs mit Innenohrschwerhörigkeit bei zwei Schwestern. Internist 13:52–56, 1972.
437. Winship I, Gericke G, Beighton P: X-linked inheritance of ocular albinism with late-onset sensorineural deafness. Am J Med Genet 19:797–803, 1984.
438. Winter RM: What's in a face? Nat Genet 12:124–129, 1996.
439. Witkop CJ Jr: Inherited disorders of pigmentation. Clin Dermatol 3:70–134, 1985.
440. Wolf B, Grier RE, Secor McVoy Jr, Heard GS: Biotinidase deficiency: novel recycling defect. J Inherit Metab Dis 8 (Suppl 1):53–58, 1985.
441. Woodhouse NJY, Sakati NA: A syndrome of hypogonadism, alopecia, diabetes mellitus, mental retardation, deafness, and ECG abnormalities. J Med Genet 20:216–219, 1983.
442. Woolf CM, Dolowitz DA, Aldous HE: Congenital deafness associated with piebaldness. Arch Otolaryngol 82:244–250, 1965.
443. Yen J, Bourke RS, Popp AJ, Worth CR: Camurati-Engelmann disease (progressive hereditary craniodiaphyseal dysplasia). J Neurosurg 48:138–142, 1978.
444. Young GF, Leon-Barth CA, Green J: Familial hemiplegic migraine, retinal degeneration, deafness, and nystagmus. Arch Neurol 23:201–209, 1970.
445. Young ID, Young EP, Mossman J, Fielder AR, Moore JR: Neuraminidase deficiency: case report and review of the phenotype. J Med Genet 24:283–290, 1987.
446. Young K, Barth CK, Moore C, Weaver DD: Otopalatodigital syndrome type II associated with omphalocele: report of three cases. Am J Med Genet 45:481–487, 1993.
447. Yumita, S, Furukawa Y, Sohn HE, Unakami H, Miura R, Yoshinaga K: Familial idiopathic hypoparathyroidism and progressive sensorineural hearing loss. Tohoku J Exp Med 148:135–141, 1986.
448. Zachmann M, Fuchs E, Prader A: Progressive high frequency hearing loss: an additional feature of the syndrome of congenital adrenal hypoplasia in gonadotrophin deficiency. Eur J Pediatr 151:167–169, 1992.
449. Ziprkowski L, Adam A: Recessive total albinism and congenital deaf-mutism. Arch Dermatol 89:151–155, 1964.
450. Ziprkowski L, Krakowski A, Adam A, Costeff H, Sade J: Partial albinism and deaf-mutism due to a recessive sex-linked gene. Arch Dermatol 86:530–539, 1962.
451. Zunich J, Esterly NB, Kaye CI: Autosomal recessive transmission of neuroectodermal syndrome. Arch Dermatol 124:1188–1189, 1988.

# III

# THE NOSE

# 10

# Embryology of the Nose and Sinuses

SAUL FRENKIEL

Nasal and sinus formation is an intricate process that begins in early embryogenesis and may not reach final development until adulthood. The formation of structures progresses through three distinct phases.[2,5,7] The preskeletal stage is marked by the emergence of mesenchymal swellings that surround the external nasal or olfactory placodes. With the appearance of the primary nasal cavity at approximately 4 weeks, development then enters the chondrocranial stage, providing the nose with its cartilaginous framework. By the end of the first trimester, the stage of ossification begins within the various bony structures of the cranial skeleton. In this dynamic process of differentiation, an influx of cellular elements occurs, along with fusion of these tissues in relation to themselves and to the entire fetus. The developing tissues possess the potential to form structures that will eventually resemble those of the biological parents, a fact that becomes most evident when one looks at the facial appearance of parents and children. Anomalies of agenesis, clefting, and cyst formation may develop when this dynamic process becomes deficient.

## Early embryology

### The presomite embryo

To appreciate the formation of definitive anatomy, a familiarity of early embryogenesis is necessary. During the second and third weeks of development, the embryoblast proceeds towards the formation of germ layers.[4] At approximately 8 days, one sees evidence of a bilaminar germ disc containing entodermal and ectodermal layers. The entoderm is composed of a layer of flattened polyhedral cells that contain large nuclei facing the primitive yolk sac. The ectodermal germ layer is composed of taller, columnar type cells that partly surround the enlarging amniotic cavity. During the third week, ectodermal cells in the caudal region proliferate and migrate medially and then caudally to form the notochordal or head process. Simultaneously, modified ectodermal cells invaginate the midline region of the caudal primitive streak and migrate between the original ecto- and entodermal layers. This mesodermal germ layer is the last embryonic tissue to develop and it leads to the formation of the trilaminar germ disc. During the third week, the ectoderm and entoderm in the cephalic region, known as the *prochordal plate,* become adherent and thinned to form the buccopharyngeal membrane. This membrane represents the forward boundary of the primitive foregut (Fig. 10–1).

### The somite embryo

The somite period occurs between the 20th and 30th developmental days and is heralded by a series of mesodermal tissue condensations on either side of the midline. In the head area, the thickened masses of tissue on either side of the notochord are termed the *paraxial mesoderm.* In terms of fetal nasal development, this emergent concentration of tissue has been classified as the preskeletal stage. It is marked by a coalescence of mesenchymal tissue in the midfacial area surrounding the ectodermal nasal placodes. This stage ends at approximately the fourth week with the disappearance of the buccopharyngeal membrane and the formation of the primitive nasal cavity.

### Dynamic morphology

Morphological growth of the germ layer involves an inherent and active movement of masses of tissue. Listed below are the important synchronous events of embryonic development in its cephalic portion.[4,8]

1. At the end of the third week, a portion of ectoderm overlying the notochord invaginates to form a neural groove and then a neural tube. The cephalic end of this tube continues to expand into the primary brain vesicles. By the fifth week, the developing brain has shown significant growth.
2. Forward development of the entodermal diverticulum into a blind pouch defines the primitive foregut. Its anterior boundary is the buccopharyngeal membrane. This membrane disintegrates by the end of week three, establishing an open communication with the amniotic cavity.
3. The paraxial mesoderm pushes laterally and cranially and continues to proliferate, forming the lateral somites. These condensations of mesoderm surround the foregut tube to become the derivatives of the pharyngeal or branchial arches. By the fourteenth somite stage, the first arch has begun to differentiate into noticeable maxillary and mandibular swellings. Cranial to the notochord, the mesoderm fuses in the midline. There is no somite development in this region, with the possible exception of the extrinsic eye muscles.
4. Synchronous with the above changes, head-folding develops for a variety of reasons. Cephalocaudal folding is caused by rapid longitudinal growth of the neural tube. Transverse or lateral folding is precipitated by rapidly growing somites. These events bring all the head structures, which were originally anterior to the prochordal plate, into a position central to the developing foregut, where they fuse with the developing septum transversum or cardiogenic region.

## The external nose

In the four-and-a-half-week-old embryo, the face forms a series of rounded swellings of proliferating mesenchyme.[4,7] A central ectodermal depression known as the *stomodeum* becomes surrounded caudally by the mandibular swellings, laterally by the maxillary swellings, and cranially by the frontal prominence. The nasal placode, a thickening of surface ectoderm, develops to either side of the frontal prominence. Even more laterally

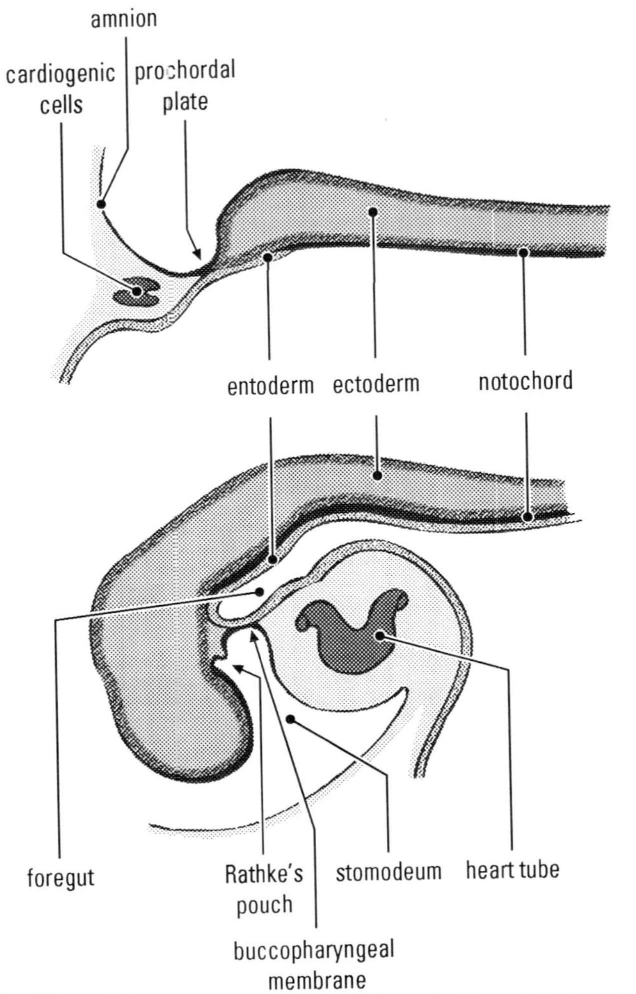


**Fig. 10–1.** Schematic representation of the cephalic end of the early embryo. These midline sagittal sections indicate developmental aspects of the stomotodeum, foregut, and rotation of the head process in relation to the heart tube.

lies the developing eye. During the fifth week, rapidly growing ridges of mesoderm known as the *medial* and *lateral swellings* surround the nasal placode which continues to invaginate as the nasal or olfactory pit. Further invagination leads to the formation of the nasal sac and eventually, the nasal cavity itself (Fig. 10–2). Facial development continues with the growth of maxillary swellings in a medial direction which merge along the way with lateral nasal swellings and finally meet in the midline with medial nasal swellings. Thus the upper lip is formed with midline fusion of this mesodermal flow of tissue. The depression separating the maxillary from the lateral nasal swellings is known as the *nasolacrimal groove*. Fusion of this overlying mesoderm will eventually form the nasolacrimal apparatus.

The middle portion of the external nose develops from the downward progression of medial nasal folds that fuse in the midline to form the frontonasal process. As part of the chondrocranial stage of development, there appear three paired chondrification centers which eventually form the lateral cartilages of the nose and the midline septum. Formation of intramembranous bone over the cartilaginous nasal capsule occurs by the eighth week, and by the beginning of the second trimester, the stage of ossification is in progress. Structural nasal support is enhanced as more of the cartilaginous capsule is replaced by intramembranous bone.

## The internal nose

### The enlarging nasal cavity

The development of the nasal cavity involves a simultaneous process of free space enlargement, degeneration of existing tissue, and an active ingrowth of mesenchymal structures. The anterior nares is formed by the nasal pits sinking into the paraxial mesoderm. The primitive nasal cavity is first characterized by a single chamber roofed by stomodeal ectoderm anterior to the line of attachment of the former buccopharyngeal membrane. Posterior to this line lies the developing entodermal foregut. At the beginning, the ectoderm of the nasal sac comes in contact with the ectoderm of the roof of the mouth to form a thickened oronasal septum. Attenuation of this structure leads

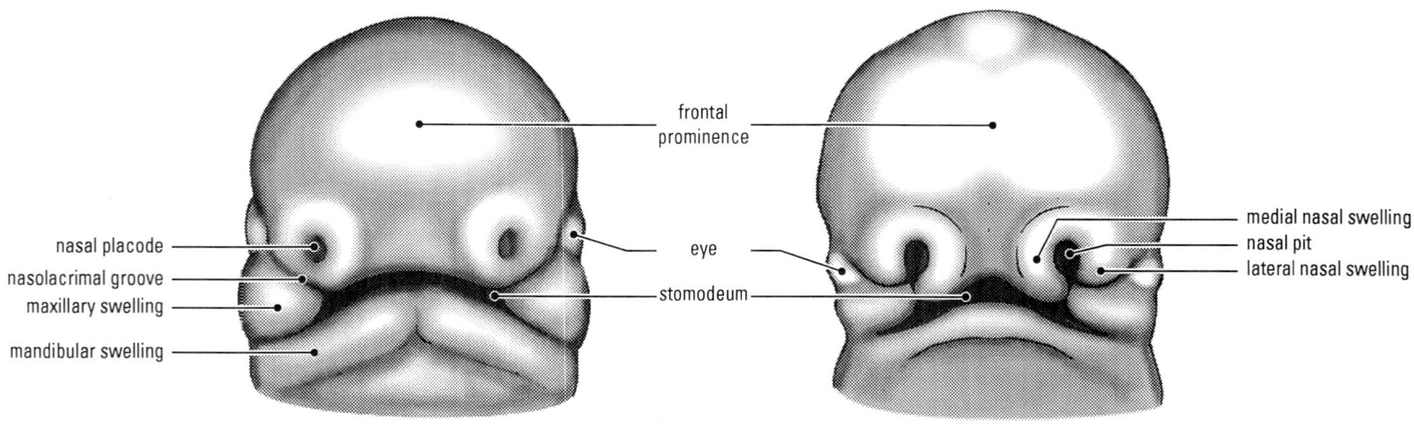


**Fig. 10–2.** Representation of facial development in the 5- to 7-week-old embryo. Note the deepening nasal chamber and external mesenchyme swellings which will form the definitive nose.

to formation of the oronasal membrane, which separates the enlarging nasal cavity from the anteriorly expanding pharynx (Fig. 10–3a). Subsequent breakdown of the membrane results in formation of the primitive choana, the communication between the nasal chamber and the oral cavity (Fig. 10–3b). With further development of the secondary palate and further deepening of the primitive nasal chambers, the definitive posterior choana become located at the junction of the nasal cavity and the most cranial portion of the developing entodermal-lined foregut, the nasopharynx (Fig. 10–3c).

### The nasal septum

In the 5-week-old embryo, delineation of the nasal septum is first seen as a condensation of paraxial mesoderm in the midline of the roof of the enlarging nasal cavity. The primitive nasal septum is formed anteriorly from the enlarging frontonasal process. It continues to grow posteriorly, meeting up with another median ridge of mesoderm known as the *tectoseptal expansion,* which emanates from the region of Rathke's pouch. The septum becomes a well-defined midline structure growing downwards and backwards until it joins up with the palatine processes that simultaneously progress to meet in the midline (Fig. 10–4). The eventual fusion of all these masses of tissue results in separation of the oral cavity inferiorly from the nasal chambers above and separation of the nasal chambers into right and left. Effectively, the developing embryo now has respiratory and digestive entrances as distinct structures. Fusion of membranes should be completed by the ninth or tenth week of development.

The nasal septum itself goes through a cartilaginous and bony stage of development. Primordial cartilage is formed through condensation and compression of interstitial tissues. Regions of ossification develop posteroinferiorly in the vomerine area and posterosuperiorly as part of the developing perpendicular plate of the ethmoid. The anterior septal portions remain cartilaginous throughout embryonic life, although some further ossification may occur into adulthood. Frequently there may persist remnants of paraseptal cartilages on either side of the nasal septum within the floor of the nose. These cartilaginous remnants are evident during the ninth week of development and run along the maxillary and vomerine bony ridges in relation to the vomeronasal organ of Jacobson.[2,3]

### The lateral nasal wall

The inferior concha is first noted in the 38–40-days old embryo as a bulge in the lateral nasal wall immediately above the developing palatine process.[1,7] With increasing height of the nasal cavity, more superiorly located ectodermal folds appear in the ethmoid region. These lateral nasal folds become further defined into the more distinct inferior, middle, and superior conchae by the ninth developmental week. In the early stages of development, the conchae do not contain cartilage or bone but merely represent folds of mesenchyme covered by ectodermal tissue. As the nasal cavity enlarges, the conchae become more prominent medially and there occurs a deepening of the grooves below each prominence, resulting in the formation of a meatus associated with each concha. A further prominence develops anterior to the ethmoidal fold, representing formation of the agger nasi or nasoturbinal. From this area emanates a

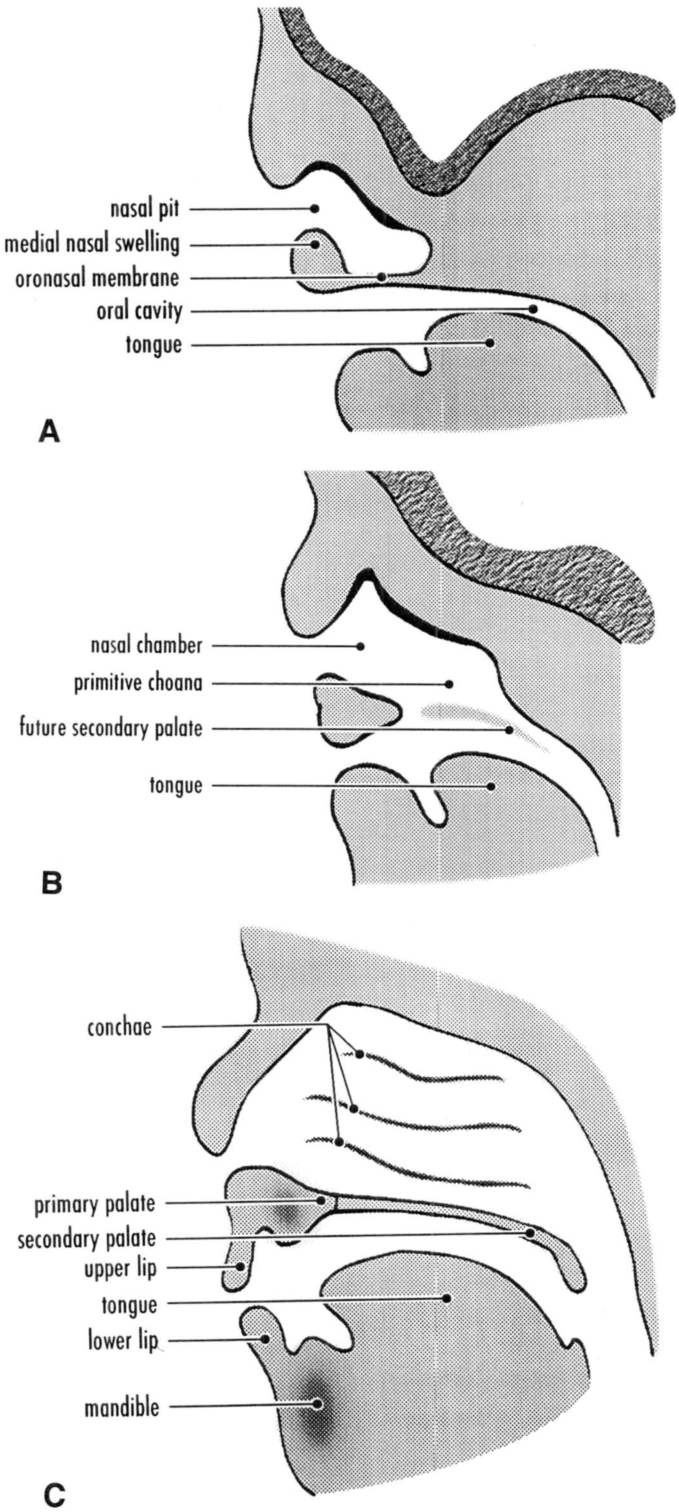


**Fig. 10–3.** Sagittal representations of the enlarging nasal cavity of the 6- to 9-week-old embryo. A: The oronasal membrane separating the nasal pit from the oral cavity. B: Breakdown of the oronasal membrane with establishment of posterior choanae. C: Maxillary and palatal development with subsequent enlargement of the nasal cavity.

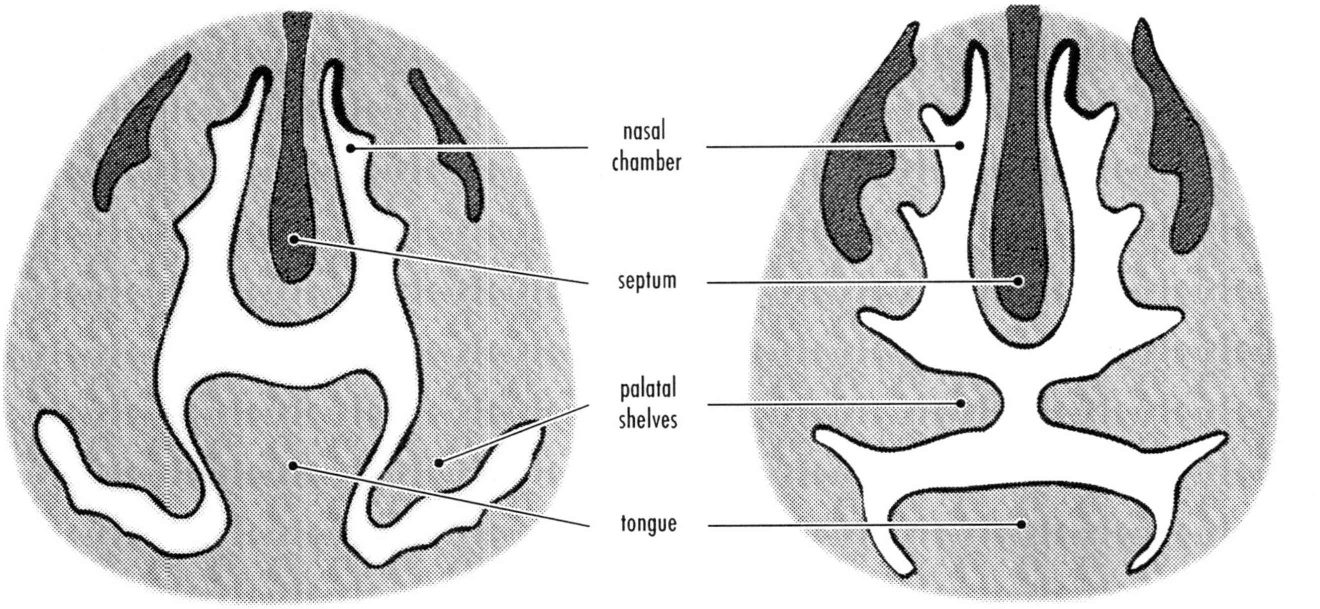


**Fig. 10–4.** Coronal representations of the nasal chambers in a 6- to 8-week-old embryo. The downward growth of the septum, inferior displacement of the tongue, and medial progression of the palatal shelves will eventually delineate the nasal cavities into right and left sides apart from the oral cavity below.

further process known as the *uncinate,* which insinuates itself into the middle meatus, along the superior portion of the inferior concha. A secondary ethmoidal fold develops in this meatus, representing the early bulla ethmoidalis. The opening between the uncinate process and the bulla ethmoidalis is known as the *hiatus semilunaris,* the entrance to the infundibulum ethmoidalae. Variations in the development of these structures can make the lateral nasal wall, and particularly the middle meatus, an interesting anatomical exercise in the adult.

The inferior concha develops as a separate bony entity termed the *inferior turbinate*. The middle and superior conchae become part of the eventual ethmoid complex. Less frequently, up to three supreme conchae may develop along with their corresponding meati. The major sinuses will take origin from these meati, which invaginate themselves into the contours of the lateral nasal wall.

## The paranasal sinuses

### The ethmoid sinus

The ethmoid sinus represents a system of air cells invaginating into the lateral masses of the ethmoid bone. Their outlines can be noticed in the latter part of the third developmental month as cylindrical extensions of mucosa, which then assume a cellular appearance by the sixth fetal month. The cellular systems having ostia within the middle meatus belong to the anterior group, while those which open into the superior meatus belong to the posterior system. As the stage of ossification progresses into the third trimester, the ethmoid air cell system becomes more defined. Development continues into the postnatal period with invasion throughout the ethmoid bone and into the orbital plate of the frontal bone. The final form of the ethmoid labyrinth may not be reached until early adulthood.[2,7]

### The frontal sinus

The frontal sinus develops with the anterosuperior expansion of the anterior ethmoidal labyrinth into the frontal bone itself. This occurs during the fourth fetal month as either a deepening of the frontal recess or directly from the ethmoid infundibulum itself. A subtle process of pneumatization of the frontal bone is frequently evident at the time of birth. The actual sinus, however, may not be demonstrable until after the first year of life. The sinus continues its vertical expansion through the frontal bone and may only reach its maximum size after puberty. Usually, one frontal sinus develops from each side, but in some cases, supernumerary sinuses may be found.[2,7]

### The maxillary sinus

In comparison to the others, the maxillary sinus displays the most consistent type of development. During the third fetal month, there is evidence of an out-pouching of mucosa in the lateral part of the ethmoid infundibulum. During the fourth month, the sinus extends laterally into the cartilaginous plate and begins to invade the maxilla shortly before birth. Further expansion occurs with resorption of cartilage, giving the sinus a slit-like appearance towards the end of fetal life. The sinus itself continues to enlarge during postnatal development as the maxilla enlarges and more particularly, as the primary and then secondary dentition erupt. Superiorly, the sinus develops in relation to the infraorbital nerve and orbital floor, while inferiorly, the downward progression of the sinus revolves around the erupting dentition, often reaching its final size towards the later teenage years.[2,7]

### The sphenoid sinus

Sphenoid sinus development differs from that of other sinuses because its origin is not from a meatus but rather from a mucosal invagination in the sphenoethmoidal recess, which can be seen in the 9–week embryo. This primitive invagination persists as the sphenoid sinus ostium. Further expansion of the sinus occurs in a downward and backward direction with formation of a pouch-like cavity within the endochondral posterior nasal capsule. Ossification of this structure occurs during the fifth fetal month and it is then that early pneumatization of the sphenoid bone occurs. Further enlargement of the air-containing space directly reflects the formation of the sphenoid bone, with its various centers of ossification and its incorporation of the bony lesser wings, greater wings, and basisphenoid. The pneumatization process is frequently localized to the midline but may expand laterally into the sphenoid wings or inferiorly into the pterygoid processes. The sphenoid sinus is evident at birth and usually reaches its mature size during the teenage years.[2,7]

## Special developmental considerations

### Epithelium

The surface lining of the nose and sinuses is of ectodermal origin and is incorporated as part of the invagination of the original nasal pit. The entranceway to the nasal cavity, an area known as the *vestibule,* is lined by keratinizing squamous epithelium containing hair appendages and sebaceous glands. Beyond the vestibule, the mucosal surface develops into a ciliated, pseudostratified columnar variety typical for the covering of the entire respiratory tract. This respiratory mucosa extends into the paranasal sinuses and to the nasopharynx until the openings of the eustachian tubes. Beyond this delineated area of the former buccopharyngeal membrane, the pharyngeal skin lining is of entodermal origin as part of foregut development.

The more specialized neurectodermal tissue is found in the roof of the nose, extending downward over the superior concha laterally and onto the top of the septum medially. Vestiges of this olfactory epithelium may also exist in the nasovomerine organ and possibly in other areas, such as the agger nasi. This epithelium consists of modified bipolar nerve cells, supporting or sustentacular nonciliated cells, and serous secreting glands to keep the area moist.[7]

### Innervation

The nerve supply of the nose and midfacial area develops in relation to the fifth cranial nerve. The ophthalmic (V-I) division supplies the region related to frontonasal development, while the maxillary (V-2) division innervates the area associated with the maxillary processes. Parasympathetic supply to the vascular and glandular elements of the mucosa comes from the preganglionic fibers carried within the facial nerve and synapsing in the sphenopalatine ganglion. The sympathetic supply enters the nose in the region of the sphenopalatine ganglion and is then distributed to the mucosa via the peripheral nervous and arterial branching. Blood supply also reflects the projection of first branchial arch development as part of the peripheral distribution of both the internal and external carotid system.

### The olfactory system

The olfactory tracts emerge from the brain as paired lateral projections of the cerebral hemispheres. This development is evident in the 8-week-old embryo. The terminal part of the tract forms a bulb that comes in contact with the roof of the enlarging nasal sac. It gives off a number of nerve bundles that penetrate the eventual cribriform plate and join the central processes of the bipolar olfactory cells.[7]

### The lacrimal system

Invagination of the nasolacrimal groove between the lateral nasal and maxillary processes during the fifth developmental week represents the beginnings of the lacrimal drainage system. First, this ectodermal tissue becomes buried as a solid cord of cells extending along the lateral border of the developing nose. In the third month, the cord of epithelial cells begins a downward canalization process and produces the lumen of the aqueduct. Canalization is usually completed at the time of birth, but its lowermost end may not be completely patent in some newborns. Areas of incomplete canalization may represent the valves seen along the course of the system.

The upper end of the system has bifurcated canaliculi that establish connections with the conjunctival sac near the inner canthus of the eye. They come together laterally to form a common canaliculus before entering the lacrimal sac. The inferior continuation of the sac is the nasolacrimal duct which courses along the lateral wall of the nose and eventually opens into the inferior meatus. The lacrimal gland also develops as an ectodermal structure from the superficial portions of the conjunctival sac in the upper, outer quadrant of the eye. The gland lies superficial to the orbital septum, receiving its secretomotor innervation from the sphenopalatine ganglion.[6,7]

### References

1. Bingham B, Wang RG, Hawke M, Kwok P: The embryonic development of the lateral nasal wall from 8 to 24 weeks. Laryngoscope 101: 992–997, 1991.
2. Davis WB: Nasal Accessory Sinuses in Man. WB Saunders, Philadelphia, 1914.
3. Delaire J, Precious D: Interaction of the development of the nasal septum, the nasal pyramid and the face. Int J Pediatr Otorhinolaryngol 12:311–326, 1987.
4. Langman J: Medical Embryology. Williams & Wilkins, Baltimore, 1963, pp 303–311.
5. Lanza DC, Kennedy DW, Koltai PJ: Applied nasal anatomy & embryology. Ear Nose Throat J 70:416–422, 1991.
6. Piest KL, Katowitz JA: Treatment of congenital nasolacrimal duct obstruction. Ophthalmol Clin North Am 4:201–209, 1991.
7. Schaeffer JP: The Nose, Paranasal Sinuses, Nasolacrimal Passageways and Olfactory Organ in Man. Blakiston, Philadelphia, 1920.
8. Wright D: Scott-Brown's Otolaryngology, Vol 1, 5th ed. Butterworths, London, 1987, pp 138–144.

# 11

# Congenital Anomalies of the Nose and Anterior Skull Base

ANTHONY G. ZEITOUNI and ROBERT S. SHAPIRO

## Nasal dermoids

Cruvier in 1817[32] was the first to describe a patient with a small hair growing out of a midline nasal pit (Fig. 11–1). The many authors who have reported on these lesions since then have used a variety of terms, such as *dermal cyst,*[32] *dermoid, dermoid cyst* and *dermoid sinus cyst*. In an effort to develop a more consistent terminology, Sessions[32] suggested that lesions without a sinus tract be referred to as *nasal dermal cysts,* and that those with a sinus tract be referred to as *nasal dermal sinus-cyst* (NDSC). These nasal cysts of dermal origin account for 3.7 to 12.6% of dermoid lesions in the head and neck, and 1.1% of all dermoids (Figs. 11–2, 11–3).

Unlike teratomas, which are derived from all three embryonic layers, these lesions are derived from ectoderm and mesoderm. They are lined with a keratinizing squamous epithelium surrounded by a fibrous capsule (Fig. 11–4). They contain adnexal structures such as hair follicles, sebaceous glands, and eccrine glands.[34] It is the presence of adnexal structures that differentiates these lesions from epidermoid cysts.

Nasal dermoids are relatively rare. In a retrospective review, Bradley found 67 dermoid and epidermoid lesions among 304,000 pediatric admissions during a 20-year period.[4] Dermal lesions, however, are the most common midline nasal anomalies.[5,19] Different reviews have alternatively reported a male preponderance,[4,23,32] or a female preponderance.[27] Familial predisposition has not been demonstrated, but several reports of families with multiple individuals affected have been published.[29] Wardinsky reported on identical triplets, each with an NDSC.[37]

### Pathogenesis

The pathogenesis of these lesions remains controversial and has generated multiple hypotheses. Sessions[32] has reviewed the different theories and divided them into two groups: those in which dermoids occur secondary to a cranial developmental error, and those which are due to a cutaneous developmental error. The theories concerning cranial development have in common the hypothesis that early in fetal development, at around 4 weeks when the anterior neuropore is closing, ectoderm is trapped outside the closing neuropore, and, with development of the fetus, forms a cyst and/or tract. In Littlewood's theory,[20] dura forms part of the middle layer of the fetal trilaminar septum. Normally the epithelial elements disappear, but in NDSC some ectodermal tissue persists. Alternatively, Grunwald in 1910[32] suggested that the dural connection existed in the "prenasal space." This space exists during embryonic life. Anterior to it lie the frontal bones and nasal bones. Inferiorly lies the cartilaginous nasal capsule. Posteriorly the space opens through the foramen cecum into the cranial cavity. In normal development, the dural connection is obliterated and the foramen cecum closes. If this fails to occur, a dermal sinus results.

In 1922, Bland Sutton,[32] proposed that dermoids result from a cutaneous developmental error. As the nasal bones develop, the cartilage of the nasal capsule is separated from the skin. In that theory, dermoids result when epithelial elements remain connected to the cartilage.

### Clinical presentation

Most cases present at birth or shortly after. Wardinsky et al. reported that 73% of cases were diagnosed within the first month.[37] Patients present with either a nasal mass, or a small midline pit if the dermal cyst is associated with a sinus tract. The mass may cause nasal obstruction. The pit may be anywhere from the base of the columella to the glabella. Bradley[4] reported that pits are most frequent in the middle third of the dorsum, while Pensler[27] described them as evenly distributed along the midline. Occasionally there are multiple pits. From the pit a "cheesy" material can often be expressed. The presence of hair growing from the pit is pathognomonic of an NDSC. Older children may present with a history of intermittent purulent discharge from the sinus opening. Most infections are limited to the sinus and cyst, but periorbital cellulitis[36] and osteomyelitis have been reported. Because the tract may extend intracranially, meningitis and brain abscess formation can occur.[27,36]

Upon physical examination, the color and consistency of the mass should be noted. Unlike encephaloceles, these masses are solid, do not enlarge with crying, and do not transilluminate.

NDSC are not associated with any syndrome. However, several reports note the presence of other anomalies of the head and neck.[23,32,34,36] The frequency of these associated anomalies has been reported to be as high as 40% by Wardinsky et al.,[37] yet in their review of the literature in 200 cases (6.5%), they found only 13 cases with associated anomalies. These anomalies tend to be variable and form no consistent pattern.

### Diagnosis

The temptation to biopsy these masses must be resisted. Instead, preoperative investigation is conducted radiographically. The most important issue to be addressed radiologically is the presence of an intracranial extension. Writing prior to the advent of computer tomography (CT), Weisman and Johnson[38] noted the following findings on plain films and tomograms of dermoids: fusiform swelling within the nasal septum, widening of the nasal vault, bifid septum, glabellar destruction, bone proliferation above the cyst, and large ethmoidal cystic spaces. In addition, enlargement of the foramen cecum and deformity of

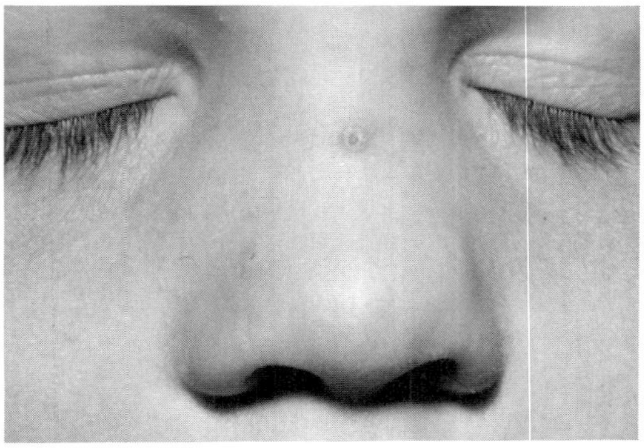

**Fig. 11–1.** Infant with midline nasal dermoid pit. (Courtesy of Dr. Steven Handler. Rudolph's Pediatrics, Appleton and Lange, 1991, with permission.)

the crista galli have been proposed as indicators of intracranial extension. However, in a study on seven patients with NDSC, foramen cecum size, bifidity of the crista galli, and interorbital distance were identical in NDSC and controls.[2] Only one patient in that study, however, had an intracranial component. On CT, the intracranial component may be hypodense or hyperdense compared to normal brain substance (Fig. 11–5).[27] Magnetic resonance imaging (MRI) will easily differentiate between dermal cyst and brain substance (Fig. 11–6).[21]

### Treatment

These lesions often become infected, and these infections must be treated prior to surgical removal. Although they are often diagnosed during infancy, surgery is usually delayed until the age of two or three, to decrease the effects on growth of the facial skeleton. However, delaying surgery must be weighed against the increased possibility of meningitis and destruction of the facial skeleton. Children with intracranial involvement should have surgery at a younger age, because of the greater risk of meningitis and intracranial abscess formation. In every case, the key to successful surgery is removal of all dermal tissue.

The type of surgery required will depend on whether the lesion is a simple nasal dermal cyst or whether there is a sinus component. If there is no sinus, a small incision over the nasal dorsum will be sufficient to excise the cyst.

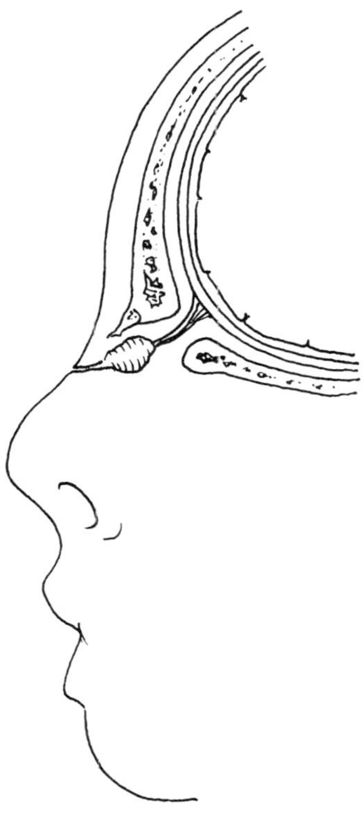

**Fig. 11–2.** Dermoid fistula with cyst.

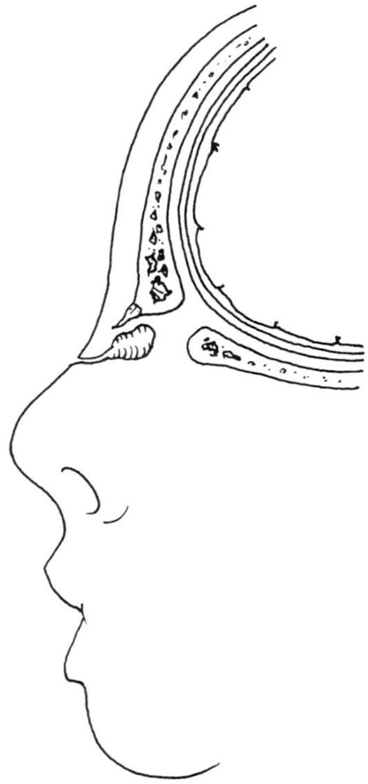

**Fig. 11–3.** Dermoid cyst with sinus; compare with MRI of dermoid in Figure 11–6.

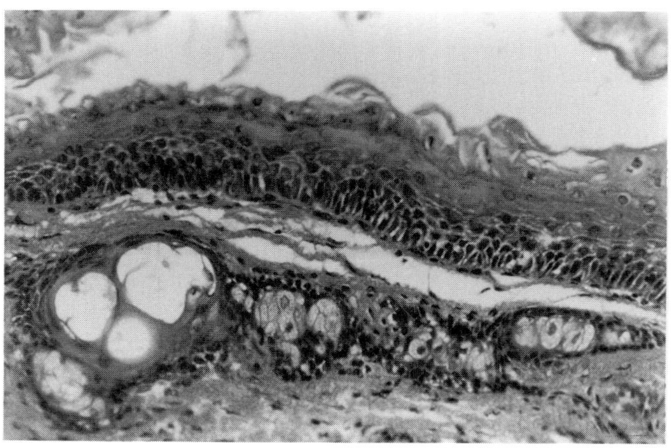

**Fig. 11–4.** Dermoid cyst. Squamous epithelium-lined cyst with skin appendages. H & E stain, magnification × 20. (Courtesy of Dr. Chantal Bernard.)

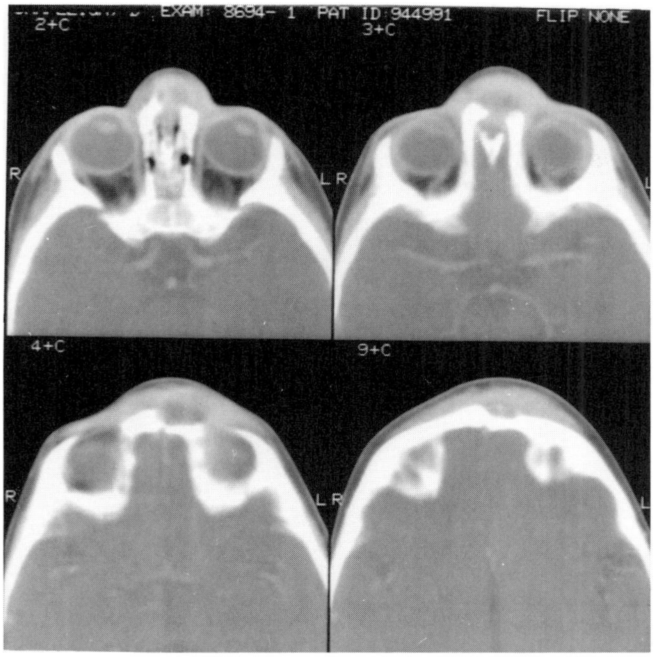


**Fig. 11–5.** CT demonstrating dermoid. Note duplication of crista galli.

For NDSC in the absence of an intracranial cyst, the entire tract from the skin to the skull base should be excised. The dissection has to be meticulous and the use of an operating microscope is necessary.[17] Methylene blue dye is used to better define the tract; however some authors avoid the use of dyes, due to concern over extravasation.[32] An ellipse is taken around the sinus opening. Since the tract[4] passes deep to the nasal bones, medial osteotomies may be required. Alternatively, lateral osteotomies can be performed and the bony nasal vault raised as a unit with the overlying skin.[16] The tract is followed superiorly until the base of the skull, where a frozen section of the most rostral part of the sinus is sent. If no dermal elements are found, then the tract is ligated.[32] It is not clear at this time whether skip lesions of dermal tissue may exist along the tract; some would suggest routine craniotomy for any dermoid with a tract extending to the skull base.

Should the preoperative investigation show an intracranial cyst, then a combined craniofacial procedure with neurosurgical consultation would be required. The role of perioperative antibiotics remains undefined because of concern that these antibiotics may select out resistant strains, leading to an intracranial infection that is more difficult to treat. A frontal craniotomy, and either an extradural or intradural approach to the intracranial cyst, is required. The objective is to deliver the intracranial component and seal the dural defect.

Recurrence is expected if any dermal tissue is left in place. One study reports a recurrence rate of 50%.[5] Rhinoplasty may be required to correct the cosmetic deformity after surgery. Wardinsky et al. reported the need for rhinoplasty in 4 of their 22 patients.[37]

## Nasopharyngeal teratoma and epignathus

Teratomas are highly unusual lesions because they contain tissues that originate from all three germ layers. They were first described by Grass, who in 1691, reported on a completely developed fetus originating from a woman's neck. With such spectacular presentation it is easy to see how these lesions acquired the name of *teratoma,* which means "monstrous" in Greek.

Most teratomas occur outside the head and neck. Teratomas of the nasopharynx are very rare. The terminology is occasionally confusing because some authors have used the term teratoma to refer to related lesions in the nasopharynx. Ewing in

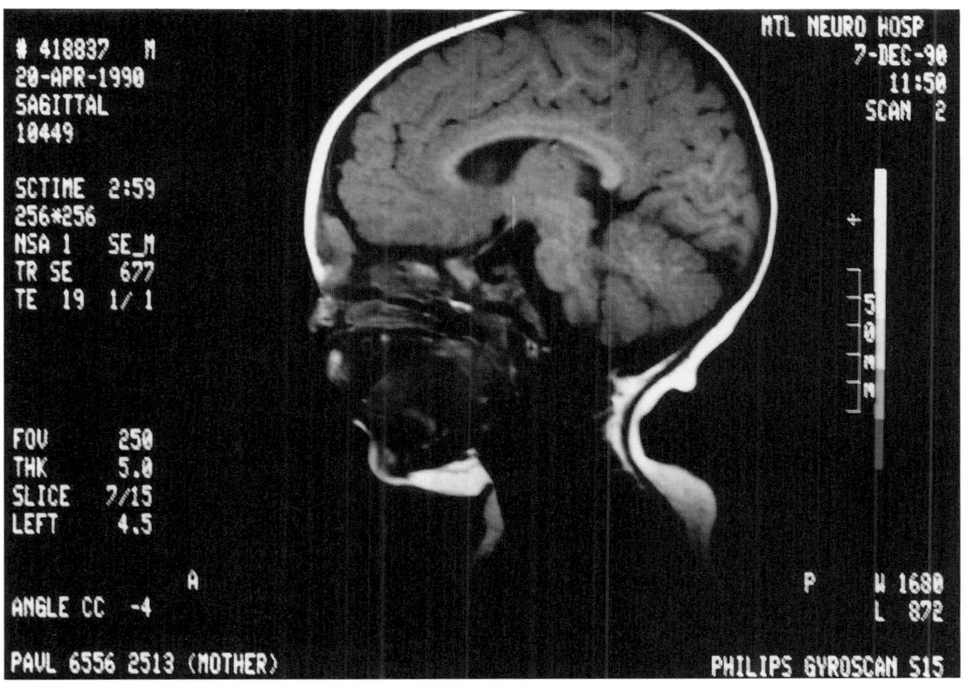


**Fig. 11–6.** MRI demonstrating dermoid. The dermoid is intracranial but separate from the brain.

1940 classified congenital nasopharyngeal masses into dermoids, teratoids, teratomas and epignathi.[26] Histologically, dermoids, or "hairy polyps," demonstrate tissue originating from ectoderm and mesoderm, but there is no evidence of endodermal tissue. Occasionally, teratomas display gross differentiation into organ systems, such as limbs, or even a homunculus. Such tumors are termed *epignathi*.

Several hypotheses to explain the origin of teratomas have been advanced, but to date, none are universally accepted.[1,30] One theory states that the teratoma is a different embryo that grows inside the body of its twin. According to this hypothesis, teratomas would be a more extreme example of conjoined twins. A different theory suggests that teratomas arise from parthenogenetic development of germ cells. While this hypothesis may explain the presence of teratomas in the ovaries and testes, it is difficult to understand how such cells would lead to head and neck teratomas. Finally, a third theory suggests that totipotential cells may escape the developing embryo's organizers and later develop into teratomas.

Infants born with nasopharyngeal teratomas usually present with severe respiratory obstruction requiring either intubation or emergency tracheostomy (Figs. 11–7, 11–8). In some cases, however, the only indication of pathology may be feeding difficulty.[26] Once the airway has been controlled, investigation to define the extent of the mass and to rule out intracranial extension is needed. CT has the advantage of accurately determining the presence of a bony defect in the sphenoid, whereas MRI may better define the relationship of the mass to the dura and the brain.

Definitive treatment consists of surgical excision. A transoral approach gives good access to the oral and oropharyngeal components of these lesions. These infants may have clefting of the palate, which facilitates a transpalatal approach to the nasopharynx. It is infrequent that nasopharyngeal teratomas have an intracranial extension,[26] but should this be detected in the preoperative investigation, a combined craniofacial procedure would be required.

There have been no reported cases of malignant transformation of nasopharyngeal teratomas; thus, with complete excision, the prognosis is good.

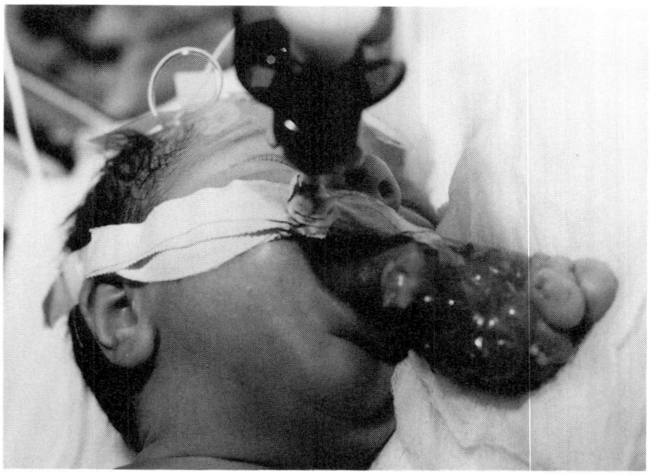

**Fig. 11–7.** Child born with large epignathus. Endotracheal intubation was essential because of complete obstruction by epignathus.

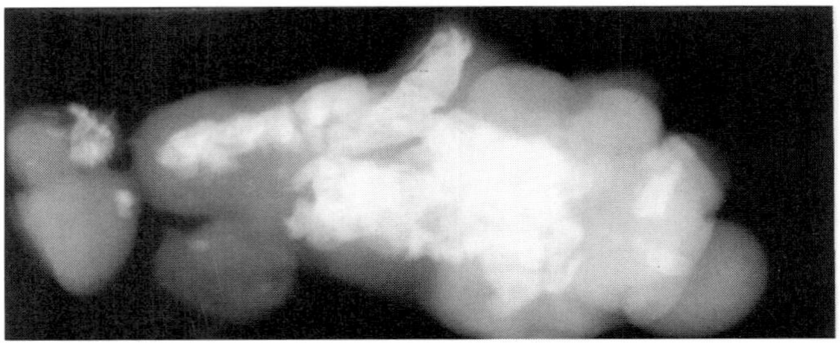

**Fig. 11–8.** Plain film demonstrating area of bone formation and teeth formation within epignathus.

## Gliomas

*Nasal gliomas* are congenital developmental anomalies where glial tissue is situated outside the central nervous system (NS), with no cerebrospinal fluid connection. They have no neoplastic potential; thus the term *glioma,* coined by Schmidt in 1900, is a misnomer. However, despite its inappropriate connotation, this term has persisted and remains in common usage. These lesions are rare. In a recent review of the literature, Younis et al. found 230 cases reported.[39] Amongst the congenital nasal anomalies, they occur less often than dermoids but more often than encephaloceles.[19,23] While Kennard and Rasmussen reported a male-to-female ratio of 3:2, Younus and Coode reported a threefold female preponderance.[19,39]

### Pathogenesis

There are three theories to account for gliomas. In the first, blastomatous cells destined to develop into glial cells become situated outside the CNS.[23] The second theory ascribes the formation of gliomas to a problem during closure of the anterior neuropore. Normally, with closure of the anterior neuropore, the neuroectoderm becomes separated from the skin, permitting the inflow of mesoderm. Failure of this mesoderm to enter the region leads to a failure of bone formation.[23] A third theory, based on studies of labelled neural crest cells, states that the fundamental problem lies in the failure of the mesoderm itself to flow into the region of the nose and anterior skull base.[16]

### Pathology

Gliomas consist of glial tissue in a connective tissue stroma. The glial tissue is composed predominantly of astrocytes, but microglia and giant cells are also commonly seen. Neurons have been reported in 10 to 60%.[19] Mitoses are rare. On electron microscopy, filaments and gap junctions characteristic of astrocytes are noted. Compared to encephaloceles, the connective tissue stroma is more abundant, and there is no evidence of a connection to the cerebrospinal fluid that characterizes encephaloceles. Most gliomas have no connection to the dura, but in 15% of cases a fibroglial stalk can be traced.

Gliomas may be characterized as intranasal or extranasal. The intranasal tumors account for 30% of all gliomas. The extranasal variety account for 60%. The remainder are combined intranasal and extranasal. While both intranasal and extranasal gliomas can have a fibrous connection to the CNS, the intracranial gliomas do so more frequently.[16]

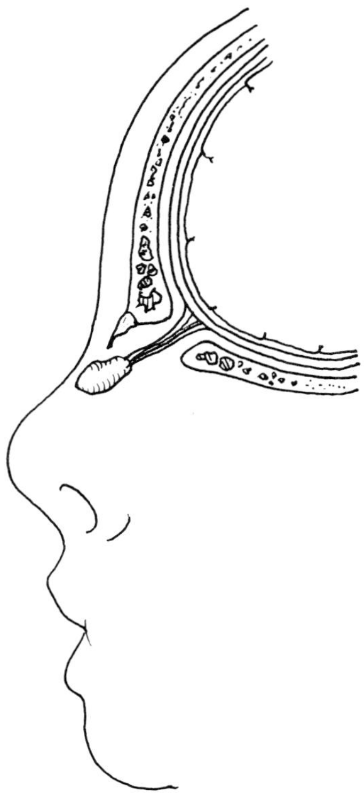

Fig. 11–9. Glioma with stalk extending intracranially. Only 15% of gliomas have connections with the dura.

## Clinical presentation

Presentation depends on site. Extracranial gliomas present as a mass on the lateral aspect of the nose. They are characteristically, but not always,[39] covered with discolored or telangiectatic skin. Rarely, they are associated with hypertelorism. The mass is smooth, firm, and noncompressible. Simultaneous bilateral digital occlusion of the patient's jugular veins does not lead to distension of the mass (Furstenberg's test). Gliomas do not transilluminate, nor do they expand with crying. These features permit differentiating these lesions from encephaloceles. Unlike dermoids, these lesions do not present in the midline (Fig. 11–9).

Intranasal gliomas usually present with unilateral nasal obstruction. They may also present with epistaxis or cerebrospinal fluid rhinorrhea. On physical examination, a nasal mass is found that may mimic the appearance of a nasal polyp. Usually they are attached to the middle turbinate but may be attached to the cribriform plate or the nasal septum. With large gliomas, the nasal bones may be splayed.[16] Hypertelorism is more common than in the extracranial type.

Although the nose is the most common site, gliomas have been reported in a wide variety of head and neck sites, such as the nasopharynx, cheek, tongue, oropharynx, and scalp.[16,19]

## Diagnosis

Although the differential diagnosis is wide (Table 11–1) biopsy of an intranasal mass in an infant or young child is to be avoided because of the possibility of producing a cerebrospinal fluid (CSF) leak or meningitis. The most valuable radiological tools are CT and MRI. On CT, a glioma may be associated with a bony defect and appear as a homogeneous soft tissue mass. The addition of a contrast agent helps to differentiate gliomas from encephaloceles. Contrast agent in the CSF will descend into an encephalocele but not into a glioma.[2] Although MRI cannot detect the possible bony defect, its superior soft tissue resolution and ability to scan the patient in any plane aid in ruling out an encephalocele by excluding brain herniation. It can also distinguish inflammatory reaction in the nose from the glioma, permitting more accurate assessment of its size.

**Table 11–1.** Differential diagnosis of pediatric nasal masses

| Congenital | Inflammatory | Neoplastic |
|---|---|---|
| Dermoid | Nasal Polyp | BENIGN |
| Glioma | Septal Abscess | Fibroma |
| Encephalocele | | Chondroma |
| Teratoma | | Neurofibroma |
| Lacrimal Cyst | | Chordoma |
| | | MALIGNANT |
| | | Neuroblastoma |
| | | Rhabdomyosarcoma |

## Treatment

Treatment of these benign lesions is surgical. Despite the preoperative investigation, the final confirmation of the nature of the lesions will occur at the time of surgery. In all these lesions neurosurgical consultation is required. The surgical approach depends on the site of the glioma. While an extranasal glioma can be removed through a standard lateral rhinotomy, the management of intranasal gliomas is more controversial, and they must be approached more cautiously. This is because the incidence of a fibroglial connection to the dura in intranasal gliomas is higher than in extranasal gliomas—35% vs. 9%, respectively.[16] This increases the chance of a dural defect and postoperative CSF leak. Two options are available. One option is to perform a routine anterior fossa exploration and lateral rhinotomy on all patients. Alternatively, some authors recommend proceeding with an extracranial approach initially, if the suspicion of an encephalocele or the possibility of a large dural connection is judged to be low after reviewing the history and radiological investigation.[16] If during surgery it becomes evident that a large dural defect exists, and that it cannot be closed from an extracranial approach, a craniotomy is performed. Hengerer and Oas[16] reviewed the literature and noted that, of 23 cases utilizing an extracranial approach, 4 developed a CSF leak. One could be closed from an extracranial approach, while the others required craniotomies. In 5 cases the treatment team elected a routine intracranial exploration; 4 were negative, and one of these cases was complicated by a subdural abscess. Hengerer and Oas conclude that, given the fact that craniotomy carries a not insignificant morbidity, and that in a large number of cases the intracranial exploration will be negative, routine craniotomy is unnecessary.

Gliomas are benign lesions. Recurrences are avoided by removing all gliomatous tissue, using careful dissection aided by the operating microscope.

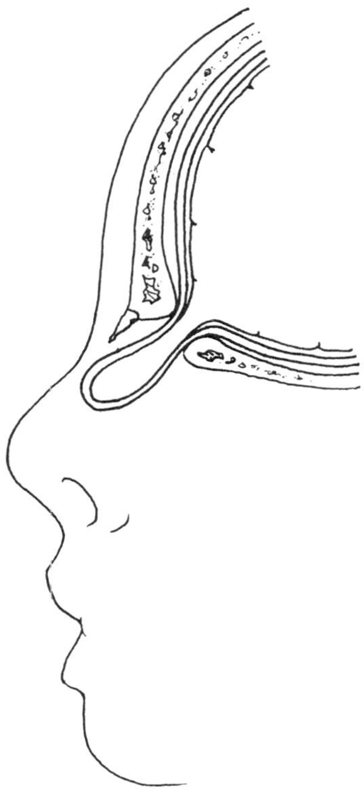

**Fig. 11–10.** Encephalocele. Herniation of brain tissue surrounded by meninges.

## Encephaloceles

*Encephaloceles* are herniations of neural tissue through a skull defect,[13] which can be congenital or acquired (Fig. 11–10). This discussion will center on congenital encephaloceles. Encephaloceles occur most frequently along the spine from the occiput to the sacrum, but between 15 and 25% occur in the anterior-frontal area.[16,40]

These lesions are diagnosed in 1/3,500 to 1/16,000 births.[13,19,40] No familial pattern has been demonstrated, but the association with diseases such as Ehlers-Danlos syndrome and syndromes such as frontonasal dysplasia and HARD-E (Hydrocephalus, Agyria, Retinal Dysplasia and Encephalocele) may suggest a genetic component.[19] The ratio of males to females appears equal.[18] The disorder may have a geographic variation, appearing more frequently in Russia and Southeast Asia.[16] In 30%–40% of cases, other brain anomalies may be found, such as microcephaly, hydrocephalus, anophthalmia, and microphthamia.[16]

### Classification

These lesions can be classified by the contents of the hernia or by the site of herniation. All are characterized by the herniation of dura and leptomeninges. If they contain nothing more, they are termed *meningoceles*. If brain is found in the hernia, it is termed an *encephalomeningocele*. Occasionally part of the ventricular system is found in the sac; this is termed an *encephalomeningocystocele*.

The classification by site is more useful clinically, as it is the site and size of the encephalocele, not the contents, that determine the symptomatology. Encephaloceles can be divided into sincipital and basal. The sincipital are the most common, accounting for 60% of encephaloceles.[23] They are further subdivided into three subtypes. The nasofrontal subtype, which exits the skull between the nasal and frontal bones, accounts for two-fifths of sincipital encephaloceles. They deform the orbit by pushing the medial orbital walls laterally. The nasoethmoidal subtype also accounts for two-fifths of sincipital encephaloceles, and exits between the nasal bones and nasal cartilages, thus leaving the nasal bones articulated to the frontal bones. The third subtype, the naso-orbital, accounts for only one-fifth of sincipital encephaloceles. They pass through a defect in the frontal process of the maxilla.[6] Basal encephaloceles are rarer, and can be divided into four subtypes. The transethmoidal and sphenoethmoidal subtypes exit the cranium through the cribriform plate, and they are the most common. They present as intranasal masses. Sphenorbital encephaloceles are very rare; they enter the orbit through the superior orbital fissure, and produce exophthalmos. Transsphenoidal encephaloceles, which are also rare, herniate in the nasopharynx through large defects posterior to the cribriform plate.

### Pathogenesis

Encephaloceles are believed to be developmentally related to gliomas. The same theories which account for gliomas account for encephaloceles, and are discussed in the section of pathogenesis of gliomas.[16]

### Pathology

Histologically these lesions are characterized by the presence of meninges, which differentiates them from gliomas. In addition, herniated neural tissue will be found if the lesion is an encephalomeningocele (Fig. 11–11).

### Clinical presentation

Sincipital encephaloceles are easier to diagnosis because they present as external masses around the nose. The diagnosis of basal encephaloceles is more difficult because of their "hidden" location and occasionally is delayed for many years.[13] In a young infant, an intranasal mass should be considered to be an encephalocele unless proven otherwise. However, even in adults, a mass resembling a simple polyp can turn out to be an encephalocele. A high index of suspicion is thus necessary at

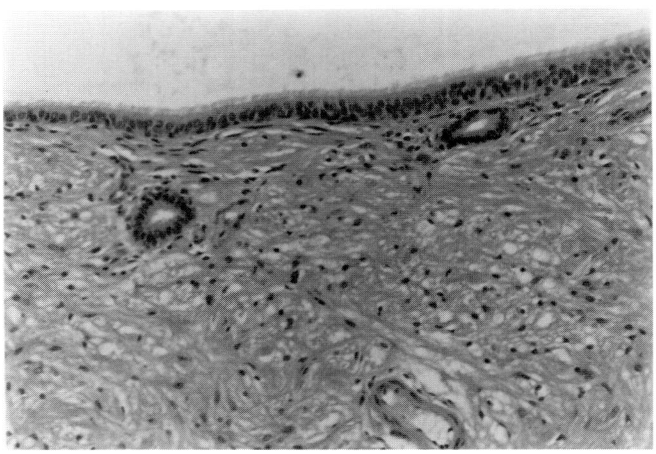

**Fig. 11–11.** Microscopic section of encephalocele. H & E stain, magnification × 20. (Courtesy of Dr. Chantal Bernard)

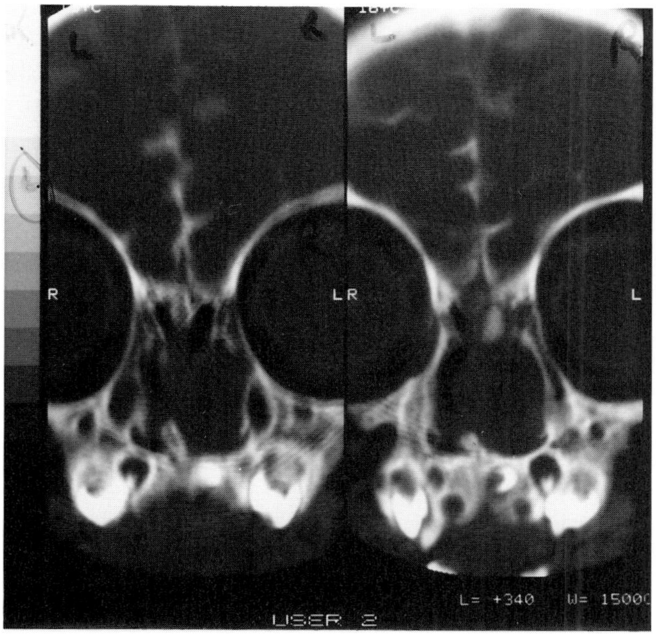


**Fig. 11–12.** CT with metrizamide demonstrating contrast in intranasal portion of encephalocele.

all times. An intranasal encephalocele usually presents as unilateral obstruction. However, with time, these lesions can push the septum over and the patient can present with bilateral obstruction. A history of rhinorrhea or recurrent meningitis should alert the physician to the possibility of an encephalocele.[7,8,13,23] Zinreich et al.[40] raised the possibility of increased susceptibility to sinusitis in these patients.

On physical examination, encephaloceles present as compressible, pulsatile masses which transilluminate. They enlarge with crying or with the Valsalva maneuver. The Furstenburg test is positive. However, all these signs are a function of the size of the communication with the subarachnoid space. In some encephaloceles this communication is small or partially scarred, and these traditional signs are not apparent. Thus, they are not totally reliable.[17] Diagnosis of an intranasal mass may be aided by gentle insertion of a probe into the nose. If the mass is an encephalocele, the probe will pass lateral, but not medial, to the mass.[22,23] Hypertelorism may be prominent in the sincipital type.

### Diagnosis

Biopsy is contraindicated. Thus, as in other congenital nasal anomalies, the investigation rests on a complete radiological study. In cases with a large bony defect, skull films may show the defect, but CT and MRI are the modalities of choice in the work-up of these patients (Fig. 11–12). While MRI can help diagnose an encephalocele by demonstrating herniation of brain tissue, CT is important because it permits preoperative assessment of the size of the bony defect. Other modalities may be useful. CT has replaced conventional tomography, but in some institutions tomography may be more readily available. Angiography may help in the diagnosis of a basal encephalocele by demonstrating displacement of small vessels into the hernia.[28] Radioactive isotopes injected by lumbar puncture have also been used successfully.[16]

### Treatment

Treatment consists of surgical excision, which should be performed early after diagnosis, because of the risk of meningitis and the increasing deformity caused by growth of the encephalocele with time. Surgery is individualized as a function of location and size of the bony defect. If there is evidence of hydrocephalus, a shunt is inserted prior to surgery.[16]

Although an extracranial approach can be used on a small sincipital encephalocele, most cases require a craniotomy. This facilitates repair of the dural and bony defects. Through the craniotomy an intradural approach is taken to the hernia sac. The herniated components are reduced or excised, and then the defect is closed. The dural defect can be closed with fascia or periosteal grafts. The bony defect is closed with bone grafts, acrylic mesh, or metallic mesh. The intranasal part of the encephalocele can then be removed extracranially. Choudhury and Taylor recommended leaving the intranasal sac, which they say will atrophy by itself.[7]

Young children appear to resolve their hypertelorism, while older children and adults who have a cosmetic deformity will require corrective surgery.

## Choanal atresia

Human infants, like other mammals, have the capacity to breathe and eat at the same time, but this is achieved at the cost of being obligate nasal breathers. In humans this capacity is lost with growth and maturation. During the period where infants are obligate nasal breathers, nasal obstruction can be catastrophic.

*Choanal atresia* is defined as a unilateral or bilateral obstruction of the posterior choanae of the nose. First reported by Johann George Roederer in 1755, this congenital anomaly occurs in 1/7,000 to 1/8,000 live births.[16,17] The unilateral form is more common. Hengerer and Oas reported a ratio of 2:1.[16] Most studies report significantly more females than males affected.[35] Curiously, the right side is involved more often then the left.[35] In up to 50% of cases, choanal atresia is associated with other anomalies.[18] The most significant association is with the CHARGE association (Table 11–2).

### Classification

In 10% of choanal atresia cases, the atresia is membranous. In the remaining 90%, the atresia is bony and can be subclassified depending on which part of the bony nasal structure is the most thickened and obstructive. In one group the lateral wall of the nose is the cause. Its increased thickness narrows or obliterates the space between the lateral wall and the vomer. This type is

**Table 11–2.** Choanal atresia: CHARGE association

| | Feature | Site |
|---|---|---|
| **C** | Coloboma | Iris, choroid, microphthalmia |
| **H** | Heart | Atrial septal defect, conotruncal lesions |
| **A** | Atresia | Membranous or bony (choanal atresia) |
| **R** | Retardation | Growth and developmental delay |
| **G** | Genitourinary | Cryptorchidism, microphallus, hydronephrosis |
| **E** | Ear | External, middle, and inner ear defect |

the most difficult to correct.[14] In other infants the vomer is thickened, leading to obstruction. Treatment consists of removing the posterior vomer, thereby advancing the posterior choanae.

### Pathogenesis

The pathogenesis of choanal atresia remains unknown. Several theories have been proposed, including persistence of the buccopharyngeal membrane, persistence of the nasobuccal membrane, or overgrowth of the horizontal and vertical processes of the palatine bone.[35] The buccopharyngeal membrane, if it were to persist, would form an obstruction posterior to the site of choanal atresia; thus, this theory is no longer favored. The mesoderm which forms the bone of the atretic plate is derived from neural crest origin. Abnormal flow or local factors in the nasal region of the developing embryo may disrupt normal development.[16]

### Diagnosis

The symptoms of unilateral and bilateral choanal atresia are different, but it is important to remember that even within each type there are marked differences in symptoms from one patient to the next.

Bilateral choanal atresia usually presents at birth as an emergency. Characteristically, infants present episodes of respiratory distress and cyanosis, relieved with crying. During crying color improves, but when crying ceases, the inspiratory effort resumes, with the lips tightly closed together, and with chest wall retraction. In addition to the airway symptoms, feeding is difficult because sucking is impaired.

Unilateral choanal atresia usually presents later in life. Cases are occasionally diagnosed in children several years old. Unilateral obstruction and chronic rhinorrhea are the cardinal symptoms. Often infants with unilateral choanal atresia escape detection until the contralateral side becomes obstructed. An association with sudden infant death syndrome is suspected for both bilateral and unilateral choanal atresia.

A quick way to diagnose choanal atresia in a neonate in respiratory difficulty is to attempt to pass a #8 French catheter intranasally. If the catheter cannot be passed deeper than 3 to 4 centimeters, the site of obstruction is localized to the nose. Other tests have been developed to document choanal atresia. Dyes such as methylene blue can be placed in the nose, and then the oropharynx observed for dye. A thin wisp of cotton held below the nose should move if there is airflow through the nose. Similarly, if the patient is breathing through the nose, the warm air will fog a mirror held below the nose. Modern fiberoptic endoscopes readily permit visualization of the atretic plate.

Radiologic investigation traditionally consisted of the installation of a radio-opaque dye into the nose, followed by multiple radiographs to observe flow of the dye (Fig. 11–13). This technique has been made all but obsolete by computer tomography, which permits documentation of the thickness of the atretic plate and permits differentiation of membranous from bony choanal atresia (Fig. 11–14).

### Treatment

Treatment must be divided into emergency and definitive. Bilateral choanal atresia in a neonate is an emergency which is best treated by inserting an oral airway. The insertion of the

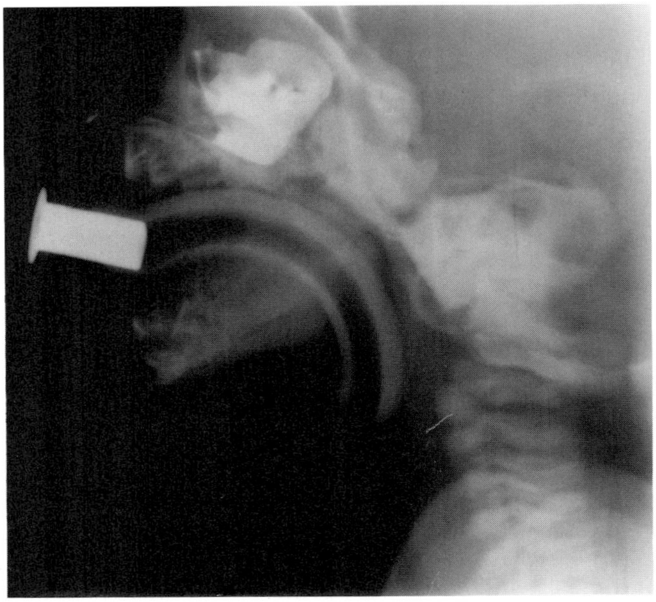

**Fig. 11–13.** Infant with choanal atresia. Note blockage of dye at level of posterior choanae.

airway breaks the seal formed by the tongue against the palate. Oral airways are readily available in a variety of sizes and are well tolerated for several weeks. Alternatively, a soft nipple, with the end hole enlarged, can be used, since it too breaks the seal between the tongue and the palate.[35] Once the airway is secure, a feeding tube can be inserted. Except in the case of a neonate with other upper airway anomalies, tracheostomy is not required.

In determining the timing of definitive surgery, the higher stenosis rate in young infants must be balanced against the increased cost and complexity of managing the infant without correction of the choanal atresia. Further complicating the issue is the variability in symptoms from one individual to the next. Jaffe[17] has proposed a three-level system for management of choanal atresia based on the severity of symptoms. Level one includes infants who have adapted well to oral breathing. These should be assisted with gavage feedings and have surgery delayed until they are 1 year old. Level two consists of patients with severe symptoms at birth but who are easily maintained on an oral airway or McGovern nipple and who convert within days to weeks to oral breathing. These patients can also have surgery delayed until 1 year of age. At level three are patients who continue to be difficult to manage in terms of airway and feedings. These infants should have early surgery.

There are three approaches to treat the choanal atresia. The oldest is the transnasal approach. It was first performed by Emmert in 1850.[35] He used a trocar to punch a hole through the atretic plate. To avoid the complications of blindly pushing a trocar, which have included damage to the brain, modifications have been proposed. It can be performed under endoscopic visualization or with the use of a carbon dioxide laser.[15] The laser technique appears to work well for membranous atresia but not for bony atresia. The transnasal approach remains limited by the high incidence of restenosis.

The transseptal approach consists of making a window in the septum anterior to a unilateral atretic plate. Air can thus flow through the window and into the normal contralateral posterior

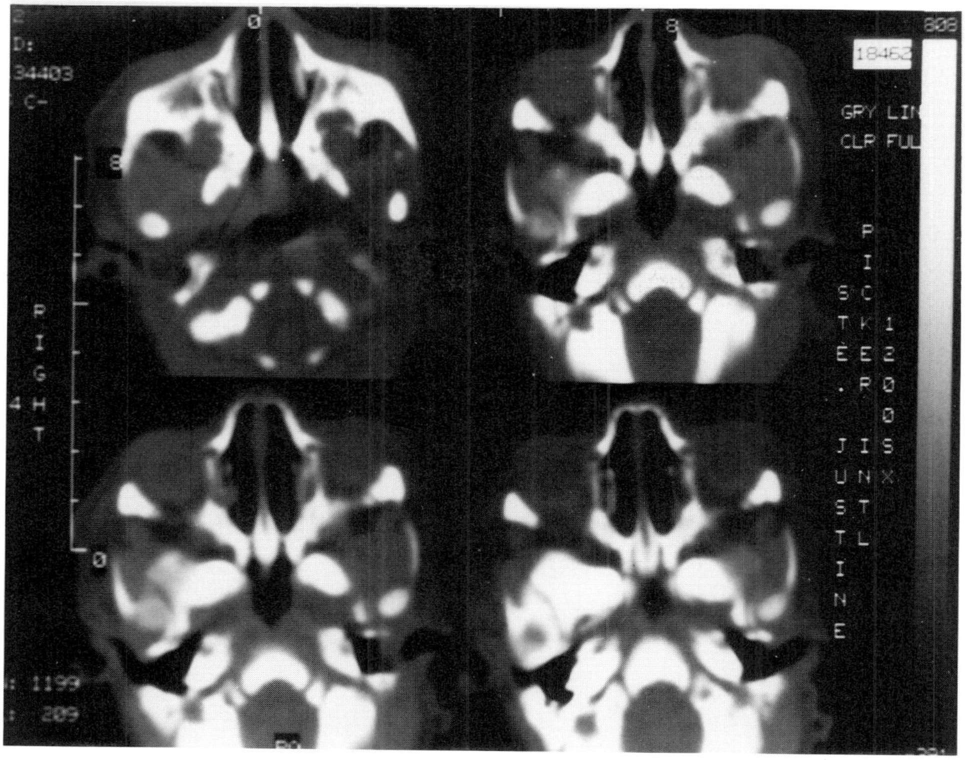

Fig. 11–14. Axial CT scan of mixed bony and membranous choanal atresia.

choana. Although the technique does not address the atresia directly, it has the advantage of being fast and simple.

The transpalatal approach remains the most popular. Although there are many variations, they all seek to expose the posterior end of the hard palate, remove it, and then excise the posterior vomer. The Owens flap[25] has the advantage of not passing over an area of bone defect, thus lessening the chance of an oronasal fistula, as seen with midline incisions (Fig. 11–15).

Whichever technique is used, the newly created posterior choanae must be stented for a period of 8 to 12 weeks.

## Median nasal cleft

Patients with median nasal cleft, also known as *bifid nose,* present with a groove separating the two halves of the nose down the midline.[10] A spectrum of severity from a shallow groove to a deep furrow, separating the nose into two halves, has been reported. This anomaly may occur individually but often occurs with hypertelorism, and clefts of the lip and palate. DeMyer[10] and Sedano et al.[31] have called attention to an association between median nasal cleft, cranium bifidum occultum, hypertelorism, cleft lip, and cleft palate. This nongenetic, congenital disorder has been referred to as *frontonasal dysplasia*[31] (see Fig. 11–16).

Upon diagnosis, the adequacy of the neonate's nasal airway must be assessed and other anomalies ruled out. If the deformity is not too pronounced, it may improve with growth of the child. More severe anomalies, where the nasal halves are separated by a wall, require cosmetic procedures later. The timing of surgery will be dictated by the severity of the defect, the reaction of the parents, and the possible effects of surgery on nasal development.

## Lateral nasal cleft

Neonates with lateral nasal cleft present with a defect of the nasal ala. The magnitude of the anomaly can vary from a small groove on the lateral aspect of the nasal ala, to a large furrow with loss of tissue all the way up to the inner canthus. Hengerer

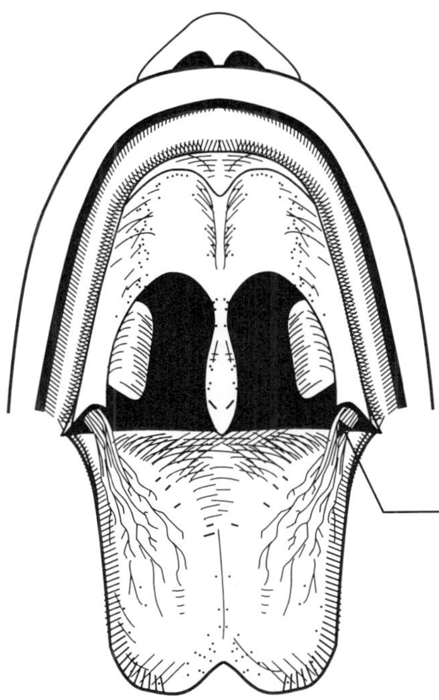


Fig. 11–15. Owens flap. Avoiding a midline incision results in a lower incidence of naso-oral fistula. The mucosa has been peeled back and the hard palate rongeured, giving access to the choanal atresia.

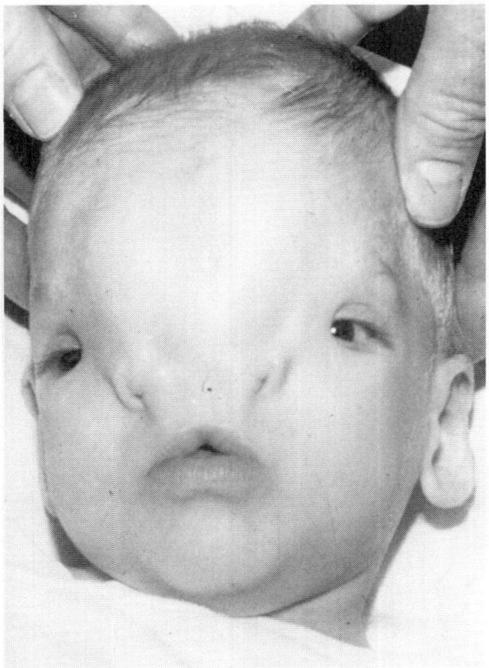

**Fig. 11–16.** Male 7-month-old infant with frontonasal dysplasia. Note the marked ocular hypertelorism, horseshoe-shaped midfacial protuberance, pronounced separation of the nostrils, and notching of the upper lip. (From Sedano et al.,[31] courtesy of Dr. Robert J. Gorlin.)

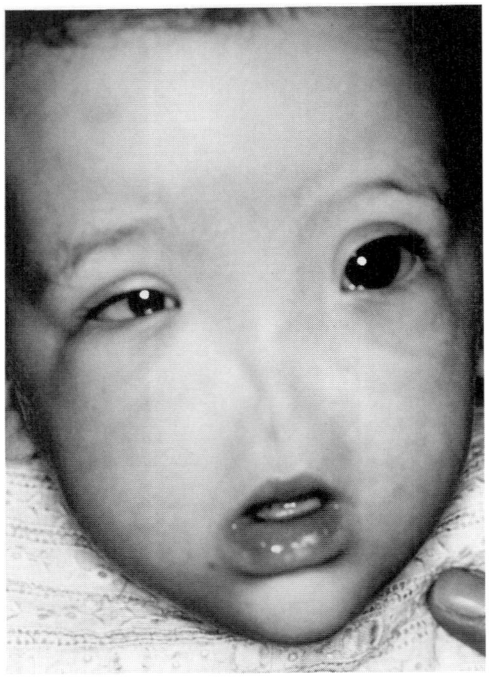

**Fig. 11–17.** Infant with arhinia. (Courtesy of Prof. Carlos Navarro Vila, M.D.[24] From Navarro-Vila et al.,[24] with permission from Georg Thieme Verlag.)

and Oas[16] believe that this anomaly is secondary to a problem of mesenchymal flow between the medial and lateral nasal processes.

The diagnosis can be readily made at birth. Since lateral nasal cleft may be associated with other anomalies, examination and work-up must be performed to rule out other congenital anomalies of the nasal region, as well as to determine patency of the nasolacrimal duct.

In planning the timing of definitive surgery to correct the defect, the severity of the cosmetic defect and the parents' attitude towards the defect must be weighed against the possible effects of early surgery on nasal development.

## Polyrhinia

Polyrhinia, or double nose, is an extremely rare anomaly in which the neonate presents with two completely formed noses. This situation is unlike median cleft, where a single nose is divided into two, each with one nostril. During embryonic development, a defect is believed to lead to duplication of the medial nasal processes.[16] Ghosh described a case which presented in association with choanal atresia.[11] Treatment consisted of transnasal correction of the choanal atresia and excision of the medial halves of each nose. One septum was preserved, following which the two lateral halves were approximated.

## Arhinia

Arhinia is a very rare condition in which there is congenital absence of the external nose, the nasal cavities, and the olfactory system (Figs. 11–17, 11–18). Although this anomaly can occur in isolation, it usually occurs in association with anomalies of the eye and the central nervous system.[33] In some cases the central nervous system anomalies may be incompatible with life.[12] Other anomalies of the midface, such as cleft lip, cleft palate, and submucous cleft palate have been reported.[24]

There are no reports of a familial pattern, but an association with anomalies of chromosome 9 has been reported. In one case, an inversion of chromosome 9 was detected,[9] while, in another, a trisomy of chromosome 9 was noted.[24] Recent

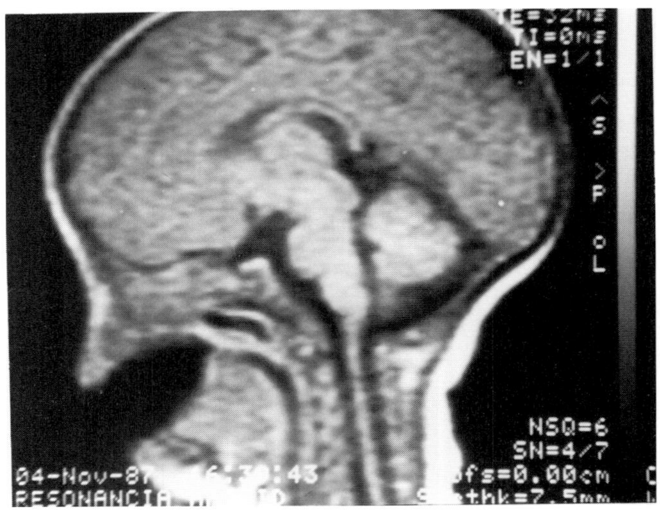


**Fig. 11–18.** MRI of infant in Figure 11–16 demonstrating congenital absence of the nose and nasal fossae. (Courtesy of Prof. Carlos Navarro Vila, M.D.[24] From Navarro-Vila et al.,[24] with permission from Georg Thieme Verlag.)

cases do not mention any relation with fetal stress during pregnancy.

The diagnosis is readily made at birth. A depression is found between the eyes, in the position of the external nose. Occasionally, a small hole or tag is found. The maxilla is underdeveloped, and intraoral examination demonstrates a high-arched palate. Neonates are obligate nasal breathers and, as one might expect, these infants may present with significant distress.[12] They should be managed in a fashion similar to those patients with choanal atresia. However, several authors have remarked that these infants quickly progress to oral breathing.[12,24] Nutritional support, using either an orogastric feeding tube or a gastrostomy, is necessary. An investigation for other congenital anomalies should be conducted.

The aptitude these neonates exhibit to develop oral breathing permits deferral of definitive surgery until the preschool years. This allows for growth of the rest of the face. Gifford et al. operated on two patients between 5 and 6 years of age, then revised the final appearance at age 15.[12] In the interim, the child should be fitted with a nasal prosthesis to minimize the psychological consequences. Surgery consists of drilling through the maxilla and then stenting the newly created nasal cavities. Local flaps and conchal cartilage can then be used to reconstruct the external nose.

## Proboscis lateralis

Proboscis lateralis, or congenital tubular nose, was first described in 1884 by Sclenkoff, but remains a very rare anomaly. The external nose fails to develop on one side; it is instead replaced with a tubular structure hanging from the inner canthus. There is no nasal cavity, but the tubular structure may contain a tract leading to the dura or skull base. Histologically, the proboscis contains sebaceous, sweat, and lacrimal gland tissue, as well as cartilage and hair.[36] In the absence of a nasal cavity, the nasolacrimal duct usually ends blindly.[3] Anomalies of the central nervous system, sometimes not compatible with life, as well as deformities of the face, are not uncommon.

During fetal development, the lateral nasal process and maxillary process fuse. The nasolacrimal duct is formed from ectoderm that becomes buried at the junction of these two processes. In proboscis lateralis the medial and lateral nasal processes are either absent or fail to develop, leading to fusion of the maxillary process with the contralateral nasal process.[3,16,36] The location of the proboscis lateralis represents the site of the embryonic suture line between the maxillary process and the contralateral nasal process.

Treatment involves rerouting the nasolacrimal duct, if necessary. The proboscis lateralis can be excised at an early age. There is insufficient data in the literature to recommend an optimal time for reconstruction, but it is the authors' belief that delaying definitive surgery until the second decade is justified.

### References


1. Ashley DJ: Origin of teratomas. Cancer 32:390–394, 1973.
2. Barkovich AJ, Vandermarck P, Edwards MS, Cogen PH: Congenital nasal masses: CT and MR imaging features in 16 cases. Am J Neuroradiol 12:105–116, 1991.
3. Binns JH: Congenital tubular nostril (proboscis lateralis). Br J Plast Surg 22:265–268, 1969.
4. Bradley PJ: Nasal dermoids in children. Int J Pediatr Otorhinolaryngol 3:63–70, 1981.
5. Bradley PJ, Singh SD: Congenital nasal masses: diagnosis and management. Clin Otolaryngol 7:87–97, 1982.
6. Charoonsmith T, Suwanwela C: Frontoethmoidal encephalomeningocele with special reference to plastic reconstruction. Clin Plast Surg 1:27–47, 1974.
7. Choudhury AR, Taylor JC: Primary intranasal encephalocele. Report of four cases. J Neurosurg 57:552–555, 1982.
8. Choudhury AR, Taylor JC: Primary intranasal encephalocele (response). J Neurosurg 59:1111, 1983.
9. Cohen DK, Goitein K: Arhinia. Rhinology 24:287–292, 1986.
10. DeMyer W: The median cleft face syndrome. Differential diagnosis of cranium bifidum occultum, hypertelorism, and median cleft nose, lip, and palate. Neurology 17:961–971, 1967.
11. Ghosh P, Dada K, Gupta S, Jamwal N, Daljit R: Double nose. J Laryngol Otol 85:963–969, 1971.
12. Gifford GH Jr, Swanson L, MacCollum DW: Congenital absence of the nose and anterior nasopharynx. Report of two cases. Plast Reconstr Surg 50:5–12, 1972.
13. Harley EH: Pediatric congenital nasal masses. Ear Nose Throat J 70:28–32, 1991.
14. Harner SG, Mcdonald TJ, Reese DF: The anatomy of congenital choanal atresia. Otolaryngol Head Neck Surg 89:7–9, 1981.
15. Healy GB, McGill T, Jako GJ, Strong MS, Vaughan CW: Management of choanal atresia with the carbon dioxide laser. Ann Otol Rhinol Laryngol 87:658–662, 1978.
16. Hengerer AS, Oas RE: Congenital Anomalies of the Nose: Their Embryology, Diagnosis and Management, 2nd ed. American Academy of Otolaryngology-Head and Neck Surgery Foundation Inc, Washington, 1987, pp 25–83.
17. Jaffe BF: Classification and management of anomalies of the nose. Otolaryngol Clin North Am 14:989–1004, 1981.
18. Kaplan LC: The CHARGE association: choanal atresia and multiple congenital anomalies. Otolaryngol Clin North Am 22:661–672, 1989.
19. Kennard CD, Rasmussen JE: Congenital midline nasal masses: diagnosis and management. J Dermatol Surg Oncol 16:1025–1036, 1990.
20. Littlewood AH: Congenital nasal dermoid cysts and fistulae. Br J Plast Surg 14:169–179, 1961.
21. Lusk RP, Lee PC: Magnetic resonance imaging of congenital midline nasal masses. Otolaryngol Head Neck Surg 95:303–306, 1986.
22. Luyendijk W, Schmidt PH: Primary intranasal encephalocele [Letter]. J Neurosurg 59:1110–1111, 1983.
23. Morgan DW, Evans JN: Developmental nasal anomalies. J Laryngol Otol 104:394–403, 1990.
24. Navarro-Vila C, Matias GC, Martinez GC, Verdaguer MJ, Acero SJ, Perez SV, Rodriguez A: Congenital absence of the nose and nasal fossae. J Craniomaxillofac Surg 19:56–60,1991.
25. Owens H: Observations in treating twenty-five cases of choanal atresia by the transpalatine approach. Laryngoscope 75:84–104, 1965.
26. Pavlin JE, O'Gorman A, Williams HB, Crépeau RJ, Shapiro RS: Epignathus: a report of two cases. Ann Plast Surg 13:452–456, 1984.
27. Pensler JM, Bauer BS, Naidich TP: Craniofacial dermoids. Plast Reconstr Surg 82:953–958, 1988.
28. Pinto RS, George AE, Koslow M, Barasch G: Neuroradiology of basal anterior fossa (transethmoidal) encephaloceles. Radiology 117:79–85, 1975.
29. Plewes JL, Jacobson I: Familial frontonasal dermoid cyst. Report of four cases. J Neurosurg 34:683–686, 1971.
30. Rybak LP, Rapp MF, McGrady MD, Schwart MR, Myers PW, Orvidas L: Obstructing nasopharyngeal teratoma in the neonate. Arch Otolaryngol Head Neck Surg 117:1411–1415, 1991.
31. Sedano HO, Cohen MM Jr, Jirasek J, Gorlin RJ: Frontonasal dysplasia. J Pediatr 76:906–913, 1970.
32. Sessions RB: Nasal dermal sinuses—new concepts and explanations. Laryngoscope 92 (Suppl 29):1–28, 1982.
33. Shubich I, Sanchez C: Nasal aplasia associated with meningocele and submucous cleft palate. Ear Nose Throat J 64:259–260, 1985.
34. Sweet RM: Lesions of the nasal radix in pediatric patients: diagnosis and management. South Med J 85:164–169, 1992.
35. Theogaraj SD, Hoehn JG, Hagan KF: Practical management of congenital choanal atresia. Plast Reconstr Surg 72:634–642, 1983.
36. Van der Meulen JC, Mazzola R, Vermey-Keers C, Stricker M, Raphael B: A morphogenetic classification of craniofacial malformations. Plast Reconstr Surg 71:560–572, 1983.
37. Wardinsky TD, Pagon RA, Kropp RJ, Hayden PW, Clarren SK: Nasal

dermoid sinus cysts: association with intracranial extension and multiple malformations. Cleft Palate Craniofac J 28:87–95, 1991.

38. Weisman PA, Johnson GF: Concealed extensions of dermoid cysts of the nose: how can the surgeon be forewarned? Plast Reconstr Surg 34:373–381, 1964.
39. Younus M, Coode PE: Nasal glioma and encephalocele: two separate entities. J Neurosurg 64:516–519, 1986.
40. Zinreich SJ, Borders JC, Eisele DW, Mattox DE, Long DM, Kennedy DW: The utility of magnetic resonance imaging in the diagnosis of intranasal meningoencephaloceles. Arch Otolaryngol Head and Neck Surg 118:1253–1256, 1992.

# Appendix C

## Syndromes and Conditions Associated with Congenital Anomalies of the Nose, Nasopharynx, and Sinuses

AHMAD S. TEEBI, TED L. TEWFIK, and VAZKEN M. DER KALOUSTIAN

**Appendix C-1** Syndromes and conditions associated with beaked nose

| Syndrome or condition | MIM No. POSSUM No.[a] | Inheritance[b] | Other ear, nose, and throat anomalies | Other manifestations |
|---|---|---|---|---|
| AD microcephaly, Bawl-Horton type[13] | 4722 | AD | | Intrauterine growth retardation (IUGR), microcephaly, deep-set eyes, mental retardation (MR) |
| Acro-cranio-facial dysostosis, Kaplan type[97] | **201050** 4407 | AR | Cleft palate, micrognathia, choanal stenosis or atresia, preauricular pits, deafness (mixed) | Craniosynostosis (coronal) hypertelorism, ptosis, hypoplastic first metatarsal or metacarpal, metatarsus adductus, MR |
| Acrocephalospondylosyndactyly, Wells type[214] | 4772 | ? | Midface hypoplasia, broad or bulbous nasal tip, hypoplastic nostrils, tracheal abnormality, short neck | Similar to Apert syndrome with spondylothoracic dysplasia, dislocated radial heads and caudal appendage |
| Alar coloboma with telecanthus or frontonasal dysplasia with alar cleft[54] | **203000** 3981 | AR | Broad nasal bridge, flattened or bifid nasal tip, coloboma of nasal cartilage; high-arched, narrow, or cleft palate | Telecanthus or hypertelorism, blepharophimosis, dental enamel defect |
| Apert syndrome or acrocephalosyndactyly type 1[30,150] | ***101200** 3007 | AD | Midface hypoplasia, small and short nose, choanal stenosis or atresia, high-arched or narrow palate (byzantine), cleft palate, low-set or anteverted ears | Craniosynostosis (coronal), "glove" and "stocking" syndactyly of fingers and toes, broad distal phalanges of thumb and big toe, cervical vertebral defects, variable MR (common) |
| Autosomal dominant trigonocephaly[59,80] | **190440** 3058 | AD | Midface hypoplasia, abnormal nasal septum or abnormal columella | Metopic suture synostosis, macrosomia, normal intelligence |
| Camptodactyly joint contractures, facial and skeletal defects, or Rozin syndrome[164] | 3641 | AR | Microstomia, high-arched and narrow palate, micrognathia, facial asymmetry | Camptodactyly, prominent eyes, joint contractures, hemihypertrophy or hemiatrophy, scoliosis, 5th finger clinodactyly, short stature |
| Chromosome abnormalities: | 3125 | | | |
| Chromosome 1, dup 1q (q32→qter)[37,169] | | | | |
| Chromosome 2, intestitial del 2(q31q33)[37] | 3685 | | | |
| Chromosome 2, partial dup 2q[37,169] | 3686 | | | |
| Chromosome 3, del 3p (pter→p25)[169] | 3520 | | | |
| Chromosome 4, partial del 4p[169] | 3069 | | | |
| Chromosome 4, partial dup 4q[169] | 3071 | | | |
| Chromosome 6, partial dup 6q[37,169] | 3689 | | | |
| Chromosome 7, partial dup 7q[169] | 3076 | | | |
| Chromosome 9, dup 9q[169] | 3117 | | | |

**Appendix C-1** Syndromes and conditions associated with beaked nose (*Continued*)

| Syndrome or condition | **MIM No.** POSSUM No.[a] | Inheritance[b] | Other ear, nose, and throat anomalies | Other manifestations |
|---|---|---|---|---|
| Chromosome 9, partial tetrasomy 9p[91] | 4534 | | | |
| Chromosome 15, dup 15q[113] | 4390 | | | |
| Chromosome 15, intestitial del 15(q13–q15)[4] | 4639 | | | |
| Chromosome 16, partial dup 16q[118,169] | 3712 | | | |
| Chromosome 18, partial dup 18q[22,169] | 3699 | | | |
| Chromosome 22, trisomy 22[187] | 3703 | | | |
| Chromosome X/Y, tetraploidy 92XXXX/XXYY[219] | 3115 | | | |
| Cleft palate, lateral synechia syndrome[43,61] | ***119550**<br>3142 | AD | Cleft lip/palate, adhesions between the lateral edge of the tongue and floor of the mouth or edge of palate, limited opening of the mouth, midface hypoplasia, micrognathia | Cryptorchidism, thumb defect, pes planus, mental retardation |
| Cloverleaf skull syndrome or Kleeblattschädel syndrome[3,27] | **148800**<br>3271 | AD | Facial clefts, low-set ears | Craniosynostosis, hydrocephalus, trilobed head enlargement, contractures of large joints, syndactyly of fingers, MR, may be associated with craniosynostosis syndrome or thanatophoric dysplasia |
| Craniomandibular dermatodysostosis or mandibuloacral dysplasia[76,147] | ***248370**<br>3161 | AR | Midface hypoplasia, limited opening of the mouth, high-arched or narrow palate, defective mandible, micrognathia, ear cartilage abnormalities, abnormal cry | Dysplastic nails, shortened distal phalanges, short limbs, stiff joints, truncal obesity, thin hair and skin, hypoplastic clavicles, delayed closure of cranial sutures, wormian bones |
| Craniosynostosis, mental retardation, and clefting syndrome in Baraitser-Rodeck-Garner syndrome[10] | **218650**<br>3559 | AR | Cleft lip/palate, anteverted ears (bat ears) | Craniosynostosis, seizures, choroidal coloboma, dysplastic kidneys, MR |
| Crouzon disease or Crouzon craniofacial dysostosis[81,106] | ***123500**<br>3158 | AD | Midface hypoplasia, high-arched or cleft palate, prognathism, atretic or small external auditory canal, conductive deafness | The most common form of inherited craniosynostosis, abnormal skull shape, exophthalmos, external strabismus, hypertelorism, upper cervical vertebral fusion, MR (germ-line mosaicism is known) |
| Cutis laxa[14,34,167] | ***123700**<br>***219100**<br>***219200**<br>***304150**<br>3180 | AD<br>AR<br>XL | Sagging cheeks, aged face, abnormal columella, abnormal cry | Lax or loose skin, hernias, hyperextensible joints, joint dislocation, recessive form may be lethal; mild autosomal recessive form is found associated with MR |
| Distal abstructive uropathy/polydactyly[73] | 4532 | ? | Ear cartilage defect, low-set ears, micrognathia | Ureteric, bladder, or urethral abnormalities, postaxial polydactyly of hand and feet, syndactyly of fingers, cryptorchidism, stillbirth |
| Dysosteosclerosis[87] | ***224300**<br>3728 | AR | High-arched or narrow palate, mandibular hyperostosis or sclerosis, micrognathia abnormal hearing, facial palsy | Short stature, short limbs, calvarial hyperostosis, sclerosis, platyspondyly, optic nerve compression, other nerve palsies, patches of skin atrophy, multiple fractures, neurological deterioration, distinguish from osteopetrosis |
| Facial dysmorphism, aortic arch anomaly, and mental retardation, or Strong syndrome[186] | **107500**<br>3448 | AD | Midface hypoplasia, mild facial asymmetry, large nose, deviated nasal septum, abnormal columella, large ears, prognathism | Right-sided aortic arch, microcephaly, mental retardation |

| Syndrome or condition | Inheritance[a] | MIM No.<br>POSSUM No.[b] | Ear, nose, and throat manifestations | Other systemic manifestations |
|---|---|---|---|---|
| Fraser-Jaquier-Chen syndrome[56] | 4306 | ? | High-arched palate, folded ear, laryngeal cleft | Short limbs (rhizomelic), postaxial polydactyly, pancreatic or renal dysplasia, imperforate anus, genital anomalies |
| Glutaric acidemia, type 2[67] | ***231680**<br>4511 | AR | Depressed nasal bridge, micrognathia | IUGR, macrocephaly, high forehead, large fontanelle, hepatomegaly, cardiomyopathy, hypotonia, seizures, MR, hypoglycemia, acidosis or hyperammonemia, organic acid disorder due to multiple acyl-Co A dehydrogenase deficiency, proposed gene location 15q23–q25 |
| Hallermann-Streiff syndrome or oculo-mandibulo-facial syndrome[26,104] | **234100**<br>3342 | ?AD<br>?AR | Small nose, hypoplastic alae nasi, microstomia, micrognathia, narrow airways (anesthetic risk), feeding problems | Sparse hair, characteristic senile facies, high forehead, microphthalmia, cataract, thin skin |
| Hoepffner-Dreyer-Rüdiger syndrome[85] | **233805**<br>4745 | AR | Microstomia, micrognathia | Lipodystrophy, joint contractures, scleroderma-like skin, hyperkeratosis, diabetes mellitus, defects in insulin-like growth factors and epidermal growth factor, growth retardation |
| Idaho 2 syndrome[25] | 3169 | | Low-set or posteriorly angulated ears, microtia, preauricular skin tags and sinuses | Craniosynostosis or antimongoloid slant of palpebral fissures, sloping shoulders with winged scapulae, MR |
| Intrauterine growth retardation, ataxia, and diabetes, or Bangstad syndrome[7] | **210740**<br>3772 | AR | Long and large nose, high nasal bridge, flared nostrils, abnormal columella, abnormal ears, conductive deafness, micrognathia | Intrauterine and postnatal growth retardation, microcephaly, long face, deep-set eyes, minor skeletal abnormality, MR, insulin-resistant diabetes, later onset of ataxia |
| Johanson-Blizzard syndrome, or nasal hypoplasia, hypothyroidism, pancreatic exocrine deficiency, and deafness[64,89] | ***243800**<br>3269 | AR | Midface hypoplasia, short nose, hypoplastic nostrils, dental anomalies, downward turned mouth angles, sensorineural deafness | Growth retardation, variable intellectual disabilities, microcephaly, scalp defect, malabsorption due to pancreatic exocrine deficiency, anal atresia, cardiac and genital defects, hypothyroidism |
| Kabuki make-up syndrome or Niikawa-Kuroki syndrome[108,172] | **147920**<br>3541 | ?AD | Bulbous or depressed nasal tip, broad nasal septum, abnormal columella; cleft, high-arched, or narrow palate; large ears, preauricular tags, conductive or sensorineural deafness, micrognathia | Microcephaly, characteristic face with long palpebral fissures, arched eyebrows, everted lateral part of the lower eyelid, brachydactyly with prominent fingertip pads, cardiac defects, moderate growth and developmental retardation |
| Lambotte syndrome[207] | **245552**<br>4785 | AR | Atresia of the external auditory canal, large and soft ears, microstomia, microretrognathia | IUGR, microcephaly, CNS anomalies, flat face, telecanthus, severe neurological impairment, preaxial polydactyly of the feet, ventricular septal defect, early lethality |
| Lowry-Maclean syndrome[121] | 3574 | ? | Cleft palate, low-set or downward folded ears, preauricular tags | Craniosynostosis, Crouzon-like face, agenesis of the corpus callosum, diaphragmatic defect, cardiac defect |
| Multiple congenital anomalies [MCA], MR, blepharophimosis, or Elliott syndrome[47] | 3863 | ? | Microstomia, high-arched or narrow palate, low-set ears, sensorineural deafness, micrognathia | IUGR, growth retardation, blepharophimosis, excessive freckling, lentigines, sparse scalp hair, skeletal defects, MR |
| MR and hypospadias, or Goldblatt syndrome[66] | **241760**<br>4398 | ?AR<br>?XLR | Midface hypoplasia, abnormal columella, high-arched or narrow palate, posteriorly-angulated ears | Microcephaly, rigid metopic sutures, synophrys, hyperextensible or hypermobile joints, hypospadias, MR |

**Appendix C-1** Syndromes and conditions associated with beaked nose (*Continued*)

| Syndrome or condition | MIM No. POSSUM No.[a] | Inheritance[b] | Other ear, nose, and throat anomalies | Other manifestations |
|---|---|---|---|---|
| MR, macrostomia, and hyperpnea, or Pitt-Hopkins syndrome[177] | 3474 | ? | Broad nasal bridge, flared nostrils, large mouth, thick lips | Short stature, coarse facies, hypertelorism, single palmar creases, terminal broadening or clubbing of fingers or toes, cardiac conduction defects, arrhythmias, irregular respiration and intermittent overbreathing, apnea, seizures, MR |
| MR, short stature, and unusual facies, or Lindström syndrome[120] | 4101 | AR | Broad nasal bridge, bifid nasal tip, cleft lip, thick lips, micrognathia, prominent ears, short neck | IUGR, short stature, hypertelorism, prominent eyes with puffy lids, hernias, camptodactyly, hypotonia, seizures, spasticity, MR |
| MR, unusual facies, Ampola type[2] | 3954 | AD | High-arched or narrow palate, anteverted, large "oval" nostrils, large ears and cartilage deficiency, micrognathia | Short stature, short limbs, frontal bossing, antimongoloid slant of palpebral fissures, strabismus, puffy eyelids, seizures, severe MR |
| MR, unusual facies, Davis-Lafer type[36] | 4086 | ?AD | Cleft palate or bifid uvula, low-set and large ears, micrognathia | Growth retardation, short stature, frontal bossing, hypertelorism, epicanthic folds, ptosis, hypospadias, cryptorchidism, fifth finger clinodactyly, hypoplastic nails, single palmar creases, hypotonia, frequent infections, MR |
| MR, unusual facies, Pitt-Rogers-Danks type[46,154] | **262350**<br>3646 | AR | Midface hypoplasia, macrostomia, flat philtrum, high-arched or narrow palate, low-set ears, abnormal hearing | IUGR, growth retardation, microcephaly, upward slanting palpebral fissures, telecanthus, prominent eyes, radioulnar synostosis, small hands, abnormal dermatoglyphics, behavior problems, MR |
| Metageria[65] | 3983 | AR | Narrow nasal bridge, thin nose, telangiectasia of ear pinna | Tall and thin stature, premature aging, absence of subcutaneous fat, telangiectasia, mottled hyperpigmentation, Raynaud's phenomenon and leg ulcers, diabetes mellitus |
| Montreal type "bird-headed" dwarfism[52] | **210700**<br>3327 | AR | Nystagmus, high nasal bridge, low-set or anteverted ears, micrognathia | Intrauterine dwarfism, microcephaly, short stature, premature graying of hair, MR (mild-borderline) |
| Osteodysplastic primordial dwarfism, type 1 or brachymelic primordial dwarfism[72,132] | ***210710**<br>4596 | AR | Prominent maxilla, high nasal bridge, micrognathia, low-set ears, short neck | IUGR, short stature, rhizomelic limb shortness, metaphyseal abnormalities, microcephaly, dislocated elbows, tapering fingers, short and broad pelvis, MR |
| Progeria or Hutchinson-Gilford syndrome[102,128] | **176670**<br>3362 | ?AD<br>?AR | Narrow nasal bridge, high-arched palate, oligodontia and hypodontia, anteverted ears, abnormal hearing, micrognathia | Growth failure, alopecia, atrophy of subcutaneous tissues (start in infancy), excessive skin wrinkling, increased skin pigmentation, aged face, atherosclerosis and hypercholesterolemia (leading to an early death) |
| Progressive macrocephaly and hamartomata, Halal-Silver type[74] | 4715 | AD | Telangiectasia of the ear pinna | Normal head circumference at birth, progressive macrocephaly, cutis marmorata, muscle wasting, multiple subcutaneous angiolipomas, broad thumb and great toe, hypotonia, delayed skeletal maturation, MR (mild) |
| Pseudoprogeria[75] | **200130**<br>3867 | AR | Short and small nose, high nasal bridge, abnormal nasal septum, microtia | Microcephaly, glaucoma, absent eyebrows and lashes, excessive skin pigmentation and freckling, progressive spastic quadriplegia, seizures, MR |

| Syndrome or condition | Inheritance[a] | MIM No. POSSUM No.[b] | Ear, nose, and throat manifestations | Other systemic manifestations |
|---|---|---|---|---|
| Pyknodysostosis or osteopetrosis acroosteolytica[181] | *265800<br>3365 | AR | Midface hypoplasia, absent or abnormal sinuses, partial absence of mandible, teeth abnormalities, micrognathia | Bony sclerosis, increased bony fragility, macrocephaly, frontal bossing, short stature, short limbs, short terminal phalanges, MR |
| Robinow-Sorauf syndrome[20] | 180750<br>3545 | AD | Depressed nasal bridge, high-arched palate, abnormal ears | Acrocephaly or turricephaly, brachycephaly, craniosynostosis, prominent eyes, hypertelorism, syndactyly of fingers and toes, bifid and broad great toe (facial features are similar to those of Saethre-Chotzen syndrome) |
| Rubinstein-Taybi syndrome[79,112] | 180849<br>3384 | AD<br>most cases are sporadic | Long and large nose, abnormal nasal septum, abnormal columella, high-arched or narrow palate, low-set ears | Short stature, narrow forehead, microcephaly, thick eyebrows, hypertelorism, antimongoloid slant of palpebral fissures, epicanthic folds, scoliosis, brachydactyly, broad and deviated thumbs/great toes, cardiac defect, hypotonia, seizures, MR (some cases have microdeletion of 16p) |
| Ruvalcaba syndrome[15] | 180870<br>3131 | AD | Small nose, thin alae nasi, broad or bulbous nasal tips, microstomia, pointed chin | IUGR, short stature, microcephaly, craniosynostosis, high forehead, high-arched eyebrows, brachyphalangy with short lateral metacarpals, epiphyseal dysplasia of the spine, urogenital and cardiac defects, MR |
| Saethre-Chotzen syndrome or acro-cephalosyndactyly type 3[141,161] | *101400<br>3009 | AD | Midface hypoplasia, deviated nasal septum, lip pits, cleft palate, microtia, abnormal helix of the ear, abnormal hearing | Variable craniosynostosis, ridged metopic suture or trigonocephaly, thickened calvarium, flat face with asymmetry, prominent eyes, hypertelorism, ptosis, brachydactyly, syndactyly of fingers and toes, single palmar creases, broad great toe/thumb, MR (mild-borderline) |
| Sakati-Nyhan syndrome or Acro-cephalopolysyndactyly, type 3[166] | 101120<br>3010 | | Midface hypoplasia, cleft lip, high-arched palate, low-set or anteverted ears, preauricular tag, short neck | Short stature, short limbs, craniosynostosis, acrocephaly or turricephaly, scalp defect, abnormal sella turcica, macrocephaly, brachydactyly, polysyndactyly; absence or hypoplasia of radius, ulna, femur, tibia, and fibula; cardiac defect |
| Say-Meyer syndrome, or trigonocephaly, short stature, and MR[168] | 314320<br>3483 | XLR | Low-set ears | Ridged metopic suture or trigonocephaly, microcephaly, short stature, hypotelorism, MR |
| Seckel syndrome or microcephalic primordial dwarfism, type 1[78] | *210600<br>3387 | AR | Prominent midface, large and long nose, micrognathia, low-set ears, abnormal ear lobe | IUGR, short stature, microcephaly, characteristic face with backward-sloping forehead, hyperextensible joints, dislocation, scoliosis, cryptorchidism, cerebral gyral or cortical defects, MR (moderate-severe) |
| Tricho-rhino-phalangeal syndrome, type 3[95,138] | 4413 | AD | Hypoplastic nostrils, abnormal columella, microstomia, downturned mouth angles, thin lips, teeth abnormalities, long philtrum, long and large ears | Growth retardation, characteristic round face, sparse scalp hair, high forehead, hypertelorism, high-arched eyebrows with lateral thinning, short fingers and toes, tapering fingers, cone-shaped epiphysis, normal intelligence |

**Appendix C-1** Syndromes and conditions associated with beaked nose (*Continued*)

| Syndrome or condition | MIM No. POSSUM No.[a] | Inheritance[b] | Other ear, nose, and throat anomalies | Other manifestations |
|---|---|---|---|---|
| Vitamin A embryopathy or retinoic acid embryopathy[1] | 3624 | Teratogenicity | Microtia, low-set ears, midface hypoplasia, flared nostrils, cleft palate or bifid uvula, atresia of external auditory canal | Microcephaly, macrocephaly, CNS defects, thymic aplasia, hypoplasia, conotruncal cardiac defects, absent or hypoplastic ulna or fibula, abnormal dermatoglyphics, hypotonia, MR, stillbirth or early death |
| Werner syndrome[69] | ***277700** 3765 | AR | Abnormal voice, telangiectasia of ear pinna | Prematurely aged face, early graying of hair, sparse scalp hair, growth failure, cataract, scleroderma-like skin changes and subcutaneous calcification, spastic paraparesis and polyneuropathy, dementia, diabetes mellitus, chromosome rearrangements in cell culture, symptoms start in young adult life |
| Wiedemann-Rautenstrauch syndrome or neonatal progeroid syndrome[143,200] | ***264090** 3721 | AR | Midface hypoplasia, nystagmus, high-arched palate, abnormal mouth, pointed chin, micrognathia, natal or neonatal teeth, low-set ears, sensorineural deafness, short neck | IUGR, short stature, aged appearance at birth, absent subcutaneous fat, frontal bossing, prominent skin vessels, blepharophimosis, joint contractures, cerebral cortex atrophy, hypotonia, MR |

**Appendix C-2** Syndromes and conditions associated with long or large nose

| Syndrome or condition | MIM No. POSSUM No.[a] | Inheritance[b] | Other ear, nose, and throat anomalies | Other manifestations |
|---|---|---|---|---|
| Acrocephalopolysyndactyly type 4 or Goodman syndrome[63] | **201020** 3818 | AR | High-arched, narrow, or short palate; flared nostrils, large ears, micrognathia | Acrocephaly, craniosynostosis, long face, camptodactyly and ulnar deviation of fingers, syndactyly of fingers and toes, postaxial polydactyly, brachydactyly, normal intelligence |
| Acro-osteolysis, short stature, MR[152] | **259610** 4491 | AR | Midface hypoplasia, broad, bulbous nasal tip | Short stature, skin wrinkling, brachydactyly, acro-osteolysis of fingers and toes, MR (borderline to mild) |
| Alagille syndrome or arteriohepatic dysplasia[41,193] | ***118450** 3019 | AD contiguous gene syndrome | Beaked nose, anteverted ears, pointed chin | Failure to thrive, characteristic facies, deep-set eyes, frontal bossing, posterior embryotoxon, jaundice with intrahepatic biliary atresia, pulmonary artery hypoplasia, vertebral defects, MR (variable), deletions of 20p |
| Blepharo-naso-facial syndrome[149] | **110050** 3039 | AD | Broad and high nasal bridge, broad and bulbous nasal tip, down-turned mouth angles | Expressionless face, telecanthus, blepharophimosis, abnormal posture and gait, movement disorder, MR |
| Broad terminal phalanges and facial anomalies or Keipert-Danks syndrome[100] | **255980** 3047 | AR | Short nasal septum and abnormal columella, flared nostrils, high-arched palate, prominent upper lip, macrostomia, sensorineural deafness | Macrocephaly, lateral facial cleft, ptosis, broad thumb and great toe, terminal broadening of fingers and toes, MR |
| Cerebro-oculo-facio-skeletal (COFS) or Pena-Shokeir syndrome, type 2[185] | **214150** 3136 | AR | Prominent premaxillary region, high nasal bridge, long philtrum, large low-set ears | Microcephaly, microphthalmia cataracts, failure to thrive, multiple joint contractures, hirsutism, urinary tract anomalies, CNS defects, hypotonia, MR |
| Chromosome abnormalities | | | | |
| Chromosome 5, interstitial del 5q[84] | 4825 | | | |

| Syndrome or condition | Inheritance[a] | MIM No. POSSUM No.[b] | Ear, nose, and throat manifestations | Other systemic manifestations |
|---|---|---|---|---|
| Chromosome 6, partial dup 6p[99] | 3075 | | | |
| Chromosome 9, dup 9q[119] | 3117 | | | |
| Chromosome 9, partial dup 9p[127] | 3079 | | | |
| Chromosome X, fra Xq27[24] | 3324 | | | |
| Chromosome 10, distal dup 10q[93] | 3083 | | | |
| Chromosome 12, del 12p13[11] | 4775 | | | |
| Chromosome 13, partial dup 13p[170] | 3119 | | | |
| Chromosome 18, i18p[5] | 3702 | | | |
| Chromosome 21, monosomy 21[12] | 3598 | | | |
| Craniofacial dysostosis, diaphyseal hyperplasia, or Dominant osteo-sclerosis, Stanescu type[77] | **122900** 3159 | AD | Midface hypoplasia, microdontia, micrognathia | Short stature, proptosis, brachycephaly, rhizomelic limb shortness, brachydactyly, dense and long bones, diaphyseal abnormality |
| Floating-Harbor syndrome[86] | **136140** 4126 | AD | Midface hypoplasia, beaked nose, broad nasal bridge, bulbous nasal tip, thin lips, macrostomia, low-set or posteriorly angulated ears, abnormal helix, short neck | IUGR, short stature, dolichocephaly, hirsutism, triangular face, deep-set eyes, small hands, hyperextensible fingers, limited elbow extension |
| Gingival fibromatosis, hepatosplenomegaly, other anomalies, or Zimmermann-Laband syndrome[153] | ***135500** 3433 | AD | High-arched palate, fissured and large tongue, thickened gingiva, protruding lips, long ear | Hepatosplenomegaly, hirsutism, absent or small nails, coarse facies, hyperextensible joints, MR |
| Hirschsprung disease, unusual facies, microcephaly, or Goldberg-Shprintzen syndrome[189] | **235730** 4119 | AR | Cleft lip, cleft soft/hard palate, anteverted ears | Microcephaly, short stature, blepharophimosis, telecanthus, Hirschsprung disease, cardiac defect, cryptorchidism, hydrocephaly, epilepsy, MR |
| Hyper IgE syndrome or Job's syndrome[68] | **147060** 4777 | ?AD | Midface hypoplasia, broad or bulbous nasal tip | Eczema, recurrent skin and respiratory infections, conjunctivitis, occasional bone or visceral infections, eosinophilia, elevated IgE and erythrocyte sedimentation rate (ESR), coarse facies, hypertelorism |
| Langer-Giedion syndrome or tricho-rhino-phalangeal syndrome, type 2[122] | ***150230** 3416 | ?AD Contiguous gene syndrome | Anteverted or small nostrils, colobomas of nostrils, abnormal columella, thin lips, long philtrum, low-set ears, conductive deafness, limited opening of mouth | Short stature, sparse, fine hair, microcephaly, thick eyebrows, multiple exostosis, multiple fractures, hypotonia, anemia, MR (variable) [deletion 8q24] |
| MR, spastic paraplegia, palmoplantar hyperkeratosis, or Fitzsimmons syndrome[53] | **309560** 3596 | ?XLR | High nasal bridge, nystagmus | Palmar or plantar hyperkeratosis, sparse scalp hair, dysplastic nails, spastic paraplegia, MR |
| Microcephaly, immunodeficiency, lymphoreticular malignancies, or Seemanová syndrome[173] | ***251260** 3176 | AR | High nasal bridge, short neck | Microcephaly with sloping forehead, bird-like facies, cellular and humoral immune deficiency, increased risk to lymphoreticular malignancies, normal intelligence |
| Nijmegen breakage syndrome[184] | ***251260** 4374 | AR | Narrow nasal bridge, low-set ears, micrognathia | Microcephaly, fine hair, telecanthus, stunted growth, café-au-lait spots, immunodeficiency, increased chromosomal breakage or rearrangements, increased sensitivity to ionizing radiation, malignancies, variable intellectual capabilities |

**Appendix C-2** Syndromes and conditions associated with long and large nose (*Continued*)

| Syndrome or condition | MIM No. POSSUM No.[a] | Inheritance[b] | Other ear, nose, and throat anomalies | Other manifestations |
|---|---|---|---|---|
| Oculo-dento-digital dysplasia or oculo-dento-osseous dysplasia[203] | ***164200** 3341 | AD | Broad nasal bridge, hypoplastic nostrils, long columella, cleft palate, dental enamel hypoplasia, broad alveolar ridge, conductive deafness | Microphthalmia, camptodactyly of 4th and 5th fingers, syndactyly of fingers and toes, macrocephaly, microcephaly, sparse hair, spasticity, symphalangism |
| Osteodysplastic primordial dwarfism, type 1[72,132] | **210710** 4596 | | See under "beaked nose" | |
| Patterson syndrome[35] | **169170** 3494 | | See under broad and bulbous nasal tip | |
| RAPADILINO syndrome RA: RAdial, PA: PAtellae and cleft or highly-arched PAlate, DI: DIarrhea and DIslocated joints, LI: Little size and LImb malformation, NO: NOse slender and NOrmal intelligence)[205] | **266280** 4733 | AR | Broad nasal bridge, cleft soft palate, high-arched palate, abnormal voice, micrognathia | Short stature, radial ray defects, small patella, dislocations, hypoplastic thumbs, hypertelorism, epicanthic folds, normal intelligence |
| Rubinstein-Taybi syndrome[79,111] | **180849** 3384 | | See under "beaked nose" | |
| Seckel syndrome[78] | **210600** 3387 | | See under "beaked nose" | |
| Short limb dwarfism resembling Grebe chondrodysplasia[194] | 4129 | ?AD | Broad and bulbous nasal tip, conductive deafness | Short stature, severe shortness of limbs—mostly mesomelic, irregular ossification, contractures, irregular length and shape of fingers and toes, round face, hypertelorism, antimongoloid slant of palpebral fissures |
| Tel-Hashomer camptodactyly[55] | ***211960** 3051 | AR | Broad nasal bridge, long philtrum, microstomia, droopy lower lip, microtia | Short stature, facial asymmetry, hypertelorism, spindle-shaped fingers, mild syndactyly, camptodactyly, muscular hypoplasia, abnormal dermatoglyphics |
| Velo-cardio-facial syndrome or Shprintzen syndrome[136] | **#192430** 3132 | AD contiguous gene syndrome | High, broad nasal bridge, abnormal nasal septum, cleft palate (may be submucous), nasal tone | Short stature, microcephaly, narrow face, cardiac defect, right-sided aortic arch, slender, tapering fingers, DiGeorge anomaly, MR, gene location 22q 11.2 |
| Winchester syndrome[215] | ***277950** 3428 | AR | Depressed nasal bridge, thick lips, thickened gingivae, atlantoaxial instability | Short stature, coarse facies, osteoporosis, carpotarsal osteolysis and progressive rheumatoid-like small joint destruction, contractures, scoliosis, corneal opacities |

**Appendix C-3** Syndromes and conditions associated with short or small nose and/or anteverted nostrils

| Syndrome or condition | MIM No. POSSUM No.[a] | Inheritance[b] | Other ear, nose, and throat anomalies | Other manifestations |
|---|---|---|---|---|
| Aarskog syndrome or facio-digito-genital syndrome[51,196] | ***305400** 3001 | XLR ?AD | Broad nasal bridge, long philtrum, low-set or posteriorly angulated ears, transverse crease below the lower lip | Short stature, round facies, hypertelorism, brachydactyly, interdigital webbing, inguinal or umbilical hernia, shawl scrotum, hyperextensible joints, normal to borderline intelligence, gene location Xp11.21 |
| Achondrogenesis, type 1[19] | ***200600** 3004 | AR | Midface hypoplasia, depressed nasal bridge, flattened nose, microstomia, long philtrum, low-set ears, short neck | Lethal short-limb dwarfism, deficient ossification of skull, vertebral bodies, and pelvic bones, severe micromelia, thin and short ribs, fractures, metaphyseal spurs |

| Syndrome or condition | Inheritance[a] | MIM No. POSSUM No.[b] | Ear, nose, and throat manifestations | Other systemic manifestations |
|---|---|---|---|---|
| Achondrogenesis, type 2[19,178] | **#200610** 3037 | AR | Flat face, depressed nasal bridge, short neck | Compared to achondrogenesis type 1: better skull ossification, less severe micromelia, partially ossified spine and ribs, no fractures, proposed gene location 12p12 |
| Achondroplasia[182] | ***100800** 3006 | AD | Midface hypoplasia, depressed nasal bridge, conductive deafness, prognathism | Short stature (may be normal at birth), macrocephaly, short limbs, trident hands, decreased interpedicular distance of lumbosacral spine, risk of spinal compression, acetabular bone spurs, homozygotes are severely affected |
| Acrocallosal syndrome[23] | ***200990** 3555 | AR | Broad nasal bridge everted lips, short philtrum, cleft palate, low-set or posteriorly angulated ears | High forehead, hypertelorism, macrocephaly, absent corpus callosum, postaxial and preaxial polydactyly, cardiac defect, MR |
| Acrodysostosis[209] | **101800** 3011 | | See under "broad and bulbous nasal tip" | |
| Acromesomelic dysplasia, Maroteaux type[115] | ***201250** 3015 | AR | Flat face or depressed maxilla | Short stature, short distal limbs (acromelic and mesomelic), brachydactyly, frontal bossing, cone-shaped epiphyses, limited elbow extension, redundant skin, lower thoracic kyphosis, normal intelligence |
| Antley-Bixler syndrome[48] | ***207410** 3570 | AR | Midface hypoplasia, choanal atresia or stenosis, long philtrum, microstomia, microtia or low-set ears | Craniosynostosis, hydrocephalus, brachycephaly, radiohumeral synostosis, joint contractures, bowed femurs, arachnodactyly, early death |
| Apert syndrome[30,150] | **101200** 3007 | | See under "beaked nose" | |
| Bloom syndrome[62] | ***210900** 3040 | AD | Midface hypoplasia, butterfly erythema on the midface and around the nose, high-pitched voice, micrognathia, anteverted ears | IUGR, short stature, microcephaly, telangiectasia, prone to infections and at increased risk of developing malignancy, mild MR, excessive chromosomal breaks in cell culture with increased frequency of sister chromatid exchanges |
| Brachmann-de Lange syndrome[90,139] | **122470** 3183 | Uncertain ?AR ?AD | Flared nostrils, thin lips and down- turned angles | IUGR, short stature, microcephaly, characteristic facies with synophrys and long eyelashes, micromelia or oligodactyly, single palmar creases, cardiac defect, severe MR, shortened survival |
| Camptomelic dysplasia or campomelic dysplasia or dwarfism[124] | ***211970** 3049 | AR | Midface hypoplasia, depressed nasal bridge, choanal atresia, micrognathia, long philtrum, cleft soft/hard palate, tracheal cartilage, hypoplasia | Short-limb dwarfism, bowed limbs, pretibial skin dimples (characteristic), hypoplastic scapulae, 11 pairs of ribs, cardiac defect, sex reversal, early death |
| Chondrodysplasia punctata[216] | ***302950** 3737 | XLR | Broad or depressed nasal bridge, sensorineural and conductive deafness, short neck | Short stature, short limbs, punctate calcification (epiphyseal stippling), terminal hypoplasia of fingers and toes, cicatricial alopecia, ichthyosis, MR, hypoplastic or cystic kidneys, proposed gene location Xp22.32 |
| Chromosome abnormalities | | | | |
| Chromosome 1, del 1q (q21→q25)[116] | 3112 | | | |

**Appendix C-3** Syndromes and conditions associated with short or small nose and/or anteverted nostrils (*Continued*)

| Syndrome or condition | MIM No. POSSUM No.[a] | Inheritance[b] | Other ear, nose, and throat anomalies | Other manifestations |
|---|---|---|---|---|
| Chromosome 3, partial dup 3p[212] | 3067 | | | |
| Chromosome 4, partial dup 4p[82] | 3070 | | | |
| Chromosome 8, partial del 8p[42] | 3691 | | | |
| Chromosome 8, partial dup 8p[107] | 3078 | | | |
| Chromosome 9, partial del 9p[195] | 3081 | | | |
| Chromosome 9, trisomy 9[183] | 3080 | | | |
| Chromosome 10, proximal dup 10q[39] | 4863 | | | |
| Chromosome 18, partial dup 18q[217] | 3699 | | | |
| Chromosome 20, partial dup 20p[70] | 3099 | | | |
| Cockayne syndrome[140] | ***216400** 3149 | AR | Nystagmus, dental caries, sensorineural deafness | Normal early growth and development, variable age of onset, progressive growth deficiency, early senile changes with dementia, retinal pigmentation, optic atrophy, cataract, corneal cloudiness, premature graying of hair, aged face, osteoporosis, hypogonadism, hypertension, proposed gene location 18q11, 10q21 |
| Coffin-Lowry syndrome[148] | ***303600** 3150 | XLR | Bulbous nose, thick nostrils and nasal septum, large mouth, thick everted lower lips, sensorineural deafness | In infancy: hypertelorism, hypotonia, spindle-shaped fingers, developmental delay. At older age: coarse facies, antimongoloid slant of palpebral fissures, ENT manifestations, tapering fingers, delayed skeletal maturation, hypotonia, MR, proposed gene location Xp22.2–p22.1 |
| Femoral hypoplasia–unusual facies syndrome[114] | **134780** 3232 | ?AD | Hypoplastic nostrils, cleft palate, long philtrum, micrognathia, thin lips | Short stature, hypoplastic or absent femur, restricted elbow movement, synostosis, vertebral segmentation defects, genitourinary abnormalities |
| Fetal alcohol syndrome[57] | ***100650** 3218 | Teratogenicity | Smooth, long philtrum, thin and smooth upper lip | Variable manifestations, facial appearance may be subtle, IUGR, microcephaly, short palpebral fissures, hirsutism, cardiac and renal defects, MR (mild to borderline), history of alcohol consumption is useful in establishing diagnosis |
| Fetal hydantoin syndrome or fetal dilantin syndrome[130] | 3221 | Teratogenicity | Broad nasal bridge, broad alveolar ridge, cleft lip/palate, short neck | Wide anterior fontanelle, metopic ridging, hypertelorism, distal digital hypoplasia, small nails (especially the 5th), hirsutism, growth deficiency, mild MR |
| Fetal trimethadione syndrome or tridione syndrome[32] | 3980 | Teratogenicity | Broad nasal bridge cleft lip/palate, folded or low-set ear | IUGR, postnatal growth deficiency, brachycephaly, V-shaped eyebrows, cardiac defects, single palmar creases, tapering fingers, ambiguous genitalia, hypospadias |

| Syndrome or condition | MIM No. POSSUM No.[b] | Inheritance[a] | Ear, nose, and throat manifestations | Other systemic manifestations |
|---|---|---|---|---|
| Fetal valproate syndrome[199] | 3650 | Teratogenicity | Broad and flat nasal bridge, long, flat philtrum, microstomia, thin upper and thick lower lips, cleft lip | Narrow forehead, epicanthic folds, long, thin fingers and toes, hyperconvex nails, radial ray defects, cardiac defects, increased risk of neural tube defects |
| Fetal warfarin syndrome or Warfarin embryopathy[218] | 3227 | Teratogenicity | Nasal hypoplasia with deep groove between the nostrils and nasal tip | Stippled epiphyses in axial skeleton, proximal femur and calcaneus, short fingers, hypoplastic nails, mild growth deficiency, mild MR |
| Fibrochondrogenesis[8] | ***228520** 3642 | AR | Marked nasal hypoplasia, absent nasal cartilage, abnormal nasal septum, microstomia, cleft palate, posteriorly angulated ears, microtia, short neck | Short-limb dwarfism (rhizomelic) short ribs, broad forehead, scalp defect, platyspondyly, coronal and saggital defects of the vertebral bodies, metaphyseal abnormality, CNS defects, early death |
| Fronto-facio-nasal dysplasia[60] | **229400** 3511 | | See under "cleft nose tip" | |
| Fryns syndrome[129] | ***229850** 3608 | AR | Broad nasal bridge, cleft lip/palate, macrostomia, thin lips, micrognathia, low-set or posteriorly angulated ears, microtia, short or webbed neck | Macrocephaly, coarse facies, distal digital hypoplasia, hypoplastic lungs, diaphragmatic hernia, intestinal and urogenital anomalies, CNS anomalies, stillbirth or early death |
| Geleophysic dysplasia or geleophysic dwarfism[180] | ***231050** 3459 | AR | Long philtrum, thick lips, micrognathia, tracheal narrowing | Coarse facies, pleasant personality, hypertelorism, short stature, progressive restriction of joint movement, brachydactyly, dysostosis multiplex, hepatomegaly, (storage of mucopolysaccarides), thickened mitral and pulmonary valves |
| Hallermann-Streiff syndrome[26,104] | **234100** 3342 | | See under "beaked nose" | |
| Johanson-Blizzard syndrome[64,89] | **243800** 3269 | | See under "beaked nose" | |
| Killian-Teschler-Nicola syndrome or Pallister-Killian syndrome[171] | 3800 | Chromosomal | Broad and depressed nasal bridge, cleft palate, macroglossia, grooved philtrum, macrostomia, down-turned mouth angles, prognathism, large, low-set ears, thickened helix, short or webbed neck, laryngeal abnormality | Short stature, coarse facies, broad and high forehead, hypertelorism, epicanthic folds, sparse scalp hair, camptodactyly, terminal hypoplasia of fingers, hypoplastic lung, cardiac defects, diaphragmatic hernia, imperforate anus, sacral dimple, caudal appendage, skin hypoplasia or pigmentary changes, hypotonia, seizures, MR, mosaic tetrasomy 12p in fibroblasts |
| Miller-Dieker syndrome[45] | 3134 | Chromosomal | Broad nasal bridge, grooved philtrum, everted lips, micrognathia, low-set or posteriorly angulated ears | IUGR, short stature, microcephaly, low anterior and posterior hair line, high forehead, bitemporal narrowing, vertical skin folds over forehead, post-axial polydactyly, single palmar creases, agenesis of corpus callosum, hypotonia, MR, deletion 17p(13.3) |
| Naguib-Richeiri-Costa syndrome[192] | **239710** 4402 | AR | Broad and depressed nasal bridge, grooved philtrum, macrostomia, droopy lower lip, anteverted ears | Normal growth and development, ptosis, hypertelorism, bifid thumb, polydactyly, cutaneous syndactyly, hypospadias, shawl scrotum |

**Appendix C-3** Syndromes and conditions associated with short or small nose and/or anteverted nostrils (*Continued*)

| Syndrome or condition | MIM No. POSSUM No.[a] | Inheritance[b] | Other ear, nose, and throat anomalies | Other manifestations |
|---|---|---|---|---|
| Osteogenesis imperfecta, type 2[21] | **#166210** 3366 | AD | Midface hypoplasia, depressed nasal bridge | Short stature, short bowed limbs, brachycephaly, large fontanelle, poorly ossified calvarium, blue sclerae, platyspondyly, osteoporosis, multiple fractures, stillbirth, early death |
| Oto-palato-digital syndrome type 1 or Taybi syndrome[83] | ***311300** 3352 | XL Semi-dominant | Broad nasal bridge, cleft soft/hard palate, microstomia, conductive deafness, low-set ears | Short stature, frontal bossing, hypertelorism, prominent supraorbital ridges, limited elbow extension, broad terminal phalanges, short nails, mild MR |
| Oto-palato-digital syndrome, type 2[156] | ***311300** 3710 | XLD | Flat and broad nasal bridge, microstomia, down-turned mouth angles, cleft palate, micrognathia, conductive or sensorineural deafness, low-set or posteriorly angulated ears, short neck | Growth deficiency, high forehead, wide anterior fontanelle and cranial sutures, hypertelorism, antimongoloid slant of palpebral fissures, overlapping fingers, polydactyly, syndactyly; long, curved clavicle; bowed forearms and legs, joint dislocations, cardiac and CNS defects |
| Pfeiffer syndrome or acrocephaly-syndactyly, type 5[28] | ***101600** 3008 | AD | Midface hypoplasia, depressed nasal bridge, choanal stenosis or atresia, long philtrum | Acrocephaly, brachycephaly, craniosynostosis, cloverleaf skull, frontal bossing, hypertelorism, antimongoloid slant of palpebral fissures, proptosis, broad thumbs and great toes, mild syndactyly of fingers and toes, 5th finger clinodactyly, seizures and MR (uncommon) |
| Robinow syndrome or fetal face syndrome[191] | ***180700** 3379 | AD AR | Depressed nasal bridge, long philtrum, triangular mouth, macrostomia, broad alveolar ridge, micrognathia, short neck | Short stature, short limbs (mesomelic), macrocephaly, fetal face with wide palpebral fissures and hypertelorism, brachydactyly, hypoplastic genitalia, normal intelligence (usually) |
| Rothmund-Thomson syndrome or Poikiloderma congenita[40,145] | ***268400** 3383 | AR | Depressed nasal bridge | Short stature, alopecia, irregular erythema, telangiectasia, cutis marmorata, irregular pigmentation, skin atrophy, photosensitivity, juvenile cataract, dysplastic nails, patchy sclerosis and abnormal trabeculation of bone, slender diaphyses, osteoporosis, limb deficiency, MR, risk of skin cancer, in vitro chromosomal instability |
| Ruvalcaba syndrome[15] | **180870** 3131 | | See under "beaked nose" | |
| Simpson-Golabi-Behmel syndrome or Golabi-Rosen syndrome[146] | ***312870** 3325 | XLR | Broad and high nasal bridge, cleft lip/palate, high-arched and narrow palate, macrostomia, everted lips, macroglossia, prognathism, preauricular skin tags | Large birth weight, coarse facies, hypertelorism, macrocephaly, tall stature, large hands, syndactyly of fingers and toes, polydactyly, advanced bone age, hypotonia, cardiac and genitourinary defects |
| Stickler syndrome or hereditary progressive arthro-ophthalmopathy[210] | ***108300** 3030 | AD | Neonate may present as Pierre Robin sequence, depressed nasal bridge, midface hypoplasia, mandibular hypoplasia, cleft soft/hard palate or uvula, sensorineural or conductive deafness | Marfanoid build, flat face, bulky joints, arthritis, coxa valga, high-grade myopia, retinal detachment scoliosis, mitral valve prolapse, spondyloepiphyseal dysplasia |
| Teebi hypertelorism syndrome[190,201] | **145420** 4539 | AD | Broad, depressed nasal bridge, midface hypoplasia, broad and bulbous nasal tip, long, grooved | Broad forehead, pronounced hypertelorism, antimongoloid slant of palpebral fissures, thick eye- |

| Syndrome or condition | Inheritance[a] | MIM No. POSSUM No.[b] | Ear, nose, and throat manifestations | Other systemic manifestations |
|---|---|---|---|---|
| | | | philtrum, high-arched and narrow palate, prognathism, posteriorly angulated ears, large ear lobule | brows, small webbed fingers, shawl scrotum, normal stature and intelligence |
| Teebi overgrowth syndrome[197] | **277590** 4738 | AR | Depressed nasal bridge, long philtrum, posteriorly angulated ears, large ear lobule, serrated gum, hoarse cry, short neck | Large birth weight, tall stature, sparse scalp hair, macrocephaly, long palpebral fissures or antimongoloid slant, loose skin, joint laxity, fifth finger clinodactyly, long great toe, advanced bone age, hypotonia, mild MR |
| Toriello-Carey syndrome[92] | **217980** 4568 | AR | Cleft soft/hard palate, glossoptosis, micrognathia, broad nasal bridge, flattened nose, low-set or posteriorly angulated ears, sensorineural deafness, laryngeal abnormality, abnormal voice | IUGR, short stature, microcephaly, blepharophimosis, telecanthus, agenesis of corpus callosum, small hands, cardiac defects, hypotonia, seizures |
| Whistling face syndrome or Freeman-Sheldon syndrome[33] | **193700** 3156 | | See under "broad and bulbous nasal tip" | |
| Williams syndrome[49,137] | **#194050** 3427 | Sporadic ?AD | Depressed nasal bridge, broad and bulbous nasal tip, macrostomia, droopy lower lip, open mouth, thick lips, dental abnormalities, long philtrum, abnormal voice | Early irritability, hypotonia, constipation and feeding difficulties, elongated, "elfin"-like facies with puffy eyelids, full cheeks, progressive joint stiffness and contractures, aortic stenosis, short stature, occasional hypercalcemia, growth and developmental delay, outgoing, happy personality, deletion in the elastin gene (7q) |

**Appendix C-4** Syndromes and conditions associated with broad or bulbous nasal tip

| Syndrome or condition | MIM No. POSSUM No.[a] | Inheritance[b] | Other ear, nose, and throat anomalies | Other manifestations |
|---|---|---|---|---|
| Acrodysostosis[209] | ***101800** 3011 | AD | Short nose, low and flat nasal bridge, long philtrum, anteverted and flared nostrils, absent nasal cartilage, abnormal septum, short columella | Short stature, short limbs (acromelic), brachydactyly, loose and wrinkled skin, progressive restriction of joint movement with arthritis, vertebral abnormalities, metaphyseal changes, cone-shaped epiphyses, MR (common) |
| Blepharo-naso-facial syndrome[149] | **110050** 3039 | AD | See under "long and large nose" | |
| Coffin-Siris syndrome[206] | **135900** 3151 | AD | Broad and depressed nasal bridge, anteverted nostrils, choanal atresia or stenosis, macrostomia, everted thick lips, short philtrum, cleft palate | IUGR, short stature, coarse facies, hirsutism with tendency to have sparse scalp hair, hypoplastic or absent 5th finger and toe nails, lax joint, small patellae, hypotonia, MR |
| Craniorhiny[135] | **123050** 4828 | AD | Prominent maxilla, nasolacrimal duct defect, short nose, anteverted nostrils, abnormal columella, long philtrum | Acrocephaly, craniosynostosis, hypertelorism, flat supraorbital ridges |
| Dwarfism with "gloomy face" or gloomy face syndrome[117] | **231520** 4886 | AR | Broad nasal bridge anteverted nostrils, thick lips, long philtrum | Pre- and postnatal growth retardation, relative macrocephaly, "gloomy face;" broad, high forehead; downward slanting palpebral fissures, small hand and feet, hyperextensible joints |
| Floating Harbor syndrome[86] | **136140** 4126 | | See under "long and large nose" | |
| Hyper IgE syndrome[68] | **147060** 4777 | | See under "long and large nose" | |

**Appendix C-4** Syndromes and conditions associated with broad or bulbous nasal tip (*Continued*)

| Syndrome or condition | MIM No. POSSUM No.[a] | Inheritance[b] | Other ear, nose, and throat anomalies | Other manifestations |
|---|---|---|---|---|
| Kabuki make-up syndrome[108,172] | **147920** 3541 | | See under "beaked nose" | |
| Noonan syndrome or Turner-like syndrome[134] | ***163950** 3335 | AD | Down-turned mouth angles, grooved philtrum, high-arched and narrow cleft palate, low-set or posteriorly angulated ears, short and broad neck with excess skin, low posterior hair line | Short stature, broad forehead, hypertelorism, antimongoloid slant of palpebral fissures, ptosis, shield chest, pectus deformity, cubitus valgus, pulmonary stenosis or other cardiac defects, cryptorchidism, normal intelligence, occasional MR, gene location 12q |
| Ohdo-blepharophimosis syndrome[133] | **249620** 3875 | | See under "abnormal columella and nasal septum" | |
| Patterson syndrome[35] | **169170** 3494 | AD | Prominent maxilla, large nose, thick lips, long and large ears, atlantoaxial instability, odontoid hypoplasia | IUGR, failure to thrive, hirsutism, lack of subcutaneous fat, redundant skin folds, particularly of limbs, joint deformities, kyphoscoliosis, large hands and feet, grossly abnormal metaphyses, noncalcified epiphyses, diabetes, cushingoid manifestations, severe MR |
| Ruvalcaba syndrome[15] | **180870** 3131 | | See under "beaked nose" | |
| Short-limb dwarf resembling Grebe chondrodysplasia[190] | 4129 | | See under "long and large nose" | |
| Smith-Lemli-Opitz syndrome[110,144] | ***270400** 3391 | AR | Broad nasal bridge, anteverted and flared nostrils, high-arched, cleft, soft/hard palate, broad alveolar ridge, low-set or posteriorly angulated ears | Short stature, failure to thrive, microcephaly, narrow forehead, epicanthic folds; ptosis, syndactyly of the second and third toes, overriding toes, polydactyly, cryptorchidism, ambiguous genitalia, hypospadias, altered tone, severe MR, defect in 7-dehydro cholesterol reductase |
| Teebi hypertelorism syndrome[195,201] | **145420** 4539 | | See under "short and small nose" | |
| Tricho-rhino-phalangeal syndrome, type 1[125] | ***190350** 3415 | AD ?AR | Pear-shaped prominent nose, broad nasal bridge, hypoplastic nostrils, abnormal columella, micrognathia, horizontal groove of the chin, large ears, deep voice, long philtrum | Short stature, sparse hair,short metacarpals and metatarsals, conoid epiphyses |
| Velo-cardio-facial syndrome[136] | | | See under "long and large nose" | |
| Weaver-Williams syndrome[213] | 4046 | ?AR | Midface hypoplasia, flat cheeks, broad nasal bridge, down-turned mouth angles, microstomia, cleft palate, micrognathia, large and anteverted ears, hearing abnormality, long neck | Thin body with failure to thrive, microcephaly, hypertelorism, osteoporosis, vertebral defects, delayed skeletal maturation, hypoplastic ulna and fibula, camptodactyly, MR |
| Whistling face syndrome or Freeman-Sheldon syndrome[33,124a] | ***193700** **277720** 3156 | AD AR | Midface hypoplasia, small and short nose, hypoplastic nostrils ± coloboma, micrognathia or retrognathia, H-shaped skin creases, microstomia, puckered appearance of the mouth, small tongue, high-arched palate, limited palatal movement and nasal speech, neck webbing | Short stature, frontal bossing, myopathic mask face, hypertelorism, downward slanting palpebral fissures, epicanthic folds, ptosis, vomiting and feeding difficulty in infancy, ulnar deviation of fingers, camptodactyly, talipes deformity, axillary webbing, kyphoscoliosis, MR |
| Williams syndrome[49,137] | **194050** 3427 | | See under "short and small nose" | |

**Appendix C-5** Syndromes and conditions associated with cleft nose or bifid tip

| Syndrome or condition | MIM No. POSSUM No.[a] | Inheritance[b] | Other ear, nose, and throat anomalies | Other manifestations |
|---|---|---|---|---|
| Alar coloboma with telecanthus or frontonasal dysplasia with alar cleft[54] | **203000** 3981 | AR | See under "beaked nose" | |
| Chromosome 6, partial dup 6p[38] | 3075 | | | |
| Craniofrontonasal dysplasia[98] | **304110** 3798 | XLD ?AD | Broad nasal bridge, high-arched, cleft palate, dental malocclusion, low-set or posteriorly angulated ears, deafness, (mixed), short or webbed neck | Acrocephaly, plagiocephaly, brachycephaly, coronal synostosis, marked hypertelorism, antimongoloid slant of palpebral fissures, facial asymmetry, high clavicles, winged scapulae, bifid thumbs, preaxial polydactyly, longitudinal splitting or grooving of nails, hypotonia, normal intelligence, MR in some cases |
| Fronto-facio-nasal dysplasia[60] | ***229400** 3511 | AR | Midface hypoplasia, broad and high nasal bridge, small nose, anteverted or hypoplastic nostrils and colobomas, abnormal columella, lateral or median cleft lip, cleft palate, nasal lipomas | Brachycephaly, frontal bossing, facial asymmetry, hypertelorism, blepharophimosis, microphthalmia, ptosis, iris coloboma, epibulbar dermoid, corpus callosum abnormality, encephalocele |
| Frontonasal dysplasia or median cleft face syndrome[58,198] | **136760** 3288 | ?AD Mostly Sporadic | Midface hypoplasia, broad nasal bridge, broad nose, coloboma of nostrils, abnormal columella, median cleft lip/palate, lateral cleft lip, oral synechiae or frenulae, low-set ears, sensorineural deafness | Cranium bifidum occultum, widow's peak, hypertelorism, central bony facial cleft, telecanthus, microphthalmia, ocular coloboma, epibulbar dermoid, agenesis or lipoma of the corpus callosum, encephalocele, cardiac defect, MR |
| Frontonasal dysplasia, congenital heart disease[131] | 4684 | ? | Similar to frontonasal dysplasia | IUGR, microcephaly, short stature, round face, cardiac defect, shawl scrotum, cryptorchidism, camptodactyly, delayed skeletal maturation, mild to borderline MR |
| Frontonasal dysplasia with MCA, Toriello type[202,208] | 4770 | AR | Similar to severe frontonasal dysplasia | Widow's peak, hypertelorism, epibulbar dermoid, tibial hypoplasia, duplicated great toes, hydrocephalus or dilated cerebral ventricles, agenesis of corpus callosum, Dandy-Walker malformation, encephalocele or meningocele |
| Hydrolethalus syndrome[174] | ***236680** 3567 | AR | Flattened nose, lateral cleft lip, cleft palate, tongue anomaly, micrognathia, laryngeal and tracheal abnormality | Macrocephaly, hydrocephalus, hypertelorism, deep-set eyes, cerebrocerebellar micropolygyria, agenesis of the corpus callosum, abnormal lung lobulation, bifid great toe, postaxial polydactyly of hands and feet, talipes deformity, cardiac defect, stillbirth or early death |
| Hypertelorism, microtia, clefting syndrome, or Bixler syndrome[17] | ***239800** 3259 | AR | Broad nasal bridge, lateral cleft lip/palate, microtia, atresia of external auditory canal, conductive deafness, microstomia | Short stature, microcephaly, marked hypertelorism and telecanthus, cardiac defect, ureteric abnormalities, horseshoe kidneys, MR |
| Oral-facial-digital, type 2, or Mohr syndrome[160] | ***252100** 3384 | AR | Low nasal bridge, broad nasal tip, midline partial cleft of lip, midline cleft tongue and uvula, tongue hamartoma, micrognathia, conductive deafness due to defect of incus, absent central incisors | Short stature, facial asymmetry, coarse hair, pre-postaxial polydactyly of hands and feet, bilateral bifid great toes, CNS anomalies, normal intelligence |

**Appendix C-6** Syndromes and conditions associated with abnormal columella or nasal septum

| Syndrome or condition | MIM No. POSSUM No.[a] | Inheritance[b] | Other ear, nose, and throat anomalies | Other manifestations |
|---|---|---|---|---|
| Acrodysostosis[209] | **101800**<br>3011 | ?AD | See under "broad and bulbous nasal tip" | |
| Alar coloboma with telecanthus[54] | **203000**<br>3981 | | See under "beaked nose" | |
| Autosomal dominant trigonocephaly[59,80] | **190440**<br>3058 | AD | See under "beaked nose" | |
| CHARGE association[111] | 3480 | | See under "choanal atresia" | |
| Chondrodysplasia punctata, mild type, or Binder syndrome[159,176] | ***302950**<br>3065<br>3330 | XLR | Midface hypoplasia, flat nose, anteverted nostrils, abnormal columella, atlantoaxial anomalies | Short stature, normal proportions, stippled epiphyses, punctate calcification, polydactyly, vertebral body clefts, diaphragmatic hernia |
| Chromosome 4, partial del 4p[169] | 3069 | | | |
| Chromosome 6, partial dup 6q[38] | 3689 | | | |
| Chromosome X, fra Xq 27[24] | 3324 | | | |
| Craniorhiny[135] | **123050**<br>4828 | ?AD | See under "broad and bulbous nasal tip" | |
| Cutis Laxa[14,34,167] | ***123700**<br>***219100**<br>***219200**<br>***304150**<br>3180 | | See under "beaked nose" | |
| Floating-Harbor syndrome[86] | **136140**<br>4126 | | See under "long and large nose" | |
| Fronto-facio-nasal dysplasia[60] | ***229400**<br>3511 | | See under "cleft nose and bifid tip" | |
| Frontonasal dysplasia[58,198] | **136760**<br>3288 | | See under "cleft nose and bifid tip" | |
| Kabuki make-up syndrome[108,172] | **147920**<br>3541 | | See under "beaked nose" | |
| Keutel syndrome[103] | ***245150**<br>3675 | AR | Flat midface, flattened nose, hypoplastic nostril, abnormal columella, macrostoma, thick lips; grooved, short philtrum; macroglossia, sensorineural deafness, anteverted ears, calcified ear cartilage, calcified larynx and tracheal rings | Hypertelorism, blepharophimosis, brachydactyly, terminal hypoplasia of fingers, peripheral pulmonary stenosis, cardiac defect, abnormal ossification and calcification, hypotonia, MR |
| Langer-Giedion syndrome[122] | **150230**<br>3416 | | See under "long and large nose" | |
| Ohdo blepharophimosis syndrome[133] | **249620**<br>3875 | AR | Flat nose, broad nasal tip, depressed nasal bridge, anteverted nostrils, abnormal columella, microstomia, everted lips; flat, long philtrum; short palate, hypoplastic teeth, low-set or anteverted ears, microtia, atresia of external auditory canal, conductive deafness | Blepharophimosis, ptosis, failure to thrive, camptodactyly, overriding toes, simian creases, cardiac defect, microcephaly, speech defect, MR |
| Perlman syndrome[71] | ***267000**<br>3643 | AR | Flat nasal bridge, short nasal septum, short nose and anteverted nostrils, everted lips, open mouth, high-arched palate, thickened gingivae, low-set ears | Hypotonic face with deep-set eyes, macrosomia, tall stature, macrocephaly, renal dysplasia, hamartoma, or Wilms tumour, hypertrophy of the islets of Langerhans, hepatosplenomegaly, cleft sternum, hypotonia, possible MR |
| Pilotto syndrome[151] | 4343 | | High nasal bridge, abnormal columella, cleft lip/palate, low-set or posteriorly-angulated ears, short neck | Short stature, microcephaly, brachycephaly, hypertelorism, facial asymmetry, retinal coloboma, vertebral defects, scoliosis, cardiac defect, mental retardation, spasticity, behavioral problems |

| Syndrome or condition | Inheritance[a] | MIM No. POSSUM No.[b] | Ear, nose, and throat manifestations | Other systemic manifestations |
|---|---|---|---|---|
| Pseudoprogeria[76] | **200130** 3867 | | See under "beaked nose" | |
| Rubinstein-Taybi syndrome[79,111] | **180849** 3384 | | See under "beaked nose" | |
| Saethre-Chotzen syndrome[141,161] | ***101400** 3009 | | See under "beaked nose" | |
| Tricho-rhino-phalangeal syndrome, type 1[125] | ***190350** 3415 | | See under "broad and bulbous nasal tip" | |
| Tricho-rhino-phalangeal syndrome, type 3[59,138] | 4413 | | See under "beaked nose" | |
| Velo-cardio-facial syndrome[136] | **#192430** 3132 | | See under "long and large nose" | |

**Appendix C-7** Syndromes and conditions associated with hypoplastic, small, flared nostrils, or coloboma of nostrils

| Syndrome or condition | MIM No. POSSUM No.[a] | Inheritance[b] | Other ear, nose, and throat anomalies | Other manifestations |
|---|---|---|---|---|
| Acrocephalopolysyndactyly type 4[63] | **201020** 3818 | | See under "long and large nose" | |
| Acrodysostosis[209] | **#101800** 3011 | | See under "broad and bulbous nasal tip" | |
| Amniotic band syndrome, including Limb-body wall complex[96,165] | 3621 4432 | Sporadic | Hypoplastic nostrils, lateral mouth cleft, cleft lip/palate | Ring constrictions, digit and limb amputations (asymmetric), syndactyly, facial clefting, evisceration of organs, scoliosis, anal atresia, anencephaly, encephalocele, holoprosencephaly, maybe stillbirth or early death, amniotic/fibrous bands may be present |
| Brachmann-de Lange syndrome[90,139] | **122470** 3183 | | See under "short and small nose" | |
| Coloboma of lens and nostrils[123] | 4182 | ? | Coloboma of nostrils | Lens coloboma, retinal dysplasia, myopia, scoliosis, vertebral defects (described in monozygotic twins) |
| Fetal warfarin syndrome[218] | 3227 | | See under "short and small nose" | |
| Fronto-facio-nasal dysplasia[60] | ***229400** 3511 | | See under "cleft nose, bifid tip" | |
| Frontonasal dysplasia | **136760** 3288 | | See under "cleft nose, bifid tip" | |
| Hallermann-Streiff syndrome[26,104] | **234100** 3342 | | See under "beaked nose" | |
| Johanson-Blizzard syndrome[64,89] | ***243800** 3269 | | See under "beaked nose" | |
| Keutel syndrome[103] | ***245150** 3675 | | See under "abnormal columella, nasal septum" | |
| Klein-Waardenburg syndrome[175] | **#148820** 3932 | | See under "absent nasal cartilage" | |
| Langer Giedion syndrome[122] | ***150230** 3416 | | See under "long, large nose" | |
| Mietens syndrome[211] | **249600** 3317 | AR | Small, narrow nose, hypoplastic, nostrils, nystagmus | Corneal opacity, flexion contractures of elbows, short radius and ulna, strabismus, borderline to mild MR |
| Oculo-dento-digital dysplasia[203] | **#164200** 3341 | | See under "long, large nose" | |
| Oral-facial-digital syndrome, type 1[9] | ***311200** 3347 | XLD | Absent lateral incisors, oral frenulae; partial clefts in mid-upper lip, tongue, and alveolar ridges; | Asymmetric shortening of digits, bifid great toe, syndactyly, clinodactyly, agenesis or hypoplasia of |

**Appendix C-7** Syndromes and conditions associated with hypoplastic, small, flared nostrils, or coloboma of nostrils (*Continued*)

| Syndrome or condition | MIM No. POSSUM No.[a] | Inheritance[b] | Other ear, nose, and throat anomalies | Other manifestations |
|---|---|---|---|---|
| | | | cleft palate, hypoplastic nostrils, hypoplastic nasal cartilage, milia of ears, choanal atresia | corpus callosum, seizures, variable MR |
| Roberts syndrome or pseudothalidomide syndrome[101,204] | ***268300** 3378 | AR | Cleft lip/palate, prominent premaxillary region, broad nasal bridge, hypoplastic nostrils, low-set or malformed ears, hypoplastic ear lobule, micrognathia | Tetramelic symmetrical limb reduction, oligodactyly, syndactyly, microcephaly, midfacial hemangioma, growth retardation, urogenital anomalies, cardiac defects, hydrocephalus, variable, MR |
| Ruvalcaba syndrome[15] | **180870** 3131 | | See under "beaked nose" | |
| Sandrow syndrome[105,126] | **135750** 4017 | AD | Broad nasal tip, abnormal columella, notched nostrils | Ulnar and fibular dimelia, supernumerary digits (mirror hands and feet), syndactyly, synostosis of phalanges, normal mental development |
| Smith-Lemli-Opitz syndrome[110,144] | ***270400** 3391 | | See under "broad, bulbous nasal tip" | |
| Tricho-rhino-phalangeal syndrome, type 1[125] | ***190350** 3415 | | See under "broad, bulbous nasal tip" | |
| Tricho-rhino-phalangeal syndrome, type 3 | 4413 | | See under "beaked nose" | |
| Velo-cardio-facial syndrome[136] | **#192430** 3132 | | See under "long, large nose" | |
| Whistling face syndrome[33,124a] | ***193700** **277720** 3156 | | See under "broad, bulbous nasal tip" | |

**Appendix C-8** Syndromes and conditions associated with choanal atresia or stenosis

| Syndrome or condition | MIM No. POSSUM No.[a] | Inheritance[b] | Other ear, nose, and throat anomalies | Other manifestations |
|---|---|---|---|---|
| Acro-cranio-facial dysostosis, Kaplan type[97] | **201050** 4407 | | See under "beaked nose" | |
| Antley-Bixler syndrome[48] | ***207410** 3570 | | See under "short, small nose" | |
| Apert syndrome[25,150] | ***101200** 3007 | | See under "beaked nose" | |
| Camptomelic dysplasia or campomelic dysplasia or dwarfism[124] | ***211970** 3049 | | See under "short, small nose" | |
| Chromosome 18, trisomy 18[22] | 3094 | | | |
| CHARGE association[111] | 3480 | Sporadic, unknown | Microtia, anteverted ears, malformed ear pinna, sensorineural or conductive deafness | **C**olobomatous malformation (common in retina) **H**eart defect **A**tresia choanae (membraneous or bony) **R**etarded growth and development **G**enital anomalies and hypogonadism **E**ar anomalies and deafness |
| Choanal atresia, lymphoedema[158] | **214800** 4265 | AR | High-arched palate | Lymphedema, hypoplastic nipples, pectus deformity |
| DiGeorge sequence[142] | ***188400** 3186 | Sporadic ?AD | Esophageal atresia | Third and fourth pharyngeal pouch abnormalities, thymic hypoplasia or aplasia with depressed cellular immunity, parathyroid hypoplasia or aplasia and hypocalcemia, aortic arch and cardiovascular abnormalities, hypertelorism, antimongoloid slant of palpebral fissures, deletion 22q11 |

| Condition or syndrome | Mode of inheritance[a] | MIM No. POSSUM No.[b] | Type of deafness[c] | Ear, nose, and throat manifestations | Other manifestations |
|---|---|---|---|---|---|
| Kaufman-McKusick syndrome[21,157] | ***236700** 3510 | | | Cleft palate, tracheal stenosis, esophageal atresia, tracheoesophageal fistula | Vaginal atresia, hydrometrocolpos, hydronephrosis, cardiac defect, postaxial polydactyly, macrocephaly, possible MR |
| Lenz-Majewski hyperostosis syndrome[163] | **151050** 3045 | AD | | Nasolacrimal duct stenosis, dysplastic enamel | Failure to thrive, macrocephaly, dense and thick bone, hypotrophic skin, symphalangism, syndactyly, sparse hair, hypertelorism, MR (absence of elastic fibers on skin biopsy) |
| Pfeiffer syndrome[28] | ***101600** 3008 | | | See under "short, small nose" | |
| Schinzel-Giedion syndrome[109] | **269150** 3025 | AR | | Midface hypoplasia, depressed nasal bridge, macroglossia, short or webbed neck | Wide fontanelles, hypertrichosis, coarse facies, proptosis, hypertelorism, mild shortness of limbs, hydronephrosis, hydroureter, genital anomalies, hypoplasia of distal phalanges, wide occipital synchondrosis, hypoplastic pubic bones, polydactyly, cardiac defect, hepatomegaly, hypotonia, MR |
| Treacher Collins syndrome or mandibulofacial dysostosis[44,162] | ***154500** 3283 | AD | | Malar hypoplasia or cleft in zygomatic bone, mandibular hypoplasia, cleft palate, macrostomia, malformed ear, conductive deafness, pharyngeal hypoplasia, tracheoesophageal fistula | Downward slanting palpebral fissures, coloboma of the lower lid, microphthalmia, heart defect, cryptorchidism, normal mental development |

**Appendix C-9** Syndromes and conditions associated with absent nasal cartilage

| Syndrome or condition | MIM No. POSSUM No.[a] | Inheritance[b] | Other ear, nose, and throat anomalies | Other manifestations |
|---|---|---|---|---|
| Acrodysostosis[209] | ***101800** 3011 | | See under broad, bulbous nasal tip | |
| Fibrochondrogenesis[8] | ***228520** 3642 | | See under short, small nose | |
| Holoprosencephaly with polydactyly or pseudotrisomy 13 syndrome[18,29] | **264480** 3982 | AR | Midline cleft lip, single nostril, cleft palate, microtia, low-set or posteriorly angulated ears, short neck | Holoprosencephaly, microphthalmia, polydactyly, limb shortness, early death (features of trisomy 13 but with normal karyotype) |
| Hypertelorism, hypospadias, tetralogy of Fallot[50] | **239711** 4776 | AR | Depressed nasal bridge, everted lips, long philtrum, dysphagia, low-set ears | Hypertelorism, hypospadias, tetralogy of Fallot, terminal broadening of phalanges |
| Klein-Waardenburg syndrome[175] | **#148820** 3932 | AD | Broad and high nasal bridge, coloboma of nostrils, droopy lower lip, sensorineural deafness | Waardenburg phenotype (telecanthus or dystopia canthorum, white forelock, partial albinism, heterochromia irides) and upper-limb musculoskeletal abnormalities, joint flexion defects, syndactyly |
| Tetra-amelia with multiple malformations[220] | **301090** 3715 | | See under anosmia | |

**Appendix C-10** Syndromes and conditions associated with anosmia

| Syndrome or condition | MIM No. POSSUM No.[a] | Inheritance[b] | Other ear, nose, and throat anomalies | Other manifestations |
|---|---|---|---|---|
| Hunter-Feldman-Miller syndrome[88] | **113480** 4632 | AD | Midface hypoplasia, short nose, hypoplastic nostrils, flat philtrum | Short stature, square and broad face, hypertelorism, hypopigmentation, cryptorchidism, hypogonadism, delayed puberty, brachydactyly, ulnar deviation of fingers (single report) |

**Appendix C-10** Syndromes and conditions associated with anosmia (*Continued*)

| Syndrome or condition | MIM No. POSSUM No.[a] | Inheritance[b] | Other ear, nose, and throat anomalies | Other manifestations |
|---|---|---|---|---|
| Ichthyosis, hypogonadism[6] | **308200**<br>3458 | XLR | Flattened nose | Ichthyosis (steroid sulphatase deficiency), hypogonadotropic hypogonadism, short stature, terminal hypoplasia of fingers, punctate calcification, spasticity, MR proposed gene location X p22.3 |
| Johnson-McMillan syndrome[94] | **147770**<br>3595 | AD | Cleft palate, large and malformed ears, stenosis or atresia of external auditory canal, conductive deafness, micrognathia | Alopecia, plagiocephaly, hypogonadism, cardiac defect, CNS anomalies, nerve palsies, MR |
| Kallmann syndrome[16,179] | ***147950**<br>***308700**<br>4216 | XLR<br>?AD | Cleft lip/palate, high-arched palate, sensorineural deafness | Short stature, obesity, hypogenitalism, hypogonadotropic hypogonadism, renal agenesis, osteoporosis, agenesis or hypoplasia of corpus callosum, cardiac defect, possible MR, proposed gene location Xp22.32 |
| Refsum syndrome[155] | ***266500**<br>3463 | AR | Nystagmus, sensorineural deafness | Retinitis pigmentosa, visual disturbances, cerebellar ataxia, peripheral neuropathy, ichthyosis, small hands and feet, phytanic acid oxidase deficiency |
| Tetra-amelia with multiple malformations or X-linked tetra-amelia syndrome[220] | **301090**<br>3715 | XLR | Absent nasal cartilage, anotia or microtia, abnormal mouth, abnormal neck | Tetra-amelia with absence or shortening of long bones, absent hands and feet, facial clefts, absent pelvic bones, hydrocephalus, septo-optic dysplasia, vertebral and rib anomalies, anal atresia, stillbirth or neonatal death |
| Usher syndrome[188] | ***276900**<br>3421 | AR | Sensorineural deafness (variable time of onset), nystagmus | Retinitis pigmentosa or pigmentary retinopathy, visual disturbances, ataxia, speech defect, behavioral problems, possible MR |

[a]MIM, *M*endelian *I*nheritance in *M*an. A Catalog of Human Genes and Genetic Disorders, by Victor A. McKusick, 11th ed, The Johns Hopkins University Press, Baltimore, 1994; POSSUM, *P*ictures *O*f *S*tandard *S*yndromes and *U*ndiagnosed *M*alformations, by Agnes Bankier et al., Murdoch Institute, Royal Children's Hospital, Victoria, Australia.
[b]AD, autosomal dominant; AR, autosomal recessive; XLR, X-linked recessive; XLD, X-linked dominant.
*confirmed gene and inheritance
#phenotype that can be caused by mutation in any of 2 or more genes

**Appendix C-11** Syndromes and conditions associated with nasal bridge abnormalities

BROAD NASAL BRIDGE SYNDROME

Aarskog syndrome
Acrocallosal syndrome
Acro-cranio-facial dysostosis, Kaplan type
Acro-fronto-facio-nasal dysostosis
Chondrodysplasia punctata, X-linked recessive
Chromosomal abnormalities
Coffin-Siris syndrome
Craniofrontonasal dysplasia
Craniometaphyseal dysplasia
Ehler-Danlos syndromes types 1, 2, 3, and 5
Fetal akinesia or hypokinesia sequence
Fetal trimethadione syndrome
Floating Harbor syndrome
Frontonasal dysplasia
Fryns syndrome
Hypertelorism-hypospadias syndrome (BBBG syndrome)
Hypertelorism, microtia, clefting syndrome (Bixler syndrome)
Jarcho-Levin syndrome
Killian-Teschler-Nicola syndrome
Maroteaux-Lamy syndrome
Miller-Dieker syndrome
Naguib-Richieri-Costa syndrome
RAPADILINO syndrome
Roberts syndrome
SCARF syndrome
Simpson-Golabi-Behmel syndrome
Teebi hypertelorism syndrome
Tel-Hashomer camptodactyly
Velo-cardio-facial syndrome
Waardenburg syndrome, types 1 and 2
Zellweger syndrome

DEPRESSED NASAL BRIDGE

Achondrogenesis, type 1
Acrodysostosis
Antley-Bixler syndrome
Börjeson-Forssman-Lehmann syndrome
Brachman-de Lange syndrome
Campomelic dysplasia
Cardio-facial-cutaneous (CFC) syndrome
Carpenter syndrome
Chondrodysplasia punctata, Conradi-Hünermann type
Chromosomal abnormalities
Coffin-Siris syndrome
Fetal hydantoin syndrome
Fetal valproate syndrome
Fetal warfarin syndrome
Frontonasal dysplasia, congenital heart disease
Glutaric aciduria, type 2
Holoprosencephaly
Hunter syndrome
Hurler syndrome
Hypertelorism-hypospadias—tetralogy of Fallot
Killian-Teschler-Nicola syndrome
Kniest dysplasia
Larsen syndrome
Mannosidosis
Marshal-Smith syndrome
Naguib-Richieri-Costa syndrome
Neu-Laxova syndrome
Oto-palato-digital syndrome, type 2
Perlman syndrome
Pfeiffer syndrome
Robinow-Sorauf syndrome
Rothmund-Thomson syndrome
Rüdiger syndrome
Teebi hypertelorism syndrome
Teebi overgrowth syndrome
Thanatophoric dysplasia
Williams syndrome

NARROW NASAL BRIDGE

Chromosome 2, interstitial deletion 2(q31–q33)
Craniofacial syndrome
Dubowitz syndrome
Ectodermal dysplasia, Rapp-Hodgkin type
Ehler-Danlos syndrome, type 4
Hallermann-Streiff syndrome
Metageria
Mietens syndrome
Nijmegen breakage syndrome
Progeria

HIGH NASAL BRIDGE

Acro-cranio-facial dysostosis, Kaplan type
Baller-Gerold syndrome
Börjeson-Forssman-Lehmann syndrome
Chromosomal abnormalities
Cohen syndrome
Dubowitz syndrome
Hypertelorism-hypospadias syndrome (BBBG syndrome)
KBG syndrome
Mandibulofacial dysostosis, Toriello type
Montreal type "bird-headed" dwarfism
Mulvihill-Smith syndrome
Nager acrofacial dysostosis
Osteodysplastic primordial dwarfism, type 1
Pilotto syndrome
Pseudoprogeria syndrome
SCARF syndrome
Seckel syndrome
Simpson-Golabi-Behmel syndrome
Treacher Collins syndrome
Trichorhinophalangeal syndrome, type 1
Velo-cardio-facial syndrome
Waardenburg syndrome types 1 and 2

## References


1. Alles AJ, Sulik KK: Retinoic-acid-induced limb-reduction defects: perturbation of zones of programmed cell death as a pathogenic mechanism. Teratology 40:163–171, 1989.
2. Ampola MG: A new familial malformation syndrome. Birth Defects 10:129–135, 1974.
3. Asku F, Mietens C: Kleeblattschädel syndrome. Klin Padiatr 191:418–428, 1979.
4. Autio S, Pihko H, Tengström C: Clinical features in de novo interstitial deletion 15q13 to q15. Clin Genet 34:293–298, 1988.
5. Back E, Toder R, Voiculescu I, Wildberg A, Schempp W: De novo isochromosome 18p in two patients: cytogenetic diagnosis and confirmation by chromosome painting. Clin Genet 45:301–304, 1994.
6. Ballabio A, Parenti G, Carrozzo R, Coppa G, Felici L, Migliori V, Silengo M, Franceschini P, Andria G: X/Y translocation in a family with X-linked icthyosis, chondrodysplasia punctata and mental retardation. Clin Genet 34:31–37, 1988.
7. Bangstad HJ, Beck-Nielsen H, Hother-Nielsen O, Nystad R, Trygstad O, Pedersen O, Aagenaes O: Primordial birdheaded nanism associated with progressive ataxia, early onset insulin resistant diabetes, goitre and primary gonadal insufficiency. Acta Paediatr Scand 78:488–493, 1989.
8. Bankier A, Fortune D, Duke J, Sillence DO: Fibrochondrogenesis in male twins at 24 weeks gestation. Am J Med Genet 38:95–98, 1991.
9. Baraitser M: The Orofaciodigital (OFD) syndromes. J Med Genet 23:116–119, 1986.
10. Baraitser M, Rodeck C, Garner A: A new craniosynostosis/mental retardation syndrome diagnosed by fetoscopy. Clin Genet 22:12–15, 1982.
11. Baroncini A, Avellini C, Neri C, Forabosco A: Distal 12p deletion in a stillborn infant. Am J Med Genet 36:358–360, 1990.
12. Bartsch O, Peterson MB, Stuhlmann I, Man G, Frantzen M, Schwinger E, Antonarakis SE, Mikkelsen M: Compensatory uniparental disomy of chromosome 21 in two cases. J Med Genet 31:534–540, 1994.
13. Bawle E, Horton M: Autosomal dominant microcephaly with mental retardation. Am J Med Genet 33:382–384, 1989.
14. Beighton PH: The dominant and recessive forms of cutis laxa. J Med Genet 9:216–221, 1972.
15. Bialer MG, Wilson WG, Kelly TE: Apparent Ruvalcaba syndrome with genitourinary abnormalities. Am J Med Genet 33:314–317, 1989.

16. Birnbacher R, Wandl-Vergesslich K, Frisch H: Diagnosis of X-recessive Kallmann syndrome in early infancy. Eur J Pediatr 153:245–247, 1994.
17. Bixler D, Christian JC, Gorlin RJ : Hypertelorism, microtia, and facial clefting. Am J Dis Child 118:495–500, 1969.
18. Boles RG, Teebi AS, Meyn MS: Pseudotrisomy 13 with bilateral limb shortness and radial hypoplasia. Am J Med Genet 44:638–640, 1992.
19. Borochowitz Z, Ornoy A, Lachman R, Rimoin DL: Achondrogenesis II—Hypochondrogenesis variability versus heterogeneity. Am J Med Genet 24:273–288, 1986.
20. Carter CO, Till K, Fraser V, Coffey R: A family study of craniosynostosis with probable recognition of a distinct syndrome. J Med Genet 19:280–285, 1982.
21. Chitayat D, Hahm SYE, Marion RW, Sachs GS, Goodman D Hutcheon RG, Weiss R, Cho S, Nitowsky HM: Further delineation of the McKusick-Kaufman hydrometrocolpos polydactyly syndrome. Am J Dis Child 141:1133–1136, 1987.
22. Christianson AL, Nelson M: Four cases of trisomy 18 syndrome with limb reduction malformations. J Med Genet 21:293–297, 1984.
23. Christianson AL, Venter PA, DuTout JL, Shipalana N, Gericke GS: Acrocallosal syndrome in two African brothers born to consanguineous parents. Am J Med Genet 51:98–101, 1994.
24. Cianchetti C, Sannio-Fancello G, Fratta A-L, Manconi F, Orano A, Pischedda M-P, Pruna D, Sinicci G, Archidiacono N, Fillippi G: Neuropsychological, psychiatric and physical manifestations in 149 members from 18 fragile X families. Am J Med Genet 40:234–243, 1991.
25. Cohen MM: Craniosynostosis and syndromes with craniosynostosis: incidence, genetics, penetrance, variability and new syndrome updating. Birth Defects 15:54, 1979.
26. Cohen MM: Hallermann-Streiff syndrome: A review. Am J Med Genet 41:488–499, 1991.
27. Cohen MM, Jr: An etiologic and nosologic overview of craniosynostosis syndrome. Birth Defects 11:137–189, 1975.
28. Cohen MM Jr: Pfeiffer syndrome update, clinical subtypes and guidlines for differential diagnosis. Am J Med Genet 45:300–307, 1993.
29. Cohen MM Jr, Gorlin RJ: Pseudotrisomy 13 syndrome. Am J Med Genet 39:332–335, 1991.
30. Cohen MM Jr, Kreiborg S: The central nervous system in the Apert syndrome. Am J Med Genet 35:36–45, 1990.
31. Cole WG, Patterson E, Bonadio J, Campbell PE, Fortune DW: The clinicopathological features of three babies with osteogenesis imperfecta resulting form the substitution of glycine by valine in the pro $\alpha$ (I) chain of type I procollagen. J Med Genet 29:112–118, 1992.
32. Dalessio DJ: Current concepts. Seizure disorders and pregnancy. N Eng J Med 312:559–563, 1985.
33. Dallapiccola B, Giannotti A, Lembo A, Sagui L: Autosomal recessive form of whistling face syndrome in sibs. Am J Med Genet 33:542–544, 1989.
34. Danks DM: Disorders of copper transport. In: The Metabolic and Molecular Bases of Inherited Disease, 7th ed, CR Scriver, AL Beaudet, WS Sly, D Valle, eds. McGraw-Hill, New York, 1995, pp 2211–2235.
35. David TJ, Webb BW, Gordon IRS: The Patterson syndrome, leprechaunism and pseudoleprechaunism. J Med Genet 18:294–298, 1981.
36. Davis JG, Lafer C: A possible new mental retardation syndrome. Birth Defects 12:235–238, 1976.
37. De Grouchy J, Turleau C: Clinical Atlas of Human Chromosomes. John Wiley and Sons, New York, 1984, pp 28–31.
38. De Grouchy J, Turleau C: Clinical Atlas of Human Chromosomes. John Wiley and Sons, New York, 1984, pp 92–95.
39. de Michelena MI, Campos PJ: A new case of proximal 10q partial trisomy. J Med Genet 28:205–206, 1991.
40. Der Kaloustian VM, McGill JJ, Vekemans M, Kopelman HR: Clonal lines of aneuploid cells in Rothmund-Thomson syndrome. Am J Med Genet 37:336–339, 1990.
41. Dhorne-Pollet S, Deleuze J-F, Hadchouel M, Bonaïti-Pellié C: Segregation analysis of Alagille syndrome. J Med Genet 31:453–457, 1994.
42. Digilio MC, Giannotti A, Marino B, Dallapiccola B: Atrioventricular canal and 8p- syndrome. Am J Med Genet 47:437–438, 1993.
43. Dinardo N, Christian JM, Bennet JA, Shutack JG: Cleft palate lateral synechia syndrome. Review of the literature and case report. Oral Surg Oral Med Oral Pathol 68:565–566, 1989.
44. Dixon MJ, Marres HAM, Edwards SJ, Dixon J, Cremers CWRJ: Treacher Collins syndrome: correlation between clinical and genetic linkage studies. Clin Dysmorphol 3:96–103, 1994.
45. Dobyns WB, Curry CJR, Hoyme HE, Turlington L, Ledbetter DH: Clinical and molecular diagnosis of Miller-Dieker syndrome. Am J Hum Genet 48:584–594, 1991.
46. Donnai D: A further patient with Pitt-Rogers-Danks syndrome of mental retardation, unusual face and intrauterine growth retardation. Am J Med Genet 24:29–32, 1986.
47. Elliott DE: Undiagnosed syndrome of psychomotor retardation, low birth weight, dwarfism, skeletal, dental, dermal and genital anomalies. Birth Defects 11:364–367, 1975.
48. Escobar LF, Bixler D, Sadore M, Bull MJ: Antley-Bixler syndrome from a prognostic perspective: report of a case and review of the literature. Am J Med Genet 29:829–836, 1988.
49. Ewart AK, Morris CA, Atkinson D, Jin W, Sternes K, Spallone P, Stock AD, Leppert M, Keating MT: Hemizygosity at the elastin locus in a developmental disorder, Williams syndrome. Nat Genet 5:11–16, 1993.
50. Farag TI, Teebi AS: Autosomal recessive inheritance of syndrome of hypertelorism, hypospadias, and tetralogy of Fallot? Am J Med Genet 35:516–518, 1990.
51. Fernandez I, Tsukahara M, Mito H, Yoshii H, Uchida M, Matsuo K, Kajii T: Congenital heart defects in Aarskog syndrome. Am J Med Genet 50:318–322, 1994.
52. Fitch N, Pinsky L, Lachance RC: A form of bird-headed dwarfism with features of premature senility. Am J Dis Child 120:260–264, 1970.
53. Fitzsimmons JS, Fitzsimmons EM, McLachlan JI, Gilbert GB: Four brothers with mental retardation, spastic paraplegia, and palmoplanter hyperkeratosis. A new syndrome? Clin Genet 23:329–335, 1983.
54. Fox JW 4th, Golden GT, Edgerton MT: Frontonasal dysplasia with alar clefts in 2 sisters: genetic considerations and surgical correction. Plast Reconstr Surg 57:553–561, 1976.
55. Franceschini P, Signorile VF, Testa A, Guala A, Franceschini D, Dalforno L: Inguinal hernia and atrial septal defect in Tel-Hashomer camptodactyly syndrome: report of a new case expanding the phenotype of the disease. Am J Med Genet 46:341–344, 1993.
56. Fraser FC, Jequier S, Chen MF: New syndrome: chondrodysplasia, situs inversus totalis, cleft epiglottis and larynx, hexadactyly of hands and feet, pancreatic cystic dysplasia, renal dysplasia/absence, micropenis and ambiguous genitalia, imperforate anus. Am J Med Genet 34:401–405, 1989.
57. Froster UG, Baird PA: Congenital defects of the limbs and alcohol exposure in pregnancy: data from a population based study. Am J Med Genet 44:782–785, 1992.
58. Fryburg JS, Persing JA, Liu KY: Frontonasal dysplasia in two successive generations. Am J Med Genet 46:712–714, 1993.
59. Frydman M, Kauschansky, Elian E: Trigonocephaly: a new familial syndrome. Am J Med Genet 18:55–59, 1984.
60. Fryer AD: Child with fronto-facio-nasal dysplasia, Hirschsprung's disease and hypospadias. Clin Dysmorphol 2:120–122, 1993.
61. Gassner I, Müller W, Rossler H, Kofler J, Mitterstieler G: Familial occurrence of syngnathia congenita syndrome. Clin Genet 15:241–244, 1979.
62. German J, Passarge E: Bloom's syndrome. XII Report from registry for 1987. Clin Genet 35:157–169, 1989.
63. Gershoni-Baruch R: Carpenter syndrome: Marked variability of expression to include the Summitt and Goodman syndromes. Am J Med Genet 35:236–240, 1990.
64. Gershoni-Baruch R, Lerner A, Braun J, Katzir Y, Iancu TC, Benderly A: Johanson-Blizzard syndrome: clinical spectrum and further delineation of the syndrome. Am J Med Genet 35:546–551, 1990.
65. Gilkes JJH, Sharvill DE, Wells RS: The premature aging syndromes. Report of eight cases and description of a new entity named metageria. Br J Dermatol 91:243–262, 1974.
66. Goldblatt J, Wallis C, Viljoen D: A new hypospadias-mental retardation syndrome in three brothers. Am J Dis Child 141:1168–1169, 1987.
67. Goodman SI, Frerman FE: Organic acidemias due to defects in lysine oxidation: 2–ketoadipic acidemia and glutaric acidemia. In: The Metabolic and Molecular Bases of Inherited Disease, 7th ed, CR Scriver, AL Beaudet, WS Sly, D Valle, eds., MacGraw-Hill, New York, 1995, pp 1451–1460.
68. Gorlin RJ, Cohen MM, Levin LS: Syndromes of the Head and Neck, 4th ed. Oxford University Press, New York, 1990, pp 909–910.
69. Goto M, Tanimoto K, Horiuchi Y, Sasazuki T: Family analysis of Werner's syndrome: a survey of 42 Japanese families with a review of the literature. Clin Genet 19:8–15, 1981.
70. Grammatico P, Cupilari F, DiRosa C, Falcolini M, Del Porto G: 20p

duplication as a result of parental translocation: familial case report and a contribution to the clinical delineation of the syndrome. Clin Genet 41:285–289, 1992.
71. Greenberg F, Copeland K, Gresik MV: Expanding the spectrum of the Perlman syndrome. Am J Med Genet 29:773–776, 1988.
72. Haan EA, Furness ME, Knowles S, Morris LL, Scott G, Svigos JM, Vigneswaren R: Osteodysplastic primordial dwarfism. Report of a further case with manifestations similar to those of types I and III. Am J Med Genet 33:224–227, 1989.
73. Halal F: Distal obstructive uropathy with polydactyly: A new syndrome? Am J Med Genet 24:753–757, 1986.
74. Halal F, Silver K: Slowly progressive macrocephaly with hamartomas: A new syndrome. Am J Med Genet 33:182–185, 1989.
75. Hall BD, Berg BO, Rudolph RS, Epstein CJ: Pseudoprogeria—Hallermann-Streiff (PHS) syndrome. Birth Defects 10:147–151, 1974.
76. Hall BD, Mier RJ: Mandibuloacral dysplasia: a rare progressive disorder with postnatal onset. Proc Greenwood Genet Center 4:125–126, 1985.
77. Hall JG: Craniofacial dysostosis—either Stanescu dysostosis or a new entity. Birth Defects 10:521–523, 1974.
78. Hayani A, Suarez CR, Molnar Z, LeBeau M, Godwin J: Acute leukaemia in a patient with Seckel syndrome. J Med Genet 31:148–149. 1994.
79. Hennekam RCM, Lommen EJP, Strengers JLM, Spijker HG, Jansen-Kokx TMG: Rubinstein-Taybi syndrome in a mother and son. Eur J Paediat 148:439–441, 1989.
80. Hennekam RCM, Van den Boogaard M-J: Autosomal dominant craniosynostosis of the sutura metopica. Clin Genet 38:374–377, 1990.
81. Hertle RW, Quin GE, Minguini N, Katowitz JA: Visual loss in patients with craniofacial synostosis. J Pediatr Ophthalmol Strabismus 28:344–349, 1991.
82. Hirsch B, Baldinger S: Pericentric inversion of chromosome 4 giving rise to dup (4p) and dup (4q) recombinants within a single kindred. Am J Med Genet 45:5–8, 1993.
83. Hoar DI, Field LL, Beards F, Hoganson G, Rollnick B, Hoo JJ: Tentative assignment of gene for oto-palato-digital syndrome to distal Xq(Xq26–q28). Am J Med Genet 42:170–172, 1992.
84. Hodgson SV, Coonar AS, Hanson P Jr, Cottrell S, Scriven PN, Jones T, Hawley PR, Wilkinson ML: Two cases of 5q deletions in patients with familial adenomatous polyposis: possible link with Caroli disease. J Med Genet 30:369–375, 1993.
85. Hoepffner HJ, Dreyer M, Reimers U, Schmidt-Preuss U, Koepp H-P, Rüdiger HW: A new familial syndrome with impaired function of three related peptide growth factors. Hum Genet 83:209–216, 1989.
86. Houlston RS, Collins AL, Dennis NR, Temple IK: Further observations on the Floating-Harbor syndrome. Clin Dysmorphol 3:143–149, 1994.
87. Houston CS, Gerrard JW, Ives EJ: Dysosteosclerosis. Am J Roentgenol 130:988–991, 1978.
88. Hunter AGW, Feldman W, Miller J: Characteristic craniofacial appearance and brachytelephalangy in a mother and son with Kallman syndrome. Am J Med Genet 24:527–532, 1986.
89. Hurst JA, Baraitser M: Johanson-Blizzard syndrome. J Med Genet 26:45–48, 1989.
90. Jackson L, Kline AD, Koch S: de Lange syndrome. A clinical review of 310 individuals. Am J Med Genet 47:940–946, 1993.
91. Jalal SM, Kukolich MK, Garcia M, Benjamin TR, Day DW: Tetrasomy 9p: an emerging syndrome. Clin Genet 39:60–64, 1991.
92. Jespers A, Buntinx I, Melis K, Vaerenberg M, Janssens G: Two siblings with midline field defects and Hirschsprung disease: variable expression of Toriello-Carey or new syndrome? Am J Med Genet 47:299–302, 1993.
93. Johnson VP, Sutliff WC: Duplication 10q confirmed by DNA in situ hybridization. Am J Med Genet 52:184–187, 1994.
94. Johnston K, Golabi M, Hall B, Ito M, Grix A: Alopecia-anosmia-deafness-hypogonadism syndrome revisited: report of a new case. Am J Med Genet 26:925–927, 1987.
95. Kajii T, Fernandez Gonzalez I, Matsuura S: Tricho-rhino-phalangeal syndrome type III. Am J Med Genet 49:349–350, 1994.
96. Kalousek DK, Bamforth S: Amnion rupture sequence and previable fetuses. Am J Med Genet 31:63–73, 1988.
97. Kaplan P, Plauchu H, Fitch N, Jequier S: A new acro-cranio-facial dysostosis in sisters. Am J Med Genet 29:95–106, 1988.
98. Kapusta L, Brunner HG, Hamel BCJ: Craniofrontonasal dysplasia. Eur J Pediatr 151:837–841, 1992.
99. Katafuchi Y, Fukuda T, Maruoka T, Tokunaga Y, Yamashita Y, Matsuishi T: Partial trisomy 6p with agenesis of the corpus callosum and choanal atresia. J Child Neurol 7:114–116, 1992.
100. Keipert JA, Fitzgerald MG, Danks DM: A new syndrome of broad terminal phalanges and facial abnormalities. Aust Paediatr J 9:10–13, 1993.
101. Keppen LD, Collin SM, Seibert JJ, Sisken JE: Roberts syndrome with normal cell division. Am J Med Genet 38:21–24, 1991.
102. Khalifa MM: Hutchinson-Gilford progeria syndrome: report of a Libyan family and evidence of autosomal recessive inheritance. Clin Genet 35:125–132, 1989.
103. Khosroshahi HE, Uluoglu O, Olgurturk R, Basaklar C, Keutel syndrome: a report of four cases. Eur J Pediatr 149:188–191, 1989.
104. Kishawi A, Malik AH, Al-Awadi SA, Teebi AS: Hallermann-Streiff syndrome. J Kwt Med Assoc 23:80–81, 1989.
105. Kogekar N, Teebi AS, Vockley J: Sandrow syndrome of mirror hands and feet and peculiar facies. Am J Med Genet 46:126–128, 1993.
106. Kreiborg S, Cohen MM Jr: Germinal mosaicism in Crouzon's syndrome. Hum Genet 84:487–488.
107. Kristoffersson U, Lagergren J, Heim S, Mandahl N: Four copies of 8p in a mentally retarded boy with mosaic karyotype. Clin Genet 34:201–203, 1988.
108. Kuroki Y, Suzuki Y, Chyo H, Hata A, Matsui I: A new malformation syndrome of long palpebral fissures, large ears, depressed nasal tip and skeletal anomalies associated with postnatal dwarfism and mental retardation. J Pediatr 99:570–573, 1981.
109. Labrune P, Lyonnet S, Zupan V, Lambert M-C, Goutieres F, Hubert P, Le Merrer M: Three new cases of Schinzel-Giedion syndrome and review of the literature. Am J Med Genet 50:90–93, 1994.
110. Lachman MF, Wright Y, Whiteman DAH, Herson V, Greenstein RM: 46, XY phenotypic female with Smith-Lemli-Opitz syndrome. Clin Genet 39:136–141, 1991.
111. Lacombe D: Facial palsy and cranial nerve abnormalities in CHARGE association. Am J Med Genet 49:351–352, 1994.
112. Lacombe D, Saura R, Taine L, Battin J: Confirmation of assignment of a locus for Rubinstein-Taybi syndrome gene to 16p13.3. Am J Med Genet 44:126–128, 1992.
113. Lacro RV, Jones KL, Mascarello JT, Jones OW, Wilson N, Jones MC: Duplication of distal 15q: report of five new cases from two different translocation kindreds. Am J Med Genet 26:719–728, 1987.
114. Lampert RP: Dominant inheritance of femoral hypoplasia-unusual facies syndrome. Clin Genet 17:255–258, 1980.
115. Langer LO Jr, Beals RK, Solomon IL, Bard PA, Bard LA, Rissman EM, Rogers JG, Dorst JP, Hall JG, Sparkes RS, Franken EA Jr: Acro mesomelic dwarfism manifestations in childhood. Am J Med Genet 1:87–100, 1977.
116. Leichtman LG, Strum D, Brothman AR: Multiple craniofacial anomalies associated with an interstitial deletion of chromosome 1(q21→q25). Am J Med Genet 45:677–678, 1993.
117. Le Merrer M, Brauner R, Maroteaux P: Dwarfism with gloomy face: a new syndrome with features of 3–M syndrome. J Med Genet 28:186–191, 1991.
118. Lessik ML, Israel J, Wong PWK, Szego K: Partial trisomy 16q secondary to a maternal 9;16 mosaicism. J Med Genet 26:63–64, 1989.
119. Lindgren V, Rosinsky B, Chin J, Berry-Kravis E: Two patients with overlapping de novo duplications of the long arm of chromosome 9, including one case with Di George sequence. Am J Med Genet 49:67–73, 1994.
120. Lindström JA: Oligophrenic, low birth weight dwarfism in sibs. Birth Defects 11:443–449, 1975.
121. Lowry RB, MacLean JR: Syndrome of mental retardation, cleft palate, eventration of diaphragm, congenital heart defect, glaucoma, growth failure and craniosynostosis. Birth Defects 13:203–228, 1977.
122. Lüdecke H-J, Johnson C, Wagner MJ, Wells DE, Turleau C, Tommerup N, Latos-Bielenska A, Sandig K-R, Meinecke P, Zabel B, Horsthemke B: Molecular definition of the shortest region of deletion overlap in the Langer-Giedion syndrome. Am J Hum Genet 49:1197–1206, 1991.
123. Magli A, François J, Pignalosa B, Reccia R: Coloboma of the lens associated with coloboma of the alar nasal cartilages in a pair of female monozygotic twins: A new syndrome? Ophthalmic Paediatr Genet 2:83–87, 1983.
124. Maraia R, Saal HM, Wangsa D: A chromosome 17q de novo paracentric inversion in a patient with campomelic dysplasia; a case report and etiologic hypothesis. Clin Genet 39:401–408, 1991.

124a. Marasovich WA, Mazaheri M, Stool SE: Otolaryngologic findings in whistling face syndrome. Arch Otolaryngol Head Neck Surg 115:1373–1380, 1989.
125. Marchau FE, Roy BCV, Parizel PM, Lambert JR, Canck ID, Leroy JG, Gevaert CM, Willems PJ, Dumon JE: Tricho-rhino-phalangeal syndrome type I (TRPI) due to an apparently balanced translocation involving 8q24. Am J Med Genet 45:450–455, 1993.
126. Martin RA, Jones MC, Jones KL: Mirror hands and feet with a distinct nasal defect, an autosomal dominant condition. Am J Med Genet 46:129–131, 1993.
127. Mastellone CB, Giovannucci Uzielli ML, Guarducci S, Nathan G: Four cases of trisomy 9p syndrome with particular chromosome rearrangements. Ann Genet 34:115–119, 1991.
128. Matsuo S, Takeuchi Y, Hayashi S, Kinugasa A, Sawada T: Patient with unusual Hutchinson-Gilford syndrome (progeria). Pediatr Neurol 10:237–240, 1994.
129. McPherson EW, Ketterer DM, Salsburey DJ: Pallister-Killian and Fryns syndromes: nosology. Am J Med Genet 47:241–245, 1993.
130. Meadow R: Anticonvulsants in pregnancy. Arch Dis Child 66:62–65, 1991.
131. Meinecke P, Blunck W: Unknown syndrome: Congenital heart disease, choanal stenosis, short stature, developmental delay, and dysmorphic facial features in a brother and sister. J Med Genet 26:407–409, 1989.
132. Meinecke P, Schaefer E, Wiedemann HR: Microcephalic osteodysplastic primordial dwarfism. Further evidence for identity of the so called types I and III. Am J Med Genet 39:232–236, 1991.
133. Melnyk AR: Blepharophimosis, ptosis and mental retardation: further delineation of Ohdo syndrome. Clin Dysmorphol 3:121–124, 1994.
134. Mendez HM, Opitz JM: Noonan syndrome: a review. Am J Med Genet 21:493–506, 1985.
135. Mindikoglu AN, Partington MW, Cohen MM Jr: Noses nobody knows—for real: riny and craniorhiny. Am J Med Genet 40:250–251, 1991.
136. Mitnick RJ, Bello JA, Shprintzen RJ: Brain anomalies in velo-cardio-facial syndrome. Am J Med Genet 54:100–106, 1994.
137. Morris CA, Thomas IT, Greenberg F: Williams syndrome: autosomal dominant inheritance. Am J Med Genet 47:478–481, 1993.
138. Nagai T, Nishimura G, Kasai H, Hasegawa T, Kato R, Ohashi H, Fukushima Y: Another family with tricho-rhino-phalangeal syndrome type III (Sagio-Kajii syndrome). Am J Med Genet 49:278–280, 1994.
139. Naguib KK, Teebi AS, Al-Awadi SA, Marafie MJ: Brachmann-de Lange syndrome in sibs. J Med Genet 24627–631, 1987.
140. Nance MA, Berry SA: Cockayne syndrome: review of 140 cases. Am J Med Genet 42:68–84, 1992.
141. Niemann-Seyde SC, Eber SW, Zoll B: Saethre-Chotzen syndrome (ACSIII) in four generations. Clin Genet 40:271–276, 1991.
142. Novak RW, Robinson HB: Coincident DiGeorge anomaly and renal agenesis and its relation to maternal diabetes. Am J Med Genet 50:311–312, 1994.
143. Obregon MG, Bergami GL, Giannotti A, Digilio MC, Virgili Q, Guadagni AM, Pompei E, Dallapiccola B: Radiographic findings in Wiedemann-Rautenstrauch syndrome. Pediatr Radiol 22:474–475, 1992.
144. Opitz JM, de La Cruz F: Cholesterol metabolism in the RSH/Smith-Lemli-Opitz syndrome: summary of an NICHD conference. Am J Med Genet 50:339–343, 1994.
145. Örstavik KH, McFadden N, Hagelsteen J, Ormerod E, van der Hagen CB: Instability of lymphocyte chromosomes in a girl with Rothmund-Thomson syndrome. J Med Genet 31:570–572, 1994.
146. Orth U, Gurrieri F, Behmel A, Genaurdi M, Cremer M, Gal A, Neri G: Gene for Simpson-Golabi-Behmel syndrome is linked to HPRT in Xq26 in two European families. Am J Med Genet 50:388–390, 1994.
147. Pallotta R, Morgese G: Mandibuloacral dysplasia: a rare progeroid syndrome. Clin Genet 26:133–138, 1984.
148. Partington MW, Mulley JC, Sutherland GR, Thode A, Turner G: A family with the Coffin Lowry syndrome revisited: localization of CLS to Xp21–pter. Am J Med Genet 30:509–521, 1988.
149. Pashayan H, Pruzansky S, Putterman A: A family with blepharo-naso-facial malformations. Am J Dis Child 125:389–396, 1973.
150. Patton MA, Goodship J, Hayward R, Lansdown R: Intellectual development in Apert's syndrome: a long term follow-up of 29 patients. J Med Genet 25:164–167, 1988.
151. Pena SD: Cleft lip and palate, congenital heart disease, scoliosis, short stature, and mental retardation: the Pilotto syndrome. Birth Defects 18: 183–186, 1982.
152. Petit P, Fryns J-P: Distal osteolysis, short stature, mental retardation, and characteristic facial appearance: delineation of an autosomal recessive subtype of essential osteolysis. Am J Med Genet 25:537–541, 1986.
153. Pina-Neto JM, Martelli Soares LR, Oliveira-Souza AH, Lopes-Petean EB, Velludo MASL, Campos de Freitas A, Ribas JP: A new case of Zimmermann-Laband syndrome with mental retardation, asymmetry of limbs and hypertrichosis. Am J Med Genet 31:691–695, 1988.
154. Pitt DB, Rogers JG, Danks DM: Mental retardation, unusual face and intrauterine growth retardation. Am J Med Genet 19:307–313, 1984.
155. Poulos A, Pollard AC, Mitchell JD, Wise G, Mortimer G: Patterns of Refsum's disease. Phytanic acid oxidase deficiency. Arch Dis Child 59:222–229, 1984.
156. Preis S, Kemperdick H, Majewski F: Oto-palato-digital syndrome type II in two unrelated boys. Clin Genet 45:154–161, 1994.
157. Pul N, Pul M, Gedik Y: McKusick-Kaufman syndrome associated with esophageal atresia and distal tracheoesophageal fistula: a case report and review of the literature. Am J Med Genet 49:341–343, 1994.
158. Qazi QH, Kanchanapoomi R, Beller E, Collins R: Inheritance of posterior choanal atresia. Am J Med Genet 13:413–416, 1982.
159. Quarell OWJ, Koch M, Hughes H: Maxillonasal dysplasia (Binder's syndrome). J Med Genet 27:384–387, 1990.
160. Reardon W, Harbord HG, Hall-Craggs MA, Kendall B, Brett EM, Baraitser M: Central nervous system malformations in Mohr's syndrome. J Med Genet 26:659–663, 1989.
161. Reid CS, McMorrow LE, McDonald-McGinn DM, Grace KJ, Ramos FJ, Zackai EH, Cohen MM, Jabs EW: Saethre-Chotzen syndrome with familial translocation at chromosome 7p22. Am J Med Genet 47:637–639, 1993.
162. Robb LJ, Fraser FC, Der Kaloustian VM: Treacher Collins-Franceschetti syndrome with tracheoesophageal fistula, rectovaginal fistula and anal atresia: variant or new syndrome? Am J Med Genet 39:119–120, 1991.
163. Robinow M, Johanson AJ, Smith TH: The Lenz-Majewski hyperostotic dwarfism. J Pediatr 91:417–421, 1977.
164. Rozin MM, Hertz M, Goodman RM: A new syndrome with camptodactyly, joint contractures, facial anomalies, and skeletal defects: a case report and review of syndromes with camptodactyly. Clin Genet 26:342–355, 1984.
165. Russo R, D'Armiento M, Angrisani P, Vecchione R: Limb body wall complex: a critical review and nosological proposal. Am J Med Genet 47:893–900, 1993.
166. Sakati N, Nyhan WL, Tisdale WK: A new syndrome with acrocephalopolysyndactyly, cardiac disease, and distinctive defects of the ear, skin, and lower limbs. J Pediatr 79:104–109, 1971.
167. Sakati NO, Nyhan WL, Shear CS, Kattan CS, Akhtar M, Bay C, Jones KL, Schackner L: Syndrome of cutis laxa, ligamentous laxity and delayed development. Pediatrics 72:850–856, 1983.
168. Say B, Meyer J: Familial trigonocephaly associated with short stature and developmental delay. Am J Dis Child 135:711–712, 1981.
169. Schinzel A: Catalogue of Unbalanced Chromosome Aberrations of Man., Walter de Gruyter, Berlin, 1984.
170. Schinzel A: Catalogue of Unbalanced Chromosome Aberrations of Man., Walter de Gruyter, Berlin, 1984, p 494.
171. Schinzel A: Tetrasomy 12p (Pallister-Killian syndrome). J Med Genet 28:122–125, 1991.
172. Schrander-Stumpel C, Meinecke P, Wilson G, Gillessen-Kaesback G, Tenschert S, Köning R, Philip N, Rizzo R, Schrander J, Pfeiffer L, Maat-Kievit A, van der Burgt I, van Essen T, Latta E, Hiling U, Verloes A, Journel H, Fryns JP: The Kabuki (Niikawa-Kuroki) syndrome: further delineation of phenotype in 29 non-Japanese patients. Eur J Pediatr 153:438–445, 1994.
173. Seemanová A, Passarge E, Beneškova D, Houťk J, Kasal P, Ševčikova M: Familial microcephaly with normal intelligence, immunodeficiency, and risk for lymphoreticular malignancies: a new autosomal recessive disorder. Am J Med Genet 20:639–648, 1985.
174. Sharma AK, Phadke S, Chandra K, Uprefi M, Khan EM, Naveed M, Agarwal SS: Overlap between Majewski and hydrolethalus syndromes: a report of two cases. Am J Med Genet 43:949–053, 1992.
175. Sheffer R, Zlotogora J: Autosomal dominant inheritance of Klein-Waardenburg syndrome. Am J Med Genet 42:320–322, 1992.
176. Sheffield LJ, Halliday JL, Jensen F: Maxillonasal dysplasia (Binder's syndrome) and chondrodysplasia punctata. J Med Genet 28:503–504, 1991.

177. Singh HA: Mental retardation, macrostomia and hyperpnoea syndrome. J Pediatr Child Health 29:156–157, 1993.
178. Soothill PW, Vuthiwong C, Rees H: Achondrogenesis type 2 diagnosed by transvaginal ultrasound at 12 weeks gestation. Prenat Diag 13:523–528, 1993.
179. Sparkes RS, Simpson RW, Paulsen CA: Familial hypogonadotropic hypogonadism with anosmia. Arch Intern Med 121:534–538, 1968.
180. Spranger J, Gilbert EF, Arya S, Hoganson GMI, Opitz JM: Geleophysic dysplasia. Am J Med Genet 19:487–506, 1984.
181. Spranger JW, Langer LO, Wiedemann HR: Bone Dysplasia. WB Saunders, Philadelphia, 1974, p 298.
182. Stanescu R, Stanescu V, Maroteaux P: Homozygous achondroplasia: morphologic and biochemical study of cartilage. Am J Med Genet 37:412–421, 1990.
183. Stoll C, Chognot D, Halb A, Luckel JC: Trisomy 9 mosaicism in two girls with multiple congenital malformations and mental retardation. J Med Genet 30:433–435, 1992.
184. Stoppa-Lyonnet D, Girault D, LeDeist F, Aurias A: Unusual T cell clones in a patient with Nijmegen breakage syndrome. J Med Genet 29:136–137, 1992.
185. Stratakis CA, Runkle B, Rennert OM: A variant of the cerebro-oculo-facio-skeletal syndrome with congenital ectropion and a case of lamellar ichthyosis in the same family. Clin Genet 45:162–163, 1994.
186. Strong WB: Familial syndrome of right sided aortic arch, mental deficiency and facial dysmorphism. J Pediat 73:882–888, 1988.
187. Sundareshan TS, Naguib KK, Al-Awadi SA, Redha MA, Hamoud MS: Apparently nonmosaic trisomy 22: clinical report and review. Am J Med Genet 36:7–10, 1990.
188. Tamayo ML, Bernal JE, Tamayo GE, Frias JL, Alvira G, Vergara O, Rodriguez V, Uribe JI, Silva JC: Usher syndrome: results of screening program in Colombia. Clin Genet 40:304–311, 1991.
189. Tanaka H, Ito J, Cho K, Mikawa M: Hirschsprung disease, unusual face, mental retardation, epilepsy and congenital heart disease: Goldberg-Shprintzen syndrome. Pediatr Neurol 9:479–481, 1993.
190. Teebi AS: Autosomal dominant syndrome resembling craniofrontonasal dysplasia. Am J Med Genet 28:581–591, 1987.
191. Teebi AS: Autosomal recessive Robinow syndrome. Am J Med Genet 35:64–68, 1990.
192. Teebi AS: Naguib-Richieri-Costa syndrome (hypertelorism-hypospadias-polysyndactyly syndrome). Am J Med Genet 44:115–116, 1992.
193. Teebi AS, Abdel-Rahim AR, Krishna-Murthy DS, Redha A: Alagille syndrome and del(20)(p11.2). Am J Med Genet 24:35–38, 1992.
194. Teebi AS, Al-Awadi SA, Opitz JM, Spranger J: Severe short limb dwarfism resembling Grebe chondrodysplasia. Hum Genet 74:386–390, 1986.
195. Teebi AS, Gibson L, McGrath JM, Meyn MS, Breg R, Yang-Feng TL: Cytogenetic and molecular characterization of 9p- anomalies. Am J Med Genet 46:288–293, 1993.
196. Teebi AS, Rucquoi J, Meyn MS: Aarskog syndrome: report of family with review and discussion of nosology. Am J Med Genet 46:561–509, 1993.
197. Teebi AS, Sundareshan TS, Hammouri MY, Al-Awadi SA, Al-Saleh QA: A new autosomal recessive disorder resembling Weaver syndrome. Am J Med Genet 33:479–482, 1989.
198. Temple IK, Brunner H, Jones B, Burn J, Baraitser M: Midline facial defects with ocular colobomata. Am J Med Genet 37:23–27, 1990.
199. Thisted E, Ebbesen F: Malformations, withdrawal manifestations and hypoglycemia after exposure to valproate in utero. Arch Dis Child 69:288–291, 1993.
200. Toriello HV: Wiedemann-Rautenstrauch syndrome. J Med Genet 27:256–257, 1990.
201. Toriello HV, Delp K: Teebi hypertelorism syndrome: report of a third family. Clin Dysmorphol 3:335–339, 1994.
202. Toriello HV, Radecki LL, Sharda J, Looyenga D, Mann R: Frontonasal "dysplasia," cerebral anomalies, and polydactyly: report of a new syndrome and discussion from a developmental field perspective. Am J Med Genet Suppl 2:89–96, 1986.
203. Traboulsi E, Faris BM, Der Kaloustian VM: Persistant hyperplastic primary vitreous and recessive oculo-dento-osseous dysplasia. Am J Med Genet 24:95–100, 1986.
204. Van Den Berg DJ, Francke U: Roberts syndrome: a review of 100 cases and a new rating system for severity. Am J Med Genet 47:1104–1123, 1993.
205. Vargas FR, de Almeida JCC, Llerena JC Jr, Reis DF: RAPADILINO syndrome. Am J Med Genet 44:716–719, 1992.
206. Verloes A, Bonneau D, Guidi O, Berthier M, Oriot D, Van Maldergem L, Koulischer L: Brachymorphism-onycho-dysplasia-dysphalangism syndrome. J Med Genet 30:158–161, 1993.
207. Verloes A, Dodinval P, Beco L, Bonnivert J, Lambotte C: Lambotte syndrome: microcephaly, holoprosencephaly, intrauterine growth retardation, facial anomalies and early lethality: a new multiple congenital anomaly/mental retardation syndrome in four sibs. Am J Med Genet 37:119–123, 1990.
208. Verloes A, Gilerot Y, Walczak E, Maldergem LV, Koulischer L: Acromelic frontonasal "dysplasia": Further delineation of a subtype with brain malformation and polydactyly (Toriello syndrome). Am J Med Genet 42:180–183, 1992.
209. Viljoen D, Beighton P: Epiphyseal stippling in acrodysostosis. Am J Med Genet 38:43–45, 1991.
210. Vintiner GM, Temple IK, Middleton-Price HR, Baraitser M, Malcolm S: Genetic and clinical heterogeneity of Stickler syndrome. Am J Med Genet 41:44–48, 1991.
211. Waring GO 3rd, Rodrigues MM: Ultrastructure and successful keratoplasty of sclerocornea in Mietens' syndrome. Am J Ophthalmol 90:469–475, 1980.
212. Watson MS, Dowton SB, Rohrbaugh: Case of direct insertion within a chromosome 3 leading to a chromosome 3 duplication in an offspring. Am J Med Genet 36:172–174, 1990.
213. Weaver DD, Williams CP: A syndrome of microcephaly, mental retardation, unusual facies, cleft palate and weight deficiency. Birth Defects 13:69–84, 1977.
214. Wells TR, Falk RE, Senac MO, Vachon L: Acrocephalospondylosyndactyly—A possible new syndrome: analysis of the vertebral and intervertebral component. Pediatr Pathol 10:117–131, 1990.
215. Winter RM: Winchester's syndrome. J Med Genet 26:772–775, 1989.
216. Wohrle D, Barbi G, Schulz W, Steinback P: Heterozygous expression of X-linked chondrodysplasia punctata. Hum Genet 86:215–218, 1990.
217. Wolff DJ, Schwartz MF, Cohen MM, Schwartz S: Precise mapping of a de novo duplication 18(q21–q22) utilizing cytogenetic, biochemical and molecular techniques. Am J Med Genet 46:520–523, 1993.
218. Wong V, Cheng CH, Chan KC: Fetal and neonatal outcome of exposure to anticoagulants during pregnancy. Am J Med Genet 45:17–21, 1993.
219. Wullich B, Henn W, Groterath E, Ermis A, Fuchs S, Zankl M: Mosaic tetraploidy in a liveborn infant with features of DiGeorge anomaly. Clin Genet 40:353–357, 1991.
220. Zimmer EZ, Taub E, Sova Y, Divon MY, Pery M, Peretz BA: Tetraamelia with multiple malformations in six male fetuses in one kindred. Euro J Pediatr 144:412–414, 1985.

# IV

## THE MOUTH, PALATE, AND PHARYNX

# 12

# Developmental Biology of the Mouth, Palate, and Pharynx

MALCOLM C. JOHNSTON

This chapter is concerned primarily with the interactions involved in embryonic development of the mouth and pharynx. There is some overlap with other chapters on development, and cross-references will be made. Developmental alterations leading to malformations such as cleft lip and palate are briefly discussed.

Surface aspects of development of the human branchial (visceral, pharyngeal) arches and primary palate are presented in Figure 12–1. The surface morphology of most lower vertebrates is almost identical and it is only in later stages (day 44 to day 50) that the human embryo acquires its distinctive appearance. The origins and developmental interactions of different epithelial and mesenchymal components have been studied primarily in lower vertebrates, but there is ample evidence that they are virtually identical in the human. Recent progress in the application of molecular methods shows great promise for a much improved understanding of the mechanisms of both normal and abnormal development.

## Early stages of development of the mouth and pharynx

Included in this section are developmental interactions from germ-layer formation through formation of the neural and pharyngeal tubes, formation and migration of neural crest cells, and formation of the olfactory and ganglionic placodes. Cell-marking studies, conducted primarily on chick and mouse embryos,[48,64,76,85] indicate that all three germ layers originate from a single embryonic layer, the epiblast, with endoderm and notochord forming from the anterior (rostral) end of the primitive streak and mesodermal cells forming from more posterior (caudal) portions of the primitive streak (Fig. 12–2A). The notochord eventually separates from the endoderm (Fig. 12–2B, C) to lie in the same plane as the mesoderm. Cells that remain in the upper layer become the ectoderm. Nonepiblast embryonic cells form the extraembryonic membranes and contribute to the placenta.

Mesodermal cells migrate from the primitive streak (Fig. 12–2A), essentially as independent cells separated by large amounts of extracellular material (not shown). This tissue arrangement is termed a *mesenchyme,* as contrasted to the compactly arranged epiblast layer, termed an *epithelium,* from which they originated. As will be seen, these two types of tissues make up the embryo from this time onward. There are other sources of mesenchyme (e.g., from the ectodermal neural crest), so the terms mesenchyme and mesoderm are *not* equivalent. Mesenchymal cells can condense to form compact epithelial tissues, such as the mesoderm in the sections illustrated in Figure 12–2B, C.

Eventually, the mesoderm (and notochord) separate the ectoderm from the underlying endoderm except for two locations: the oral plate or buccopharyngeal membrane (Figs. 12–2A, 12–3A–D) and the anal plate or cloacal membrane (Fig. 12–3A–C), the structures of which initially block opposite ends of the developing digestive tract. Unsupported by mesenchyme with its developing vascular system, these membranes eventually break down.

As has been shown by experimental separation of mesoderm (and notochord) from the ectoderm and endoderm (see Holfreter and Hamburger[29]), the mesoderm and notochord are capable of differentiating on their own into somites and other specialized embryonic tissues, as illustrated in Fig. 12–2C. Also shown experimentally through tissue transplantation and recombination in culture, initially in amphibian[83] and later in other embryos (including mammals[3]), the notochord and associated "paraxial" mesoderm are responsible for "inducing" neural plate formation (Fig. 12–2A,B) in the overlying ectoderm. Through this initial epithelial–mesenchymal interaction, the "chorda-mesoderm" also specifies regional specialization in the neural plate, such as the neural crest at its edges, the eye fields and, apparently, the olfactory placodes (Fig. 12–2A). The placodes eventually separate from the neural plate and, as will be seen, are major players in primary plate formation.

The neural plate rolls up to form the neural tube (Fig. 12–2B,C) and eventually separates from the surface ectoderm. Initially, the buccopharyngeal membrane and heart primordium are in front of the neural plate (Figs. 12–2A, 12–3A), but rapid growth of the forebrain (Figs. 12–2B; 12–3B,C) results in the heart and buccal plate assuming an increasingly caudal position relative to the forebrain. This relative retropositioning is also responsible for forming the floor (ventral portion) of the pharynx (Fig. 12–3B-D).

Before or after the neural folds make contact, neural crest cells migrate from the ectodermal neural folds (which have the compact epithelial configuration). They form another group of mesenchymal cells that migrate to almost all parts of the embryo, eventually forming the melanocytes responsible for skin and iris pigmentation, most of the cells of the peripheral nervous system and, of most importance to this chapter, almost all of the skeletal and connective tissues of the face and anterior neck (Fig. 12–4). Although this latter contribution of crest cells was well documented from early studies on amphibians (reviewed by Hörstadius[30]), it was not until the development of cell-marking procedures suitable for higher vertebrate embryos, principally in avian embryos[34,35,49,50,65,66] and the rat and mouse,[6a,43,68,77,86,87] that it was accepted by investigators working on normal and abnormal development of the head and neck in humans.

In addition to the peculiar origin of skeletal and connective

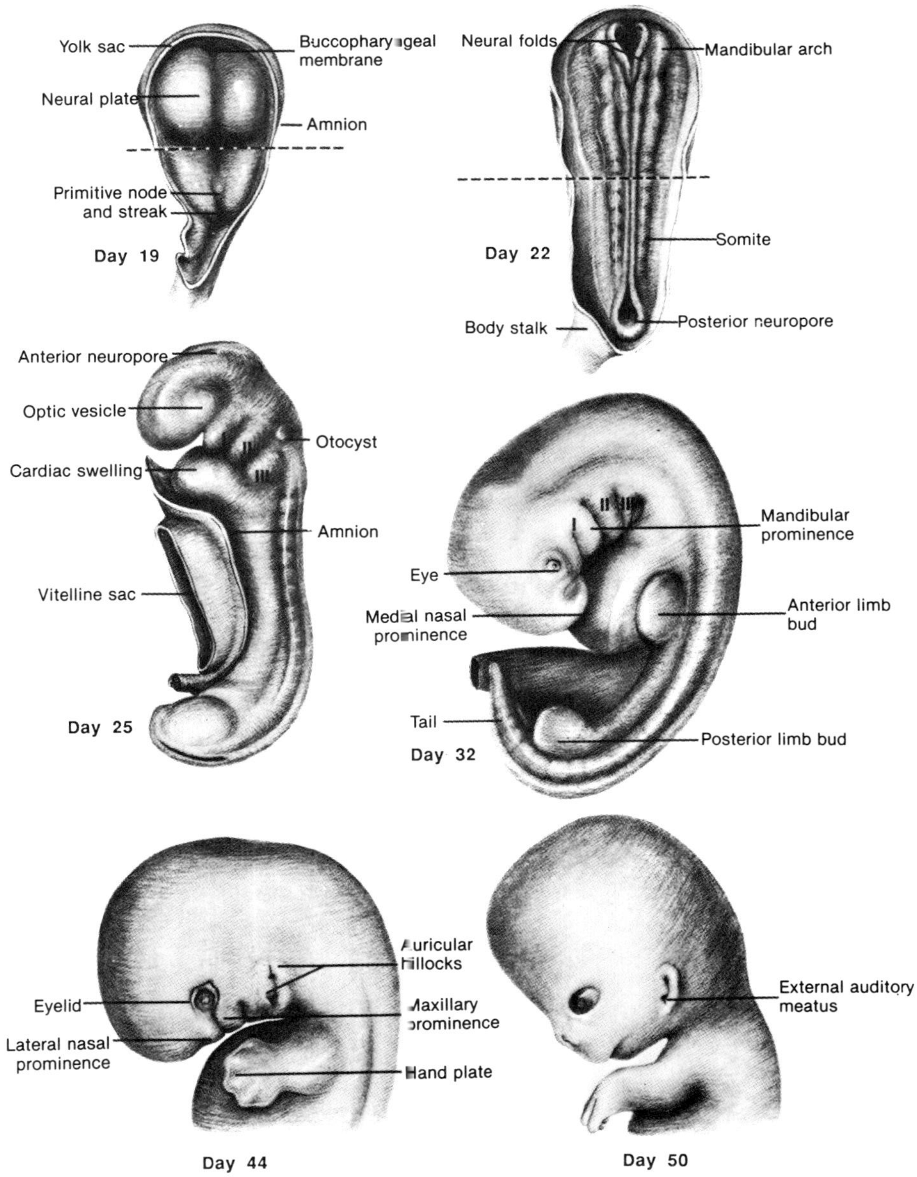


**Fig. 12–1.** Development of the human embryo from the germ-layer stage (day 19), almost to the end of the embryonic period (day 50). The pharyngeal (visceral, branchial) arches are numbered by Roman numerals. Development of the primary palate (primitive roof of the mouth) is underway by day 32 and development of the secondary palate shortly after day 50. Through day 32, surface features of the human embryo are very similar to those of other higher vertebrates, indicating similar developmental mechanisms. (From Johnston and Sulik,[41] with permission.)

tissues in the head and anterior neck is the placodal origin of many of the neuroblasts in the cranial sensory ganglia[11,38] including virtually all of the ganglionic neurons of the acoustico-vestibular ganglia (Fig. 12–4C-E, Fig. 6–8, Chapter 6), in contrast to more caudal sensory ganglia where all of the neurons are of neural crest origin. The induction of the ganglionic placodes is largely unknown, although there is some evidence that crest cells may be involved[31] (see section on homeobox genes below), and, at least for the VIIth, IXth, and Xth nerve ganglia, there is some evidence that pharyngeal pouch endoderm is involved.[10] Certainly, these placodes form in direct contact with the endoderm.

## Pharyngeal (visceral, branchial) arches and tongue

The pharyngeal arches are illustrated in Figure 12–1 at days 25 and 32. They are frequently also referred to as *branchial arches* or *visceral arches*. They are created by invagination of the surface ectoderm, usually termed *pharyngeal clefts* or *pouches* and the pharyngeal endoderm, usually termed *visceral pouches*. The first evidence of segmentation is the formation of the pharyngeal pouches which contact the surface ectoderm at the proximal ends of the pharyngeal arches very early (before the arrival of crest cells). While the mechanisms of pharyngeal segmentation are largely unknown, it seems probable that the organizing influences are in the mesoderm and notochord, as is the case for neural segmentation (see below). In fish and larval amphibia, the ectodermal–endodermal contact breaks down to form gill slits. In higher vertebrates, the ectoderm and endoderm become separated by mesenchyme. Occasionally, this fails to occur, leading to the formation of branchial clefts or cysts.

Even before crest cells begin their migration they show evidence of segmentation that coincides with the segmentation of the hindbrain into rhombomeres, with the pattern of homeobox gene expression largely similar in both the rhombomeres and their derived crest cells (Figs. 12–5, 12–6). There is now considerable evidence (e.g. Fietz et al.)[17] that the control for segmentation of the neural plate is largely dependentant on the underlying notochord, its anterior extension, the prechordal plate, and associated paraxial mesoderm. First arch crest cells are derived from rhombomeres 1 and 2, second arch crest cells from rhombomere 4, while third and fourth arch crest cells are derived from rhombomeres 6 and 7 (see Lumsden et al.[53]; Fig. 12–5). Although crest cells form in rhombomere 3, they apparently undergo cell death,[22] effectively separating the first and second arch crest into two streams (Figs. 12–5A,C). Few crest cells develop from rhombomere 5 and this, in combination with the otic placode that is tightly sealed to the brain, effectively separates second from third arch crest. Thus, when the crest cells enter the arches between pharyngeal pouch endoderm–ectoderm contacts (D. Noden, personal communication), first, second, and third arch crest cells are already travelling in separate streams. Separation of third and fourth arch may depend at least partly on the contact to second pouch and the surface ectoderm, but each crest cell population is apparently already expressing its peculiar pattern of homeobox gene activity that will determine its response to inductive influences emanating from pharyngeal arch structures (e.g., pharyngeal endoderm).[24,30] For example, when 1st arch (or more rostral) crest is substituted for second arch crest, a duplicate mandibular arch skeletal apparatus forms.[66] When a homeobox gene (*Hoxa-2*) normally expressed in hyoid and more caudal arch crest is "knocked out" in transgenic mice, the first arch skeletal apparatus is duplicated in the second arch region.[20,71] Other Hox genes are added in the more caudal arches and some of them are presumably responsible for converting the responses of third and fourth arch crest to form skeletal elements appropriate for those arches. (For reviews on *Hox* genes and head segmentation see Noden,[67] Morriss-Kay,[62] Krumlauf,[46] Wilkinson,[95] and Johnston and Bronsky[36]).

When crest cells reach the individual arches, they surround the mesoderm already present, converting it to core-like structures (Figs. 12–4). This mesoderm is apparently responsible for forming the endothelia of blood vessels (Fig. 12–7, 12–8, 12–9) such as that of the aortic arch blood vessels and appears to consist almost entirely of endothelially lined vesicles containing developing blood cells.[40] In the face and anterior neck other (nonendothelial) components of the blood vessel walls (e.g., fibroblast and smooth muscle cells) are formed by crest cell mesenchyme.

Once the pharyngeal arches are vascularized, it appears that the remaining mesodermal core cells die[40] and are replaced by

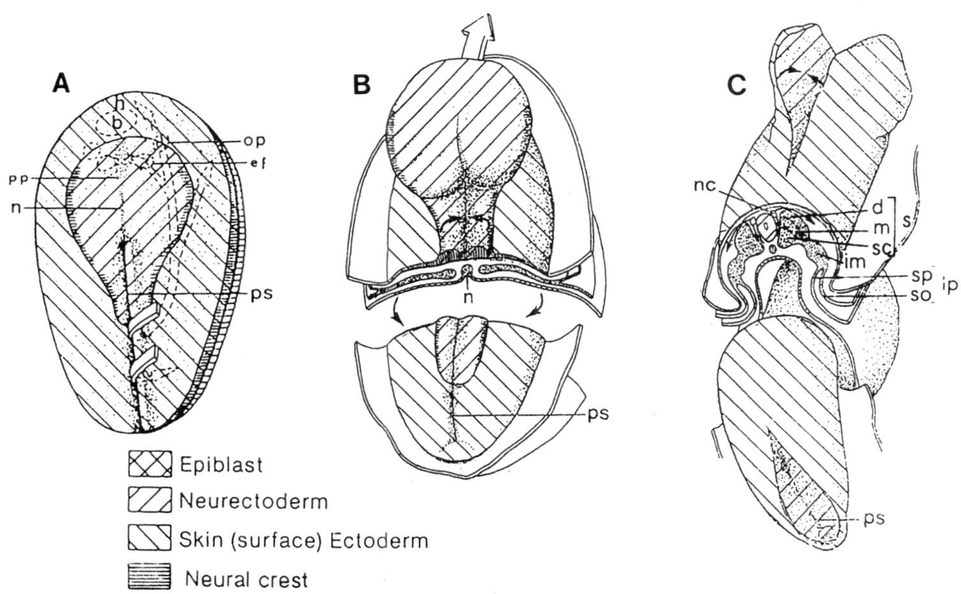


**Fig. 12–2.** Sketches summarizing development from germ-layer formation through formation of the neural and gastrointestinal tubes. Cell-marking procedures now indicate that the entire embryo develops from a single layer (see text). The notochord (n) and the endoderm form as a single layer from the anterior end of the primitive streak (ps). Mesodermal cells migrate through the lateral edges of the primitive streak, eventually separating the remaining surface cells from the endoderm and lying in the same plane as the notochord after it becomes separated from the endoderm (B and C). Two areas where the ectoderm and endoderm remain fused are at the buccal (oral) plate (b in A) and the anal plate (not shown). The notochord (n, and its anterior extension, the prechordal plate, pp) and a portion of the associated mesoderm induce the neural plate and associated structures, apparently including the olfactory (nasal) placodes (op in A) as well as the eye fields (ef) and neural crest (nc in C). Rapid growth of the neural plate and anterior neural tube moves them over and anterior to the buccal plate and heart (h) so that the latter become relatively more caudally located. The mesoderm organizes itself into the dermatome (d), myotome (m) and sclerotome (sc) of the somite (s), the intermediate mesoderm (im), and the splanchnopleure (sp) and somatopleure (so) of the lateral plate (lp). (Modified from Johnston and Sulik,[42] with permission.)

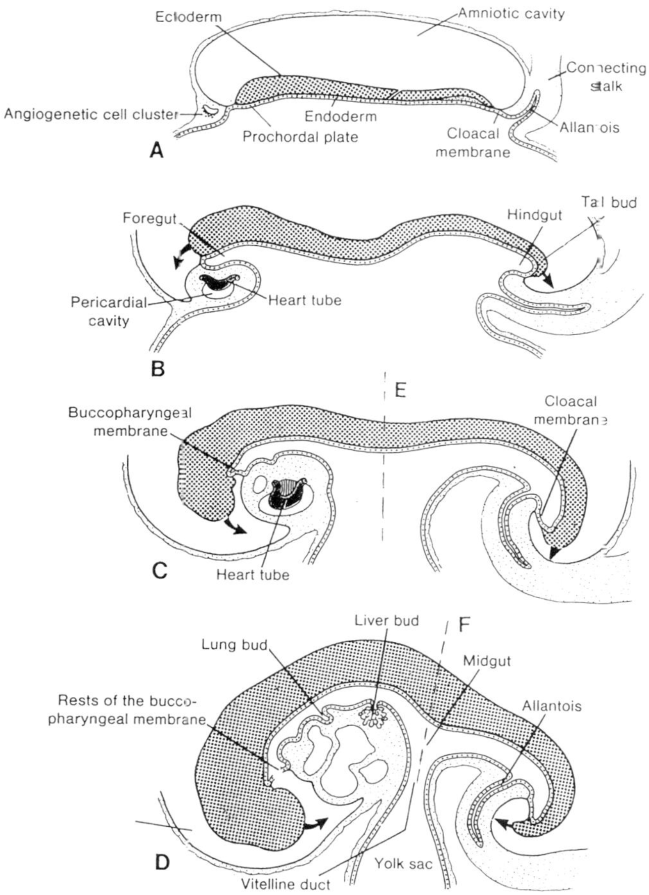


**Fig. 12–3.** Longitudinal sections through the developing human embryo illustrating the manner in which differential growth and folding movements from about day 17 to day 36 create the fore- and hindguts (compare to Fig. 12–2B, C). Primarily because of rapid growth of the anterior neural plate and tube, the buccopharyngeal membrane and heart become relatively more ventrally and caudally positioned so that they form the floor of the foregut. (Modified from Sadler,[74] with permission.)

new mesodermal cells which migrate from paraxial mesoderm (somites and somitomeres, see Figs. 12–5, 12–10) and form the contractile myoblasts of skeletal voluntary muscle (Fig. 12–10). It appears that the myotomes of somites (Fig. 12–2C) or comparable structures rostral to the ear are the only structures capable of forming these particular muscle cells. They have to undergo sometimes long, complex migrations, such as those that form the myoblasts of the tongue and other hypoglossal musculature (see Hazelton;[26] Fig. 12–10). The migrating muscle masses somehow take with them axons of the appropriate motor nerve (e.g. the hypoglossal nerve). The pharyngeal muscle masses are innervated by the VIth, VIIth, IXth, and Xth nerves. After arrival in the visceral arches, many of the myoblasts split off from these so-called muscle plates and migrate as groups of cells, taking with them branches of motor nerve. When they finally settle down to form the definitive muscles, the connective tissues are derived from the local mesenchyme (which is almost entirely of crest origin in the face and anterior neck).

The initial bilateral lingual swellings of the tongue (Fig. 12–8E,F) presumably result from arrival of the hypoglossal myoblasts (Fig. 12–10). The nature of other swellings, such as the tubercular impar (Fig. 12–8E), is not clear. The foramen cecum, which forms at the junctions of the anterior and posterior parts of the tongue, marks the invagination of the endodermal primordium of the thyroid gland.

The formation of the thyroid and other pharyngeal glands in the chick and human is illustrated in Figure 12–9. In general, the human primordia tend to migrate to the midline. Initially, the endodermal primordia invaginate crest cell mesenchyme, which eventually forms most of the connective tissue component of the glands.

Rapid proliferation of crest cells in each individual arch is apparently responsible for longitudinal swellings, and this results in further accentuation of the ectodermal clefts and pharyngeal grooves (Figs. 12–8, 12–9, 12–11A). Growth of the arches and other facial outgrowths is apparently dependent on epithelial–mesenchymal interactions (for reviews see Minkoff,[60] and Richman[70]). These interactions may be mediated in part by a mesenchymal cell process meshwork (Fig. 12–11C). There is some evidence that growth factors, such as fibroblast growth factor (FGF), are produced by the epithelia and, by diffusion, may stimulate mesenchymal cell prolifera-

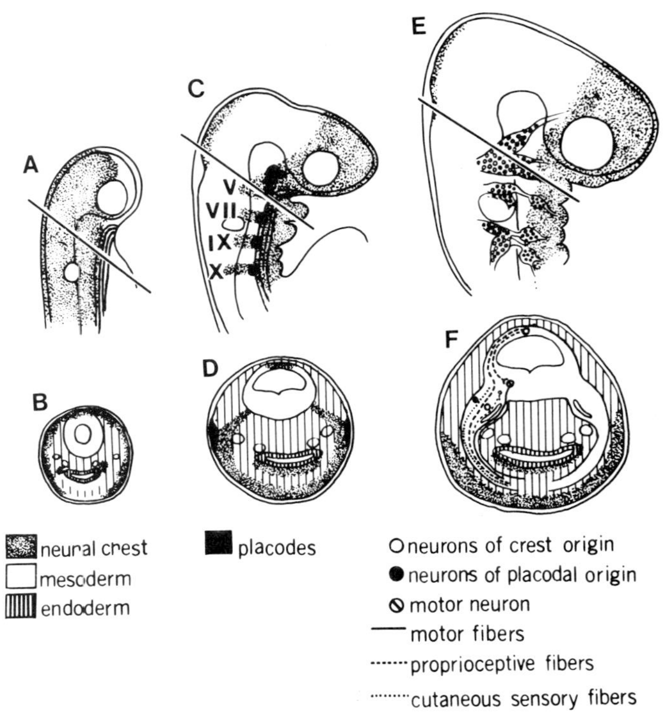


**Fig.12–4.** Migration of neural crest cells to the facial region (A,B; roughly day 22 to day 25) where they assume their final positions (C,D). Cords of crest cells remain attached to the neural tube (C,D) and these will form the initial primordia of cranial general sensory ganglia. Ganglionic placodes ("thickenings" of ectodermal epithelia) contribute the earliest differentiating neurons to the distal ends of the ganglia (C,E). Neural crest cells form the remaining neurons and all of the supporting cells. The final, or nearly final, distribution of crest and placodal neurons is illustrated in E. Motor neurons in the neural tube send their fibers with migrating myoblasts (Fig. 12–8) and become closely associated with those of the sensory neurons entering each of the pharyngeal arches. This basic pattern is repeated for all the pharyngeal arches. (From Johnston and Hazelton,[38] with permission.)

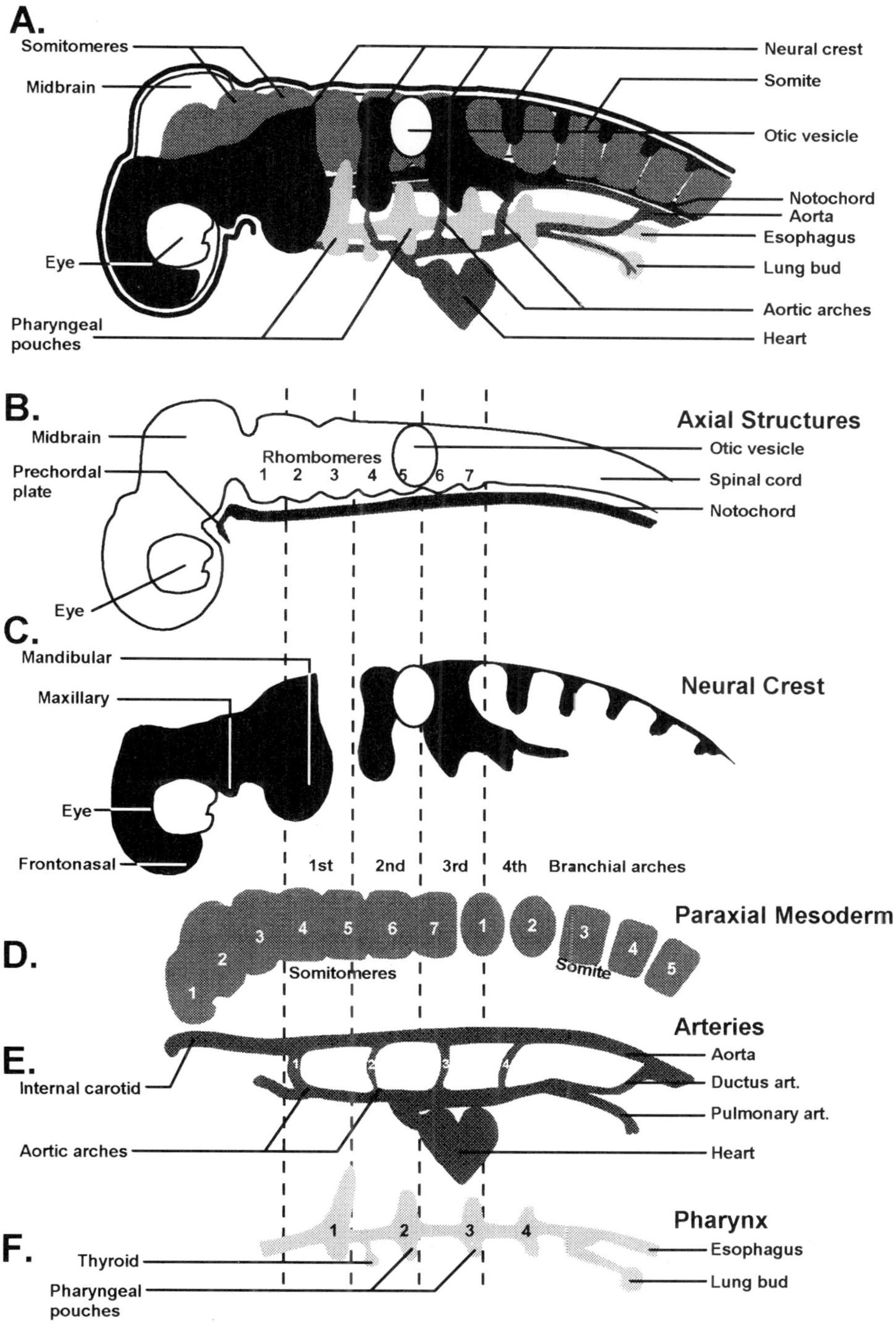


**Fig. 12–5.** Schematic diagrams depicting the segmental origins of different cell populations giving rise to the head and neck (redrawn from Noden[67]). In B–F the different components have been separated ("exploded"), with vertical lines showing the segmental relationships. The initial segmental control may lie in the notochord and its rostral (anterior) extension, the prechordal plate, but by the stages of development illustrated, segmental control lies principally in the rhombomeres (hindbrain neuromeres in B) and the segmented pharynx (F). The neural crest (C) is derived from the neuromeres (e.g., second or hyoid arch crest from rhombomere 4) and migrates into the immediately ventral pharyngeal (branchial, visceral) arches. At these stages, blood is carried from the heart to the rest of the embryo through the aortic arch blood vessels (E). The endothelial cells are derived from mesoderm but, in the face and anterior neck, other elements in the vessel wall (e.g., fibroblasts and smooth muscle cells) are derived from the neural crest, as are almost all other skeletal and connective tissues except the enamel of the teeth. Skeletal and connective tissues in other portions of the head and neck are derived from mesodermal somites and somitomeres (D), as are all the myoblasts of "voluntary" muscles (e.g., the masseter muscles).

tion.[70] A peculiar feature of the first and second arches is the organization of growth centers at their distal ends (Figs. 12–11B), which grow forward over the developing heart, eventually merging with their opposite members in the ventral midline (Fig. 12–11C). Failure of completion of this phenomenon may be responsible for malformations sometimes referred to as *cleft mandibles* or *cleft chins*.

## Development of the primary palate

The principal components of the primary palate are the olfactory placode and the associated covering epithelia of the medial and lateral nasal prominences with their associated frontonasal crest mesenchyme, as well as the maxillary prominences and their associated neural crest mesenchyme (Fig. 12–11). The

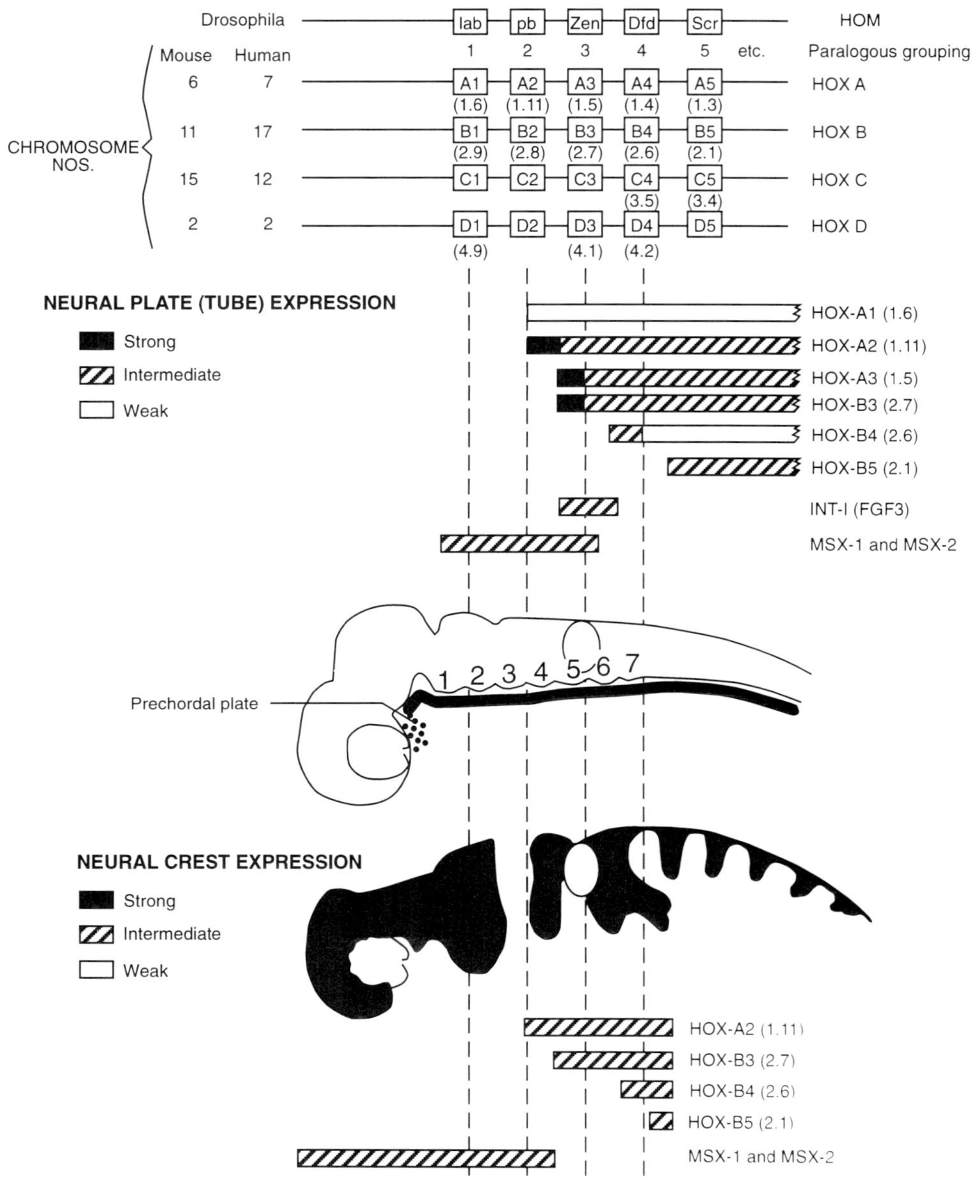


**Fig. 12–6.** *Hox* and other homeobox genes involved in head development, with emphasis on the pharynx and other craniofacial tissues. Homeobox genes dictate the synthesis of proteins that bind to DNA and alter the activity of other genes. Our understanding of the control of head segmentation in embryos has been greatly enhanced by the discovery that the same set of genes involved in the regulation of head segmentation in *Drosophila* also functions in vertebrates. These genes are arranged on a single chromosome in *Drosophila* in a head-to-tail (lab→Scr, etc.) sequence. This block of genes (now termed *Hox* genes) has been duplicated on four different chromosomes in the mouse and human, as indicated. Their expression patterns (usually detected as radiolabeled mRNA) in mouse (and chick) embryo neural plate (and tube) and neural crest are indicated (see text for details). The older mouse designations for the genes are given in parenthesis (e.g., the old *Hox-1.6* is now *Hox-a1*). Other homeobox genes, some of which used to be called *Hox* genes, have been given other names (e.g., the old *Hox-7* and *Hox-8* are now termed *Msx-1* and *Msx-2*). The expression of *Msx-1* and *Msx-2*, which have major involvement in facial development, and *Int-2*, which is involved in ear development, are indicated as examples of non-*Hox* homeobox genes. (Diagram modified from Noden,[67] with permission.)

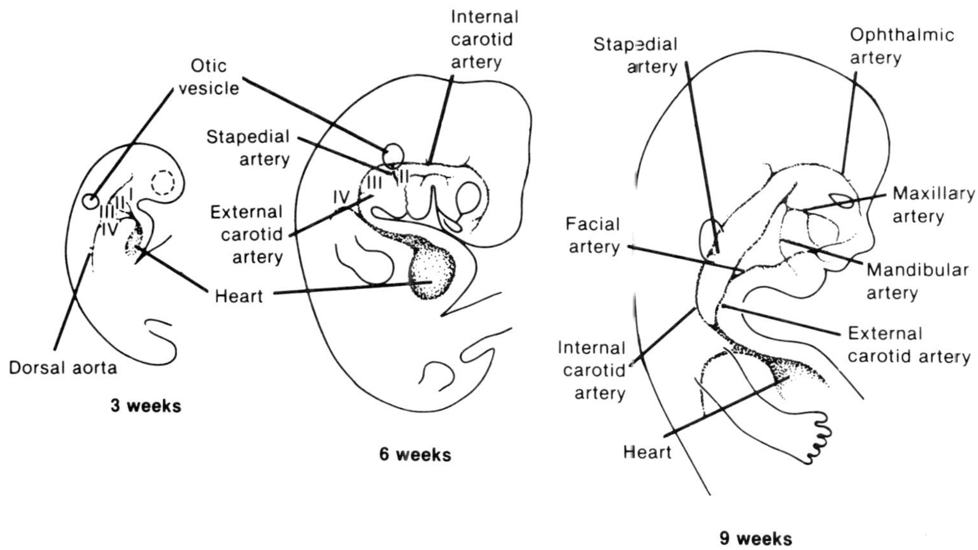


**Fig. 12–7.** Development of the vascular system in the face and neck of the human embryo. (From Ross and Johnston,[72] with permission.)

maxillary prominence (MxP) merges with the lateral nasal prominence (LNP), and then both of them contact and fuse with the medial nasal prominence (the epithelial seam breaks down; see Figs. 12–12B, 12–13).

When the premigratory frontonasal and maxillary neural crest is substituted experimentally for hyoid crest, it responds the same way as mandibular arch crest (i.e., it produces mandibular skeletal structures).[66] In normal development, this "ground plan" of the crest mesenchyme migrating into areas rostral to the mandibular arch appears to be modified by interactions with tissues they encounter: principally the forebrain, eye, and olfactory placode. Eventually, these crest cells will form the skeletal and connective tissues associated with these structures. While the nature of the tissue interaction is still largely unknown, there are some fascinating clues as to what it may be (for review see Johnston and Bronsky).[36]

*Msx-1* and *Msx-2* homeobox genes are active in crest cells before,[22] during, and after[54,55] crest cell migration, particularly in the distal portions of the arches and the epithelia and mesenchyme of the developing teeth. A knockout for *Msx-1*[75] shows failed or arrested tooth development and (secondarily?) malformations such as cleft palate.

There is also some evidence for growth factor involvement in epithelial/mesenchymal interactions. The apparent ability of FGF to at least partially support the development of facial prominence mesenchyme in culture has already been noted. Specific variants of FGF (e.g., FGF-8)[9a] have been noted in specific areas of the olfactory placode and in epithelia associated with the developing visceral arches. The olfactory placode also shows very high levels of another growth factor, BMP-3,[27] a member of the TGF$\beta$ family.

Retinoic acid (RA) apparently also plays a major role in primary palate development. Retinoic acid receptors (RARs) are present[94] and double RAR$\alpha$-RAR$\gamma$ knockouts show defects in primary palate development.[51]

The descriptive aspects of primary palate formation are now fairly well established and some insight into the underlying mechanism has been gained. It appears that the olfactory placodes are derived from the anterior neural folds[9,29] (Fig. 12–2A) from which they eventually separate. After the prospective placodal epithelium becomes underlain by neural crest cells, it begins to thicken, chiefly through its cells assuming a columnar configuration. The lateral edge of the placode begins to curl forward (Figs. 12–11, 12–12), which appears to at least partly involve a morphogenetic movement,[82] together with high rates of cell proliferation.[60] The maxillary prominence grows under the eye and merges with the lateral nasal prominence. Both the maxillary and lateral nasal prominences make contact with the medial prominence with an epithelial seam between them (Figs. 12–12, 12–13). Before contact is made, a layer of surface peridermal cells is lost[58] and the underlying epithelial cells appear to actively participate in the contact and adhesion between the prominences,[58] as has been well documented for the epithelia of the contacting palatal shelf edges in secondary palate formation.[93] In both primary (Figs. 12–12, 12–13) and secondary palate formation, a portion of the contacting epithelium "breaks down" so that the underlying mesenchyme becomes confluent. There is very good evidence from cell marking and cytological studies on secondary palate formation (see below) that such contacting epithelial cells transform into mesenchyme cells and actively participate in this fusion; this presumably will also be found to be the case for primary palate formation.

In primary palate formation, a portion of the epithelial seam behind the fusion area persists. It hollows out to form a channel connecting the olfactory pit with the oral cavity (Figs. 12–12, 12–13), thus giving rise to the primitive nasal cavity.

Failure of primary palate formation leads to clefts of the lip with or without cleft palate CL(P); Fig. 12–16, by far the most common severe human craniofacial malformation. (For reviews see Ross and Johnston,[72] Fraser,[19] and Johnston and Bronsky.[36]) Most human "nonsyndromic" CL(P) (i.e., those not associated with malformations that are part of a known syndrome) are probably multifactorial (i.e., result from a combination of genetic and environmental factors) in each individual case. Why there is sometimes an associated cleft palate is not clear, although a number of ideas have been put forward.[36,81,90] Experimentally, clefts of the lip with or without associated cleft palate can be produced by interfering with

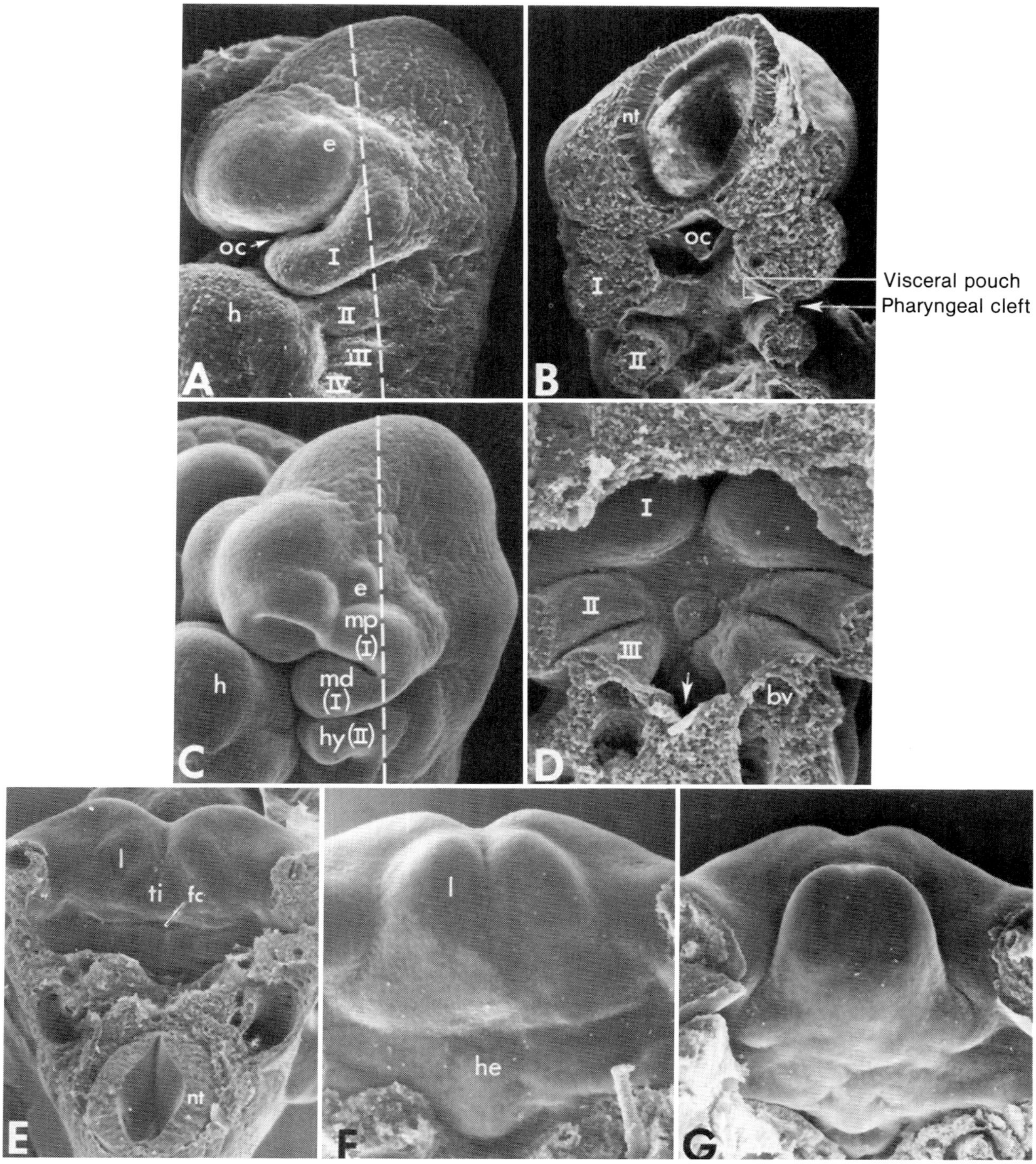


**Fig. 12-8.** Scanning electron micrographs of the developing pharyngeal arches and tongue of mouse embryos. At the stages in development illustrated in A (roughly equivalent to human day 26), the first arch has largely separated from the heart (h) and by the stage of development equivalent to human day 32, in C, the second arch has largely separated from the heart. The planes of section for the specimens depicted in B and D are illustrated in A and C. These specimens show sectioned arches and the floor of the pharynx. Roman numerals identify each arch and the arrow in D indicates the entrance into the esophagus. Development of the tongue is illustrated in E–G. The development of the lingual swellings (l in E and F) presumably corresponds to the arrival of the hypoglossal cord myoblasts (Fig. 12–11). Other structures indicated are the foramen cecum (fc in E), a remnant of the invaginating thyroid epithelium, tubercular impar (ti in E), and the hypobranchial eminence (he in F), the function of which is unknown. bv, blood vessel; hy, hyoid arch; md, mandibular arch; mp, maxillary prominence; nt, neural tube; oc, oral cavity. (From Johnston and Sulik,[42] with permission.)

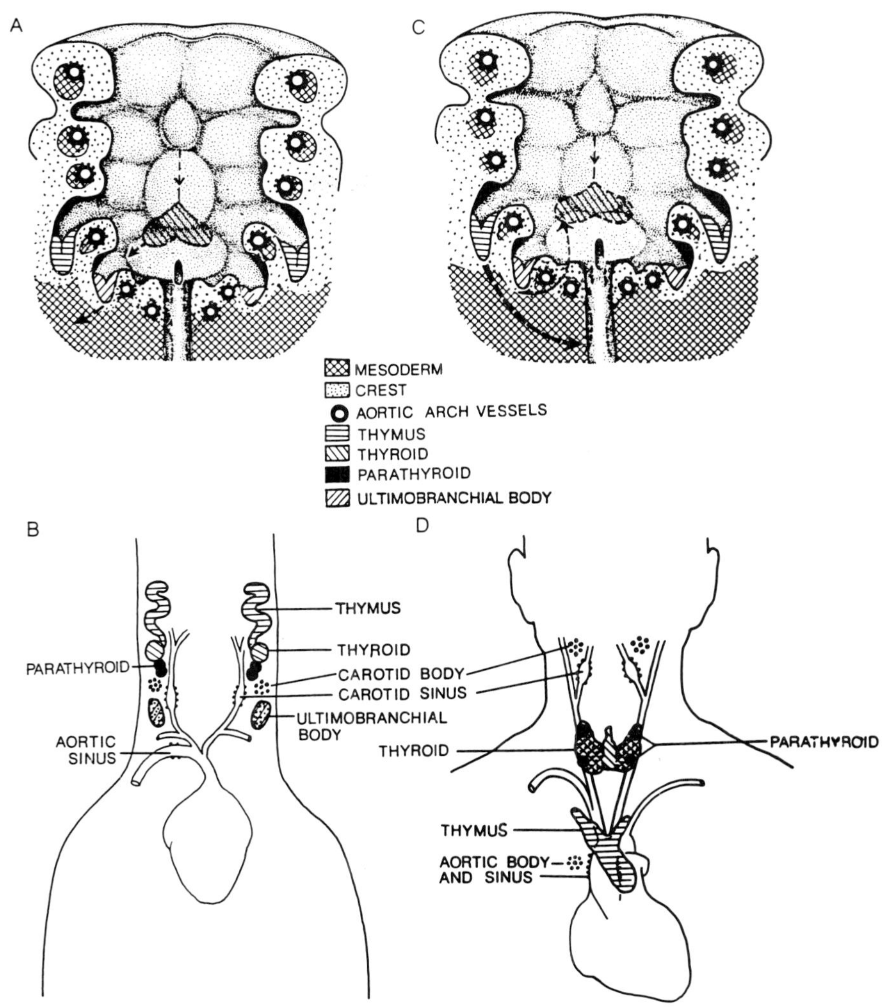


**Fig. 12–9.** Comparative development of the pharyngeal glands in the chick (A,B) and human (C,D) embryos. In the human embryo, the glands move toward the midline and the ultimobrancial body fuses with the thyroid gland (thereby bringing crest-derived c cells into the thyroid gland). (From Johnston et al.,[35] with permission.)

many aspects of primary palate formation,[36,72] even by removing crest cells prior to their migration.[33,56,92]

Predisposing genetic factors may consist of narrow medial nasal prominences (MNPs) in both humans[12,36,39] and other animals.[89] In the A/J mouse, a single gene (leading to narrow MNPs?) may cause CL(P) by itself on the appropriate genetic background.[44] Similar ideas have been put forward for a large portion of human CL(P)s (see Chung et al.[8]), although most investigators feel that pedigree data are more consistent with multifactorial inheritance.[19,36]

A major breakthrough came with the application of techniques of molecular genetics to CL(P) populations. Based on observations of TGF-$\alpha$ (the embryonic form of epidermal growth factor) in secondary palate formation,[69] Ardinger et al.[1a] examined blood samples from CL(P) patients for evidence of unusual variants of genes producing TGF$\alpha$s and found them to be present in high frequencies. Their findings have been confirmed by numerous other investigators.[7,28,32,73] Pedigree studies indicate, however, that other genetic and/or environmental factors are probably essential in most cases.[15] TGF-$\alpha$ plays a major role in embryonic development, particularly in the regulation of epithelial differentiation. The very high spontaneous incidence of CL(P) in CL/Fr mice may be partly attributed to abnormalities in differentiation of fusion epithelia.[36,57] Other unusual variations in the genes for developmentally important regulatory molecules have also been found (e.g., RAR$\alpha$,[7,73] NADH dehydrogenase,[73] and cytochrome P450).[73]

The strongest environmental factor in human CL(P) appears to be cigarette smoking (see Erikson et al.,[14] Keels[45]). Although smoking has many physiological effects, most investigators (e.g., Longo[52]) feel that the most significant prenatal effects are caused by carbon monoxide, which leads to embryonic and fetal hypoxia. Embryonic tissue levels of $O_2$ are critical for normal functioning of the electron transport chain and ATP formation. Many popular CL(P) teratogens in animals also seem to act by producing ATP deficiency, including maternal hypoxia[59] and 6–amino-nicotinamide (6–AN).[91] The latter also acts by interfering with the electron transport chain function by altering NADH dehydrogenase, the first enzyme in the chain to accept electrons from high-energy intermediates. The incidence of primary palate clefts induced by 6–AN in the chick embryo can be decreased by the use of high energy intermediates that donate electrons further down the chain,[47] by-passing the nonfunctional NADH dehydrogenase. High ATP levels may be particularly critical for primary palate development both be-

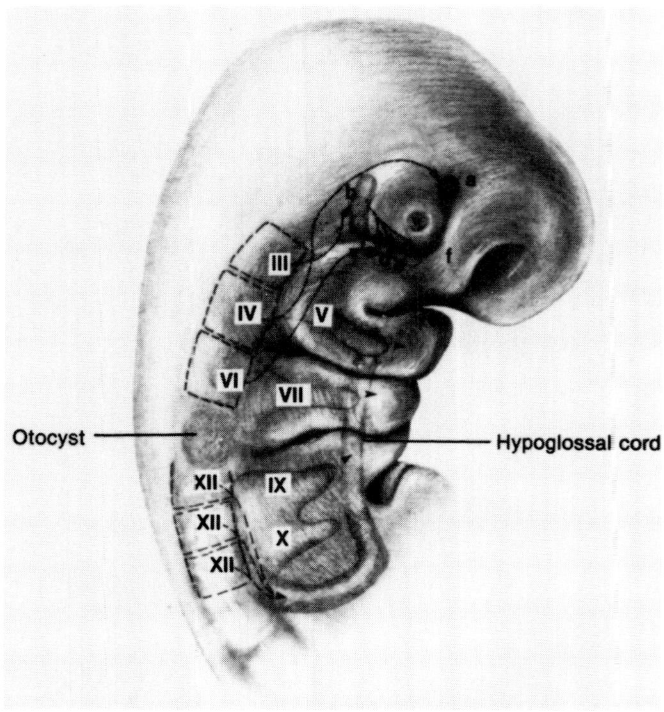


**Fig. 12–10.** All, or almost all, of the myoblasts of skeletal voluntary muscle throughout the body arise from the myotomes of postotic somites (Figs. 12–2C and 12–5D) or from comparable structures in preotic somitomeres (Fig. 12–5D). They undergo primary migrations into staging areas such as the cores of the visceral arches or the embryonic tongue as shown, with secondary migrations to the locations of individual muscles (not shown). The cranial nerves providing motor innervation are indicated by roman numerals. Extrinsic ocular muscle primordia are indicated by a–f. For details, see text. (From Johnston and Sulik,[41] with permission.)

cause of the high proliferation rates[60] and the morphogenetic movement[6,82] involved.

Other environmental factors that may be important to CL(P) formation include low folate levels,[2,5,63,88] presumably on account of high primary palate proliferation rates. Folate supplements have been shown to reduce the incidence of neural tube defects (anencephaly and spina bifida)[63] and similar reductions for CL(P) may be possible.[5,88] The anticonvulsant drug phenytoin (Dilantin) has also been implicated.[1,25,84]

The importance of a combination of genetic and environmental factors in individual cases is indicated by the very high incidence of CL(P) found in children with a TGF$\alpha$ variant who are born to mothers who smoke cigarettes.[32] It seems certain that nonsyndromic clefts result from these and other such combinations.

On the other hand, syndromic CL(P) is often associated with single major genes (see Gorlin et al.,[21] and Appendix D, Syndromes and Conditions Associated with Congenital Anomalies of the Mouth, Palate, and Pharynx, p. 263). Examples are CL(P)s associated with the van der Woude syndrome and hemifacial microsomia, although in the latter case, environmental factors may also play a role.[36] Similarly, major environmental factors may produce CL(P) associated with syndromes such as fetal alcohol syndrome (FAS) and fetal hydantoin (phenytoin) syndrome (FHS).

Also, numerous associated malformations were found in a large prospective study of CL(P) born to mothers who smoke.[45] Maternal cigarette smoking sufficient to cause CL(P) apparently also frequently causes other developmental alterations that are not recognized as belonging to known syndromes.

## Secondary palate formation

Figure 12–14 depicts the major features involved in secondary (hard and soft) palate formation that normally takes place be-

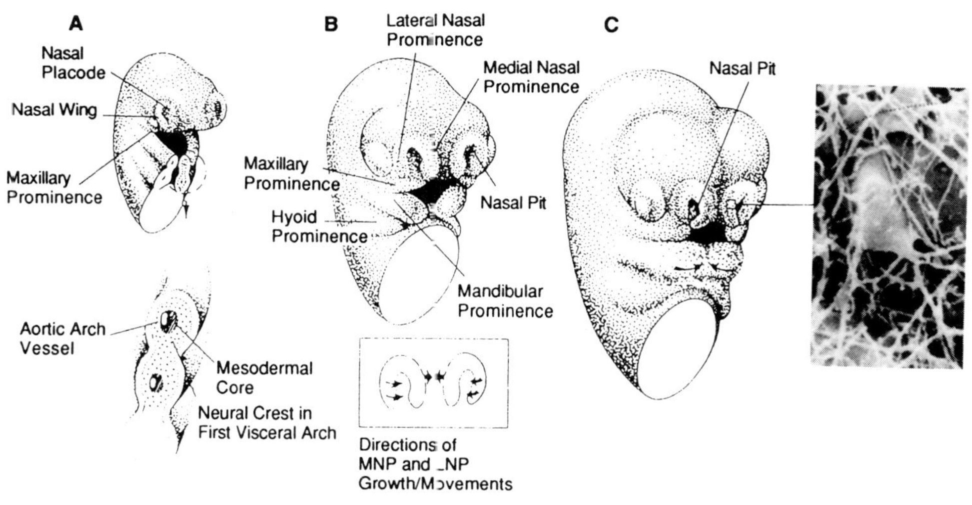


**Fig. 12–11.** At the completion of their migration (Fig. 12–4), crest cells surround the mesodermal cores in the pharyngeal arches (A, detail) and form all the mesenchyme between the covering epithelium and underlying brain and eye in portions of the face above the oral cavity. Maintenance of high rates of proliferation in the mesenchyme is dependent on the overlying epithelia and is possibly mediated through the mesenchymal cell process meshwork underlying the epithelium, which has been removed in the scanning electron micrograph in C. These epithelial effects apparently involve growth factors (see text). Major morphogenetic movements (summarized in inset in B) are also involved in facial prominence formation. Contact between the prominences (B and C) initiates separation of the developing oral and nasal cavities. Failure of this contact and subsequent fusion leads to a cleft lip. (Modified from Johnston and Sulik,[41] with permission.)

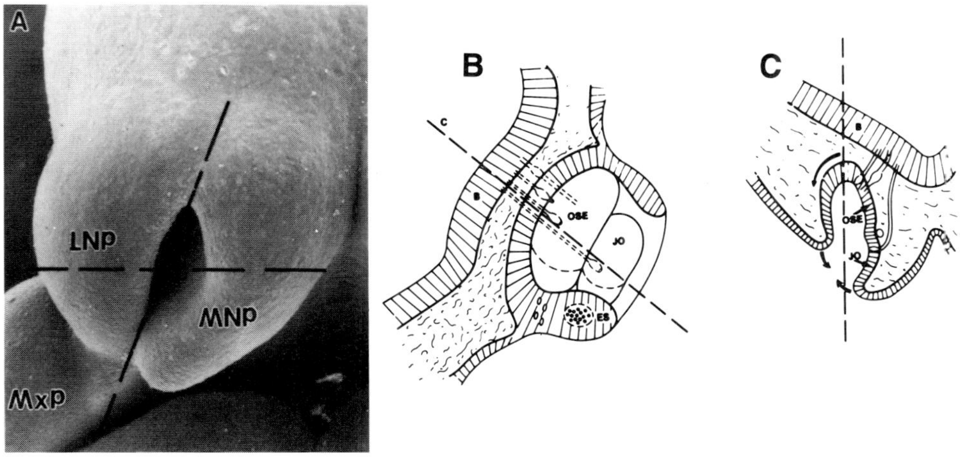


**Fig. 12–12.** Components involved in primary palate formation. A: Scanning electron micrograph of the right side of the developing primary palate of a 39 somite mouse embryo (equivalent to a day 34 human embryo) depicting the lateral nasal (LNP), medial nasal (MNP) and maxillary (MxP) prominences. The section planes for the diagrams in B and C are indicated. B: Schematic diagram of a sectioned primary palate and associated forebrain (plane indicated in A and C). The epithelia are indicated by cross-hatching and the intervening mesenchyme by scroll. The epithelial surface of the medial aspect of the nasal pit and representative neurons are depicted. Many of the neurons of the olfactory sensory epithelium (OSE) and Jacobsen's organ (JO) have already differentiated and sent processes into the brain. Some neuronal cell bodies have moved into the olfactory nerve from the placode. The epithelial seam (ES) formed between the facial prominences is "breaking down" in one area (stipple), and will be replaced by mesenchymal "penetration," and cavitation in another area (open circles) where the nasal passage connecting the olfactory pit and oral cavity will form. C: Section plane (illustrated in A and B) indicating (long arrow) that the curling of the olfactory placode and associated mesenchyme movement is nearing completion (see in Fig. 12B and the text). Largely because of these morphogenetic movements, the olfactory sensory epithelium (OSE) will be finally located at the top of the nasal cavity. The medial nasal prominence appears to bend laterally in the horizontal plane as well as in the coronal plane. (From Bronsky and Johnston,[6] with permission.)

tween days 50 and 60 in the human. The epithelial changes are well documented (see Waterman and Meller)[93] and involve death and shedding of the surface epithelial cells (pericytes), as illustrated in Figure 12–15. The underlying basal epithelial cells actively participate in contact and adhesion.[93]

Recent studies using rat palatal shelves in culture suggest strongly (on the basis of cytological changes[18] and cell marking)[80] that most of these basal cells survive and eventually transform into mesenchymal cells. Basal epithelial cells in primary palate formation may also have a similar fate.

Cleft palate (CP; see Fig. 12–16), while not as common or as well studied in humans, has been very extensively studied in animals.[4,19,23,96] Genetic predisposition in the human may involve increased tongue size,[39] small mandibles,[19,36,72,79] tongue-tie (abnormally short lingual frenulum)[61] and other anatomical variations that may inhibit withdrawal of the tongue from between the palatal shelves (Fig. 12–14). In different mouse strains, increased incidence of CP is associated with delayed palate shelf elevation.[90] The increased incidence of unusual TGF$\alpha$ variants in CP patients[78] suggests that interference with epithelial differentiation could also be a predisposing factor.

The molecular mechanisms involved in normal secondary palate formation in animals have been very extensively studied (see Zimmerman,[96] Ferguson,[16] and Greene and Weston[23] for reviews). Much information has accumulated about the potential roles of extracellular molecules, growth factors, and other molecules.

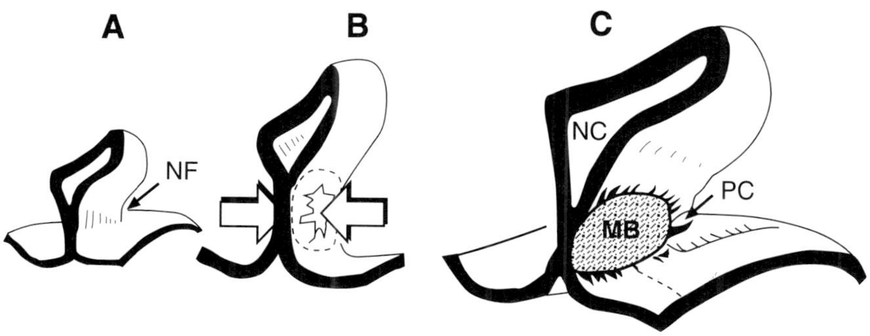


**Fig. 12–13.** Three-dimensional depiction of sectioned (coronal plane) developing human primary palates viewed from the front. The intact nasal fin (NF = epithelial seam) is indicated in A, the onset of epithelial breakdown and mesenchymal penetration (arrows) in B and the formation of the mesenchyme bridge (MB) in C. Cavitation of the nasal fin (epithelial seam) behind the mesenchymal bridge (Fig. 12–12B) will lead to formation of the nasal passage connecting the nasal cavity (NC) to the roof of the oral cavity at the posterior choana (PC). (From Diewart and Wang,[13] with permission.)

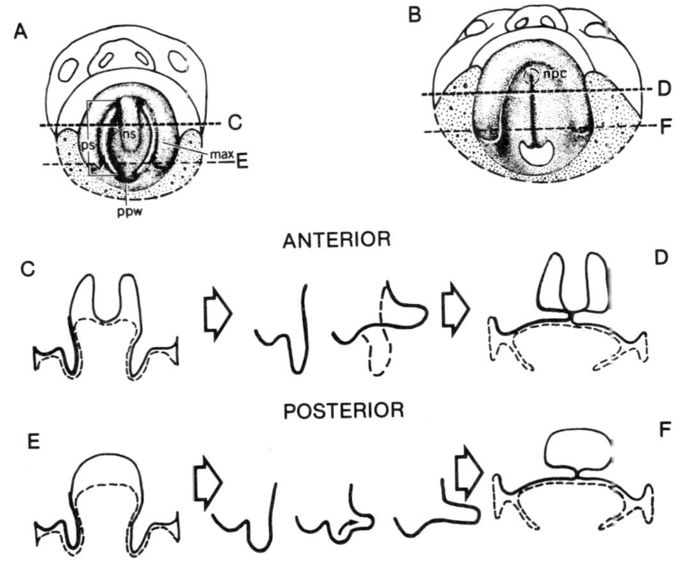


**Fig. 12–14.** Secondary palate formation before (A,C,E) and after (B,D,F) palatal shelf elevation. Shelf elevation appears to involve "barn door" rotation for the anterior (hard palate) region and tissue translocation in the posterior (soft palate) region. (From Johnston et al.,[37] with permission.)

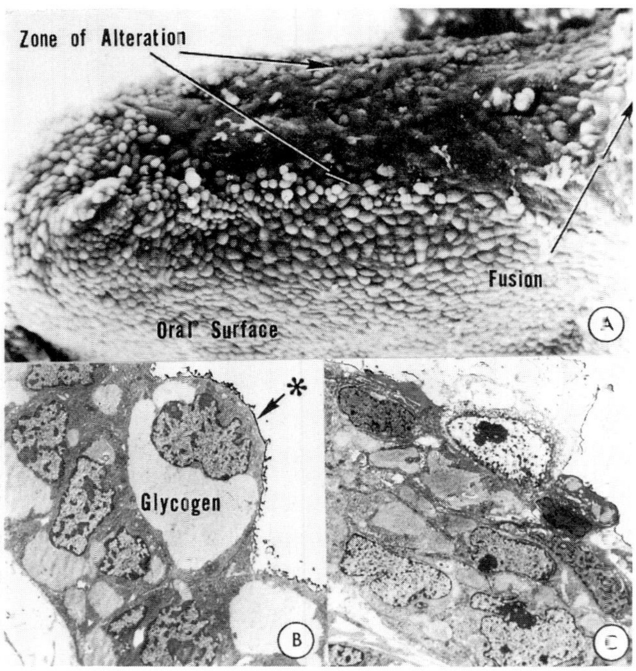


**Fig. 12–15.** Scanning (A) and transmission (B,C) electron micrographs (EMs) of the same human palatal shelf, approximately day 56. The metal coating necessary for the scanning EM is indicated by an asterisk in the section through the oral surface epithelium in B. In the section (C) through the future fusion epithelium (zone of alteration in A), surface epithelial cells are dying and being shed. The underlying basal epithelial cells participate actively in the formation of the epithelial seam and it appears that many of them transform into mesenchymal cells during epithelial breakdown (for details, see text). (From Waterman and Meller,[93] with permission.)

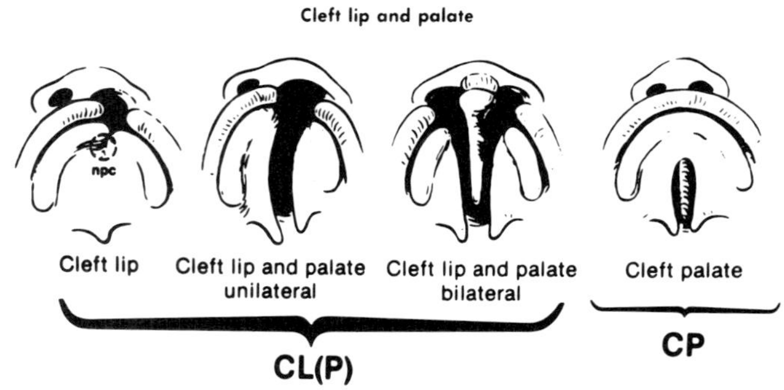


**Fig. 12–16.** Principal variations of clefts of the lip and/or palate (From Ross and Johnston,[72] with permission.)

There is little evidence for the role of environmental factors in human CP. Again, the incidence is increased in children born to mothers who smoke cigarettes.[45] An extremely large number of environmental agents have been shown to be cleft palate teratogens in animals (for reviews see Zimmerman,[96] and Greene and Weston[23]) but their human relevance has not been determined.

## References

1. Abrishamchian AR, Khoury MJ, Calle EE: The contribution of maternal epilepsy and its treatment to the etiology of oral clefts: a population based case-control study. Genet Epidemiol 11:343–351, 1994.

1a. Ardinger HH, Buetow KH, Bell GI, Bardach J, VanDemark DR, Murray JC: Association of genetic variation of the transforming growth factor-alpha gene with cleft lip and palate. Am J Med Genet 45:348–353, 1989.

2. Asling CW: Congenital defects of the face and palate following maternal deficiency of pteroylglutamic acid. In: Congenital Anomalies of the Face and Associated Structures, S Pruzansky, ed. Charles C Thomas, Springfield, 1961, pp 173–187.

3. Beddington RS: Induction of a second neural axis by the mouse node. Development 120:613–620, 1994.

4. Bonner JJ, Slavkin HC: Cleft palate susceptibility linked to histocompatibility—2(H-2) in the mouse. Immunogenetics 2:213–218, 1975.

5. Briggs RM: Vitamin supplementation as a possible factor in the incidence of cleft lip/palate deformities in humans. Clin Plast Surg 3:647–652, 1976.

6. Bronsky PT, Johnston MC: Morphogenetic movements involved in normal primary palate development and cleft lip formation (in preparation).

6a. Chan W, Tam PPL: A morphological and experimental study of the mesencephalic neural crest cells in the mouse embryo using wheat germ agglutinin—gold conjugate as the cell marker. Development 102:427–442, 1988.

7. Chenevix-Trench G, Jones K, Green AC, Duffy DL, Martin NG: Cleft lip with or without cleft palate: associations with transforming growth factor alpha and retinoic acid receptor loci. Am J Hum Genet 51:1377–1385, 1992.

8. Chung CS, Bixler D, Watanabe T, Koguchi H, Fogh-Anderson P: Segregation analysis of cleft lip with or without cleft palate: a comparison of Danish and Japanese data. Am J Hum Genet 39:603–611, 1986.

9. Couly G, Le Douarin NM: The fate map of the cephalic neural primordium at the presomitic to the 3-somite stage in the avian embryo. Development 103 (Suppl):101–113, 1988.

9a. Crossley PH, Martin GR: The mouse Fgf8 gene encodes a family of polypeptides and is expressed in regions that direct outgrowth and patterning in the developing embryo. Development 121:439–451, 1995.

10. Damas H: Observations sur le développement des ganglions crâniens chez *Lamperta fluviatilus*. Arch Biol 62:65–95, 1951.

11. D'Amico-Martel A, Noden DM: Contributions of placodal and neural crest cells to avian cranial peripheral ganglia. Am J Anat 166:445–468, 1983.

12. Diewert VM, Shiota K: Morphological observations in normal primary palate and cleft lip embryos in the Kyoto collection. Teratology 41:663–677, 1990.
13. Diewert VM, Wang KY: Recent advances in primary palate and mid-face morphogenesis research. Crit Rev Oral Biol Med 4:111–130, 1992.
14. Ericson A, Kallen B, Westerholm P: Cigarette smoking as an etiologic factor in cleft lip and palate. Am J Obstet Gynecol 135:348–351, 1979.
15. Farrall M, Buetow KH, Murray JC: Resolving an apparent paradox concerning the role of TGFA in CL/P. Am J Hum Genet 52:434–436, 1993.
16. Ferguson MWJ: Palate development. Development 103(Suppl):41–60, 1988.
17. Fietz MJ, Concordet J-P, Barbosa R, Johnson R, Krauss S, McMahon AP, Tabin C, Ingham PW: The *hedgehog* gene family in *Drosophila* and vertebrate development. Development (Suppl):43–51, 1994.
18. Fitchett JE, Hay ED: Medial edge epithelium transforms to mesenchyme after embryonic palatal shelves fuse. Dev Biol 131:455–474, 1989.
19. Fraser FC: The multifactorial threshold concept—uses and misuses. Teratology 14:267–280, 1976.
20. Gendron-Maguire M, Mallo M, Zhang M, Gridley T: Hoxa-2 mutant mice exhibit homeotic transformation of skeletal elements derived from cranial neural crest. Cell 75:1317–1331, 1993.
21. Gorlin RJ, Cohen MM, Levin KS: Syndromes of the Head and Neck, 3rd ed. Oxford University Press, New York, 1990, p 977.
22. Graham A, Heyman I, Lumsden A: Even-numbered rhombomeres control the apoptotic elimination of neural crest cells from odd-numbered rhombomeres in the chick hindbrain. Development 119:233–245, 1993.
23. Greene RM, Weston WM: Craniofacial embryology. In: Mastery of Surgery, M Cohen, ed. Little, Brown and Co, New York, 1994, pp 457–470.
24. Hall BK, Hörstadius S: The Neural Crest. Oxford University Press, London, 1988.
25. Hansen DK, Hodes ME: Comparative teratogenicity of phenytoin among several inbred strains of mice. Teratology 28:175–179, 1983.
26. Hazelton RD: A radioautographic analysis of the migration and fate of the occipital somites of the chick embryo with specific reference to the hypoglossal musculature. J Embryol Exp Morphol 24:455–466, 1970.
27. Hogan BL, Blessing M, Winnier GE, Suzuki N, Jones CM: Growth factors in development: the role of TGF-$\beta$ related polypeptide signalling molecules in embryogenesis. Development (Suppl):53–60, 1994.
28. Holder SE, Vintiner GM, Farren G, Malcolm S, Winter RM: Confirmation of an association between RFLPs at the transforming growth factor-alpha locus and nonsyndromic cleft lip and palate. J Med Genet 29:390–392, 1992.
29. Holtfreter J, Hamburger V: Amphibians. In: Analysis of Development, Willyer DH, Weiss PA, B Hamburger, eds. WB Saunders, Philadelphia, 1955, pp 230–296.
30. Hörstadius S: The Neural Crest. Oxford Press, Oxford, U.K., 1950.
31. Hunt P, Wilkinson D, Krumlauf R: Patterning the vertebrate head: murine Hox 2 genes mark distinct subpopulations of premigratory and migrating cranial neural crest. Development 112:43–50, 1991.
32. Hwang SJ, Beaty TH, Panny SR, Street NA, Joseph JM, Gordon S, McIntosh I, Francomano CA: Association study of transforming growth factor alpha (TGF$\alpha$)taq 1 polymorphism and oral clefts: indication of gene-environment interaction in a population-based sample of infants with birth defects. Am J Epidemiol 141:629–636, 1995.
33. Johnston MC: Facial malformations in chick embryos, resulting from removal of neural crest. Preprinted abstr, Annu Meeting, Int Assoc Dental Res, Los Angeles, CA, J Dent Res 43:822, 1964.
34. Johnston MC: A radioautographic study of the migration and fate of cranial neural crest cells in the chick embryo. Anat Rec 156:143–156, 1966.
35. Johnston MC, Bhakdinaronk A, Reid YC: An expanded role for the neural crest in oral and pharyngeal development. In: Oral Sensation and Perception-Development in the Fetus and Infant, JF Bosma, ed. U.S. Govt Printing Office, Washington DC, 1974, pp 37–52.
36. Johnston MC, Bronsky PT: Prenatal craniofacial development: new insights on normal and abnormal mechanisms. Crit Rev Oral Biol Med 6:25–79, 1995.
37. Johnston MC, Hassell JR, Brown KS: The embryology of cleft lip and cleft palate. Clin Plast Surg 2:195–203, 1975.
38. Johnston MC, Hazelton RB: Embryonic origins of facial structures related to oral sensory and motor function. In: Oral Sensory Perception, JF Bosma, ed. Charles C Thomas, Springfield, 1972, pp 96–97.
39. Johnston MC, Hunter WS, Niswander DF: Facial morphology in twins discordant for clefts of the lip and palate: a pilot study (in preparation).
40. Johnston MC, Listgarten MA: The migration, interaction and early differentiation of oro-facial tissues. In: Developmental Aspects of Oral Biology, HS Slavkin, LA Bavetta, eds. Academic Press, New York, 1972, pp 55–80.
41. Johnston MC, Sulik KK: Development of the face and oral cavity. In: Orban's Oral Histology and Embryology, 9th ed, SV Bhaskar, ed CV Mosby, St. Louis, 1980, pp 1–23.
42. Johnston MC, Sulik KK: Embryology of the head and neck. In: Pediatric Plastic Surgery, NG Serafin, ND Georgiade, eds. CV Mosby, St. Louis, 1984, pp 184–215.
43. Johnston MC, Vig KN, Ambrose LJ: Neurocristopathy as a unifying concept: clinical correlations. Adv Neurol 29:97–104, 1981.
44. Juriloff DM, Mah DG: The major locus for multifactorial non syndromic cleft lip maps to mouse chromosome 11. Mamm Genome 6:63–69, 1995.
45. Keels MA: The Role of Maternal Cigarette Smoking in the Etiology of Cleft Lip With or Without Cleft Palate. PhD Dissertation, University of North Carolina, 1991.
46. Krumlauf R: Hox genes and pattern formation in the branchial arches of the vertebrate head. Trends Genet 9:106–112, 1993.
47. Landauer W, Sopher D: Succinate, glycerophosphate and ascorbate as sources of cellular energy and as antiteratogens. J Embryol Exp Morphol 24:189–202, 1970.
48. Lawson KA, Meneses JJ, Pedersen RA: Clonal analysis of epiblast fate during germ layer formation in the mouse embryo. Development 113:891–911, 1991.
49. Le Douarin N: The Neural Crest. Cambridge University Press, Cambridge, U.K., 1983.
50. LeLièvre: Rôle des cellules mesectodermiques issues des crêtes neurales céphaliques dans la formation des arcs branchiaux et du squelette viscéral. J Embryol Exp Morphol 31:453–477, 1974.
51. Lohnes D, Mark M, Mendelsohn C, Dollé P, Dierich A, Gorry P, Gansmuller A, Chambon P: Function of retinoic acid receptors (RARs) during development (I). Craniofacial and skeletal abnormalities in RAR double mutants. Development 120:2723–2748, 1994.
52. Longo LD: Environmental pollution and pregnancy: risks and uncertainties for the fetus and infant. Am J Obstet Gynecol 137:162–173, 1980.
53. Lumsden A, Sprawson N, Graham A: Segmental origin and migration of neural crest cells in the hindbrain of the chick embryo. Development 113:1281–1291, 1991.
54. MacKenzie A, Ferguson MW, Sharpe PT: Hox-7 expression during murine craniofacial development. Development 113:601–611, 1991.
55. MacKenzie A, Ferguson MWJ, Sharpe PT: Expression patterns of the homeobox gene, Hox-8, in the mouse embryo suggest a role in specifying tooth initiation and shape. Development 115:403–420, 1992.
56. McKee GJ, Ferguson MW: The effects of mesencephalic neural crest cell extirpation on the development of chicken embryos. J Anat 139:491–512, 1984.
57. Millicovsky G, Ambrose LJH, Johnston MC: Developmental alterations associated with spontaneous cleft lip and palate in CL/Fr mice. Am J Anat 164:29–44, 1982.
58. Millicovsky G, Johnston MC: Active role of embryonic facial epithelium: new evidence of cellular events in morphogenesis. J Embryol Exp Morphol 63:53–66, 1981.
59. Millicovsky G, Johnston MC: Hyperoxia and hypoxia in pregnancy: simple experimental manipulation alters the incidence of cleft lip and palate in CL/Fr mice. Proc Natl Acad Sci USA 78:5722–5723, 1981.
60. Minkoff R: Cell proliferation during formation of the embryonic facial primordia. J Craniofac Genet Dev Biol 11:251–261, 1991.
61. Moore GE, Williamson R, Jensson O, Chambers J, Takakubo F, Newton R, Balacs MA, Ivens A: Localization of a mutant gene for cleft palate and ankyloglossia in an X-linked Icelandic family. J Craniofac Genet Dev Biol 11:372–376, 1991.
62. Morriss-Kay G: Retinoic acid and craniofacial development: molecules and morphogenesis. Bioessays 15:9–15, 1993.
63. [MRC] Medical Research Council Vitamin Study Research Group: Prevention of neural tube defects: results of the medical research council vitamin study. Lancet 338:131, 1991.
64. Nicolet G: Analyse autoradiographique de la localisation des différentes ébauches présomptives dans la ligne primitive de l'embryon de poulet. J Embryol Exp Morphol 23:79–108, 1970.

65. Noden DM: An analysis of the migratory behaviour of avian cephalic neural crest cells. Dev Biol 42:106–130, 1975.
66. Noden DM: The role of the neural crest in patterning of avian cranial skeletal, connective, and muscle tissues. Dev Biol 96:144–165, 1983.
67. Noden DM: Vertebrate craniofacial development: the relation between ontogenetic process and morphological outcome. Brain Behav Evol 38:190–225, 1991.
68. Osumi-Yamashita N, Ninomiya Y, Doi H, Eto K: The contribution of both forebrain and midbrain crest cells to the mesenchyme in the frontonasal mass of mouse embryos. Dev Biol 164:409–419, 1994.
69. Pratt RM: Role of epidermal growth factor in embryonic development. In: Current Topics in Developmental Biology, A Moscona, A Monroy, eds. Academic Press, New York, 1987, pp 175–193.
70. Richman JM: The role of retinoids in normal and abnormal embryonic craniofacial morphogenesis. Crit Rev Oral Biol Med 4:93–109, 1992.
71. Rijli FM, Mark M, Lakkaraju S, Dierich A, Dolle P, Chambon P: A homeotic transformation is generated in the rostral branchial region of the head by disruption of Hoxa-2, which acts as a selector gene. Cell 75:1333–1349, 1993.
72. Ross RB, Johnston MC: Cleft Lip and Palate. Williams & Wilkins, Baltimore, 1972.
73. Rosvold EA, Gasser DL, Rhodes M, Buetow KH: Association of detoxification enzyme polymorphisms with cleft lip and palate. Am J Hum Genet 55(Suppl):A48, 1994.
74. Sadler TW: Langman's Medical Embryology, 6th ed. Williams & Wilkins, Baltimore, 1990.
75. Satokata I, Maas R: Msx1 deficient mice exhibit cleft palate and abnormalities of craniofacial and tooth development. Nat Genet 6:348–356, 1994.
76. Schoenwolf GC, Garcia-Martinez V, Dias MS: Mesoderm movement and fate during avian gastrulation and neurulation. Dev Dyn 193:235–248, 1992.
77. Serbedzija GN, Bronner-Fraser M, Fraser SE: Vital dye analysis of cranial neural crest cell migration in the mouse embryo. Development 116:297–307, 1992.
78. Shiang R, Lidral AC, Ardinger HH, Murray JC, Buetow KH: Association of TGFA DNA variants with cleft lip and palate (OFC2). Cytogenet Cell Genet 58:1872, 1992.
79. Shibasaki Y, Ross RB: Facial growth in children with isolated cleft palate. Cleft Palate J 6:290–302, 1969.
80. Shuler CF, Halpern DE, Guo Y, Sank AC: Medial edge epithelium fate traced by cell lineage analysis during epithelial-mesenchymal transformation in vivo. Dev Biol 154:318–330, 1992.
81. Smiley GR, Vanek RJ, Dixon AD: Width of the craniofacial complex during formation of the secondary palate. Cleft Palate J 8:371–378, 1971.
82. Smuts MK: Rapid nasal pit formation in mouse stimulated by ATP-containing medium. J Exp Zool 216:409–414, 1981.
83. Spemann H, Mangold H: Induction of embryonic primordia by implantation of organizers from a different species. In: Foundations of Experimental Embryology, BH Willier, JM Oppenheimer, eds. Hafner, New York, 1924, pp 144–184.
84. Sulik KK, Cook CS, Webster WS: Teratogens and craniofacial malformations: relationships to cell death. Development 103 (Suppl):213–231, 1988.
85. Sulik K, Dehart DB, Inagaki T, Carson JL, Vrablic T, Gesteland K, Schoenwolf GC: Morphogenesis of the murine node and notochordal plate. Dev Dyn 201:260–278, 1994.
86. Tam PPL, Beddington RSP: The formation of mesodermal tissues in the mouse embryo during gastrulation and early organogenesis. Development 99:109–126, 1987.
87. Tan SS, Morriss-Kay G: The development and distribution of cranial neural crest in the rat embryo. Cell Tissue Res 240:403–416, 1985.
88. Tolarova M: Periconceptional supplementation with vitamins and folic acid to prevent recurrence of cleft lip. Lancet 2:217, 1982.
89. Trasler DG: Pathogenesis of cleft lip and its relation to embryonic face shape in A/J and C57Bl mice. Teratology 1:33–49, 1968.
90. Trasler DG, Fraser FC: Role of the tongue in producing cleft palate in mice with spontaneous cleft lip. Dev Biol 6:45–60, 1963.
91. Trasler DG, Rearden CA, Rajchgot H: A selection experiment for distinct types of 6–aminonicotinamide-induced cleft lip in mice. Teratology 18:49–54, 1978.
92. van Limborgh J, Lieuw Kie Song SH, Been W: Cleft lip and palate due to deficiency of mesencephalic neural crest cells. Cleft Palate J 20:251–259, 1983.
93. Waterman RE, Meller SM: Alterations in the epithelial surface of human palatal shelves prior to and during fusion: a scanning electron microscopic study. Anat Rec 180:111–135, 1974.
94. Wedden SE: Effects of retinoids on chick face development. Craniofac Genet Dev Biol 11:326–337, 1991.
95. Wilkinson DG: Molecular mechanisms of segmental patterning in the vertebrate hindbrain and neural crest. Bioessays 15:499–505, 1993.
96. Zimmerman EF (ed): Palate Development: Normal and Abnormal, Cellular and Molecular Aspects. In: Current Topics in Developmental Biology, Vol 19. Academic Press, New York, 1984.

# 13

# Congenital Anomalies of the Mouth, Palate, and Pharynx

TASSOS DIONISOPOULOS and H. BRUCE WILLIAMS

Most of this chapter will deal with cleft lip and palate and immediately related issues such as secondary deformities and velopharyngeal insufficiency. The field is colossal. Therefore, an in-depth discussion of surgical techniques and areas of controversy is precluded. The interested reader is encouraged to consult the references for further information. The remainder of the chapter will discuss briefly the miscellaneous deformities such as vascular malformations, tumors, and disorders of the tongue, with a strong emphasis on the experience of the authors.

The current surgical procedures available for cleft lip and palate have been refined to such an extent that their results and revisions are deemed highly acceptable and reproducible. All this is attained with a mortality that approaches zero. Paralleling the improvements in surgical correction of the deformity has been the evolution of diagnostic and therapeutic techniques concerned with the management of the associated disorders of speech, hearing, and dentition. We feel that the next era of surgical advances will come from eliminating scarring which plays a role in the development of secondary cleft deformities and compromises velar function after repair.

## Cleft lip and palate

### History

Clefting of the lip is the most common facial congenital anomaly. Evidence of its existence in prehistoric man is sparse. The deformity has been identified among mummies from thousands of years ago and has been represented in the ceramic sculpture of the Andes dating to around the time of Christ. The Chinese referred to the deformity as "harelip" as early as 400 A.D.[67] In the West, Galen was the first of the early Greek physicians to mention the cleft lip deformity, referring to it as a "coloboma."[65,67]

Repair of the cleft lip lagged behind the description of the deformity. Ancient peoples dealt with malformed children through infanticide. Although the Chinese of the Tsin Dynasty had similar attitudes, there is evidence that they had attempted closure of the clefts. Western attempts surfaced around 1000 A.D. and are continuing to this day. Current procedures, timing, and improved neonatal medical care have resulted in a significantly improved outlook for these patients with respect to attaining near normal appearance and function.

As the anatomy of the defect began to be understood, methods for the closure of cleft lips evolved rapidly from the early techniques which consisted of paring of the cleft edges and straight line closure. The concept of transposing full thickness tissue from the lateral side of the cleft was used by Mirault[70] in his triangular flap method (see later). This technique brought in the excess tissue from the relatively abundant lateral lip element into the area of the lip that was deficient. Le Mesurier[56] popularized a quadrilateral flap method of lip repair in which a Cupid's bow was surgically created for the first time. Randall[82] modified Tennison's[102] triangular flap design, making the procedure easier and more reproducible. Accurate measurements from the normal side were used as a reference to achieve intraoperative symmetry. Both the Le Mesurier and Tennison-Randall repairs have disadvantages in their outcome. Millard's[64] rotation-advancement technique is presently the most popular method of lip closure (Fig. 13–1).

### Epidemiology and genetics

The deformity termed cleft lip +/− palate (CL/P) can be distinguished from that of an isolated cleft palate (CP). On the basis of epidemiologic, embryologic, and genetic factors, the belief is that these two conditions are different.[39]

Approximately one-third of the clefting occurs as an isolated deformity involving the palate alone while in two-thirds the clefting involves the lip with or without the palate (CL/P). Among the CL/P group as a whole, there is a marked predominance of males (60%–80%), while the opposite holds true in the isolated CP deformity.[20] The majority of patients have combined lip and palate deformities. The association of a cleft palate with a cleft lip deformity is strongest among infants with bilateral cleft lips (approximately 86% of cases), while in the unilateral cases it falls to 68%.[39] The unilateral cleft occurs most commonly on the left side.

There are also interracial differences in the incidence of CL/P versus CP. The mean incidence of CL/P among Orientals is 2.1/1,000 live births while in Caucasians it is 1/1,000 and in Blacks, 0.41/1,000.[34] Relatively high rates are also seen in some North American populations of Asian descent as in Indians of the southwest United States and the west coast of Canada. The incidence of isolated CP is constant among the three racial groups at 0.5/1,000 births. The incidence of CL/P is believed to increase with increasing parental age, with the father's age having a greater influence than the mother's.[35,116] The incidence of CP is higher in children of older mothers with higher parity.[73a]

As expected, the incidence of CL/P in relatives of children with CL/P is significantly increased; however, isolated CP alone occurs in this group at the same frequency as in the general population. Similarly, the relatives of children with isolated cleft palates have a higher risk of recurrence of that deformity without an increased incidence of the CL/P deformity.[116]

Most cases of CL/P or CP without associated malformations have a multifactorial etiology. However, it may be hard to distinguish these from situations where a major gene is acting with reduced penetrance, influenced by polygenic variation. In CL/

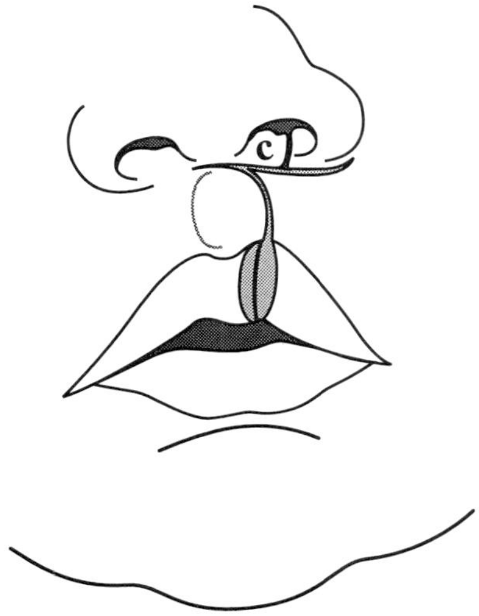


**Fig. 13–1.** Millard rotation advancement repair. See text for details.

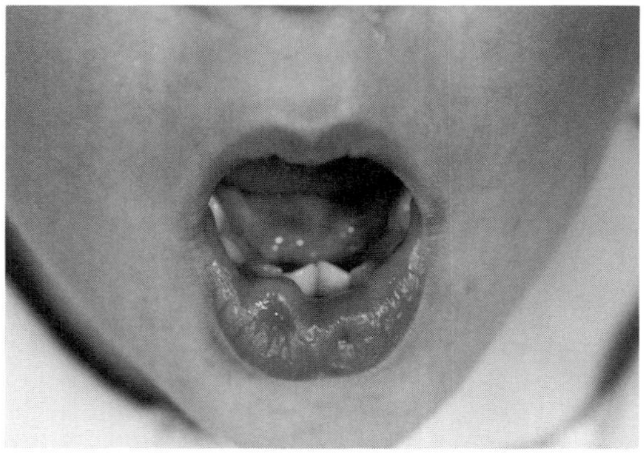

**Fig. 13–2.** Van der Woude syndrome. Note presence of lower lip pits. See text for details.

P the recurrence risk is higher in the sibs of female probands than of male probands, in the sibs of patients with a severe defect than in those with a mild form, and after two affected sibs than after one.[73a] In CP the recurrence risks are higher for sibs of male probands (6.3%) than for sibs of female probands (2.3%). Moreover, environmental influences are higher in the causation of CP than CL/P.[73a] Until better insight into the basis of the defect is gained, we have to depend on empiric risk figures as guidelines for genetic counseling (Table 13–1).

Identifiable syndromes are thought to make up approximately 5% of the group and are more common among isolated cleft palate patients.[34,73a] More than 140 syndromes involve orofacial cleft. Of these, around 100 are monogenic. An example is the van der Woude syndrome which is characterized by the presence of lower lip pits, isolated CP or CL/P, and an autosomal dominant pattern of inheritance with a high degree of penetrance (Fig. 13–2).[28]

Cleft lip and/or palate may occur also in chromosomal syndromes, especially trisomy 13 and trisomy 18.

## Embryology

The embryology of the developing primary and secondary palates is covered in more detail in chapter 12; however, certain aspects deserve reiteration, not only for their importance but also because they emphasize the differences between the deformity of CL/P from isolated CP.

The overall development of this region of the face includes formation of the primary palate followed by formation of the secondary palate. Primary palate formation occurs at approximately 30–37 days gestational age (Fig. 13–3) by the growth and fusion of the medial nasal, lateral nasal, and maxillary processes. The maxillary process develops from the proximal half of the first arch which grows to meet and fuse with the nasal processes that have grown and moved in association with the olfactory placode.[50] Most researchers believe that mesodermal penetration is the process underlying the assembly of the primary palate.[99] The basic theory emphasizes the importance of mesodermal reinforcement along the lines of fusion of the migrating processes. Epithelial breakdown and clefting will result from this lack of reinforcement. The associated cleft of the hard and soft palates is presumed to occur as a result of the tongue which protrudes into the lip cleft and impedes the elevation of the palatine shelves.[50] The secondary palate arises from the two palatal shelves that are wedged in a vertical direction by the interposed tongue (Fig. 13–4). As the head extends at about week 7[92] and the mandible grows,[50] the tongue is withdrawn and the shelves can then swing to a midline position for the hard palate, or they can mold as in the soft palate and then fuse.

## Classification of CL/P

A system of classification should ideally comprise simple terms that would completely describe and categorize the deformity. It should be easily used by the clinician, yet at the same time allow accurate communication between treating professionals. Various schemes of classification have been offered over the last 70 years but few have received wide clinical acceptance. In this section, we will highlight four of the more popular.

In 1922, Davis and Ritchie presented their scheme which divided the deformity into three groups based on the location of the cleft with respect to the alveolus.[25] Group I comprised clefts anterior to the alveolus (i.e., lip, either unilateral, median, or bilateral). Group II clefts contained postalveolar clefts (i.e., of the palate alone). Subdivisions in this group included those of the soft palate alone, of the soft and hard palates, or

**Table 13–1.** Rates (%) of recurrence in a child of given relationship to an affected person

| | Affected Relative(s) | | | | | | | |
|---|---|---|---|---|---|---|---|---|
| | Parent | Brother | Sister | Sib | 2 Sibs | Parent + Sib | 2nd Degree | 3rd Degree |
| Cleft lip ± palate | 4.0 | 3.9 | 5.0 | 4.3 | 9 | 15? | 0.7 | 0.4 |
| Cleft palate | 5.8 | 6.3 | 2.3 | 2.9 | | 15? | 0.4 | 0.3 |

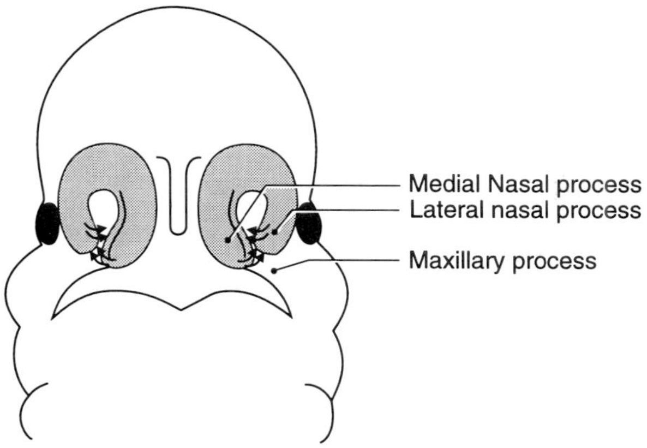


**Fig. 13–3.** Formation of the primary palate: fusion of the lateral nasal, medial nasal, and maxillary prominences.

simply a submucous cleft. Each subgroup was further subdivided as to the extent of the cleft: 1/3, 1/2, etc. The last group contained clefts extending from the lip, through the alveolus, into the hard and soft palates.

Veau proposed a numerical grouping of clefting of the lip and palate (Fig. 13–5, A to D).[104] Group I (A) involved a defect in the soft palate only. Group II (B) involved both the soft and hard palates. In Group III (C) the cleft went from the soft palate through the alveolus and usually involved the lip. Complete bilateral clefts were placed in Group IV (D). (See Veau classification in cleft palate section). The weakness of this classification scheme lies in ignoring clefts of the lip and alveolus without associated palatal clefts.

The next major comprehensive classification system was put forth by Kernahan and Stark in 1958.[52] Paul Fogh-Anderson had previously described the importance of the incisive foramen as a boundary marker in his morphologic classification of CL/P.[33] Kernahan and Stark again highlighted this embryologic landmark in their system.[52] The primary palate consists of the lip, anterior septum, and premaxilla up to the incisive foramen. Clefts in this area are termed *clefts of the primary palate* and usually occur during weeks 4–7 of embryonic life. The secondary palate consists of the roof of the mouth from the incisive foramen to the uvula. Clefts of this area are termed *clefts of the secondary palate* and occur at 7–12 weeks gestation, later than those of the primary palate. Further subdivisions include complete and incomplete as well as uni- and bilateral clefts.

Kernahan subsequently provided a graphic classification scheme using a *Y* configuration (Fig. 13–6).[51] The *Y* was divided into 9 segments representing normal anatomy. Areas 1+4 represent the lip; 2+5 the alveolus; 3+6 the palate between the alveolus and the incisive foramen; 7+8 the hard palate; and area 9 the soft palate. This simplified scheme has become popular, especially with further modifications in Millard's text *Cleft Craft*.[66] Among these are the placement of triangles over the limbs to represent the nares and nasal deformities as well as an *O* in the center to denote the premaxilla and its degree of protrusion.

The International Confederation of Plastic and Reconstructive Surgery has adopted the following scheme. It again uses an embryological framework to divide clefts into four groups, with further subdivisions denoting uni- or bilaterality as well as the extent of the cleft. The first group includes defects of the lip, or alveolus. The second comprises clefts of the secondary palate (i.e., of the soft or hard palate or both). The third group contains any combination of clefts involving the primary and secondary palates. In the last group are the rare facial clefts which will be discussed elsewhere.

#### Functional anatomy of cleft lip and palate

Central to understanding the surgical correction of clefts of the lip and palate is an understanding of the anatomic deformity. The following section will describe the anatomic abnormalities existing among CL/P by discussing the individual components: the muscles of the lip, their neurovascular structures, the structural abnormalities, and the cleft lip nasal deformities in both unilateral and bilateral clefts.

In general, functional derangement in clefts of both lip and palate lies in the failure of the muscles to meet their counterparts during embryologic development. Instead, nonfunctional substitute attachments are found and can result in atrophy of the muscle units or maladaptive attempts at accommodation.[32] Reconstruction of the underlying musculature by detachment from their atypical insertions underlies a modern principle in CL/P repairs.

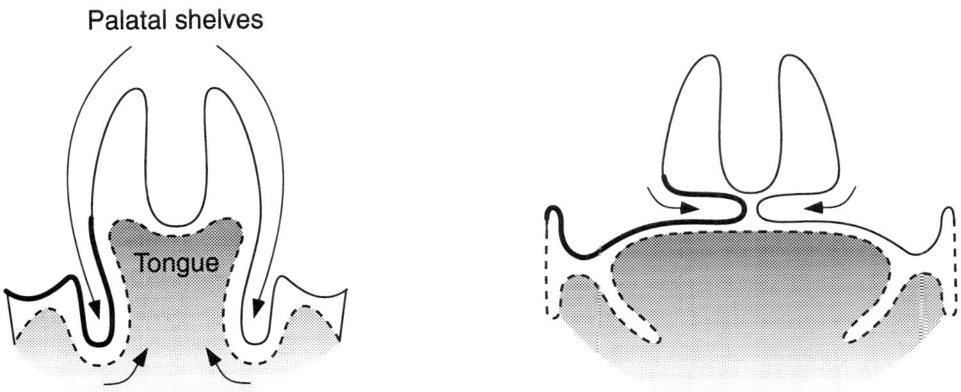


**Fig. 13–4.** Formation of the secondary palate: palatal shelf elevation and fusion. (After MC Johnston et al., Clin Plast Surg 2:195, 1975,[50a] with permission.)

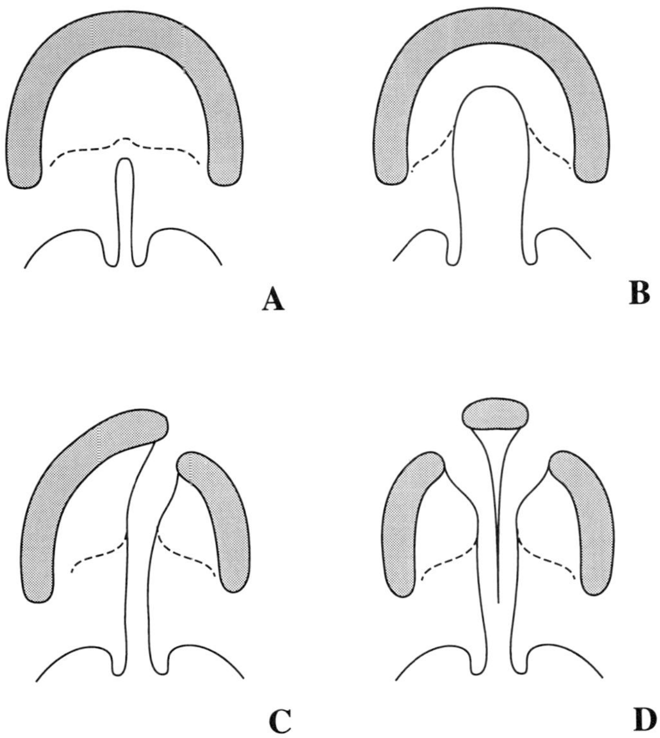


**Fig. 13–5.** Veau classification of cleft lip/palate. In A, the cleft is in the soft palate alone. Type B (B) is a cleft of the entire hard palate. A unilateral cleft of both soft and hard palates makes up type C (C). Type D (D) is a bilateral cleft lip and palate.

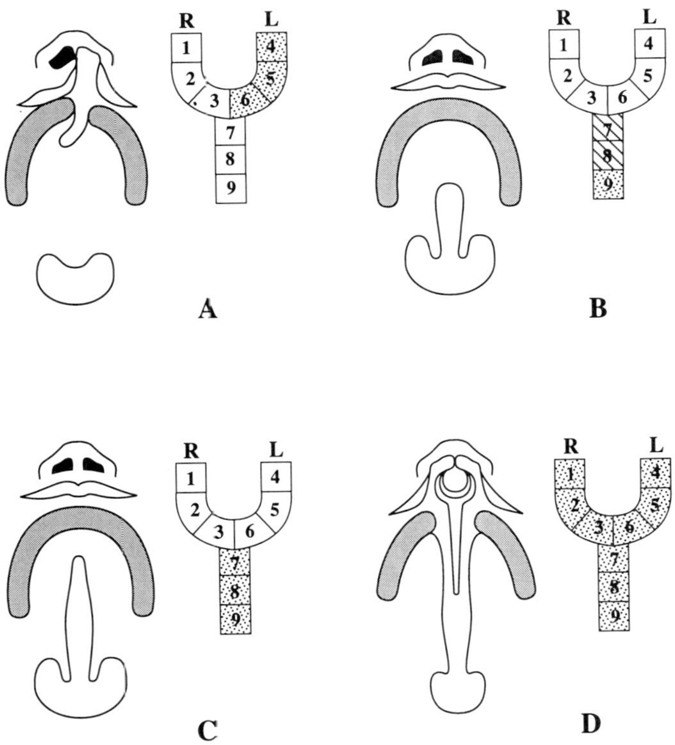


**Fig. 13–6.** Classification after Kernahan and Stark, including symbolic classification. The striped Y allows for rapid documentation and description of the deformity. (After Kernahan, 1971,[51] with permission.)

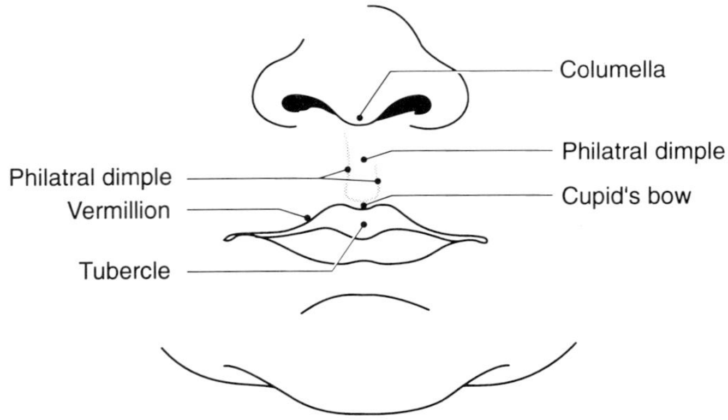


**Fig. 13–7.** Normal child showing landmarks: cupids bow, tubercle vermillion, philtral columns, and columella.

### Cleft lip

The normal surface anatomy of the lower face of the infant is highlighted in Figure 13–7. The border between the white lip and the red vermillion is termed the *white roll* or the *mucocutaneous ridge*. In the midline, a dip in the roll forms the Cupid's bow below which projection of the vermillion forms the tubercle. From each peak of the Cupid's bow, a vertical ridge termed the *philtral column* sweeps towards the columella. Lying between these philtral columns is a depression termed the *philtral dimple*. The philtrum is normally one quarter the width of the mouth.[66] The average vertical height of the lip in the newborn as measured from the peak of the Cupid's bow to the nasal base is 10 mm.

The musculature of lip and cleft is shown in Figure 13–8. The orbicularis oris (oo) is the prime muscle comprising the lip and is divided both functionally and anatomically into two parts. The deep component works in concert with other oropharyngeal muscles in swallowing and serves as a sphincter. The superficial oo deals with facial expression, inserting into the anterior nasal spine, sill and alar base, as well as inserting into the skin to form the philtral ridges. In a complete cleft lip, the fibers of the deep oo are interrupted on their way around the mouth by the cleft and end on either side of the defect. The superficial component turns upward, running along the margins of the cleft to end beneath either the ala or the columella. Incomplete clefts behave similarly, except in cases where the cleft is less than two-thirds the height of the lip. Here the muscle fibers run along the margins of the cleft, then change direction and run horizontally over the top of the cleft. These fibers, however, are interspersed with connective tissue.[32] The arterial supply to the lip in cleft cases parallels the events occurring with the muscles. The vessels course along the margins of the cleft towards either the columella or the alar bases where they form anastomoses with nearby vessels.

In bilateral deformity, the degree of completeness of the cleft and its symmetry are the variables determining the anatomic characteristics in each case. The cleft may involve the primary palate alone or with the secondary palate. The prolabium will vary in size but appears to be deficient in resurfacing in the central portion of the lip because it is retracted and lacks any muscle fibers. There appears to be no columella and in some cases the prolabium seems to be attached to the tip of the nose. The size and the position of the premaxilla are also variable. The alveolar arch may have collapsed, effectively excluding the premaxilla.

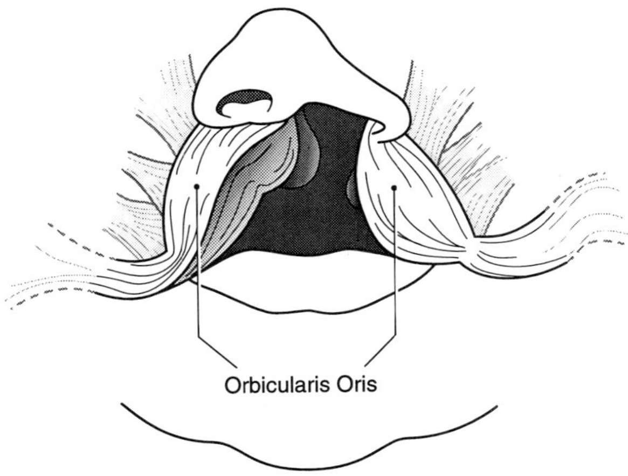


**Fig. 13–8.** Muscular defects in the unilateral deformity. See text for details.

In complete bilateral clefts the muscle fibers and vessels in the lateral lip elements behave as in unilateral cases; however, the prolabium lacks muscle fibers and is composed only of fibrous connective tissue. Its blood supply is via septal and columellar vessels. When the bilateral cleft lip is incomplete, the muscle bundles cross over into the prolabium and fill it to a greater extent than in the equivalent unilateral case. The skin appendages are lacking or at least deficient in the prolabium.

The nasal deformity associated with a cleft lip varies in severity from case to case but its appearance is characteristic. In the unilateral deformity, the normal side serves to highlight the anomaly and serves as the model for the correction. Huffman and Lierle[46] have listed the following deformities that may be present: (1) deflection of the nasal tip towards the noncleft side; (2) retroplacement of the cleft alar cartilage dome; (3) presence of an obtuse angle between the medial and lateral crura of the lower lateral cartilage on the cleft side; (4) buckling of the ala on the cleft side; (5) absence of the alar-facial groove on the cleft side and attachement of the ala to the face at an obtuse angle; (6) presence of an apparent or real bony deficiency of the maxilla on the cleft side; (7) larger nares on the cleft side; (8) shorter columella on the cleft side, positioning the entire columella at a slant towards the noncleft side; (9) displacement of the medial crus inferiorly within the columella; (10) dislocation of the caudal portion of the septum to the noncleft side from the nasal spine; and (11) downward rotation of the alar cartilage on the cleft side. In the bilateral deformity both alae are rotated downward and spread apart, giving the nasal tip a large, flat, and bifid appearance.[66] The columella may be so short in the bilateral cleft that the prolabium may appear to be attached directly to the nasal tip. The nostrils are wide, the alar bases flared, and the alar rims hooded.

There is controversy surrounding the origin of the cleft lip nasal deformity.[62] Theories include a tissue deficiency due to deficient mesodermal penetration, a deformity resulting from the abnormal stresses imposed by the presence of orbicularis and alveolar clefts, or a combination of the above.

### Cleft palate

The key landmark in the bony palate is the incisive foramen. Anterior to it lies the premaxilla which includes the two premaxillary bones, the alveolus, and the incisors. The premaxilla can vary in size, composition, and configuration, ranging from being well developed and containing eight teeth (four primary and four secondary) to being small with only two incisors. The unrestrained premaxilla can protrude from the arch and rotate in response to tongue movements both intrauterine and neonatal. The maxillary arches may collapse to a point where the premaxilla may be excluded from the arch, especially in complete bilateral clefts of the arch. Soft tissue structures in this primary palate include the nasal tip and the upper central lip. Posterior to the incisive foramen lies the secondary palate consisting of the hard and soft palates. The hard palate (Fig. 13–9) is formed by the palatine processes of the maxilla and the palatine bones which form its most posterior edge. The palatine bones also contain foramina for the egress of the palatine neurovascular supply of the overlying mucoperiosteum.

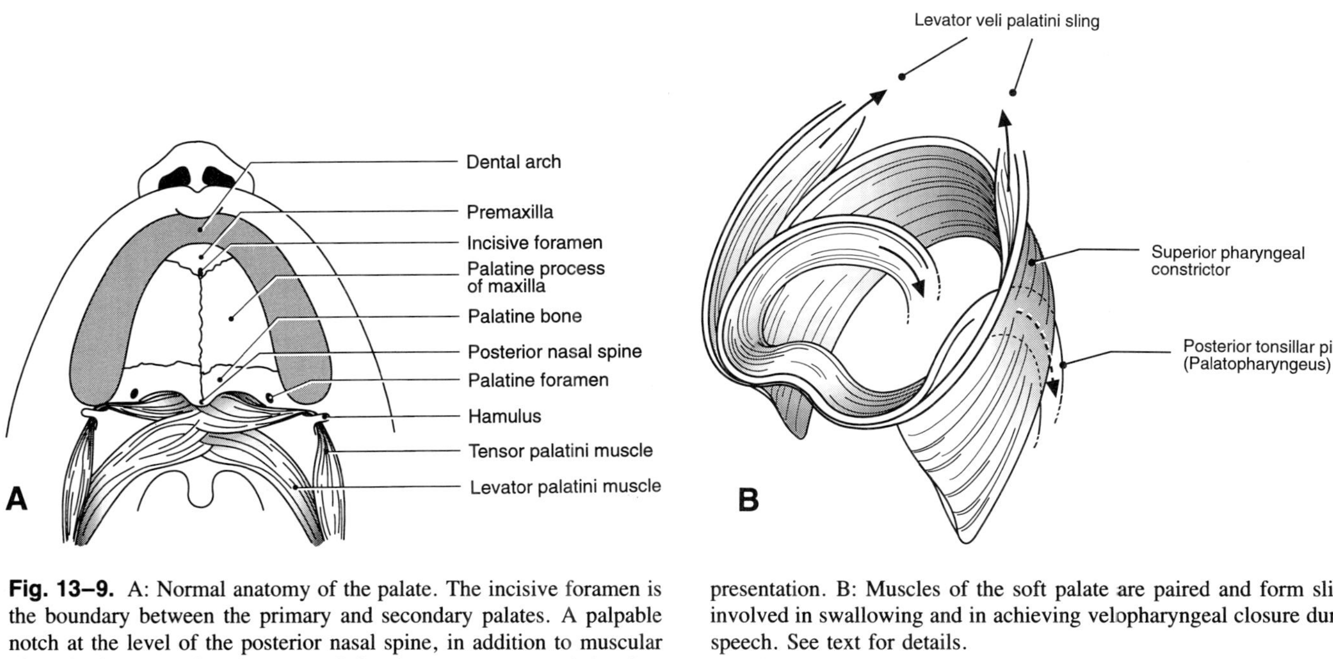


**Fig. 13–9.** A: Normal anatomy of the palate. The incisive foramen is the boundary between the primary and secondary palates. A palpable notch at the level of the posterior nasal spine, in addition to muscular diastasis, is present in submucous clefts, the most common cleft palate presentation. B: Muscles of the soft palate are paired and form slings involved in swallowing and in achieving velopharyngeal closure during speech. See text for details.

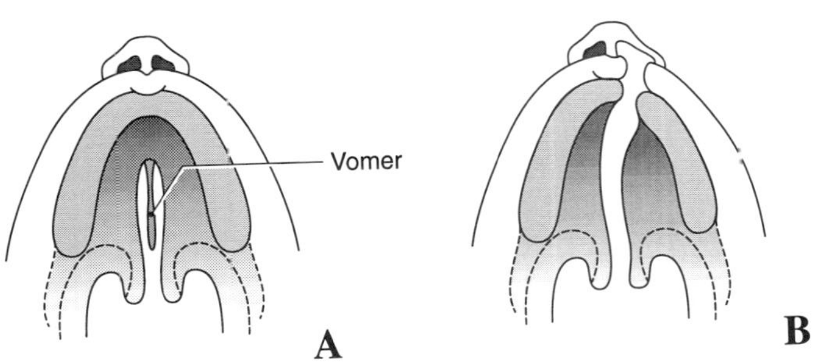


**Fig. 13–10.** Cleft palate variations. A: Complete cleft of the secondary palate. B: Unilateral complete cleft of the primary and secondary palates.

The soft palate lies immediately posterior to the bony palate and plays an important role in speech and swallowing. The musculature of the soft palate (Fig. 13–9B) consists of paired muscles on either side of the midline. The levator veli palatini are the most important muscles involved in the production of speech and velopharyngeal competence. From their origin on the undersurface of the temporal bone, the paired muscles meet at an aponeurosis across the middle of the soft palate and work as a sling by elevating it towards the posterior wall of the pharynx. Posterior movement of the palate is supplemented by the contraction of the palatopharyngeus which inserts into the posterior tonsillar pillar. Further narrowing of the velopharyngeal port is attained by the contraction of the superior pharyngeal constrictor which decreases the dimensions through posterior and lateral wall movement (Fig. 13–9B). The role of the tensor veli palatini is felt to be primarily one of dilating the eustachian tube and maintaining its integrity.[45] The contribution of the uvular muscles to normal speech is considered to be minimal.[12]

A cleft of the palate results in structural and soft tissue abnormalities and may exist as an isolated deformity or with a cleft of the primary palate. Whereas clefts limited to the secondary palate are midline defects (Fig. 13–10), those which include a prepalatal component are asymmetric with the vomer left attached to the bony palate on the noncleft side. The dental arch on the noncleft side usually splays outward because of the lack of a restraining force from the lip, while the palate itself is usually shortened in the anteroposterior direction. Bilateral complete clefts allow the entire premaxilla to protrude from the adjacent alveolar ridges. In addition to being displaced and possibly rotated, its return to the arch may be prevented by the collapse of the palatine shelves behind it, leaving it attached only by the vomer.

The soft tissue defect in the cleft palate results in hypoplasia of the velar musculature as well as a derangement in the insertion of its muscular components (Fig. 13–11). The normal midline insertion and transverse orientation of the levator palatini is disturbed and the fibers now pass longitudinally to insert along the bony cleft margin and the posterior aspect of the palatine bones. Similar derangements occur in the other palatal muscles. Dysfunction occurs in speech with velopharyngeal incompetence and in eustachian tube obstruction with middle ear effusions, infections, and possibly, hearing loss.

### Fetal surgery

Experimental work and human clinical experience in fetal surgery has shown that the fetus responds uniquely to injury by healing more rapidly and without the formation of scar.[58,59] The reasons for scarless healing in the fetus are unknown at the present time but progress has been made in understanding how it differs from wound healing which occurs in the postnatal period.

The differences are felt to lie in either the properties of fetal cells, the uterine environment, or a combination of the two.[58,59] Early postulations implicated the minimal inflammatory response of the fetus to injury and the sterile amniotic fluid as possible mechanisms.[1,73] However, it has been shown that isolating the fetal wound from the amniotic fluid still results in a scarless wound.[58,59] It is known that there is a transition to a postnatal mode of wound healing occurring at some point in utero. In the sheep model it is during the third trimester, but the transition point in humans is unknown.[2]

The phenomenon of scarless healing may be more appropriately linked to the macromolecular organization of the fetal extracellular matrix.[2] The hyaluronic acid–rich environment is thought to facilitate cellular movement and proliferation.[96] The early deposition of fibronectin and related factors in addition to interstitial matrix structure may be the cause of the observed rapid epithelialization.[111] A scarless fetal wound would then be the result of a more effective organization at a macromolecular level of the lower amounts of connective tissue deposited after injury.[96]

There have been several papers in the plastic surgery literature which discuss in utero cleft lip repair.[19,23,30,41,101] The potential benefits of achieving this type of healing in the patient with craniofacial anomalies extends beyond achieving an invisible scar. Secondary cleft deformities that are often caused by the effects of wound contraction and scar formation can theoretically be prevented. These include deformities of the lip and nose and maxillary growth disturbances.

With prenatal ultrasound and an experienced specialist, the diagnosis of cleft lip and palate can be made between 12 and 20 weeks gestational age. The technical and ethical implications are great. The safe window period in which this surgery could be performed is felt to be between 22 and 30 weeks gestational age.[19] The miscarriage rate is higher if performed earlier, while the incidence of preterm labour is very high if performed later.[23] The operative intervention contemplated is technically perfect cleft lip and/or palate repair. Anything less would require a postnatal revision, which would negate the benefit sought in this experimental surgery.

The implication for the mother lies in the fact that she would

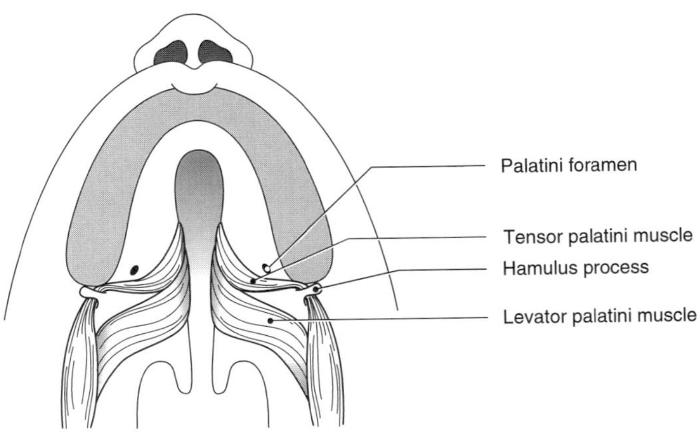


**Fig. 13–11.** The underlying defect in the musculature of a cleft palate. Note the abnormal insertions and orientation of the velar muscles.

have to undergo two surgical procedures. In order to gain access to the fetus, a vertical hysterotomy would be required, followed by a cesarean section to deliver the child at term.[23] Recently, a transuterine endoscopic technique has been used successfully in experimental in utero fetal lamb cleft lip repair.[30] This may obviate the need for an ex utero repair with the associated complications to both mother and child.

Further issues to be considered include the ethics of deciding to perform this type of experimental surgery as well as reconciling the interests of mother and fetus. Issues of informed consent and the rights of the fetus will figure prominently in our medicolegal climate, as will the economics of such a costly intervention.

More research on fetal wound healing is required before it can be considered for human cleft repair. Indeed, the subsequent understanding of wound healing mechanisms may allow for the pharmacologic manipulation of such a repair during postnatal repair, thereby attaining a scarless wound in an inviolate fetus. At the present time, fetal surgery is reserved for life-threatening anomalies such as congenital diaphragmatic hernias and lung malformations.

### Neonatal management

In a small percentage of cases, particularly those associated with the Robin sequence, the airway is at risk and the priority is to relieve respiratory distress. For most newborns, however, the earliest physical problem involves feeding. Despite having normal sucking and swallowing reflexes, the cleft hampers their attempts to generate enough negative pressure to nurse. Whether breast milk or formula, the child's nutrition must then be delivered through bottle feeding, with nipples having larger holes cut into the top, making delivery of the food effortless. The nurses play a role in teaching the mother proper feeding techniques.

A multidisciplinary approach is required to integrate the complex features involved in the care of these children and their families. This is best accomplished in the setting of a cleft palate team which includes pediatricians, plastic surgeons, otolaryngologists, pedodontists, orthodontists, nurses, speech therapists, audiologists, and social workers. Consultants are the radiologists, geneticists, and neurologists. The purpose of the team is to evaluate and treat children referred with cleft lip and/or palate or those children felt to have excessive nasality. The multidisciplinary composition ensures that each patient and the family will receive the most comprehensive care plan utilizing all available resources from birth into adolescence. It also provides a tool for clinical research.

The birth of an infant with an anomaly evokes a variety of feelings in the parents, most of which are negative. An important component of care provided by the team lies in the area of education and emotional support to the parents. Parental support through regular home contact is provided and access to the team coordinator is available in the event questions arise while the child is at home.

### Repair of the cleft lip and palate deformity

#### Unilateral cleft lip

Most surgeons would agree that repair of the lip should be performed within the first year of life. Although some would advocate an immediate repair, the majority follow the Rules of Ten: hemoglobin greater than 10 gm, age greater than 10 weeks, and a weight greater than 10 lbs. The concern is for the safety of the infant undergoing general anaesthesia. In addition, the procedure is made simpler and more accurate for the surgeon after the child has grown.

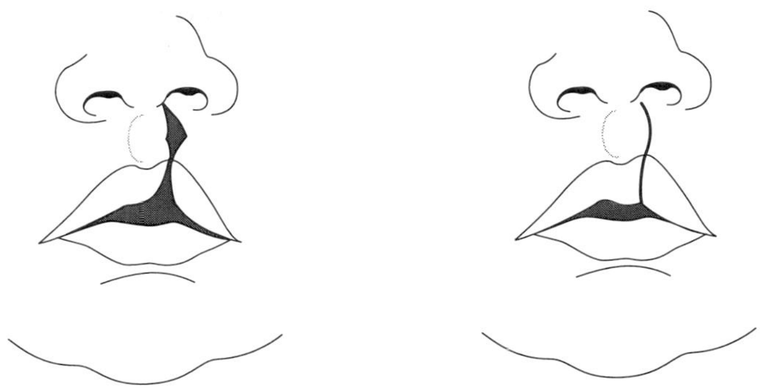

**Fig. 13–12.** Rose-Thompson unilateral cleft lip repair. Scar contracture results in notching of the lip.

The earliest cleft lip repair recorded was in the fourth century A.D. by an unidentified Chinese surgeon. Their technique of paring the edges of the cleft and suturing it closed persisted into the day of Ambroise Paré, who coined the term *harelip* and closed the wound by using a long needle through both lip elements and a figure-of-eight thread.

The vertical deficiency which resulted from this closure was addressed by Rose and Thompson in 1891 and 1912, respectively.[66] They were able to lengthen the edges of the cleft by concave excisions along the edges of the cleft which resulted in a straight line when the wound was closed (Fig. 13–12). A deficiency in the Rose-Thompson repair was in producing a conspicuous straight-line scar which caused noticeable notching with subsequent scar contracture. Horizontal shortening would result from excising and discarding tissue along the cleft margins.

Malgaigne[60] was the first to introduce the concept of transferring local flaps for closure of the cleft. This technique was modified soon after by Mirault,[70] who brought in a lateral flap to fill in the medial deficit. Brown further modified the size of the flap and developed a technique that brought in tissue to deficient areas and disrupted the straight line closure at the vermilion (Fig. 13–13).[17]

Le Mesurier[56] popularized the quadrilateral flap which had been first described in 1884 by Hagedorn.[40] Its significance lies in that, for the first time, a Cupid's bow had been created. This was done by transposing the quadrilateral flap into a releasing incision in the medial lip element (Fig. 13–14).

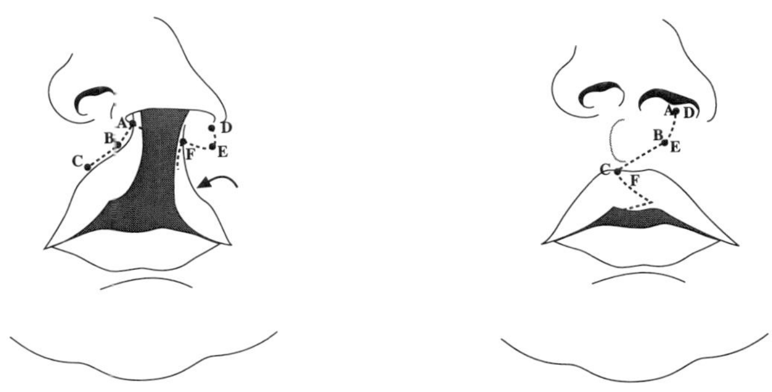


**Fig. 13–13.** Mirault-Blair-Brown unilateral cleft lip repair. Although the scars are better camouflaged, a Cupid's bow was still lacking.

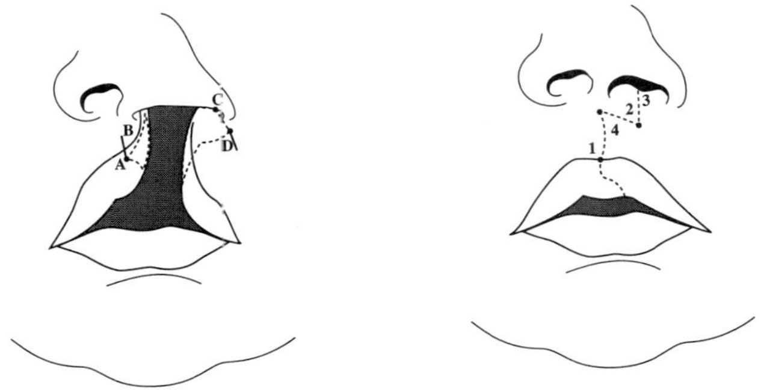

Fig. 13–14. Le Mesurier unilateral cleft lip repair. Although a Cupid's bow is created, the resulting midline scar is noticeable.

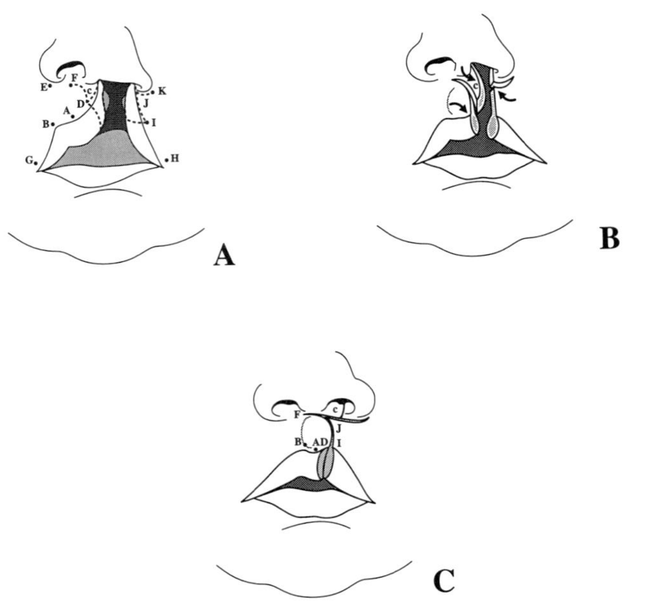


Fig. 13–16. A–C: Millard rotation-advancement unilateral cleft lip repair. See text for details.

Further advances included the Z-plasty technique developed by Tennison, in which the Cupid's bow was conserved and placed in a more normal position.[102] In his modification of the Tennison repair, Randall refined the flaps, defined the mathematics of the design, and reconstructed the fibers of the orbicularis (Fig. 13–15A,B).[82] The scarring, however, was still quite evident on the cleft side. Skoogs' method was similar, but as a double Z-plasty (Fig. 13–15C).[97,98]

The most popular method of closure of the unilateral cleft lip was developed by Millard.[64] The concept was an advancement of a lateral flap into the upper portion of the lip, combined with a downward rotation of the medial segment, hence the name *rotation-advancement* lip repair (Fig. 13–16).

This technique provides several benefits. Rotation of the medial lip element reorients the fibers of the orbicularis. The patient's Cupid's bow and philtral dimple are preserved and rotated down to a normal position. The donor area in the upper lip is then filled with the advancement flap fashioned through a relaxing incision in the lateral lip element. This advancement places the tension of the closure under the alar base, narrowing the vestibule and promoting the alignment of the maxillary arches. This technique also partially corrects the cleft lip nasal deformity because it allows the columella on the cleft side to be lengthened. The repositioning of the alar base further reconstructs the nasal floor and nostril sill.

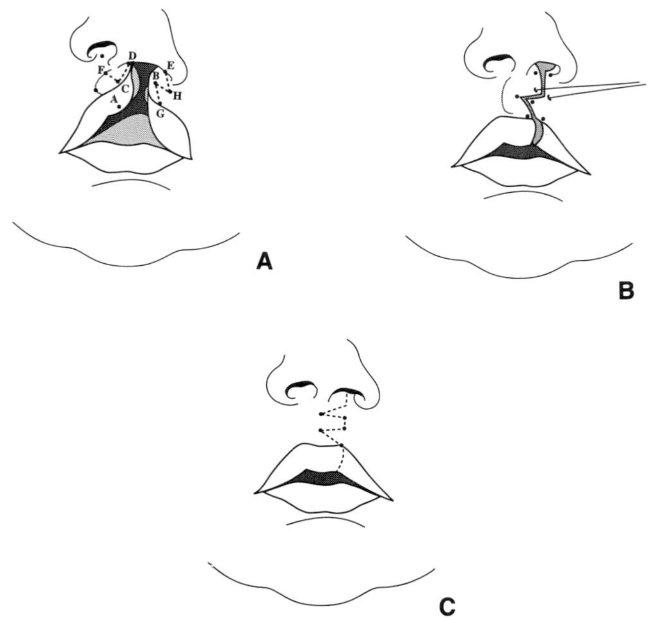


Fig. 13–15. A, B: Randall modification of the Tennison Z-plasty unilateral cleft lip repair. C: Skoog method. Both methods disrupt the philtral column of the cleft side.

Beginning around the Cupid's bow (Fig. 13–16), the landmarks used in the technique are as follows:[66] the center and the peak of the bow on the noncleft side is marked on the vermilion ridge; that length is then transferred to the cleft side vermilion ridge to mark the proposed site of the new peak on the cleft side, point 3. The rotation incision mimics a philtral ridge and so begins from point 3 and curves to the base of the columella and extends across approximately two-third's of the columellar width to point 5. A back cut *X* is often used to gain more length and facilitate the rotation. An incision along the membranous septum frees the "c"-flap that results from these incisions. This flap is then advanced into the columella.

The peak of the bow on the cleft side is marked relative to the commissure using the length measurement obtained from the noncleft side commissure to peak (7 to 8 = 2 to 6). These measurements have been shown to be important in analyzing the final results of these techniques.[112] The height of the lip on the cleft side (8 to 9) must equal the height on the rotation side (3 to X). An incision along the alar base and upper sulcus (9–10) will free the lateral flap and allow it to advance into the gap created after the medial flap is rotated. The muscle in the lateral flap is similarly freed in order to realign the fibers and provide another layer for closure.

Millard emphasizes the importance of having the maxillary arches aligned before definitive lip closure since they are the platform on which the lip and nose rest. If the cleft extends through the alveolus and palate, asymmetry of the medial and lateral maxillary elements can occur. Commonly, there is an outward rotation of the noncleft arch and an inward collapse of the cleft arch to varying degrees. Definitive lip closure at this stage would subject the healing wound to a great deal of tension, with a poorer scar as a result. Correction of the maxillary asymmetry can be accomplished with either lip adhesion as a first stage or presurgical orthodontics.

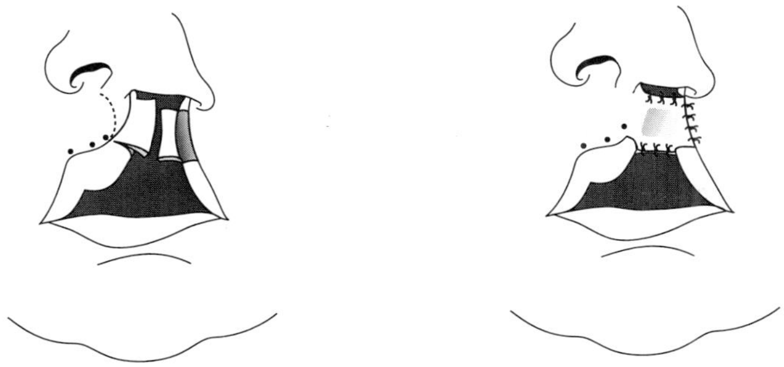

**Fig. 13–17.** The technique of lip adhesion in wide clefts. Note the preservation of landmarks that will be used for subsequent rotation advancement.

## Presurgical orthodontics

This involves the use of an appliance to gently reposition the palatal segments into normal alignment. The simplest device is adhesive tape across the prolabium and each cheek in bilateral clefts.[90] Other devices can be splints to maintain the alignment or adjustable appliances to reposition the segments into a normal arch. Similarly, the principle of lip adhesion can provide a correcting force across the cleft and convert a wide complete cleft into an incomplete one while awaiting definitive lip repair 3 to 6 months later (Fig. 13–17). Introducing scar into the area in addition to the high incidence of wound dehiscence are criticisms of preliminary lip adhesion.

Closure of the alveolar cleft is most often deferred until later in childhood, usually in the form of cancellous bone grafting of the residual cleft during the period of mixed dentition. Millard has been evaluating gingivoperiosteoplasty during primary lip repair. This technique involves bridging the residual gap in an alveolar cleft with local alveolar and mucoperiosteal flaps, forming a tunnel that will fill with blood and later form bone.[68]

## Bilateral cleft lip

The two factors unique to bilateral cleft lip deformity that can affect its management and ensuing results are the status of the premaxillary segment, and the degree of symmetry and completeness of the deformity. There are several surgical goals in correcting a bilateral cleft. The lip cleft and nasal deformity must certainly be repaired, but in conjunction with the establishment of a normal relationship between the premaxilla and alveolar arches.

Presurgical orthodontics are used to attain a normal arch alignment and thereby reduce the amount of tension placed on the lip closure. They can also be used to expand the maxillary arches if they have collapsed behind the premaxilla. The prominent premaxilla can often be returned by using a head bonnet elastic traction device. Surgical approaches can include either a staged lip closure or, alternatively, a lip adhesion. Intraoral devices that can simultaneously retract the premaxilla and expand the palatal shelves in a short period of time (7–10 days) are advocated by some surgeons.[37,90]

Further principles of bilateral cleft lip repair include having the prolabium provide the full vertical dimension of the central lip.[21] Earlier repairs transferred flaps from lateral elements to increase the vertical height of the prolabium, but this resulted in trapping of the prolabium in contracting scar.[7] Therefore, no lateral lip elements should be used below the prolabium. The vermilion of the prolabium is too thin and therefore is best turned down as lining, while the central vermilion is augmented, using flaps containing vermilion and muscle from the lateral lip elements.

The simplest of the lip closures and one that can produce acceptable results is the Veau straight line closure (Fig. 13–18).[105] It is especially indicated when the prolabium is not ex-

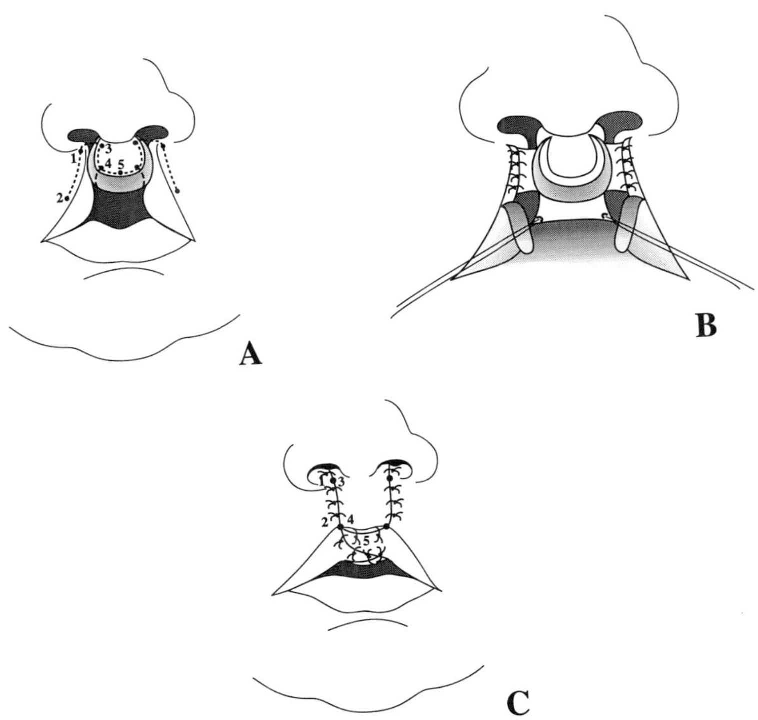


**Fig. 13–18.** A–C: Veau straight line repair for bilateral cleft lip.

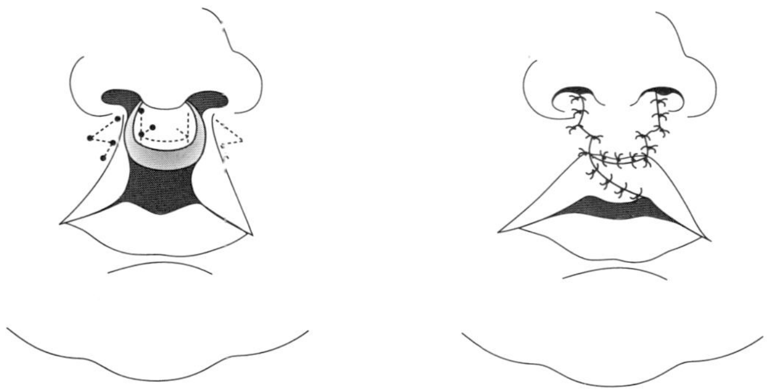

**Fig. 13–19.** Triangular closure for bilateral cleft lip.

tremely small. The vermilion ridge of the prolabium is completely excised and replaced by using turned down flaps of white roll from the lateral lip elements. The remainder of the red lip from the prolabium is turned down to provide additional projection for the tubercle. Flaps of skin are raised from the lateral margins of the prolabium and turned inward to line the buccal surface of the lip. Flaps of prolabial skin can also be raised along the lateral margins of a very wide prolabium as fork flaps and banked in the nasal floor. A columellar lengthening can then be done before the child starts school.[22]

There are a number of variations on the theme of camouflaging the scars.[8,102] The Tennison adaptation of the unilateral triangular flap technique can provide a more natural philtral dimple. However, scars may be more evident, and certainly revisions are made more difficult by the resulting zig-zag scarring (Fig. 13–19).

Millard has applied his rotation advancement principle to the treatment of complete and incomplete bilateral clefts. Complete clefts are treated in two stages. In the first, the lip is closed and lateral prolabial flaps are stored as fork flaps in the floor of the nose. Later, usually before the child begins school, a columella lengthening is accomplished by advancing the banked flaps into the columella (Fig. 13–20 A,B). A large prolabium is obviously required in this technique.

The width of the Cupid's bow is marked to be approximately 6–8 mm. Fork flaps based on the columella are raised from the excess lateral prolabium and sutured to the alar base flaps. This leaves a visible mound in each naris until the second stage when a V-Y advancement of this banked tissue is performed to lengthen the columella (Fig. 13–20B) The vermilion (Fig. 13–20A) on the prolabium is turned down as a flap to augment the tubercle while its new white roll is carried by the advancing lateral lip flaps. The muscles in the lateral lip flaps are sutured together behind the prolabium. With incomplete clefts the columella is usually of adequate length. The procedure involves releasing the prolabium from the columella to lengthen the central lip and fill in the defect by advancing the lateral lip flaps, which carries the vermilion ridge.

Mulliken's experience with the Millard technique has suggested further modifications.[72] He reports a 2.5–fold increase in size of the prolabial segment as a result of the closure and modifies the prolabial flap into a biconcave shape whose columellar base is 2 mm wide and 4–5 mm at the Cupid's bow. The lateral alar cartilages are dissected and advanced and the forked flaps stored in the nasal floor.

## Cleft palate

The timing of surgical intervention with cleft palate remains controversial. The goals of repair with closure of the defect are to achieve normal speech and hearing, normal dental occlusion, and normal facial and palatal growth. Timing of operative intervention must take into consideration what is known and what is postulated about facial growth and speech development.

The exact growth center of the midface has not yet been elucidated. It is felt, however, that the center shifts to the cranial base from the vomer at about 5 years of age. It has been observed that patients with nonoperated clefts exhibit normal maxillary growth.[26,76] There have been several studies indicating that midface underdevelopment has less to do with the age at which a child is operated on than with the trauma associated with the surgical intervention itself.

As for speech, it is known that vocalization begins with birth and that an intact speech mechanism is needed to ensure that the correct neural programming required to integrate the muscular actions involved in speech is set. This is thought by speech pathologists to occur certainly within the first year of life. Once compensatory speech patterns are established, they are difficult to correct.

It is generally held that early palatal repair is associated with better speech results and hearing but at the risk of having negative effects on facial growth. The additional problem lies in the inherent difficulty for the surgeon to operate on structures so small. Studies of speech comparing different ages at which surgery was performed have generally shown that earlier correction results in better speech.[6,26,31,85] Speech production was shown to be abnormal in only 10% of children undergoing repair under 12 months of age as opposed to over 80% in those operated on after 12 months of age.[26] Additional benefits include less middle ear disease because of earlier protection of the eustachian tube.[85]

Traditionally, clefts of the palate were closed between 18 and 24 months of age. The trend is towards earlier intervention because of the benefits to speech as discussed above; however, the most appropriate early age has not yet been determined. Some authors would prefer to close the cleft between 3 and 9 months of age;[84] however, a definitive study has yet to be done. Most centers in North America close the cleft between the ages of 12 and 18 months. It is felt that, in a child in that age group, the structures have become larger and more manageable intraoperatively, and that the correction is performed early enough not to impede the development of normal speech.

## Surgical procedures

Techniques used in repairing cleft palate fall essentially into one of two categories. In the first are all the one-stage procedures in which the entire defect in the palate is closed, usually with mucoperiosteal flaps. These will be described subsequently. The alternative is a multistage approach in which the velum is closed initially, followed by a delayed hard palate repair. The defect in the hard palate may or may not be obturated during the interval between stages.

Staged repair of the palate is the oldest form of cleft palate correction and dates back over 100 years. Schweckendiek reports normal bony growth with early (8 months) soft palate repair, followed by obturation of the hard palate defect until definitive repair occurs at adolescence.[94] However, a long-term

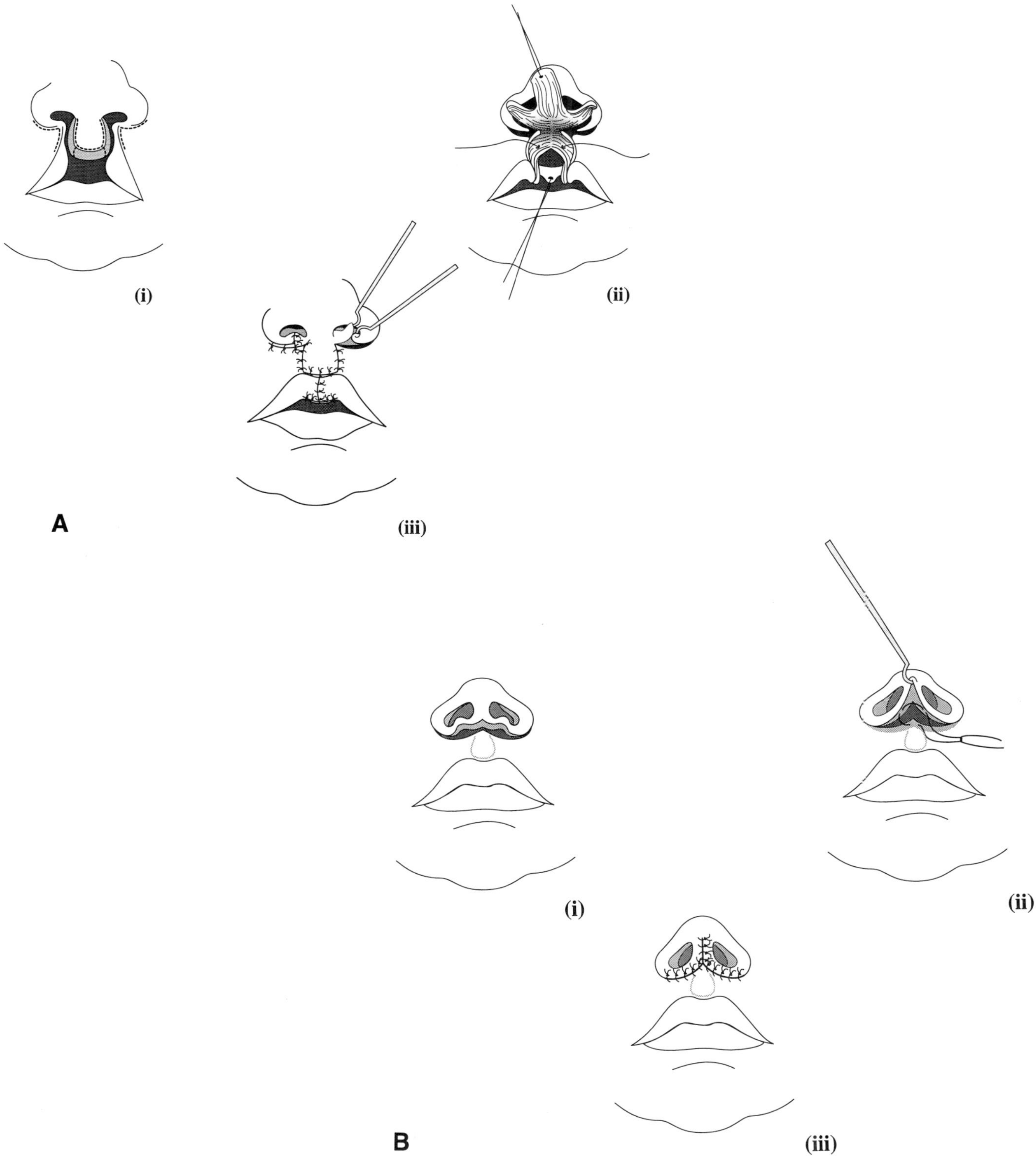


**Fig. 13–20.** Millard repair for the bilateral deformity. A: First stage; B: Second stage. See text for details.

assessment of patients having undergone this approach revealed a high incidence of short and poorly mobile palates, which led to a high incidence of velopharyngeal incompetence.[4]

Many European centers follow another two-stage approach described by Perko in which the velum is closed at 18 months of age and the hard palate is closed between 5 and 8 years of age.[80] Perko reports, and another study confirms, that speech development is not disturbed by the remaining hard palate cleft. The patients had an adequate velopharyngeal mechanism with fewer maladaptive articulation errors than with the Schwecken-diek approach.[103]

The most common approach is a single-stage, soft and hard

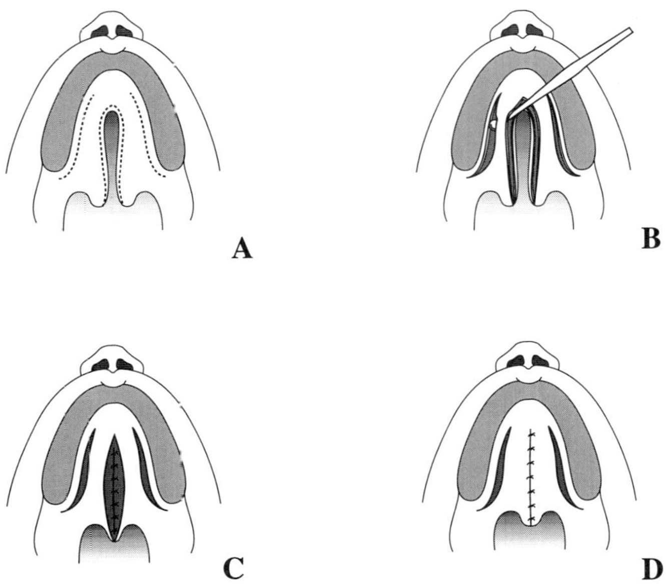


**Fig. 13–21.** Von Langenbeck cleft palate repair. A: The incisions are indicated. B: Lateral relaxing incisions allow mobilization of the palatal mucoperiosteum as a bipedicled flap based on the greater palatine vessels. C: The nasal mucosa is closed. D: Completed repair. The raw donor areas are allowed to heal secondarily.

palate closure done when the child is between 6 and 18 months of age. A primary palatal cleft, if present, is closed when the child is between the ages of 3 and 6 months.

### Specific procedures

*The Von Langenbeck palatoplasty.* The Von Langenbeck palatoplasty is the oldest of the more popular techniques. Essentially it involves the creation of bipedicled mucoperiosteal flaps on either side of the defect via relaxing incisions which border the defect and the lingual side of the alveolar ridge (Fig. 13–21) The resulting flaps are approximated in a side-to-side manner across the cleft after the abnormally inserted levators are freed from their bony attachments. A vomer flap can be used to provide a second layer for closure. Advantages of the Von Langenbeck include less dissection and movement of the mucoperiosteum than other procedures. It fails to provide additional length to the palate.

*The Veau-Wardill-Kilner palatoplasty.* Wardill[108] and Kilner[53] each devised a procedure basically similar to but more extensive than the one used by Veau[105] several years earlier. It has become in essence a V-Y push back of hard palate mucoperiosteal flaps that results in palatal lengthening. Figure 13–22 illustrates the Oxford modification as well as the basic principles.[79] Although the area of raw bone closes within 2 weeks, it is felt that growth and occlusal abnormalities may result from scarring in that area of the anterior palate.[5] Modifications of the technique have been proposed to decrease the scar contracture, such as elevating the flap above the periosteum in order to leave the bone covered.[80] However, these dissections are difficult and may risk compromising the blood supply to the flap.

*The Furlow double opposing Z-plasty.* A new palatoplasty has recently been described by Furlow and termed the *double opposing Z-plasty technique*.[36] The procedure is illustrated in Figure 13–23. It involves the creation of doubly reversing Z-plasties on the oral and nasal sides of the soft palate. This procedure allows the palate to be lengthened without raising extensive mucoperiosteal flaps from the hard palate. In addition, it allows for a simpler reorientation of the levators transversely and overlapped across the defect. The closure also avoids a straight line scar which has the potential to contract and shorten the palate.

The operation consists of designing two Z-plasties: one on the oral side and the other on the nasal side of the palate. Beginning on the oral side, the muscle is contained in the posteriorly based flap of each Z, which is dissected off the palatine shelf and raised as a mucomuscular flap. Elevating the flaps on the oral surface reveals the deeper plane where the second Z-plasty will be fashioned. These flaps are designed in the opposite direction to the more superficial ones, resulting in the levator veli palatini again being contained in the posteriorly based flap, which this time is lined by nasal mucosa. Each Z is closed separately, resulting in palatal lengthening and anatomic reconstruction of the levator sling. The defect in the hard palate is closed by using a vomer flap, usually in two layers.

*Intravelar veloplasty.* The abnormal orientation and substitute insertions of the levator veli palatini muscles must be addressed in the repair of palatal clefts. At a minimum they must be detached from the posterior edge of the hard palate and reoriented in a transverse direction to mimic the normal musculature of the palate. Other surgeons advocate suturing the muscles end-to-end or even overlapping them to achieve a tighter sling.[16,54] The importance of muscular reconstruction is emphasized by many authors who argue for attempting to duplicate the levator loop to attain a dynamic functioning unit as opposed to simply repositioning the muscles (Fig. 13–9B).[81,89] In fact, comparative studies do exist reporting better speech results and improved velopharyngeal function with careful reconstruction of the levator sling.[16,27] Although there are also studies show-

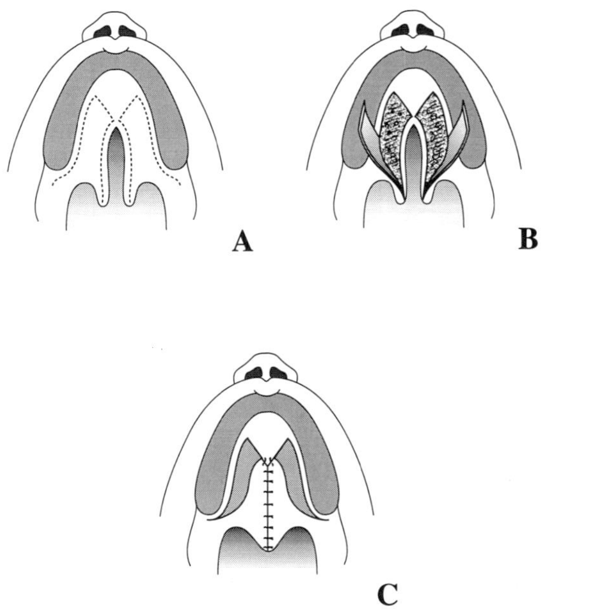


**Fig. 13–22.** Veau-Wardill-Kilner procedure. A: The incisions are indicated. B: Unipedicled mucoperiosteal flaps are raised based on the greater palatine vessels. Velar musculature is detached from its abnormal insertion on the edge of the bony cleft and reoriented. C: Result after nasal and oral closure.

ing no beneficial effect of intravelar veloplasty on velopharyngeal competence, most surgeons include a levator sling reconstruction as part of their cleft closure.[61]

## Velopharyngeal insufficiency

### Clinical manifestations

Normal speech requires a competent velopharyngeal mechanism. The velopharyngeal sphincter is conceptualized as functioning in concert with the larynx and mouth to produce speech. The palate forms a part of the velopharyngeal sphincter which functions to separate the nasal cavity from the vocal tract for the formation of consonants and vowels and to integrate the nasal cavity and vocal tract in the formation of nasal consonants. Malfunction of this mechanism, such as the inability to close the sphincter completely, is termed *velopharyngeal insufficiency* (VPI). It is characterized by hypernasality, nasal emissions, and adaptive changes and inarticulations such as pharyngeal fricatives, sound substitution, and glottal stops.

In a general sense, surgery aims to produce a mechanism which will restore the development of normal speech. Calnan has classified the causes of VPI as anatomic and neuromuscular in origin.[18] An understanding of the anatomy and physiology of the velopharyngeal port is essential to understanding the treatment.

As stated earlier, the purpose of the sphincter is to separate and/or couple the oral and nasal cavities to provide for accurate phonation. This is accomplished by soft palate movement (tension and elevation) as well as by lateral and posterior pharyngeal wall movement to narrow the lumen. As speech begins, the soft palate rises and tenses. Complete closure is essential in the production and release of consonants, especially the plosives (e.g., *p*ie, *t*ie, *c*at) and the fricatives *th*in, *s*in, *f*an). An open sphincter is necessary for the production of nasal sounds (e.g., *m*e, *n*o, si*ng*). Tensing and raising of the soft palate with or without full sphincter closure produces vowels. The degree to which the sphincter is opened or closed, the size of the pharynx, and tension of its underlying musculature also work to produce different vowels.

An incompetent sphincter will allow air to escape through the nose during attempts to produce the consonants, requiring a build-up of intraoral breath pressure. The child will use other components of the vocal tract in an attempt to compensate. Examples include using glottal stops to substitute for a plosive (unable to say "dog" the child will say "gog"). Being unable to produce the normal fricatives, he may use pharyngeal fricatives which are produced by constricting the air stream by the tongue and posterior pharyngeal wall. Nasal snorting or velar fricatives may also be used in substitutions. These and other substitutions and maladaptive patterns are noted in children as young as 3 years of age. The least affected are the vowels and nasal consonants.

At the present time, most techniques of palate repair, despite their best intentions, yield an incidence of VPI of approximately 20%–30%.[71,86] One of the difficulties in arriving at precise data lies in the fact that there is no uniform, reproducible method of recording the results. The evaluation of success of any given procedure relies on the assessment of the patients' speech postoperatively. For the most part this assessment has been largely clinical, relying on the judgment of the trained ears of the speech pathologist and plastic surgeon as well as the other members of the cleft palate team. Various other modalities have been developed to objectively assess speech quality and velopharyngeal function postoperatively.

Articulation tests have been designed in which the absence or presence of velopharyngeal closure is determined using words requiring oral pressure build-up for their correct pronunciation. Other tests try to determine the substitutions used by the child to accommodate for having VPI. Sound spectrographic analysis has attempted to correlate the auditory perception with an objective tool, but it is not considered a useful test for VPI. Once the screening tests have shown the presence of VPI, it is helpful to quantitate the characteristics to facilitate an objective comparison of the pre- and postoperative results.

### Diagnostic methods

Pressure and air flow measurements, both oral and nasal, can be used to determine the effectiveness of velopharyngeal closure. A number of appliances exist, ranging from simple mirrored surfaces to complex devices, for measuring nasal air flow and pressure. A nasal air flow rate of 125 cc/sec is associated with VPI, as is a finding of a differential in nasal and oral pressure measurements.[55] These measurements are useful. However, only as screening tests and no details of sphincter function can be obtained.

As the velopharyngeal mechanism comprises many different movement patterns, its imaging requires it to be assessed in a three-dimensional fashion. Imaging studies add more information and consist of radiologic and endoscopic assessments.

#### Radiologic methods

Standard soft tissue radiographs are able to provide a two-dimensional assessment of the relationship between the soft palate and the posterior pharyngeal wall. However, cine and videofluoroscopy are required for an evaluation of the movement of the pharyngeal walls and the palate itself. Barium coating as well as various projections are needed for an accurate

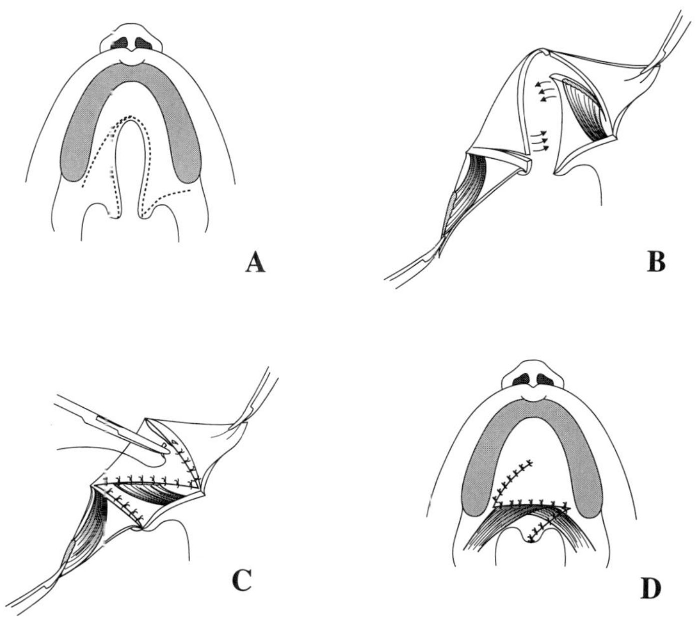


**Fig. 13–23.** A–D: Furlow double Z-plasty repair, after Furlow, 1986.

assessment. The experience of the radiologist with these techniques clearly comes into play in the diagnosis of VPI. Computed tomography (CT) scanning combined with endoscopy has been proposed as another method, but it too is limited for evaluating a dynamic event.[44]

### Endoscopic methods

Nasendoscopy allows for direct observation of the components of the velopharyngeal sphincter. Both flexible and rigid scopes are available, although the rigid ones are preferred because of the better optics they provide. When combined with a lateral cinefluoroscopy, a dynamic assessment can be made.

## Surgery for VPI

Velopharyngeal insufficiency may be treated surgically using pharyngeal flaps, pharyngeal sphincter reconstruction (pharyngoplasty), or pharyngeal wall implants. Currently, a pharyngeal flap is the most popular option.

### Pharyngeal flap

Essentially two types have been described: an inferiorly based flap and a superiorly based one. Although studies comparing the results of the two techniques have not yielded an advantage of one over the other, the superiorly based flap is used more often.[15,110] The soft palate is divided and separated in the midline, allowing access to the posterior pharyngeal wall. The flap is outlined and then elevated above the level of the prevertebral fascia, containing mucosa and superior constrictor muscle. The flap is then placed and sutured above and behind the velum, which is then closed. Obturation of the velopharyngeal port is thus achieved. The nasopharyngeal space is decreased in both the anteroposterior and circumferential dimensions. Communication between the nasopharynx and the rest of the upper airway occurs through the openings allowed lateral to the flap. The donor site may be left open or closed.

Technical considerations in pharyngeal flap surgery include placing the base of the flap at a high level in the pharynx where the sphincter is actually working, so that any lateral pharyngeal wall movement would close the gaps. This is felt to be a key maneuver to achieving success. Preoperative assessment using nasendoscopy and videofluoroscopy is also felt to be important in tailoring the flap size to match the defect in the port.[95] Turnover flaps of nasal mucosa are used to line raw surfaces of the flap to prevent it from becoming fibrotic and distorted.

### Pharyngoplasty

The Hynes pharyngoplasty involves elevating two superiorly based flaps consisting of mucosa and salpingopharyngeus muscle and overlapping them transversely across the midline (Fig. 13–24).[47] This produces a ridge which brings the posterior wall of the pharynx closer to the soft palate. Closing the donor site effectively narrows the pharynx.

Orticochea has described a dynamic muscle sphincter procedure in which lateral pharyngeal flaps containing the palatopharyngeus muscles are sutured to an inferiorly based pharyngeal flap.[74] These muscles course through the posterior tonsillar pillar and help pull the soft palate posteriorly. Their innervation is kept relatively intact as their innervation enters in a centromedial direction allowing their transposition. Experience with this technique and its modifications has been positive.[74,87]

### Retropharyngeal implants

These procedures date back to the last century in early attempts to augment the posterior wall of the pharynx. A number of materials have been used, some autogenous and some synthetic. Injectable Teflon®,[10,11] Proplast®,[115] and Silastic®[13] have been used but have been plagued with problems of migration and extrusion.

The goal of surgical intervention in VPI is to attain acceptable speech. There is, however, no uniform tool for assessing this end point. Acceptability of speech can vary in different languages and even among different groups speaking the same language. Different researchers have measured speech adequacy in various ways, some being objective and others subjective. In addition, there are a number of other variables such as patient specifics, severity of the speech defect, details of the procedure, etc., that must be accounted for in comparing treatment modalities. Gross estimates of *improved* speech however range from 50%–95%.[24] One large long-term study has yielded satisfactory speech results in 80% of patients; 15% of these patients were further improved with speech therapy while the remainder required further surgery.[15]

## Secondary deformities

Although a complete discussion of secondary deformities is beyond the mandate of this chapter, it is important to touch upon certain aspects of these deformities to appreciate the long-term commitment involved in the care of these children. Most infants born with clefts will require more than one operation in their lifetime to correct the primary deformity or the consequences of attempts at correction of the primary defect. Examples in the three components of lip, nose, and bony framework will be discussed.

Many of the deformities of the lip apply to both unilateral and bilateral clefts and include unacceptable scarring, tissue deficiencies (vertical or horizontal), vertical tissue excess, landmark abnormalities, and mucosal abnormalities. Scar revisions for wide or otherwise unacceptable scars along the lines of closure should be done later in adolescence to avoid the clinical observation of hypertrophic scar tendency of children. Techniques involve basic plastic surgical principles and tension-free wound closure and can include simple excision and Z-plasty and W-plasty methods to break up the tendency towards scar contracture. Notching at the vermilion border, which is common among straight line closures, is amenable to correction by Z-plasty lengthening.

As mentioned earlier, the Tennison-Randall and Le Mesurier repairs were prone to lengthen with time and secondary revisions are often necessary. Correction of the long lip is difficult and involves a full thickness excision in the perialar portion of the upper lip.[109]

A short lip can occur after repair of a wide cleft by using the Millard technique. Often the condition corrects with time. However, failure to do so requires operative correction. In many cases, this is best achieved with a full thickness redo of the rotation-advancement, combined with excision of the vertical scar in an elliptical fashion to gain further lip elongation. Diastasis or similar functional abnormalities of the orbicularis

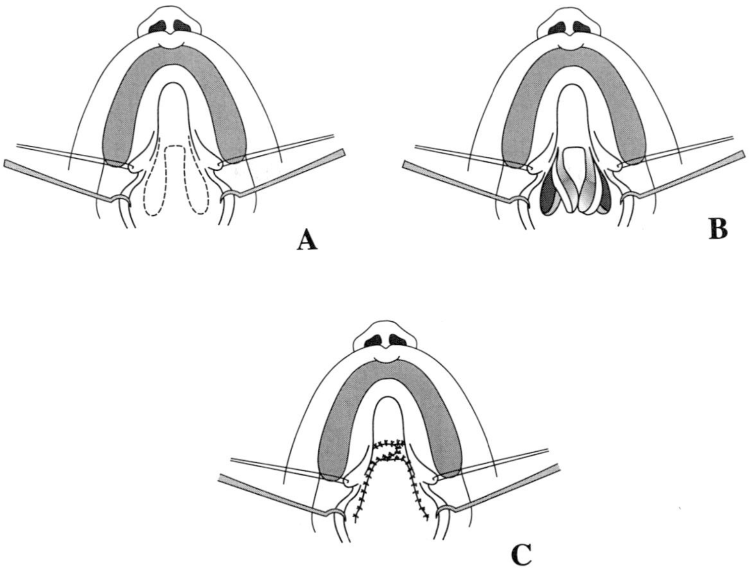

**Fig. 13–24.** A–C: Hynes pharyngoplasty. See text for details.

can be corrected at this time. The presence of such muscular abnormalities frequently leads to unsatisfactory scarring, as the tension is transferred to the skin closure.

Secondary deformities requiring revision are more common among the bilateral cleft lip group for a number of reasons, including the greater amount of scarring present and the deficiency of tissue that is inherent in that deformity. An example would be a lip which is tight horizontally. An Abbé lip switch would provide the composite tissue required and improve lip function.[48]

The cleft lip nasal deformity remains a surgical challenge. The pathologic anatomy of the primary deformity is discussed elsewhere. The nose can be repaired in association with the lip deformity as an infant, as a preschooler, as an adolescent, or as an adult. Controversy surrounds the timing of surgical intervention for its correction with respect to the effects of surgery on future growth of the involved structures.

Advocates of primary lip and nose repair report that the good results obtained in this period persist and that growth is not adversely affected when careful surgery is performed.[3,14,62,63,91] Millard waits until the child is ready for school before performing an alar lift, arguing that the cartilages are too delicate to manipulate in an infant.[69] A rim incision is used to gain access to the displaced cartilage, freeing it from the skin and lining (Fig. 13–25). It is then lifted and fixed to its normal position with the use of slowly absorbable polyglycolic acid on nonabsorbable sutures.

There exists a multitude of techniques for the correction of the cleft lip nasal deformity.[43,66] The goal is to achieve a symmetrically appearing nose. Access to the deformity may be gained through an intranasal incision; in severe, previously operated noses or in bilateral deformities, however, an external incision is preferred. The displaced and deformed alar cartilages are mobilized and repositioned in a supermedial direction. Although formal rhinoplasty has been performed between the ages of 8 and 12 years with no alteration of facial or nasal growth, most surgeons would wait until patients are in their teens.[75] Maxillary surgery should precede definitive rhinoplasty.

Secondary deformities associated with a bilateral cleft lip are often centered around a short columella, blunt nasal tip, and flared alar bases. A Cronin-type columellar lengthening advances nasal floor tissue medially into the columella and simultaneously corrects the alar flare.[21] Forked flaps can be raised from the lip during a secondary revision and advanced into the columella. The second stage of Millard's bilateral complete cleft repair similarly advances forked prolabial flaps that were banked in the nostril floors at the time of primary lip repair.[65]

Oronasal fistulae, whether they be through the soft or hard palates or the alveolar ridge, as well as dental abnormalities, are other complications requiring secondary procedures. The incidence of palatal fistula after cleft repair can range from 10% to 50%. They occur most frequently after repair of complete clefts of the primary and secondary palates as opposed to isolated cleft palates.

Anterior and alveolar palatal fistulae are repaired either when secondary lip revisions are performed or during bone grafting of the alveolar cleft. This is most commonly performed using autogenous cancellous bone grafts covered with mucoperiosteal and gingival flaps. Closing the fistula without bone grafting results in a higher incidence of failure.[49] Closure of small asymptomatic fistulae may be deferred for a long time or not closed at all. Symptoms include leakage of food and liquids through the nose, nasal irritation, and odors. Larger fistulae can produce speech problems such as hypernasality.

Closure of oronasal and nasolabial fistulae is done using two layers. A nasal layer is reconstructed by turnover flaps from circumscribing the fistula while the oral layer is fashioned from mucoperiosteal flaps. Larger fistulae require the elevation of buccal flaps for secure closure.

Posterior palatal fistulae can be closed by similar techniques, i.e., using local tissue in the form of mucoperiosteal flaps. Inability to close the defect using mucoperiosteal flaps because of excessive scarring, and previous unsuccessful operations may require the use of tongue flaps[38] or pedicled nasal septal flaps.[29] Defects in the soft palate are closed when symptomatic through using a two-layer closure and relaxing incisions. The

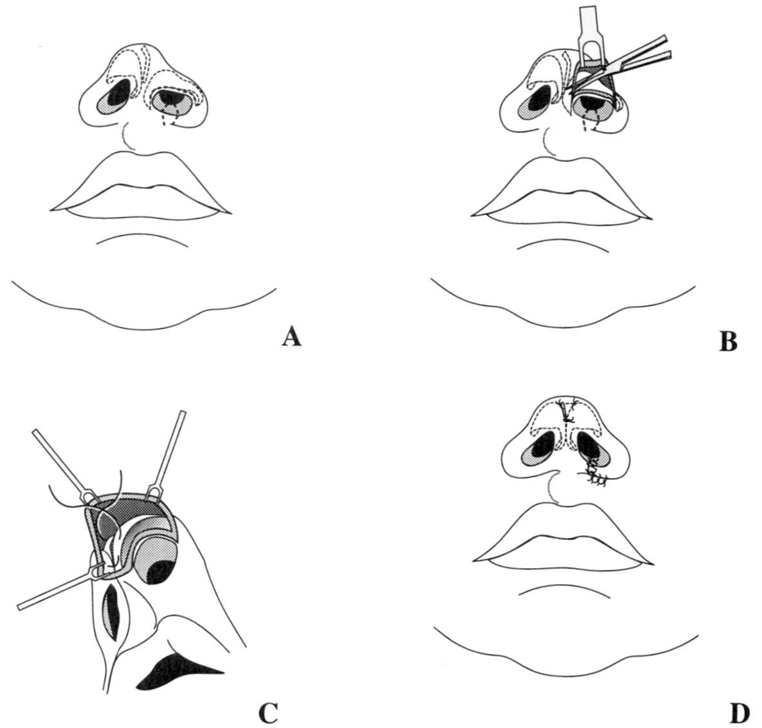


**Fig. 13–25.** A–D: Alar lift after Millard, 1982.[69]

presence of velopharyngeal insufficiency in addition to a large fistula requires a pharyngeal flap.

There are wide differences in the approach towards management of alveolar clefts. Early reports of successful primary bone-grafting during lip closure resulted in wide acceptance of this technique during the 1950s and 60s. It was felt that this approach would not only prevent collapse of the maxilla but that it may normalize craniofacial development as well as possibly stimulating maxillary growth.[114] Later there were numerous reports of growth disturbances after large groups of these patients had been followed through their growth phase. Class III malocclusion and midface retrusion was seen to be the result of this disturbance in maxillary growth. This approach has largely been abandoned by most centers in Canada and the U.S.

Skoogs' periosteoplasty resulted in bone formation in the cleft after transferring local flaps containing periosteum.[98] Follow-up studies indicate acceptable bone formation without negative effects on subsequent maxillary growth.[42] This is similar to Millard's gingivoperiosteoplasty performed at the time of the lip closure.

Most centers perform secondary bone grafting between the ages of 6 and 11 years, which is the period of mixed dentition. At that stage, the sagittal and transverse growth of this portion of the maxilla have largely been completed. Vertical growth is felt to occur mainly by the addition of alveolar bone, which is itself stimulated by the eruption of permanent dentition.[100] By closing the cleft through bone-grafting and later orthodontically guiding the permanent tooth into the area, alveolar bone is formed which contributes to the vertical dimensions of the maxilla.[9] Additional benefits include stabilizing the maxillary arch, especially in bilateral clefts, as well as having the bone graft in the cleft provide stability for the remaining teeth on either side of the cleft.

Sources for bone graft are many and include tibia, rib, cranium, and iliac crest. In general, cancellous bone is preferred because of its rapid incorporation and its accommodation to the subsequent translocation of teeth. The authors favor the use of iliac crest as a donor site because of its exclusive cancellous content and reliability as compared to calvarial sites.

## Miscellaneous:

### Robin sequence

Retrognathism, which is a feature of the Pierre Robin sequence, results in a functional abnormality of the tongue and its musculature. The risk to the newborn lies in the potential for airway obstruction which often manifests during sleep when the tongue is at rest and the mandible retropositioned. Respiratory difficulties and the associated cleft palate can further lead to feeding difficulties and failure to thrive.

Treatment is prioritized according to the severity of airway compromise followed by the extent of feeding difficulties. Conservative treatment consists of placing the infant prone in addition to intensive nursing monitoring. Although these maneuvers may be adequate in mild cases, surgery is indicated if there is no improvement after 7 days.[77] Other indications for surgery include a mandibular arch greater than 1 cm behind the maxillary arch and repeated episodes of cyanosis or pneumonia.[83] However, most of the cases are managed in pediatric intensive care units, without surgery.

Although tongue repositioning and K-wire fixation have been described as a method of management,[93] the most appropriate surgical treatment consists of a tongue-lip adhesion. Currently, a modification[83] of the Routledge[88] procedure is a popular method (Fig. 13–26). To prevent dehiscence, the stay sutures are kept for 2 weeks while the adhesion itself is kept until the time of the palate repair, usually at around 12 to 18 months of age. With this technique there is no obstruction of the salivary ducts or interference with dentition.

## Macroglossia

Several classification schemes for macroglossia have been proposed.[106,107] Congenital macroglossia may be due to tumours such as dermoids, muscular hypertrophy or hyperplasia as in the Beckwith-Wiedemann syndrome, and hemihypertrophy. More commonly, it is due to vascular malformations. Macroglossia may interfere with speech or deglutition. The exposed tongue can dry, fissure, and ulcerate. Further problems include oral hygiene and drooling.

The most common vascular malformations of the tongue are lymphatic, often called *lymphangiomas of the tongue*.[113] Extensive, mixed, capillary-cavernous lymphangiomas or lymphangioma circumscriptum of the entire thickness of the tongue are difficult problems to manage. Massive swelling of the tongue with the subsequent inability to close the mouth, or even airway compromise, can occur after surgical biopsy or relatively minor trauma. Superimposed lymphangitis can compound the swelling. Conservative treatment is recommended in the early years of life and consists of avoiding trauma and prompt antibiotic therapy at the earliest sign of infection. Surgery should be delayed until the child is older, (4–5 years) to lessen the chances of postoperative airway problems.[113]

Macroglossia is a prominent feature of Down syndrome. In these cases, the glossoptosis is a combination of a small oral cavity and a large tongue. The enlarged tongue is felt to be a reactive hypertrophy due to the muscular hypotonia present in these children.[57]

Partial resection will usually succeed in returning the tongue to the mouth and remove this visible stigma of retardation. The parents usually report improvements in speech and this undoubtedly aids in attempts at integrating these children into society.

The $CO_2$ laser has proved to be a very effective tool in performing partial glossectomy, especially by decreasing blood loss. Patients undergoing the procedure for lymphangiomas must be covered perioperatively with antibiotics effective

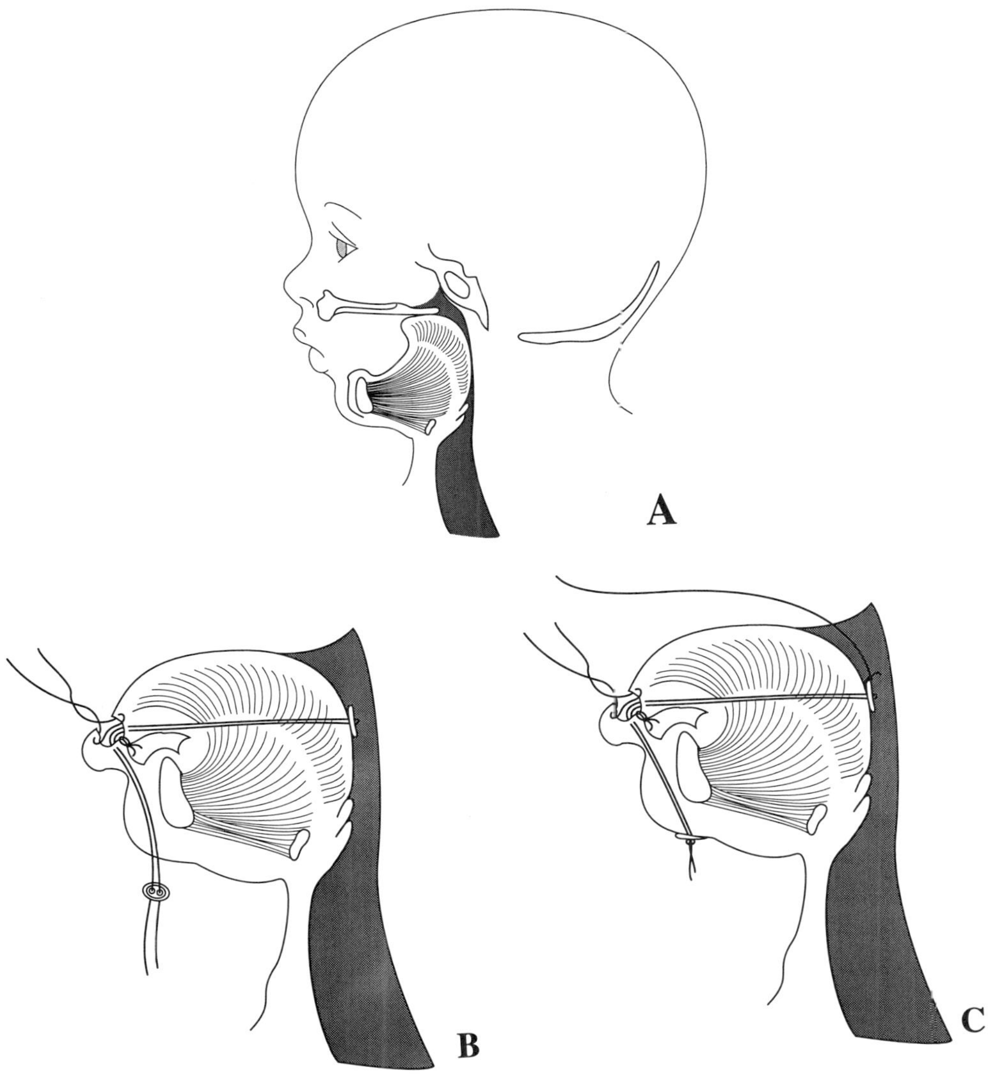


**Fig. 13–26.** Modified Routledge procedure. Adhesion of the tongue to the lip is performed and reinforced by a heavy suture through the repair and tied over buttons at the base of the tongue and externally under the chin (A–C). A separate suture is tied to the button at the base of the tongue to allow for it to be retrieved at a later date.

against streptococcal infection. A moderate amount of swelling can be expected postoperatively; however, most children usually resume at least a liquid diet by the first postoperative day. Down syndrome patients should similarly be covered perioperatively with antibiotics. They have a slower postoperative recovery, often requiring several days of intravenous fluid before they begin to take food by mouth.

## Ankyloglossia

Commonly known as *tongue-tie,* ankyloglossia is manifested by the presence of a frenulum tethering the tip of the tongue to the floor of the mouth. Articulation errors are uncommon. However, surgical treatment is indicated when the tip of the tongue is severely restricted or at the request of the parents. Any technique, particularly in a small child, should be performed under general anaesthesia and not as an office procedure. Care must be taken to avoid injuring Wharton's ducts. The release may be a simple division of the band or a Z-plasty lengthening.

## Epignathus

Epignathi are rare teratomas that present dramatically at birth where they are seen to protrude from the mouth and compromise the airway. Grossly, they are covered with skin and mucosa and seem to arise from the palate or pharynx, filling the oral cavity. Bony tissue is often palpable within these masses. Although one theory holds that they are parasitic fetuses, the more popular theory is that they arise from pluripotential stem cells from the region of Rathke's pouch.[78]

Histology reveals well-differentiated tissue from all three germ-cell lines.

Management consists of immediately securing an airway by intubation or even tracheostomy. Once encephalocele and intracranial extension have been ruled out with a high-resolution CT scan, an oral approach is used to excise the tumour.[78]

The mucosal origin of the tumour is left to granulate or is closed primarily. This management sequence has resulted in the salvage of neonates that otherwise would have succumbed to asphyxiation.

## References


1. Adzick NS, Harrison MR, Glick PL, Beckstead JH, Villa RL, Scheuenstuhl H, Goodson WH 3d: Comparison of fetal, newborn, and adult wound healing by histologic, enzyme-histochemical, and hydroxyproline determinations. J Ped Surg 20:315–319, 1985.
2. Adzick NS, Longaker MT: Scarless fetal healing: therapeutic implications. Ann Surg 215:3–7 1992.
3. Anderl H: Simultaneous repair of lip and nose in the unilateral cleft (A long term report). In: Recent Advances in Plastic Surgery, IT Jackson, BC Sommerlad, eds. Churchill Livingstone, Edinburgh, 1985, p 1.
4. Bardach J, Morris HL, Olin WH: Late results of primary veloplasty: the Marburg Project. Plast Reconstr Surg 73:207–218, 1984.
5. Bardach J, Salyer K: Surgical Techniques in Cleft Lip and Palate. Year Book Medical Publishers, Chicago, 1987.
6. Barimo JP, Habal MB, Scheuerle J, Ritterman SI: Postnatal palatoplasty, implications for normal speech articulation—a preliminary report. Scand J Plast Reconstr Surg Hand Surg 21:139–143, 1987.
7. Barsky AJ: Principles and Practice of Plastic Surgery. Williams and Wilkins, Baltimore, 1950.
8. Bauer TB, Trusler HM, Tondra JM: Changing concepts in the management of bilateral cleft lip deformities. Plast Reconstr Surg 24:321–332, 1959.
9. Bergland O, Semb G, Abyholm FE: Elimination of the residual alveolar cleft by secondary bone grafting and subsequent orthodontic treatment. Cleft Palate J 23:175–205, 1986.
10. Bluestone CD, Musgrave RH, McWilliams BJ, Crozier PA: Teflon injection pharyngoplasty. Cleft Palate J 5:19–22, 1968.
11. Bluestone CD, Stool SE (eds): Pediatric Otolaryngology, vol 2. WB Saunders Co, Philadelphia, 1983.
12. Boorman JG, Sommerlad BC: Musculus uvulae and levator palati: their anatomical and functional relationship in velopharyngeal closure. Br J Plast Surg 38:333–338, 1985.
13. Brauer RO: Retropharyngeal implantation of silicone gel pillows for velopharyngeal incompetence. Plast Reconstr Surg 51:254–262, 1973.
14. Broadbent TR, Woolf RM: Cleft lip nasal deformity. Ann Plast Surg 12:216–234, 1984.
15. Bronsted K, Liisberg WB, Orsted A, Prytz S, Fogh-Andersen P: Surgical and speech results following palatopharyngoplasty operations in Denmark, 1959–1977. Cleft Palate J 21:170–179, 1984.
16. Brown AS, Cohen MA, Randall P: Levator muscle reconstruction: does it make a difference? Plast Reconstr Surg 72:1–8, 1983.
17. Brown JB, McDowell F: Small triangular flap operation for primary repair of single cleft lips. Plast Reconstr Surg 5:392–402, 1950.
18. Calnan J: Surgery for speech. In: Recent Advances in Plastic Surgery. Churchill Livingstone, Edinburgh, 1976.
19. Christ JE: Fetal surgery: a frontier for plastic surgery. Plast Reconstr Surg 77:645–647, 1986.
20. Cohen MM Jr: Syndromes with cleft lip and palate. Cleft palate J 15:306, 1978.
21. Cronin TD: Lengthening columella by use of skin from nasal floor and alae. Plast Reconstr Surg 21:417–426, 1958.
22. Cronin TD: Surgery of the double cleft lip and protruding premaxilla. Plast Reconstr Surg 19:389–400, 1958.
23. Dado DV, Kernahan DA, Gionopoulos JG: Intrauterine repair of cleft lip: what's involved. Plast Reconstr Surg 85:461–465, 1990.
24. Dalston RM, Stuteville OH: A clinical investigation of the efficacy of primary nasopalatal pharyngoplasty. Cleft Palate J 12:177–192, 1975.
25. Davis JS, Ritchie HF: Classification of congenital clefts of the lip and palate. JAMA 79:1323–1327, 1922.
26. Dorf DS, Curtin JW: Early cleft palate repair and speech outcome. Plast Reconstr Surg 70:74–81, 1982.
27. Dreyer TM, Trier WC: A comparison of palatoplasty techniques. Cleft Palate J 21:251–253, 1984.
28. Eastman JR, Bixler D, Escobar V: Linkage studies in Van der Woude syndrome. J Med Genet 15:217–218, 1978.
29. Edgerton MT, Devito RV: Closure of palatal defects by means of a hinged nasal septum flap. Plast Reconstr Surg 31:537–541, 1963.
30. Estes JM, Whitby DJ, Lorenz HP, Longaker MT, Szabo Z, Adzick NS, Harrison MR: Endoscopic creation and repair of fetal cleft lip. Plast Reconstr Surg 90:743–746, 1992.
31. Evans D, Renfrew C: The timing of primary cleft palate repair. Scand J Plast Reconstr Surg 8:153–155, 1974.
32. Fára M: The musculature of cleft lip and palate. In: Plastic Surgery, vol 4, JG McCarthy, ed. WB Saunders, Philadelphia, 1990, pp 2598–2626.
33. Fogh-Andersen P: Inheritance of Harelip and Cleft Palate. Nyt Nordisk Forlag, Arnold Busck, Copenhagen, 1942.
34. Fraser FC: The genetics of cleft lip and cleft palate. Am J Hum Genet 22:336–352, 1970.
35. Fraser GR, Calnan JS: Cleft lip and palate: seasonal incidence, birth weight, birth rank, sex, site, associated malformations and parental age: A statistical survey. Arch Dis Child 36:420–423, 1961.
36. Furlow LT Jr: Cleft palate repair by double opposing Z-plasty. Plast Reconstr Surg 78:724–738, 1986.
37. Georgiade NG, Mason R, Riefkohl R, Georgiade G, Barwick W: Preoperative positioning of the protruding maxilla in the bilateral cleft lip patient. Plast Reconstr Surg 83:32, 1983.
38. Guerrero-Santos J, Altamirano JT: The use of lingual flaps in repair of fistulas of the hard palate. Plast Reconstr Surg 38:123–128, 1966.
39. Habib Z: Genetic counselling and genetics of cleft lip and cleft palate. Obstet Gynecol Surg 33:441, 1978.
40. Hagedorn M: Über eine Modifikation der Hasenschartenoperation, Zentralbl Chir 11:756, 1884.
41. Hallock GG: In defence of intrauterine repair of cleft lip. Plast Reconstr Surg 85:801–802, 1990.
42. Hellquist R, Ponten B: The influence of infant periosteoplasty on facial growth and dental occlusion from five to eight years of age in cases of complete unilateral cleft lip and palate. Scand J Plast Reconstr Surg 13:305–312, 1979.

43. Hobar PC, Rohrich RJ: Cleft lip II: secondary deformites. Selected Readings in Plastic Surgery 6:1–26, 1991.
44. Honjo I, Mitoma T, Ushiro K, Kawano M: Evaluation of velopharyngeal closure by CT scan and endoscopy. Plast Reconstr Surg 74:620–627, 1984.
45. Honjo I, Okazaki N, Kumazawa T: Experimental study of eustachian tube function with regard to its related muscle. Acta Otolaryngol 87:84–89, 1979.
46. Huffman WC, Lierle DM: Studies on the pathologic anatomy of the harelip nose. Plast Reconstr Surg 4:225–234, 1949.
47. Hynes W: Pharyngoplasty by muscle transplantation. Br J Plast Surg 3:128–135, 1950.
48. Jackson IT, Soutar DS: The sandwich Abbe flap in secondary cleft lip deformity. Plast Reconstr Surg 66:38–45, 1980.
49. Johanson B, Ohisson A, Friede H, Ahlgren J: A follow-up study of cleft lip and palate patients treated with orthodontics, secondary bone grafting, and prosthetic rehabilitation. Scand J Plast Reconstr Surg 8:121–135, 1974.
50. Johnston MC, Sulik KK: Embryology of the head and neck. In: Pediatric Plastic Surgery, D Serafin, NG Georgiade, eds. CV Mosby, St. Louis, 1984.
50a. Johnston MC, Hassell JR, Brown KS: The embryology of cleft lip and cleft palate. Clin Plast Surg 2:195–203, 1975.
51. Kernahan DA: The striped Y—A symbolic classification for cleft lip and palate. Plast Reconstr Surg 47:469–470, 1971.
52. Kernahan DA, Stark RB: A new classification for cleft lip and cleft palate. Plast Reconstr Surg 22:435–441, 1958.
53. Kilner TP: Cleft lip and palate repair technique. St. Thomas's Hospital Reports 2:127–140, 1937.
54. Kriens O: Anatomy of the velopharyngeal area in cleft palate. Clin Plast Surg 2:261–288, 1975.
55. Laine T, Warren DW, Dalston RM, Morr KE: Screening of velopharyngeal closure based on nasal airflow rate measurements. Cleft Palate J 25:220–225, 1988.
56. Le Mesurier AB: A method of cutting and suturing the lip in the treatment of complete unilateral clefts. Plast Reconstr Surg 4:1–12, 1949.
57. Lemperle G, Radu D: Facial plastic surgery in children with Down's Syndrome. Plast Reconstr Surg 66:337–345, 1980.
58. Longaker MT, Adzick NS: The biology of fetal wound healing: a review. Plast Reconstr Surg 87:788–798, 1991.
59. Longaker MT, Burd DA, Gown AM, Yen TS, Jennings RW, Duncan BW, Harrison MR, Adzick NS: Midgestational excisional fetal lamb wounds contract in utero. J Ped Surg 26:942–947, 1991.
60. Malgaigne JF: Manuel de Médecine Opératoire, 4th ed. Paris, 1843.
61. Marsh JL, Grames LM, Holtman B: Intravelar veloplasty: a prospective study. Cleft Palate J 26:46–50, 1989.
62. McComb H: Primary repair of the bilateral cleft lip nose: a 10–year review. Plast Reconstr Surg 77:701–716, 1986.
63. McComb H: Primary repair of the cleft lip nose. In: Plastic Surgery, vol 4, JG McCarthy, ed. WB Saunders, Philadelphia, 1990, pp 2708–2722.
64. Millard DR Jr: Refinements in rotation-advancement cleft lip technique. Plast Reconstr Surg 33:26–38 1964.
65. Millard DR Jr: Closure of bilateral cleft lip and elongation of columella by two operations in infancy. Plast Reconstr Surg 47:324–331, 1971.
66. Millard DR Jr: The unilateral deformity. In: Cleft Craft I. Little, Brown & Co, Boston, 1976, pp 153–177.
67. Millard DR Jr: Bilateral and rare deformities. In: Cleft Craft II. Little, Brown & Co, Boston, 1977, pp 89–97.
68. Millard DR Jr: Alveolar and palatal deformities. In Cleft Craft III, Little, Brown & Co, Boston, 1980 pp 249–262.
69. Millard DR Jr: Earlier correction of the unilateral cleft lip nose. Plast Reconstr Surg 70:64–73, 1982.
70. Mirault G: Deux lettres sur l'opération du bec-de-lièvre considéré dans ses divers états de simplicité et complication. J Chir 2:257, 1844.
71. Moss ALH, Pigott RW, Albery EH: Hynes pharyngoplasty revisited. Plast Reconstr Surg 79:346–353, 1987.
72. Mulliken JB: Principles and techniques of bilateral complete cleft lip repair. Plast Reconstr Surg 75:477–486, 1985.
73. Mulvihill SJ, Stone MM, Fonkalsrud EW, Debas HT: Trophic effect of amniotic fluid on fetal gastrointestinal development. J Surg Res 40:291–296, 1986.
73a. Nora JJ, Fraser FC, Bear J, Greenberg CR, Patterson D, Warburton D: Medical Genetics: Principle and Practice, 4th ed. Lea & Febiger, Philadelphia, 1994, pp 270–279.
74. Orticochea M: A review of 236 cleft palate patients treated with dynamic muscle sphincter. Plast Reconstr Surg 71:180–188, 1983.
75. Ortiz-Monasterio F, Olmedo A: Corrective rhinoplasty before puberty: a long-term follow-up. Plast Reconstr Surg 68:381–391, 1981.
76. Ortiz-Monasterio F, Rebeil AS, Valderrama M, Cruz R: Cephalometric measurements on adult patients with non–operated cleft palates. Plast Reconstr Surg 24:53–61, 1959.
77. Parsons RW, Smith DJ: Rule of thumb criteria for tongue-lip adhesion in Pierre Robin anomalad. Plast Reconstr Surg 70:210–212, 1982.
78. Pavlin JE, O'Gorman A, Williams HB, Crépeau RJ, Shapiro RS: Epignathus: a report of two cases. Ann Plast Surg 13:452–456, 1984.
79. Peet E: The Oxford technique of cleft palate repair. Plast Reconstr Surg 28:282–294, 1961.
80. Perko MA: Two stage closure of cleft palate. J Maxillofac Surg 7:46–80, 1979.
81. Pigott RW: Objectives for cleft palate repair. Ann Plast Surg 19:247–259, 1987.
82. Randall P: A triangular flap operation for the primary repair of unilateral clefts of the lip. Plast Reconstr Surg 23:331–347, 1959.
83. Randall P: The Robin sequence: micrognathia and glossoptosis with airway obstruction. In: Plastic Surgery, vol. 4, JG McCarthy, ed. WB Saunders, Philadelphia, 1990, pp 2123–3134.
84. Randall P, LaRossa D: Cleft palate. In: Plastic Surgery, Vol 4, JG McCarthy, eds. WB Saunders, Philadelphia, 1990, pp 2723–2752, 1990.
85. Randall P, LaRossa DD, Fakraee SM, Cohen MA: Cleft palate closure at 3 to 7 months of age: a preliminary report. Plast Reconstr Surg 71:624–628, 1983.
86. Riski JE, Georgiade NG, Serafin D, Barwick W, Georgiade GS, Riefkohl R: The orticochea pharyngoplasty and primary palatoplasty: an evaluation. Ann Plast Surg 18:303–309, 1987.
87. Riski JE, Serafin D, Riefkohl R, Georgiade GS, Georgiade NG: A rationale for modifying the site of insertion of the Orticochea pharyngoplasty. Plast Reconstr Surg 73:882–894, 1984.
88. Routledge RT: The Pierre Robin Syndrome: a surgical emergency in the neonatal period. Br J Plast Surg 13:204–218, 1960.
89. Ruding R: Cleft palate: anatomic and surgical considerations. Plast Reconstr Surg 33:132–147, 1964.
90. Rutrick R, Black PW, Jurkiewicz MJ: Bilateral cleft lip and palate: presurgical treatment. Ann Plast Surg 12:105–117, 1984.
91. Salyer KE: Correction of the unilateral cleft lip nose: a 15–year experience. Plast Reconstr Surg 77:558–566, 1986.
92. Sando WC, Jurkiewicz MJ: Cleft palate. In: Plastic Surgery: Principles and Practice. MJ Jurkiewicz, TJ Krizek, Mathes SJ, Ariyan S, eds. CV Mosby, St. Louis, MO, 1990, pp 81–97.
93. Schatten WE, Tidmore TL Jr: Airway management in patients with Pierre Robin syndrome. Plast Reconstr Surg 38:309–311, 1966.
94. Schweckendiek W, Doz P: Primary veloplasty: long term results without maxillary deformity. A 25 year report. Cleft Palate J 15:268–274, 1978.
95. Shprintzen RJ, Lewin ML, Croft CB, Daniller AI, Argamaso RV, Ship AG, Strauch B: A comprehensive study of pharyngeal flap surgery: tailor made flaps. Cleft Palate J 16:46–55, 1979.
96. Siebert JW, Burd AR, McCarthy JG, Weinzweig J, Ehrlich HP: Fetal wound healing: a biochemical study of scarless healing. Plast Reconstr Surg 85:495–502, 1990.
97. Skoog T: A design for the repair of unilateral cleft lips. Am J Surg 95:223–226, 1958.
98. Skoog T: The use of periosteum and Surgicel for bone restoration in congenital clefts of the maxilla. A clinical report and experimental investigation. Scand J Plast Reconstr Surg 1:113–130, 1967.
99. Stark RB: The pathogenesis of harelip and cleft palate. Plast Reconstr Surg 13:20–39, 1954.
100. Steedle JR, Proffit WR: The pattern and control of eruptive tooth movements. Am J Orthod 87:56–66, 1985.
101. Sullivan WG: Intrauterine repair of cleft lip: what's involved. Discussion. Plast Reconstr Surg 85:466–467, 1990.
102. Tennison CW: The repair of the unilateral cleft lip by the stencil method. Plast Reconstr Surg 9:115–120, 1952.
103. Van Demark DR, Gnoinski W, Hotz MM, Perko M, Nussbaumer H: Speech results of the Zürich approach in the treatment of unilateral cleft lip and palate. Plast Reconstr Surg 83:605–613, 1989.
104. Veau V: Division Palatine: Anatomie, Chirurgie, Phonétique. Masson et Cie, Paris, 1931.

105. Veau V: Operative treatment of complete double harelip. Ann Surg 76:143–156, 1922.
106. Velcek FT, Klotz DH, Hill CH, Ladogana LE, Kottmeier PK: Tongue lesions in children. J Ped Surg 14:238–246, 1979.
107. Vogel JE, Mulliken JB, Kaban LB: Macroglossia: a review of the condition and a new classification. Plast Reconstr Surg 78:715–723, 1986.
108. Wardill WEM: The techniques of operation for cleft palate. Br J Surg 25:117–130, 1937.
109. Webster JP: Crescentic perialar cheek excision for upper lip flap advancement with a short history of upper lip repair. Plast Reconstr Surg 16:434–464, 1955.
110. Whitaker LA, Randall P, Graham WP 3rd, Hamilton RW, Winchester R: A prospective and randomized series comparing superiorly and inferiorly based posterior pharyngeal flaps. Cleft Palate J 9:304–311, 1972.
111. Whitby DJ, Longaker MT, Harrison MR, Adzick NS, Ferguson MW: Rapid epithelialisation of fetal wounds is associated with the early deposition of tenascin. J Cell Sci 99:583–586, 1991.
112. Williams HB: A method of assessing cleft lip repairs: comparison of LeMesurier and Millard techniques. Plast Reconstr Surg 41:103–107, 1968.
113. Williams HB: Vascular neoplasms. Clin Plast Surg 7:397–411, 1980.
114. Wolfe SA, Price GW, Stuzin JM, Berkowitz S: Alveolar and anterior palatal clefts. In: Plastic Surgery, vol 4, JG McCarthy, ed. WB Saunders, Philadelphia, 1990, pp 2753–2770.
115. Wolford LM, Oelschlaeger M, Deal R: Proplast as a pharyngeal wall implant to correct velopharyngeal insufficiency. Cleft Palate J 26:119–126, 1989.
116. Woolf CM, Woolf RM, Broadbent TR: Genetic and nongenetic variables related to cleft lip and palate. Plast Reconstr Surg 32:65–74, 1963.

# Appendix D

## Syndromes and Conditions Associated with Congenital Anomalies of the Mouth, Palate, and Pharynx

TED L. TEWFIK, AHMAD S. TEEBI, and VAZKEN M. DER KALOUSTIAN

| Syndrome or condition | Inheritance[a] | MIM No. POSSUM No.[b] | Ear, nose, and throat manifestations | Other manifestations |
|---|---|---|---|---|
| Aase syndrome (Blackfan-Diamond syndrome)[98] | AR | **205600** 3002 | Cleft upper lip, cleft palate, webbed neck | Congenital hypoplastic anemia, triphalangeal thumbs, absent or hypoplastic thumb, symphalangism, radioulnar synostosis, radial hypoplasia, abnormal palmar dematoglyphics, cyanotic or acyanotic heart disease, short stature |
| Aase-Smith syndrome (hydrocephalus, cleft palate, digital anomalies)[152,171] | AD | ***147800** 3829 | Micrognathia, cleft hard palate, limited opening of the mouth, dysplastic ear pinna | Ptosis, short palpebral fissures, contractures of large joints, camptodactyly, mental retardation, Dandy-Walker malformation, hydrocephalus, holoprosencephaly or arhinencephaly, adrenal tumors |
| Abruzzo-Erickson syndrome | | | See Cleft palate, eye coloboma, short stature, hypospadias | |
| Acrocallosal syndrome or Schinzel syndrome[65,84] | AR | ***200990** 3555 | Cleft palate, broad nasal bridge, anteverted nostrils, posteriorly angulated ears | Macrocephaly, hypotelorism, agenesis of corpus callosum, downward slanting palpebral fissures, preaxial or postaxial polydactyly, short or bifid great toes, cardiac defects, moderate to severe mental retardation, anal atresia or stenosis, cryptorchidism |
| Acrocephalosyndactyly type III (see Saethre-Chotzen syndrome) | | | | |
| Acro-cranio-facial dysostosis, Kaplan type[106] | AR | **210050** 4407 | Cleft palate, preauricular tags or pits, low-set malformed ears, atresia of the external canal, choanal atresia, deafness, short neck | Microcephaly, sutural synostosis, large fontanelles, myopia, ptosis, short phalanges, ulnar deviation of fingers, coxa valga, short great toe, mental retardation |
| Acrofacial dysostosis, cleft lip/palate and/or triphalangeal thumbs[183] | AR | **154400** 3610 | Cleft upper lip (non-midline), cleft palate, bifid uvula, malar hypoplasia, micrognathia | Hypoplastic triphalangeal thumbs, hypertelorism, deep-set eyes |
| Acro-fronto-facio-nasal dysostosis[182] | AR | **201180** 3695 | Cleft upper lip (non midline) cleft palate, bifid nasal tip | Hypertelorism, short stature, mental retardation, camptodactyly, brachydactyly, syndactyly, postaxial polydactyly, carpal synostosis, hypoplastic or absent tibia and fibula |
| Adducted thumb syndrome (Christian syndrome)[116] | AR | ***201550** 3591 | Open mouth appearance, micrognathia, cleft palate, cleft uvula, tracheolaryngeal abnormalities, depressed nasal bridge, dysplastic/low-set ears or posteriorly angulated ears, torticollis | Generalized hirsutism, telecanthus, craniosynostosis, adducted thumbs, camptodactyly, squint, contracture of large joints, mental retardation, hypotonia, talipes equinovarus |

**Appendix D** Syndromes and conditions associated with congenital anomalies of the mouth, palate, and pharynx (*Continued*)

| Syndrome or condition | Inheritance[a] | MIM No. POSSUM No.[b] | Ear, nose, and throat manifestations | Other manifestations |
|---|---|---|---|---|
| Aicardi syndrome, papilloma of choroid plexus, cleft lip, cleft palate[188] | | 3018 | Cleft lip and/or palate | Callosal agenesis, chorioretinopathy, microphthalmia, porencephaly, corticoheterotopias, Arnold-Chiari malformation, lissencephaly, Dandy-Walker malformation |
| Alar coloboma with telecanthus (alar clefts hypertelorism syndrome)[61] | AR | **203000** 3981 | Cleft palate or high-arched palate, beaked short nose, coloboma of nostrils, abnormal columella | Short palpebral fissures, defect of enamel development |
| Allanson clefting syndrome or clefting, ectropion and conical teeth[5] | AD | **119580** 3667 | Cleft upper lip (non-midline), cleft palate, conical teeth | Ectropion of the eyelids, hypertelorism, absent or decreased eyelashes or brows, alopecia of the scalp |
| Amnion rupture sequence[27] | Mostly sporadic | 3621 | Cleft lip, cleft palate, facial clefts, choanal atresia, unilateral proboscis, nasal disruptions, Robin sequence | Microcephaly, microphthalmia, limb amputations, abdominal wall defects |
| Anencephaly and/or cleft lip-palate[110] | Mostly sporadic | 5378 | Cleft lip and/or palate | Anencephaly |
| Ankyloblepharon filiforme adnatum or cleft lip/palate, filiform fusion of eyelids[3,74,194,237] | AD | **106250** 3139 | Significantly abnormal facies, lower lip pits, cleft lip (unilateral or bilateral), cleft palate | Lid adhesions, cardiovascular anomalies |
| Ankyloglossia, camptomelic variant[210] | Uncertain | | Adhesion of the tongue to the palate, depressed or flat nasal bridge | Hypertelorism, bowed femur/humerus, radius/tibia, mesomelia of upper and/or lower limbs, short stature, multiple fractures, platyspondyly, talipes equinovarus |
| Ankyloglossia, clasped thumbs, iris heterochromia[199] | Uncertain | 4492 | Broad nasal bridge, cleft palate, speech defect | Heterochromia irides, camptodactyly, ulnar deviation of fingers, adducted thumbs |
| Ankyloglossia, cleft palate[21, 150] | XLR | | Tongue tie, cleft palate or submucous cleft, small or absent uvula | |
| Atelosteogenesis, type I (spondylo-humero-femoral hypoplasia)[91,216] | AD Uncertain | **108720** 3552 | Micrognathia, depressed nasal bridge, microstomia, cleft palate, tracheal abnormality | Short stature, short limbs, macrocephaly, delayed ossification of spine, multiple joint dislocations, vertebral clefts, bowed or abnormal long bones |
| Atelosteogenesis type III[209] | Uncertain | 4761 | Midface hypoplasia, micrognathia, depressed nasal bridge, cleft palate, microstomia, dysphagia, laryngeal abnormality, atretic auditory canal | Short stature, short limbs, multiple joint dislocations, hypertelorism, absent fibula, atlantoaxial instability, inguinal hernia, camptodactyly, syndactyly, hydrocephalus, hypotonia |
| Baller-Gerold syndrome or craniosynostosis, radial aplasia syndrome | | | See Part II, Appendix B | |
| Baraitser syndrome[14] | AR? | **218650** 3559 | Cleft lip/palate, prominent ears | Craniosynostosis, mental retardation, seizures, choroidal colobomas, mild mesomelic shortening of the extremities, cystic dysplastic kidneys |
| Bartsocas-Papas syndrome or popliteal pterygium syndrome, lethal type[137,169] | AR | ***263650** | Cleft upper lip (non-midline), cleft palate, notched hypoplastic alae nasi, small nose | Popliteal pterygium, microcephaly, absent or hypoplastic thumbs, syndactyly of fingers and toes, synechiae/fused eyelids, corneal ulceration |
| Beare-Stevenson syndrome[16,211] | ?Sporadic ?AD | **123790** 3831 | Cleft palate | Cutis gyratum, acanthosis nigricans, hypertelorism, bifid scrotum |
| Bencze syndrome[19,117] | AD | ***141350** 2364 | Submucous cleft palate | Mild facial asymmetry, esotropia, amblyopia |

| Syndrome or condition | Inheritance[a] | MIM No. POSSUM No.[b] | Ear, nose, and throat manifestations | Other manifestations |
|---|---|---|---|---|
| Blepharophimosis, cleft palate[113] | AD | 4062 | Depressed nasal bridge, long philtrum, cleft palate, posteriorly angulated ears | Microcephaly, hypertelorism, syndactyly of fingers, single palmar creases, cyanotic heart disease |
| Brachial plexus neuropathy, characteristic facies, cleft palate[2,95] | AD | ***162100** 3811 | Cleft palate, bifid uvula, hoarseness (? involvement of recurrent laryngeal nerve) | Sudden attacks of pain in shoulder, radiating to arms and hands; partial denervation of several muscles of upper extremities |
| Branchio-oculofacial syndrome[63,125] | AD | ***113620** 3618 | Branchial clefts or sinuses, broad nasal bridge, abnormal nasal septum, short philtrum, cleft palate, median cleft lip, down-turned angles of mouth, oral synechiae, conductive deafness, dysplastic posteriorly angulated ears | Short stature, frontal bossing, aged face, defects of the lacrimal system, microphthalmos; colobomas of iris, retina and choroid, myopia, polydactyly, mental retardation |
| Branchio-skeleto-genital (BSG) syndrome (el-Sahy-Waters syndrome)[55] | AR | **211380** 3946 | Midface hypoplasia, relative prognathism, mandibular cysts, triangular face, nystagmus, broad nose, winged alae, cleft palate, abnormal voice | Hypertelorism, nystagmus, pectus excavatum, ptosis, squint, fused vertebral spinous processes, bony cysts, hypospadias |
| Campomelic dysplasia (Campomelic dwarfism)[129,133] | AR | ***211970** 3049 | Flat face, small, flat nose, anteverted nostrils, long philtrum, cleft palate, short neck, tracheal cartilage hypoplasia and airway obstruction | Pectus excavatum, kyphoscoliosis, abnormal pelvis, short limbs, brachydactyly, hydrocephalus, mental retardation, sex reversal (XY female) |
| Cantrell's pentalogy (Defects of sternum, abdominal wall, diaphragm, pericardium, heart)[136] | Uncertain | 3248 | Cleft palate and lip, upper respiratory tract anomalies | Sternal fusion, defects of anterior diaphragm, omphalocele, ectopia cordis, spina bifida |
| Catel-Manzke syndrome (palatodigital syndrome)[50] | Uncertain | **302380** 3557 | 90% have cleft palate and micrognathia | Bilateral clinodactyly (radial angulation) of the index finger, talipes equinovarus in 30%, congenital heart defect |
| Cerebro-costo-mandibular syndrome[54,102] | AD AR | **117650** 3056 | Cleft palate, glossoptosis, triangular facies, micrognatia, conductive deafness, tracheal anomaly, dysphagia, speech defect | Short stature, microcephaly, lax skin, chest asymmetry, pectus carinatum, abnormal rib number, delayed ossification of pelvis |
| CHARGE association (**C**oloboma of iris, **H**eart defect, **A**tresia of choanae, **R**etardation, **G**enital anomalies, **E**ar anomalies) | Uncertain | **214800** 3480 | See Part II, Appendix A | |
| Charlie M. syndrome[70,105] | Sporadic | 3182 | Cleft palate, hypertelorism, facial paralysis, absent or conically crowned incisors | Hypodactyly of hands and feet |
| Chitayat-Azouz syndrome (Robin sequence with facial and digital anomalies)[36] | XLR | **311895** 4932 | Midface hypoplasia, micrognathia, Robin sequence, broad nasal bridge, cleft hard palate, glossoptosis | High hairline, frontal bossing, puffy eyelids, pectus excavatum, delayed skeletal maturation, hypoplastic phalanges, clinodactyly of 5th fingers, overlapping toes with syndactyly |
| Chondrodysplasia punctata, rhizomelic type[66,87,178] | AR | ***215100** 3064 | Cleft palate and submucous palatal cleft | Frontal bossing, cataracts, ichthyosis, severe congenital rhizomelic shortening of the extremities, contractures |
| Chromosome 2, interstitial deletion 2(q31q33)[180] | | 3685 | Midface hypoplasia, nystagmus, beaked nose, cleft palate, posteriorly angulated ears | Small for gestational age, short stature, microcephaly, blepharophimosis, ptosis, microphthalmos, cataract, squint, camptodactyly, syndactyly, mental retardation, hypotonia, abnormal gait |
| Chromosome 3, dup 3p[31] | | | 30% have cleft lip with or without cleft palate, prominent philtrum, large mouth, micrognathia | Short neck, brachycephaly, frontal bossing; possibly 10% associated with holoprosencephaly |

**Appendix D** Syndromes and conditions associated with congenital anomalies of the mouth, palate, and pharynx (*Continued*)

| Syndrome or condition | Inheritance[a] | MIM No. POSSUM No.[b] | Ear, nose, and throat manifestations | Other manifestations |
|---|---|---|---|---|
| Chromosome 3, partial dup 3q[93,229] | | 3688 | Micrognathia, small nose, cleft palate, preauricular tags, abnormal orientation of ears, short neck | Resembles de Lange syndrome with frequent brain, limb, cardiac anomalies; short stature, increased body hair, microphthalmos, iris coloboma, abnormal rib number, hypospadias, mental retardation |
| Chromosome 4, partial del 4p (Wolf-Hirschhorn syndrome)[151] | | 3069 | Cleft lip and palate (10%), cleft palate (40%), micrognathia (50%); wide nasal bridge with prominent glabella; ears have lobeless pinnae and may have preauricular dimple or skin tag | Very severe psychomotor and growth retardation, high forehead; 35% have coloboma of the iris |
| Chromosome 4, partial del 4q[124] | | 3072 | Cleft palate with or without cleft lip is common; low-set, posteriorly angulated ears with malformed helices, short nose, anteverted nostrils, micrognathia | Microcephaly, cardiac lesions (atrial and ventricular septal defect), limited extension of elbows, clinodactyly, tapering fingers |
| Chromosome 5, del 5p (cri-du-chat syndrome)[155] | | | Downward slanting palpebral fissures, hypertelorism, epicanthal folds, posteriorly angulated ears, preauricular tags, broad nasal bridge with prominent nasal root and micrognathia | Mental retardation, microcephaly, talipes, dislocated hips, inguinal hernia |
| Chromosome 6, partial del 6q | | 4051 | See Part II, Appendix A | |
| Chromosome 7, terminal del 7q[24] | | 4663 | Micrognathia, optic nerve anomalies, nystagmus, anteverted nostrils, tented upper lip, cleft palate/lip, abnormal ear helix, conductive deafness | Holoprosencephaly, mental retardation, prominent forehead, hypotelorism, squint, herniae, hypospadias, small penis, missing fingers, syndactyly, ureteric anomalies |
| Chromosome 7, partial dup 7q[160] | | | Cleft palate, short nose, long philtrum, thin vermilion, tented upper lip, micrognathia | Large fontanels, square prominent forehead, short, downward slanting palpebral fissures |
| Chromosome 8, trisomy 8 mosaicism (Warkany syndrome)[121] | | 3077 | Micrognathia, cleft palate, macrostomia, thick lips, conductive deafness, tracheoesophageal fistula, short neck | Deep palmar and plantar creases, frontal bossing, deep-set eyes, microphthalmos, iris coloboma, hypospadias, developmental retardation |
| Chromosome 8, partial dup 8q | | 3120 | See Part II, Appendix A | |
| Chromosome 8, partial dup 8p[59,235] | | 3078 | Cleft palate and/or bifid uvula, low nasal bridge, anteverted nostrils, wide mouth, large ear lobes | High forehead, frontal and parietal bossing, round face, severe mental retardation, various congential heart malformations |
| Chromosome 9, partial dup 9p[96] | | 3079 | Prominent nose, short neck, down-turned mouth angles, cleft lip/palate | Brachycephaly, severe mental retardation, hypertelorism, deep-set eyes, microcephaly, hydrocephalus, frontal bossing, iris coloboma, myopia, squint, thoracolumbar kyphosis, delayed skeletal maturation, carpal fusion, hydrocephalus |
| Chromosome 9, trisomy[122] | | 3080 | Midface hypoplasia, micrognathia, microphthalmos, high nasal bridge, flared nostrils, cleft hard palate, low-set ears, ear cartilage hypoplasia, preauricular tags, short neck | Early lethality, mental retardation, microcephaly, deep-set eyes, narrow palpebral fissures, coloboma of iris, kyphoscoliosis, delayed ossification of pelvic bones, arachnodactyly, adducted thumbs, polycystic kidneys, cardiac anomalies, hypotonia |
| Chromosome 10, partial dup 10p[68] | | 3084 | Cleft lip/palate noted in over 40%, ears often low-set | Severe mental and motor retardation, dolichocephaly, prominent forehead, wide-open sutures and |

| Syndrome or condition | Inheritance[a] | MIM No. POSSUM No.[b] | Ear, nose, and throat manifestations | Other manifestations |
|---|---|---|---|---|
| | | | | anterior fontanel; elbows, wrists, and fingers often hyperextensible, kidneys tend to be cystic |
| Chromosome 10, distal dup 10q[48] | | 3083 | Flat face, tented upper lip, small nose, prominent philtrum, cleft palate, low-set ears | Severe mental retardation, microcephaly, high-arched eyebrows, pectus excavatum, cryptorchidism, abnormalities of the cardiovascular system |
| Chromosome 11, partial dup 11q[47] | | | Cleft palate, large and beaked nose, preauricular tags or pits | Low birth weight, mental retardation, hypertonia, microcephaly, genitourinary anomalies, imperforate anus, cryptorchidism |
| Chromosome 13, del 13q (q12q14→q14q31)[22] | | 3125 | Broad nasal bridge, cleft palate, low-set ears, conductive deafness | Mental and growth retardation associated with retinoblastoma, epicanthal folds, microphthalmos, iris coloboma, small hands, brachydactyly, single palmar creases, hypotonia |
| Chromosome 13, del 13q (q22 or 31→qter)[224] | | 3091 | Cleft or high-arched palate, high nasal bridge, micrognathia | Severe mental retardation, brain and heart defects, colobomatous microphthalmia, sloping forehead, abnormal teeth, ambiguous genitalia |
| Chromosome 13, partial dup 13q[158,205] | | 3690 | Large nose, micrognathia, thin lips, long philtrum, cleft palate, low-set ears, prominent antihelix, short neck | Short stature, microcephaly, mental retardation, epicanthal folds, persistence of fetal hemoglobin, cryptorchidism |
| Chromosome 13, trisomy 13 syndrome[17,38] | | | Cleft palate, lateral or median cleft lip, micrognathia | Moderate microcepahly, microphthalmia, ulnar hexadactyly, skin defect at vertex of skull, severe developmental retardation, variable degrees of holoprosencephaly, congenital heart disease, cryptorchidism |
| Chromosome 14, trisomy 14 mosaic[127,228] | | 4389 | Wide nasal bridge, micrognathia, short neck, cleft hard and/or soft palate in 40% | Growth and mental retardation, pectus excavatum, hypertelorism, single palmar creases, dislocated hips, seizures, malplaced anus, tetralogy of Fallot, body asymmetry |
| Chromosome 14, partial dup 14q[159] | | | Cleft palate in 50%, broad nose, carp mouth, micrognathia, posteriorly angulated ears with prominent antitragus | Mental retardation, growth retardation (pre- and postnatal), large face, chubby cheeks, high and widely placed nipples, hypogenitalism; brain, lung, and heart defects |
| Chromosome 15, partial dup 15q (trisomy for the proximal long arm of chromosome 15)[132] | | | Cleft palate, micrognathia, bulbous nose, long philtrum, malformed pinnae | Microdolichocephaly, occasionally hydrocephaly, downward slanting palpebral fissures |
| Chromosome 17, del 17 (p11.2p11.2) (Smith-Magenis syndrome)[39,149] | | 4368 | Flat face, prominent jaw, broad nasal bridge, cleft hard palate, low-set ears, hoarse voice, speech defects, conductive deafness, dysphagia, delayed dentition | Growth and mental retardation, flat occiput, epicanthal folds, terminal clubbing of fingers, short hands, cerebral cortex atrophy, seizures, onychotillomania |
| Chromosome 17, partial dup 17q[162] | | 4727 | Depressed nasal bridge, macrostomia, short neck | Microcephaly, mental and growth retardation, frontal bossing, syndactyly of fingers, ureteric anomalies, polydactyly |
| Chromosome 18, tetrasomy 18p | | | See Part II, Appendix A | |
| Chromosome 18, partial del 18p[154,173] | | 3095 | Broad face, broad nasal bridge, nystagmus, cleft palate, low-set ears, ear cartilage hypoplasia, short neck | Growth and mental retardation, irregular teeth, skeletal and genital defects, decreased skin pigmentation, hypertelorism, ptosis, mi- |

**Appendix D** Syndromes and conditions associated with congenital anomalies of the mouth, palate, and pharynx (*Continued*)

| Syndrome or condition | Inheritance[a] | MIM No. POSSUM No.[b] | Ear, nose, and throat manifestations | Other manifestations |
|---|---|---|---|---|
| | | | | crophthalmos, cataract, iris coloboma, visual loss, squint, kyphoscoliosis, umbilical hernia, hypospadias, large hands, coxa vara, dislocated hips, endocrine defects |
| Chromosome 18, partial del 18q[202] | | 3096 | Carp-like mouth, cleft lip, cleft palate, prominent antihelix or antitragus, stenotic ear canals, impaired hearing, broad nasal bridge | Hypotonia, mental retardation, abnormal genitalia, tapered fingers, microcephaly, strabismus, nystagmus, coloboma of iris |
| Chromosome 19, partial dup 19q[203] | | | Cleft palate, short nose, short philtrum | Mental retardation, low birth weight and length, hypotonia, duplicated thumb |
| Chromosome 21, trisomy 21[73] | | 3598 | Small mouth, protruding tongue, small ears, depressed bridge of the nose, epicanthic folds, cleft palate (rare) | Mental deficiency, congenital heart disease, excessive nuchal skin folds, single palmar crease, narrow and upward slanting palpebral fissures, short stature |
| Chromosome tetraploidy (92, XXXX/XXYY)[120,240] | | 3115 | Flat face, beaked nose, broad and high nasal bridge, cleft palate, low-set ears | Stillbirth, short stature, microcephaly, large fontanelle, abnormal sella turcica, pectus excavatum, ambiguous genitalia, missing toes, cerebral cortex atrophy, seizures, hypotonia |
| Chromosome triploidy (69 XXX/XXY)[139] | | 3114 | Structural asymmetry of face, micrognathia, choanal stenosis, cleft palate, low-set ears, short neck, abnormal esophagus | Stillbirth, asymmetry of body, microcephaly, poorly ossified calvarium, microphthalmos, corneal clouding, retinal coloboma, ambiguous genitalia, syndactyly, missing toes, thymic aplasia, Arnold-Chiari malformation, moderate to severe mental retardation, adrenal malformation |
| Cleft lip with or without cleft palate (nonsyndromic)[147] | | | | Presence of a CL ± P susceptibility locus on the long arm of chromosome 4 |
| Cleft lip/palate, ectrodactyly[189] | Uncertain | 3834 | Cleft upper lip (non-midline), cleft palate, dysplastic ears | Oligodactyly, split hands and/or feet, brachydactyly, syndactyly of fingers and toes |
| Cleft lip/palate-pituitary deficiency[18] | Uncertain | 3833 | Cleft upper lip (non-midline or midline), cleft palate | Hypopituitarism, isolated growth hormone deficiency, short stature, mental retardation |
| Cleft palate, lateral oral synechiae[51] | AD | **109550** 3142 | Cleft upper lip, cleft uvula, cleft palate, beaked nose, oral synechiae, prominent everted lower lip | Blepharophimosis or blepharospasm, blocked or absent nasolacrimal ducts, trismus, mental retardation |
| Cleft palate, omphalocele[44] | AR | **258320** 3835 | Bifid uvula, cleft palate | Omphalocele, internal hydrocephalus, uterine abnormalities |
| Cleft lip and palate, contractures, agenesis of fibula and ulna[174] | ?AR | | Cleft lip and palate | Two siblings with consanguineous parents; oligodactyly or polydactyly and aplasia of nails |
| Cleft lip/palate and extrathoracic ectopia of the heart[146] | Sporadic | | Cleft lip and/or palate | Extrathoracic heart |
| Cleft lip and palate, abnormal ears, congenital heart defect skeletal abnormalites[233] | ?AR | | Bilateral cleft lip/palate, micrognathia, malformed pinnae, absent external meatus | Cryptorchidism, persistent truncus arteriosus, bilobed lungs, parathyroid aplasia, lethal |
| Cleft lip/palate, posterior keratoconus, short stature, mental retardation and genitourinary anomalies[6] | ?AR | 3109 | Cleft lip/palate, prominent nose | Two siblings with keratoconus, retinal colobomas, short stature, mental retardation, vertebral segmentation and fusion anomalies |

| Syndrome or condition | Inheritance[a] | MIM No. POSSUM No.[b] | Ear, nose, and throat manifestations | Other manifestations |
|---|---|---|---|---|
| Cleft lip/palate, urogenital anomalies, somatic and mental retardation[131] | ?AR | | Cleft lip/palate | Six sibs in an inbred Gypsy family; somatic and mental retardation; unilateral aplasia or bilateral hypoplasia of kidney; ectopia or malrotation of kidney, vesicoureteral reflux, bladder diverticulosis, penoscrotal hypospadias |
| Cleft palate, dwarfism, trichodysplasia, and unusual facies[103] | | | Cleft palate, micrognathia, prominent pinnae | Coarse and brittle hair, narrow palpebral fissures, growth retardation |
| Cleft palate, ectodermal dysplasia, growth failure, and apparent pancreatic insufficiency[52] | ?AR | | V-shaped cleft palate, micrognathia | Growth failure, eczema, pancreatic insufficiency, diarrhea |
| Cleft palate, eye coloboma, short stature, and hypospadias (Abruzzo-Erickson syndrome)[1] | ?XLR<br>?AR | **214800**<br>2365 | Cleft palate, deafness choanal atresia | Short stature, hypospadias, radial synostosis, eye colobomas |
| Cleft palate, hypotonia, and mental retardation[46] | ?AR | | Cleft palate | Brother and sister with mental retardation, hypotonia, failure to thrive, frontal bossing, epicanthal folds |
| Cleft palate, macular coloboma, short stature, and skeletal anomalies (Phillips-Griffiths syndrome or Sorsby syndrome)[175,220] | ?AR | **120400**<br>3282 | Cleft palate, sensorineural deafness, nystagmus | Brother and sister with bilateral macular colobomas, hallus valgus, flexion deformities of interphalangeal joints of fifth fingers, growth retardation, hypoplastic kidneys |
| Cleft palate, microcephaly, mental retardation, and musculoskeletal mass deficiency (Weaver-Williams syndrome)[236] | ?AR | 4046 | Cleft palate, midface hypoplasia, small down-turned mouth | Mental retardation, microcephaly in a sister and brother |
| Cleft palate, micrognathia, talipes equinovarus, atrial septal defect, and persistence of left superior vena cava[71] | ?XLR | | Cleft palate, micrognathia | Talipes equinovarus, atrial septal defect, left superior vena cava, cardiac conduction anomaly |
| Cleft palate, stapes fixation, and oligodontia[77] | ?AR | **216300**<br>3145 | Cleft palate, conductive deafness, oligodontia, absent alveolar ridges | Coalition of all cuneiform bones in two sisters |
| Cleft palate, unusual facies, conductive hearing loss, and male pseudohermaphroditism[92] | ?AR | | Cleft palate, conductive deafness | Male and female sibs with intrauterine growth retardation, failure to thrive, severe mental retardation, hypotonia, pulmonary hypertension with pulmonary disease, anemia (PDA), hypospadias, cryptorchidism |
| Cleft palate, ventricular septal defect, persistent truncus arteriosus, and intrauterine death[128] | ?AR | | Cleft palate | Sibs with persistent truncus arteriosus and abnormal right pulmonary artery |
| Cleft uvula, deafness, nephrosis, congenital urinary tract, and digital anomalies[15] | ?XLR<br>?AR | | Cleft uvula, conductive deafness | Nephrosis, shortening and broadening of distal portion of thumbs and great toes |
| Clefting-premaxillary agenesis[135] | AD | | Cleft lip/palate | Hypotelorism, premaxillary agenesis, antimongoloid slant of palpebral fissures, microcephaly, mental retardation |
| Cleidocranial dysplasia[153] | AD | ***119600**<br>3146 | Submucous cleft palate and complete cleft of hard and soft palates, supernumerary teeth with anomalies, underdeveloped or absent paranasal sinuses and mastoids | Large skull, wormian bones, hypoplastic or absent clavicles, mapped at 6p21 |
| Congenital myopathy, malignant hyperthermia, and cleft palate (King syndrome)[212,213] | ?AR | **145600**<br>4183 | Cleft palate | Congenital myopathy, malignant hyperthermia, skeletal anomalies, kyphoscoliosis |

**Appendix D** Syndromes and conditions associated with congenital anomalies of the mouth, palate, and pharynx (*Continued*)

| Syndrome or condition | Inheritance[a] | MIM No. POSSUM No.[b] | Ear, nose, and throat manifestations | Other manifestations |
|---|---|---|---|---|
| Crane-Heise syndrome[40] | ?AR | **218090** | Cleft lip/palate, micrognathia | Agenesis of clavicles and cervical vertebrae, talipes equinovarus |
| Craniofrontonasal dysplasia | | | See Part II, Appendix B | |
| Craniosynostosis, fibular aplasia (Lowry syndrome)[37] | AR AD | **218550** 3171 | Cleft hard palate, low-set ears, short neck | Stillbirth, large fontanelle, craniosynostosis, prominent eyes, cryptorchidism, small penis, absent fibulae, single palmar creases, contracture of large joints |
| Crouzon craniofacial dysostosis[100,112,170] | AD | ***123500** 3158 | Midface hypoplasia, prognathism, beaked nose, short philtrum, cleft palate, high palate, macroglossia, choanal atresia or stenosis, atresia of the external auditory meatus, conductive deafness | Acrocephaly, sutural synostosis, frontal bossing, hypertelorism, flat supraorbital ridges, prominent eyes, iris coloboma, malocclusion, borderline mental retardation, seizures, mapped on chromosomes 10q and 4p and due to FGFR II and III mutations |
| Cryptophthalmos, multiple congenital anomalies syndrome (Fraser syndrome) | | | See Part II, Appendix B | |
| Deafness, myopia, cataract, saddle nose | | | See Part II, Appendix B | |
| Diastrophic dysplasia[185] | AR | ***222600** 3185 | Cleft palate (25%–50%), characteristic external ear deformities (cauliflower ears) | Micromelic dwarfism, progressive scoliosis, deformites of extremities, hitchhiker thumbs |
| Distal arthrogryposis, type II (arthrogryposis, Gordon type)[181,186,219] | AD | **108130** 3166 | Cleft palate | Camptodactyly, talipes, scoliosis, short stature |
| Dyssegmental dysplasia, Silverman-Handmaker type[4] | AR | **224400** 4281 | Flat face, micrognathia, cleft palate, short neck, microstomia | Encephalocele (common), short limbs, short and bowed trunk, microcephaly, prominent eyes, short ribs, multiple vertebral malsegmentation, hemivertebrae, dextrocardia, cardiac anomalies, cerebellar hypoplasia, stillbrith or early death |
| Dyssegmental dysplasia, Rolland-Desbuquios type I[4] | AR | **224400** 4282 | Cleft palate, micrognathia, short neck | Short and bowed limbs, short stature; thick, wide, and short ribs; platyspondyly, vertebral segmentation defects |
| Ectodermal dysplasia, autosomal recessive (Bustos type or Margarita type)[29] | AR | **225060** 4936 | Abnormal facies, midfacial hypoplasia, cleft lip/palate; long, pointed ears | Decreased body hair, hyperkeratosis, hypoplastic nails, microdontia, syndactyly of fingers |
| Ectodermal dysplasia, Rapp-Hodgkin type[196] | AD | ***129400** 3137 | Small, narrow nose; cleft lip/palate, hypoplastic alae nasi | Short stature, dry skin, coarse and sparse hair, hypoplastic nails, defects of the lacrimal system, microdontia, hypospadias |
| (Ectrodactyly-ectodermal dysplasia-clefting (EEC) syndrome)[89,192] | AD | **129900** 3211 | Cleft lip palate (75%), nasolacrimal duct obstruction, conductive hearing loss (30%) | Lobster-claw anomaly of the hands and feet, nail dysplasia; scalp hair, lashes, and eyebrows are nearly always sparse; pigmented nevi in 12%, mental retardation in 10%, genitourinary system anomalies in 20% |
| Ectrodactyly-cleft palate (ECP) syndrome[164] | AD | **129830** 4213 | Cleft palate | Ectrodactyly involving hands and feet |
| Facio-auriculo-vertebral or oculo-auriculo-vertebral (OAV) spectrum (Goldenhar syndrome or Hemifacial microsomia) | | | See Part II, Appendix B | |

| Syndrome or condition | Inheritance[a] | MIM No. POSSUM No.[b] | Ear, nose, and throat manifestations | Other manifestations |
|---|---|---|---|---|
| Femoral hypoplasia-unusual facies syndrome[8] | ? | **134780** 3232 | Cleft palate (80%), micrognathia (80%), mildly dysmorphic pinnae (45%), short nose with hypoplastic alae (65%) | Hypoplastic femur, upper extremities and shoulder girdle affected (75%), cardiac anomalies (20%), genitourinary anomalies (60%) |
| Fetal alcohol syndrome[72,165] | | 3218 | Prominent lateral palatine ridges, cleft lip or cleft palate, small teeth with faulty enamel, hearing disorder, flat midface | Ptosis, strabismus, epicanthic folds, congenital heart disease, hypospadias, hydronephrosis, cutaneous hemangioma |
| Fetal aminopterin syndrome[101] | | 3219 | Midface hypoplasia, micrognathia, broad nasal bridge, low-set ears, cleft palate | Stillbirth, short stature, microcephaly, sutural synostosis, hypertelorism, prominent eyes, short limbs, rudimentary nails, coxa vara, dislocated hip, dextrocardia, mental retardation, hypotonia |
| Fetal hydantoin syndrome[83] | | 3221 | Clefts of the lip and/or palate, hypoplastic midface, short nose, broad and low nasal bridge, mild micrognathia | Microcephaly, mental retardation, ptosis, strabismus, distal phalangeal hypoplasia |
| Fetal trimethadione syndrome[107] | | 3980 | Broad nasal bridge, cleft lip/palate, posteriorly angulated ears, conductive deafness, webbed neck, speech defect | Growth and mental retardation, cardiac defects, V-shaped eyebrows, cryptorchidism, tapered fingers |
| Fibrochondrogenesis[239] | AR | ***228520** 3640 | Cleft palate present in several patients | Lethal short-limb dwarfism, abnormal vertebrae |
| Filiform adhesions of the eyelids and cleft/lip palate | | | See Ankyloblepharon filiform adnatum | |
| Focal dermal hypoplasia (Goltz-Gorlin syndrome)[28] | 95% Sporadic | **305600** 3204 | Cleft lip and/or palate have been described | Thin skin with linear or reticular hyperpigmentation and telangiectasia, focal absence of skin at birth, anomalies of eyes in 40% (microphthalmia, strabismus, ectopia lentis), mental retardation, syndactyly, polydactyly, oligodactyly |
| Fontaine syndrome[60] | AD | **183700** 3880 | Submucous cleft palate, cleft uvula, microretrognathia, dysmorphic pinnae | Ectrodactyly of the hands and feet |
| Fronto-facio-nasal dysplasia[238] | AR | ***229400** 3511 | Midline facial defect, bifid nose, cleft lip/palate, abnormal sinuses | Hypertelorism, encephalocele, flat occiput, ptosis, coloboma of eyelids, decreased lashes, cataract, microcornea, epibulbar dermoid, microphthalmos |
| Frontonasal dysplasia (Median cleft face syndrome)[49] | AD | **136760** 3288 | Median cleft of the upper lip present in severe cases, rarely with cleft palate; flattened nose, widely spaced nostrils, broad nasal root, clefting of nose or notching of nasal alae, preauricular tags, conductive hearing loss | Hypertelorism, occasional mental deficiency, preaxial polydactyly with or without tibial hypoplasia |
| Fryns syndrome[41,109] | AR | ***229850** 3608 | Coarse facies, cleft lip/palate, micrognathia, large nose with anteverted nostrils, thin lips, low-set ears, short neck, tracheal anomalies, poorly-shaped auricles with attached earlobes | Distal digital hypoplasia or rudimentary nails, urogenital and intestinal defects, microphthalmos, corneal clouding, chest asymmetry, short ribs, cyanotic heart disease, absent or hypoplastic diaphragm, diaphragmatic hernia, hypoplastic lungs, hypoplastic corpus callosum |
| Genito-palato-cardiac syndrome (Gardner-Silengo-Wachtel[79] syndrome) | AR | **231060** 4209 | Micrognathia, cleft palate, low-set ears, webbed neck | Male pseudohermaphroditism, renal and cardiac anomalies, flexion deformity of thumbs, malrotation of gut |
| Glossopalatine ankylosis syndrome[34] | Sporadic | | Cleft palate | Limb anomalies |

**Appendix D** Syndromes and conditions associated with congenital anomalies of the mouth, palate, and pharynx (*Continued*)

| Syndrome or condition | Inheritance[a] | MIM No. POSSUM No.[b] | Ear, nose, and throat manifestations | Other manifestations |
|---|---|---|---|---|
| Gordon syndrome[186] | AD | ***114300** 3166 | Cleft palate | Camptodactyly, talipes, scoliosis |
| Hay-Wells syndrome[80] | AD | 3524 | Celft palate, rarely cleft lip | Congenital ankyloblepharon, absent or dystrophic nails, coarse and wiry sparse hair, hypohidrosis |
| Hirschsprung disease, unusual facies, microcephaly[12,114] | AR | **235730** 4119 | Submucous cleft | Microcephaly, short stature, thick eyebrows, coloboma of iris, oligodontia, hydrocephalus, mental retardation |
| Hypertelorism-microtia-clefting syndrome (Bixler syndrome)[13] | AR | **239800** 3259 | Cleft lip/palate, microtia | Two sisters with hypertelorism, short stature, mild psychomotor retardation, ectopic kidneys, congenital heart defects |
| Hypoglossia-hypodactylia syndrome[225] | Sporadic | **103300** 3537 | Celft palate, hypoglossia, absent mandibular incisors | Variable limb anomalies |
| Hypogonadotropic hypogonadism with cleft lip and/or palate[226] | | | Celft lip and/or palate | Low urinary gonadotropin levels |
| Hypoplastic right heart and microcephaly[9] | Uncertain | 3955 | Micrognathia, cleft hard and/or soft palate, low-set ears | Holoprosencephaly |
| Hypothalamic-hamartoblastoma syndrome (ano-cerebro-digital syndrome or Pallister-Hall syndrome) (see p 509) | | | | |
| Hypothyroidism, cleft palate, spiky hair[11] | AD | **241850** 4622 | Cleft palate, choanal atresia, bifid epiglottis | Congenital athyroidal hypothyroidism, spiky hair in two male sibs |
| Ichthyosis, mental retardation, macrosomia, colobomata syndrome (CHIME syndrome or Zunich-Kaye syndrome)[241] | AR | **280000** 3605 | Conductive deafness, depressed nasal bridge, macrostomia, cleft hard and/or soft palate | Seizures, retinal colobomas, fine sparse hair, hyperkeratosis of palms and soles, tall stature, hypertelorism, dental malocclusion, brachydactyly, cyanotic heart disease, autism, MR |
| Kabuki make-up syndrome[157] | ?AR ?AD | **147920** 3541 | Cleft lip and/or palate or submucous cleft palate in 40%, retrognathia | Strikingly unusual facies reminiscent of make-up used in Kabuki theatre, short stature (80%), short fifth fingers (90%), scoliosis (50%), dislocation of hips (35%), rib anomalies (20%), spina bifida occulta (15%), mental retardation |
| Kallmann syndrome[20,85] | XLR | ***308700** 4216 | Anosmia, cleft lip/palate, sensorineural deafness | Hypogonadotrophic hypogonadism, cryptorchidism, small penis, diffuse osteoporosis, diabetes mellitus |
| Kaufman-McKusick syndrome (hydrometrocolpos, polydactyly, congenital heart defect)[35,234] | AR | ***236700** 3510 | Choanal stenosis, cleft hard and/or soft palate, laryngeal anomaly | Partial vaginal atresia or imperforate hymen, hydronephrosis, hydrometrocolpos, malrotation of the gut, Hirschsprung disease, urogenital anomalies, anal stenosis or atresia, postaxial polydactyly |
| Klippel-Feil syndrome (see p 481) | | | | |
| Kniest dysplasia (metatropic dysplasia, type II)[177,208] | AD | **156550** 3272 | Cleft palate, flat midface, depressed nasal bridge | Club foot, short trunk, kyphoscoliosis, prominent knees, severe myopia (40%), restricted joint movement |
| Larsen syndrome[214] | AD AR | ***150250** 3275 | Flat face, midface hypoplasia, small nose, long philtrum, cleft palate, mixed hearing loss | Multiple joint hypermobility or dislocations, vertebral anomalies, kyphosis of the cervical spine, cardiovascular anomalies, genital malformations, talipes varus or valgus, bifid calcaneus and advanced bone age in the carpals |

| Syndrome or condition | Inheritance[a] | MIM No. POSSUM No.[b] | Ear, nose, and throat manifestations | Other manifestations |
|---|---|---|---|---|
| Laryngeal cleft, laryngeal web, cleft palate[227] | ? | **181450** 4156 | Cleft lip/palate, cleft larynx | Congenital heart anomalies, urogenital anomalies |
| Lateral palatal synechiae and cleft palate[64] | AD | | Bands of mucosa (unilateral or bilateral) extend from the edges of palatal cleft to lateral margins of tongue or oral floor | |
| Lateral proboscis, cleft lip/palate[76] | | 4890 | Cleft nose, bifid tip, unilateral absence of nose, cleft lip/palate, oblique facial cleft | Coloboma of lids and/or iris, defects of the lacrimal system, anencephaly |
| Lenz microphthalmia syndrome (microphthalmia, digital anomalies, or anophthalmia and associated anomalies)[223] | XLR | ***309800** 3302 | Depressed premaxillary region, flattened nose, cleft lip/palate, crowded or wide-spaced teeth, simple ears, webbed neck, speech defect | Mild to severe microphthalmia with colobomas, blepharoptosis, epicanthic folds, ptosis, mental retardation, skeletal and urogenital anomalies; may present as Potter sequence with renal agenesis, umbilical hernia, syndactyly, genu valgum, intestinal atresia |
| Lymphedema of pubertal onset and cleft palate[58] | ?AD | | Cleft palate | Lymphedema of pubertal onset largely in legs |
| Macrosomia, microphthalmia, cleft palate syndrome (Teebi macrosomia syndrome)[215] | AR | **248110** 4692 | Median cleft palate | Severe microphthalmia, large birth weight, recurrent infections, early death |
| Marden-Walker syndrome (blepharophimosis, joint contractures, hypotonia)[78,94] | AR | ***248700** 3284 | Microstomia, cleft or high-arched palate, low-set ears, flat nasal bridge | Blepharophimosis, hypertelorism, small for gestational age, microcephaly, hypospadias, camptodactyly, cardiac conduction defects, hypoplastic kidneys, pyloric stenosis, abnormal electromyography |
| Marfan syndrome[145,179] | AD | **#154700** 3285 | High-arched or cleft palate | Tall stature, long limbs, scoliosis, pectus carinatum/excavatum, hypermobile joints, large hands, arachnodactyly, flat foot, aortic dilatation and aneurysms, aortic or mitral regurgitation, diaphragmatic hernia, lens dislocation, skin striae, death usually due to cardiovascular cause |
| Maternal PKU syndrome (phenylketonuria embryopathy)[138,191] | | ***261600** 3533 | Round face, depressed nasal bridge, cleft hard and/or soft palate | Microcephaly, mental retardation, congenital heart disease, seizures |
| Meckel syndrome[198] | AR | ***249000** | Cleft lip/palate | Microcephaly, encephalocele, microphthalmia, congenital heart defects, postaxial polydactyly, polycystic kidneys |
| Mental retardation, cleft lip/palate, ectodermal dysplasia, syndactyly syndrome (Zlotogora-Oğur syndrome)[161,190] | AR | ***225000** 3141 | Microstomia, cleft hard and/or soft palate, small nose, abnormal size of ear lobe, micrognathia | Sparse scalp and body hair, dry skin, blepharophimosis, corneal clouding, tooth discoloration, abnormal female genitalia, cryptorchidism, syndactyly, mental retardation |
| Microcephalic primordial dwarfism type III (Osteodysplastic primordial dwarfism type III)[143,144] | AR | **210730** 4146 | Micrognathia, prominent nose, thick lips, cleft palate, low-set ears, short neck | Seckel-like intrauterine dwarf, severe microcephaly, platyspondyly, long clavicles, pelvic anomalies, dislocated elbows and hips, retinal aplasia, brachydactyly, single palmar creases, moderate to severe mental retardation |
| Microcephaly, cleft palate, chorioretinopathy (Halal syndrome)[81] | AD | **156590** 3600 | Cleft palate, prognathism, midface hypoplasia, horizontal nystagmus | Two sisters and their mother reported—microcephaly, mild hypotelorism, maxillary hypoplasia, abnormal retinal pigmentation |
| Multiple pterygium syndrome (see p 496) | | | | |

**Appendix D** Syndromes and conditions associated with congenital anomalies of the mouth, palate, and pharynx (*Continued*)

| Syndrome or condition | Inheritance[a] | MIM No. POSSUM No.[b] | Ear, nose, and throat manifestations | Other manifestations |
|---|---|---|---|---|
| Nager syndrome[67,82] | Mostly sporadic | **154400** 3143 | Cleft palate, maxillary hypoplasia, micrognathia, laryngeal and epiglottal hypoplasia | Colobomas of lower eyelids in 20%, hypoplastic thumb, radial hypoplasia in 50%, genitourinary abnormalities |
| Nance Sweeney syndrome (chondrodystrophy with sensorineural deafness) | | | See Part II, Appendix A | |
| Nevoid basal cell carcinoma syndrome (Gorlin syndrome)[73a] | AD | **109400** 3527 | Cleft lip and/or palate in about 5%, exaggerated length of mandible | Nevoid basal cell carcinomas, odontogenic keratocysts, skeletal anomalies, intracranial calcifications, corneal opacity, cataract, retinitis pigmentosa |
| Neu-Laxova syndrome[195] | AR | ***256520** 3326 | Small and flattened nose, macrostomia, cleft hard and/or soft palate, cleft lip, short neck | Joint contractures, severe intrauterine growth retardation, collodion skin, retracted eyelids, microphthalmos, cryptorchidism, small penis, syndactyly, hypoplastic kidneys, liver anomalies, hypoplasia of corpus callosum, hypoplastic cerebellum and lissencephaly, microcephaly |
| Oculo-palato-cerebral dwarfism[62] | AR | **257910** 3993 | Cleft palate, long and large ears | Microcephaly, mental retardation, spasticity, short stature, smooth and doughy skin, microphthalmos, corneal opacity, scoliosis, small hands and feet |
| Odontotrichomelic hypohidrotic dysplasia (tetramelic deficiency, ectodermal dysplasia, prominent ears)[172] | AR | **273400** 3355 | Large nose, paramedian cleft lip, cleft hard and/or soft palate, dental malocclusion, prominent and simple ears | Dry skin, small nails, small penis, abnormal teeth, short limbs, hypoplastic radius/ulna, missing fingers and toes, seizures and EEG abnormalities |
| Orocraniodigital syndrome (Juberg-Hayward syndrome)[75,232] | AR | **216100** 3138 | Midline cleft lip, cleft hard palate, submucous cleft, broad nasal bridge, hypoplasia of the alae nasi and columella | Microcephaly, hypertelorism, hypoplastic and distally displaced thumbs, hypoplasia of radius, short limbs, restricted joint mobility, camptodactyly, irregular shape of toes, ectopic kidneys, borderline mental retardation |
| Orofaciodigital syndrome type I (OFD I)[126,197,221] | XLD | ***311200** 3347 | Upper lip pits, midline cleft lip, cleft alveolus and/or palate, oligodontia, oral frenulae, tongue lobulation, hypoplasia of the alar cartilage and narrow nostrils, broad nasal bridge | Dry skin, coarse hair, hypertelorism, bifid great toe, upward slanting palpebral fissures, polydactyly of hallux, brachydactyly and skin syndactyly of hands, brachydactyly of toes, polycystic kidneys, hydrocephalus, mental retardation |
| Orofaciodigital syndrome type II (Mohr syndrome or OFD II) | | | | |
| Orofaciodigital syndrome type IV[141] | AR | **258860** 3147 | Lobulated tongue, cleft hard and/or soft palate, conductive deafness, laryngeal anomaly | Short limbs, polydactyly, syndactyly, talipes varus/valgus, cyanotic heart disease, imperforate anus, Dandy-Walker malformation, mental retardation |
| Orofaciodigital syndrome type V (Turston syndrome)[59] | AR | | Median cleft of upper lip | Postaxial polydactyly of hands and feet |
| Osteopathia striata with cranial sclerosis[111,176] | AD | ***166500** 4249 | Facial palsy, abnormal sinuses, depressed nasal bridge, cleft palate | Macrocephaly, frontal bossing, linear striations in metaphyses and diaphyses |
| Otopalatodigital syndrome type I | | | See Part II, Appendix B | |

| Syndrome or condition | Inheritance[a] | MIM No. POSSUM No.[b] | Ear, nose, and throat manifestations | Other manifestations |
|---|---|---|---|---|
| Otopalatodigital syndrome type II[26] | XLR | **311300** 3710 | Cleft palate, bifid uvula, midface hypoplasia, low-set ears, micrognathia, microstoma | Short stature, abnormal ribs and vertebrae; bowed humeri, radii, femora, tibiae |
| Palant cleft palate syndrome[166] | AR | **260150** 3144 | Significantly abnormal facies, bulbous nasal tip, cleft soft and/or hard palate | Mental retardation, microcephaly, short stature, almond-shaped and deep-set eyes, upward eye slant and narrow fissures, scoliosis, camptodactyly of fingers, clinodactyly and syndactyly of toes, firm and non-bony prominence on the anteromedial surface of both wrists |
| Pallister-W syndrome (W syndrome)[167] | XLR | **311450** 3357 | Midline craniofacial defects, broad nasal tip, cleft lip/palate congenitally absent upper central incisors | Mental retardation, seizures, spasticity, hypertelorism, squint, camptodactyly, cubitus valgus, subluxation at the proximal radioulnar joints |
| Patellar aplasia and cleft palate[104] | | | Cleft palate, slender nose, small chin | Radial and patellar aplasia and/or hypoplasia and short stature |
| Pena-Shokeir phenotype (Fetal akinesia-hypokinesia sequence)[56,163] | AR | ***208150** 3135 | Microstomia, cleft hard palate, low-set ears, flat nose, short and webbed neck | Small for gestational age, poor muscle build, hypertelorism, prominent eyes, bell-shaped chest, cryptorchidism, multiple ankyloses, camptodactyly, abnormal palmar dermatoglyphics, rocker bottom feet, hydrocephalus, seizures, pulmonary hypoplasia, early death |
| Polydactyly-cleft lip or Varadi-Papp syndrome[221] | AR | **277170** | Midline cleft upper lip, oral frenulae, wide-spaced teeth | Postaxial polydactyly of fingers and toes, psychomotor retardation |
| Popliteal pterygium syndrome[90,142] | AD | ***119500** 3360 | Cleft lip/palate, gingival synechiae, lip pits | Popliteal pterygium, syndactyly, genital hypoplasia, discolored nails, symphalangism, small patellae |
| Postaxial acrofacial dysostosis (Miller syndrome, Wildervanck-Smith syndrome, Genée-Wiedemann syndrome)[73b] | AR | ***263750** 3487 | Cleft lip and/or palate, cup-shaped pinnae, malformed external auditory canals and middle ears | Downward slanting palpebral fissures, eyelid colobomas, postaxial agenesis of digit of hands and feet, abnormal thumbs (50%), radioulnar synostosis, congenital heart defects |
| Posterior palatal synechiae and cleft palate[7] | Sporadic | | Cleft palate with membranous extension to base of the tongue | |
| Potter sequence or bilateral renal agenesis/oligohydramnios sequence | | | See Part II, Appendix A | |
| Pseudodiastrophic dysplasia[57] | AR | **264180** 4177 | Cleft palate, submucous cleft palate, bifid uvula, flat nasal bridge, midface hypoplasia, no cystic enlargement of pinnae | Rhizomelic shortening of limbs, elbow dislocated, no hitchhiker's thumb |
| Pseudotrisomy 13 syndrome (holoprosencephaly with polydactyly)[148,231] | AR | 3982 | Midline cleft lip, micrognathia, depressed premaxillary region, choanal atresia or stenosis, microstomia, microtia, short neck | Holoprosencephaly, polydactyly, microcephaly, ambiguous genitalia, polydactyly, pulmonary atresia, hypoplastic kidneys, imperforate anus, malrotation of the gut, limb shortness, normal chromosomes |
| Retinoblastoma and cleft palate[25] | ? | | Cleft palate | Retinoblastoma |
| Rhizomelic chondrodysplasia punctata (see Chondrodysplasia, rhizomelic type) | | | | |
| Ring-shaped skin creases and cleft palate[115] | AD | ***156610** 4404 | Cleft hard palate, abnormal ear structure | Marked annular skin creases with underlying lipomatoses, hemihy- |

**Appendix D** Syndromes and conditions associated with congenital anomalies of the mouth, palate, and pharynx (*Continued*)

| Syndrome or condition | Inheritance[a] | MIM No. POSSUM No.[b] | Ear, nose, and throat manifestations | Other manifestations |
|---|---|---|---|---|
| | | | | pertrophy, borderline mental retardation, seizures (the term *Michelin tire baby* is pejorative and should be abandoned) |
| Roberts syndrome (pseudothalidomide syndrome)[88,108,193] | AR | ***268300**<br>3378 | Cleft hard and/or soft palate, midline cleft lip, prominent premaxillary region, micrognathia, broad nasal bridge, low-set ears | Tetramelic symmetrical limb reduction, radial defects, oligodactyly, syndactyly, microcephaly, small nails, hypertelorism, microcornea, cryptorchidism, large penis, uterine and/or vaginal abnormalities, ectopic/cystic kidneys, congential heart defects, hydrocephalus, mental retardation |
| Robin sequence | | | Cleft palate, small mouth, micrognathia | See also Part II, Appendix B |
| Robin sequence, congenital heart defect[71] | XLR | **311900**<br>4012 | Cleft hard palate, glossoptosis | Vascular structural defects (persistance of left superior vena cava and ASD), talipes equinovarus |
| Robin sequence-oligodactyly[187] | Uncertain<br>?AD | **172880**<br>3851 | Cleft hard palate, glossoptosis, micrognathia, dental malocclusion | Pre- and postaxial oligodactyly, clinodactyly, metacarpal synostosis |
| Robinow syndrome[30] | AD<br>AR | **180700**<br>3379 | Cleft lip and palate (10%), gingival enlargement (65%), bifid or hypoplastic uvula (20%), fetal face | Developmental delay (20%), short stature, mesomelic shortening of extremities, micropenis |
| Rüdiger syndrome (mental retardation, coarse face, limb hypoplasia, stenotic urethra)[217] | | | See Part II, Appendix A | |
| Russell-Silver syndrome[45,53] | AD<br>AR | **270050**<br>3385 | Triangular face, thin lips, cleft hard palate, posteriorly angulated ears, prominent ears | Intrauterine and postnatal growth retardation, thin build, increased body hair, large fontanelle, thick eyelashes, body asymmetry, genitourinary anomalies, normal mental development |
| Saethre-Chotzen syndrome (acrocephalosyndactyly type III)[99,156] | AD | ***101400**<br>3009 | Midfacial asymmetry, beaked nose, deviated nasal septum, lip pits, cleft hard palate, microtia, prominent antihelix | Variable craniosynostosis (commonly coronal), broad forehead, sclerotic calvarium, abnormal sella turcica, ptosis, optic nerve anomaly, small hands, skin syndactyly, coxa valga, borderline mental retardation, short stature |
| Say syndrome[200] | ?AD | 4496 | Cleft palate, large ears, micrognathia | Microcephaly, short stature, hypoplastic toenails and nipples, hypoplastic distal phalanges and tapering fingers |
| Schinzel syndrome (see Acrocallosal syndrome) | | | | |
| Schisis association[43] | | 4137 | Oral clefts (lip/palate), abnormal esophagus (TE fistula) | Neural tube defects, diaphragmatic hernia |
| Short rib, polydactyly syndrome (Majewski type)[33,218] | AR | ***263520**<br>3389 | Depressed nasal bridge, midline cleft lip, cleft hard palate, low-set ears, short neck, laryngeal anomaly | Short stature, short limbs, macrocephaly, brachydactyly, postaxial polydactyly, hypoplastic kidneys, abnormal pancreas |
| Short rib syndrome, Beemer-Langer type[10,123] | AR | ***269860**<br>3586 | Cleft lip, oral frenulae, flat face, depressed nasal bridge, cleft hard palate, webbed neck | Short lower limbs, polydactyly, pyloric stenosis, macrocephaly, small scapula, high clavicles, ambiguous genitalia, brachydactyly |
| Short stature, mental retardation cleft lip/palate, eye anomalies[184] | | 4952 | Midface hypoplasia, nystagmus, paramedial cleft lip, cleft palate | Microcephaly, deep-set eyes, microphthalmia, coloboma of retina, squint, mental retardation of any degree |

| Syndrome or condition | Inheritance[a] | MIM No. POSSUM No.[b] | Ear, nose, and throat manifestations | Other manifestations |
|---|---|---|---|---|
| Shprintzen syndrome (see Velocardiofacial syndrome) | | | | |
| Simpson-Golabi-Behmel syndrome | | | See Part II, Appendix A | |
| Smith-Lemli-Opitz syndrome[97,119,168] | AR | ***270400** 3391 | Broad nasal bridge, broad tip, anteverted nostrils, micrognathia, cleft hard and/or soft palate, low-set ears, dysphagia | Mental retardation, microcephaly, ptosis, partial syndactyly of 2nd and 3rd toes, polydactyly, ambiguous genitalia (diagnosis in a female may be difficult), glaucoma, cataract, small hands, abnormal palmar dermatoglyphics, pyloric stenosis, moderate to severe mental retardation, hypotonia, low plasma cholesterol, accumulation of 7-dehydrocholesterol, defect in 7-dehydrocholesterol reductase |
| Smith-Lemli-Opitz syndrome type II[42,140] | AR | ***268670** 3645 | Small tongue, cleft palate, low-set ears, short neck, laryngeal anomaly | Lethal multiple congenital anomalies, short limbs, polydactyly, ambiguous genitalia, cataracts, heart defects, unilobar lungs, mental retardation |
| Sorsby syndrome (macular coloboma and brachydactyly)[220] | AD | **120400** 3282 | Cleft palate, nystagmus, sensorineural deafness | Bilateral macular colobomata, scoliosis, symphalangism, clinodactyly of fingers, hypoplastic kidneys |
| Spondyloepimetaphyseal dysplasia with joint laxity (SEMDJL)[222] | AR | ***271640** 4257 | Cleft hard palate, long philtrum | Severe progressive kyphoscoliosis, high and broad forehead, hyperelastic skin, prominent eyes, blue sclerae, abnormal vertebrae, diffuse osteoporosis, dislocated hip, talipes varus/valgus |
| Spondyloepiphyseal dysplasia (SED) congenita[130] | AD | **#183900** 3394 | Cleft palate, abnormal hearing | Short trunk, short limbs with epiphyseal abnormalities, myopia, retinal detachment, odontoid hypoplasia, kyphoscoliosis, delayed skeletal maturation, coxa vara, genu varum, pectus carinatum |
| Spondylometaepiphyseal dysplasia, Strudwick type (Z syndrome)[134,206] | AR | **#184250** 3561 | Cleft hard palate | Short limbs with metaphyseal abnormalities, odontoid hypoplasia, atlantoaxial instability, abnormal vertebrae, genu valgum, flat foot, ureteric anomalies |
| Sprengel anomaly[86] | Sporadic AD | ***184400** 4092 | Cleft hard palate, short neck | Scapula is elevated and hypoplastic, shoulder muscle hypoplasia, multiple vertebral segmentation defects, rib abnormalites, scoliosis |
| Stickler syndrome | | | See Part II, Appendix B | |
| Submucosal cleft palate, hypotelorism, and hypospadias[201] | AD | | Submucosal cleft palate | Blepharophimosis, upward slanting palpebral fissures, hypospadias, mild cutaneous syndactyly of 3rd and 4th fingers |
| Thrombocytopenia, absent radius, van Haeringen type[230] | ? | 4348 | Cleft palate, microtia, micrognatia, short neck, tracheal anomalies | Intermittent thrombocytopenia, short stature, short limbs, absent radius/ulna, microcephaly, chromosome breaks with X-rays; may be part of thrombocytopenia absent radius (TAR) syndrome |
| Tibial hemimelia, cleft lip/palate[204] | AR | **275220** 4395 | Cleft hard palate, paramedian cleft lip | Short stature, short limbs, abnormal knee, abnormal ankle |
| Toriello-Carey syndrome | | | See Part III, Appendix C-4 | |

**Appendix D** Syndromes and conditions associated with congenital anomalies of the mouth, palate, and pharynx (*Continued*)

| Syndrome or condition | Inheritance[a] | MIM No. POSSUM No.[b] | Ear, nose, and throat manifestations | Other manifestations |
|---|---|---|---|---|
| Treacher Collins syndrome (Mandibulofacial dysostosis or Franceschetti-Zwahlen-Klein syndrome) | | | See Part II, Appendix B | |
| Van der Woude syndrome (cleft lip/palate, lip pits)[23,118] | AD | ***119300** 3140 | Lower lip pits, paramedial cleft lip, cleft hard and/or soft palate | Oligodontia |
| Velo-cardio-facial syndrome (Shprintzen syndrome)[207] | AD | **192430** 3132 | Cleft palate (often submucous), high nasal bridge and large nose, nasal speech, notched or hypoplastic alae nasi, deafness, micrognathia | Short stature, microcephaly, mental retardation; long,thin, and hyperextensible fingers, VSD, pulmonary stenosis, right aortic arch, ocular abnormalities, deletion of 22q11 |
| Walker-Warburg syndrome (HARD-E syndrome or **H**ydrocephalus, **A**gyria, **R**etinal **D**ysplasia, **E**ncephalocele) | | | See Part II, Appendix A | |
| Weaver-Williams syndrome (see Cleft palate, microcephaly, mental retardation, and musculoskeletal mass deficiency) | | | | |
| Weissenbacher-Zweymüller syndrome[32] | AR | **277610** 3097 | Midface hypoplasia, micrognathia, cleft hard palate, glossoptosis | Short limbs, wide metaphyses, hypotonia, coronal clefts of vertebrae, retinal detachment |
| Wildervanck syndrome (Cervico-oculo-acoustic syndrome) | | | See Part II, Appendix A | |
| Zlotogora-Oğur syndrome (see mental retardation, cleft lip/palate, ectodermal dysplasia, syndactyly syndrome) | | | | |

[a]AD, autosomal dominant,; AR, autosomal recessive; XLR, X-linked recessive; XLD, X-linked dominant.
[b]MIM, *M*endelian *I*nheritance in *M*an. A Catalog of Human Genes and Genetic Disorders, by Victor A. McKusick, 11th ed, The Johns Hopkins University Press, Baltimore, 1994; POSSUM, *P*ictures *O*f *S*tandard *S*yndromes and *U*ndiagnosed *M*alformations, by Agnes Bankier et al., Murdoch Institute, Royal Children's Hospital, Victoria, Australia.
*confirmed gene and inheritance
#phenotype that can be caused by mutation in any of 2 or more genes

## References


1. Abruzzo MA, Erickson RP: Re-evaluation of new X-linked syndrome for evidence of CHARGE syndrome or X association. Am J Med Genet 34:397–400, 1989.
2. Airaksinen EM, Iivanainen M, Karli P, Sainio K, Haltia M: Hereditary recurrent brachial plexus neuropathy with dysmorphic features. Acta Neurol Scand 71:309–316, 1985.
3. Akkermans CH, Stern LM: Ankyloblepharon filiforme adnatum. Br J Ophthalmol 63:129–131, 1979.
4. Aleck KA, Grix A, Clericuzio C, Kaplan P, Adomian GE, Lachman R, Rimoin DL: Dyssegmental dysplasias: clinical, radiographic and morphologic evidence of heterogeneity. Am J Med Genet 27:295–312, 1987.
5. Allanson JE, McGillivray BC: Familial clefting syndrome with ectropion and dental anomaly without limb anomalies. Clin Genet 27:426–429, 1985.
6. Anyane-Yeboa K, Mackay C, Taterka P, Merkrebs A, Allendorf D: Cleft lip and palate, corneal opacities and profound psychomotor retardation. A newly recognized genetic syndrome. Cleft Palate J 20:246–250, 1983.
7. Arcand P, Haikal J: Persistent buccopharyngeal membrane. J Otolaryngol 17:125–127, 1988.
8. Assemany SR, Muzzo S, Gardner LI: Syndrome of phocomelic diabetic embryopathy (caudal dysplasia). Am J Dis Child 123:489–491, 1972.
9. Baetz-Greenwalt B, Ratliff NB, Moodie DS: Hypoplastic right-sided heart complex: a cluster of cases with associated congenital birth defects. A new syndrome? J Pediatr 103:399–401, 1983.
10. Balçi S, Erçal MD, Onol B, Çağlar M, Doğan A, Doğruel N: Familial short rib syndrome, type Beemer, with pyloric stenosis and short intestine, one case diagnosed prenatally. Clin Genet 39:298–303, 1991.
11. Bamforth JS, Hughes IA, Lazarus JH, Weaver CM, Harper PS: Congenital hypothyroidism, spiky hair and cleft palate. J Med Genet 26:49–51, 1989.
12. Bankier A: Hirschsprung's disease, distinctive facies, and microcephaly. J Med Genet 26:287–288, 1989.
13. Baraitser M: The hypertelorism-microtia-clefting syndrome. J Med Genet 19:387–388, 1982.
14. Baraitser M, Rodeck C, Garner A: A new craniosynostosis/mental retardation syndrome diagnosed by fetoscopy. Clin Genet 22:12–15, 1982.
15. Barakat AY, D'Albora JB, Martin MM, Jose PA: Familial nephrosis, nerve deafness, and hypoparathyroidism. J Pediatr 91:61–64, 1977.
16. Beare JM, Dodge JA, Nevin NC: Cutis gyratum, acanthosis nigricans, and other congenital anomalies: a new syndrome. Br J Dermatol 81:241–247, 1969.
17. Beer S, Fried K, Krespin HI, Rosenblatt M, Tieder M: Trisomy 13 mosaic presenting as cleft lip and palate. Hum Hered 26:321–323, 1976.
18. Ben-Amitai D, Rachmel A, Levy Y, Sivan Y, Nitzan M, Steinherz R: Hypodipsic hypernatremia and hypertriglyceridemia associated with

cleft lip and cleft palate: a new hypothalamic dysfunction syndrome? Am J Med Genet 36:275–278, 1990.
19. Bencze J, Schintzler A, Walawska J: Dominant inheritance of hemifacial hypoplasia associated with strabismus. Oral Surg 35:489–500, 1973.
20. Bick DP, Schorderet DF, Price PA, Campbell L, Huff RW, Shapiro LJ, Moore CM: Prenatal diagnosis and investigation of a fetus with chondrodysplasia punctata, ichthyosis, and Kallmann syndrome due to an Xp deletion. Prenat Diagn 12:19–29, 1992.
21. Björnsson A, Arnason A, Tippet P: X-linked cleft palate and ankyloglossia in an Icelandic family. Cleft Palate J 26:3–8, 1989.
22. Blanquet V, Creau-Goldberg N, de Grouchy J, Turleau C: Molecular detection of constitutional deletions in patients with retinoblastoma. Am J Med Genet 39:355–361, 1991.
23. Bocian M, Walker AP: Lip pits and deletion 1q32→41. Am J Med Genet 26:437–443, 1987.
24. Bogart MH, Cunniff C, Bradshaw C, Jones KL, Jones OW: Terminal deletions of the long arm of chromosome 7: five new cases. Am J Med Genet 36:53–55, 1990.
25. Bonaiti-Pellie C, Briard-Guillemot ML, Feingold J, Frezal J: Associated congenital malformations in retinoblastoma. Clin Genet 7:37–39, 1975.
26. Brewster TG, Lachman RS, Kushner DC, Holmes LB, Isler RJ, Rimoin DL: Oto-palato-digital syndrome, type II—an X-linked skeletal dysplasia. Am J Med Genet 20:249–254, 1985.
27. Broome DL, Ebbin AJ, Jung AL, Feinauer LR, Madsen M: Aberrant tissue bands and craniofacial defects. Birth Defects 12:65–79, 1979.
28. Bucci E, Lo Muzio L, Mignogna MD: Oral and dental anomalies in Goltz syndrome. J Pedodont 13:161–168, 1989.
29. Bustos T, Simosa V, Pinto-Cisternas J, Abramovits W, Jolay L, Rodriguez L, Fernandez L, Ramela M: Autosomal recessive ectodermal dysplasia I. An undescribed dysplasia/malformation syndrome. Am J Med Genet 41:398–404, 1991.
30. Butler MG, Wadlington WB: Robinow syndrome: report of two patients and review of literature. Clin Genet 31:77–85, 1987.
31. Charrow JM, Cohen MM, Meeker D: Duplication of 3p syndrome: report of a new case and review of the literature. Am J Med Genet 8:431–436, 1981.
32. Chemke J, Carmi R, Galil A, Bar-Ziv Y, Ben Ytzhak I, Zwrowski L: Weissenbacher-Zweymüller syndrome: a distinct autosomal recessive skeletal dysplasia. Am J Med Genet 43:989–995, 1992.
33. Chen H, Yang SS, Gonzalez E, Fowler M, Al Saadi A: Short rib-polydactyly syndrome, Majewski type. Am J Med Genet 7:215–222, 1980.
34. Chicarelli ZN, Palayes IM: Oromandibular limb hypogenesis syndromes. Plast Reconstr Surg 76:13–24, 1985.
35. Chitayat D, Hahm SY, Marion RW, Sachs GS, Goldman D, Hutcheon RG, Weiss R, Cho S, Nitowsky HM: Further delineation of the McKusick-Kaufman hydrometrocolpos-polydactyly syndrome. Am J Dis Child 141:1133–1136, 1987.
36. Chitayat D, Meunier CM, Hodgkinson KA, Azouz ME: Robin sequence with facial and digital anomalies in two half-brothers by the same mother. Am J Med Genet 40:167–172, 1991.
37. Cohen MM Jr: Craniosynostosis and syndromes with craniosynostosis: incidence, genetics, penetrance, variability, and new syndrome updating. Birth Defects 15:13–63, 1979.
38. Cohen MM Jr: Perspectives on holoprosencephaly. Part I. Epidemiology, genetics, and syndromology. Teratology 40:211–235, 1989.
39. Colley AF, Leversha MA, Voulaire LE, Rogers JG: Five cases demonstrating the distinctive behavioural features of chromosome deletion 17(p11.2p11.2) (Smith-Magenis syndrome). J Paediatr Child Health 26:17–21, 1990.
40. Crane JB, Heise RL: New syndrome in three affected siblings. Pediatrics 68:235–237, 1981.
41. Cunniff C, Jones KL, Saal HM, Stern JH: Fryns syndrome: an autosomal recessive disorder associated with craniofacial anomalies, diaphragmatic hernia, and distal digital hypoplasia. Pediatrics 85:499–504, 1990.
42. Curry CJ, Carey JC, Holland JS, Chopra D, Fineman R, Golabi M, Sherman S, Pagon RA, Allanson J, Shulman S, Barr M, McGravey V, Dabiri C, Schimke N, Ives E, Hall BD: Smith-Lemli-Opitz syndrome—type II: multiple congenital anomalies with male pseudohermaphroditism and frequent early lethality. Am J Med Genet 26:45–57, 1987.
43. Czeizel A: Schisis-association. Am J Med Genet 10:25–35, 1981.
44. Czeizel A: New lethal omphalocele-cleft palate syndrome? Hum Genet 64:99, 1983.
45. Davies PS, Valley R, Preece MA: Adolescent growth and puberty progression in the Silver-Russell syndrome. Arch Dis Child 63:130–135, 1988.
46. Davis JG, Lafer C: A possible new mental retardation syndrome. Birth Defects 12:235–238, 1976.
47. De France HF, Beemer FA, Senders RC, Gerards LJ, Cats BP: Partial trisomy 11q due to paternal t(11q;18p); further delineation of the clinical picture. Clin Genet 25:295–299, 1984.
48. De Grouchy J, Turleau C: Clinical Atlas of Human Chromosomes. John Wiley & Sons, New York, 1984, pp 176–181.
49. De Moor MM, Baruch R, Human DG: Frontonasal dysplasia associated with tetralogy of Fallot. J Med Genet 24:107–109, 1987.
50. Dignan PS, Martin LW, Zenni EJ Jr: Pierre Robin anomaly with an accessory metacarpal of the index fingers. The Catel-Manzke syndrome. Clin Genet 29:168–173, 1986.
51. Dinardo NM, Christian JM, Bennett JA, Shutack JG: Cleft palate lateral synechia syndrome. Review of the literature and case report. Oral Surg Oral Med Oral Pathol 68:565–566, 1989.
52. Donlan MA: Growth failure, cleft palate, ectodermal dysplasia and apparent pancreatic insufficiency—a new syndrome. Birth Defects 13:230–231, 1977.
53. Donnai D, Thompson E, Allanson J, Baraitser M: Severe Silver-Russell syndrome. J Med Genet 26:447–451, 1989.
54. Drossou-Agakidou V, Andreou A, Soubassi-Griva V, Pandouraki M: Cerebro-costo-mandibular syndrome in four sibs, two pairs of twins. J Med Genet 28:704–707, 1991.
55. El-sahy NI, Waters WR: The branchio-skeleto-genital syndrome. A new hereditary syndrome. Plast Reconstr Surg 48:542–550, 1971.
56. Erdl R, Schmidtke K, Jakobeit M, Nerlich A, Schramm T: Pena-Shokeir phenotype with major CNS malformations: clinicopathological report of two siblings. Clin Genet 36:127–135, 1989.
57. Eteson DJ, Beluffi G, Burgio GR, Belloni C, Lachman RS, Rimoin DL: Pseudodiastrophic dysplasia: a distinct newborn skeletal dysplasia. J Pediatr 109:635–641, 1986.
58. Figueroa AA, Pruzansky S, Rollnick BR: Meige disease (familial lymphedema praecox) and cleft palate: report of a family and review of the literature. Cleft Palat J 20:151–157, 1983.
59. Fineman RM, Ablow RC, Breg WR, Wing SD, Rose JS, Rothman SL, Warpinski J: Complete and partial trisomy of different segments of chromosome 8: Case report and review. Clin Genet 16:390–396, 1979.
60. Fontaine G, Farriaux JP, Delattre P, Gidlecki Z, Poupard B, Durieux G, Piquet JJ: Une observation familiale du syndrome ectrodactylie et dysostose mandibulofaciale. J Génét Hum 22:289–307, 1974.
61. Fox JW, Golden GT, Edgerton MT: Frontonasal dysplasia with alar clefts in two sisters. Genetic considerations and surgical correction. Plast Reconstr Surg 57:553–561, 1976.
62. Frydman M, Kauschansky A, Leshem I, Savir H: Oculo-palato-cerebral dwarfism: a new syndrome. Clin Genet 27:414–419, 1985.
63. Fujimoto A, Lipson M, Lacro RV, Shinno NW, Boelter WD, Jones KL, Wilson MG: New autosomal dominant branchio-oculo-facial syndrome. Am J Med Genet 27:943–951, 1987.
64. Gassner I, Müller W, Rossler H, Kofler J, Mitterstieler G: Familial occurrence of syngnathia congenita syndrome. Clin Genet 15:241–244, 1979.
65. Gelman-Kohan Z, Antonelli J, Ankori-Cohen H, Adar H, Chemke J: Further delineation of the acrocallosal syndrome. Eur J Pediatr 150:797–799, 1991.
66. Gilbert EF, Opitz JM, Spranger JW, Langer LO Jr, Wolfson JJ, Viseskul C Chondrodysplasia punctata-rhizomelic form. Eur J Pediatr 123:89–109, 1976.
67. Goldstein DJ, Mirkin LD: Nager acrofacial dysostosis: evidence for apparent heterogeneity. Am J Med Genet 30:741–746, 1988.
68. Gonzalez CH, Billerbeck AEC, Takayama LC, Wajntal A: Duplication 10p in a girl due to a maternal translocation t(10;14)(p11:12). Am J Med Genet 14:159–167, 1983.
69. Gopalakrishna A, Thatte RL: Median cleft lip associated with bimanual hexadactyly and bilateral accessory toes: another case. Br J Plast Surg 35:354–355, 1982.
70. Gorlin RJ: Some facial syndromes. Birth Defects 5:65–76, 1969.
71. Gorlin RJ, Cervenka J, Anderson RC, Sauk JJ, Bevis WD: Robin's syndrome. A probably X-linked subvariety exhibiting persistence of left superior vena cava and atrial septal defect. Am J Dis Child 119:176–178, 1970.
72. Gorlin RJ, Cohen MM Jr, Levin LS: Syndromes of the Head and Neck, 3rd ed. Oxford University Press, New York, 1990, pp 16–17.
73. Gorlin RJ, Cohen MM Jr, Levin LS: Syndromes of the Head

and Neck, 3rd ed. Oxford University Press, New York, 1990, pp 33–40.
73a. Gorlin RJ,Cohen MM Jr, Levin LS: Syndromes of the Head and Neck, 3rd ed. Oxford University Press, New York, 1990, pp 372–380.
73b. Gorlin RJ,Cohen MM Jr, Levin LS: Syndromes of the Head and Neck, 3rd ed. Oxford University Press, New York, 1990, pp 654–655.
74. Gorlin RJ, Cohen MM Jr, Levin LS: Syndromes of the Head and Neck, 3rd ed. Oxford University Press, New York, 1990, p 721.
75. Gorlin RJ, Cohen MM Jr, Levin LS: Syndromes of the Head and Neck, 3rd ed. Oxford University Press, New York, 1990, p 749.
76. Gorlin RJ, Cohen MM Jr, Levin LS: Syndromes of the Head and Neck, 3rd ed. Oxford University Press, New York, 1990, pp 775–776.
77. Gorlin RJ, Schorf RA, Paparella MM: Cleft palate, stapes fixation and oligodontia—a new autosomal recessive inherited syndrome. Birth Defects 7:87–88, 1971.
78. Gossage D, Perrin JM, Butler MG: A 26 month-old child with Marden-Walker syndrome and pyloric stenosis. Am J Med Genet 26:915–919, 1987.
79. Greenberg F, Gresik MV, Carpenter RJ, Law SW, Hoffman LP, Ledbetter DH: Gardner-Silengo-Wachtel or genito-palato-cardiac syndrome: male pseudohermaphroditism with micrognathia, cleft palate, and conotruncal cardiac defect. Am J Med Genet 26:59–64, 1987.
80. Greene SL, Michels VV, Doyle JA: Variable expression in ankyloblepharon-ectodermal defects—cleft lip and palate syndrome. Am J Med Genet 27:207–212, 1987.
81. Halal F: Dominantly inherited syndrome of microcephaly and cleft palate. Am J Med Genet 15:135–140, 1983.
82. Hall BD: Nager acrofacial dysostosis: Autosomal dominant inheritance in mild to moderately affected mother and lethally affected phocomelic son. Am J Med Genet 33:394–397, 1989.
83. Hanson JW: Teratogen update: fetal hydantoin effects. Teratology 33:349–353, 1986.
84. Hendricks HJ, Brunner HG, Haagen TA, Hamel BC: Acrocallosal syndrome. Am J Med Genet 35:443–446, 1990.
85. Hipkin LJ, Casson IF, Davis JC: Identical twins discordant for Kallmann's syndrome. J Med Genet 27:198–199, 1990.
86. Hodgson SV, Chiu DC: Dominant transmission of Sprengel's shoulder and cleft palate. J Med Genet 18:263–265, 1981.
87. Hoefler G, Hoefler S, Watkins PA, Chen WW, Moser A, Baldwin V, McGillivray B, Charrow J, Friedman JM, Rutledge L, et al: Biochemical abnormalities in rhizomelic chondrodysplasia punctata. J Pediatr 112:726–733, 1988.
88. Holmes-Siedle M, Seres-Santamaria A, Crocker M, Hall JG, Gourchman M: A sibship with Roberts/SC phocomelia syndrome. Am J Med Genet 37:18–22, 1990.
89. Hoyme HE, Jones KL, Nyhan WL, Pauli RM, Robinow M: Autosomal dominant ectrodactyly and absence of long bones of upper or lower limbs: further clinical delineation. J Pediatr 111:538–543, 1987.
90. Hunter A: The popliteal pterygium syndrome: report of a new family and review of the literature. Am J Med Genet 36:196–208, 1990.
91. Hunter AG, Carpenter BF: Atelosteogenesis I and boomerang dysplasia: a question of nosology. Clin Genet 39:471–480, 1991.
92. Ieshima A, Koeda T, Inagaki M: Peculiar face, deafness, cleft palate, male pseudohermaphroditism, and growth and psychomotor retardation; a new autosomal recessive syndrome? Clin Genet 30:136–141, 1986.
93. Ismail SR, Koussef BG, Kotb SM, Kholeif SF: Duplication 3q(q21→qter) without limb anomalies. Am J Med Genet 38:518–522, 1991.
94. Jaatoul NY, Haddad NE, Khoury LA, Afifi AK, Bahuth NB, Deeb ME, Mikati MA, Der Kaloustian VM: Brief clinical report and review: the Marden-Walker syndrome. Am J Med Genet 11:259–271, 1982.
95. Jacob JC, Andermann F, Robb JP: Heredofamilial neuritis with brachial predilection. Neurology 11:1025–1033, 1961.
96. Jones KL: Smith's Recognizable Patterns of Human Malformation, 5th ed. WB Saunders, Philadelphia, 1996, p 50.
97. Jones KL: Smith's Recognizable Patterns of Human Malformation, 5th ed. WB Saunders, Philadelphia, 1996, p 112–13.
98. Jones KL: Smith's Recognizable Patterns of Human Malformation, 5th ed. WB Saunders, Philadelphia, 1996, p 324.
99. Jones KL: Smith's Recognizable Patterns of Human Malformation, 5th ed. WB Saunders, Philadelphia, 1996, p 412.
100. Jones KL: Smith's Recognizable Patterns of Human Malformation, 5th ed. WB Saunders, Philadelphia, 1996, p 420–421.
101. Jones KL: Smith's Recognizable Patterns of Human Malformation, 5th ed. WB Saunders, Philadelphia, 1996, p 570.
102. Jones KL: Smith's Recognizable Patterns of Human Malformation, 5th ed. WB Saunders, Philadelphia, 1996, p 596.
103. Jorgenson RJ, Bick D: A new syndrome of dwarfism, trichodysplasia, cleft palate and unusual facies. Presented at March of Dimes Clinical Genetics Conference, Baltimore, 1988.
104. Kääriäinen H, Ryöppy S, Norio R: RAPADILINO syndrome with radial and patellar aplasia/hypoplasia as main manifestations. Am J Med Genet 33:346–351, 1989.
105. Kaplan P, Cummings C, Fraser FC: A "community" of face-limb malformation syndromes. J Pediatr 89:241–247, 1976.
106. Kaplan P, Plauchu H, Fitch N, Jéquier S: A new acro-cranio-facial dysostosis syndrome in sisters. Am J Med Genet 29:95–106, 1988.
107. Kelly TE: Teratogenicity of anticonvulsant drugs. I: Review of the literature. Am J Med Genet 19:413–434, 1984.
108. Keppen LD, Gollin SM, Siebert JJ, Sisken JE: Roberts syndrome with normal cell division. Am J Med Genet 38:21–24, 1991.
109. Kershisnik MM, Craven CM, Jung AL, Carey JC, Knisely AS: Osteochondrodysplasia in Fryns syndrome. Am J Dis Child 145:656–660, 1991.
110. Khoury MJ, Cordero JF, Mulinare J, Opitz JM: Selected midline defect association: A population study. Pediatrics 84:266–272, 1989.
111. Kornreich L, Grunebaum M, Ziv N, Shuper A, Mimouni M: Osteopathia striata, cranial sclerosis with cleft palate and facial nerve palsy. Eur J Pediatr 147:101–103, 1988.
112. Kreiborg S, Cohen MM Jr: Germinal mosaicism in Crouzon syndrome. Hum Genet 84:487–488, 1990.
113. Krieble BF, Bixler D: Autosomal dominant blepharophimosis with multiple congenital anomalies. J Clin Dysmorphol 2:24–29, 1984.
114. Kumasaka K, Clarren SK: Familial patterns of central nervous system dysfunction, growth deficiency, facial clefts and congenital megacolon: a specific disorder? Am J Med Genet 31:465–466, 1988.
115. Kunze J: The "Michelin tire baby syndrome": an autosomal dominant trait. Am J Med Genet 25:169–171, 1986.
116. Kunze J, Park W, Hansen KH, Hanefeld F: Adducted thumb syndrome. Report of a new case and a diagnostic approach. Eur J Pediatr 141:122–126, 1983.
117. Kurnit D, Hall JG, Shurtleff DB, Cohen MM Jr: An autosomal dominantly inherited syndrome of facial asymmetry, esotropia, and amblyopia, and submucous cleft palate (Bencze syndrome). Clin Genet 16:301–304, 1979.
118. Kuster W, Lambrecht JT: Cleft lip and palate, lower lip pits, and limb deficiency defects. J Med Genet 25:565–567, 1988.
119. Lachman MF, Wright Y, Whiteman DA, Herson V, Greenstein RM: Brief clinical report: a 46,XY phenotypic female with Smith-Lemli-Opitz syndrome. Clin Genet 39:136–141, 1991.
120. Lafer CZ, Neu RL: A liveborn infant with tetraploidy. Am J Med Genet 31:375–378, 1988.
121. Lessick M, Israel J, Szego K, Wong P: Leiomyosarcoma in a patient with trisomy 8 mosaicism. J Med Genet 27:643–644, 1990.
122. Levy I, Levy Y, Mammon Z, Nitzan M, Steinherz R: Gastrointestinal abnormalities in the syndrome of mosaic trisomy 9. J Med Genet 26:280–281, 1989.
123. Lin AE, Doshi N, Flom L, Tenenholz B, Filkins KL: Beemer-Langer syndrome with manifestations of an orofaciodigital syndrome. Am J Med Genet 39:247–251, 1991.
124. Lin AE, Garver KL, Diggans G, Clemens M, Wenger SL, Steele MW, Jones MC, Israel J: Interstitial and terminal deletions of the long arm of chromosome 4: further delineation of phenotypes. Am J Med Genet 31:533–548, 1988.
125. Lin AE, Losken HW, Jaffe R, Biglan AW: The branchio-oculo-facial syndrome. Cleft Palate Craniofac J 28:96–102, 1991.
126. Lipp MJ, Lubit EC: The oral-facial digital syndrome: case report of a mother and daughter. Cleft Palate J 27:311–316, 1990.
127. Lipson MH: Trisomy 14 mosaicism syndrome. Am J Med Genet 24:541–544, 1987.
128. Lowry RB, Miller JR: Cleft palate and congenital heart disease. Lancet 1:1302–1303, 1971.
129. Macpherson RI, Skinner SA, Donnenfeld AE: A campomelic dysplasia. Pediatr Radiol 20:90–93, 1989.
130. Macpherson RI, Wood BP: Spondyloepiphyseal dysplasia congenita. A cause of lethal neonatal dwarfism. Pediatr Radiol 9:217–224, 1980.

131. Malpuech G, Demeocq F, Palcoux JB, Vanlieferinghen P: A previously undescribed autosomal recessive multiple congenital anomalies/mental retardation (MCA/MR) syndrome with growth failure, lip/palate cleft(s), and urogenital anomalies. Am J Med Genet 16:475–480, 1983.
132. Mankinen CB, Hold JG, Sears JW: Partial trisomy 15 in a young girl. Clin Genet 10:27–32, 1976.
133. Maraia R, Saal HM, Wangsa D: A chromosome 17q de novo paracentric inversion in a patient with campomelic dysplasia; case report and etiologic hypothesis. Clin Genet 39:401–408, 1991.
134. Maroteaux P, Spranger J: The spondylometaphyseal dysplasias. A tentative classification. Pediatr Radiol 21:293–297, 1991.
135. Martin AO, Perrin JCS, Muir WA: An autosomal dominant midline cleft syndrome resembling familial holoprosencephaly. Clin Genet 12:65–72, 1977.
136. Martin RA, Cunniff C, Erickson L, Jones KL: Pentalogy of Cantrell and ectopia cordis, a familial developmental field complex. Am J Med Genet 42:839–841, 1992.
137. Martinez-Frias ML, Frias JL, Vazquez I, Fernandez J: Bartsocas-Papas syndrome: Three familial cases from Spain. Am J Med Genet 39:34–37, 1991.
138. Matalon R, Michals K, Blau N, Rouse B: Hyperphenylalaninemia due to inherited deficiencies of tetrahydrobiopterin. Adv Pediatr 36:67–89, 1989.
139. McFadden DE, Kalousek DK: Two different phenotypes of fetuses with chromosomal triploidy: correlation with parental origin of the extra haploid set. Am J Med Genet 38:535–538, 1991.
140. McKeever PA, Young ID: Smith-Lemli-Opitz syndrome. II: A disorder of the fetal adrenals? J Med Genet 27:465–466, 1990.
141. Meinecke P, Hayek H: Orofaciodigital syndrome type IV (Mohr-Majewski syndrome) with severe expression expanding the known spectrum of anomalies. J Med Genet 27:200–202, 1990.
142. Meinecke P, Menzel J, Froster-Iskenius U: Kniepterygium-Syndrom bei einem Neugeborenen. Monatsschrift Kinderheilkunde 137:228–230, 1989.
143. Meinecke P, Passarge E: Microcephalic osteodysplastic primordial dwarfism type I/III in sibs. J Med Genet 28:795–800, 1991.
144. Meinecke P, Schaefer E, Wiedemann HR: Microcephalic osteodysplastic primordial dwarfism: further evidence for identity of the so-called types I and II. Am J Med Genet 39:232–236, 1991.
145. Milewicz DM, Pyeritz RE, Crawford ES, Byers PH: Marfan syndrome: defective synthesis, secretion, and extracellular matrix formation of fibrillin by cultured dermal fibroblasts. J Clin Invest 89:79–86, 1992.
146. Millhouse RF, Joos HA: Extrathoracic ectopia cordis: Report of cases and review of literature. Am Heart J 57:470–476, 1959.
147. Mitchell LE, Healey SC, Chenevix-Trench G: Evidence for an association between nonsyndromic cleft lip with or without cleft palate and a gene located on the long arm of chromosome 4. Am J Hum Genet 57:1130–1136, 1995.
148. Moerman P, Fryns JP: Holoprosencephaly and postaxial polydactyly: another observation. J Med Genet 25:501–502, 1988.
149. Moncla A, Livet MO, Auger M, Maltei JF, Matei MG, Giraud F: Smith-Magenis syndrome: a new contiguous gene syndrome. Report of three new cases. J Med Genet 28:627–632, 1991.
150. Moore GE, Ivens A, Chambers J, Farral M, Williamson R, Page DC, Björnsson A, Arnason A, Jennson O: Linkage of an X-chromosome cleft palate gene. Nature 326:91–92, 1987.
151. Morishita M, Shiba R, Chiyo H, Furuyama J, Fujita H, Atsumi Y: The oral manifestations of 4p- syndrome. J Oral Maxillofac Surg 41:601–605, 1983.
152. Muis N, Beemer FA, van Dijken P, Klep-de Pater JM: The Aase-Smith syndrome. Case report and review of the literature. Eur J Pediatr 145:153–157, 1986.
153. Mundlos S, Mulliken JB, Abramson DL, Warman ML, Knoll JH, Olsen BR: Genetic mapping of cleidocranial dysplasia and evidence of a microdeletion in one family. Hum Mol Genet 4:71–75, 1995.
154. Münke M: Clinical cytogenetic, and molecular approaches to the genetic heterogeneity of holoprosencephaly. Am J Med Genet 34:237–245, 1989.
155. Niebuhr E: The cri-du-chat syndrome. Hum Genet 42:143–152, 1978; 44:227–275, 1978.
156. Niemann-Seyde SC, Eber SW, Zoll B: Saethre-Chotzen syndrome (ACS III) in four generations. Clin Genet 40:271–276, 1991.
157. Niikawa N, Kuroki Y, Kajii T, Matsuura N, Ishkiriyama S, Tonoki H, Ishikawa N, Yamada Y, Fujita M, Umemoto H, et al: Kabuki make-up (Niikawa-Kuroki) syndrome: a study of 62 patients. Am J Med Genet 31:565–589, 1988.
158. Nikolis J, Ivanovic K, Diklic V: Partial trisomy 13q resulting from a paternal reciprocal Yq;13q translocation. J Med Genet 28:425–426, 1991.
159. Nikolis J, Ivanovic K, Kosanovic M: Tandem duplication of chromosome 14(q24→q32) in male newborn with congenital malformations. Clin Genet 23:321–324, 1983.
160. Novales MA, Fernandez-Novoa C, Hevia A, San Martin V, Galera H: Partial trisomy for the long arm of chromosome 7. Hum Genet 62:378–381, 1982.
161. Oğur G, Yüksel M: Association of syndactyly, ectodermal dysplasia, and cleft lip and palate: report of two sibs from Turkey. J Med Genet 25:37–40, 1988.
162. Ohdo S, Madokoro H, Sonoda T, Ohba K: Sibs lacking characteristic features of duplication of distal 17q. J Med Genet 26:465–468, 1989.
163. Ohlsson A, Fong KW, Rose TH, Moore DC: Prenatal sonographic diagnosis of Pena-Shokeir syndrome type I, or fetal akinesia deformation sequence. Am J Med Genet 29:59–65, 1988.
164. Opitz JM, Frias JL, Cohen MM Jr: The ECP syndrome, another autosomal dominant case of monodactylous ectrodactyly. Eur J Pediatr 133:217–220, 1980.
165. Ouellette EM, Rosett HL, Rosman NP, Weiner L: Adverse effects on offspring of maternal alcohol abuse during pregnancy. N Engl J Med 297:528–530, 1977.
166. Palant DI, Feingold M, Berkman MD: Unusual facies, cleft palate, mental retardation, and limb abnormalities in siblings: a new syndrome. J Pediatr 78:686–689, 1971.
167. Pallister PD, Herrmann J, Spranger JW, Gorlin RJ, Langer LO, Opitz JM: The W syndrome. Studies of malformation syndromes of man XXVIII. Birth Defects 10:51–60, 1974.
168. Pankau R, Partsch CJ, Funda J, Sippell WG: Hypothalamic pituitary-gonadal function in two infants with Smith-Lemli-Opitz syndrome. Am J Med Genet 43:513–516, 1992.
169. Papadia F, Longo N: Nosological difference between the Bartsocas-Papas syndrome and lethal multiple pterygium syndrome [letter]. Am J Med Genet 29:699–700, 1988.
170. Park W-J, Bellus GA, Jabs EW: Mutations in fibroblast growth factor receptors: phenotypic consequences during eukaryotic development. Am J Hum Genet 57:748–754, 1995.
171. Patton MA, Sharma A, Winter RM: The Aase-Smith syndrome. Clin Genet 28:521–525, 1985.
172. Pavone L, Rizzo R, Tine A, Micali G, Sorge G, Neri G: A case of the Freire-Maia Odontotrichomelic syndrome: nosology with EEC syndrome. Am J Med Genet 33:190–193, 1989.
173. Pearl W: Heart disease associated with deletion of the short arm of chromosome 18. Pediatr Cardiol 10:174–176, 1989.
174. Pfeiffer RA, Stoss H, Voigt HJ, Wundisch GF: Absence of fibula and ulna with oligodactyly, contractures, right-angle bowing of femora, abnormal familial morphology, cleft lip/palate and brain malforamtion in two sibs: a possibly new lethal syndrome. Am J Med Genet 29:901–908, 1988.
175. Phillips CI, Griffiths DL: Macular coloboma and skeletal abnormalities. Br J Ophthalmol 53:346–349, 1969.
176. Piechowiak H, Goebel FD, Hirche U, Tyrell R: Cranial sclerosis with striated bone disease (osteopathia striata). Klin Pediatr 198:418–424, 1986.
177. Poole AR, Pidoux I, Reiner A, Rosenberg L, Hollister D, Murray L, Rimoin D: Kniest dysplasia is characterized by an apparent abnormal processing of the C-propeptide of type II cartilage collagen resulting in imperfect fibril assembly. J Clin Invest 81:579–589, 1988.
178. Poulos A, Sheffield L, Sharp P, Sherwood G, Johnson D, Beckman K, Fellenberg AJ, Wraith JE, Chow, CW, Usher S et al: Rhizomelic chondrodysplasia punctata. Clinical, pathological and biochemical findings in two patients. J Pediatr 113:685–690, 1988.
179. Pyeritz RE, Fishman EK, Bernhardt BA, Siegelman SS: Dural ectasia is a common feature of the Marfan syndrome. Am J Hum Genet 43:726–732, 1988.
180. Ramer JC, Mowrey PN, Robins DB, Ligato S, Towfighi J, Ladda RL: Five children with del(2)(q31q33) and one individual with dup(2)(q31q33) from a single family: review of brain, cardiac, and limb malformation. Am J Med Genet 37:392–400, 1990.
181. Reiss JA, Sheffield LJ: Distal arthrogryposis type II: a family with varying congenital abnormalities. Am J Med Genet 24:255–267, 1986.

182. Richieri-Costa A, Colletto GM, Gollop TR, Masiero D: A previously undescribed autosomal recessive multiple congenital anomalies/mental retardation (MCA/MR) syndrome with fronto-nasal dysostosis, cleft lip/palate, limb hypoplasia, and postaxial polysyndactyly: acro-fronto-facio-nasal dysostosis syndrome. Am J Med Genet 20:631–638, 1985.
183. Richieri-Costa A, Gollop TR, Colletto GM: Syndrome of acrofacial dysostosis, cleft lip/palate and triphalangeal thumb in a Brazilian family. Am J Med Genet 14:225–229, 1983.
184. Richieri-Costa A, Guion-Almeida ML: Short stature, mental retardation, eye anomalies, and cleft lip/palate. Am J Med Genet 42:449–452, 1992.
185. Rintala A, Marttinen E, Rantala SL, Kaitila I: Cleft palate, in diastrophic dysplasia. Morphology, results of treatment and complications. Scand J Plast Surg 20:45–49, 1986.
186. Robinow M, Johnson GF: The Gordon syndrome: autosomal dominant cleft palate, camptodactyly and club feet. Am J Med Genet 9:139–146, 1981.
187. Robinow M, Johnson GF, Apesos J: Robin sequence and oligodactyly in a mother and son. Am J Med Genet 25:293–297, 1986.
188. Robinow M, Johnson GF, Minella PA: Aicardi syndrome, papilloma of the choroid plexus, cleft lip, and cleft of the posterior palate. J Pediatr 104:404–405, 1984.
189. Rodini ESO, Fretas JAS, Richieri-Costa A: Ectrodactyly, cleft lip/palate syndrome. Am J Med Genet 38:539–541, 1991.
190. Rodini ESO, Richieri-Costa A: Autosomal recessive ectodermal dysplasia, cleft lip/palate, mental retardation, and syndactyly: the Zlotogora-Oğur syndrome. Am J Med Genet 36:473–476, 1990.
191. Rohr FJ, Doherty LB, Waisbren SE, Bailey IV, Ampola MG, Benacerraf B, Levy HL: The New England Maternal PKU Project: prospective study of untreated and treated pregnancies and their outcomes. J Pediatr 110:391–398, 1987.
192. Rollnick BR, Hoo JJ: Genitourinary anomalies are a component manifestation in the ectodermal dysplasia, ectrodactyly, cleft lip/palate (EEC) syndrome. Am J Med Genet 29:131–136, 1988.
193. Romke C, Froster–Iskenius U, Heyne K, Hohn W, Hof M, Grzejszczyk G, Rauskolb R, Rehder H, Schwinger E: Roberts syndrome and SC phocomelia. A single genetic entity. Clin Genet 31:170–177, 1987.
194. Rosenman Y, Ronen S, Eidelman AI, Schimmel MS: Ankyloblepharon filiforme adnatum: congenital eyelid-band syndromes. Am J Dis Child 134:751–753, 1980.
195. Russo R, D'Armiento M, Martinelli P, Ventruto V: Neu-Laxova syndrome: pathological, radiological, and prenatal findings in a stillborn female. Am J Med Genet 32:136–139, 1989.
196. Salinas CF, Montes GM: Rapp-Hodgkin syndrome: observations on ten cases and characteristic hair changes (pili canaliculi). Birth Defects 24:149–168, 1988.
197. Salinas CF, Pai GS, Vera CL, Militinovic J, Hagerty R, Cooper JD, Cagna DR: Variability of expression of the orofaciodigital syndrome type I in black females: six cases. Am J Med Genet 38:574–582, 1991.
198. Salonen R: The Meckel syndrome: clinicopathologic findings in 67 patients. Am J Med Genet 18:671–689, 1984.
199. Sato T, Iida M, Yamaguchi Y: A family with hereditary ankyloglossia complicated by heterochromia irides and a congenital clasped thumb. Int J Oral Surg 12:359–362, 1983.
200. Say B, Barber DH, Hobbs J, Coldwell JG: A new dominantly inherited syndrome of cleft palate. Humangenetik 26:267–269, 1975.
201. Schilbach U, Rott H-D: Ocular hypotelorism, submucosal cleft palate, and hypospadias: a new autosomal dominant syndrome. Am J Med Genet 31:863–870, 1988.
202. Schinzel A, Hayashi K, Schmid W: Structural aberrations of chromosome 18. II. The 18q- syndrome. Report of three cases. Humangenetik 26:123–132, 1975.
203. Shmid W: Trisomy for the distal third of the long arm of chromosome 19 in brother and sister. Hum Genet 46:263–270, 1979.
204. Schoenecker PL, Capelli AM, Millar EA, Sheen MR, Haher T, Aiona MD, Meyer LC: Congenital longitudinal deficiency of the tibia. J Bone Joint Surg 71:278–287, 1989.
205. Schwartz S, Harris M, Ehrenpreis R, Zaslav A, Raffel LJ, Schwartz MF, Lieber E, Cohen MM: De novo 13q partial duplication identified by cytogenetic, biochemical and molecular approaches. Clin Genet 40:417–422, 1991.
206. Shebib SM, Chudley AE, Reed MH: Spondylometepiphyseal dysplasia congenita, Strudwick type. Pediatr Radiol 21:298–300, 1991.
207. Shprintzen RJ, Siegel-Sadewitz VL, Amato J, Goldberg RB: Anomalies associated with cleft lip, cleft palate, or both. Am J Med Genet 20:585–595, 1985.
208. Spranger J, Maroteaux P: La maladie de Kniest. Arch Fr Pédiatr 30:735–750, 1973.
209. Stern HJ, Graham JM Jr, Lachman RS, Horton W, Bernini PM, Spiegel PK, Bodurtha J, Ives EJ, Bocian M, Rimoin DL: Atelosteogenesis type III: a distinct skeletal dysplasia with features overlapping atelosteogenesis and oto-palato-digital syndrome type II. Am J Med Genet 36:183–195, 1990.
210. Stevenson RE: Campomelia, prenatal fractures, and ankyloglossia superior. Proc Greenwood Center 1:47–51, 1982.
211. Stevenson RE, Ferlauto GJ, Taylor HA: Cutis gyratum and acanthosis nigricans associated with other anomalies: a distinctive syndrome. J Pediatr 99:950–952, 1978.
212. Stewart CR, Kahler SG, Gilchrist JM: Congenital myopathy with malignant hyperthermia and cleft palate: King syndrome? Neurology 37:(Suppl 1):201, 1987.
213. Stewart CR, Kahler SG, Gilchrist JM: Congenital myopathy with cleft palate and increased susceptibility to malignant hyperthermia: King syndrome? Pediatr Neurol 4:371–374, 1988.
214. Strisciuglio P, Sebastio G, Andria G, Maione S, Raia V: Severe cardiac anomalies in sibs with Larsen syndrome. J Med Genet 20:422–424, 1983.
215. Teebi AS, al-Saleh QA, Hassoon MM, Farag TI, al-Awadi SA: Macrosomia, microphthalmia, +/− cleft palate and early infant death: a new autosomal recessive syndrome. Clin Genet 36:174–177, 1989.
216. Temple K, Hall CA, Chitty L, Baraitser M: A case of atelosteogenesis. J Med Genet 27:194–197, 1990.
217. Temtamy S, McKusick V: The Genetics of Hand Malformations, Birth Defects OAS XIV(3). Alan R Liss, New York, 1978, pp 264–265.
218. Temtamy S, McKusick V: The Genetics of Hand Malformations, Birth Defects OAS XIV(3). Alan R Liss, New York, 1978, p 429–437.
219. Temtamy S, McKusick V: The Genetics of Hand Malformations, Birth Defects OAS XIV(3). Alan R Liss, New York, 1978, p 457.
220. Thompson EM, Baraitser M: Sorsby syndrome: a report on further generations of the original family. J Med Genet 25:313–321, 1988.
221. Toriello HV: Heterogeneity and variability in the oral-facial-digital syndromes. Am J Med Genet Suppl 4:149–159, 1988.
222. Torrington M, Beighton P: The ancestry of spondyloepimetaphyseal dysplasia with joint laxity (SEMDJL) in South Africa. Clin Genet 39:210–213, 1991.
223. Traboulsi EI, Lenz W, Gonzales-Ramos M, Siegel J, Macrae WG, Maumenee IH: The Lenz microphthalmia syndrome. Am J Ophthalmol 105:40–45, 1988.
224. Tranebjaerg L, Nielsen KB, Tommerup N, Warburg M, Mikkelsen M: Interstitial deletion 13q: further delineation of the syndrome by clinical and high-resolution chromosome analysis of five patients. Am J Med Genet 29:739–753, 1988.
225. Tuncbilek E, Yalcin C, Atasu M: Aglossia-adactylia syndrome (special emphasis on the inheritance pattern). Clin Genet 11:421–423, 1977.
226. Tuohy PG, Franklin RC: Cleft palate and gonadotropin deficiency. Arch Dis Child 59:580–582, 1984.
227. Tyler DC: Laryngeal cleft: report of eight patients and review of the literature. Am J Med Genet 21:61–75, 1985.
228. Vachvanichsanong P, Jinorose U, Sangnuachua P: Trisomy 14 mosaicism in a 5-year-old boy. Am J Med Genet 40:80–83, 1991.
229. Van Essen AJ, Kok K, van den Berg A, de Jong B, Stellink F, Bos AF, Scheffer H, Buys CH: Partial 3q duplication syndrome and assignment of D3S5 to 3q25–3q28. Hum Genet 87:151–154, 1991.
230. Van Haeringen A, Veenstra F, Maaswinkel-Mooij PD, van de Kamp JJP: Intermittent thrombocytopenia and absent radii: report of a patient with additional unusual manifestations. Am J Med Genet 34:202–206, 1989.
231. Verloes A, Aymé S, Gambarelli D, Gonzales M, Le Merrer M, Mulliez N, Philip N, Roume J: Holoprosencephaly-polydactyly ('pseudotrisomy 13') syndrome: a syndrome with features of hydrolethalus and Smith-Lemli-Opitz syndromes. A collaborative multicentric study. J Med Genet 28:297–303, 1991.
232. Verloes A, Le Merrer M, Davin JC, Wittamer P, Abrassart C, Bricteux G, Briard ML: The orocraniodigital syndrome of Juberg and Hayward. J Med Genet 29:262–265, 1992.
233. Verloove-Vanhorick SP, Brubakk AM, Ruys JH: Extensive congenital malformations in two siblings: Maternal prediabetes or a new syndrome? Acta Paediatr Scand 70:767–769, 1981.

234. Vince JD, Martin NJ: McKusick-Kaufman syndrome: report of an instructive family. Am J Med Genet 32:174–177, 1989.

235. Walker AP, Bocian M: Partial duplication 8q12→q21.1 in two sibs with maternally derived insertional and reciprocal translocations: case reports and review of partial duplications of chromosome 8. Am J Med Genet 27:3–22, 1987.

236. Weaver DD, Williams CPS: A syndrome of microcephaly, mental retardation, unusual facies, cleft palate and weight deficiency. Birth Defects 13:69–84, 1977.

237. Weiss AH, Riscile G, Koussef BG: Ankyloblepharon filiforme adnatum. Am J Med Genet 42:369–373, 1992.

238. White EW, Figueroa R, Flannery DB: Frontofacionasal dysplasia. Am J Med Genet 40:338–340, 1991.

239. Whitley CB, Langer LO Jr, Ophoven J, Gilbert EF, Gonzalez CH, Mammel M, Coleman M, Rosemberg S, Rodriques CJ, Sibley R, et al: Fibrochondrogenesis: lethal, autosomal recessive chondrodysplasia with distinctive cartilage histopathology. Am J Med Genet 19:265–275, 1984.

240. Wullich B, Henn W, Groterath E, Ermis A, Fuchs S, Zankl M: Mosaic tetraploidy in a liveborn infant with features of the DiGeorge anomaly. Clin Genet 40:353–357, 1991.

241. Zunich J, Esterly NB, Holbrook KA, Kaye CI: Congenital migratory ichthyosiform dermatosis with neurologic and ophthalmologic abnormalities. Arch Dermatol 121:1149–1156, 1985.

# V

## THE CRANIUM AND FACE

# 14

# Embryology of the Face

ROBERT J. GORLIN and HAROLD C. SLAVKIN

The prospects for advances in craniofacial developmental biology over the next decade are unprecedented and should lead to a fresh outlook on the interrelationship between the clinical and basic sciences. The same kind of effective union between internal medicine and oncology on the one hand and biochemistry, immunology, microbiology, and pharmacology on the other can be anticipated between developmental biology and pediatrics, otolaryngology, neurology, and maxillofacial plastic surgery. The advances in early detection, prevention, and effective treatment of craniofacial disorders should result in a significant decrease in human suffering and relief from the enormous burdens of lifelong disability.

Embryologists have clearly defined the central problems of developmental biology. These questions include how information encoded within DNA is sequentially expressed to give rise to cell lineages that form tissues and organs, and how the patterns of morphogenesis are created and sustained during development. How does the fertilized egg give rise to the adult organism?

In recent years, molecular biology and genetics have been applied to the problems of embryology, and these collaborations have led to a new intellectual synthesis regarding human development. This chapter provides a primer towards understanding the morphogenetic development of the human face. Our purpose is twofold: (1) to describe highlights of the morphogenetic processes associated with embryonic craniofacial development; and (2) to indicate the advances being made towards a molecular knowledge of how the human face is formed.

## Early craniofacial development

The basic embryology of craniofacial formation has been extensively studied in many species and will only be briefly described here. For more extensive information, the reader is referred to works on the embryological origins of the face[2,7,11,18,28,51,61,62,64,71,79] and the mechanisms of pattern formation of the craniofacial complex.[18,29–31,43,44,47,52,57–59,80,81,89]

The earliest craniofacial formation is directly related to the mechanism of anterior–posterior (A-P) specification of the vertebrate body axis and to the organization of a repetitive body pattern that is a fundamental aspect of embryonic development. Both invertebrate and vertebrate embryonic development includes morphological subdivisions into specialized cephalic segments and trunk segments.[10,28,30,31,42,47,54,60,74,89,90]

In the hierarchy of processes required for early craniofacial embryology, the allocation of specific cell lineages during gastrulation, such as the cephalic axial mesoderm, which gives rise to the notochord, and the morphogenetic gradients during neurulation, result in the formation of the A–P gradient. Morphological characteristics indicate the general subdivision of the anterior neural plate into the forebrain, midbrain, and hindbrain, and the discrete subdivisions into eight rhombomeres (cephalic segments or somitomeres) which subdivide the midbrain (rhombomeres 1 and 2) and hindbrain (rhombomeres 3–8). The hindbrain as a segmented structure may have an extended function in the general patterning of regional diversity within the branchial arches. These cephalic subdivisions appear as morphological bulges as the occipital somites and branchial arches form and the subsequent subdivision of the trunk advances into increasing somite pairs.[30,31,47,54]

Whereas in the trunk the A–P gradient within the paraxial mesoderm is a significant intrinsic source of patterning information for vertebrae and ribs appropriate to their site of origin, in the cephalic or head formation, the specialized neuroectoderm appears to be the source of dorsoventral patterning information for the branchial arches and their special derivatives.[43,44,47,60] How do the A–P and dorsoventral morphogenetic gradients encoded within each rhombomere translate into first branchial arch morphogenesis and the formation of the face?

## Cephalic neural crest

During neurulation, which produces the forebrain, midbrain and hindbrain divisions, the posterior extension of the midbrain forms two morphological bulges called *rhombomeres 1 and 2,* whereas *rhombomeres 3–8* are sequentially generated as subdivisions of the hindbrain.[29–31,47,62,63,87] In tandem, the first branchial arch forms adjacent to rhombomeres 1 and 2. Cell lineage analyses indicate that each rhombomere as well as the sequence of rhombomeres reflects the A–P gradient and also encodes the early prepattern information for the subsequent embryology of the face.[44,54,60,69,74] The lateral margins of the neural plate related to rhombomeres 2, 4, and 6 give rise to the cephalic neural crest cells uniquely associated with the branchial arches and their derivatives.[30,31,74] The cranial neural crest appears to be imprinted with its regional identity prior to cell migrations, and this positional information within neuroectoderm is then translocated from the A–P and dorsoventral gradients within rhombomere segments to the forming branchial arches.[48] These remarkable distinctions between cephalic and trunk segmentation, the cephalic dependence upon neuroectoderm in contrast to the trunk paraxial mesoderm prepatterns, appear to be highly conserved and encoded within regulatory genes called *homeotic genes* which will be considered in more detail in subsequent sections of this chapter.

The basic embryonic morphology of the head is distinct from

that of the trunk. The earliest demarcation of the cephalic end of the embryo is marked by the appearance of the prochordal plate, the fusion of the ectoderm and endoderm that constitutes the buccopharyngeal membrane. In the human embryo, by the end of the third week, the conversion of the inner cell mass into an embryo with three primary germ layers has been completed, and the anteroposterior axis has become established within the primitive ectoderm by formation of the primitive streak at the caudal end of the embryo. This is followed by formation of the neural plate, the neural folds, and, finally, the neural tube, and it is from the ends of the neural folds that the neural crest cells arise.[5,7,24,30,43,44,60,90]

In human neurulation (i.e., formation of the neural tube from the neural plate), closure at the rostral neuropore occurs around the 25th day with closure of the caudal neuropore around the 27th day.[57–59] At about the time of closure, cranial neural crest cells from the dorsal portion of the neural tube separate from the neural plate neuroectoderm and from each other. They disrupt the basement membrane and migrate from rhombomeres 1 and 2 into the underlying extracellular, matrix-rich space between the neuroectoderm and paraxial mesoderm. There, structure and function are as mesenchymal cells, hence the term *ectomesenchyme*. These crest-derived mesenchymal cells invade the forming pharyngeal arches and travel along several stereotypic routes to various locations in the forming face. Crest cells, according to position, have been classified by either their location with respect to A–P segment—cranial, vagal, truncal, and lumbosacral—or with more precise localization to A–P rhombomeres and somites. Each group of crest cells has specific neuronal and non-neuronal derivatives and each has specific potential.

Neural crest cells possess both signalling and receptor systems for intereacting with other cell phenotypes and extracellular matrix molecules. For example, integrin receptors, present on some neural crest cells, adhere preferentially to both fibronectin and laminin. Numerous other cell surface adhesion and substrate molecules (CAMs and SAMs), including proteoglycans, syndecans, heparan sulfate, hyaluronate, glycosyltransferases, and tenascin, are present in the extracellular matrix and mediate cell–cell interactions. Some of these proteins guide crest cell migration.[13]

Onset of neural migration is related to a decrease or loss of particular CAMs and an increase in cell surface (e.g., integrin) receptors for specific extracellular matrix molecules such as fibronectin. These receptors are essential and function in the selective attachments to fibronectin; the glycoprotein forms an open meshwork through which the neural crest cells migrate.[5,74] The space between the network is occupied by hyaluronic acid. Critical is the composition of the extracellular matrix: neural crest cells have a predilection for migration on fibronectin, tenascin, and laminin, but avoid areas rich in chondroitin sulfate proteoglycans.[56]

Interest in the neural crest and its determining role in craniofacial development has been greatly enhanced during the last two decades by the use of such techniques as quail-chick chimeras, fluorescent dye marking, the use of monoclonal antibodies against specific neural crest cells in birds, transgenic mutants, and studies of extracellular matrices against which crest cells interact.[5,24,26,40,49,74,86]

Among its many derivatives, the most rostral neural crest cells (rhombomeres 1 and 2) migrate to populate the frontonasal prominence. They are later joined by cells from the anterior mesencephalic crest. Cells come from the posterior mesencephalic region to populate the maxillae. The mandibular primordia arise from cells derived from both the posterior mesencephalic region and anterior rhombencephalon.[14] These then give rise to the cartilage and bone of the upper face, maxilla, and mandible, to all dental tissues except the enamel, and to cranial sensory ganglia.[92] Crest cells immediately anterior to the otic placode supply second arch structures while crest cells arriving at occipital somites 1–5 (rhombencephalic crest) populate the third, fourth, and sixth pharyngeal arches as well as the nonendothelial layers of the arteries of the branchial arches. There is a small region near the junction of metencephalon and myelencephalon where no neural crest cells migrate.[58] Cells that participate in conotruncal septation migrate ventrally. Trunk crest cells give rise to pigment cells, sensory and sympathetic ganglia, enteric ganglion cells, and adrenomedullary cells. There is patterning such that the more anterior (rostral) elements of the craniofacial skeleton have their origin in the more rostral regions of the neural crest, i.e., migration occurs along specific pathways determined in large part by the axial level of origin. Cranial neural crest cells give rise to cartilage, while truncal neural crest cells do not have this ability, even when grafted to the head. However, when grafted to the more caudal vagal level, vagal derivatives are produced.[34]

The fate of certain cranial neural crest cells seems to depend upon the sequence of their interactions (epigenetic cascades) with other crest cells, prechordal plate, pharyngeal/stomodeal endoderm, other epithelia, mesenchyme, and the developing neural and vascular systems.[75] For example, the interaction of certain neural crest cells, interacting with oral ectoderm, causes the induction of enamel-forming cells, (i.e., ameloblasts) to be differentiated, which in turn causes odontoblasts to be differentiated from the dental papilla, etc. (Tables 14–1 and 14–2).[37,43,84] The same applies to Meckel's cartilage, chon-

**Table 14–1.** Neural derivatives of neural crest cells

| Tissue or structure | Cranial crest derivative | Trunk crest derivative |
|---|---|---|
| Sensory ganglia | Trigeminal (V) | Spinal ganglia |
| | Geniculate (VII) | |
| | Superior (root IX) | |
| | Jugular or vagal (root X) | |
| Parasympathetic | Ciliary | Pelvic plexus |
| | Ethmoid lingual | Remak's ganglion |
| | Otic | |
| | Sphenopalatine | Enteric system (Meissner's and Auerbach's plexi) |
| | Submandibular | Visceral intrinsic |
| | Enteric system | |
| Sympathetic neurons | — | Superior cervical |
| | | Paravertebral chain |
| | | Celiac, mesenteric, adrenal, retroaortic complexes |
| Accessory cells | Glial cells | — |
| | Schwann sheath cells | |
| | Some meningeal cells | |

Based on Slavkin[79] and Jones.[34]

**Table 14–2.** Non-neural derivatives of cranial and trunk neural crest cells

| General cell types | Specific cell types |
|---|---|
| Secretory cells | ACTH-secreting corticotrophic cells |
| | Adrenal medullary chromaffin cells |
| | Thyroid C cells (calcitonin) |
| | Carotid body type I cells |
| | MSH-secreting cells |
| Skeletal and connective tissues (cranial-derived only) | Anterior trabecular cartilage |
| | Chondroblasts in visceral cartilages (e.g., Meckel's cartilage) |
| | Chondroblasts in chondrocranial cartilages |
| | Connective tissue components of adenohypophysis, salivary gland, parathyroids, thyroid, thymus |
| | Connective tissue support of striated muscle |
| | Part of dermis of craniofacies |
| | Osteoblasts in membranous bones |
| | Osteoblasts in alveolar bone |
| | Part of basal plate |
| | Sclera and choroid optic coats |
| Teeth | Dental papilla mesenchyme |
| | Odontoblasts |
| | Cementoblasts |
| | Periodontal ligament fibroblasts |
| Pigmented cells | Melanocytes of skin, hair, irides |
| Muscles | Ciliary muscles |
| | Cranial vasculature |
| | Dermal smooth muscle |
| | Few striated muscles |
| Mesenchyme | Corneal endothelium and stromal fibroblasts |

Based on Slavkin[79] and Jones.[34]

droblasts, osteoblasts, etc.[24–26,83] Meckel's cartilage is derived across all vertebrate species from neural crest cells located at the mesencephalic level of the developing neural tube (rhombomeres 1 and 2). Chondrification of Meckel's cartilage occurs *only* after interaction with oral ectoderm-derived epithelium. In this epithelial–mesenchymal interaction, some element in the basal lamina of the extracellular basement membrane of the epithelium signals cells in the ectomesenchyme to respond to signals that may be hundreds of microns distant.[25] The time when this occurs is species specific (heterochrony). In birds, cranial neural crest cells interact with cranial ectoderm next to the neural tube, and in mammals the mandibular epithelium comes into contact with postmigration crest cells that have reached the arch. Signals from one tissue (e.g., growth and differentiation factors) thus influence proximate tissues to enter specific developmental pathways by signal transduction. Tissue-inductive processes depend upon a plethora of signals (e.g., retinoic acid, epidermal growth factor, insulin-like growth factors, fibroblast growth factors) and their cognate receptors.[80–82] Some of these involve cell–matrix interactions, others cell–cell interactions, while still others involve diffusible molecules, including growth factors (e.g., transforming growth factor isoforms).[3,12,18,66,91] Some interactions stimulate, others inhibit. For example, there is now ample experimental evidence to indicate that growth factors elaborated by the notochord inhibit neural crest cell migration.

Paraxial and lateral plate mesoderm yield cephalic derivatives such as the bones of the calvaria, myoblasts of the branchial arches, extrinsic eye muscles, and hypoglossal muscles.[58,88] Although facial muscles have mesodermal origin, their patterning is specified by the cranial neural crest-derived ectomesenchyme that forms their connective tissue sheaths.[59]

## Embryology of the face

By the end of the fourth week, the anterior neuropore has closed. The forming face consists of a large frontal prominence that constitutes the upper boundary of the stomodeum (primitive mouth) and results from ectodermal proliferation ventral to the developing brain. The primary mouth is separated from the foregut by the buccopharyngeal membrane that undergoes selective cell death (apoptosis) and ruptures at this time in development (Fig. 14–1).[7] On each side of the lower aspect of the frontonasal prominence, the nasal placodes are forming. These bilateral circular structures, located just above the primary mouth, are represented by local thickenings of the surface ectoderm. Rapid proliferation of ectomesenchyme results in nasal swellings both lateral and medial to the nasal placodes. By means of selective cell death, active invagination of epithelia at the base of the olfactory placodes, and greater proliferation of surrounding mesenchymal tissues, the nasal or olfactory pits are formed and extend into the primitive mouth. These are the primitive nostrils. Sulik and Schoenwolf (1985)[85] have elegantly illustrated these changes by scanning electron microscopy (SEM) (Fig. 14–2).

Extremely active growth occurs during the fifth and sixth weeks. The maxillary swellings, which represent the upper anterior portion of the first pharyngeal arch, enlarge considerably, again through ectomesenchymal proliferation.

Around the 7th week, the facial prominences become smooth, the lateral nasal and maxillary prominences forming the lateral wall of the nose. The frontal prominence and maxillary prominences form the eyelids. The nasal pit epithelium burrows to the roof of the stomodeum. The fused epithelia separating them, i.e. the oronasal membrane, degenerates to form the primitive choanae. Failure to do so, due to ingrowth of ectomesenchyme, results in choanal atresia.

The eyes, initially laterally situated and separated by a considerable distance, migrate toward the midline, while the median nasal prominence moves forward and is reduced in width. The central facial T zone (philtrum, columella, nose and interorbital distance) then remains unchanged at 20% of facial width. At about the same time, the median nasal prominences, fuse with the maxillary prominences, forming the upper lip.

During the sixth and seventh weeks, the medial nasal prominences merge with each other and with the bilateral maxillary prominences derived from the first branchial arch. Thus, the upper lip is formed laterally by the maxillary prominences and medially by the fused medial nasal prominences. It should be emphasized that the lateral nasal prominences play no role in formation of the upper lip but form the alae or wings of the

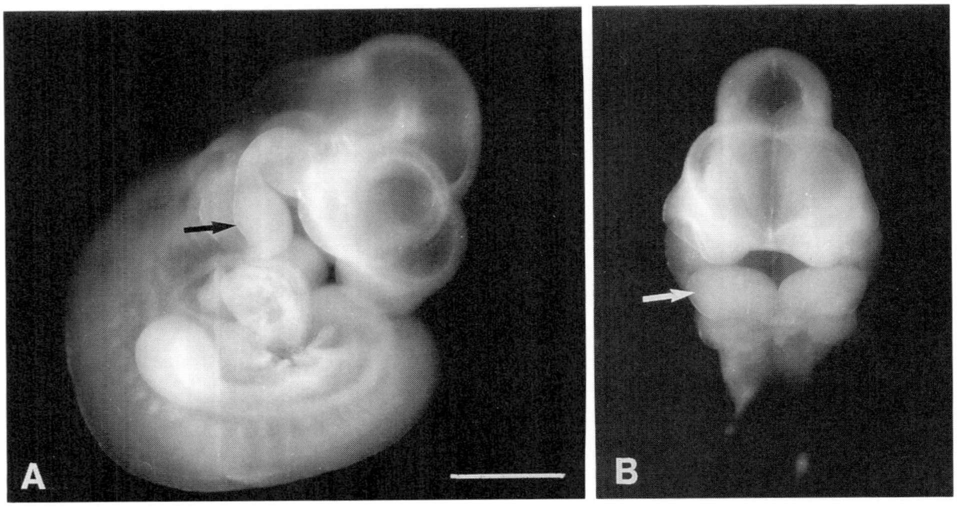


**Fig. 14–1.** The major features of craniofacial morphogenesis are evident during early mammalian development. A: Lateral view of mouse embryo illustrating the first branchial arch-derived mandibular process (arrow). B: Frontal view showing the mandibular process (arrow), stomodeum, maxillary, and nasal processes. Bar line = 1 mm.

nose. The philtral ridges have nothing to do with facial prominences. They do not appear until the third to fourth embryonal month. The mesenchymal continuity of the various prominences (maxillary, lateral nasal, medial nasal) comes together at the base nasal pit, but their free frontal edges undergo epithelial fusion following specialized surface changes in the covering cells, cell death, and alterations in the underlying ectomesenchyme.[28,50,85] The facial groove most marked by these mergings is between the lateral nasal prominence and the maxillary prominence. This is the nasolacrimal groove. The epithelium entrapped in the floor of the groove detaches from the overlying epithelium, canalizes, and becomes the nasolacrimal duct, the upper end of which becomes the lacrimal sac. The canal will ultimately connect the inner canthus of the eye and the inferior meatus of the nasal cavity. The mandibular processes, constituting most of the first arch, merge with each other in the midline. The lower lip is formed entirely from the mandibular process.

## Embryology of the palate

The *primary palate* or premaxillary palate consists of the two merged medial nasal prominences that bulge and coalesce at about the 40th postovulatory day. These form the intermaxillary segment which, in turn, consists of two portions: (1) a labial component that forms the philtrum of the upper lip, that is, the indented area flanked by roughly parallel ridges that run from the columella of the nose to the middle of the upper lip; and (2) the triangular palatal component of bone that includes

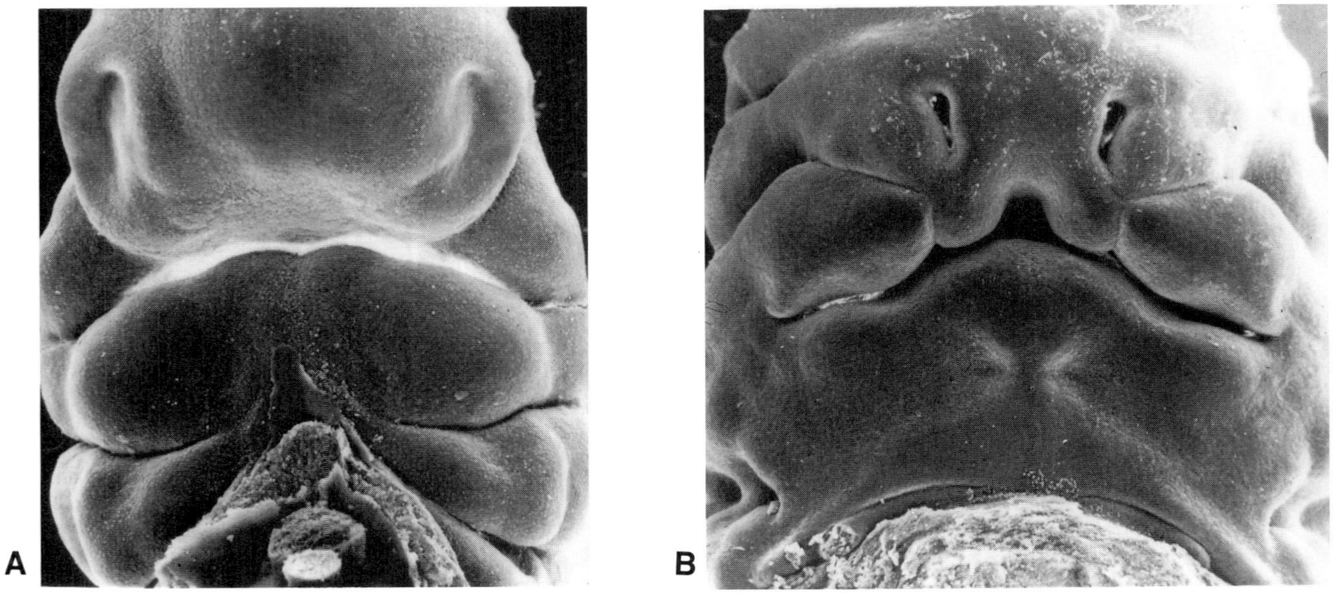


**Fig. 14–2.** (A) Scanning electron micrograph (SEM) of face of a 5-week-old mouse embryo. Note olfactory pits developing on lateral portions of frontonasal prominence. B: SEM of a 6-week-old embryo. Upper lip formed from fusion between notched median nasal prominence has not yet fused with maxillary processes. (A and B courtesy of K. Sulik, Chapel Hill, North Carolina.)

the four maxillary incisor teeth. The primary palate extends posteriorly to the incisive foramen or, clinically, to the incisive papilla. Cranially, the intermaxillary segment is continuous with the rostral part of the nasal septum which is derived from the frontal prominence.[15–17]

The *secondary palate* comprises at least 90% of the hard and soft palates, that is, all except the anterior portion (primary palate) that holds the incisor teeth. Its development appears to be somewhat more complicated than originally thought. The palatal shelves originate as swellings or shelf-like burgeonings of the medial surfaces of the maxillary prominences. They appear in the sixth week. As they encounter the tongue, they are deflected vertically down the sides of the tongue. Elevation of the palatal processes to a horizontal plane is rapid, being more vigorous anteriorly, that is, in the part nearer the primary palate. Elevation begins about the 56th postovulatory day (Fig. 14–3A–D).

What promotes the elevation has been called *intrinsic shelf force* and is associated with local synthesis of growth and differentiation factors as well as glycosaminoglycans, especially hyaluronic acid within the shelf mesenchyme. This causes water imbibition. The force appears to be directed by alignment of collagen fibrils and palatal mesenchyme cells and by epithelial tension, and is possibly mediated by neurotransmitters (e.g., serotonin). Elevation of the shelves is associated with an increase in vertical dimension of the oronasal complex and a widening and forward growth of the mandible, allowing the tongue to drop. Female human embryos elevate their palatal shelves approximately 1 week later than males.[8]

However, whereas programmed cell death has been used to describe the developmental program for the fate of the medial-edge epithelial cells during secondary palate fusion, recent cell lineage analyses provide new evidence for both medial-edge epithelial migrations away from the fusion area and actual transdifferentiation resulting in ectodermallyderived, medial-edge epithelia becoming mesenchymal cells.[15–18,20,77,78] Therefore, palatal fusion appears to involve epithelial cell death, cell migrations, and transdifferentiation, resulting in the final phase of palate formation.

Once the shelves are elevated to the horizontal plane, there is continued differentiation and regional specialization of epithelium. The nasal surface becomes mucus secreting and of a pseudostratified, ciliated columnar nature, while the oral surface becomes keratinized. However, programmed cell death oc-

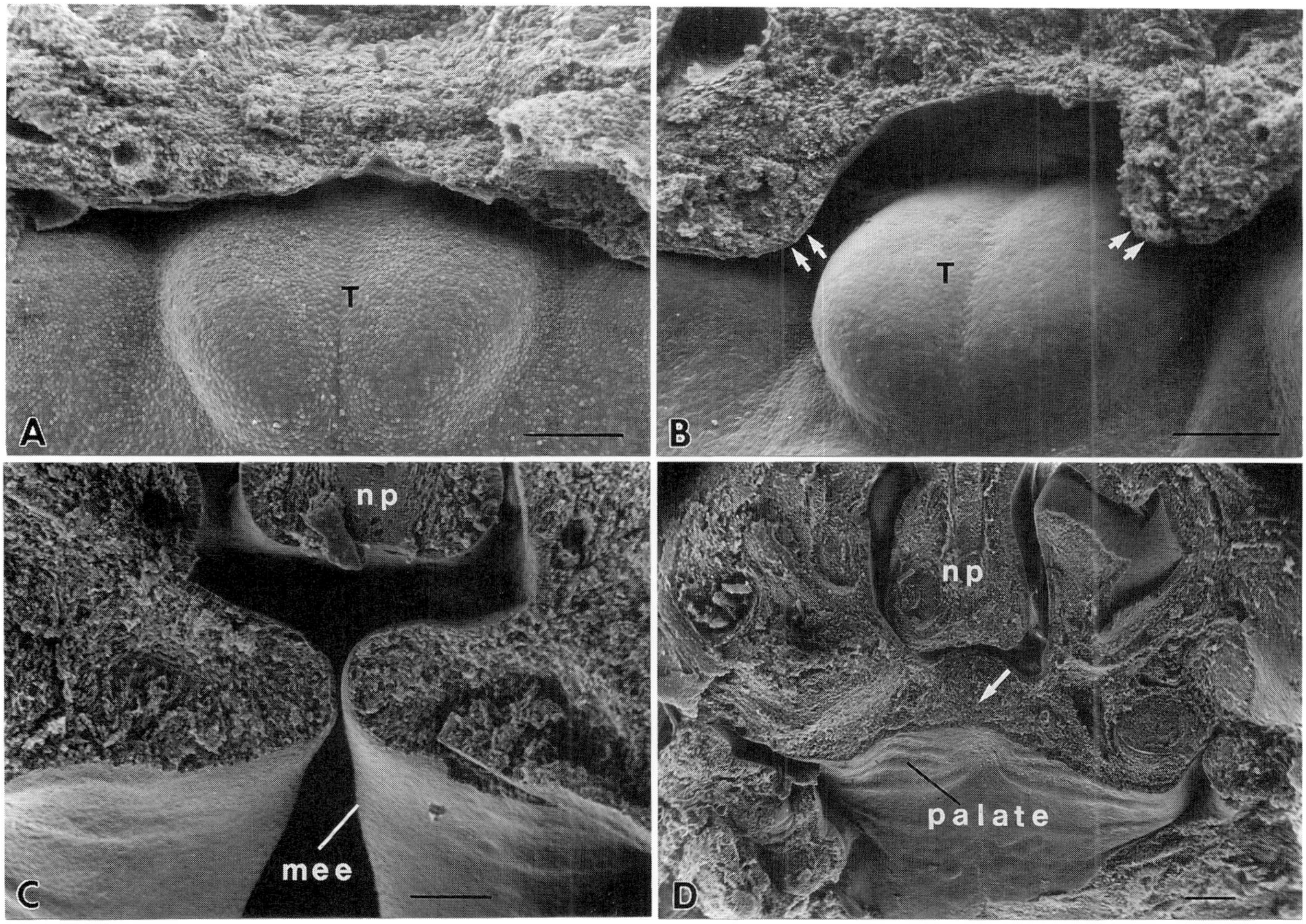


**Fig. 14–3.** Scanning electron micrograph showing major features of secondary palate morphogenesis. Using mouse embryonic specimens, fracture planes were created to visualize the developmental processes associated with secondary palate fusion. A: Prior to intial palatal process formation, the primitive tongue (T, tuberculum impar) is evident and associated with the mandibular process. B: Double arrows indicate forming palatal processes, prior to tongue (T) elevation. C: Medial edge epithelia (mee) approximate and fuse at midline. After fusion, medial edge epithelial cells transform or transdifferentiate into mesenchyme-like cells (see Fitchett and Hay, 1989[20]; Shuler et al, 1992[78]). Note position of nasal process at midline. D: Survey of closed palatal shelves forming the complete palate. Arrow indicates midline of the secondary palate. Note position of nasal process. Bar line = 100 $\mu$m.

curs on the medial edge of each palatal shelf and on the lower edge of the nasal septum. When the palatal shelf and nasal septum edges touch, the epithelium has thinned, forming a seam that has undergone advanced stages of degeneration allowing ectomesenchyme from each side to join in the midline. The mesenchymal cells underlying the epithelium develop extended cell processes and desmosomes develop between contacting epithelial cells. All of these changes are mediated by complex interactions between transmembrane and soluble growth factors, and extracellular matrix molecules.[66,80,81,91] Palatal bone formation is initiated and complete fusion is effected by the tenth week. Final closure, by fusion, occurs somewhat later in females than in males. The soft palate and uvula are formed by merging, not fusion, of two growth centers at the caudal end of the hard palate. Excellent reviews of secondary palate formation are those of Slavkin, (1979),[79] and Ferguson, (1987, 1988).[16,17] In some infants, there is cystic degeneration of the epithelial remnants that produces evanescent midline palatal microcysts (Epstein's pearls).[6,36]

## Genes controlling the geometry of the human face

There are several approaches to identify the developmental control genes for the human face. First, abnormal phenotypes of a mouse mutant can provide clues for specific genes required for craniofacial morphogenesis. For example, the *Patch* (Ph) mutation in mice is a deletion of the gene encoding the platelet-derived growth factor receptor $\alpha$ subunit (PDGFR$\alpha$), which, in homozygous mutant embryos, results in defects in craniofacial structures. Second, one can tag a chromosomal region by insertion of a transgene or retrovirus into the germ line of a mouse.[49] This approach provides a methodology to identify craniofacial malformations after breeding transgenic mice to homozygosity. For example, malformed craniofacial skeletal structures could indicate that the transgene was inserted into a genetic locus essential for normal first branchial arch-derived maxillary and mandibular formations. [29,35,42,54] Finally, human and mouse genes can be identified and characterized by utilizing information from genetically more accessible organisms such as *Drosophilia melanogaster* (fruit fly). This approach has discovered a number of transcriptional control genes associated with early postimplantation processes, including neurulation and branchial arch and limb formations.[73] The result has been the identification of human homeobox (HOX), paired-box (PAX) and pituitary-specific (POU) transcription factor genes.[1,35,73]

A *homeobox* is a region of 183 base pairs that encodes a DNA-binding domain of 61 amino acids and functions as a transcription factor. It appears to be present in three major classes of developmental control genes in *Drosophila,* namely maternal effect genes (e.g., *bicoid),* segmentation genes (e.g., *fushi tarazu*) and homeotic genes (e.g., *antennapedia* and *msh,* muscle-segmentation genes). In mouse, and presumably human, these homeotic genes are organized in four clusters, each spanning more than 100 kilobases on five different chromosomes (i.e., in mouse, *Hox-1* to chromosome 6, *Hox-2* to chromosome 11, *Hox-3* to chromosome 15, *Hox-4* to chromosome 2, and *Hox-7/8* to chromosome 5) (Fig. 14–4).

By examination of the temporal and spatial expression of these transcription factor genes, as well as analysis of several transgene mutants, a number of generalizations can now be made. First, a characteristic of *Hox* and *Pax-1* expression patterns is their transcription during the formation of the anterior–posterior axis in the forming neural plate producing subdivisions or segmented tissue boundaries termed *somitomeres* or *rhombomeres* within the midbrain and hindbrain, and their expression within the paraxial mesoderm resulting in the A–P–segmented somite structures. *HOX-1, -2, -3* and *-4* are all expressed in the forming central nervous tissue and in most somites and their derivatives.[29–31,47] The neuroectoderm of rhombomeres 1 and 2 gives rise to cranial neural crest cells that express *HOX-7* and *HOX-8* transcripts (i.e., related to *Drosophila msh*-genes) during their migrations and within the first branchial arch derivatives (e.g., mandible, tooth organs) and forelimb buds (Fig. 14–5).[18,45,46] *Hox-7* and *Hox-8* genes are candidates for tooth formation and possibly as mutant genes in Treacher Collins syndrome.[18]

Most homeobox genes in mice and humans are organized in four gene clusters on four different chromosomes: *HOX1* on human chromosome 7p21–p14, *HOX2* on human chromosome 17q21–q22, *HOX3* on human chromosome 12q12–q13, and *HOX4* on 2q31–q37. Presumably, these homeobox genes evolved from those of lower organisms by repeated gene duplication and divergence. Homeobox genes are transcribed in early development of conversion of the inner cell mass into a three–germ layer embryo. Expression is continued through midgestation in segmented tissues in the *HOX2* cluster and possibly in others. The domain of expression of any one homeobox gene correlates with its chromosome location, each successive gene being expressed in a zone with a boundary closer to the anterior end of the developing embryo. A homeobox mutation in *MSX2* has been shown to be responsible for Boston-type craniosynostosis.[33]

Lately, other homeobox-containing genes have been isolated that appear to have more divergent sequences and, in contrast to those mentioned above, appear to play a significant role in cell differentiation and organogenesis. One of these, *Hox-7* mapped to chromosome 4p16.1, has been found in the craniofacial processes of mice embryos. Because of its spatial and temporal expressions, it may play a role in cellular differentiation of a number of craniofacial structures such as the anterior pituitary, external ear, and skull bones.[27,32,45,46] Especially interesting papers regarding this differentiation are those of Finkelstein and Boncinelli[19] and Krumlauf.[38]

## Growth and differentiation factors in craniofacial development

Growth and differentiation factors have become epigenetic metaphors for molecular determinants that signal positional information during development.[23,66,91] Many factors and their cognate receptors have been identified and characterized and found to have broad tissue distributions and to elicit biological activities when present at pico- or nanomolar concentrations (e.g., vitamin D metabolites, retinoic acid, and growth and differentiation polypeptide factors). The obvious ubiquity of these signals suggests that processes other than simple diffusion are likely required to regulate the signalling of discrete populations of cells for a specific duration by a specific growth factor. In fact, most growth factors do not passively diffuse from their site of secretion to interact with the nearest cell surface receptor. Rather, these epigenetic regulatory factors contain structural motifs that either inhibit or activate biological activity, or motifs that provide unique binding to substrate adhesion or

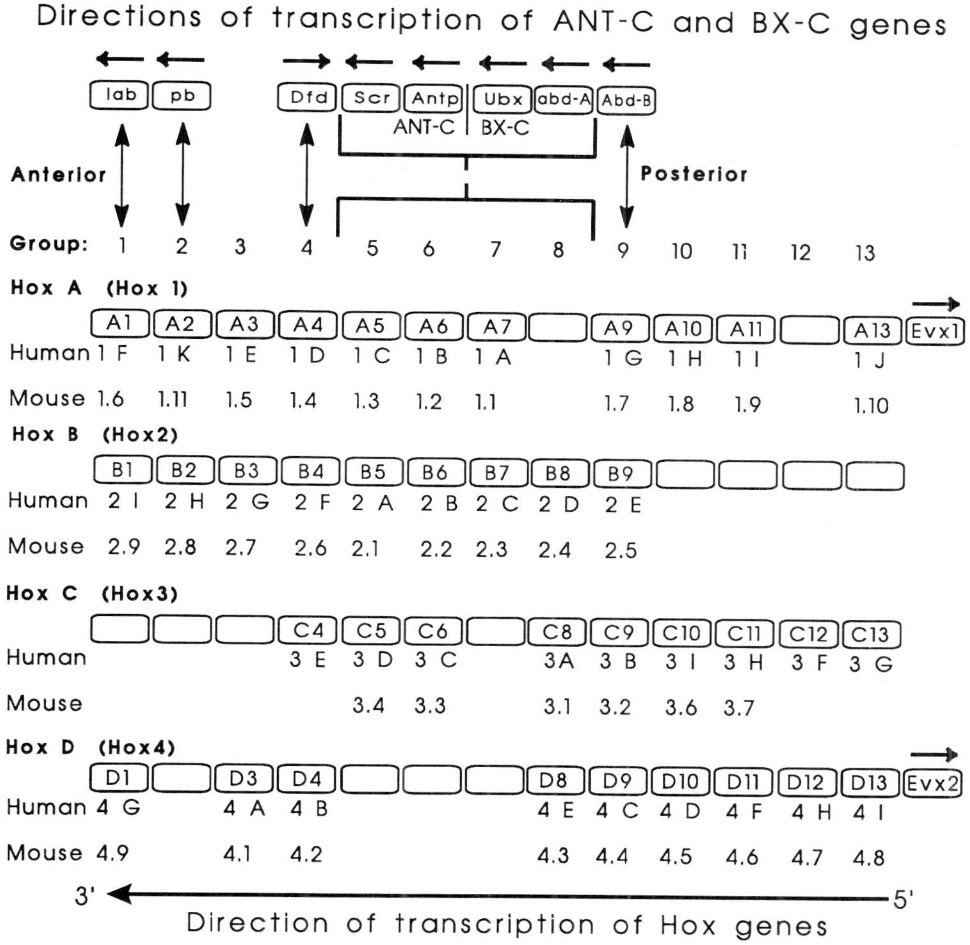


**Fig. 14–4.** New nomenclature for four major mammalian *Hox* complexes (human and mouse) aligned with *Drosophila* genes that established the highly conserved sequence similarity and expression patterns for the relatedness of these transcription regulatory factors. The new nomenclature are single letters (A, B, C, and D) followed by a number from 1 to 13. Empty ovals indicate that no gene has as yet been identified. (Figure redrawn and modifed from Scott, 1992.[73])

extracellular matrix molecules. Such physical properties within the primary structure of these signals provide confinement for growth and differentiation factors to function at precise times and positions during development.[82] Therefore, the specificity of growth factor signalling is derived from its binding to cell surface receptors and/or with motifs within the extracellular matrix molecules. These properties and the specificity of cell adhesion molecules (CAMs, e.g., L-CAM, N-CAM) provide a basis for generating morphogenetic boundaries that precede the genesis of tissue compartments.

What mechanisms control growth factor signalling in time and space? The initiation of growth factor activity can be controlled by two levels of regulation: (1) intracellular processing (e.g., transcription, translation, and secretion from the synthetic cell); and (2) extracellular processing (e.g., activation of the growth factor bioactivity from a latent form [transforming growth factor $\beta$] (TGF-$\beta$), or released from a complex formed with the extracellular matrix [insulin-like growth factors (IGFs), heparin-binding epidermal growth factor (EGF)]. Such processes produce fine and coarse levels to control changes in the concentration of growth factor availability to bind to cognate receptors.

During early embryology of the face (i.e., neurulation, cranial nerve development, cranial neural cell migrations, ganglia formations, branchial arch formations, vascularization, and instructive epithelial–mesenchymal interactions) numerous regionally specified growth and differentiation factors are expressed.[18] Often the key issue is presentation of the bioactivity. How is the regulation of growth factor activity controlled in time and space? There are essentially two strategies: (1) transmembrane domains within the growth factor to anchor the factor in the plasma membrane, allowing the bioactive domain to reside in the extracellular microenvironment (e.g., EGF, TGF-$\alpha$); and (2) soluble growth factors with motifs that bind the growth factors to extracellular matrix components (e.g., heparin-binding EGF, basic fibroblast growth factors [BFGFs], platelet-derived growth factor $\alpha$ [PDGF-$\alpha$]).[82] In both strategies, extracellular proteases provide specific cleavage to liberate or activate the growth factor activity at close range between cells or between cells and their extracellular matrixes.[3,12,21,39,66,91,94]

During craniofacial embryogenesis, these signalling molecules provide cues for the increase or decrease of cell division and DNA synthesis, stimulate postmitotic differential gene expression, induce programmed cell death, inhibit cell migrations, or enhance transdifferentiation. The available evidence argues for multiple growth and differentiation signals rather than one discrete morphogen for each morphogenetic process.

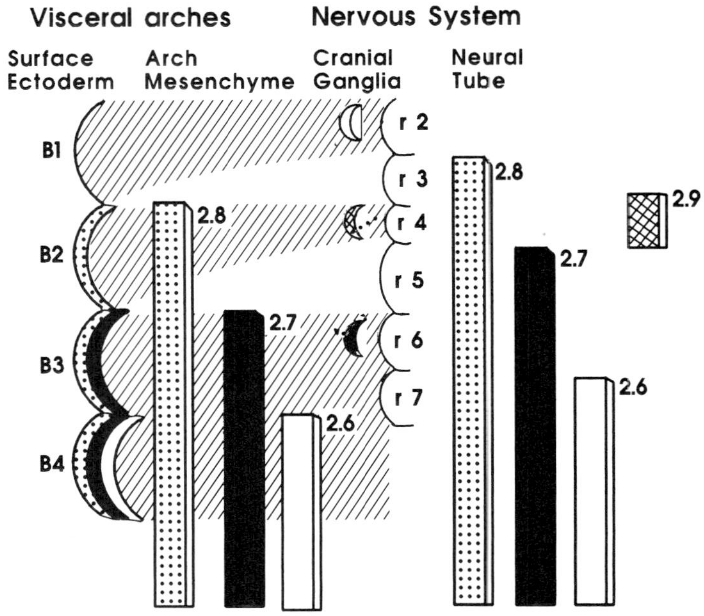


**Fig.14–5.** Schematic representation of cranial neural crest cell migrations, rhombomeres, visceral or branchial arches, and *Hox* 2.6–2.9 gene expression along the cephalic–caudal or anteroposterior axis in mouse embryonic craniofacial development. Diagonal lines indicate migratory pathways for crest cells from neuroectoderm associated with rhombomeres 2, 4, and 6 and branchial arches 1–4. The expression of *Hox* 2.6–2.9 genes is indicated within the neural tube, associated cranial ganglia, and branchial arches 2–4. Drawing is based on the evidence from Hunt et al., 1991.[31] In addition, *Hox* 7 and 8 genes are expressed in the first branchial arch (MacKenzie et al., 1991[45,46]).

For example, IGFs, fibroblast growth factors (FGFs), EGF, and TGF-$\beta$ isoforms all appear to regulate first branchial arch morphogenesis, including cell division, cell migrations, and the timing and position of the craniofacial skeletal constituents.[65,67,72] Recently, Murray and colleagues demonstrated linkage of Rieger syndrome to the region of the EGF gene on chromosome 4.[55] (See summary of Rieger syndrome in Gorlin et al.[22])

Various point mutations within fibroblast growth factor receptors (FGFR) 1 and 2 have been shown to be responsible for a group of craniosynostoses. There are four FGFRs that are membrane-spanning tyrosine kinases. So far, no disorder has been mapped to FGFR4 but achondroplasia, hypochondroplasia, and the thanatophoric dysplasias have been shown to be due to mutations in FGFR3.[4,68,76] Crouzon syndrome, Apert syndrome, Jackson-Weiss syndrome, and Pfeiffer syndrome in some patients are due to various amino acid substitutions in FGFR2.[41,70,93] Still other patients with Pfeiffer syndrome have a mutation in FGFR1.[53] Where different amino acid substitutions cause the same disorder, certain mutations cause different degrees of expression. In Apert syndrome, for example, one substitution effects more severe syndactyly.[9]

## Summary

Pattern formation describes the emergence of temporal and spatial biological organization during development. The mechanisms by which patterns are controlled appear to enlist the integration of many developmental problems, including the control of cell growth, the allocation and determination of specific phenotypes, cell–cell communication, tissue-specific differentiation, differential gene expression, and morphogenesis. The embryology of the human face provides a number of opportunities to understand normal and abnormal development and to discover the remarkable interrelationships between the formation of the midface and lower face structures. Further, it is becoming evident that a prepattern is encoded within the neuroectoderm of the forming cephalic neural plate and that this developmental information resides in the early rhombomeres of the midbrain. It is also evident that cranial neural crest cells from rhombomeres 1 and 2 translocate the encoded information to the perimeter of the first branchial arch and its derivatives. The encoded information, which is translocated from the midbrain rhombomeres to the branchial arch, is related to discrete patterns of homeotic gene expression, retinoic acid receptors, specific growth and differentiation factors and their cognate receptors, and a host of fine controls within cell adhesion, substrate adhesion, and extracellular matrix molecules. Simple diffusion of soluble growth and differentiation factors does not explain the fine controls for craniofacial morphogenesis. Rather, unique intracellular and/or extracellular processing of growth factors provides the controls for time and positional information in the form of patterns of signalling. These patterns are determined and maintained through subtle and sequential cell–extracellular matrix interactions resulting in discrete boundary conditions and subsequent histogenesis. The embryology of the face clearly represents a classical model for pattern formation.

### References

1. Akam M: Hox and HOM: homologous gene clusters in insects and vertebrates. Cell 57:347–349, 1989.

2. Arey LB: Developmental Anatomy, 7th ed. WB Saunders, Philadelphia, 1965.
3. Ayer-le Lievre C, Stahlbom PA, Sara VR: Expression of IGF-I and -II mRNA in the brain and craniofacial region of the rat fetus. Development 111:105–115, 1991.
4. Bellus GA, McIntosh I, Smith EA, Aylesworth AS, Kaitila I, Horton WA, Greenhaw GA, Hecht JT, Francomano CA: A recurrent mutation in the tyrosine kinase domain of fibroblast growth factor receptor 3 causes hypochondroplasia. Nat Genet 10:357–359, 1995.
5. Bronner-Fraser M: Experimental analyses of the migration and cell lineage of avian neural crest cells. Cleft Palate J 27:110–120, 1990.
6. Burdi AR: Distribution of midpalatine cysts: a reevaluation of human palatal closure mechanisms. J Oral Surg 26:41–45, 1968.
7. Burdi AR, Lawton TJ, Grosslight J: Prenatal pattern emergence in early human facial development. Cleft Palate J 25:8–15, 1988.
8. Burdi AR, Silvey RG: Sexual differences in closure of the human palatal shelves. Cleft Palate J 6:1–7, 1969.
9. Cohen MM Jr: Craniosynostoses: phenotypic/molecular correlations. Am J Med Genet 56:334–339, 1995.
10. Conlon RA, Rossant J: Exogenous retinoic acid rapidly induces anterior ectopic expression of murine Hox-2 genes in vivo. Development 116:357–368, 1992.
11. de Beer GR: The Development of the Vertebrate Skull. Clarendon Press, Oxford, 1937, pp 354–373.
12. Dixon MJ, Ferguson MWJ: The effects of epidermal growth factor, transforming growth factors alpha and beta and platelet-derived growth factor on murine palatal shelves in organ culture. Arch Oral Biol 37:395–410, 1992.
13. Duband JL, Thiery JP: Distribution of laminin and collagen during avian neural crest development. Development 101:461–478, 1987.
14. Erickson CA: Morphogenesis of the avian trunk neural crest: use of morphological techniques in elucidating the process. Microsc Res Tech 26:329–351, 1993.
15. Ferguson MWJ: Palatal shelf elevation in the Wistar rat fetus. J Anat 125:555–577, 1978.
16. Ferguson MWJ: Palate development: mechanisms and malformations. Ir J Med Sci 156:309–315, 1987.
17. Ferguson MWJ: Palate development. Development 103:41–60, 1988.
18. Ferguson MWJ: The orofacial region. In: Textbook of Fetal and Perinatal Pathology, Vol 2, JS Wigglesworth, DB Singer, eds. Blackwell Scientific Publications, Boston, 1991, pp 843–880.
19. Finkelstein R, Boncinelli E: From fly head to mammalian forebrain: the story of otd and Otx. Trends Genet 10:310–315, 1994.
20. Fitchett JE, Hay ED: Medial edge epithelium transforms to mesenchyme after embryonic palatal shelves fuse. Dev Biol 131:455–474, 1989.
21. Fitzpatrick DR, Denhez F, Kondaiah P, Akhurst RJ: Differential expression of TGF beta isoforms in murine palatogenesis. Development 109:585–595, 1990.
22. Gorlin RJ, Cohen, MM Jr, Levin LS: Syndromes of the Head and Neck, 3rd ed. Oxford University Press, New York, 1990, pp 859–860.
23. Gurdon JB: Embryonic induction—molecular prospects. Development 99:285–306, 1987.
24. Hall BK: The Neural Crest. Oxford University Press, London, 1988.
25. Hall BK: The embryonic development of bone. Am Sci 76:174–181, 1988.
26. Hall, BK: Evolutionary issues in craniofacial biology. Cleft Palate J 27:95–100, 1990.
27. Hill RE, Jones PF, Rees AR, Sime CM, Justice MJ, Copeland NG, Jenkins NA, Graham E, Davidson DR: A new family of mouse homeo box-containing genes: molecular structure, chromosomal location and developmental expression of Hox 7.1. Genes Dev 3:26–37, 1989.
28. Hinrichsen K: The early development of morphology and patterns of the face in the early human embryo. Adv Anat Embryol Cell Biol 98:1–79, 1985.
29. Holland PWH: Homeobox genes and the vertebrate head. Development 103(Suppl):17–24, 1988.
30. Hunt P, Gulisano M, Cook M, Sham MH, Faiella A, Wilkinson D, Boncinelli E, Krumlauf R: A distinct Hox code for the branchial arch region of the vertebrate head. Nature 353:861–864, 1991.
31. Hunt P, Whiting J, Muchamore I, Marshall H, Krumlauf R: Homeobox genes and models for patterning the hindbrain and branchial arches. Development 1:187–196, 1991.
32. Ivens A, Flavin N, Williamson R, Dixon M, Bates G, Buckingham M, Robert B: The human homeobox gene HOX 7 maps to chromosome 4p16 and may be implicated in Wolf-Hirschhorn syndrome. Hum Genet 84:473–476, 1990.
33. Jabs EW, Müller U, Li X, Ma L, Luo W, Haworth IS, Klisak I, Sparkes R, Warman ML, Mulliken JB, Snead ML, Maxson R: A mutation in the homeodomain of the human *MSX2* gene in a family affected with autosomal dominant craniosynostosis. Cell 75:443–450, 1993.
34. Jones MC: The neurocristopathies: reinterpretation based upon the mechanism of abnormal morphogenesis. Cleft Palate J 27:136–140, 1990.
35. Kessel M, Gruss P: Murine developmental control genes. Science 249:374–379, 1990.
36. Kitamura H: Epithelial remnants and pearls in the secondary palate in the human abortus: a contribution to the study of the mechanism of cleft palate formation. Cleft Palate J 3:240–257, 1966.
37. Kollar EJ: Epithelial-mesenchymal interactions in the mammalian integument: tooth development as a model for instructive induction. In: Epithelial-Mesenchymal Interactions in Development, RH Sawyer, JF Fallon, eds. Praeger Publishing, New York, 1983, pp 27–49.
38. Krumlauf R: Hox genes in vertebrate development. Cell 78:191–201, 1994.
39. Lamson G, Giudice LC, Rosenfeld RG: Insulin-like growth factor binding proteins: structural and molecular relationships. Growth Factors 5:19–28, 1991.
40. Le Douarin NM: Cell recognition based on natural morphological nuclear markers. Med Biol 52:281–319, 1974.
41. Li X, Lewanda AF, Eluma F, Jerald H, Choi H, Alozie I, Proukakis C, Talbot CC Jr, Kolk CV, Bird LM, Jones MC, Cunningham M, Clarren SK, Pyeritz RE, Weissenbach J, Jackson CE, Jabs EW: Two craniosynostotic syndrome loci, Crouzon and Jackson-Weiss, map to chromosome 10q23–q26. Genomics 22:418–424, 1994.
42. Lufkin T, Dierich A, LeMeur M, Mark M, Chambon P: Disruption of the Hox 1.6 homeobox gene results in defects in a region corresponding to its rostral domain of expression. Cell 66:1105–1119, 1991.
43. Lumsden AGS: Spatial organization of the epithelium and the role of neural crest cells in the initiation of the mammalian tooth germ. Development 103:155–169, 1988.
44. Lumsden A, Sprawson N, Graham A: Segmental origin and migration of neural crest cells in the hindbrain region of the chick embryo. Development 113:1281–1291, 1991.
45. MacKenzie A, Ferguson MWJ, Sharpe PT: Hox-7 expression during murine craniofacial development. Development 113:601–611, 1991.
46. MacKenzie A, Leeming GL, Jowett AK, Ferguson MWJ, Sharpe PT: The homeobox gene Hox 7.1 has specific regional and temporal expression patterns during early murine craniofacial embryogenesis, especially tooth development in vivo and in vitro. Development 111:269–285, 1991.
47. Maden M, Hunt P, Eriksson U, Kuroiwa A, Krumlauf R, Summerbill D: Retinoic acid-binding protein, rhombomeres and the neural crest. Development 111:35–43, 1991.
48. Maderson PFA: Development and Evolutionary Aspects of the Neural Crest. John Wiley and Sons, New York, 1987.
49. Mansour SL, Goddard JM, Capecchi MR: Mice homozygous for a targeted disruption of the proto-oncogene *int-2* have developmental defects in the tail and inner ear. Development 117:13–28,1993.
50. Millikovsky G, Johnston MC: Active role of embryonal facial epithelium: new evidence of cellular events in morphogenesis. J Embryol Exp Morphol 63:53–66, 1981.
51. Moore KL: The Developing Human: Clinically Oriented Embryology, 3rd ed. WB Saunders, Philadelphia, 1982, pp 179–215.
52. Morriss-Kay G, Tucket F: Early events in mammalian craniofacial morphogenesis. J Craniofac Genet Dev Biol 11:181–191, 1991.
53. Muenke M, Schell T, Hehr A, Robin NH, Losken HW, Schinzel A, Pulleyn LJ, Rutland P, Reardon W, Malcolm S, Winter RM: A common mutation in the fibroblast growth factor receptor 1 gene in Pfeiffer syndrome. Nat Genet 8:269–273, 1994.
54. Murphy P, Hill RE: Expression of the mouse labial-like homeobox-containing genes, Hox 2.9 and Hox 1.6, during segmentation of the hindbrain. Development 111:61–74, 1991.
55. Murray JC, Bennett SR, Kwitek AE, Small KW, Schinzel A, Alward WLM, Weber JL, Bell GI, Buetow KH: Linkage of Rieger syndrome to the region of the epidermal growth factor gene on chromosome 4. Nat Genet 2:46–49, 1992.
56. Newgreen DF, Erickson CA: The migration of neural crest cells. Int Rev Cytol 103:89–145, 1986.
57. Noden DM: The role of the neural crest in patterning of avian cranial skeletal, connective and muscle tissues. Dev Biol 96:144–165, 1983.
58. Noden DM: Origins and patterning of craniofacial mesenchymal tissues. J Craniofac Genet Dev Biol (Suppl) 2:15–31, 1986.

59. Noden DM: Patterning of avian craniofacial muscles. Dev Biol 116:347–356, 1986.
60. Noden DM: Cell movements and control of patterned tissue assembly during craniofacial development. J Craniofac Genet Dev Biol 11:192–213, 1991.
61. O'Rahilly R: The timing and sequence of events in the development of the human eye and ear during the embryonic period proper. Anat Embryol 168:87–99, 1983.
62. O'Rahilly R, Gardner E: The timing and sequence of events in the development of the human nervous system during the embryonic period proper. Z Anat Entwickl Gesch 134:1–12, 1971.
63. O'Rahilly R, Müller F: Neurulation in the normal human embryo. In: Neural Tube Defects (Ciba Foundation Symposium 181), G Bock, J Marsh, eds. John Wiley and Sons, Chichester, 1994, pp 70–89.
64. Patten BM: Human Embryology, 2nd ed. Blakiston, (Division of McGraw-Hill), New York, 1953.
65. Pelton RW, Hogan BLM, Miller DA, Moses HL: Differential expression of genes encoding TGFs b1, b2, and b3 during murine palate formation. Dev Biol 141:456–460, 1990.
65a. Przylepa KA, Paznekas W, Zhang M, Golabi M, Bias W, Manshad MJ, Carey JC, Hall BD, Stevenson R, Orlow SJ, Cohen MM Jr, Jabs EW: Fibroblast growth factor receptor 2 mutations in Beare-Stevenson cutis gyrata syndrome. Nat Genet 13:492–494, 1996.
66. Rosenblum IY, Heyner S: Growth Factors in Mammalian Development. CRC Press, Boca Raton, 1989.
67. Rotwein P: Structure, evolution, expression and regulation of insulin-like growth factors I and II. Growth Factors 5:3–18, 1991.
68. Rousseau F, Saugier P, LeMerrer M, Munnich A, Delezoide A-L, Maroteaux P, Bonaventure J, Narcy F, Sanak M: Stop codon *FGFR3* mutations in thanatophoric dwarfism type 1. Nat Genet 10:11–12, 1995.
69. Ruberte E, Dolle P, Chambon P, Morris-Kay G: Retinoic acid receptors and cellular retinoid binding proteins. Their differential pattern of transcription during early morphogenesis in mouse embryos. Development 111:45–60, 1991.
70. Rutland P, Pulleyn LJ, Reardon W, Baraitser M, Hayward R, Jones B, Malcolm S, Winter RM, Oldridge M, Slaney SF, Poole MD, Wilkie AOM: Identical mutations in the *FGFR2* gene cause both Pfeiffer and Crouzon syndrome phenotypes. Nat Genet 9:173–176, 1995.
71. Sadler TW: Langman's Medical Embryology, 6th ed. Williams & Wilkins, Baltimore, 1990.
72. Sara VR, Hall K: Insulin-like growth factors and their binding proteins. Physiol Rev 70:591–614, 1990.
73. Scott MP: Vertebrate homeobox gene nomenclature. Cell 71:551–553, 1992.
74. Serbedzija GN, Bronner-Fraser M, Fraser SE: Vital dye analysis of cranial neural crest cell migration in the mouse embryo. Development 116:297–307, 1992.
75. Sharpe PM, Ferguson MWJ: Mesenchymal influences on epithelial differentiation in developing systems. J Cell Sci (Suppl)10:195–230, 1988.
76. Shiang R, Thompson LM, Zhu Y-Z, Church DM, Fielder TJ, Bocian M, Winokur ST, Wasmuth JJ: Mutations in the transmembrane domain of FGFR3 cause the most common genetic form of dwarfism, achondroplasia. Cell 78:335–342, 1994.
77. Shuler CF, Guo Y, Majumder A, Luo RY: Molecular and morphologic changes during the epithelial-mesenchymal transformation of palatal shelf medial edge epithelium in vitro. Int J Dev Biol 35:463–472, 1991.
78. Shuler CF, Halpern DE, Guo Y, Sank AC: Medial edge epithelium fate traced by cell lineage analysis during epithelial-mesenchymal transformation in vivo. Dev Biol 154:318–330, 1992.
79. Slavkin HC: Craniofacial Developmental Biology. Lea & Febiger, Philadelphia, 1979.
80. Slavkin HC: Cellular and molecular determinants during craniofacial development. In: Craniofacial Malformations, M Stricker, J Van der Meulen, B Raphael, R Mazzola, eds. Churchill Livingstone, Edinburgh, 1990, pp 15–26.
81. Slavkin HC: Regulatory issues during early craniofacial development: a summary. Cleft Palate J 27:101–109, 1990.
82. Slavkin HC: Perspective on morphogenesis. In: Fundamentals of Bone Growth: Methodology and Applications, AD Dixon, BG Sarnat, DAN Hoyte, eds. CRC Press, Boca Raton, 1991, pp 23–33.
83. Smith L, Thorogood P: Transfilter studies on the mechanism of epitheliomesenchymal interaction leading to chondrogenic differentiation of neural crest cells. J Embryol Exp Morphol 75:165–168, 1983.
84. Smith MM, Hall BK: Development and evolutionary origins of vertebrate skeletogenic and odontogenic tissues. Biol Rev 65:277–373, 1990.
85. Sulik KK, Schoenwolf GC: Highlights of craniofacial morphogenesis in mammalian embryos as revealed by scanning electron microscopy. Scanning Electron Microsc 4:1735–1752, 1985.
86. Tan SS, Morriss-Kay G: The development and distribution of the cranial neural crest in the rat embryo. Cell Tissue Res 240:403–416, 1985.
87. Tan SS, Morriss-Kay G: Analysis of cranial neural crest cell migration and early fates in postimplantation rat chimaeras. J Embryol Exp Morphol 93:21–58, 1986.
88. Thorogood P: The developmental specification of the vertebrate skull. Development 103 (Suppl 1):141–153, 1988.
89. Veermeij-Keers C: Craniofacial embryology and morphogenesis: normal and abnormal. In: Craniofacial Malformations, M Stricker, JC Van der Meulen, B Raphael, R Mazzola, eds. Churchill Livingstone, Edinburgh, 1990, pp 27–60.
90. Verwoerd CDA, van Oostrom CG: Cephalic neural crest and placodes. Adv Anat Embryol Cell Biol 58:1–75, 1979.
91. Waterfield MD: Growth factors in cell and developmental biology. Cell Sci 13 (Suppl):1–208, 1990.
92. Wedden SE, Ralphs JR, Tickle C: Pattern formation of the facial primordia. Development 103 (Suppl):31–40, 1988.
93. Wilkie AOM, Slaney SF, Oldridge M, Poole MD, Ashworth GJ, Hockley AD, Hayward RD, David DJ, Pulleyn LJ, Rutland P, Malcolm S, Winter RM, Reardon W: Apert syndrome results from localized mutations of *FGFR2* and is allelic with Crouzon syndrome. Nat Genet 9:165–172, 1995.
94. Williams JM, Robinson RA, Solursh M: Immunohistochemical localization of TGF-$\beta_1$ during morphogenetic movements of the developing mouse palate. J Craniofac Gen Dev Biol 11:138–145, 1991.

# 15

# Major Craniofacial Anomalies

MARIE-LUCIE LESSARD and JOHN B. MULLIKEN

The incidence of major craniofacial anomalies is 1:5,000 to 1:100,000 live births, compared to 1:1,000 for cleft lip/palate and 0.4/1,000 for cleft palate. Many of these are genetic in origin; most cases are sporadic, the result of a spontaneous mutation. Many are also syndromic, i.e., associated with developmental errors outside the craniofacial region. The specialty of craniofacial surgery was fathered by Paul Tessier during the last quarter century. Now the major craniofacial malformations can be surgically mended, with varying success, based on the principles and techniques of Tessier and his disciples. As this century ends, another epoch in craniofacial biology is beginning: the search for the molecular basis of normal and abnormal craniofacial development.

This is a review of the uncommon craniofacial anomalies. The most important conditions are discussed in order of incidence, from the most to the least frequent. The disorders are listed and illustrated with drawings of the bony and soft tissue abnormalities in Figures 15–1, 15–2 and 15–3: the malformations are listed from high to low incidence, from top to bottom. The unique and very rare are omitted by necessity of space. Robin sequence is discussed elsewhere in this text. The principles of operative treatment are given for each subgroup whereas operative techniques are referenced.

## Multidisciplinary craniofacial team

Surgical correction of major craniofacial deformities requires answers to the following questions: what to do, when to do it, how much to do, and how to assess the outcome. Experience in planning procedures and handling intra- and postoperative complications is critical. One craniofacial team is probably adequate for a population of 10–20 million.[87] With the growth of the specialty, the patient population is, in several geographic areas, insufficient to maintain surgical expertise and to support clinical research. There are 228 craniofacial and cleft lip teams listed in 36 centers of the United States.[128]

Children with major craniofacial anomalies deserve to be evaluated and cared for in university-based referral centers. Typically, the craniofacial teams see patients on a weekly or biweekly basis. Furthermore, most teams find that separate meetings are necessary for orthodontic and surgical planning, communication with referring physicians, dental colleagues and patients, as well as for review of clinical and basic research projects. Each craniofacial unit varies depending on the particular specialty interests and expertise. The ideal craniofacial program might include the following specialists, listed in alphabetic order. An asterisk indicates team members who are usually present at clinical sessions.

- Anesthesiologist (pediatric)
- Anthropologist
- Audiologist*
- Dentist or orthodontist*
- Epidemiologist
- Geneticist or dysmorphologist*
- Neurologist
- Neuroradiologist
- Neurosurgeon
- Nurse practitioner*
- Ophthalmologist
- Oral and maxillofacial surgeon*
- Otolaryngologist*
- Pediatrician
- Plastic surgeon*
- Psychiatrist or psychologist*
- Social worker*
- Speech therapist*
- Statistician
- Team coordinator*

## Craniofacial surgery—general concepts

Proper diagnosis is fundamental to any treatment plan. Other components that influence decision-making include facial growth chronology, bone thickness for bone grafting, and adequate fixation. All these aspects are applicable to the congenital malformations being discussed. Concepts are presented separately prior to the description of each entity.

The surgical techniques have been grouped following description of the syndromic and nonsyndromic craniosynostoses. Hemifacial microsomia, Treacher Collins syndrome, and orbital hypertelorism are different and have specific surgical strategies.

The following subjects are summarized prior to describing the syndromic and nonsyndromic malformations: (1) craniofacial growth; (2) Le Fort terminology; (3) bone grafting; and (4) plating systems.

### Craniofacial growth

Surgical planning takes into account the accelerated cranial growth that parallels brain growth during the first 2 years of life. At birth the cranium is already 65% of adult size; it reaches 85% by age 3–4 and 95% by 10 years. On the other hand, the facial skeleton at birth is only 40%–45% of its adult size, and only 65% at 10 years of age.[95] Midfacial and maxillary projection is completed in adolescence; mandibular growth accelerates at age 12 and is not completed until age 15–16 in girls and age 17–18 in boys. As a basic principle, cranial anomalies that restrict brain growth should be operated upon between 3 and 8 months of life to avoid brain compression and allow normal growth and shape. Most facial deformities can be corrected later, unless there are functional consequences.

# Non-Syndromic craniosynostoses (NSC)

## Scaphocephaly

(Dolichocephaly)

- 21-57% of NSC
- Incidence: 1:4200-8500
- Rarely familial
- "Boat-like" skull shape
- Frontal and occipital bossing
- Increased intracranial pressure (20%)

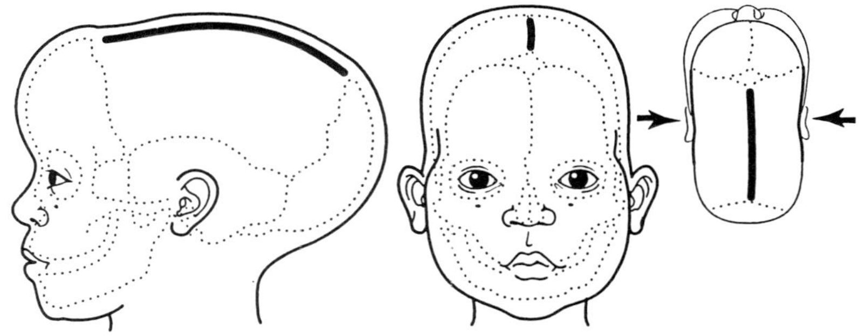

*Premature fusion of sagittal suture*

## Synostotic Frontal Plagiocephaly (SFP)

(Unilateral coronal synostosis)

- 10-20% of NSC
- Incidence: 1:10,000
- Rarely familial
- Increased intracranial pressure (14%)
- Ipsilateral flattened forehead brow elevation, and wide palpebral fissure
- Contralateral frontal bossing
- Ipsilateral deviation of nasal root
- Anteriorly displaced ipsilateral auricle
- Contralateral head-tilt / "ocular torticollis" (14%)
- X-Ray: "harlequin sign" (elevated lesser wing of sphenoid)

* SFP to be differentiated from DFP (DFP = deformational frontal plagiocephaly)

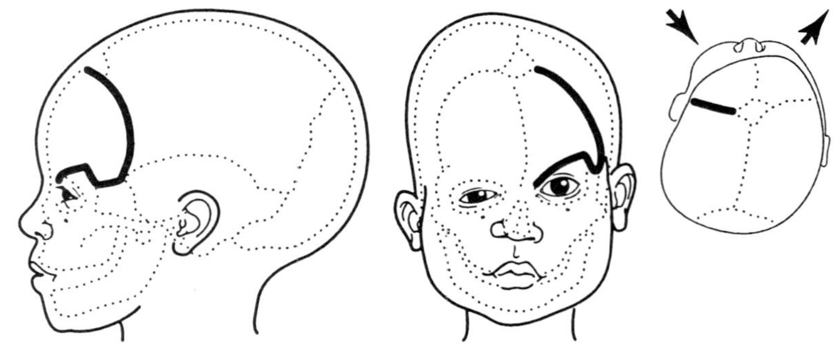

*Premature fusion of coronal suture*

## Brachycephaly

- 6-12% of NSC
- Skull: short anteroposterior diameter
- Acrocephaly (oxycephaly)
- Compensatory increase in bitemporal width
- Supraorbital recession

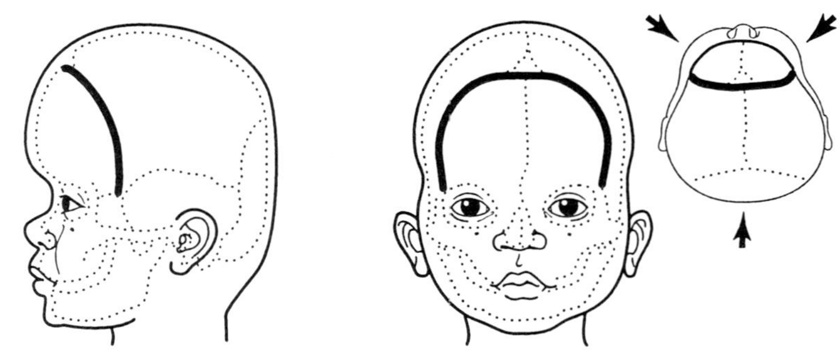

*Premature fusion of coronal suture*

## Trigonocephaly

- 4-5% of NSC
- Triangular forehead
- Rarely genetic: 9p- & trisomy 13 syndromes
- Metopic "keel" ridge
- Hypotelorism (decreased inter-orbital distance)

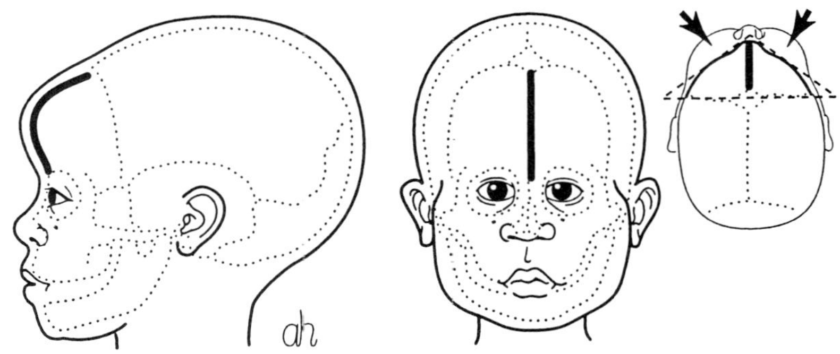


*Premature fusion of metopic suture*

**Fig. 15–1.** Non-syndromic craniosynostoses.

# Syndromic craniosynostoses

*Premature fusion of skull base*

## Saethre-Chotzen Syndrome

- **Chromosome:** 7p (7p21-p22)
- **Gene:** unknown
- **Autosomal dominant**
- Incidence: very common craniosynostosis
- Brachyturricephaly
- Low frontal hairline
- Blepharoptosis (85%)
- Tear duct stenosis
- Minor auricular anomalies (80%)
  - low set rotated ears
  - prominent helical crus
- Beaked nose: depressed nasofrontal region with septal deviation
- No maxillary hypoplasia
- Congenital heart defect (33%)
- **Hand Anomalies:** brachysyndactyly, index and middle fingers

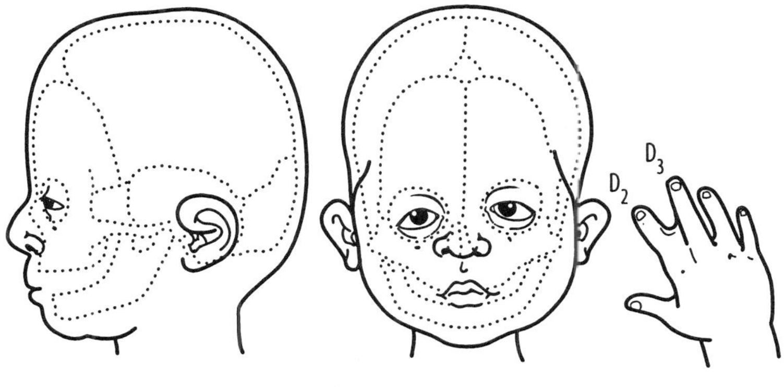


## Crouzon Syndrome

- **Chromosome:** 10q (10q25.3-q26)
- **Gene:** FGFR2
- **Autosomal dominant**
- Most cases sporadic, 10 % familial
- Incidence: 1:25,000
- Brachycephaly
- Exorbitism: (75%)
- Maxillary hypoplasia
- Relative mandibular prognathism
- Conductive hearing loss (50%)
- Cervical spine anomalies
- Chiari I malformation (30%) and cervical syringomyelia (10%)
- **No hand anomalies in most cases**

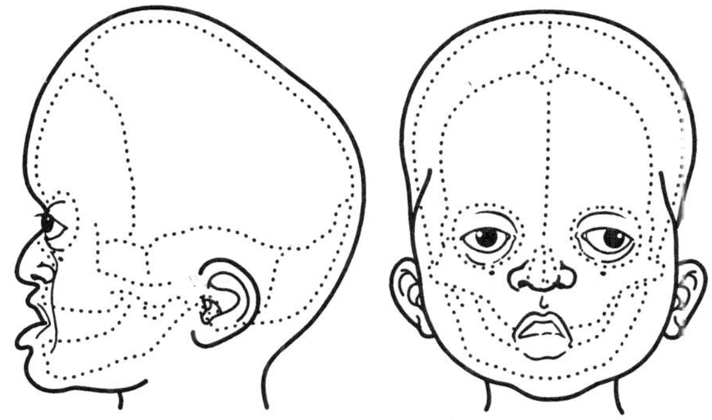

## Apert Syndrome

- **Chromosome:** 10q (10q25.3-q26)
- **Gene:** FGFR2
- **Autosomal dominant**
- Most cases sporadic
- Incidence: 1:72,990
- 4.5% of all craniosynostoses
- Oxycephaly, brachycephaly
- Exorbitism, hypertelorism
- Maxillary hypoplasia +/- V-shaped dental arch
- Relative mandibular prognathism: Class III malocclusion
- Acne vulgaris (70%)
- Cardiovascular and genito-urinary anomalies (10%)
- Cervical spine anomalies C5-C6
- **Hand Anomalies:** complex syndactyly
- **Foot Anomalies:** complex syndactyly

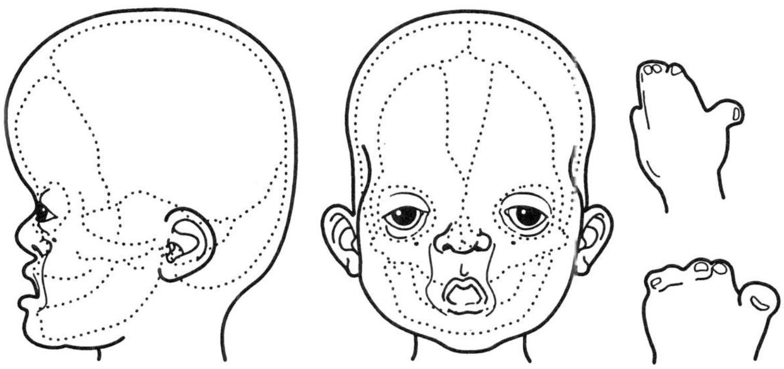

## Pfeiffer Syndrome

- **Chromosome:** 8p (8p11.2-p12) **Gene:** FGFR1
  10q (10q25.3-q26) **Gene:** FGFR2
- **Autosomal dominant**
- Incidence: unknown
- Turribrachycephaly
- Ocular proptosis
- Downslanting palpebral fissures
- Midface hypoplasia variable, Class III malocclusion
- Cervical spine anomalies
- **Hand anomalies:** broad thumbs variable
- **Foot anomalies:** broad great toes

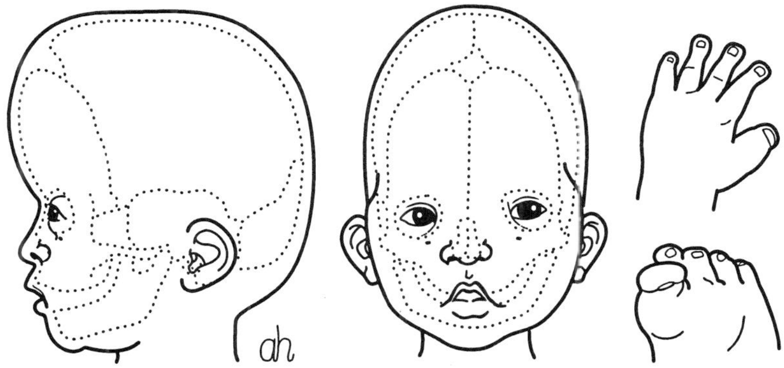

**Fig. 15–2.** Syndromic craniosynostoses.

## Carpenter Syndrome

- **Chromosome:** unknown
- **Autosomal recessive**
- Incidence: rare
- Craniosynostosis
- Tower-shaped skull (oxycephaly)
- Telecanthus
- Mental retardation
- Congenital heart disease
- Coxa valga/pes varus
- Hypogenitalism
- **Hand anomalies:**
  clinodactyly & short digits (D3 & D4)
- **Foot anomalies:**
  preaxial polysyndactyly

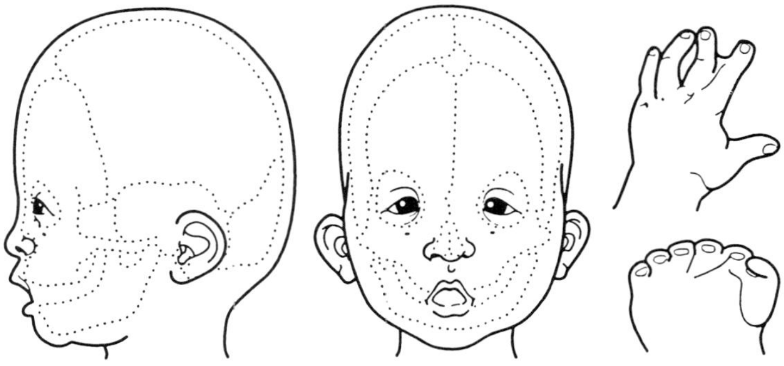

# Other craniofacial anomalies

## Hemifacial Microsomia
(Oculoauriculovertebral spectrum/Otomandibular dysostosis/
1st & 2nd branchial arch anomaly)

- **Chromosome:** unknown
- **Gene:** unknown
- Inheritance: sporadic
- Etiology: heterogeneous
- Incidence: 1: 5000
- Unilateral (85%)
- Underdevelopment of temporal bone & zygoma
- Epibulbar dermoids (20%)
- Microtia, preauricular skin tags (40%)
- Mandibular hypoplasia to absent ramus (100%)
- Abnormal glenoid fossa in severe cases
- Unilateral macrostomia (40%)
- Facial nerve palsy (10-50%)
- Extra-craniofacial anomalies:
  skeletal, cardiac, pulmonary, renal, GI

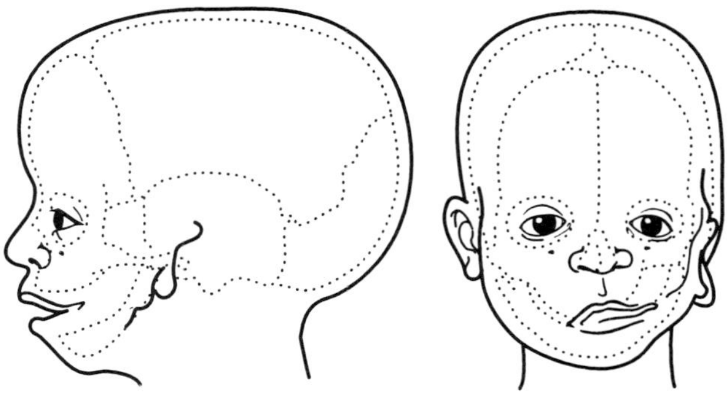

## Treacher Collins Syndrome
(Franceschetti-Zwahlen-Klein syndrome / Mandibulofacial dysostosis *)

- **Chromosome:** 5q (5q32-q33.1)
- **Autosomal dominant**
- **Gene:** unknown
- Incidence: 1:3500-5642
- 2:1 male to female ratio
- Absence or hypoplasia of zygomas
- Coloboma (notching of the lateral lower eyelids)
- Missing eyelashes, medial third
- Microtia & middle ear anomalies
- Choanal stenosis
- Mandible: micrognathia & microgenia
- Macrostomia: bilateral
- Cleft palate: 1/3 cases
- X-Ray: cleft of the inferolateral orbit
- Normal intelligence
- No facial nerve weakness

*Always symmetric

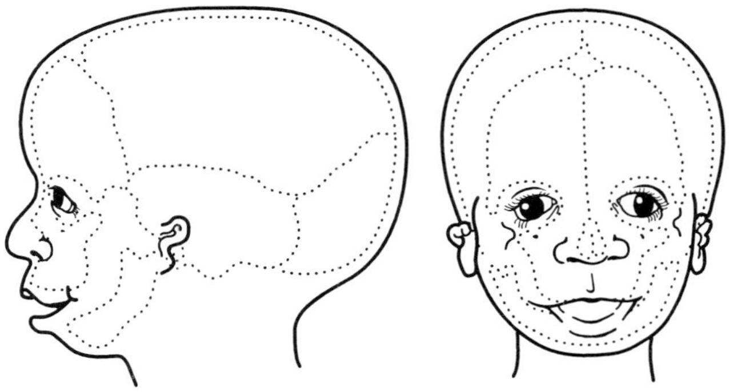

## Orbital Hypertelorism
( A physical finding, not a syndrome )

- Incidence: 1:25,000
- Generic term, present in many syndromes
- Major categories:
  - craniosynostoses
  - frontonasal dysplasia
  - median cleft face
  - nasofrontal encephalocele
- Possible increase of intracranial pressure
- Nasofrontal dysplasia (0-14 Tessier Cleft)
- Cribriform plates: low
- Ethmoid sinuses: abnormal
- Nasal malformation, duplication or medial cleft
- Short nose

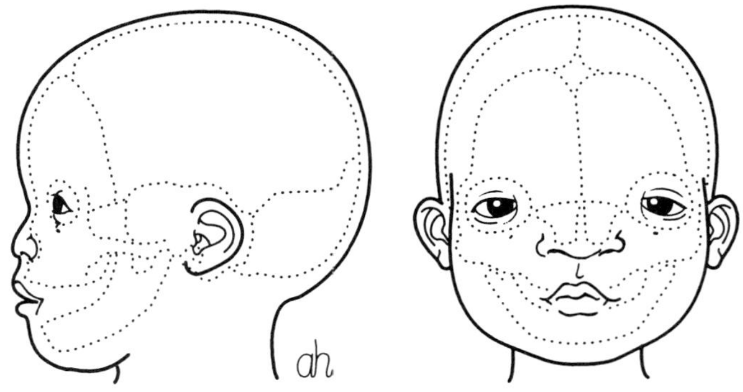

**Fig. 15–3.** Other craniofacial anomalies.

In addition to the differences in growth between the facial and the cranial skeleton, predictions of normal growth are not always valid in craniofacial patients. Patients can respond differently to surgical intervention because of abnormal growth related to a specific craniofacial disorder or syndrome.[95]

### Le Fort terminology

The name *Le Fort* is widely used in craniofacial surgery and refers to the different levels and severity of facial fractures; Le Fort I, II, and III, with the latter being a complete craniofacial dysjunction. This terminology of Le Fort I, II, and III was first described for facial fractures by Le Fort (1901), who completed a set of experiments that demonstrated the areas of structural weakness of the maxilla.[65]

In this text, the terms *Le Fort I, II, and III* refer to the controlled osteotomies used in the correction of various congenital deformities of the face. The Le Fort I, II, and III osteotomies (surgically created fracture lines) create skeletal segments that can be mobilized for advancement or setback in both vertical and/or horizontal planes.[65,71]

### Bone grafting

Bone grafting is used in four basic ways in craniofacial surgery: (1) onlay, (2) inlay, (3) interposition for stabilization and, (4) construction (when an anatomic structure is absent). Early in the specialty, rib and iliac bone were the most frequently used grafts. Rib grafts have the advantage in that they can be split and can then be easily bent to achieve contour, but like iliac bone grafts, they tend to resorb, unless firmly secured to adjacent bone. Iliac bone is useful where thick interpositional blocks or a large quantity of cancellous bone is necessary.

Craniofacial surgeons favor cranial bone grafts over iliac and rib for several reasons. The cranial donor site is in the same surgical field, thus avoiding another operative site with its potential complications. Cranial bone has more cortex than marrow and it maintains its volume as a graft, especially when rigidly fixed.[105] Early publications suggested that calvaria, which is of membranous origin, did better in the craniofacial area as compared to iliac and rib grafts which are of endochondral origin.[164] Recently, it has been demonstrated that the calvaria maintains its volume because it is comprised of a higher proportion of cortical bone.[8] In short, the architecture or proportion of cortical-to-cancellous bone is more important for successful grafting than embryonic origin.

### Plating systems

Rigid fixation with plates and screws is often used for stabilization in the craniofacial skeleton. Miniaturized plates and screws have been developed for infants and children. These systems should not be left in young pediatric patients. The plates and screws can migrate from an extra- to intracranial position. Furthermore, it is well documented that plates interfere with facial growth.[67,68] Growth restriction has been found to be directly proportional to the amount of fixation hardware. Interosseous stainless steel wire fixation is often used for craniofacial procedures in infants and young children. If rigid fixation in an infant requires microplates and screws, the hardware is removed a few months later. It is best to use the least amount of fixation possible to provide adequate three-dimensional control and stability. Removal of microfixation plates after bone healing, but prior to completion of skull growth, allows for resumption of normal growth.[163]

Artifacts on radiographic imaging is another drawback of metallic plating systems. These artifacts seen on computed tomography (CT) and magnetic resonance (MR) imaging are described respectively as *starbursts* and *black holes*. They can interfere with radiological interpretation especially in follow-up or after excision of tumor. In a study of several metallic craniofacial plating systems, titanium caused fewer artifacts than stainless steel or vitallium.[30,31]

Biodegradable fixation plates and screws are currently under study in clinical trials.

## Skeletal malformations

### Craniosynostosis

*Craniosynostosis* is the term applied to a variety of cranial deformities that appear to result from abnormal development of the calvarial sutures. Although commonly conceived to be either agenesis or premature closure of sutures, the pathogenesis of craniosynostosis is unknown. Cohen believes that craniosynostosis is both etiologically and pathogenetically heterogeneous.[10,11] Primary forms manifest either in a sporadic or familial (genetic) pattern, with craniosynostosis as the predominant abnormality. Both autosomal dominant and autosomal recessive inheritance is described.[10,11] Secondary craniosynostosis can occur in various rare hematological and metabolic disorders and with intrauterine constraint of the fetal skull.[11] Environmental insults such as trauma, drugs, and intrauterine infection are also associated with premature closure of the cranial sutures.[40]

In the past, the craniosynostoses have been classified by the particular abnormal cranial morphology, as related to the degree and extent of involvement of various sutures. The anatomic manifestations include *turribrachycephaly* (coronal sutures), *synostotic plagiocephaly* (frontal: unilateral coronal suture or posterior: lambdoid suture), *scaphocephaly* (sagittal suture), and multiple craniosynostoses, usually associated with skull-base sutural synostoses. The syndromic craniosynostoses are recognized by proper names, the most common being Saethre-Chotzen, Apert, Crouzon, Pfeiffer and Jackson-Weiss. These eponymous craniosynostotic syndromes are inherited in an autosomal dominant pattern except Carpenter syndrome which is an autosomal recessive disorder. With advances in molecular genetics, classification based on gene location is possible.

The various craniosynostoses are presented below in decreasing order of incidence (Figs. 15–1, 15–2, 15–3).

### Nonsyndromic craniosynostoses

#### Scaphocephaly and dolichocephaly (sagittal synostosis)

The incidence of this isolated craniosynostotic malformation varies from 1:4,200[51] to 1:8,500.[21] It is the most frequent type of craniosynostosis. Males are more often affected than females, in a gender ratio of 4:1. In relation to all synostoses, it varies from 21%–57%, depending on the series.[29,81] The majority of these cases are sporadic; however, familial cases do occur (2%–4%). The term *scaphocephaly* was first used by Von Bauer to describe the elongated, narrow, "boat-like" cra-

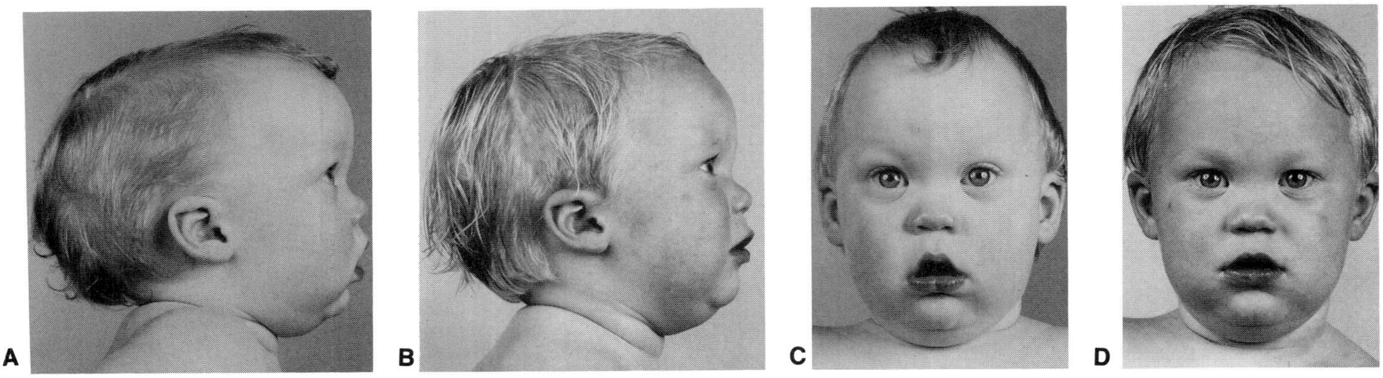

**Fig. 15–4.** Scaphocephaly–dolichocephaly (sagittal synostosis). A: Lateral view of 10-month-old baby with sagittal synostosis. Bossing of forehead and occiput produces the "boat-like" shaped head (scaphocephaly). B: Lateral view after cranioplasty, including 2 cm reduction in anteroposterior dimension. C, D: Frontal view before and after surgical correction. Temporoparietal cranium expanded using a "barrel-stave" technique. (Courtesy of Dr. Claes Lauritzen.)

nial shape. Premature fusion of the sagittal suture is accompanied by excessive compensatory anteroposterior cranial growth (Fig. 15–4).

Complete sagittal synostosis, in addition to biparietal narrowing, causes frontal bossing and occipital bulging. If only the anterior sagittal portion is fused, frontal bossing and bicoronal expansion predominate. With posterior sagittal fusion, the distortion presents in the occipital region, with expansion at the lambdoid sutures and with minimal frontal bossing.[94]

*Treatment.* Surgical strategies for sagittal synostosis can be categorized according to age: (1) patients less than 1 year old, (2) patients 1–3 years old, and (3) patients older than 3 years with end-stage scaphocephaly.[94]

If the correction is undertaken within the first few months of life, a wide sagittal craniectomy gives quite satisfactory results. By 1 year of age, strip craniectomy alone does not predictably result in normal cranial shape. Extended craniotomy cuts are needed to widen the biparietal distance. If a child presents with end-stage scaphocephaly, extensive cranial modeling is needed to achieve biparietal widening and shortening of the anteroposterior cranial dimension. Objective studies comparing extended strip craniectomy vs. calvariectomy with remodeling have shown that normalization of calvarial width-to-length ratio is more likely with the more extensive procedure than following simple strip craniectomy.[73]

### Plagiocephaly

*Plagiocephaly* is a generic term used to describe congenital asymmetry of the cranium. The first step in diagnosis is to categorize plagiocephaly as predominantly frontal or posterior. The second step is to separate pathogenetically plagiocephaly as either synostotic or deformational.[4] This differentiation is crucial to the care of the infant because synostotic plagiocephaly requires surgical correction whereas deformational plagiocephaly usually does not (Fig. 15–5).

*Synostotic frontal plagiocephaly (SFP).* This results from unilateral synostosis of the "coronal ring" that includes sphenofrontal, sphenoethmoid, sphenozygomatic and frontoethmoid sutures.[44] Fusion first manifests in the inferior frontoparietal suture and spreads superiorly along the frontoparietal ("coronal") suture and medially to involve the anterior cranial base. An estimate of the prevalence of unilateral coronal synostosis is 1:10,000 births; it constitutes 10%–20% of all forms of craniosynostosis.[4,89] Most cases of SFP are sporadic and nonsyndromic. Intracranial pressure is elevated above 15mm Hg in only 14% of SFP infants.[119,120]

There is frequently a contralateral *ocular torticollis* (14%) in synostotic frontal plagiocephaly. This term, however, is a misnomer because there is no shortening of neck muscles. In SFP patients, there is a head tilt towards the normal side in an attempt to correct for diplopia; it is secondary to relative overactivity of the ipsilateral inferior rectus muscle. The head-tilt mimics a lateral rectus palsy but the mechanism is more complex. This head tilt is present in 45%–60% of children with SFP.[122]

*Deformational frontal plagiocephaly (DFP).* This is secondary to compressive and restrictive forces acting either *in utero,* at birth, or postnatally. It is very common and presents in 5%–48% of otherwise healthy newborns.[156] Its mildest form is head molding that occurs during vaginal delivery. More severe deformation results from restriction of cranial growth by rigid intrauterine structures or by the pelvis. There is typical flattening and compensatory overgrowth in the nonrestricted cranial region. DFP is left sided in 73% of cases. This is logical since 85% of vertex presentation are in the left occiptoanterior position (LOA).[4] These same prenatal forces also cause other deformational abnormalities in association with DFP: torticollis, talipes, dislocated hip, scoliosis, prominent ears, and micrognathia.[156]

There is a "true" torticollis, a head tilt toward the abnormal side in 64% of these children.[4] DFP has also been called *torticollis with plagiocephaly.* The question of which came first, the ipsilateral torticollis or DFP, remains unanswered.

*Differentiation between deformational and synostotic frontal plagiocephaly by physical examination (Fig. 15–5).* Palpable coronal ridging is not pathognomonic of SFP. It is found in only 7% of all patients with unilateral coronal synostosis.[63] Radiographic findings can be unreliable in the first 3 months of life.[29] Nevertheless, physical examination does serve to distinguish the two major types of frontal plagiocephaly.

The first step in differentiating between SFP and DFP is to determine which side of the forehead is flattened. This is best noted by observing the child from the front and from above, from a "bird's eye" view.

The ipsilateral orbital rim is higher in SFP and there is a compensational expansion of the contralateral forehead. In DFP, in contrast, the ipsilateral superior orbital rim and eyebrow are lower than the normal side. Often the palpebral fissure is narrowed on the flattened side in DFP. There is a characteristic anterior displacement of the ipsilateral ear in SFP, whereas in DFP there is posteroinferior displacement of the ipsilaterally involved ear. The nasal root is deviated to the ipsilateral side in virtually all patients with SFP, whereas it is straight in DFP. Two-thirds of infants with DFP have a torticollis on the affected or flattened side of the forehead and face; often the chin point is slightly deviated to the same side. In contrast, there is often a minor deviation of the chin to the normal side in SFP. Sometimes the child holds the head tilted to the normal side, the so-called *ocular torticollis,* referred to above.

Computed tomography with three-dimensional reformatting is useful for research but probably unnecessary for diagnosis or

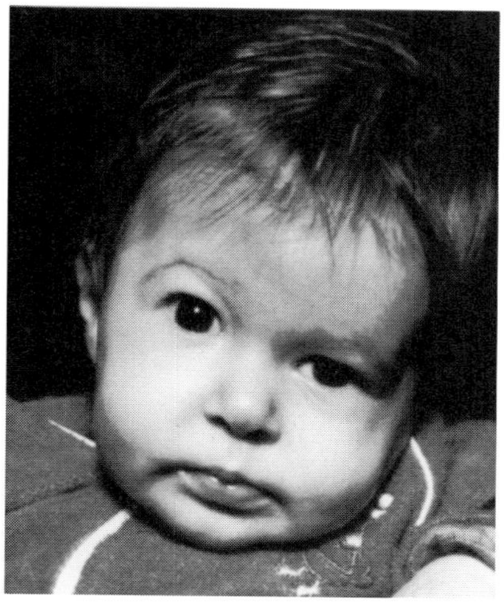

A

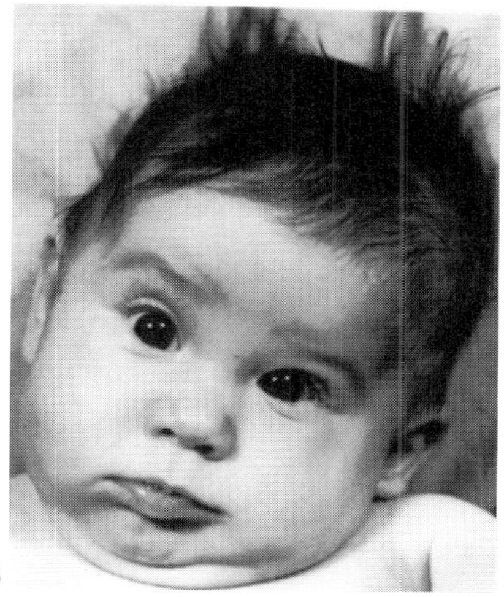

B

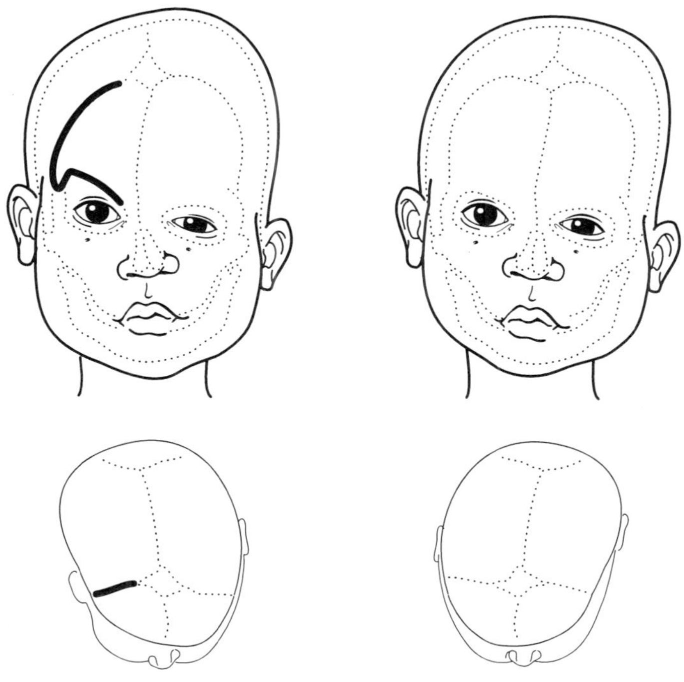

| Anatomic Features | Right Synostotic | Left Deformational |
|---|---|---|
| Ipsilateral superior orbital rim | • Superior | • Inferior |
| Ipsilateral ear | • Anterior/superior | • Posterior/inferior |
| Nasal root | • Ipsilateral deviation | • Midline |
| Ipsilateral cheek | • Forward | • Posterior |
| Chin deviation | • Contralateral | • Ipsilateral |
| Ipsilateral palpebral fissure | • Wide | • Narrow |

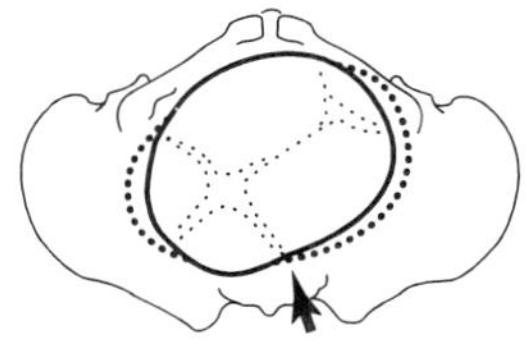

**Fig. 15–5.** Anatomical features that differentiate synostotic (SFP) from deformational (DFP) frontal plagiocephaly. Frontal views comparing SFP (A) and DFP (B) are shown. In the lower right corner, a drawing depicts the maternal pelvis with the fetal head in the most frequent vertex presentation which is the left occipitoanterior position (LOA). This is the probable basis for the left DFP and more common right deformational posterior plagiocephaly (DPP).

management of frontal plagiocephaly. In SFP, there is a "harlequin" sign, seen on plain anteroposterior skull radiograph. This sign is due to ipsilateral elevation and posterior displacement of the lesser wing of the sphenoid. Radiologic study is used to confirm the clinical impression of unicoronal synostosis. Keep in mind that early in the course of this disorder, the suture line can still be visible, so the diagnosis of unilateral coronal synostosis cannot be excluded.

*Posterior plagiocephaly: synostotic vs. deformational.* Synostotic posterior plagiocephaly (SPP) and deformational posterior plagiocephaly (DPP) have similar anatomic features.[21] The occipitoparietal flattening and secondary deformities are typically more pronounced in true synostosis of the lambdoid suture. The ipsilateral ear is anteriorly displaced and there is ipsilateral frontal bossing, along with bulging of the contralateral parieto-occipital area. Synostotic posterior plagiocephaly, caused by lambdoid synostosis, is an extremely rare condition. In contrast, DPP is very common and becoming more so since pediatricians now recommend that infants be positioned on their back during sleep to minimize the chances of sudden infant death syndrome.

Treatment

*Deformational plagiocephaly.* It is critical to distinguish between deformational plagiocephaly and synostotic plagiocephaly since deformational flattening is usually self-correcting and does not require surgical intervention.

Nonsurgical management consists of positioning, helmeting, and physiotherapy if there is associated torticollis. Positioning involves placing the child so that the head lies on the bulged side. A helmet is used for both frontal and posterior deformational plagiocephaly. A custom-made helmet accelerates the modeling process. Helmeting, however, requires an expert orthotist. This conservative management should be started early, in the first 3–6 months of life.[121] If this treatment is not available and/or is impossible, good results are still expected.[9,121]

*Synostotic plagiocephaly.* Synostotic frontal plagiocephaly must be corrected surgically and this is best accomplished in early to mid-infancy. There are two concepts that guide the surgical treatment of SFP. The first is early release of the synostotic cranium to allow the expanding brain to correct the residual deformity.[130,131] The second and contradictory view is that one cannot rely completely on brain growth to expand the flattened forehead. Rather, the fronto-orbital elements must be positioned firmly and symmetrically. The original type of correction of unilateral coronal craniosynostosis is rarely used, i.e., simple strip craniectomy, with or without alloplastic silicone sheathing, to isolate bone edges from the dura. This technique rapidly releases intracranial pressure but does not reliably produce upper craniofacial symmetry. This is due to rapid reossification of the craniotomy gap. Furthermore, involvement of the anterior cranial base is not addressed by strip craniectomy.

The current surgical strategy for SFP is fronto-orbital advancement. There is, however, controversy over bilateral vs. unilateral approaches. Some surgeons still use a unilateral procedure, a variant of the *lateral canthal advancement* described first by the neurosurgeons Hoffman and Mohr.[47] Whitaker and colleagues improved the unilateral frontal advancement procedure by stabilization of the supraorbital bar with a tongue-in-groove technique.[159] Most surgeons favor a bilateral approach described by Marchac,[72] which is based on the fact that the contralateral forehead is abnormally bossed, a compensation for the restricted growth on the synostotic side. With Marchac's technique, the entire supraorbital bar is mobilized and interosseous wires are used to attach a single piece of skull of optimal shape above it, to construct a symmetric forehead. Mulliken includes a closing nasal osteotomy just below the nasofrontal suture to correct the nasal deviation, as part of bilateral correction.[44]

The surgical approach is different when SFP presents in end-stage or unoperated patients. After 5 years, brain growth no longer helps to correct frontal asymmetry. At this age, the deformity is not only cranial but also craniofacial. Therefore, complex orbital osteotomies, rhinoplasty, maxillary osteotomy (Le Fort I), and bone grafting are necessary to provide symmetry. Minor contouring and masking operations can also be done to give the appearance of symmetry.

The diagnosis of synostotic posterior (lambdoid) synostosis requires radiographic confirmation, either with plain films or CT scans. This subject is confusing because some surgeons believe that a functional lambdoid synostosis can occur even with a radiographically and histologically open lambdoid suture.[79] Surgical strategies range from extended strip craniectomy to more complicated biparieto-occipital cranioplasty, depending on the time of intervention.

### Brachycephaly and bilateral coronal synostoses

Brachycephalic children present with abnormal fusion of the coronal ring but with normal midfacial development and usually normal extremities. The cranium is shortened in the sagittal axis with compensatory increase in the bitemporal and bicoronal distance. Delayed closure of the anterior fontanelle can cause the vertex of the cranium to become pointed (oxycephaly). Exorbitism is obvious, but it is not as severe as in patients with associated midfacial retrusion. These children do not fit into well-recognized categories of craniosynostotic syndromes. Nevertheless, these cases are likely to be genetic (probably single-gene) disorders and with advances in craniofacial molecular genetics, their specific molecular diagnosis will be established.

*Treatment.* The treatment is fronto-orbital advancement and modeling.

### Trigonocephaly or metopic synostosis

Trigonocephaly (the term stems from the Greek *trigonos,* or triangular, + *kephalē,* or head) results from premature fusion of the metopic (interfrontal) suture. It is infrequent; the incidence is less than 10% of all craniosynostoses.[28,131]

The characteristics of this fronto-orbital malformation are prominent frontal keel, narrow forehead, and closely set eyes (orbital hypotelorism). The triangular-shaped forehead manifests decreased bifrontal and bicoronal width and increased biparietal width (Fig. 15–6). This malformation is usually isolated and nonsyndromic; however, it can be seen in trisomy 13 and other chromosomal disorders, such as 9p deletion.[153] Prominent metopic ridging can be a normal familial variant that corrects itself with time.

*Treatment.* For years this disorder was treated with linear strip craniectomy to alleviate increased intracranial pressure. At the present time it is either managed by complete bilateral fronto-orbital reshaping, or rarely by contour burring, or not treated at all in mild cases. Fronto-orbital modeling only partially corrects the hypotelorbitism.[74] There is no consensus about surgically widening the interorbital distance. Some cra-

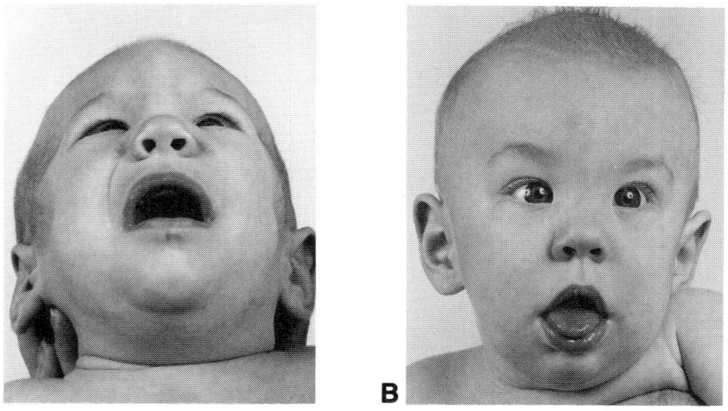

A B

**Fig. 15–6.** Trigonocephaly (metopic synostosis). A: Submental view of a 3-month-old boy with premature closure of interfrontal suture. B: Frontal view showing associated hypotelorism and decreased bifrontal width.

niofacial surgeons favor it,[28,108] others do not.[37] The surgical time-frame is 3–6 months of age; but some authors recommend observation for up to 18 months to 2 years of age if the deformity is minor.[28]

Some authors question the necessity for operative correction of trigonocephaly since a certain degree of self-correction occurs.[26,33,98] It is rare to see an adolescent or adult with uncorrected trigonocephaly. Friede and colleagues[37] documented 11 infants by cephalometry, including 5 minor cases that were not operated. In the untreated group, there was improvement of forehead contour with growth, but ultimately it remained narrower than normal. In the treated group, their findings support the clinical impression that normalization of the forehead ridge does occur with a slight reduction of epicanthal folds. Posnick et al.[108] analyzed pre- and postoperative CT scan images in a group of 10 patients, aged between 6 and 48 months, and found that their operation corrected the intercanthal distance (101% of normal), undercorrected the interorbital distance (90% of normal), and decreased medial wall protrusion (90% of normal), whereas frontal and supraorbital rim contours remained corrected with growth.[108]

## Syndromic craniosynostoses

*Craniofacial dysostosis* is a generic term used to describe familial forms of synostosis involving not only the cranial vault but also various cranial base sutures and midfacial deformities. The familial craniofacial dysostoses were described by Carpenter in 1901,[6] Apert in 1906,[1a] Crouzon in 1912,[19] Saethre,[125a] and Chotzen[8a] in 1931, and 1932 and Pfeiffer in 1964.[109] Another term frequently used in association with these anomalies is *kleeblattschädel,* referring to the cloverleaf shape of the skull that occurs when multiple cranial vault and cranial base sutures fuse prematurely.

### Saethre-Chotzen syndrome

This disorder may be the most common of the syndromic craniosynostoses because of the high incidence of familial cases. The condition was first described in 1931 by Saethre[125a] and in 1932 by Chotzen.[8a] The most common physical characteristics are blepharoptosis (85%), minor auricular anomalies (80%), beaked nose (70%), deviated nasal septum (65%), high-arched palate (60%), class I occlusion (50%), and class III occlusion (45%).[99] It is also characterized by coronal synostosis, low frontal hairline with up-turned hair follicles, small ears with prominent helical crura, tear duct stenosis, dermatoglyphic alterations, brachydactyly, and partial syndactyly or webbing. Partial cutaneous syndactyly can occur between the second and third toes and occasionally involves other toes.[11] Syndactyly is not an obligatory anomaly of Saethre-Chotzen syndrome.

This syndrome is underrecognized because some cases are very mild and even the severe cases usually do not have major neurologic symptoms or intracranial hypertension. It is commonly misdiagnosed as synostotic frontal plagiocephaly or Crouzon syndrome.

It is an autosomal dominant disorder with high penetrance and variable expressivity.[100] The responsible gene lies on chromosome 7 (7p21–p22).[3,66,116,150] However, there may be more than one locus for Saethre-Chotzen syndrome on 7p.[118]

Saethre-Chotzen patients rarely need complicated operative correction since they do not have major esthetic or functional problems. Fronto-orbital advancement in infancy is usually indicated. Surgical correction is necessary only if blepharoptosis is severe, or for nasal septal deviation.

### Crouzon syndrome

Crouzon syndrome is an autosomal dominant disorder. Most cases are sporadic. The incidence is reported to be from 1:25,000 to 1:60,000.[11,14a] The classic findings are coronal synostosis, maxillary hypoplasia and exorbitism[19,21] (Fig. 15–7). Additional features include minor orbital hypertelorism with exotropia, calcification of the stylohyoid ligament, cervical spine anomalies, fused vertebrae, Chiari I malformation, syringomyelia, elbow stiffness, and acanthosis nigricans, the latter in an atypical periorbital/perioral/cervical distribution.

The most common cranial shape is either brachycephaly or oxycephaly (pointed skull). The eyes are proptotic in 75% of cases, secondary to the shallow orbits; the midface is retruded with malocclusion (angle classification, class III). Besides proptosis, optic atrophy is documented in 25% and blindness in 5% of patients. Otolaryngological anomalies include narrowed external auditory canal in 15% of the cases, conductive hearing loss in approximately 50%, and deviated nasal septum in 35% of patients. The mandible appears prominent because of the hypoplastic maxilla (relative prognathism). It grows normally and may become secondarily deformed with a vertically long chin.

Crouzon syndrome is a genetically heterogeneous disorder. The responsible (10 q) chromosome was first identified by link-

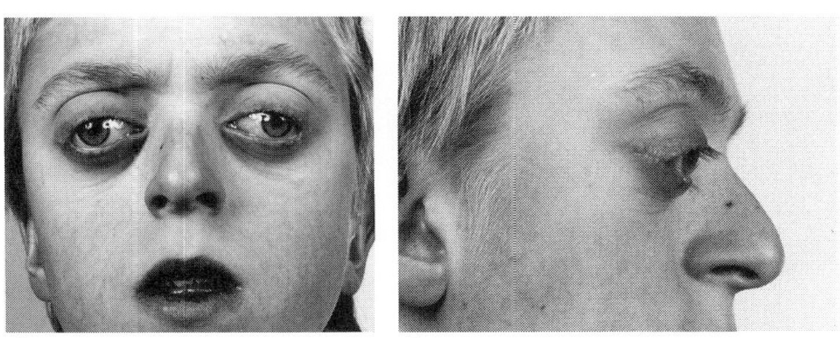

A B

**Fig. 15–7.** Crouzon syndrome. A, B: Anteroposterior (AP) and lateral photograph demonstrating brachycephaly, exorbitism, and midfacial retrusion. (Courtesy of Dr. Claes Lauritzen.)

age analysis using the candidate gene approach.[113] A few months later, the gene itself was identified to be fibroblast growth factor receptor 2 (FGFR2). Many mutations have been documented within the *FGFR2* gene.[101,117,160] There is also locus heterogeneity for Crouzon syndrome with acanthosis nigricans which occurs by mutation of the *FGFR3* gene on chromosome 4, the same as for achondroplasia.[93a] (See also Chapters 1 and 14 and Section IX)

Surgical intervention involves fronto-orbital and midfacial advancement, usually done in stages in childhood. The occlusion is corrected adequately with orthodontics and final maxillary advancement after skeletal growth is completed.

### Apert syndrome

Apert syndrome occurs in 1.5:100,000 births.[16,39] Because of the high neonatal mortality rate, the true prevalence is closer to 1:2,000,000.[42] Familial cases are rare. This is probably explained by sexual unattractiveness and the relatively high frequency of mental retardation. Apert syndrome accounts for approximately 4.5% of all cases of craniosynostosis.

The characteristic features of this syndrome are craniosynostosis, midfacial hypoplasia, and/or retrusion, as well as symmetric complex syndactyly of the hands and feet (Fig. 15–8). The term *premature synostosis* is a misnomer in Apert syndrome since a proper metopic suture never actually forms. A large gap in the midline of the forehead gradually closes.[14] The orbital physical characteristics are shallow orbits, orbital hypertelorism, downward slanting palpebral fissures, and strabismus (Fig. 15–8A,B).

Midface retrusion and/or hypoplasia results in relative mandibular prognathism and a beaked nose. Approximately 30% of patients have cleft of the soft palate or bifid uvula. Other oral findings are V-shaped maxillary dental arch, enlarged palatal shelves, severe crowding, and malocclusion.[103] Acne vulgaris appears in adolescence in more than 70% of patients; comedones and pustules are major problems.[133,134] Rhizomelic shortening of the limbs (upper and lower) and progressive or generalized skeletal dysplasia with limitation of motion at the elbows, shoulders, hips, and knees are all part of this syndrome. A number of these patients evidence minor to significant mental retardation. All infants with Apert syndrome should have a baseline CT and an MRI to define possible CNS abnormalities, especially if a neurosurgical procedure is planned.[14] Diagnostic investigation should also include a search for cardiovascular and genitourinary anomalies that occur in 10% and 9.6% of patients, respectively.[15]

The gene for Apert syndrome also lies in the extracellular immunoglobulin domain of FGFR2.[160] Whereas Crouzon syndrome patients have multiple allelic mutations in *FGFR2,* Apert syndrome patients typically have two mutations in adjacent *FGFR2* residues with frequencies of 66.7% and 30%, respectively.[156] To date, only one patient does not have either mutation.[102,160]

### Pfeiffer syndrome

The original description of this syndrome dates to 1964.[104] The incidence is not precisely documented; it is probably similar to that for Crouzon and Apert syndromes. Pfeiffer syndrome patients have a tall skull (turribrachycephaly) with a flattened occiput due to bilateral coronal synostosis. The forehead is large and the eyes slant downward with minor exorbitism. Midfacial retrusion is variable. The disorder is usually, but not always, characterized by broad thumbs and broad great toes, partial soft tissue syndactyly, and symphalangism of the hands.[46,126] The mean great toe/second toe ratio is 1.91(n:21) with a range of 1.72–2.23.[13]

Cohen proposed three clinical subtypes for this syndrome: type 1 is the minor phenotype described above; type 2 consists of cloverleaf skull with "Pfeiffer hands" and feet, together with ankylosis of the elbows; and type 3 is similar to type 2 but without the cloverleaf skull.[13] The anterior cranial base is short and there is ocular proptosis. These three subtypes have important prognostic implications: type 1 has a good outcome and normal intelligence; types 2 and 3 have severe neurological problems, poor prognosis, and usually early death.[13]

Pfeiffer syndrome is an autosomal dominant disorder with complete penetrance and variable expressivity. Linkage studies, using microsatellite markers, mapped this disorder to chromosome 8p11.2–p12 near the centromere in several families with a mutation in *FGFR1*.[82,123,127] However, not all families linked to chromosome 8, suggesting that at least one other genetic locus can cause this disorder (genetic or locus heterogeneity). A second locus for Pfeiffer syndrome is a mutation in *FGFR2,* on chromosome 10q (10q25.3–q26), the same gene responsible for Crouzon syndrome.[124,127]

### Carpenter syndrome

This is the only known autosomal recessive craniosynostotic syndrome. This rare disorder, originally described by Carpenter in 1901,[6] is characterized by craniosynostosis, often with preaxial polysyndactyly of the feet. The fingers are short with clinodactyly (3rd and 4th fingers) and with variable soft tissue syndactyly. The cranium has a tower shape (turricephaly) as well as oxycephaly (pointed skull). Coxa valga, pes varus, congenital heart disease, mental retardation, hypogenitalism, and mild obesity have been associated with this condition. The dystopia canthorum (primary telecanthus) is nearly a constant feature. However, the interpupillary and interorbital distances are normal.[22,42] The chromosomal locus has not been mapped.

### Cloverleaf skull, kleeblattschädel anomaly, and triphyllocephaly

This is not a specific disorder but an etiologically and pathogenetically diverse condition. It represents the most extreme form of cranio-orbitofaciostenosis and is often associated with hydrocephalus.[49] It is a familiar term in the craniofacial literature used to describe a trilobular skull secondary to complex or pancraniosynostosis. The cloverleaf skull may occur as an isolated event or in association with bony ankylosis of the limbs, in Crouzon, Carpenter, Pfeiffer, and Apert syndromes, and in thanatophoric dysplasia.[42] Sporadic thanatophoric dysplasia, the most common lethal cause of neonatal dwarfism, has been shown to be the result of mutations in *FGFR3*.[137] Achondroplasia, the most common form of dwarfism, also is caused by a mutation in *FGFR3* on chromosome 4p.[129]

### Other rare craniosynostosis syndromes

In craniosynostosis, Boston type, the mutation was found to be in the homeodomain of the human *MSX2* gene.[54,83,154]

Another rare craniosynostosis, Adelaide type, is inherited as

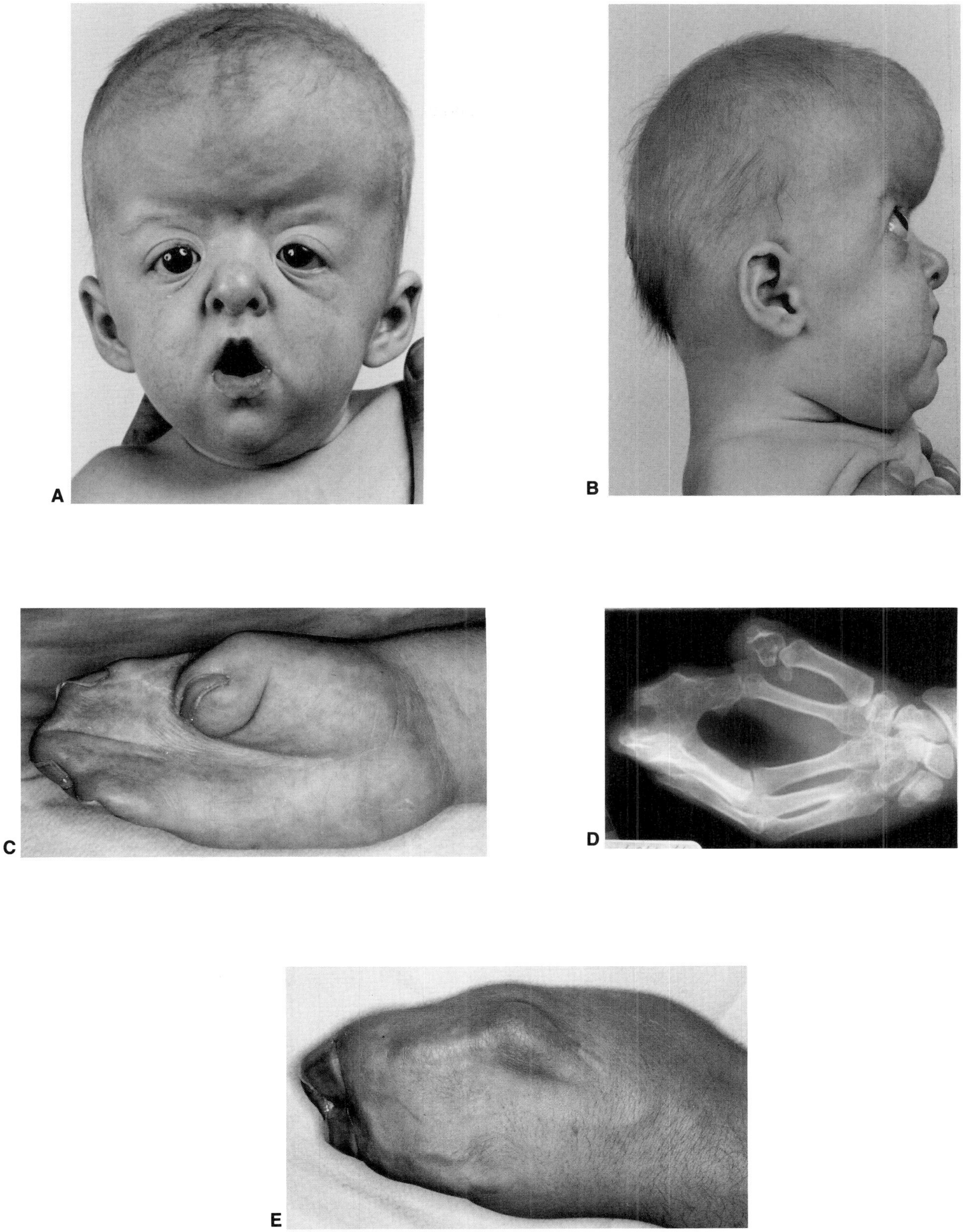

**Fig. 15–8.** Apert syndrome. A: Apert baby: note midfacial hypoplasia and retrusion, exorbitism and brachycephaly (short anteroposterior cranial distance). B: Lateral view showing exorbitism and forehead deformity. (Courtesy Dr. Claes Lauritzen) C, D, E: Complex syndactyly-typical "mitten hands." (Courtesy of Dr. J. Upton.)

an autosomal dominant and associated with digital abnormalities. Its gene localizes to 4p16.[48]

The Jackson-Weiss syndrome is a very rare condition characterized by craniosynostosis and foot anomalies. Mutations in the same region of *FGFR2* as for certain cases of Crouzon syndrome have been identified.[53] This is also the case of the Beare-Stevenson cutis gyrata syndrome, an autosomal dominant condition characterized by craniosynostosis, craniofacial dysmorphism, furrowed skin disorder of cutis gyrata, acanthosis nigricans and other congenital anomalies.[113a]

### General guidelines for surgical correction of syndromic craniosynostoses

The indications, timing, and strategies for surgical correction of the various craniosynostotic syndromes are still in evolution. The surgical strategy must take into account functional problems, abnormal and normal craniofacial growth, and possible complications at different ages.

*In infancy: primary cranio-orbital decompression and modeling.* Elevated intracranial pressure is a potential concern in any infant or child with craniosynostosis. Renier et al.[120] determined that 42% of untreated children with more than one suture synostosis and 14% of those with just one fused suture have significantly elevated intracranial pressure (>15 mm Hg).

The initial surgical treatment generally involves suture release, simultaneous cranial vault, and upper orbital osteotomies, with shaping and advancement, accomplished between 6 and 10 months of age. The depth of the upper orbits is increased and proptosis corrected. Advancement at the anterior cranial base is typically between 1.5 and 2.5 cm. A degree of sagittal overcorrection of the supraorbital ridge is needed, depending on the particular syndrome.

*In young children: fronto-orbital advancement or posterior decompression.* The child is followed clinically and by CT scanning as indicated. If signs of increased intracranial pressure appear, urgent decompression and reshaping is indicated. A second craniotomy is always more challenging and needs to be done with care because there is a higher incidence of dural tear and more blood loss than in the primary procedure. In some instances, posterior decompression and expansion are required if pressure mounts in the presence of a deformed and/or constricted posterior cranial vault.

*In childhood: Midfacial advancement.* Monobloc or subcranial (Le Fort III) midfacial advancement and/or facial bipartition are surgical options to correct the abnormal midface, depending on whether there is associated orbital hypertelorism. The type of surgical procedure is determined by the deformity and functional problems. The indications for midfacial advancement are either respiratory compromise, exorbitism, midfacial retrusion, and/or the accompanying psychosocial implications.

Sleep apnea is more frequent in Apert than in Crouzon syndrome. However, improvement in the airway after midfacial advancement is unpredictable in syndromic craniosynostoses. One reason is that the etiology of obstructive sleep apnea syndrome (OSAS) is multifactorial in children with craniosynostosis. There can be narrowing of the nasopharyngeal space (choanal stenosis) associated with midfacial hypoplasia, or there can be lower airway pathology, laryngotracheomalacia, or cartilaginous fusion, particularly in Apert and Crouzon syndromes. The most dangerous period is between 3 and 5 years of age, with enlargement of the adenoids and tonsils causing compromise of an already narrowed nasopharyngeal space. In this situation, combined adenoidectomy-tonsillectomy should be considered. As noted above, midfacial advancement is not necessarily the answer. Studies have shown that it is often ineffective when done primarily to correct obstructive sleep apnea.[27] Alternative procedures to open the airway include uvulopalatopharyngoplasty (UPPP), wedge resection at the base of the tongue, or creation of a cleft of the soft palate. Tracheostomy should be used whenever necessary. In older patients, continuous positive air pressure (CPAP) is an alternative.[27,125]

The first surgical corrections for Apert and Crouzon syndromes were described by Tessier 25 years ago. He devised single-stage extra- and intracranial frontofacial advancement, Le Fort III advancement, and frontal bone advancement.[139] His disciples developed a monobloc osteotomy to advance simultaneously the orbits and midface.[96,149] Tessier refined vertical splitting and shaping of the monobloc, a procedure now known as facial bipartition. Monobloc advancement carries a higher risk of complications, such as intracranial infection, bone loss, etc., although some surgeons prefer this procedure.[92]

Staged fronto-orbital advancement and subcranial midfacial advancement carries a lower risk and permits proper adjustment of the upper and midfacial elements.[80] The midface should be maximally advanced, depending on the sagittal relationship of the orbits to the globes. It is usually difficult to adjust simultaneously the orbits and the occlusion. A separate Le Fort I osteotomy and advancement with genioplasty is often required in adolescence after completion of skeletal growth.

The approach for correction of craniofacial deformity is different if there is associated orbital hypertelorism. In Apert syndrome, a frequently considered option is facial bipartition osteotomy. This involves a midline facial split so that the medial and lateral orbital rims can be medially rotated and transposed while the posterior maxillary arch is widened.[84,146] Bipartition is usually not required for Crouzon and Pfeiffer patients because orbital hypertelorism is minor in these patients.

*In adolescence: Management of orthognathic problems.* Patients with craniofacial synostosis, despite frontal advancement and midfacial advancement, usually require correction of end-stage malocclusion (prognathism). Skeletal maturity occurs around age 14–16 years in females and 16–18 years in males. Only then can elective jaw surgery be performed in conjunction with orthodontic treatment with a minimal risk of relapse. A Le Fort I maxillary advancement is needed as the mandible grows normally and produces an anterior cross-bite or open-bite.[5] Bilateral sagittal split osteotomy of the mandible is sometimes required. Stabilization is achieved with miniplates and screws with or without intermaxillary fixation (IMF) to give jaw harmony.

## Other craniofacial anomalies

### Hemifacial microsomia (HFM): oculoauriculovertebral spectrum

There is a litany of terms for hemifacial microsomia (HFM): the oculoauriculovertebral spectrum, first and second branchial arch syndrome, craniofacial microsomia, oral-mandibular-auricular syndrome, otocraniocephalic syndrome, auriculobranchiogenic dysplasia, otomandibular dysostosis, lateral facial dysplasia, necrotic facial dysplasia, intrauterine facial necrosis, hemignathia and microtia syndrome, unilateral facial agenesis, and Goldenhar syndrome.[17]

Analysis of statistical correlations of anomalies in HFM fails to substantiate Goldenhar syndrome as a distinct variant.[152] This fact was first noted by Gorlin and Pinborg (1964)[41] and substantiated by Cohen,[12] who prefers the term *oculoauriculovertebral spectrum*. The term *hemifacial microsomia* is mellifluous and has become ingrained in medical parlance. Extracraniofacial anomalies, if present, can be designated *HFM plus* to designate the expanded spectrum.[50] The incidence of HFM is approximately 1:5,000 births.[43] Hemifacial microsomia is the second most common facial anomaly syndrome after cleft lip and/or cleft palate. A male-to-female ratio of 2:1 has been documented.[43] However, a later study[152] did not confirm this predominance among males. Bilateral mandibular hypoplasia is found in 16% of patients.

Grabb noted a 2% empirical risk that a family with one affected child could have another with the same condition.[43] Most syndromologists believe that it is not a familial disorder; nevertheless, there are very rare, well-documented familial cases.

HFM is a spectrum of variable malformations occurring during development of the first two visceral or pharyngeal arches, the intervening first pharyngeal pouch and first branchial cleft, as well as the temporal primordia. The etiology and pathogenesis are considered to be heterogeneous, thus accounting for the wide range of phenotypic expression. One theory of pathogenesis involves vascular disruption with hemorrhage and hematoma formation.[109,112] Another pathogenic theory impugns disruption of migration and distribution of neural crest cells responsible for the pharyngeal arches and midline somatic structures.[57]

Several classifications for HFM have been proposed.[20,64,85,114,115,152] The most inclusive and flexible is OMENS. The acronym represents each one of the five major manifestations of HFM: *O* for orbital distortion, *M* for mandibular hypoplasia, *E* for ear anomaly, *N* for nerve involvement and *S* for soft tissue deficiency (Fig. 15–9).[152] The term *OMENS-plus* is used to include the expanded spectrum: cardiac, skeletal, pulmonary, renal, gastrointestinal, and limb anomalies.[50]

One hundred and fifty-four patients with HFM classified using OMENS and analyzed statistically showed a positive association between the severity of the mandibular hypoplasia and the severity of orbital, auricular, neural, and soft tissue involvement. This study documented that HFM was associated with macrostomia (62%); facial nerve involvement (45%); ear tags (40%); palatal deviation to the normal side (39%); epibulbar dermoids (20%); horizontal discrepancy of the orbits (15%); and deformational frontal plagiocephaly (5%).[152]

*Treatment*. The management of hemifacial microsomia exemplifies the need for an interdisciplinary approach to craniofacial anomalies. In the past, there has been a tendency for each specialist to concentrate on his or her own particular area of interest or expertise. The infant or child with HFM presents not only with congenital anomalies but with the result of abnormal growth and the potential interference of prior treatment. A systematic approach focuses on the hypoplastic mandible as the key to management of the deformity.

In infancy, treatment includes excision of preauricular tags, closure of macrostomia, and transposition of the microtic ear lobule if it is located low and anteriorly on the cheek.

It is useful to type or grade the mandibular deformity as first proposed by Pruzansky[114,115] and later modified.[93,136,152] Type I is a miniature mandible with identifiable anatomy; type II is a functioning temporomandibular joint (TMJ) but with an abnormal shape and glenoid fossa. Type II is subcategorized as either type IIA if the glenoid fossa is in an acceptable functional position (in reference to the opposite TMJ) or type IIB if the TMJ is abnormally placed and cannot be incorporated in the surgical construction.[58] Type III deformity indicates an absent ramus and nonexistent glenoid fossa.

The concept for treatment of the child with HFM is elongation of the affected ramus (types I, II) or construction of a ramus and condyle if it is missing (type III). Elongation or construction of the ramus creates an open bite on the affected side. This space is slowly closed over a period of 2 years with gradual reduction of an orthodontic splint. This appliance regulates eruption of maxillary teeth and thereby stimulates maxillary (midfacial) growth. The goal is to achieve a horizontal occlusal plane.

*Type I*, a mini-mandible skeletal deformity, can often be managed with a functional orthodontic appliance called an activator. This device can be placed by age 3 years. If the appliance fails to prevent obliquity of the occlusal plane, then elongation of the ramus or mandibular distraction is indicated between 6 and 12 years, during mixed dentition. If a type I deformity presents late in adulthood, then bilateral mandibular osteotomies are required to prevent abnormal forces from acting on the normal TMJ. A Le Fort I maxillary osteotomy can also be necessary.

*Type II* mandible can also be treated for a time with a functional appliance; however, all type II children require mandibular elongation. Type IIA children have a well-placed, but short ramus. They are candidates for a vertical osteotomy and elongation or a simple oblique or transverse corticotomy and gradual mandibular distraction.

In *type IIB* or *type III* mandible, construction of the ascending ramus is needed, usually when the child has a full complement of deciduous teeth. TMJ reconstruction has been done on some patients as early as age 2 years[85] and on others between 6 and 12 years.[76,91] Type III patients rarely present in adulthood. These patients require full construction of the mandible, TMJ, zygomatic arch, and in some cases, a leveling orbital osteotomy. Le Fort I or maxillary osteotomy is required to give a level occlusal plane and symmetry. The condyle is constructed with costal cartilage and bone graft is used to construct the glenoid fossa. Sliding genioplasty is often necessary in combination, with or without a mandibular procedure as the final surgical step for the young adult with HFM.[90]

Ear construction must be conceptualized prior to mandibular correction to avoid improper placement of incisions and scarring. In high-grade mandibular deformity, i.e., type IIB or type III, it is usually best to defer ear construction until skeletal symmetry is achieved. In low-grade mandibular hypoplasia, the ear construction can be done anytime after age 6 years, when the costochondral elements are large enough to build an autogenous auricular framework.

Soft tissues can be hypoplastic in HFM. In rare cases, after restoration of the skeletal framework, soft tissue must be added. Onlay bone grafts to the ramus usually give symmetric lateral facial contour. Free tissue transfer by microsurgical techniques is another option. In minor cases, a dermal graft can be sufficient.

Mandibular distraction is a new method for ramus elongation for type I, type IIA, and some type IIB mandibles. This technique was originally described for long bones by Ilizarov in Russia. It involves an osteotomy (corticotomy) and placing me-

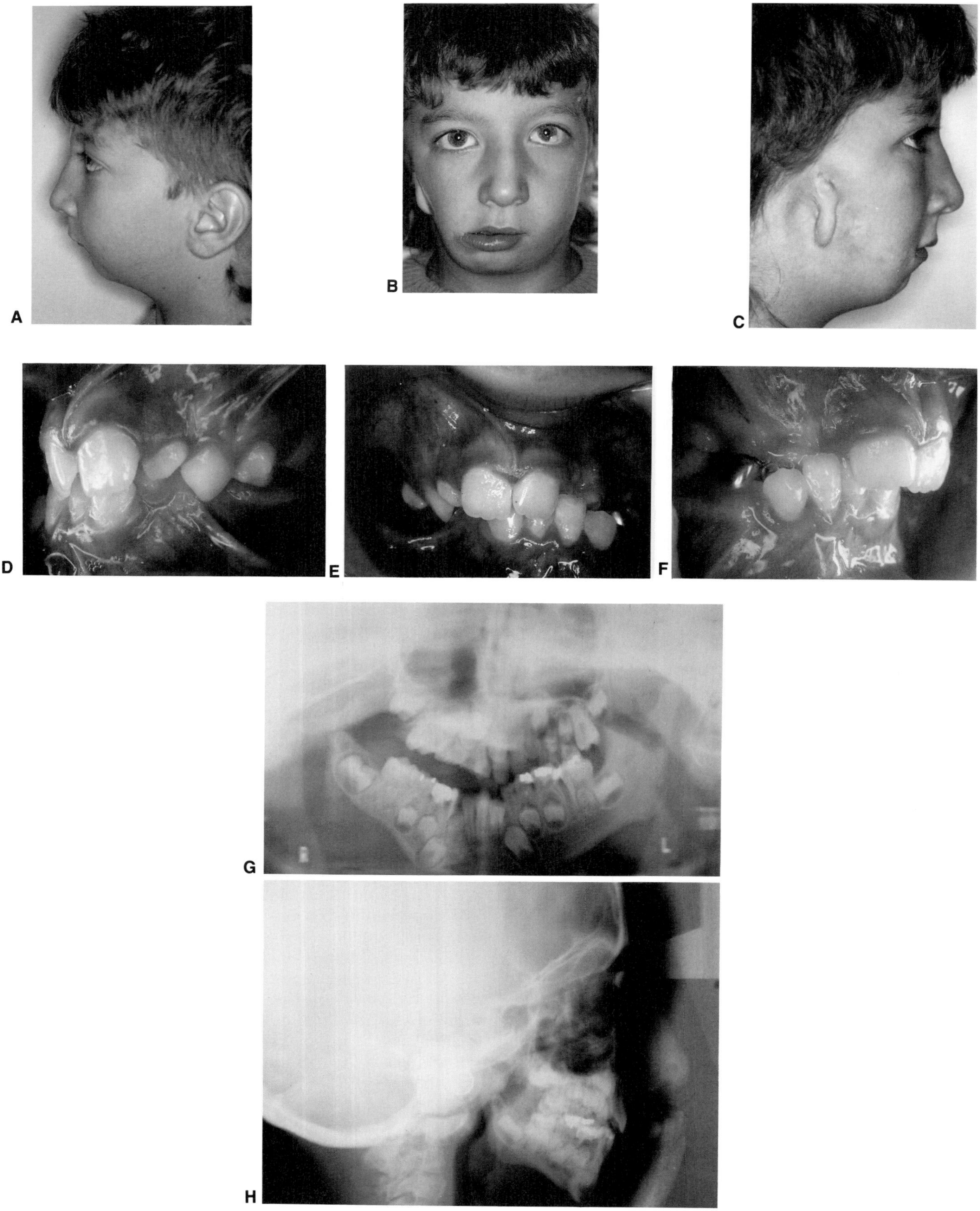

**Fig. 15–9.** Hemifacial microsomia (oculoauriculovertebral spectrum). A–C: Lateral and frontal views of a 7-year-old boy with mandibular asymmetry and chin deviation toward the side of the hypoplastic ramus, epibulbar dermoid (O.S.), and grade III microtia. D–F: Intraoral views demonstrate the mandibular shift resulting in a lingual crossbite on the right and a buccal crossbite on the left. (Courtesy of Dr. Stehane Schwartz.) G, H: Panographic and lateral cephalographs show the hypoplastic ramus and absence of the right temporomandibular joint (OMENS classification: $O_0$ $M_3$ $E_3$ $N^7_2$ $S_2$).

tallic pins through the hypoplastic ramus on each side of the osteotomy. The distraction device is attached, secured to the pins, and the device is turned 1 mm per day.[59,60,75] The mean amount of lengthening or distraction is 24.5 mm at a rate of 1 mm/day. It can be done as early as 2 years of age. Distraction osteogenesis gives more mandibular bone than with elongation by sliding vertical osteotomy or rib graft construction.[77,138] Careful follow-up documentation of the ramus height and occlusal plane is necessary. Nevertheless, the concept and possibilities for skeletal distraction are very promising for the ramus and for correction of other craniofacial skeletal abnormalities.

### Mandibulofacial dysostosis (Treacher Collins or Franceschetti syndrome)

*Franceschetti-Zwahlen-Klein syndrome or mandibulofacial dysostosis* (MFD) are the terms used for this disorder in European publications[34–36]. In the English-American literature, most authors credit the English ophthalmologist, Treacher Collins, as the author of the seminal paper.[148] Berry, however, described this entity earlier.[2]

The incidence is from 1:3,500 to 1:5,642 live births.[43,110,111] A positive family history is found in approximately 50% of cases.[151] Inheritance follows an autosomal dominant pattern. There is no racial predilection. The gene lies on the long arm of chromosome 5 at 5q32–q33.1.[23–25,52,69]

Theories on the pathogenesis of this malformative syndrome include failure of mesoderm differentiation in the first and second branchial arches, defective ossification of the facial bone, and tissue ischemia resulting from hypoplasia of the stapedial artery.[70,80]

Five categories are described by Franceschetti,[35] depending on the number of features present. In Tessier's classification, the complete form of the syndrome manifests craniofacial clefts 6, 7, and 8.[140]

These patients have a complex craniofacial malformation involving the middle and lower part of the face and affecting both bony structures and soft tissues. The deformity is *always* bilateral and *nearly always* symmetric.[89] They have downward sloping palpebral fissures, depressed cheekbones, deformed pinnas, a receding chin, and wide oral commissures (macrostomia) (Fig. 15–10A–C). This syndrome can be mistaken for bilateral hemifacial microsomia. The degree of symmetry and normal facial nerve function are important distinguishing characteristics of Treacher Collins syndrome.

Plain radiographs reveal the malar hypoplasia, tear drop–shaped orbits, and partial or complete absence of the zygomatic arches (Fig. 15–10D,E). In severe cases there is absence of the lateral wall and the floor of the orbits, i.e., a clefting of the inferolateral orbit extending into the sphenomaxillary (inferior orbital) fissure. Mandibular retrognathism is present, with shortening of the body and the ramus of the mandible. The chin is retruded severely and the nasomaxillary area is relatively prominent.[38] These children usually have normal intelligence.

Narrowing of the upper airway and hearing impairment are major issues in infancy. These infants are prone to obstructive sleep apnea and sudden infant death syndrome.[56] The size of the nasopharynx in children with Treacher Collins syndrome is about 50% smaller than normal.[132]

Treatment

*Infancy.* Skin tags should be excised during infancy. Some authors advocate correction of the coloboma in the first year of life.[38] Usually, however, there is no functional reason to do this in infancy as the upper eyelid offers adequate protection of the globes. With a tiny mandible, the upper airway has to be evaluated and, if necessary, secured with a tracheostomy.[89] It is very important to assess speech development and hearing. Middle ear anomalies are frequently associated with this syndrome. These children need to be fitted with an appropriate hearing aid, usually a bone conduction device over the mastoid.

The surgical plan for Treacher Collins syndrome must be tailored to the patient's specific deformities, taking into consideration facial growth and psychosocial impact. The surgical correction can be separated into procedures for the upper face and those for the jaws or lower face.

*Surgical plan: Skeletal correction of zygomas and orbits.* Skeletal correction includes construction or augmentation of the zygomatic arches and infraorbital rims. Clefts in the orbital floors must be bone grafted to correct the inferolateral orbital deficiency.[145] The downward slope of the superolateral orbital rim is corrected by a semilunar ostectomy and contour burring. Notwithstanding the near absence of the lateral canthal tendons, a concerted effort at lateral canthoplasty is required.

The upper facial skeleton can be corrected as early as age 5 or 6 years. Some authors recommend surgery at 3 years of age, as soon as the cranium is thick enough.[89] Various tissues (cartilage, dermal grafts, temporalis muscle, and split ribs) have been used to build up the hypoplastic zygomas in Treacher Collins syndrome patients. The cranium is now the preferred donor site. There is less resorption of its volume compared to other donor sites, less morbidity, and easy access to an area which is already in the operative field.[78,164] Theoretically, vascularized cranial bone should maintain volume better than a graft.[78] Other authors prefer bone grafts covered with a pericranial flap,[7] citing the fact that it is practically impossible to rely on the vascularity of cranial bone flaps. It is also difficult to maintain the muscle in contact with underlying bone. In short, the benefits of a vascularized cranial bone transfer and the added time for such an operation are difficult to justify.

*Eyelid deformities.* The downward slope of the palpebral fissures is due to abnormal inclination of the lateral orbital wall and the lateral ptotic canthal tendon. This can be corrected, in part, by altering the orbital skeleton and lateral canthopexy. The superolateral orbital rim is contoured, and split-thickness cranial grafts are used to construct and elevate the orbital floor. The lateral canthus can be positioned upward into drill holes in the newly reconstructed orbital rim or to temporal fascia. Many techniques have been described for correction of lower eyelid coloboma and/or hypoplasia: flap transposition from the upper to the lower eyelid, full-thickness skin grafts, intermarginal adhesions, the Kuhnt-Szymanowski procedure, Z-plasties, and lateral tarsorrhaphies. All too often the result is incomplete correction and scarring of the lower eyelid.[86]

Tessier and Tulasne[147] describe a method of correcting a major coloboma by marginal excision, Z-plasty for cutaneous lengthening, overlapping and suturing of the preseptal orbicularis muscle, as well as final transposition of the skin flaps and lateral canthopexy.[140] For less severe cases, Munro suggests simple vertical excision of the lateral eyelid only and superior reattachment of the residual lid to the lateral canthus.[89]

*Mandibular hypoplasia.* Micrognathia and microgenia with shortened posterior vertical height of both maxilla and mandible are consistent features. The facial profile is abnormally convex. In older patients, angle class II malocclusion and open bite are common presenting problems.

Tessier and Tulasne[147] propose a type of Le Fort II osteotomy to intrude the nasofrontal angle and lower the maxillary tuberosity; this is combined with mandibular osteotomy. More

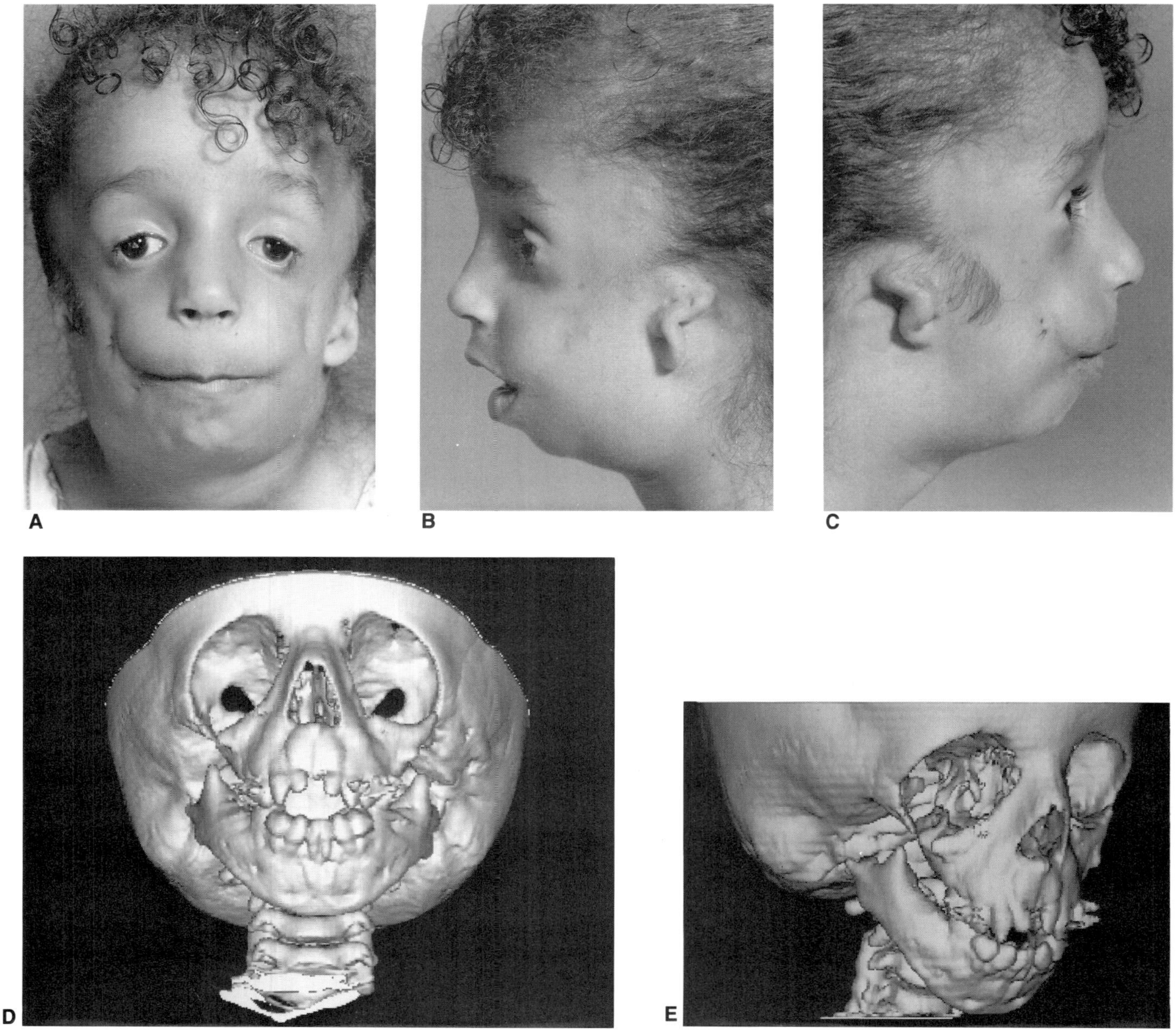

**Fig. 15–10.** Mandibulofacial dysostosis or Treacher Collins syndrome. A–C: Frontal and lateral views of a 6-year-old female with Treacher Collins syndrome. Note the symmetry in the downward slant of the eyes, missing lower (medial one-third) eyelashes, hypoplastic malar eminences, bilateral macrostomia, relatively broad nasal pyramid, decreased vertical height of the lower face, and bilateral microtia. D, E: Computerized tomography (CT) with 3D reconstruction demonstrates absence of the zygomas, clefting of the inferolateral orbits, and diminished height of posterior maxilla and rami. Although the child has a symmetric deformity, the CT study revealed slight asymmetry of orbital clefting.

commonly, Le Fort I osteotomy is done to lengthen the posterior maxillary height in severe cases of anterior open bite, combined with bilateral mandibular sagittal split osteotomies and genioplasty.[89] Bilateral mandibular distraction in early childhood, recently described, shows remarkable results.[80a] Many of these patients have a prominent nose and benefit from reduction rhinoplasty. Fuente del Campo proposed nasomaxillary osteotomies (flattening of the centrofacial region) at the age of 5 years to reduce nasal overprojection.[38]

*Adjunctive procedures.* Ear construction can be done after 6 years of age when there is sufficient costal cartilage to make the framework. Male patients can benefit from transposition of sideburns. Females may chose simple excision or depilation of the abnormal preauricular hair. There is no acceptable procedure to add the missing eyelashes along the medial lower lids.

## Midline anomalies: orbital hypertelorism

The term *hypertelorism* means an increased distance between two structures. In the past, the expression *ocular hypertelorism* was used for wide-spaced eyes, but this is inaccurate since the distance between the eyes does not necessarily correspond to the interorbital width. To avoid this confusion, Tessier[144] proposed the term *orbital hypertelorism,* which is synonymous with *hyperteleorbitism*. By definition, this term means an increased interorbital distance, as measured between the dacryons on radiological assessment and manifested clinically by the appearance of the eyes being too far apart. However, purely soft tissue problems, due to congenital anomalies or traumatic detachment of the canthal tendons, can give a similar impression. This is *telecanthus:* an increased distance between the medial canthi with a normal inter- or intraorbital distance.

Orbital hypertelorism is not a syndrome or a diagnosis but rather an anatomical finding associated with a number of craniofacial conditions. The most common causes are craniosynostotic conditions, particulary the Apert syndrome; other causes are frontal encephalocele, frontonasal dysplasia, craniofrontonasal dysplasia, and median facial cleft. Orbital hypertelorism and midline clefts are probably due to an arrest in embryonic development.

*Classification*. The severity of the orbital hypertelorism is graded: first degree is 30–34 mm interorbital distance (IOD); second degree is 34 to 40 mm IOD; third degree is greater than 40 mm IOD.[141] The normal values are 24–32 mm for adult males and 22–28 mm for adult females.[45] Tables for interorbital distance for children and even fetuses are available.[18,55]

Patients with orbital hypertelorism often have a short nose, a broad nasal root, bifid nasal tip, or cleft of the nose and upper lip (Fig. 15–11A,B).

*Treatment*. If the interorbital space is wide, this central complex must be resected; 360° orbital osteotomies permit translocation of the orbits medially. This is the classic correction originally described by Tessier.[142] A facial bipartition procedure is considered if the midface is abnormal with an inverted V-shaped maxilla and alveolar ridge, as in median cleft face or craniofrontonasal dysplasia (Fig. 15–9C–E).

Tessier wisely said: "the surgery of hypertelorbitism is surgery of the nose."[86] In severe cases, total nasal construction with a forehead flap is required, with prior tissue expansion if necessary.[97] Multiple procedures on the nasal complex is a common scenario.[86]

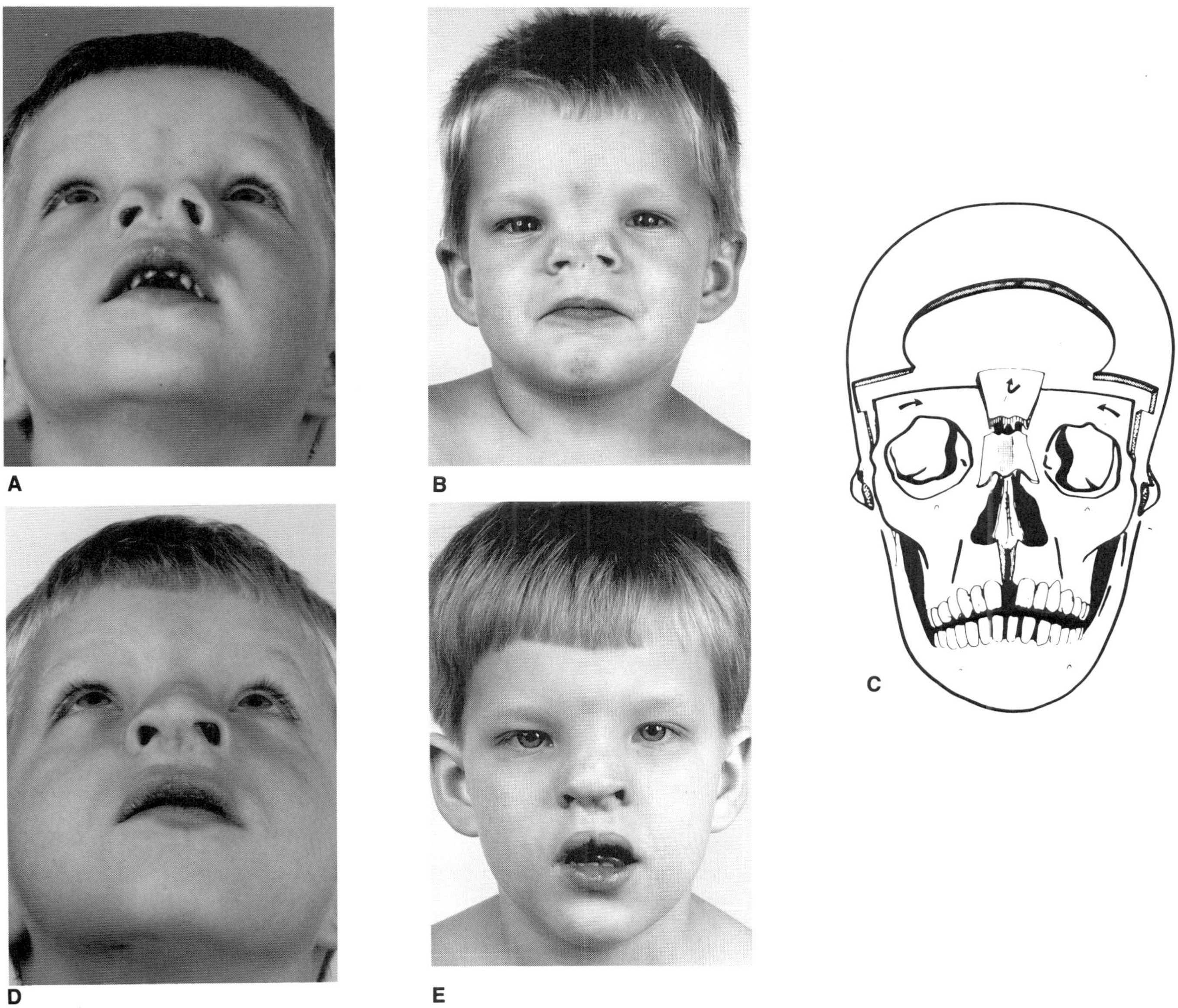

**Fig. 15–11.** Orbital hypertelorism (0–14 Tessier cleft). A, B: Preoperative submental and frontal views of a 4-year-old child with hyperteleorbitism, showing a bifid nose and an inverted V–shaped palate. C: Facial bipartition surgical correction. (Drawing is courtesy of Dr. C. Lauritzen.) D, E: Submental and frontal views of the post-facial bipartition procedure. (Courtesy of Dr. Claes Lauritzen.)

Surgical correction of orbital hypertelorism requires a combined, intracranial–extracranial approach. Some minor anomalies can be corrected via a subcranial approach or by transposition of the medial orbits. The low anatomic level of the cribriform plates must always be kept in mind. In young children, orbital transposition adds potential risk to the permanent dentition which is very high in the maxilla and very close to the orbital rim. There is evidence that standard orbital osteotomies for orbital hypertelorism can interfere with anterior facial growth.[86]

Minor hypertelorbitic anomalies do not require surgical correction. For this reason, it is best to defer surgical correction of orbital hypertelorism until the patient is 8–12 years of age, unless it is a grotesque deformity, e.g., grade III or median cleft face.

### Rare facial clefts

The true incidence of rare craniofacial clefts is not known; however, there is a reported 0.3%–1% frequency of facial clefts.[32,106,107] Tessier[143] (1973) presented his classification based on extensive personal experience. Clefts are numbered from 0 to 14 and follow vertical lines with axes through the eyebrows or eyelid, the maxilla, nose, and lip (Fig. 15–12). These numbers are distributed along a "northbound" and "southbound" hemisphere, according to the anatomical location of the clefts.[61]

## Complications in craniofacial surgery

Fifteen years ago, the combined complication rate at six craniofacial centers was 25.7% for intracranial and orbital procedures, in contrast to 8.8% for extracranial and orbital procedures.[157] The complication rate decreased from 22.3% in 1971–75 to 5.4% over the next decade.[88] This decrease is due in part to shortening the operating time by 50%–70%. Advances in anesthetic techniques and improved radiologic planning have also probably made a difference.[135]

In the past, the most common complications were infection (6.2%), cerebrospinal fluid (CSF) leakage (3.2%), and death (2.2%).[158] Whitaker et al. reviewed 164 consecutive patients and found 8% major complications and 11% minor complications.[157] A more recently published[135] complication rate of 8.6% is similar to that in other analyses. The most common complications were still infection (23%), CSF leakage (14%), misdiagnosis (1.4%), and death (0.5%).[135]

Mucosal tears increase the risk of infection due to intracranial contamination from the sinuses and nasal cavities.[88] They should be avoided. If they occur, they can be repaired, e.g., with galeal flap to minimize nasoethmoidal communication into the anterior cranial fossa.

Closed suction drains are used beneath the scalp flap. There is no evidence that drains act as a tract for bacteria. If tracheostomy is needed and justified, it should be done at the beginning of the procedure to avoid bacterial colonization and potential nosocomial infections.

To "shave or not to shave" prior to a coronal incision has been a subject of lively debate. Neurosurgeons usually prefer to shave the head, while craniofacial surgeons prefer not to. Clinical and laboratory studies support the concept that shaving increases the number of bacteria on the skin within several hours.[1] Studies by a neurosurgeon[161,162] document that avoiding shaving does not increase the risk of the infection whereas shaving does. However, cleansing of the hair before the operation is very important. Clipping hair does not significantly increase surface bacterial counts.

The major reasons for a low postoperative complication rate are operative experience and close interaction between involved specialties.

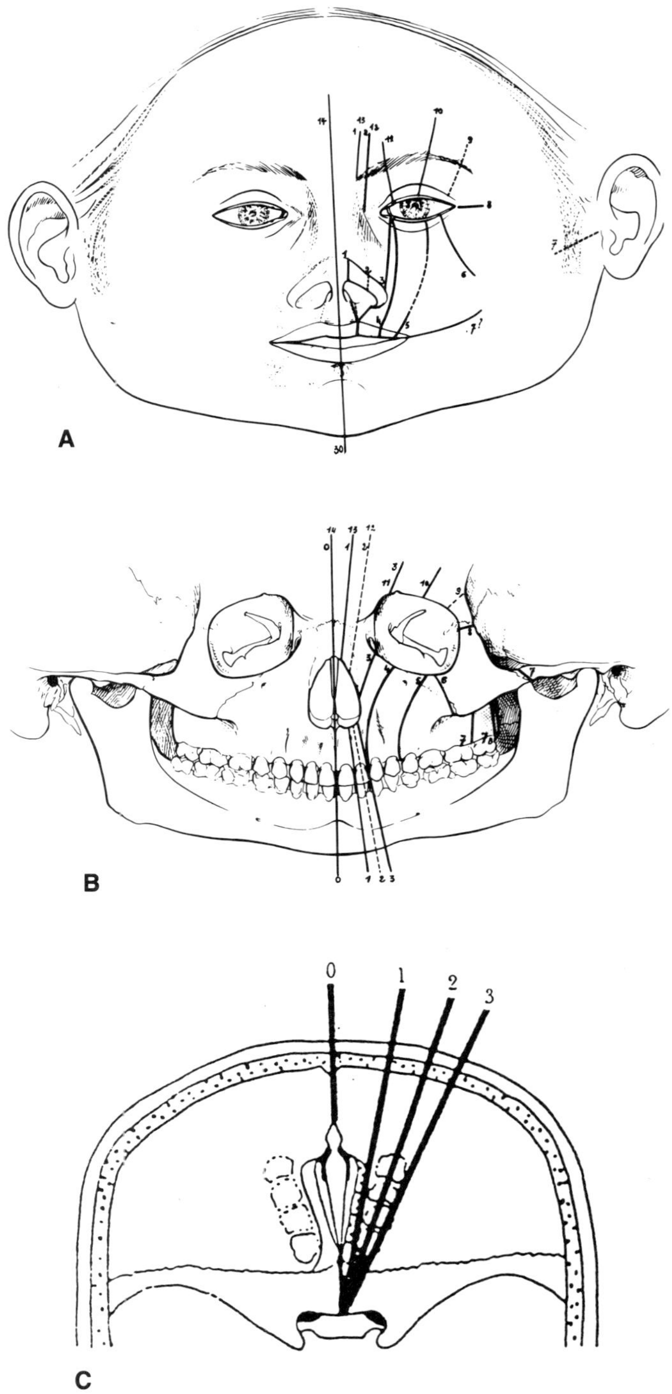


**Fig. 15–12.** Classification of rare facial clefts. A–C: Geographic pattern of facial clefts numbered according to Tessier: soft tissue, bony, and anterior skull base, #0 to #14.

## Epilogue

It is daunting to try and imagine the future of a discipline as young as craniofacial surgery. It is easier to envision technological changes than the more distant impact of molecular genetics.

The present epoch of craniofacial surgery, fathered by Tessier in the last quarter century, focuses on the operative correction of malformations. Permutations of his surgical procedures can be simulated using computer technology. Furthermore, computerized three-dimensional data can be used to study postoperative skeletal and soft tissue alterations and changes with craniofacial growth. Some day, surgical procedures will be image-guided, i.e., intraoperative computers will be used to enhance reality and to document the placement of skeletal segments and monitor soft tissue changes.

Rigid fixation with metal plates and screws is, undoubtedly, a major advance in craniofacial surgery. Biodegradable systems are under study in animal models and clinical trials are in progress. Bone segments will be secured with biocompatible glue. Osteodistraction has proven useful in long bones and for lengthening the hypoplastic mandible. Other bones in the craniofacial skeleton, e.g., a retruded midface or forehead, can also be moved forward using distraction techniques. The currently available distraction devices are clumsy; internal or integrated hardware is needed.

Fetal epidemiologic studies show that one-third of all embryos with cleft lip/palate are lost by spontaneous abortion.[62] These fetuses often have multiple malformations, putting them at high risk for intrauterine death, a process of natural selection called *terathanasia*.[155]

Nevertheless, exciting possibilities exist for intrauterine repair of major craniofacial anomalies and particularly the minor anomalies, cleft lip/palate. Studies in fetal wound-healing will surely benefit surgical procedures in many specialties. Craniofacial surgical procedures rely on healing of translocated bone segments and transplanted bone grafts. In the future, osteoinductive (growth) factors will be given to accelerate bony healing. Animal studies have demonstrated the potential for tissue engineering, i.e., building living constructs of cultured cells attached to a biodegradable matrix. In this way, a patient's own bony or cartilaginous framework can be prefabricated in the laboratory and transferred in vivo. Craniofacial surgeons have always favored fresh bone grafts, and there is solid experimental evidence for the superiority of such grafts. Future alloplastic implants will be more acceptable to both surgeon and recipient.

Another epoch is just beginning—the search for the molecular basis of craniofacial dysmorphism. Advances in molecular genetics have brought us to the horizon of understanding the precise mechanisms of human malformations. Soon, the genes for all the major craniofacial disorders will be known. The next step will be to unravel just how gene mutations affect craniofacial development and morphogenesis. Genetically engineered animal models are already facilitating this journey.

Some surgeons might ask whether future insights in craniofacial genetics will result in fewer anomalies for surgical correction! But, isn't this the dream of every physician devoted to the care of children with these deformities? Surgeons should have a love–hate relationship with the birth defects they struggle to mend. Because the majority of craniofacial defects are sporadic in occurrence, it is unlikely that their frequency can be significantly reduced in the near future. Early prenatal testing is possible for families affected by a disorder for which the gene is known. It is also likely that advances in preimplantation diagnosis and, perhaps some day, gene therapy, will be available for families affected with hereditary craniofacial disorders.

The most important advances will occur at the interface between specialties involved in the treatment of craniofacial disorders. Molecularly-oriented surgeons will then benefit from working with colleagues in the basic sciences.

*Acknowledgments*—The authors are grateful to the Shriners Hospital for Children, Montreal, for their support.

### References

1. Alexander JW, Fischer JE, Boyajian M, Palmquist J, Morris MJ: The influence of hair-removal methods on wound infections. Arch Surg 118:347–352, 1983.

1a. Apert E: De l'acrocéphalosyndactylie. *Bull Soc Med Paris* 23:1310–1330, 1906.

2. Berry GA: Note on a congenital defect (coloboma) of the lower lid. Lond Ophthalmol Hosp Rep 12:255, 1889.

3. Brueton LA, van Herwerden L, Chotai KA, Winter RM: The mapping of a gene for craniosynostosis: evidence for linkage of the Saethre-Chotzen syndrome to distal chromosome 7p. J Med Genet 29: 681–685, 1992.

4. Bruneteau RJ, Mulliken JB: Frontal plagiocephaly: synostotic, compensational, or deformational. Plast Reconstr Surg 89:21–31, 1992.

5. Bu BH, Kaban LB, Vargervik K: Effect of LeFort III osteotomy on mandibular growth in patients with Crouzon and Apert syndromes. J Oral Maxillofac Surg 47:666–671, 1989.

6. Carpenter G: Two sisters showing malformations of the skull and other congenital abnormalities. Rep Soc Study Dis Child (London) 1:110–118, 1901.

7. Casanova R, Cavalcante D, Grotting JC, Vasconez LO, Psillakis JM: Anatomic basis for vascularized outer-table calvarial bone flaps. Plast Reconstr Surg 78:300–308, 1986.

8. Chen NT, Glowacki J, Bucky LP, Hong H-Z, Kim WK, Yaremchuk MJ: The roles of revascularization and resorption on endurance of craniofacial onlay bone grafts in the rabbit. Plast Reconstr Surg 93:714–722, 1994.

8a. Chotzen F: Eine eigenartige familiäre Entwicklungsstörung. (Akrocephalosyndaktylie, Dysostosis craniofacialis und Hypertelorism us). *Monatschr Kinderheilkd* 55:97–122, 1932.

9. Clarren SK, Smith DW, Hansen JW: Helmet treatment for plagiocephaly and congenital muscular torticollis. J Pediatr 94: 43–46, 1979.

10. Cohen MM Jr: Craniostenoses and syndromes with craniosynostosis. Incidence, genetics, penetrance, variability and new syndrome updating. Birth Defects 15:13–63, 1979.

11. Cohen MM Jr: History, terminology, and classification of craniosynostosis. In: Craniosynostosis. Diagnosis, Evaluation, and Management. MM Cohen Jr, ed. Raven Press, New York, 1986, pp 1–20.

12. Cohen MM Jr: Discussion: The OMENS classification of hemifacial microsomia. Cleft Palate Craniofac J 28:77, 1991.

13. Cohen MM Jr: Pfeiffer syndrome update, clinical subtypes, and guidelines for differential diagnosis. Am J Med Genet 45: 300–307, 1993.

14. Cohen MM Jr, Kreiborg S: The central nervous system in the Apert syndrome. Am J Med Genet 35:36–45, 1990.

14.a Cohen MMJr, Kreiborg JS: Birth prevalence studies of the Crouzon syndrome: comparison of direct and indirect methods. Clin Genet 41:12–15, 1992.

15. Cohen MM Jr, Kreiborg S: Visceral anomalies in the Apert syndrome. Am J Med Genet 45:758–760, 1993.

16. Cohen MM Jr, Kreiborg S, Lammer EJ, Cordero JF, Mastroiacovo P, Erickson JD, Roeper P, Martínez-Frias ML: Birth prevalence study of the Apert syndrome. Am J Med Genet 42:655–659, 1992.

17. Cohen MM Jr, Rollnick BR, Kaye CI: Oculoauriculovertebral spectrum: an updated critique. Cleft Palate J 26:276–286, 1989.

18. Costaras M, Pruzansky S, Broadbent BH Jr: Bony interorbital distance (BIOD), head size, and level of the cribriform plate relative to orbital height: I. Normal standards for age and sex. J Craniofac Genet Dev Biol 2:5–18, 1982.

19. Crouzon O: Dysostose craniofaciale héréditaire. Bull Mem Soc Med Hôpital Paris 33:545–555, 1912.
20. David DJ, Mahatumarat C, Cooter RD: Hemifacial microsomia: a multisystem classification. Plast Reconstr Surg 80:525–535, 1987.
21. David JD, Poswillo D, Simpson D: The Craniosynostoses: Causes, Natural History and Management. Springer-Verlag, New York, 1982, pp 1–331.
22. Der Kaloustian VM, Sinno AA, Nassar SI: Carpenter's syndrome (acrocephalopolysyndactyly Type II). Am J Dis Child 124:716–718, 1972.
23. Dixon MJ, Dixon J, Houseal T, Bhatt M, Ward DC, Klinger K, Landes GM: Narrowing the position of the Treacher Collins syndrome locus to a small interval between three new microsatellite markers at 5q32–33.1. Am J Hum Genet 52:907–914, 1993.
24. Dixon MJ, Marres HA, Edwards SJ, Dixon J, Cremers CW: Treacher Collins syndrome: correlation between clinical and genetic linkage studies. Clin Dysmorphol 3:96–103, 1994.
25. Dixon MJ, Read AP, Donnai D, Colley A, Dixon J, Williamson R: The gene for Treacher Collins syndrome maps to the long arm of chromosome 5. Am J Hum Genet 49:17–22, 1991.
26. Dominguez R, Oh KS, Bender T, Girdany BR: Uncomplicated trigonocephaly—a radiographic affirmation of conservative therapy. Radiology 140:681–688, 1981.
27. Edwards TJC, David DJ, Martin J: Aggressive surgical management of sleep apnea syndrome in the syndromal craniosynostoses. J Craniofac Surg 3:8–10, 1992.
28. Eppley BL, Sadove AM: Surgical correction of metopic suture synostosis. Clin Plast Surg 21:555–562, 1994.
29. Fernbach SK, Naidich TP: Radiological evaluation of craniosynostosis. In: Craniosynostosis: Diagnosis, Evaluation and Management. MM Cohen Jr, ed. Raven Press, New York, 1986, pp 191–214.
30. Fiala TGS, Novelline RA, Yaremchuk MJ: Comparison of CT imaging artifacts from craniomaxillofacial internal fixation devices. Plast Reconstr Surg 92:1227–1232, 1993.
31. Fiala TGS, Paige KT, Davis TL, Campbell TA, Rosen BR, Yaremchuk MJ: Comparison of artifact from craniomaxillofacial internal fixation devices: magnetic resonance imaging. Plast Reconstr Surg 93:725–731, 1994.
32. Fogh-Andersen P: Rare clefts of the face. Acta Chir Scand 129:275–281, 1965.
33. Foltz EL, Loeser JD: Craniosynostosis. J Neurosurg 43:48–57, 1975.
34. Franceschetti A, Klein D: Mandibulo-facial dysostosis: new hereditary syndrome. Acta Ophthalmol 27:143–224, 1949.
35. Franceschetti A, Klein D, Brocher JEW: La dysostose mandibulofaciale dans le cadre des syndromes du premier arc branchial. Schweiz Med Wochenschr 89:478–483, 1959.
36. Franceschetti A, Zwahlen P: Un syndrome nouveau: la synostose mandibulo-faciale. Bull Schweiz Akad Med Wiss 1:60–66, 1944.
37. Friede H, Alberius P, Lilja J, Lauritzen C: Trigonocephaly: clinical and cephalometric assessment of craniofacial morphology in operated and non treated patients. Cleft Palate J 27:362–367, 1990.
38. Fuente del Campo A, Martinez Elizondo M, Arnaud E: Treacher Collins syndrome (mandibulofacial dysostosis). Clin Plast Surg 21:613–623, 1994.
39. Gorlin RJ: Classification of craniosynostosis syndromes. In: Scientific Foundations and Surgical Treatment of Craniosynostosis, JA Persing, MT Edgerton, JA Jane, eds. Williams & Wilkins, Baltimore, 1989, pp 1–8.
40. Gorlin RJ: Syndromes with craniosynostosis: general aspects and well-known syndromes. In: Syndromes of the Head and Neck, 3rd ed, RJ Gorlin, MMJ Cohen, LS Levin, eds. Oxford University Press, New York, 1990, pp 519–539.
41. Gorlin RJ, Pindborg JJ, eds. Syndromes of the Head and Neck. McGraw-Hill, New York, 1964.
42. Gorlin RJ, Pindborg JJ, Cohen MM Jr (eds): Syndromes of the Head and Neck, 2nd ed. McGraw-Hill, New York, 1976.
43. Grabb WC: The first and second brachial arch syndrome. Plast Reconstr Surg 36:485–508, 1965.
44. Hansen M, Mulliken JB: Frontal plagiocephaly. Diagnosis and treatment. Clin Plast Surg 21:543–553, 1994.
45. Hansman CF: Growth of interorbital distance and skull thickness as observed in roentgenographic measurements. Radiology 86:87–96, 1966.
46. Hodach RJ, Viseskul C, Gilbert EF, Herrmann JP, Wolfson JJ, Kaveggia EG, Opitz JM: Studies of malformation syndromes in man XXXVI: the Pfeiffer syndrome, association with Kleeblattschädel and multiple visceral anomalies. Case report and review. Z Kinderheilkunde 119:87–103, 1975.
47. Hoffman HJ, Mohr G: Lateral canthal advancement of the supraorbital margin. A new corrective technique in the treatment of coronal synostosis. J Neurosurg 45:376–381, 1976.
48. Hollway GE, Phillips HA, Ades LC, Haan EA, Mulley JC: Localization of craniosynostosis Adelaide type to 4p16. Hum Mol Genet 4:681–683, 1995.
49. Holtermüller K, Wiedemann HR: Kleeblattschädel-Syndrom. Med Monatsschr 14:439–446, 1960.
50. Horgan JE, Padwa BL, LaBrie RA, Mulliken JB: OMENS-plus—analysis of craniofacial and extracranial facial anomalies in hemifacial microsomia. Cleft Palate Craniofac J, 32:405–412, 1995.
51. Hunter AGW, Rudd NL: Craniosynostosis. I. Sagittal synostosis: Its genetics and associated clinical findings in 214 patients who lacked involvement of the coronal suture(s). Teratology 14:185–193, 1976.
52. Jabs EW, Li X, Lovett M, Yamaoka LH, Taylor E, Speer MC, Coss C, Cadle R, Hall B, Brown K, et al: Genetic and physical mapping of the Treacher Collins syndrome locus with respect to loci in the chromosome 5q3 region. Genomics 1:7–13, 1993.
53. Jabs EW, Li X, Scott AF, Meyers G, Chen W, Eccles M, Mao JI, Charnas LR, Jackson CE, Jaye M: Jackson-Weiss and Crouzon syndromes are allelic with mutations in fibroblast growth factor receptor 2. Nat Genet 8:275–279, 1994.
54. Jabs EW, Müller V, Li X, Ma L, Luo W, Haworth IS, Klisak I, Sparkes R, Warman ML, Mulliken JB, et al: A mutation in the homeodomain of the human MSX2 gene in a family affected with autosomal dominant craniosynostosis. Cell 75:443–450, 1993.
55. Jeanty P, Dramaix-Wilmet M, Van Gansbeke D, Van Regemorter N, Rodesch F: Fetal ocular biometry by ultrasound. Radiology 143:513–516, 1982.
56. Johnston C, Taussig LM, Koopmann C, Smith P, Bjelland J: Obstructive sleep apnea in Treacher Collins syndrome. Cleft Palate J 18:39–44, 1981.
57. Johnston MC: Embryology of the head and neck. In: Plastic Surgery, JG McCarthy, JW May Jr, JW Little, eds. WB Saunders, Philadelphia, 1990, pp 2451–2495.
58. Kaban LB, Moses MH, Mulliken JB: Surgical correction of hemifacial microsomia in the growing child. Plast Reconstr Surg 82:9–19, 1988.
59. Karp NS, McCarthy JG, Schreiber JS, Sissons HA, Thorne CH: Membranous bone lengthening: a serial histological study. Ann Plast Surg 29:2–7, 1992.
60. Karp NS, Thorne CH, McCarthy JG, Sissons HA: Bone lengthening in the craniofacial skeleton. Ann Plast Surg 24:231–237, 1990.
61. Kawamoto HKJr: The kaleidoscopic world of rare craniofacial clefts; order out of chaos (Tessier classification). Clin Plast Surg 3:529–572, 1976.
62. Kraus BS, Kitamura H, Ooe T: Malformations associated with cleft lip and palate in human embryos and fetuses. Am J Obstet Gynecol 86:321–328, 1963.
63. Laitinen L: Craniosynostosis. Ann Paediatr Fenniae 2(Suppl 6):1–130, 1956.
64. Lauritzen C, Munro IR, Ross RB: Classification and treatment of hemifacial microsomia. Scand J Plast Surg 19:33–39, 1985.
65. Le Fort R: Etude expérimentale sur les fractures de la mâchoire supérieure. Rev Chir 23:208–227; 360–379; 479–507, 1901.
66. Lewanda AF, Cohen MM Jr, Jackson CE, Taylor EW, Li X, Beloff M, Day D, Clarren SK, Ortiz R, Garcia C, et al: Genetic heterogeneity among craniosynostosis syndromes: mapping the Saethre-Chotzen syndrome locus between D7S513 and D7S516 and exclusion of Jackson-Weiss and Crouzon syndrome loci from 7p. Genomics 19:115–119, 1994.
67. Lin KY, Bartlett SP, Yaremchuk MJ, Fallon M, Grossman RF, Whitaker LA: The effect of rigid fixation on the survival of onlay bone grafts: an experimental study. Plast Reconstr Surg 86:449–456, 1990.
68. Lin KY, Bartlett SP, Yaremchuk MJ, Grossman RF, Udupa JK, Whitaker LA: An experimental study on the effect of rigid fixation on the developing craniofacial skeleton. Plast Reconstr Surg 87:229–235, 1991.
69. Loftus SK, Edwards SJ, Scherpbier-Heddema T, Buetow KH, Wasmuth JJ, Dixon MJ: A combined genetic and radiation hybrid map surrounding the Treacher Collins syndrome locus on chromosome 5q. Hum Mol Genet 2:1785–1792, 1993.
70. Mann I, Kilner TP: Deficiency of the malar bones with defect of the lower eyelids. Br J Ophthalmol 27:13–20, 1943.
71. Manson PN: Facial injuries. In: Plastic Surgery, Vol 2, JG McCarthy, ed. WB Saunders, Philadelphia, 1990, pp 867–1141.

72. Marchac D: Radical forehead remodelling for craniostenosis. Plast Reconstr Surg 61:823–835, 1978.
73. Marsh JL, Jenny A, Galic M, Picker S, Vannier MW: Surgical management of sagittal synostosis. A quantitative evaluation of two techniques. Neurosurg Clin North Am 2:629–640, 1991.
74. Marsh JL, Schwartz HG: The surgical correction of coronal and metopic craniosynostoses. J Neurosurg 59:245–251, 1983.
75. McCarthy JG: The role of distraction osteogenesis in the reconstruction of the mandible in unilateral craniofacial microsomia. Clin Plast Surg 21:625–630, 1994.
76. McCarthy JG, Grayson BH, Coccaro PJ, Wood-Smith D: Craniofacial microsomia. In: Plastic Surgery, Vol 4, Cleft Lip & Palate and Craniofacial Anomalies. JG McCarthy, JW May, Jr, JW Littler, eds. WB Saunders, Philadelphia, 1990, pp 3054–3100.
77. McCarthy JG, Schreiber J, Karp N, Thorne CH, Grayson BH: Lengthening the human mandible by gradual distraction. Plast Reconstr Surg 89:1–8, 1992.
78. McCarthy JG, Zide BM: The spectrum of calvarial bone grafting; introduction of the vascularized calvarial bone flap. Plast Reconstr Surg 74:10–18, 1984.
79. McComb JG: Treatment of functional lambdoid synostosis. Neurosurg Clin North Am 2:665–672, 1991.
80. McKenzie J, Craig J: Mandibulofacial dysostosis (Treacher Collins Syndrome). Arch Dis Child 30:391–395, 1955.
80a. Molina F, Ortiz Monasterio F: Mandibular elongation and remodeling by distraction: a farewell to major osteotomies. Plast Reconstr Surg 96:825–840, 1995.
81. Montaut J, Stricker M: Les dysmorphies cranio-faciales: les synostoses prématurées (craniosténoses et faciosténoses). Masson, Paris, 1977.
82. Muenke M, Schell U, Hehr A, Robin NH, Losken HW, Schinzel A, Pulleyn LJ, Rutland P, Reardon W, Malcolm S, et al: A common mutation in the fibroblast growth factor receptor 1 gene in Pfeiffer syndrome. Nat Genet 8:269–274, 1994.
83. Müller U, Warman ML, Mulliken JB, Weber JL: Assignment of a gene locus involved in craniosynostosis to chromosome 5qter. Hum Mol Genet 2:119–122, 1993.
84. Mulliken JB, Bruneteau RJ: Surgical correction of the craniofacial anomalies in Apert syndrome. Clin Plast Surg 18:277–289, 1991.
85. Mulliken JB, Kaban LB: Analysis and treatment of hemifacial microsomia in childhood. Clin Plast Surg 14:91–100, 1987.
86. Mulliken JB, Kaban LB, Evans CA, Strand RD, Murray JE: Facial skeletal changes following hypertelorbitism correction. Plast Reconstr Surg 77:7–16, 1986.
87. Munro IR: Craniofacial surgery. In: Plastic Surgery, 3rd ed, WC Grabb, JW Smith, eds. Little, Brown, Boston, 1979, pp 131–160.
88. Munro IR, Sabatier RE: An analysis of 12 years of craniomaxillofacial surgery in Toronto. Plast Reconstr Surg 76:29–35, 1985.
89. Munro IR, Kay PP, Randall P, Ruff GL, Siebert JW: Craniofacial syndromes. In: Plastic Surgery, Vol 4, Cleft Lip & Palate and Craniofacial Anomalies. JG McCarthy, JW May, Jr, JW Littler, eds. WB Saunders, Philadelphia, 1990, pp 3101–3123.
90. Munro IR, Lauritzen CGK: Periorbital tumors. In: Craniofacial Surgery, EP Caronni, ed. Little, Brown & Co, Boston, 1985, pp 329–344.
91. Munro IR, Lauritzen CGK: Classification and treatment of hemifacial microsomia. In: Craniofacial Surgery, EP Caronni, ed. Little, Brown & Co, Boston, 1985, pp 391–400.
92. Munro IR, Raposo do Amaral CM, Carroni EP, Chen Y-R, Habal MB, Wolfe SA, Whitaker LA: The round table session on craniofacial surgery. J Craniofac Surg 4:64–66, 1993.
93. Murray JE, Kaban LB, Mulliken JB: Analysis and treatment of hemifacial microsomia. Plast Reconstr Surg 74:186–199, 1984.
93a. Meyers GA, Orlow SJ, Munro IR, Przylepa KA, Jabs EW: Fibroblast growth factor receptor 3 *(FGFR3)* transmembrane mutation in Crouzon syndrome with acanthosis nigricans. Nat Genet 11:462–464, 1995.
94. Ocampo RV Jr, Persing JA: Sagittal synostosis. Clin Plast Surg 21:563–574, 1994.
95. Ohman JC, Richtsmeier JT: Perspectives on craniofacial growth. Clin Plast Surg 21:489–499, 1994.
96. Ortiz-Monasterio F, Fuente del Campo AF, Carrillo A: Advancement of the orbits and the midface in one piece, combined with frontal repositioning, for the correction of Crouzon's deformities. Plast Reconstr Surg 61:507–516, 1978.
97. Ortiz-Monasterio F, Molina F: Orbital hypertelorism. Clin Plast Surg 21:599–612, 1994.
98. Ousterhout DK, Peterson-Falzone SJ: Long-term follow-up on a case of untreated trigonocephaly. Cleft Palate J 27:72–75, 1990.
99. Padwa BL, Warman ML, Whiteman DAH, Mulliken JB: Anthropometric analysis of the phenotypic spectrum in Saethre-Chotzen syndrome in five families. In: Proceedings of the Fifth International Congress of the International Society of Craniofacial Surgery, FO Monasterio, HC Monduzzi, ed. Bologna, 1994, pp 157–158.
100. Pantke OA, Cohen MM Jr, Witkop CJJr, Feingold M, Schaumann B, Pantke HC, Gorlin RJ: The Saethre-Chozen syndrome. Birth Defects 11:190–225, 1975.
101. Park W-J, Meyers GA, Li X, Theda C, Day D, Orlow SJ, Jones MC, Jabs EW: Novel *FGFR2* mutations in Crouzon and Jackson-Weiss syndromes show allelic heterogeneity and phenotypic variability. Hum Mol Genet 4:1229–1233, 1995.
102. Park W-J, Theda C, Maestri NE, Meyers GA, Fryburg JS, Dufresne C, Cohen MM Jr, Jabs EW: Analysis of phenotypic features and FGFR2 mutations in Apert syndrome. Am J Hum Genet 57:321–328, 1995.
103. Peterson SJ, Pruzansky S: Palatal anomalies in the syndromes of Apert and Crouzon. Cleft Palate J 11:394–403, 1974.
104. Pfeiffer UJ: Dominant erbliche Akrocephalosyndaktylie. Z Kinderheilkunde 90:301–320, 1964.
105. Phillips JH, Rahn BA: Fixation effects on membranous and endochondral onlay bone graft revascularization and bone deposition. Plast Reconstr Surg 85:891–897, 1990.
106. Pitanguy IHJ: Facial clefts as seen in a large series of untreated adults and their later management. In: Craniofacial Anomalies. JJ Longacre, ed. Lippincott, Philadelphia, 1968, p 167.
107. Popescu V: Despicaturile congenitale transversale ale fetei. Stomatologia 15:139–152, 1968.
108. Posnick JC, Lin KY, Chen P, Armstrong D: Metopic synostosis: quantitative assessment of presenting deformity and surgical results based on CT scans. Plast Reconstr Surg 93:16–24, 1994.
109. Poswillo D: The pathogenesis of the first and second branchial arch syndrome. Oral Surg 35:302–328, 1973.
110. Poswillo DE: Orofacial malformations. Proc R Soc Med 67:343–349, 1974.
111. Poswillo D: Otomandibular deformity: pathogenesis as a guide to reconstruction. J Maxillo Fac Surg 2:64–72, 1974.
112. Poswillo D: Hemorrhage in development of the face. Birth Defects 11:61–81, 1975.
113. Preston RA, Post JC, Keats BJ, Aston CE, Ferrell RE, Priest J, Nouri N, Losken HW, Morris CA, Hurtt MR, et al: A gene for Crouzon craniofacial dysostosis maps to the long arm of chromosome 10. Nat Genet 7:149–153, 1994.
113a. Przylepa KA, Paznekas W, Zhang M, Golabi M, Bias W, Bamshad MJ, Carey JC, Hall BD, Stevenson R, Orlow SJ, Cohen MMJr, Jabs EW: Fibroblast growth factor receptor 2 mutations in Beare-Stevenson cutis gyrata syndrome. Nat Genet 13:492–494, 1996.
114. Pruzansky S: Not all dwarfed mandibles are alike. Birth Defects 1(2):120–129, 1969.
115. Pruzansky S: The challenge and opportunity in craniofacial anomalies. Cleft Palate J 8:239–250, 1971.
116. Reardon W, McManus SP, Summers D, Winter RM: Cytogenetic evidence that the Saethre-Chotzen gene maps to 7p21.2. Am J Med Genet 47:633–636, 1993.
117. Reardon W, Winter RM, Rutland P, Pulleyn LJ, Jones BM, Malcolm S: Mutations in the fibroblast growth factor receptor 2 gene cause Crouzon syndrome. Nat Genetics 8:98–103, 1994.
118. Reid CS, McMorrow LE, McDonald-McGinn DM, Grace KJ, Ramos FJ, Zackai EH, Cohen MM Jr, Jabs EW: Saethre-Chotzen syndrome with familial translocation at chromosome 7p22. Am J Med Genet 47:637–639, 1993.
119. Renier D, Saint-Rose CH, Marchac D: Intracranial pressure in craniostenoses. 302 recordings. In: Craniofacial Surgery: Proceedings of the 1st Congress of the International Society of Craniomaxillofacial Surgery, D Marchac, ed. Springer-Verlag, Heidelberg, 1987, pp 110–113.
120. Renier D, Sainte-Rose C, Marchac D, Hirsch JF: Intracranial pressure in craniostenosis. J Neurosurg 57:370–377, 1982.
121. Ripley CE, Pomatto J, Beals SP, Joganic EF, Manwaring KH, Moss SD: Treatment of positional plagiocephaly with dynamic orthotic cranioplasty. J Craniofac Surg 5:150–159, 1994.
122. Robb RM, Boger WP 3d: Vertical strabismus associated with plagiocephaly. J Pediatr Ophthalmol Strabismus 20:58–62, 1983.
123. Robin NH, Feldman GJ, Mitchell HF, Lorenz P, Wilroy RS, Zackai EH, Allanson JE, Reich EW, Pfeiffer RA, Clarke LA, Warman ML, Mulliken JB, Brueton LA, Winter RM, Price RA, Gasser DL, Muenke M: Linkage of Pfeiffer syndrome to chromosome 8 centro-

mere and evidence for genetic heterogeneity. Hum Mol Genet 3:2153–2158, 1994.

124. Rutland P, Pulleyn LJ, Reardon W, Baraitser M, Hayward R, Jones B, Malcolm S, Winter RM, Oldridge M, Slaney SF, et al: Identical mutations in the FGFR2 gene cause both Pfeiffer and Crouzon syndrome phenotypes. Nat Genetics 9:173–176, 1995.
125. Sadove AM: Commentary on aggressive surgical management of sleep apnea syndrome in the syndromal craniosynostoses. J Craniofac Surg 3:11, 1992.
125a. Saethre H: Ein Beitrag zum Turmschädelproblem. (Pathogenese, Erblichkeit und Symptomalogie). *Dtsch Z Nervenheilkd* 117:533–555, 1931.
126. Saldino RM, Steinbach HL, Epstein CJ: Familial acrocephalosyndactyly (Pfeiffer syndrome). Am J Roentgenol 116:609–622, 1972.
127. Schell U, Hehr A, Feldman GJ, Robin NH, Zackai EH, de Die-Smulders C, Viskochil DH, Stewart JM, Wolff G, Ohashi H, et al: Mutations in FGFR1 and FGFR2 cause familial and sporadic Pfeiffer syndrome. Hum Mol Genet 4:323–328, 1995.
128. Scheuerle J, Pannbacker M: Responses to telephone inquiries made to craniofacial treatment teams. J Craniofac Surg 5:143–145, 1994.
129. Shiang R, Thompson LM, Zhu YZ, Church DM, Fielder TJ, Bocian M, Winokur ST, Wasmuth JJ: Mutations in the transmembrane domain of FGFR3 cause the most common genetic form of dwarfism, achondroplasia. Cell 78:335–342, 1994.
130. Shillito J Jr: A plea for early operations for craniosynostosis. Surg Neurol 37:182–188, 1992.
131. Shillito JJ, Matson DD: Craniosynostosis: a review of 519 surgical patients. Pediatrics 41:829–853, 1968.
132. Shprintzen RJ, Croft C, Berkman MD, Rakoff SJ: Pharyngeal hypoplasia in Treacher Collins syndrome. Arch Otolaryngol 105:127–131, 1979.
133. Solomon LM, Fretzin D, Pruzansky S: Pilosebaceous abnormalities in Apert's syndrome. Arch Dermatol 102:381–385, 1970.
134. Steffen C: Acneform eruption in Apert's syndrome. Arch Dermatol 118:206–208, 1982.
135. Stieg PE, Mulliken JB: Neurosurgical complications in craniofacial surgery. Neurosurg Clin North Am 2:703–708, 1991.
136. Swanson LT, Murray JE: Asymmetries of the lower part of the face. In: Symposium on Reconstruction of Jaw Deformity, 6th ed, LA Whitaker, P Randall, eds. CV Mosby, St. Louis, 1976, pp 171–195.
137. Tavormina PL, Shiang R, Thompson LM, Zhu Y-Z, Wilkin DJ, Lachman RS, Wilcox WR, Rimoin DL, Cohn DH, Wasmith JJ: Thanatophoric dysplasia (types I and II) caused by distinct mutations in fibroblast growth factor receptor 3. Nat Genetics 9:321–328, 1995.
138. Taylor GI: Discussion: McCarthy JG, Schreiber J, Karp N: Lengthening the human mandible by gradual distraction. Plast Reconstr Surg 89:9–10, 1992.
139. Tessier P: Ostéotomies totales de la face: Syndrome de Crouzon, syndrome d'Apert: oxycéphalies, scaphocéphalies, turricéphalies. Ann Chir Plast 12:273–286, 1967.
140. Tessier P: Relationship of craniostenoses to craniofacial dysostoses and to faciostenoses: a study with therapeutic implications. Plast Reconstr Surg 48:224–237, 1971.
141. Tessier P: Orbital hypertelorism. I. Successive surgical attempts. Material and methods. Causes and mechanisms. Scand J Plast Reconstr Surg 6:135–155, 1972.
142. Tessier P, Guiot G, Derome P: Orbital hypertelorism II. Definitive treatment of orbital hypertelorism by craniofacial or by extracranial osteotomies. Scand J Plast Reconstr Surg 7:39–58, 1973.
143. Tessier P: Anatomical classification of facial, cranio-facial and latero-facial clefts. J Maxillofac Surg 4:69–92, 1976.
144. Tessier P: The definitive treatment of hypertelorism by craniofacial and laterofacial clefts. J Maxillofac Surg 4:69–92, 1979.
145. Tessier P: Plastic Surgery of the Orbit and Eyelids. Masson, New York, 1981, pp 169–170.
146. Tessier P: Apert's syndrome: acrocephalo-syndactyly type I. In: Craniofacial Surgery, EP Caronni, ed. Little, Brown & Co, Boston, 1985, pp 280–303.
147. Tessier P, Tulasne JF: Treacher Collins syndrome. Combined rotation of the midfacial segment and mandibular lengthening. In: Proceedings of the First International Congress of the International Society of Craniofacial Surgery, D Marchac, ed. Springer-Verlag, Berlin, 1987, p 369.
148. Treacher Collins E: Case with symmetrical congenital notches in the outer part of each lid and defective development of the malar bones. Trans Ophthalmol Soc UK 20:190–191, 1900.
149. Van der Meulen JCH: Medial faciotomy. Br J Plast Surg 32: 339–342, 1979.
150. van Herwerden L, Rose CSP, Reardon W, Brueton LA, Weissenbach J, Malcolm S, Winter RM: Evidence for locus heterogeneity in acrocephalosyndactyly: a refined localization for the Saethre-Chotzen syndrome locus on distal chromosome 7p- and exclusion of Jackson-Weiss syndrome from craniosynostosis loci on 7p and 5q. Am J Hum Genet 54:669–674, 1994.
151. Vatré JL: Etude génétique et classification clinique de 154 cas de dysostose mandibulo-faciale—syndrome de Franceschetti avec description de leurs associations malformatives. J Genet Hum 19:17–100, 1971.
152. Vento AR, LaBrie RA, Mulliken JB: The O.M.E.N.S. classification of hemifacial microsomia. Cleft Palate Craniofac J 28:68–76, 1991.
153. Wagstaff J, Hemann M: A familial "balanced" 3;9 translocation with cryptic 8q insertion leading to deletion and duplication of 9p23 loci in siblings. Am J Hum Genet 56:302–309, 1995.
154. Warman ML, Mulliken JB, Hayward PG, Müller U: Newly recognized autosomal dominant disorder with craniosynostosis. Am J Med Genet 46:444–449, 1993.
155. Warkany J: Terathanasia. Teratology 17:187–192, 1978.
156. Watson GH: Relation between side of plagiocephaly, dislocation of hip scoliosis, bat ears and sternomastoid tumors. Arch Dis Child 46:203–210, 1971.
157. Whitaker LA, Bartlett SP, Schut L, Bruce D: Craniosynostosis: an analysis of the timing, treatment and complications in 164 consecutive patients. Plast Reconstr Surg 80:195–212, 1987.
158. Whitaker LA, Munro IR, Salyer KE, Jackson IT, Ortiz-Monasterio F, Marchac D: Combined report on problems and complications in 793 craniofacial operations. Plast Reconstr Surg 64:198–203, 1979.
159. Whitaker LA, Schut L, Kerr LP: Early surgery for isolated craniofacial dysostosis. Improvement and possible prevention of increasing deformity. Plast Reconstr Surg 60:575–581, 1977.
160. Wilkie AOM, Slaney SF, Oldridge M, Poole MD, Ashworth GJ, Hockley AD, Hayward RD, David DJ, Pulleyn LJ, Rutland P, Malcolm S, Winter RM, Reardon W: Apert syndrome results from localized mutations of FGFR2 and is allelic with Crouzon syndrome. Nat Genet 9:165–172, 1995.
161. Winston KR: Hair and neurosurgery. Neurosurgery 31:320–329, 1992.
162. Winston KR: Comments. Neurosurgery 34:770, 1994.
163. Wong L, Woodberry K, Richtsmeier JT, Dufresne CR, Manson PN: Modifying the effects of rigid fixation on craniofacial growth. Paper presented at the 37th annual meeting, Plastic Surgery Research Council Toronto, April 1992, 69–71.
164. Zins JE, Whitaker LA: Membranous versus endochondral bone: implications for craniofacial reconstruction. Plast Reconstr Surg 72:778–784, 1983.

# VI

# THE NECK

# 16

# Embryology of the Neck

EUGENE DANIELS

The early development of the neck region is usually described together with the head region because their basic components develop from few pharyngeal structures (pharyngeal apparatus) in a craniocaudal sequence. This chapter will focus on dynamic changes in the embryonic neck (cervical) region that influence the anatomical relationships seen in the definitive neck, as well as the localization of abnormal structures that may form during development.

The contoured neck is discernible when the head is demarcated from the trunk during the seventh and eighth weeks.[12] However, definition of cervical structures begins much earlier when the developing hindbrain and somites are first patterned. It is the precocious development of the brain and associated somites (compared to trunk regions) that determines the early complex relationships of many normal and abnormal structures in the embryonic cervical region.

## Terminology

During the third week of development, the flat trilaminar embryo undergoes spectacular head–tail and lateral foldings to form a cylindrical embryo, and is for the first time more recognizable as a human form. However, at this time the head and neck region resembles that of a fish embryo of comparable stage with laterally placed clefts (Fig. 16–2). These clefts resemble gill clefts, hence the term *branchial clefts* (from the Greek *Branchia,* meaning "gills"). Considering biodynamic mechanisms, Blechschmidt[2] suggests that these clefts are the result of "flexion folds," a consequence of head–tail folding within an enveloping but restricted amniotic cavity. The basic tissues (ectoderm, neuroepithelium, intraembryonic mesenchyme, endoderm) which form the head and neck region are initially organized into a primitive pattern of similar segmented structures termed the *pharyngeal apparatus.* The term *pharyngeal apparatus,* which consists of pharyngeal arches, pouches, membranes, and clefts, will be used in this description of the human neck.

## Early definition of a cervical region

### Origin of cells and tissues of the cervical region

The earliest morphogenetic event that marks the allocation of head and neck cell precursors is the cranial migration of primitive intraembryonic mesenchyme during gastrulation (approximately day 14). The primitive mesenchyme forms an axially placed notochord and loose mesenchyme. The notochord induces the neural plate, and demarcation of a cephalic neural plate defines the brain–cervical spinal cord junction.

The rostral mesenchyme rapidly becomes organized into paired aggregates, or somites, on either side of the notochord. As neurulation proceeds, active migration of cephalic neural crest cells from the junction of the surface ectoderm and induced neuroectoderm occurs (note arrows in Fig. 16–1). The site of rhombomeres, which appear as periodic bulges of the hindbrain region, is in close spatial relationship with the pharyngeal arches. Neural crest cells from the hindbrain region contribute a significant population of cells to the developing head and anterior neck region.[9,15] Muscle components are derived from the early intraembryonic mesenchyme.[15]

Lumsden and Keynes[17] analyzed segmental patterns in the chick hindbrain. These authors reported that each of the three principal pharyngeal arches lie in register with the hindbrain segments. In mammalian embryos it appears that the neural crest cells from rhombomeres 2 and 4 contribute to most structures in pharyngeal arches I and II, respectively.[11]

Studies[5] involving the formation of chick-quail chimeras suggest that the superficial ectoderm covering the pharyngeal arches appears to represent early anteroposterior segments (ectomeres) that coincide with the spacial distribution of neural crest cells arising from specific levels of the neural fold. The ectoderm of the arches therefore appears to show an early segmented pattern which parallels that described for the neural crest and hindbrain.

In the primitive pharyngeal region, complex cellular interactions occur between neuroepithelium, neural placode, surface ectoderm, migratory neural crest cells, pharyngeal endoderm, and intra-embryonic mesoderm. While it appears to be too complex to unravel the genes involved in primary and subsequent cellular interactions, there is considerable evidence from mouse embryo studies that the orderly expression of homeobox genes appears to have a primary involvement in pharyngeal arch development.[11,16,18] Similar genes have been described in human embryos, and there is considerable similarity in early development of mouse and human craniofacial and neck anomalies.

The observation that segment-restricted patterns of homeobox gene expression in the rhombomeres (hindbrain) are also observed in the cranial ganglia, surface ectoderm, and mesectoderm of specific pharyngeal arches,[11] suggests that the cranial neural crest may be instructed with developmental cues (molecular prepatterning) necessary for specific cellular interactions in the pharyngeal tissues. Studies with mutant embryos suggest that the expression of genes during the earliest phases of head and neck formation play an essential role in the patterning of the pharyngeal apparatus.[4]

### Trilaminar embryo phase

The essential tissues of the cervical region are formed in the flat trilaminar embryo (days 22–24)[1] before the head–tail and lateral folding have progressed.

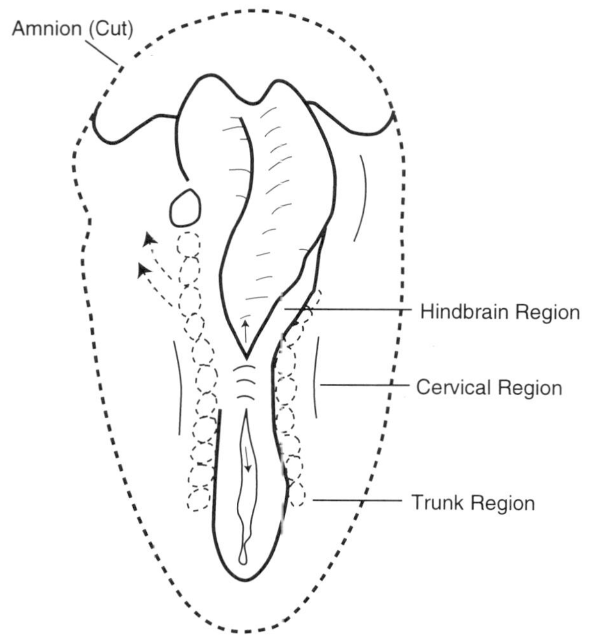


**Fig. 16–1.** A dorsal view of a trilaminar stage embryo seen in an opened amniotic sac. Note the advanced stage of development of the cervical region compared to the trunk region. Occipital and cervical somites have formed, and neural crest cells from the hindbrain region have migrated (interrupted arrows) to form the anlagen of the pharyngeal arches. The arrows indicate the cranial and caudal direction of neurulation.

Studies on the expression of homeobox genes in the hindbrain region also provide convincing evidence that structures destined to develop in the future head and neck region are specified before the cylindrical embryo is formed.[11]

Neural crest cell migrations and cell aggregations to form somites have already been initiated during this phase. In figure 16–1 note that the enlarged brain region of the central nervous system is clearly defined and that somites are distinguishable in the region of the brain–spinal cord junction. This junction will mark the site of the cervical flexure of the central nervous system (CNS).

Very rapid growth ensues, and within a period of a few days (between days 20 and 30), many primordial structures in the head and neck region are actively formed. Table 16–1 lists the sequence of formation of significant embryonic structures related to cervical development.

**Table 16–1.** Timetable of significant embryonic events during early cervical development

| |
|---|
| DAYS 20–21: LENGTH 1.0–1.5 mm: |
| 1–3 paired somites. |
| Trilaminar embryo (Fig. 16–1) |
| Development of intraembryonic mesoderm derived from primitive streak |
| Notochord induces neuroepithelium and neural folds present |
| Intraembryonic vessels appear |
| DAY 22 ±1: LENGTH 1.5–2.0 mm: |
| 4–12 paired somites |
| Cylindrical embryo |
| Foregut, midgut, and hindgut formed during head-tail and lateral folding |
| Brain (forebrain, midbrain, hindbrain) distinguishable from spinal cord in open neural tube |
| Fusion of neural folds near hindbrain region |
| I and II pharyngeal arches distinguishable (neural crest cell infiltration) |
| 1st and 2nd pharyngeal grooves present |
| DAY 24 ±1: LENGTH 2.0–3.0 mm: |
| 13–20 paired somites |
| 2 pharyngeal pouches and pharyngeal membranes |
| Shallow otic pit |
| Neural crest proliferation to form ganglia (V, VII, VIII) |
| Buccopharyngeal membrane breaks down |
| DAY 26 ±1: LENGTH 3.5 mm: |
| 21–29 paired somites |
| Upper limb buds appear |
| 3 pharyngeal arches |
| 4 pharyngeal pouches |
| Closure of anterior neuropore |
| Thyroid diverticulum in pharynx floor |
| Laryngotracheal groove |
| Prominent heart |
| DAY 28 ±1: LENGTH 4.0–5.0 mm: |
| 30–35 somites. |
| Marked midbrain flexure (no distinct hindbrain and cervical flexures) |
| Identification of cervical sinus as depression caudal to hyoid arch |
| Free otocyst in mesenchyme |
| Most of 1st pharyngeal artery degenerates |
| Lower limb buds |
| Primary lung buds |
| DAYS 28–30: LENGTH 6.0–7.0 mm: |
| 38 paired somites |
| 3 pairs of pharyngeal arches |
| Distinct midbrain, hindbrain, and cervical flexures |
| Cervical sinus deepens |
| Roof of IV ventricle thins |
| Branches to intersegmental arteries to upper limb bud form primordia of subclavian arteries |
| 3rd, 4th, and 6th aortic arteries persist |
| Primary bronchi appear |
| Otocyst with aggregating mesenchymal capsule |

Adapted from Blechschmidt,[1] Davis,[6] and Gasser.[7]

### External appearance of a discernible neck region

A cylindrical embryo is formed after head–tail and lateral folding of the trilaminar embryo, and for the first time, the region of the future neck is identifiable (Fig. 16–2).

This dynamic folding also results in the formation of a primitive gut and umbilical cord, as well as the positioning of the

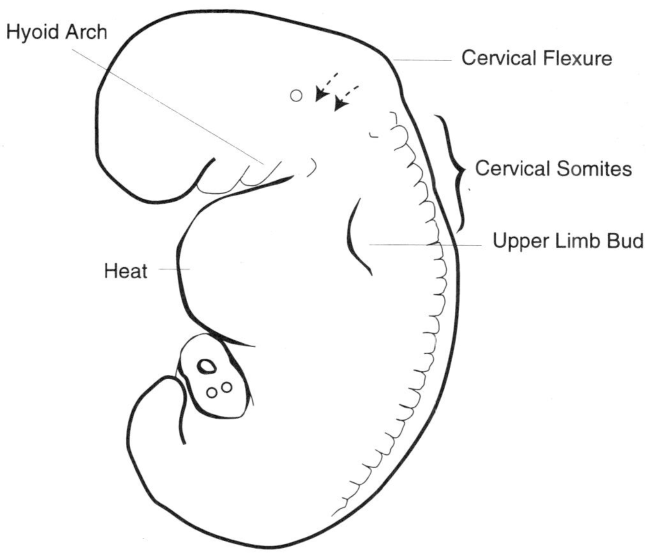


**Fig. 16–2.** An external view of a human embryo at about 26 days. The position of the developing cervical flexure is indicated, and the head region is flexed onto the relatively large ventral heart. The posterior cervical region is defined by the eight cervical somites. The arrows indicate the close proximity of migratory paths from the hindbrain to pharyngeal arch sites II (hyoid arch) and III (glossopharyngeal arch).

pericardium and septum transversum in a more ventral cervical region. As a consequence of the head–tail folding, the cranial region of the foregut assumes a flattened shape and the face region is squeezed onto the pericardial region (Fig. 16–2). The early foregut may be divided into two regions, the anterior and posterior parts of the pharynx.

The anterior part of the pharynx is flattened and medially related to the paired aortic arches which arise from the aortic sac. Four pairs of pharyngeal pouches squeeze laterally between the paired aortic arches, which are surrounded by neural crest cells. The neural crest cells contribute to the cartilagenous rudiment of each pair of pharyngeal arches. The four pairs of pouches become related caudally to the first four pairs of pharyngeal arches.

The posterior part of the pharynx contributes to the formation of the oesophagus and laryngotracheal segment. In the early phase of the cylindrical embryo, no contoured neck is evident. Therefore, it is appropriate to refer to this area as the *cervical region*. This region is primarily defined by the eight cervical somites that have been previously established in the trilaminar embryo and contribute to the cervical vertebrae characterized by the absence of ribs (in contrast to the 12 thoracic somites). The most reliable indicator of the cervical region in the early embryo (35 days) is the CNS with its enlarged brain, cervical flexure, and developed somites with established cervical ganglia. The cylindrical embryo assumes a C-shape within the confined space of the amniotic sac. The C-shaped neural tube, with enlarging brain, shows two sharp ventral bends, namely, the cephalic flexure near the midbrain region and a cervical flexure at the brain–spinal cord junction (Fig. 16–2). In Figure 16–2, the future definitive neck region is clearly defined in the dorsal aspect. Dorsally, the cervical flexure of the spinal cord marks the cephalic limits of the neck, whereas the upper limb bud marks the approximate eighth (or lower) cervical somite. There is no appreciable ventral neck region at this phase due to the head flexure onto the pericardial region. The heart is very close to the hyoid region and is therefore in intimate proximity to the pharyngeal floor filled with subpharyngeal mesenchyme.

Externally, the pharyngeal arches and clefts are gradually modified, due to relative growth changes. Figure 16–3 shows external changes in the cervical region of the embryo.

In the anterolateral aspect, the neck region is defined by the relatively enlarged hyoid arch and the epipericardial ridge. The smaller III and IV arches, second, third, and fourth clefts and membranes lie buried in a depression between the hyoid and epipericardial ridge called the *cervical sinus* (of His) (also clearly shown in a coronal section in Figure 16–5).

The hyoid arch and epipericardial ridge are significant embryonic structures that define the anterolateral aspect of the neck in later development. The primordial aortic arch, cartilage, muscle, and nerve of each pharyngeal arch develop into specific structures during this period. Table 16–2 summarizes the skeletal and muscular structures that will form from these arches.

While the arches are formed predominantly from neural crest cells, the epipericardial ridge is emphasized by the cervical flexure onto the heart as well as the migration of cervical myoblasts which form the sternocleidomastoid and trapezius muscles. Figure 16–3 also indicates the relative migratory paths of myoblasts and accompanying nerves into the anterior and lateral neck regions. Note that the occipital and cervical somites are in close proximity to the floor of the pharynx (migratory path 1 to tongue region), lateral aspect of the neck (migratory path 2 towards hyoid arch), epipericardial ridge (migratory path 3 by sternomastoid myoblasts), diaphragm (migratory path 4), and upper limb bud (migratory path 5). Innervation by the hypoglossal, cervical plexus, accessory, phrenic, and brachial plexus is established. At this phase in development, the sternocleidomastoid with accessory nerve (C2–3), hypoglossal nerve (XII), and vagus nerve (X) are structurally related within the epipericardial region. A significant relationship of these structures is also established during this critical phase in development. The cervical sinus, containing clefts and arches III and IV, lies anterior to the epipericardial ridge containing the sternocleidomastoid muscle. In addition, the enlarged hyoid arch contains platysmal myoblasts superficially as it enlarges toward the epipericardial ridge region (clavicular region; Fig. 16–5). Closure of the cervical sinus to form a cervical cyst would be anterior to the sternocleidomastoid muscle and deep to the platysma.

### Internal relationships of pharyngeal components in the embryonic neck region

Figures 16–4 and 16–5 show the intimate relationships of the various components of the pharyngeal apparatus. In Figure 16–4, the surface ectoderm has been removed to show the persisting arteries in pharyngeal arches III, IV, and VI.

The cervical flexure and prominent heart result in an intimate structural relationship formed between the pharyngeal components such as the pouches, arches, and subpharyngeal mesenchyme (Fig. 16–4). The ventral aspect of the pharynx represents a strategic cervical site, immediately under the pharyngeal floor, which contains the aortic sac and is infiltrated with mesenchyme (subpharyngeal mesenchyme). The floor of the pharynx is therefore separated from the roof of the pericardium by a subpharyngeal plane of loose mesenchyme in which the aortic

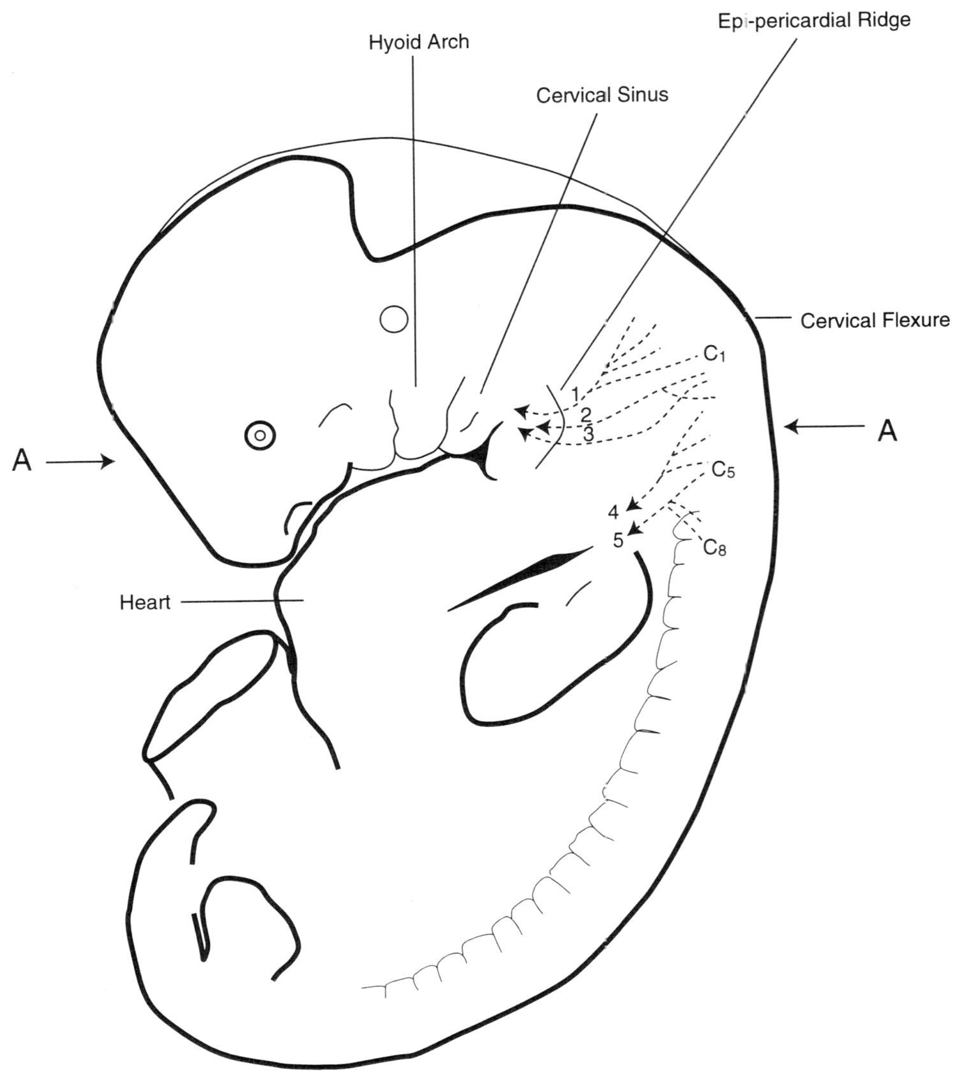


**Fig. 16–3.** An external view of a human embryo at about 35 days. A lateral bulge (epi-pericardial ridge) is formed between the cervical flexure and enlarged heart. The left hyoid arch is enlarged and overlaps the smaller third and fourth arches to enclose an ectodermal depression called the *cervical sinus*. The epi-pericardial ridge also marks the migratory routes (interrupted arrows) of (1) the occipital myoblasts to the ventral pharyngeal region; (2) cervical myoblasts to the infrahyoid region (cervical plexus); and (3) sternocleidomastoid myoblasts from cervical somites. Cervical myoblasts from somites 3–5 and 5–8 migrate into the closely approximated regions of the developing diaphragm (4) and upper limb bud (5), respectively. A, level of embryonic pharynx.

sac and vessels develop. As can be seen in Figure 16–4, the subpharyngeal mesenchymal site is (1) a restricted space in the embryo and (2) conveniently positioned to allow neural crest cell (NCC) infiltration during interaction with the developing pharyngeal pouches as well as with the cardiac outflow tract.[14]

The flexed head–neck region on the pericardium formed lateral epipericardial ridges (shown in Fig. 16–3) which represent sites through which mesenchyme migrate to enter the subpharyngeal tongue region and hyoid arch. The confined subpharyngeal site (stippled area in Fig. 16–4) will eventually enlarge and contribute appreciably to the development of the anterior neck region. It is in this site that the endodermal pouch components—the thyroid, parathyroids, and thymus—become associated with the developing great vessels—aorta, carotid, and pulmonary arteries. Note that a laterally placed epipericardial ridge is located just caudal to the arch area. Occipital and cervical somite mesoderm and hypoglossal nerves take this route to the tongue region in the floor of the pharynx and anterior neck region. The subpharyngeal mesenchyme is also the site were the hyoid arch (II) and glossopharyngeal arch (III) contribute to the development of the hyoid body that demarcates the mouth floor from the anterior neck. Later, the descent of the heart from this region facilitates further development of the anterior neck region as well as downward displacement of pharyngeal endodermal derivatives such as the thyroid, thymus, and parathyroids (as described below).

## Early association of pouch derivatives with cardiovascular structures in the neck

The endodermal components of the thyroid gland arise from the midpharyngeal floor marked by the foramen cecum, just anterior to the body of the developing hyoid bone (Fig. 16–5).

In the subpharyngeal mesenchyme, the thyroid diverticulum forms a thyroglossal duct in the midline and is in close proximity to the aortic sac. In a 19 mm embryo,[6] the gland lies ventral to the skeletal arch derivatives, arches II and III, but deep to the infrahyoid muscles. As described earlier, these muscles are not arch derivatives but migrate from cervical myotomes through the epipericardial ridge (Fig. 16–3).

In human embryos, the endoderm from the third ventral (and possibly the fourth) pharyngeal pouches contribute to the formation of the thymus.[13] The thymic primordium interacts with surrounding mesenchyme which develop from neural crest cells derived from the hindbrain region.[3,15] The paired developing rudiments are closely attached to the third aortic arches, or future internal carotids, and aortic sac, and hence become associated with the displacement of the heart (along with the aorta and internal carotids) into the superior mediastinum of the thorax (described below). The parathyroid glands of the third pouches are associated with the cranial end of the thymus, whereas those of the fourth pouch lie in close proximity to the lateral lobe of the thyroid gland.

## Formation of the cervical skeleton and musculature

The most rostral somites—four occipital and eight cervical—are the first to form and differentiate. The somites in these regions give rise to firm posterior skeletal structures, the base of the skull and cervical vertebrae, whereas the pharyngeal arches form the cartilagenous skeleton, the hyoid and thyroid cartilages, in the anterior aspect of the neck.

### Derivatives of occipital somites

The first occipital somite rapidly disperses and appears to form no definitive structure, whereas the three remaining occipital somites lose their segmented arrangement and contribute to three sclerotomal cell masses, fusing to form a condensed mass attached to the cartilagenous basal plate of the developing skull. This assimilation into the base of the skull makes occipital somite nerve components, the hypoglossal nerve, a part of the cranial nerve series. Thus, chondrification extends from the base of the skull into this occipital region which in turn extends dorsally around the foramen magnum as the occipital tectum (tectum posterius), which shows similarity to a neural arch of a vertebra. Evidence of the origin of the hypoglossal nerve is suggested by the grouping of its rootlets into two to four bundles through separate openings in the dura mater and sometimes through divided bony hypoglossal canals.[10]

The three occipital somites that fuse with sclerotomal cell masses also contribute to occipital myotomes, which migrate into the ventral pharyngeal region where the tongue develops (described earlier).

On the basis of comparative anatomy and functional innervation, the ventral divisions of the three occipital myotomes 2–4 are thought to give rise to the intrinsic and extrinsic muscles of the tongue. This interpretation is considered reasonable because the embryonic muscle masses receive their motor innervation very early in embryogenesis and retain their innervation regardless of how far they migrate during development, according to the law of original innervation.

The hypoglossal nerve is associated with these myotomes very early during embryogenesis and supplies the musculature

**Table 16–2.** Development of pharyngeal arches and pouches

| Arch | | | | | Pouch |
|---|---|---|---|---|---|
| Number | Skeletal derivatives | Muscles | Nerve | Artery | |
| I. Mandibular | Meckel's cartilage<br>Malleus, incus<br>Anterior ligament of malleus<br>Sphenomandibular ligament | Muscles of mastication<br>Mylohyoid and anterior belly of digastric<br>Tensor palati<br>Tensor tympany | V<br>Trigeminal | Contribution to maxillary artery | 1. Eustachian tube<br>Middle ear |
| II. Hyoid | 1. Stapes<br>2. Styloid process<br>3. Stylohyoid ligament<br>4. Lesser cornu and upper part of body of hyoid bone | 1. Stapedius<br>2. Posterior belly of digastric<br>3. Stylohyoid<br>4. Muscles of facial expression (including buccinator, extrinsic and intrinsic auricular muscles, occipitofrontalis, platysma | VII<br>Facial | Stapedial | 2. Palatine tonsil |
| III. Glossopharyngeal | Greater cornu and lower part of body of hyoid bone | Stylopharyngeus | XI<br>Glossopharyngeal | Common carotid and part of Internal carotid | 3. Thymus, Inferior parathyroid |
| IV. Plus | Thyroid cartilage,<br>Laryngeal cartilages | Pharyngeal constrictors, Laryngeal muscles | X<br>Vagus (superior, laryngeal and pharyngeal branches) | Aorta | 4. Superior parathyroid |

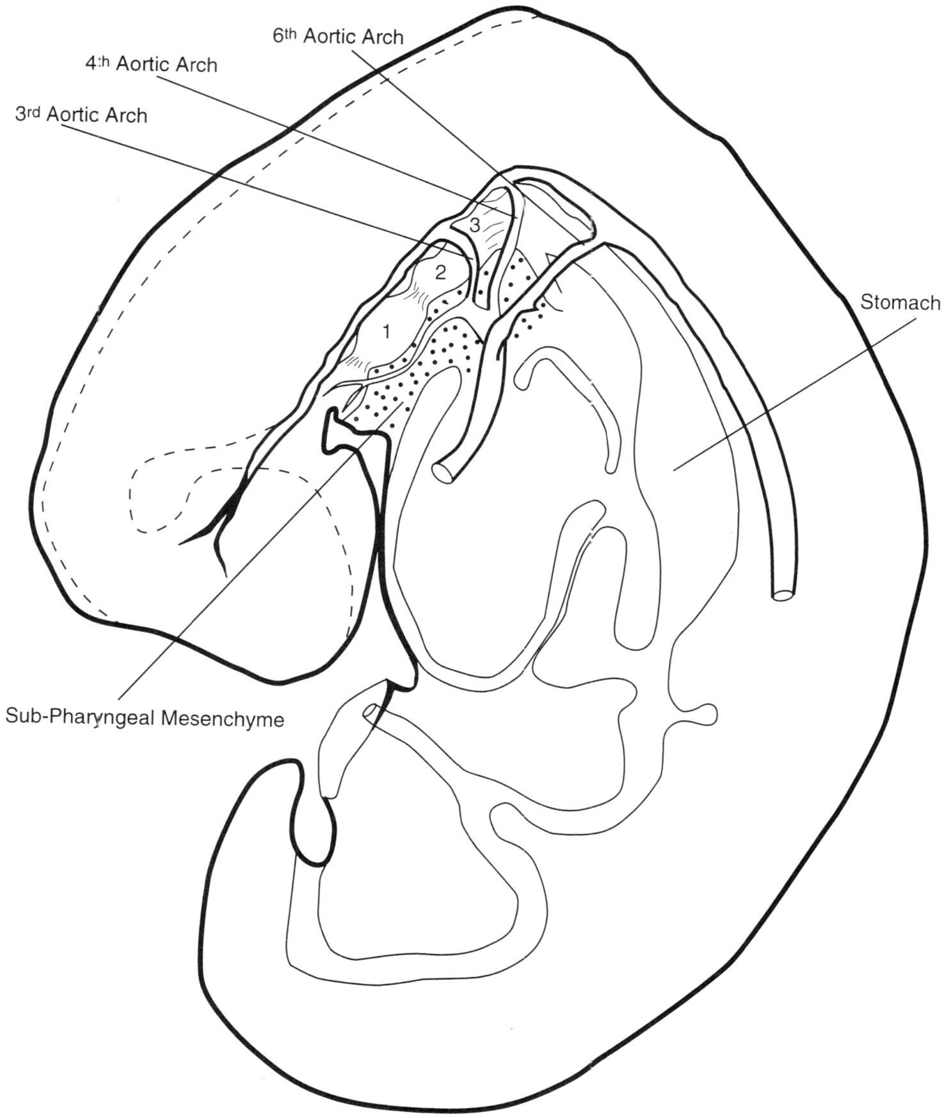


**Fig. 16–4.** A parasagittal view of the left pharyngeal pouches (1–3) and their spatial relationships to the floor of the pharynx and aortic arches (35-day embryo). The pharyngeal arches between the pouches have been dissected away leaving only the vascular portions (aortic arches) intact. Note that the anterior pharynx is flattened due to the cervical flexure and project four lateral pharyngeal pouches (1–3 shown). The floor of the pharynx (stippled area, sub-pharyngeal mesenchyme) is small but is destined to form the floor of the mouth and anterior neck region. Note the close proximity of the sub-pharyngeal mesenchyme to the pharyngeal pouches and aortic sac.

of the tongue. The hypoglossal nerve passes to the developing tongue musculature via the epipericardial ridge and hence is closely associated with cervical nerves with which it forms a plexiform connection. At this site the ansa hypoglossae is formed (Fig. 16–3). As described below, the cervical myoblasts also migrate through the epipericardial ridge and distribute between the ridge and hyoid arch as precursors of the-infrahyoid muscles, cervical somites 2–4. The physical communication of ventral divisions of the cervical nerves and the hypoglossal nerve is established during their common development through the epipericardial ridge (note migatory paths shown in Fig. 16–3).

### Derivatives of cervical somites

The cervical somites differentiate into dermatome, myotome, and sclerotomal components initially in a segmental fashion. However, the distribution and development of these components show unique features because of the pharyngeal arch derivatives in the anterior neck region and the upper limb bud with scapula formation.

Sclerotomal cells from the ventromedial portion of the somites lose their epithelial-like organization and migrate medially around the notochord to contribute to the vertebra and intervertebral discs. From the eight cervical somites, seven cervical vertebrae are differentiated. The cranial half of the first cervical sclerotome is displaced cranially and joins the fourth occipital somite.[6] Lateral extensions of (cervical) sclerotomal cells are short and remain attached to the vertebrae, following its complete ossification. The vertebral artery develops as a longitudinal anastomosis between the seventh and first intersegmental arteries and becomes associated with the cervical transverse processes.

The dorsolateral portion of the somite, the dermomyotome,

differentiates into connective tissue and muscle. Mesenchymal cells spread beneath the overlying ectoderm to form the dermis and subcutaneous tissues (posterior head, neck, and most of upper limb). Cervical dermatomes C2–C4 distribute to the occipital and neck regions, up to the suprasternal region, whereas dermatomes C5–C8 contribute to the developing upper extremity.

The myotomal cells spread dorsally, flanking the developing vertebrae, and ventrally, where they extend into the somatopleure, or lateral plate mesoderm. By the fifth to sixth week, when the embryo is 7–8 mm, the longitudinal separation of myotomes into dorsal (epaxial) and ventral (hypoaxial) portions is distinguished by a slight longitudinal constriction.[10] This division is associated with three organizations: (1) the primary branching of cervical spinal nerves into dorsal and ventral primary rami; (2) the plane of formation of the transverse processes of the cervical vertebrae; and (3) the first intermuscular septum of the fascia of the neck, which corresponds to the lumbodorsal fascia of the trunk. After the appearance of the transverse process, rib primordia are not normally formed.

The epaxial divisions of the myotome, or epimeres, contribute to the medial and lateral groups of extensors of the vertebral column and are supplied by the medial and lateral branches of the posterior primary ramus. The medial group contributes to the short oblique muscles semispinalis, multifidus, rotatores, and the spinalis. The lateral group fuses into a larger number of segments to contribute to the iliocostalis longissimus and splenius.

The hypaxial division of the myotome, the hypomere, develops atypically, due to the development of scapulae and limbs, visceral arches, and descent of pericardium. Myoblasts contribute to the flexors of the cervical vertebral column, the prevertebral longus capitis and cervicis, and scalenes, as well as to the infrahyoid muscles (plus geniohyoid), upper limb, and diaphragmatic muscles. The ventral divisions of cervical nerves accompany these myoblasts and account for innnervation of the cervical and brachial plexus as well as the diaphragm.

The upper limb bud develops in a region near the cervicothoracic junction, with mesenchymal contributions from cervical somites C5–C8 and a thoracic somite. This is reflected in

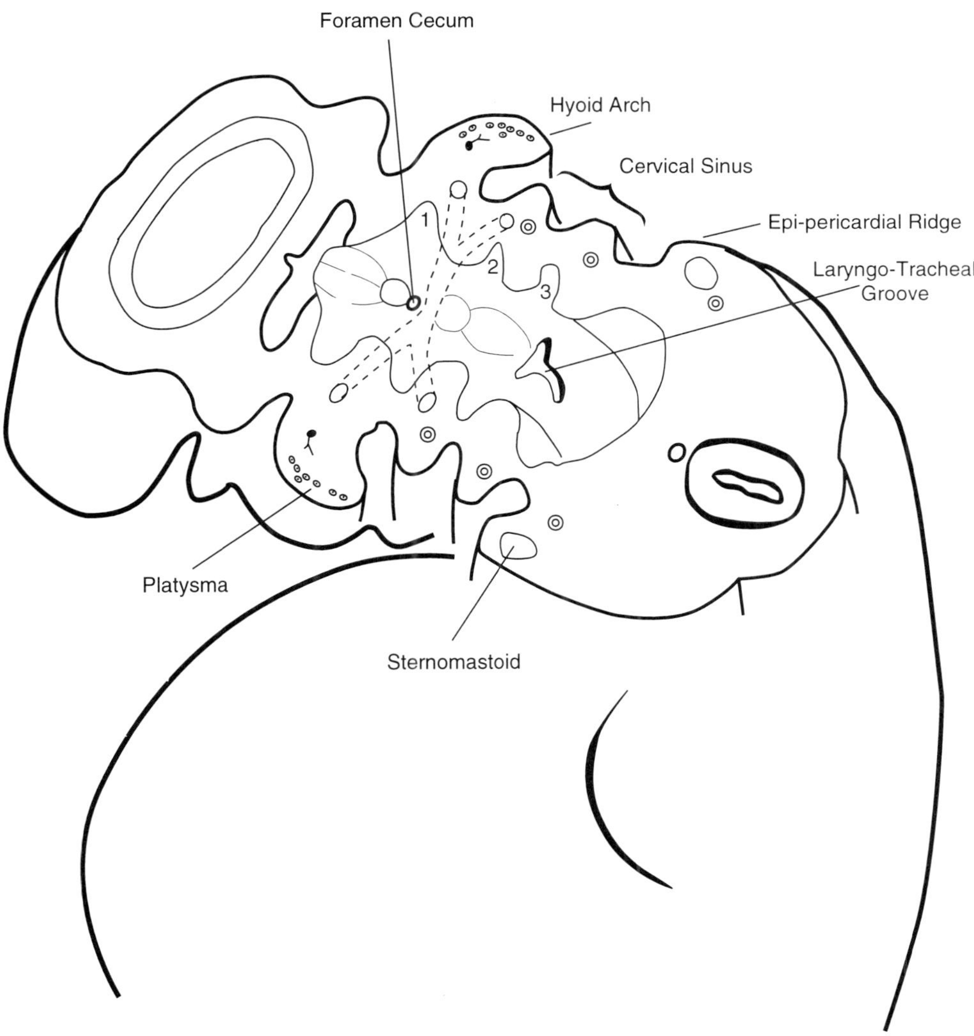


**Fig. 16–5.** Coronal section through the embryonic pharynx (section A in Fig. 16–3) showing the endodermally lined pharyngeal floor and laterally extending pouches (1–3). Note the foramen cecum just anterior to the body of the developing hyoid bone (II and III arch derivatives). The laryngo-tracheal groove lies medial to the third and fourth pouch positions. Note the relative positions of the hyoid (with platysmal myoblasts and VIIth nerve), ectodermally lined cervical sinus and epi-pericardial ridge containing sternocleidomastoid myoblasts. The small IIIrd arch, seen within the cervical sinus, contains the third aortic arch (future internal carotid artery).

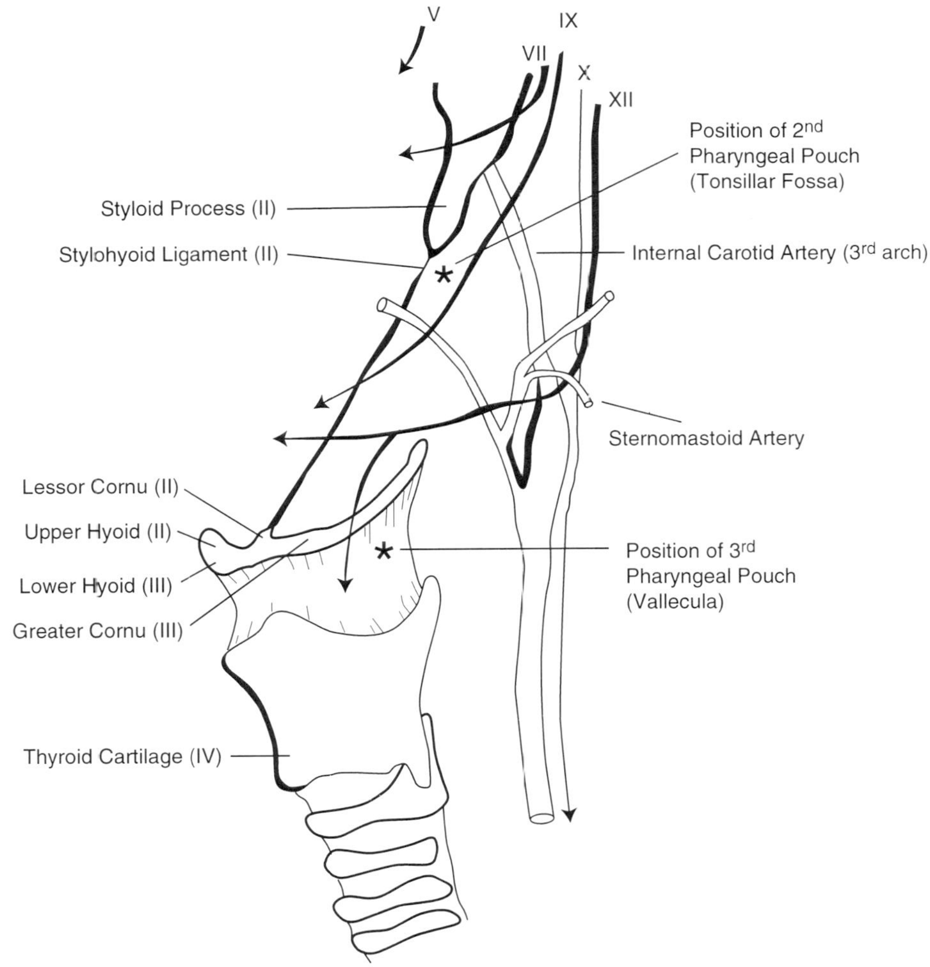


**Fig. 16–6.** Relationships of definitive neck structures derived from arches II–IV. Note the displacement of the nerves cranially but maintaining their relationship lateral to the internal carotid artery (third aortic arch). This displacement includes the hypoglossal nerve. The relative sites of the pharyngeal pouches 2 and 3 are shown in relation to their arch derivatives.

the contribution of corresponding nerves to the brachial plexus (according to the law of original innervation). The abnormal development of cervical ribs is frequently observed when the plexus is prefixed, arising from C4–C8 segments. In a postfixed plexus, the first rib is abnormal, incomplete, or absent.[20] Movement of the root origin of the plexus cranially or caudally by one segment determines whether the first rib that is allowed to form will articulate with the seventh (cervical) or eighth (first thoracic) vertebra in the series. Cervical ribs may be unilateral or bilateral. Neural crest cells in the cervical region contribute to the cervical sympathetic ganglia. While all roots of the brachial plexus convey postganglionic cervical sympathetic fibers peripherally, it appears that more (25%–45%) postganglionic fibers pass via the eighth cervical root.[20]

## Retained embryonic relations in the definitive neck

The displacement of the heart and great vessels into the thoracic region results in complex, shifting relations of the original embryonic structures formed in the cervical region. The arch derivatives of II, III, and IV form distinguishable supporting skeletal structures and fixed locations, whereas the soft tissues comprising vessels and glands are dynamically modified and displaced.

Deducing the origin of isolated cysts in the neck can be very difficult in the absence of specific tissue antigenic markers because of the complicated and shifting configurations during neck formation. There are, however, certain embryonic relations that are well preserved during neck formation which can assist us in understanding the organization of neck viscera and possibly the embryonic origin of certain cystic anomalies.

The definitive anatomical relationships of the neck structures are determined by (1) the early established embryonic relation of the arch nerves to the aortic arches, (2) modifications of the original aortic arches, (3) the epipericardial ridge structures, and (4) early association of pouch derivatives (thymus, parathyroids, thyroid) to the developing heart and great vessels in the cervical region.

### Relations of nerves and arteries

In the embryonic phase, the arch nerves (V, VII, IX) and the hypoglossal nerve (XII) enter the appropriate arches and epipericardial ridge lateral to the primitive dorsal aorta. With the displacement of the heart into the thoracic region, the third aortic arch and cranial dorsal aorta form the elongated internal carotid artery. Concurrently, towards the base of the skull, there is a cranial displacement of the arch nerves (V, VII, IX) that remain lateral to the elongated internal carotid artery (Fig. 16–6). The superior laryngeal branch of X is also displaced cranially and descends posteriorly to the internal carotid artery.

Figure 16–6 shows the hypoglossal nerve also being cranially displaced from its original epipericardial ridge position. This nerve maintains its position lateral to the internal carotid artery, but its upward displacement is stopped as it hooks around a small branch of the external carotid artery, the inferior sternomastoid branch of the occipital artery. Note in Figure 16–6 the approximate position of the hypoglossal nerve near the hyoid bone as the nerve forms the characteristic L-shaped bend toward the suprahyoid (tongue) region. Since the hypoglossal nerve initially develops in the epipericardial ridge, which is caudally related to the embryonic cervical sinus or cyst (Fig. 16–5), a true cervical cyst or internal sinus and fistula would theoretically always pass cranial to the L-shaped loop of the hypoglossal nerve before opening into the pharynx.[6,8] For example, an abnormal cervical sinus maintaining a communication with the second pharyngeal pouch would pass cranial to the hypoglossal nerve, between the carotid arterial fork, over the IXth nerve (third arch derivatives) and pass below the stylohyoid ligament (second arch derivative) to open into the palatine tonsillar region (note site in Fig. 16–6).

### Relations of arches to pouches

The cervical sinus is structurally related to pharyngeal pouch internal clefts 2, 3 and 4 (Fig. 16–5). The approximate pharyngeal sites for these clefts can be identified because of the skeletal structures derived from their adjacent arches. Figure 16–6 indicates that the second pouch internal cleft is located below the second arch derivatives (styloid process, stylohyoid ligament, lesser cornu, upper body of hyoid) and localized in the palatine tonsillar region (second pouch derivative). The third internal pouch cleft is located below the third arch derivative, or lower body of hyoid, greater cornu, in the vallecula region deep to the thyrohyoid membrane.

### Relations of pouch derivatives to arteries

The epithelial organs derived from the third and fourth pouches are closely associated with the aortic sac and third aortic arch in the subpharyngeal mesenchyme (Figs. 16–4, 16–5). This subpharyngeal plane of loose mesenchyme facilitates the differential growth that causes the downward displacement of the pericardium (and septum transversum) and formation of distinct pharynx and neck regions. The thymus (or ventral horn of the third pouch) is displaced caudally into the superior mediastinal region and draws with it parathyroid 3, resulting in its ultimate positioning in a more inferior aspect of the thyroid gland.

The thyroglossal duct of the thyroid gland appears to be associated with this differential growth as well. During the fourth week, the duct passes anterior to the developing body of the hyoid (second and third arches) in the midline. This midline relationship is constant; however, there are occasional instances when the duct or its remnants pass through the body of the hyoid bone or lie behind it.[19] The thyroglossal duct is reduced and its area of attachment to the forming isthmus of the thyroid is indicated by a pyramidal lobe. A pyramidal lobe is present in about 50% of individuals and a fibrous remnant of the thyroglossal duct is usually present.[8]

## Summary of critical events related to cervical development

Structures that are destined to be localized in the definitive neck region are allocated during the earliest trilaminar embryonic phases. Recent studies provide strong evidence that early expression of homeobox genes in a spatiotemporal sequence is a significant critical phase in the formation of the pharyngeal apparatus.

Chisaka and Capecchi[4] reported that many of the tissues and organs that are deficient in a Hox-1.5$^-$ / Hox-1.5$^-$ mouse are derived from the pharyngeal arches and pharyngeal pouches, therefore suggesting that *Hox-1.5* may play a role in the early patterning of tissues in the pharyngeal arches and pouches. The homozygotes were athymic and aparathyroid, and had reduced thyroid and submaxillary tissue as well as heart and great vessel anomalies. The phenotypic set of deficiencies seen in the Hox-1.5$^-$ homozygous recessive mouse is remarkably similar to that in the human congenital DiGeorge syndrome. This similarity, however, appears to be confined only to a common developmental pathway that assured the similar, eventual defects.

The migration of cervical somitic components and their contributions to the upper limb bud also represent a critical phase that determines the normal development of musculoskeletal structures and innervation patterns in the neck and upper limb.

A second critical phase during later cervical development is the differential growth of tissues and organs and the displacement of heart and great vessels from cervical to thoracic region. The anlagen have been formed, so that only abnormal sizes and ectopic locations may result. Development of the hyoid and cervical sinus formation and degeneration are significant events during this phase.

### References


1. Blechschmidt E: The Stages of Human Development Before Birth. WB Saunders, Philadelphia, 1961.
2. Blechschmidt E: The Beginnings of Human Life. Springer-Verlag, New York, 1977.
3. Bockman DE, Kirby ML: Dependence of thymus development on derivatives of the neural crest. Science 223:498–500, 1984.
4. Chisaka O, Capecchi MR: Regionally restricted developmental defects resulting from targeted disruption of the mouse homeobox gene hox-1.5. Nature 350:473–479, 1991.
5. Couly G, LeDouarin NM: Head morphogenesis in embryonic avian chimeras: evidence for a segmental pattern in the ectoderm corresponding to the neuromeres. Development 108: 543–558, 1990.
6. Davis J: Human Developmental Anatomy. Ronald Press, New York, 1963.
7. Gasser RF: Atlas of Human Embryos, Harper & Row, Maryland, 1975.
8. Gray SW, Skandalakis JE: Embryology for Surgeons: The Embryological Basis for the Treatment of Congenital Defects. WB Saunders, Philadelphia, 1972.
9. Hall BK: Developmental and Cellular Skeletal Biology. Academic Press, New York, 1978, pp 37–54.
10. Hamilton WJ, Boyd JD, Mossman HW: Human Embryology, 3rd ed. W Heffer & Sons, Cambridge, 1962.
11. Hunt P, Krumlauf R: Deciphering the Hox code: clues to patterning branchial regions of the head. Cell 66:1075–1078, 1991.
12. Keith A: Human Embryology and Morphology, 6th ed. Williams & Wilkins, Baltimore, 1948.

13. Kendall MD: Functional anatomy of the thymic microenvironment. J Anat 177:1–29, 1991.
14. Kirby ML, Gale TF, Stewart DE: Neural crest cells contribute to normal aorticopulmonary septation. Science 220:1059–1061, 1983.
15. Le Douarin N: The Neural Crest. Cambridge University Press, Cambridge, 1982.
16. Lufkin T, Dierich A, LeMeur M, Mark M, Chambon P: Disruption of Hox-1.6 homeobox gene results in defects in a region corresponding to its rostral domain of expression. Cell 66:1105–1119, 1991.
17. Lumsden A, Keynes R: Segmental patterns of neuronal development in the chick hindbrain. Nature 337: 424–428, 1989.
18. Mackenzie A, Leeming GL, Jowett AK, Ferguson MW, Sharpe PT: The homeobox gene Hox 7.1 has specific regional and temporal expression patterns during early mouse craniofacial embryogenesis, especially tooth development in vivo and in vitro. Development 111:269–285, 1991.
19. Sgalitzer KE: Contribution to the study of the morphogenesis of the thyroid gland. J Anat 75:389–405, 1941.
20. Sunderland S: Nerves and Nerve Injuries. Churchill Livingstone, Edinburgh and New York, 1978.

# 17

# Congenital Anomalies of the Neck

DANIEL J. KELLEY and CHARLES M. MYER, III

Congenital neck anomalies are a complex but fascinating area for clinicians involved in the treatment of disorders of the head and neck. The wide range of presentations of these varied lesions are challenging to even the most skilled and experienced physicians. A thorough understanding of the complex embryology involved in the pathogenesis of congenital neck anomalies is an essential prerequisite to any discussion of this topic. In this chapter we will discuss the most common neck anomalies with an emphasis on etiology, evaluation, and management.

## Branchial anomalies

Branchial anomalies are a common cause of congenital neck masses. *Branchial* is derived from the Greek word for gills.[52] Cervical fistulas have been attributed to abnormalities in the branchial system since 1832.[173] Between 90 and 95% of congenital anomalies of the branchial structures are from second arch, pouch, and cleft lesions.[56,76,228] First branchial anomalies represent less than 1% of all branchial anomalies.[64] Third and fourth branchial anomalies are extremely rare.[228]

Anomalies related to branchial development include cysts, sinuses, and fistulae.[56] Cystic lesions derived from the branchial system develop from embryologic rests trapped within developing tissue.[234] The cysts have a mucosal or epithelial lining and no external opening.[151] Sinuses and fistulae arise from incomplete closure of branchial cleft structures.[234] A branchial fistula involves remnants of both the pouch and cleft.[76] A sinus is a tract open either to the pharynx or skin, but not both.[83]

### Embryology and etiology

During embryologic development, the branchial apparatus resembles primitive gill slits.[56] It consists of five paired mesodermic arches separated by four pairs of invaginations of ectoderm, known as *branchial clefts,* and endoderm, known as *branchial pouches*. Each arch is supplied by its own artery and nerve and develops into skeletal muscle and connective tissue.[148] Differentiation usually begins between the sixth and seventh week of fetal development.[56] The second branchial arch grows caudally, covering the third arch and fusing with the fourth arch.[173] The second, third, and fourth branchial clefts eventually fuse into a structure known as the *cervical sinus of His*.[148,173] The downward growth of the second arch, which later develops into the platysma muscle, explains why all branchial anomalies other than first branchial anomalies are located deep to the platysma muscle. The majority of branchial tissue has differentiated by day 45 of fetal development. Failure of obliteration of the cervical sinus of His gives rise to the various branchial cleft anomalies.[148]

There are currently three theories that attempt to explain the etiology of branchial anomalies. The most widely held theory proposes that they arise from anomalous development of the branchial apparatus.[52] First branchial anomalies are the result of incomplete fusion between the first and second branchial arches.[64] Second branchial anomalies are thought to be the most common because the second cleft has the greatest depth and persists the longest during embryologic development.[56] Arguments against the branchial origin of lateral cervical cysts include their presentation later in life and the presence of lymphoid tissue within the cyst wall, which suggests a lymph node origin.[77] An alternate theory proposes that squamous epithelium migrates from the pharynx via the lymphatic system to regional lymph nodes in response to recurrent infection.[52] The epithelial lining of lateral cervical cysts is similar to upper aerodigestive tract epithelium.[77] Rests of salivary tissue trapped within lymph nodes is another possibility.[21,52,95] Lateral cervical cysts could be derived from a combination of salivary inclusions and branchial remnants.[95] Persistence of the thymopharyngeal duct has also been offered as the source of these lesions.

### Classification

In 1972, Work classified first branchial anomalies into types I and II. Type I first branchial anomalies are duplications of the membranous external auditory canal. They are located in the postauricular region and can extend medial and anterior to the external auditory canal. These anomalies are lateral to the facial nerve and can end in a blind pouch at the level of the tympanic membrane (Fig. 17–1).[257]

Type II first branchial anomalies are duplications of the external auditory canal and auricle.[234] They consist of components of both the first and second arch as well as a portion of the branchial cleft. These anomalies are not to be confused with pretragal cysts or sinuses, which arise from a failure of fusion of the auricular helix around the first branchial arch dorsum. These pretragal lesions are not related to the external auditory canal, although they are always lateral to the facial nerve. Type II first branchial anomalies extend medial and inferior to the external auditory canal and can be medial or lateral to the facial nerve. The sinus tract or mass can be located inferior to the angle of the mandible and along the anterior border of the sternocleidomastoid muscle (Fig. 17–1).[64]

Second branchial anomalies are classified into four different categories based on their anatomic location along the branchial tract.[11,138] The majority of second branchial anomalies are types I, II, or III.[228] Type I second branchial anomalies are located along the anterior border of the sternocleidomastoid muscle, deep to the platysma muscle and cervical fascia. The

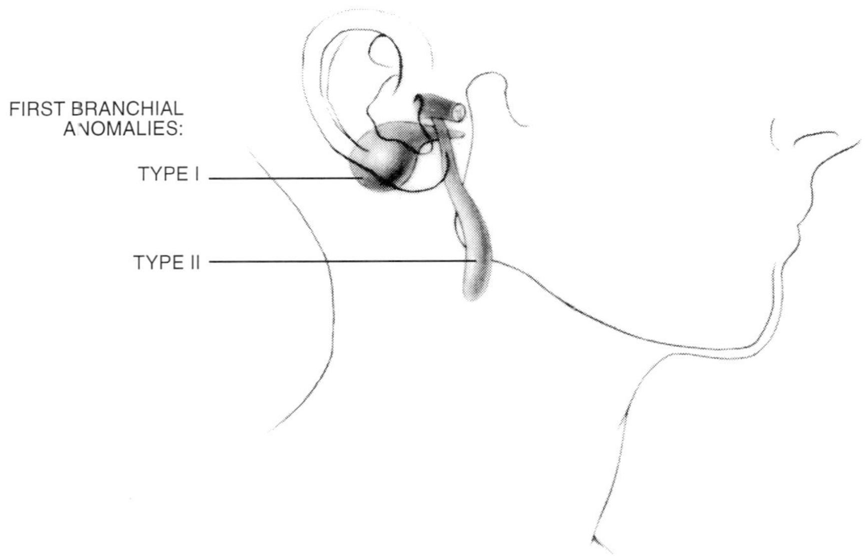


**Fig. 17–1.** First branchial anomalies can present in the periauricular region with a typical pattern for type I and type II anomalies and they can have a variable relationship to the facial nerve.

type II anomaly, the most frequent type, lies in contact with the great vessels. Type III second branchial anomalies pass medial between the internal and external carotid arteries and extend to the lateral pharyngeal wall.[138,228] They are found superior to the glossopharyngeal and hypoglossal nerves and inferior to the stylohyoid ligament (Fig. 17–2).[151] Type IV cysts are located adjacent to the pharyngeal wall and medial to the great vessels, usually at the level of the tonsillar fossa.[138,228] This latter group is considered very unusual.[248] The tract can enter anywhere from the nasopharynx to the hypopharynx, but most commonly involves the tonsillar fossa.[151]

Third branchial anomalies are located along the anterior border of the sternocleidomastoid muscle but typically pass posterior to the great vessels and inferior to the glossopharyngeal nerve. It remains superior to the hypoglossal and superior laryngeal nerves (Fig. 17–3).[137]

Fourth branchial anomalies originate at the apex of the pyriform sinus.[153,228] From the pyriform sinus, a fistula tract travels anteriorly and inferiorly to the cricothyroid muscle and thyroid cartilage, both of which are fourth arch structures. In the right neck, it is located superior to the recurrent laryngeal nerve, a sixth branchial arch structure, and inferior to the superior laryngeal nerve, which is the fourth branchial arch nerve.[90,228] A right-sided lesion would pass underneath the right subclavian artery before ascending into the neck. In the left neck, the fistula tract would travel inferiorly to the posterior aspect of the aortic arch, also of fourth branchial arch derivation. At this point, it should loop anteriorly under the aorta and course superiorly in the neck just posterior to the common carotid artery. The fistula travels superior to the hypoglossal nerve and then descends in the neck to end along the anteroinferior sternocleidomastoid muscle.[228] Fourth branchial anomalies often termi-

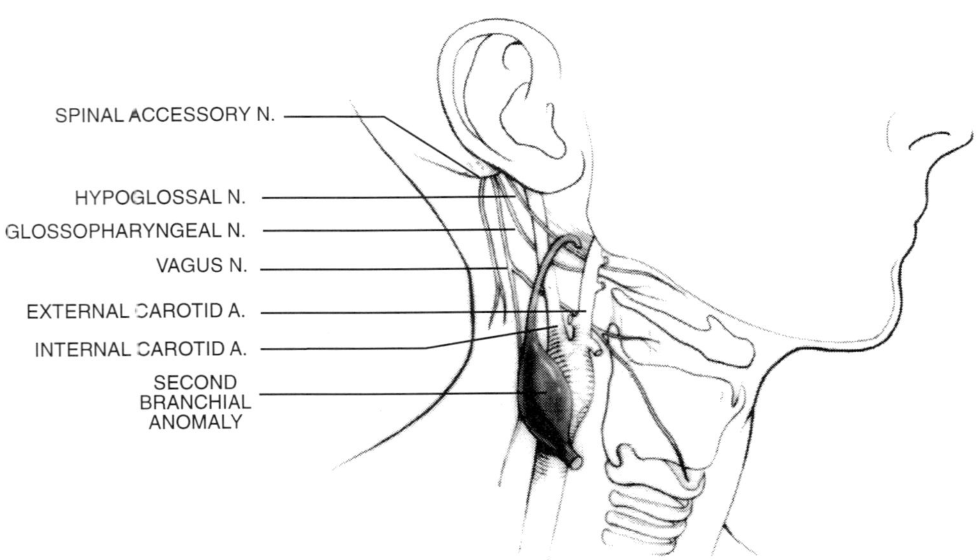


**Fig. 17–2.** Relationship of a second branchial anomaly to the great vessels and cranial verves.

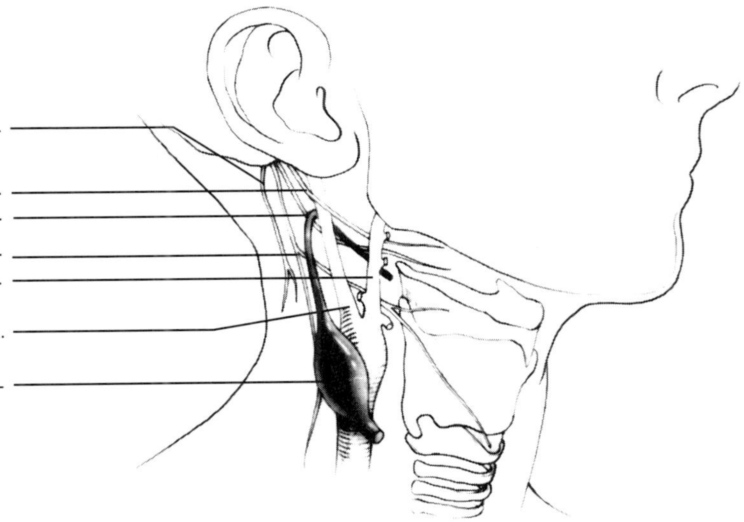


**Fig. 17–3.** Relationship of a third branchial anomaly to the great vessels and cranial nerves.

nate in the perithyroid space, thyroid gland, or cervical esophagus.[151,153] Cysts are usually located between the larynx and great vessels.[153] A fourth branchial fistula has not been demonstrated completely in a surgical specimen.[151]

### Clinical presentation

Signs and symptoms of first branchial anomalies include recurrent pre- and postauricular swelling, a fistula within the external auditory canal presenting as drainage, or a fistula below the angle of the mandible.[52,64] Typically, a fistula is located below the angle of the mandible and along the anterior border of the sternocleidomastoid muscle. Lesions of type I first branchial anomalies may present posteriorly, adjacent to the pinna and concha as a cystic mass or fistula (Fig. 17–4A). A common occurrence is infection followed by drainage. They can terminate near a bony plate at the level of the mesotympanum.[64]

Type II first branchial anomalies are more common than type I lesions.[64] They often present with a fistula from the concha, external auditory canal, or neck (Fig. 17–4B). A sinus tract extends medial and inferior to the external auditory canal.[64] There is often one opening in the floor of the external auditory canal and an additional opening along the lower border of the mandible.[234] They are commonly associated with the parotid gland. Type II lesions can pass either medial or lateral to the facial nerve and frequently accompany the digastric muscle. Involvement of the pes anserinus is not unusual. Termination is usually at the anterior border of the sternocleidomastoid muscle.[64]

In the majority of cases of first branchial anomalies, the middle ear and tympanic membrane are unaffected. There are case reports of involvement of the tympanic membrane and middle ear space. However, a recurrent abscess in the neck can be found in combination with a cystic lesion on the tympanic membrane or in the middle ear.[234] First branchial anomalies can occur within the parotid gland and present with facial paralysis. They are associated with hemifacial microsomia.[33,227] The course of the tract is different in the presence of hemifacial microsomia due to the associated altered development.[227]

Second branchial anomalies occur bilaterally in 2% of cases. Cystic lesions are three times as common as fistulae.[56] When

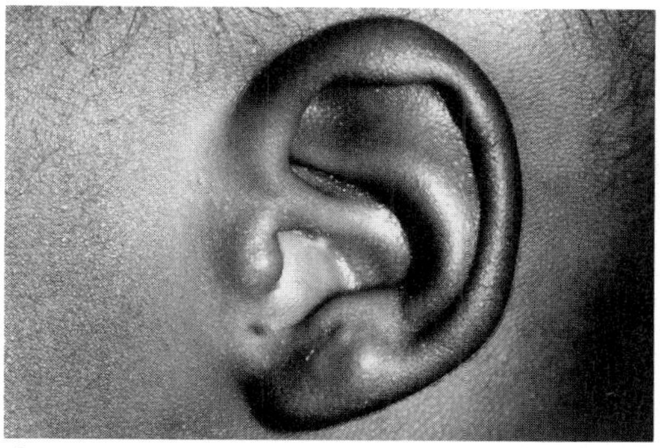

A

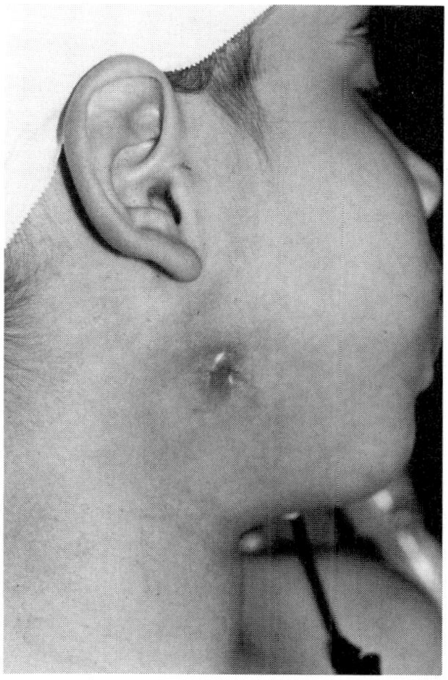

B

**Fig. 17–4.** A type I first branchial anomaly often presents at the base of the concha (A) while a type II first branchial anomaly usually presents at the angle of the mandible (B).

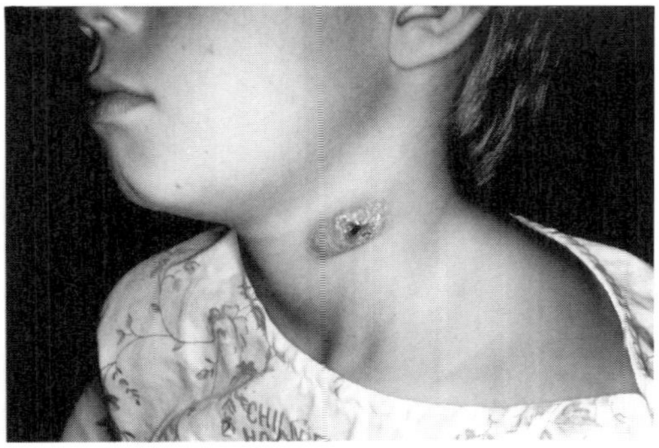

**Fig. 17–5.** Typical presentation of an infected second branchial anomaly.

cystic, they often present as a smooth, soft mass in the lateral neck, anterior and deep to the sternocleidomastoid muscle.[52,112] The most common time of presentation is during the second decade of life.[52] Second branchial anomalies can present in the neonate, but this is rare.[211] Without an external fistula tract, the diagnosis of a second branchial anomaly in a newborn is difficult.[56,148]

Any fistula or cyst below the level of the digastric muscle should be considered of second branchial origin. They often become apparent following an upper respiratory tract infection.[64] Changes in size associated with upper respiratory infections are noted in 25% of patients with branchial cysts.[56] Abscess or fistula formation may be a complication of this process (Fig. 17–5).[72] Pharyngeal cysts near the tonsillar fossa can result from second branchial anomalies but are unusual. A cystic mass with a smooth mucosal surface on the posterior wall of the oropharynx is the most common presentation of pharyngeal branchial anomalies.[228]

Neonates can develop airway obstruction due to third branchial anomalies.[148] Parapharyngeal abscess also can be the initial presentation. Branchial cysts within the parapharyngeal space range from 0.7 to 3% of lesions in this space. There are three cases in the literature of a branchial cyst in the parapharyngeal space presenting as an abscess.[165] Infected third branchial anomalies are also associated with hypoglossal nerve palsy. The etiology of this paralysis is thought to be due to a local neuritis caused by the influence of toxins. In addition, compression and distention of the nerve due to local inflammation and enlargement of the cyst exacerbates local inflammation. It is more likely that acute distention rather than gradual enlargement will cause compression.[72]

Unlike second branchial anomalies, fourth branchial anomalies usually present during childhood. A lateral cervical cyst with an internal fistula in the pyriform sinus is a common occurrence.[98,168] If there is a connection to the skin, it is usually secondary to a rupture of an abscess cavity.[98] In the neonate, obstructive symptoms such as respiratory difficulty and dysphagia can occur.[153] The fistula tract can end in either the perithyroid space or within the thyroid gland.[228] In older children, recurrent abscesses in the lateral neck as well as acute suppurative thyroiditis are the most common forms of presentation.[98,168] Perithyroid space abscess and retropharyngeal space abscess can be associated with fourth branchial anomalies.[109,228] Recurrence of infection appears to be a common feature.[168] There are case reports of fourth branchial sinus tracts extending under the clavicle near the subclavian vessels.[76,201,228] Abscess and granulation tissue within the mediastinum and supraclavicular regions have been reported as well. Fourth branchial sinuses are located almost exclusively on the left side.[228]

## Diagnosis

Any cystic neck mass necessitates a thorough medical history and physical examination, including careful otologic examination.[234] A Lempert or Vienna bivalve ear speculum can help visualize the cartilagenous external auditory canal for these anomalies. Placing the patient in the Trendelenburg position can sometimes make a branchial anomaly more noticeable.[64] The appearance of methylene blue from an external sinus after swallowing can help confirm the presence of an internal fistula tract.[153] Endolaryngeal examination or endoscopy of the upper aerodigestive tract with particular attention to the pyriform sinus is recommended in these cases to identify the location of the internal fistula.[90,153] Evaluation of branchiogenic carcinoma includes panendoscopy with biopsies from the tonsil region, base of tongue, and nasopharynx.[112]

Aspiration of the mass should be undertaken if the diagnosis is unclear.[64] The cyst may contain yellow fluid and occasionally cholesterol products.[212] High levels of salivary amylases, even in cysts lacking salivary gland tissue, have been demonstrated.[95] Aspiration may aid in the diagnosis by showing squamous ciliated columnar or pseudostratified epithelial cells.[173] Appropriate laboratory studies should be obtained on the aspirate to rule out an infectious or neoplastic etiology.[64]

Patients suspected of pyriform sinus fistulae and presenting with acute thyroiditis, thyroid abscess, or thyroid cyst should undergo a barium esophagogram after administration of intravenous antibiotics and resolution of inflammation.[90] A barium esophagogram can often demonstrate the presence of a sinus tract from the pyriform sinus. This examination will fail to demonstrate the sinus when the contrast material does not enter the sinus tract. Barium can be injected through a catheter placed in the pyriform sinus. In addition, ultrasound examination of the thyroid gland can show changes in echogenicity of the gland and edema of the surrounding soft tissues in cases of fourth branchial anomalies.[109] A thyroid scan may show diminished uptake in the involved lobe in these cases.[109,153]

Computed tomography (CT) has been considered the radiologic procedure of choice in the evaluation of branchial anomalies.[64] Branchial cysts are typically located along the anterior border of the sternocleidomastoid muscle and demonstrate a homogeneous mass with low attenuation in the central region and a smooth enhancing rim along the periphery. During acute infection, the cyst wall is less well defined. Differentiation from a necrotic node is based on the thicker, irregular rim that can also enhance with extracapsular spread of tumor. CT can sometimes identify the internal course of second branchial anomalies as it passes between the internal and external carotid arteries at the bifurcation and terminates in the tonsillar fossae.[33,212] Injection of radiopaque material will aid in their demonstration.[33] CT has failed in some cases to identify branchial anomalies presenting as cystic structures within the parapharyngeal space.[165] CT evaluation from the base of skull to the larynx is recommended in patients with branchiogenic carcinoma.[112]

Magnetic resonance imaging(MRI) may be a better test because of its soft tissue resolution.[130] MRI typically demonstrates a low T1 weighted image and a high T2 weighted signal. With high protein content in the cyst, a high T1 weighted image is possible.[212]

### Histology

Type I first branchial anomalies are typically lined by squamous epithelium.[257] There are no mesodermal structures, such as cartilage, contained within the wall of the type I first branchial anomaly. It is considered a purely ectodermal lesion. Type II anomalies contain both ectodermal and mesodermal structures, such as skin, adenexa, and cartilage. Type II anomalies sometimes do not contain mesodermal elements, making histologic analysis of these specimens potentially difficult.[64]

Second branchial anomalies can be lined by either stratified squamous or pseudostratified columnar epithelium.[112] Endodermally derived respiratory type epithelium is also possible as a remnant of the internal pharyngeal duct.[228] Between 8 and 10% of branchial anomalies are lined by ciliated columnar epithelium.[33] Ciliated cystic lesions of the lateral neck are sometimes called *bronchogenic cysts,* based on their histologic features which are similar to respiratory bronchioles. It is more likely that these are derived from branchial clefts containing mesodermal remnants.[41]

Branchial anomalies often have a sparse mononuclear inflammatory infiltrate.[41,173] Lymphoid tissue with and without germinal centers in the subepithelium is a characteristic of these cysts.[95,112] This can be confused with cystic changes within lymph node epithelium.[228] Occasionally, salivary tissue, sebaceous glands, or cholesterol clumps can be found within the epithelial lining of a branchial anomaly.[77,95] A branchial cyst containing gastric epithelium has been reported. Gastric epithelium within a branchial cyst suggests the possibility of differentiation of epithelium contained within these anomalies.[77] Histologic evidence for a third branchial anomaly would include the presence of thymic tissue within the cyst wall.[90]

Branchiogenic carcinoma was first suggested by Volkmann in 1882. Several cases of primary branchial carcinoma were reported from 1926 to 1935.[112] Martin in 1950 reviewed 250 cases of branchial cyst carcinoma and felt that only three cases could be considered legitimate, thus leading him to propose the following criteria for the diagnosis of branchial carcinoma. There must be a malignancy that develops in an epithelial cyst in the lateral neck. The location of the mass must be along a line extending from a point anterior to the tragus to the anterior border of the sternocleidomastoid muscle.[134] Histologic examination of the mass must be consistent with a branchial anomaly and demonstrate a cystic structure lined with squamous or pseudostratified columnar epithelium displaying atypia, dysplasia, and carcinoma.[112,134] While lymphoid elements can be present, the presence of perinodular sinuses, intranodular trabeculae, or peripheral lobulation would argue for a metastatic lymph node rather than a primary carcinoma.[112]

The most controversial criterion is patient survival for at least 5 years without any other primary malignancy of the head and neck that might explain a malignant cystic neck mass.[134] The mortality rate associated with carcinoma in the neck and the fact that radiation therapy can control occult primaries leave few candidates for this diagnosis. Therefore, absence of any identifiable primary in the head and neck and clear histologic identification of the nature of the tumor are considered the most important criteria for diagnosis.[112]

### Treatment

Branchial anomalies are best treated by complete excision.[109] Quite often patients have had previous incision and drainage before the diagnosis of a branchial anomaly is made.[64] Recurrent infection can make excision of these lesions difficult due to the formation of fibrosis around vital structures. The injection of methylene blue into internal or external fistula tracts has been used in the past to aid in surgical excision, but this can stain surrounding tissues.[60] Paraffin and polymers have been injected into sinus tracts to aid in dissection.[60,261] Lacrimal duct dilators, wire stylettes, and arterial intimal strippers also have been used intraoperatively to identify fistula tracts (Fig. 17–6).[46,60] This is a blind maneuver and can create false passages and damage adjacent structures. These techniques are considered of limited usefulness.[60]

Surgical approaches to first branchial anomalies must include the possibility of facial nerve exposure and protection.[64] Excision of these anomalies in children is somewhat more difficult because the facial nerve is smaller and more superficial, its landmarks less well defined, and its relationship to first branchial anomalies more variable when compared to adults. Adequate exposure and protection of the facial nerve is essential (Fig. 17–7). If the tract involves the cartilagenous external auditory canal, the cartilage and overlying skin should be excised with the main specimen. Any tract entering the temporal bone should be dissected to its entrance to the bone and then amputated. The portion within the tympanic membrane or middle ear space should be removed separately. This may require removal of part of the tympanic membrane. Curettage of the bone at the entry site is considered adequate. It is not recommended that the bone be drilled or excised.[234] Both superficial parotidectomy and careful enucleation have been successful. Following resection, the external auditory canal should be packed for a period of 3–4 weeks to avoid canal stenosis.[64]

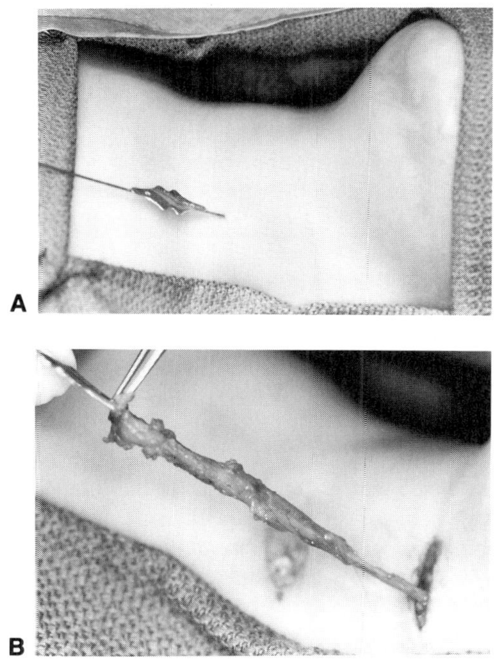


**Fig. 17–6.** Lacrimal probes may aid in the identification (A) and dissection (B) of the sinus tract of branchial anomalies.

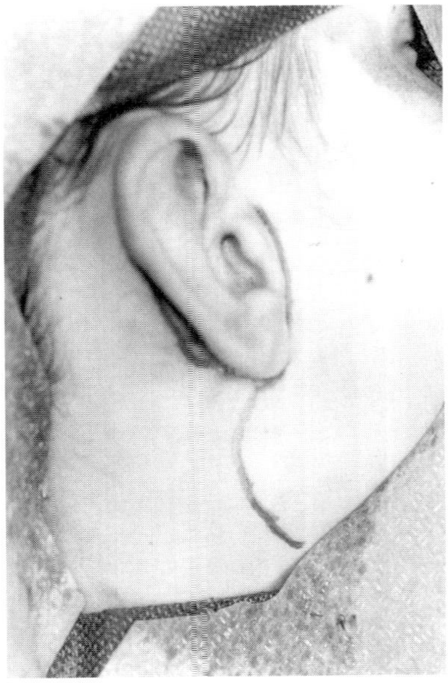

**Fig. 17–7.** Surgical incisions used in the excision of first branchial anomalies.

Second branchial anomalies are approached best through an incision along the anterior border of the sternocleidomastoid muscle, parallel to the natural skin folds. This anomaly usually travels along the carotid sheath and bisects the external and internal carotid artery just above the bifurcation. It also travels lateral and superior to the hypoglossal and glossopharyngeal nerves and terminates in the tonsillar fossa.[33] Second branchial anomalies presenting as pharyngeal cysts can be excised via an intraoral approach with no complications.[52,228]

Third branchial anomalies can be approached through a neck incision as well. They travel posterior to the internal carotid artery and superior to the hypoglossal nerve, but inferior to the glossopharyngeal nerve, remaining superficial to the vagus nerve as it enters the pyriform sinus.[33] Respiratory distress secondary to a third branchial anomaly may require urgent surgical therapy.[148] Excision can be undertaken successfully in the neonate, especially in cases of upper aerodigestive tract obstruction.[211] Needle aspiration of the mass can temporarily improve respiratory symptoms.[148] An external approach for branchial anomalies of the parapharyngeal space also is recommended.[165]

Surgical excision of fourth branchial anomalies presenting with suppurative thyroiditis should occur at 4 to 8 weeks following treatment of the acute infection. The incision should be via a standard thyroidectomy collar incision with identification and protection of the recurrent laryngeal nerve. Partial or total ipsilateral thyroid lobectomy is completed and left attached to the branchial anomaly. After identification and retraction of the carotid sheath, the tract is followed along the inferior constrictor to the pyriform sinus. Retraction of the thyroid ala and possible resection to facilitate exposure are completed. The sinus tract is divided at the pyriform sinus.[90] A modified hemithyroidectomy is sometimes necessary to achieve adequate resection.[56a,153] Placement of a Fogarty catheter through the pyriform apex can aid in dissection. In addition, an esophageal bougie may make palpation of the inflated Fogarty catheter balloon easier.[76]

Complications

Recurrence rates for resection of branchial anomalies is approximately 3% with no prior surgery or infection. This figure increases to 20% when complicated by prior surgical intervention or inflammation. Potential sources of morbidity include all of the neurovascular structures within the field of resection.[151,153]

## Thyroglossal duct anomalies

Thyroglossal duct anomalies are the most commonly occurring congenital anomaly of the neck.[137,242] Remnants of the thyroglossal duct are reported in 7% of the population.[147,235] Approximately 25%–30% of all persons have a pyramidal lobe of the thyroid, considered by some to be the inferior extent of the thyroglossal tract.[147] Thyroglossal duct anomalies make up between 2 and 4% of all neck masses.[242] They are second only to enlarged cervical lymph nodes as a cause of neck masses in children and occur twice as often as branchial anomalies.[120,253] When growths of lymphatic origin are excluded, thyroglossal duct cysts are responsible for 40% of neck masses and 70% of congenital neck anomalies.[75,209,235,246] They are the most common cause of midline neck masses between the ages of 6 months and 15 years.[10,75] Anomalous development of the thyroid gland can give rise to masses in the neck as well. Aberrations range from ectopic thyroid tissue to complete failure of the thyroid to descend. Thyroid tissue is present at the base of tongue in 10% of the normal population.[264]

Thyroglossal duct cysts (TGDC) are congenital anomalies that arise from persistence of an epithelial tract between the thyroid gland and the origin of the foramen cecum.[4,108] TGDC are not considered to be inherited. However, there are case reports of three and four consecutive generations of females in the same family with a thyroglossal duct cyst.[242] There are no known sexual, racial, or geographic predilections.[108,168]

### Embryology and etiology

The primordial thyroid gland first appears during the third week of fetal development.[171] Immediately after the mandibular arch reaches the midline, a median bud evaginates from the foramen cecum and descends from the pharynx into a loose subpharyngeal mesoderm ventral and caudal to the developing second arch.[49,147,253] This bilobed diverticulum descends into the neck as a hollow tube, forming a tract known as the *thyroglossal duct*.[49,171] The thyroid primordium attaches to the ventral aortic stem and moves caudally with the evolving vasculature. After fusing with the lateral aspect of the fourth branchial pouches, the association of the thyroid gland with the aortic sac involutes. Parafollicular C-cell precursors become incorporated at this time.[147]

In normal development, the thyroglossal duct tract is situated between the first branchial arch structures and elements derived from the other arches, such as the hyoid bone, thyrohyoid membrane, and thyroid cartilage, which are posterior to the tract.[24] The hyoid bone is derived from the second branchial arch and develops after the descent of the thyroid gland.[49,253] During the second gestational month, it divides the thyroglossal tract into infrahyoid and suprahyoid segments.[49,97] The tract usually descends anterior to the thyroid and cricoid cartilages, as well as the developing hyoid bone.[128,253] It can, however, pass posteriorly or through the hyoid bone or surround it and TGDC remnants can be trapped within the hyoid bone.[24,49,128,253] By 8 weeks gestational age, the tract between the foramen cecum and the thyroid gland usually is obliterated. Persistence of the duct can give rise to cysts, sinuses, or fistulae.[24,128,253] Accessory thyroid tissue also can arise anywhere along this tract.[128]

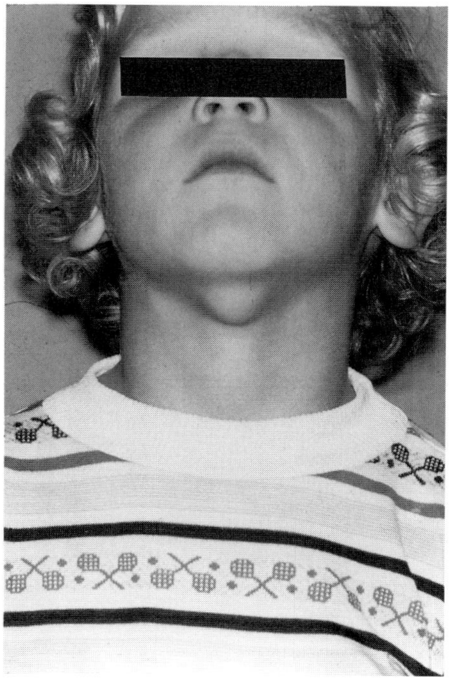

A

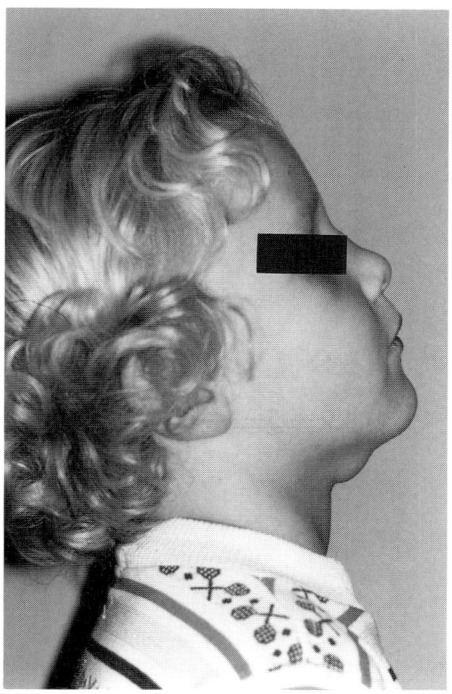

B

**Fig. 17–8.** Typical appearance of a thyroglossal duct cyst from an anteroposterior (A) and lateral view (B).

## Clinical presentation

TGDC are most commonly discovered in the first decade of life and there is no sex predilection.[75,242] Half of these anomalies present before the age of 10 years and almost 70% present before the age of 30 years.[48,235] Presentation in an adult at any age is possible.[75,108] Most TGDC present as an asymptomatic, painless midline neck mass (Fig. 17–8).[75,108,253] The mass can be firm or hard.[48]

It is located lateral to the midline in approximately 10%–29% of patients.[10,32,48] The paramedian position is attributed to the presence of the levator glandulae thyroidae muscle or normal thyroid tissue.[11,75] Sixty-five percent of these lesions are infrahyoid, 20% are suprahyoid, and 15% are juxtahyoid.[3,75,209,235] The majority are in close approximation to the hyoid bone.[10] An intralingual location is found in about 2% of patients.[3,235] Suprasternal thyroglossal duct cysts occur in about 10% of cases.[3,32]

The cysts are usually freely mobile and nontender.[75] Movement of the mass with swallowing or tongue protrusion is common.[75,108,213,242] These lesions become symptomatic due to inflammation and infection, with possible progression to cellulitis and abscess formation.[32,48] Patients can present with dysphagia, dysphonia, dyspnea, a draining sinus, or a change in size of the mass.[48,108,253] A history of recurrent infection is also possible.[121,255] A sinus tract is found in 35% of cases.[75,168,235] This can involve the anterior tongue, the anterior neck skin, or the foramen cecum.[242] TGDC can also present in combination with a dermoid cyst.[10,49]

Upper respiratory tract obstruction is possible with thyroglossal duct anomalies.[32] Individuals with intralingual thyroglossal duct anomalies are particularly at risk.[32,88] Laryngeal involvement by TGDC is well reported.[209] Extrinsic compression, invasion into the pre-epiglottic space with presentation as a submucosal supraglottic mass, or erosion through the thyroid cartilage can occur.[163,209,249] Sudden infant death, secondary to upper airway obstruction, has been associated with histologically confirmed thyroglossal duct remnants.[32,88] A TGDC lined by gastric epithelium theoretically could produce acid and result in ulceration, tracheal penetration, hemorrhage, and even death.[36]

The clinical presentation of thyroglossal duct carcinoma is identical to that of the benign cyst.[69,128,235,246]

## Diagnosis

Patient evaluation should include a complete history and physical examination, including indirect or direct laryngoscopy.[108,128] Radiographic evaluation may include plain films that can show a mass anterior to the pharynx. A lateral view will determine its relationship to the hyoid bone.[75] Plain films of the neck are usually negative with thyroglossal duct cysts, although hyoid displacement can be seen occasionally.[27] Some authors also recommend a preoperative chest Xray in the evaluation of any midline neck mass.[103] Thyroid function tests are typically normal.

Computed tomography or ultrasound should be the primary investigative tool in the evaluation of thyroglossal duct anomalies.[69] Ultrasound can be used to determine whether the mass is cystic or solid and, if cystic, to determine the characteristics of the fluid and cyst wall.[27,69,168] Typically, the thyroglossal duct cyst contains fluid with multiple internal echos.[75] The typical radiographic appearance on CT is a smooth, well-circumscribed, low-density lesion with peripheral rim enhancement and occasional internal septations following injection of contrast material.[24,27,69,75] The density of this tissue is usually less than that of the surrounding musculature.[75] The mass is usually nonenhancing on contrast injection.[24] Thick, nodular walls of the cyst or soft tissue density within or adjacent to the cyst reflect a history of inflammation or possible malignancy.[65,75,203] Computed tomography also can help identify the extent of the lesion and aid in treatment planning.[24,27,209] The location of the duct within the hyoid bone can be determined by CT (Fig. 17–9).[171] A contrast agent can be injected into the lesion to determine extension to the foramen cecum.[129]

A thyroid scan is recommended by some authors as part of a normal preoperative evaluation, given that the only functional thyroid tissue in a patient may be removed along with the TGDC.[27,108] Although thyroid scans are usually normal, they will confirm the presence of normal thyroid tissue and show foci of ectopic thyroid tissue within the cyst.[75] A radioisotope scan demonstrates functioning thyroid tissue within a TGDC in only one-third of cases.[27,235]

Fine needle aspiration is used routinely by some authors as a preoperative test.[103,108,128,129] Aspiration of mucinous material of a midline neck mass can be considered diagnostic of a TGDC.[242] Measurement of thyroglobulin concentrations can be used to confirm the thyroid origin of the lesion.[110] Occasionally, aspiration for diagnosis of a thyroglossal duct cyst will result in permanent decompression.[108] Diagnosis of a cyst containing carcinoma is a further benefit of fine needle aspiration.[108] Preoperative incisional biopsy has also been used to diagnose thyroglossal duct carcinoma prior to surgery.[129] Even after an extensive preoperative evaluation, the diagnosis often remains uncertain until histologic examination is completed.[27]

### Histology

Because the foramen cecum occurs at a junction of ectoderm and endoderm, a variety of epithelial linings are possible for thyroglossal duct cysts.[49] Stratified squamous, pseudostratified, cuboidal, columnar, and transitional epithelium within the cyst have been described.[128,129,238,253] Pseudostratified columnar epithelium of the respiratory type and stratified squamous epithelium are the most common epithelial linings.[238] Columnar epithelium has been found in 50% of specimens in some series. The next most common pattern is squamous epithelium.[97] Gastrointestinal epithelium lining a thyroglossal duct cyst has also been reported.[36,101]

Skin appendages within TGDC are probably the result of ectodermal cells within the tract.[49] Cartilage within a TGDC has also been described. It is possible that groups of cartilagenous cells can be entrapped by the thyroglossal duct during its descent near the hyoid bone. Metaplasia of fibroblast cells in response to recurrent infection and inflammation can also explain the presence of cartilage within the cyst.[236]

Histologic diagnosis of a thyroglossal duct cyst is based on the identification of normal thyroid follicles in the cyst wall.[245] Thyroid tissue within the cyst cavity can be found between 1.5% and 62% of specimens.[103,129,213,235] The incidence of thyroid tissue within the thyroglossal duct ranges from 5 to 75%, depending on the extent of histologic examination.[128] The absence of thyroid tissue within a midline cyst does not exclude the diagnosis of a thyroglossal duct cyst. A close association of the cyst tract to the hyoid bone is a common finding.[108,242]

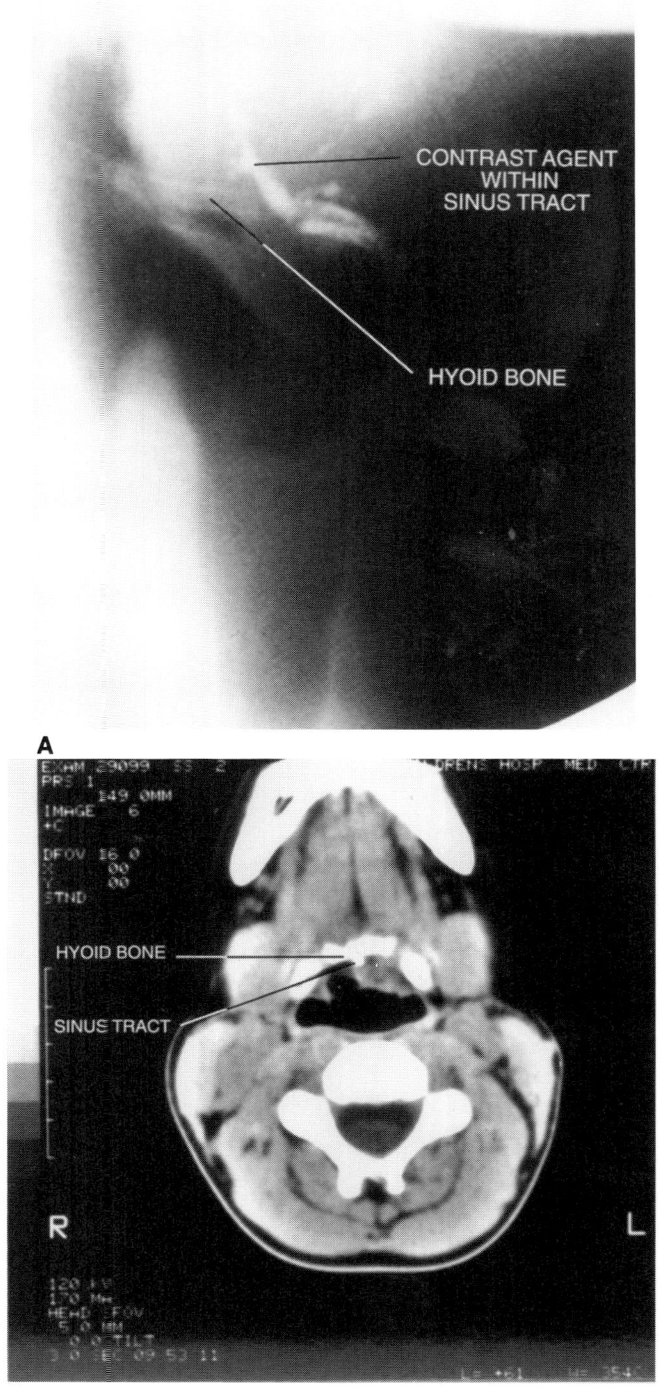


**Fig. 17–9.** A: Radiographic demonstration of the relationship of a thyroglossal duct cyst to the hyoid bone seen by injection of contrast agent into the sinus tract. B: CT scan demonstrating the relationship of the sinus tract to the hyoid bone.

Malignant transformation of thyroglossal duct cysts is well reported, but it is exceedingly rare.[69,75,103,128,246,254] The diagnosis of carcinoma in a thyroglossal duct cyst is made usually at postoperative histologic examination.[129] As of 1988, 150 cases of carcinoma had been reported within the thyroglossal anomalies. However, only 3 of these patients were less than 10 years of age.[103] Lingual ectopic thyroid can also undergo malignant transformation, as can nonlingual ectopic thyroid tissue.[264] The risk of carcinoma is less than 1%.[48,120] Carcinomas are thought to arise from the thyroid tissue rather than from the duct or cyst epithelium.[69,75] Malignant tumors within the cyst encompass all of the histologic diagnoses possible with primary thyroid carcinoma except medullary carcinoma, which arises from parafollicular cells.[103,128,253] The diagnosis is based on three criteria: normal epithelium containing thyroid follicles, identification of carcinoma within the duct epithelium, and no evidence of carcinoma within the thyroid gland.[99]

The vast majority of carcinomas are papillary thyroid carcinomas and they appear similar to papillary neoplasms within the thyroid gland proper.[75,108,120,128,246] Between 6 and 9% of cases of malignant thyroglossal duct cysts are squamous cell carcinomas.[106,129,152] The presence of a TGDC, histologic diagnosis of squamous cell carcinoma arising from the cyst, and the exclusion of metastases from other regions must be determined before making a diagnosis of squamous cell carcinoma arising from a TGDC.[129] Mixed papillary-follicular carcinoma, adenocarcinoma, Hurthle cell neoplasm, and follicular carcinoma have all been reported.[237,246]

### Differential diagnosis

Some series report a 31% incidence of pathologies other than thyroglossal duct cysts for midline neck masses.[10,49] Dermoid cysts are the second-most common pathologic diagnosis in this location.[10] Some dermoid cysts move with swallowing, are attached to the hyoid bone, and demonstrate a tract during excision.[49] Also included in the differential diagnosis of the thyroglossal duct cyst are ectopic thyroid tissue, branchial anomalies, sebaceous cyst, cystic hygroma, lymphadenitis, lymphadenopathy, hemangioma, benign intralaryngeal tumors, sialadenitis, lingual or submental abscess, lipoma, and tuberculosis.[27,32,168] Some reticuloendothelial diseases can present with a midline neck mass.[168] Cases of fibromatosis and *Mycobacterium intracellulare* are reported in this location.[10] Tophaceous gout has been reported as presenting as a midline neck mass.[118] Laryngeal hemangiopericytoma, laryngeal saccular cyst, or laryngocele can present in a similar manner. In adults, the differential diagnosis must include malignancy, and the patient must be aware of the need for more extensive surgery based on intraoperative frozen sections.[27] In patients with a large midline mass of the thyrohyoid area with distortion of the laryngeal lumen, one must entertain the possibility of epidermoid carcinoma, sarcoma, or salivary gland neoplasm.[48]

## Treatment

Historically, thyroglossal duct cysts were treated by incision and drainage.[168] Incision and drainage is now considered inadequate therapy and reserved only for acute infections.[10,168] Simple excision of a thyroglossal duct cyst should be avoided.[10] The treatment of choice is the Sistrunk procedure which consists of an en bloc resection of the midportion of the hyoid in addition to the cyst and tract.[49,75,108,168] Excision of the central portion of the hyoid bone and complete dissection of the duct was first described by Shlange in 1893.[10] Sistrunk popularized the technique in 1920, recommending excision of the central part of the hyoid bone and a cuff of muscle around the duct as well.[10,205]

The Sistrunk procedure begins with a transverse skin incision approximately 4–5 cm in length, slightly inferior to the neck mass (Fig. 17–10A, B).[246] An elliptical incision is incorporated around a sinus tract, if present.[168,246] The skin, subcutaneous tissues, and platysma are reflected and the midline fascia incised to expose the cyst (Fig. 17–10C).[168] The duct can divide into several branches and is sometimes difficult to find.[10] The cyst and sinus tract are dissected to the midportion of the hyoid bone which is then resected (Fig. 17–10D).[246] By dissecting medial to the lesser cornu, the stylohyoid musculature, and fascial slings, the digastric muscles are not interrupted. Approximately 1.5–2 cm of the hyoid bone should be removed. Retrohyoid and intrahyoid localization of a thyroglossal duct cyst supports the necessity of a Sistrunk procedure in virtually all cases of thyroglossal anomalies.[24] The soft tissues lying between the hyoid and the foramen cecum are resected also.[246] Removal of a generous amount of tissue around the tract helps prevent avulsion of this structure.[97] A finger placed intraorally to push the foramen cecum anteriorly will aid in the dissection (Fig. 17–10E). The oral cavity mucosa can be excised or left intact. Any defect in the mucosa created during the procedure should be closed with absorbable suture (Fig. 17–10F).[168]

Modifications of the Sistrunk procedure include excision of 3–4 cm of the midportion of the hyoid bone and inferior dissection beginning immediately superior to the thyroid isthmus (Fig. 17–11).[10,141,182] It is possible to excise an extensive tract through multiple stairstep incisions.[10] Excision of a thyroglossal duct cyst may occasionally require an anterior neck dissection because of its extension into surrounding structures.[141] In addition, a tongue-splitting procedure can be utilized to approach a fistula between the tongue base and the cyst. Drainage of the operative site is recommended.[168]

The intraoperative differentiation of midline neck cysts is important. The second-most common midline neck mass, a dermoid cyst, can be treated with simple excision.[49] Frozen section of the mass can be obtained prior to excision of the hyoid bone in the event that the mass is suspected to be a dermoid, or in those cases appearing suspicious for carcinoma.[108,129] Intraoperative aspiration of the cyst is another way to aid in the determination of histology. Those cysts which cannot be aspirated can be bisected.[115] In this way, the surgeon can avoid a more extensive resection in cases of midline dermoid cysts.

Other authors feel that the distinction between thyroglossal duct cysts and dermoid cysts in midline cervical neck masses is not important in the surgical care of the patient. They do not recommend aspiration or opening of the cyst intraoperatively because of the possibility of misidentification of the cyst contents and inadvertent incomplete resection.[49] They recommend that all midline cervical cysts be treated with the Sistrunk procedure to avoid inadequate excision and recurrence.[10,49] Even if it contains the patient's only thyroid tissue, resection is advised because of the cyst's tendency toward infection and progressive enlargement and because this ectopic thyroid tissue is often insufficient for normal endocrine function.[108]

Thyroglossal duct anomalies presenting in adult life are an absolute indication for surgery because of the possibility of malignancy.[213] Following excision, thyroglossal duct cysts can be opened and examined. If a mass is found within the cyst, frozen section should be obtained. If frozen section evaluation confirms the presence of carcinoma, the thyroid gland and neck should be evaluated carefully. Biopsy of any palpable thyroid mass should be performed intraoperatively.[128]

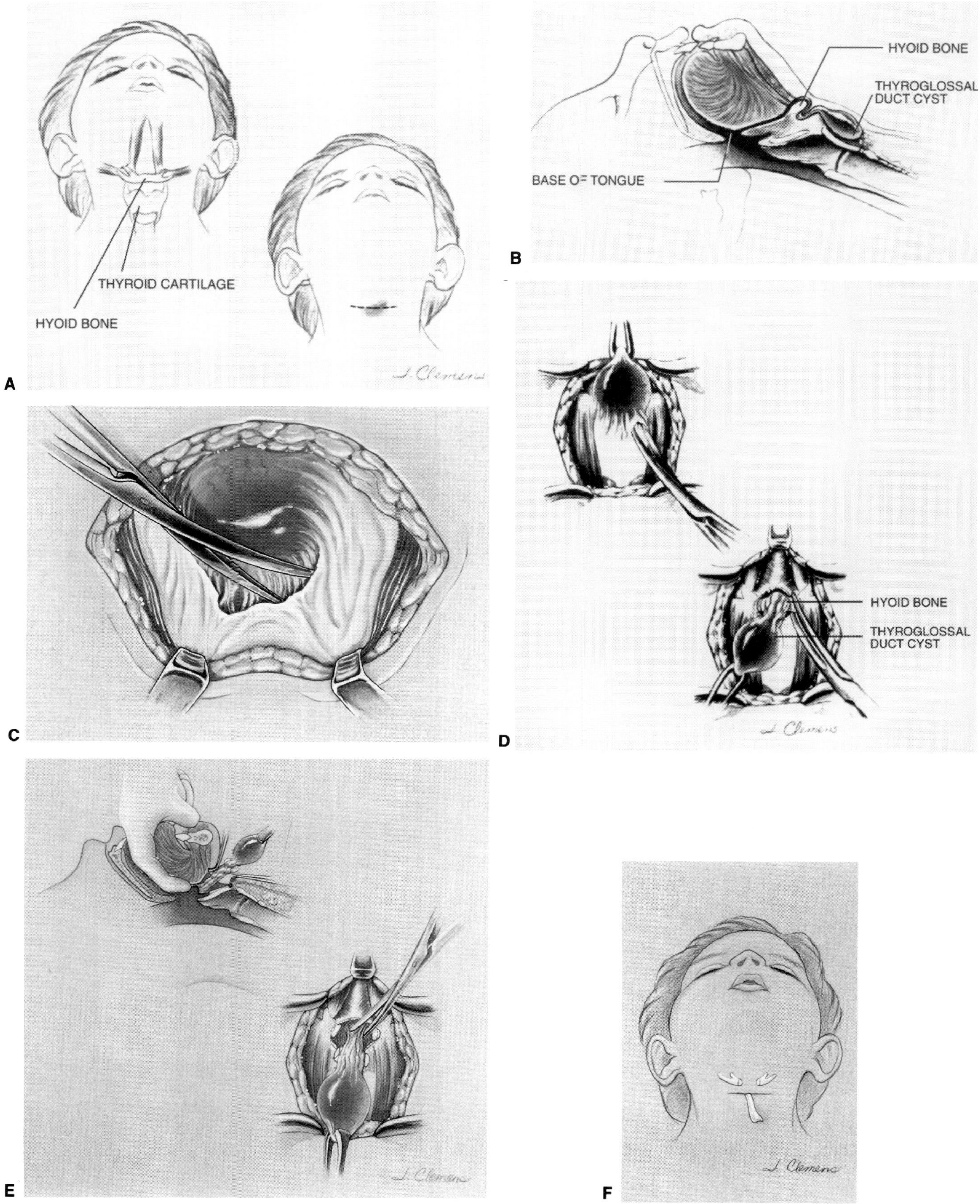


**Fig. 17–10.** Excision of a thyroglossal duct cyst by the Sistrunk procedure. A: Anteroposterior view demonstrating the hyoid bone (left) and incision (right). B: Lateral view showing the relationship of the thyroglossal duct cyst to the hyoid bone. C: Dissection around the cyst. D: Mobilization of the cyst, leaving it pedicled to the hyoid bone and division of the hyoid bone. E: Placement of a finger in the vallecula and completion of dissection across the base of the tongue. F: Completed procedure with central core of the hyoid bone removed.

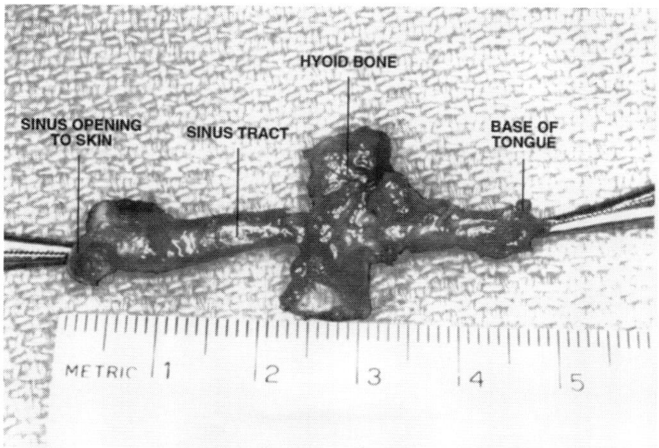


**Fig. 17–11.** Resected specimen with segment of hyoid.

### Complications

Prior to the description of the Sistrunk procedure in 1920, recurrence rates as high as 70%–80% were associated with simple excision. Following Schlange's report in 1893 advocating excision of the cyst and the central portion of the hyoid bone, recurrence rates dropped to 20%. The Sistrunk procedure has reduced recurrence rates to 3%–5%.[168] Multiple operations, recurrent infection, young age, and the presence of a sinus tract increase the risk of recurrence.[10,75,97,209] Previous surgery contributes to recurrence by obscuring the sinus tract and encouraging multiple sinus tracts.[10] Thyroglossal remnants in continuity with the isthmus of the thyroid gland can be another source of recurrent disease.[182] The surgical management of recurrent thyroglossal duct disease consists of wide excision of the pharyngeal mucosa and wider resection of the midportion of the hyoid bone. The best opportunity for curative excision occurs at the time of initial presentation.[97]

## Hemangiomas

Hemangiomas are the most common human congenital anomalies.[207] The reported incidence of hemangiomas, excluding salmon patch, ranges from 0.3 to 2% of births.[17,86] Salmon patch is reported in 40% of neonates.[70] By the first year of life, 10% of children have at least one visible hemangioma.[207] Approximately 16% of patients have hemangiomas in multiple locations.[86] Between 15 and 35% of hemangiomas are located in the head and neck.[17,172] Females are affected three times as frequently as males.[86,172]

### Etiology

Hemangiomas result from failed embryologic development of vascular cells.[65] The vascular system develops from a meshwork of endothelial lakes into a series of capillary channels with a muscular layer. These eventually become mature vessels. Each of the stages of development is named according to the degree of differentiation that occurs during that stage. Abnormalities during the endothelial stage result in cavernous or capillary hemangiomas while abnormalities in a retiform stage will produce an arteriovenous (AV) fistula or a mixed hemangioma.[166] Intramuscular hemangiomas most likely result from mesodermal arrests of vasoformative tissue.[220] Nevus flammeus is thought to result from loss of sympathetic neurons or altered nervous function of the vascular plexus.[197]

### Classification

Hemangiomas are classified within the spectrum of vascular tumors, ranging from AV malformations to lymphangiomas.[17,172] Edgerton has classified these lesions into one of the more useful systems currently employed.[70] Type 1 hemangiomas include forms of neonatal staining, such as nevus flammeus simplex, also referred to as *erythema nuchae* or *stork bite*.[70,197] Type 2 lesions, termed *intradermal capillary hemangiomas,* include salmon patches, port wine stains, and spider angiomas. Juvenile capillary hemangiomas, including strawberry marks, strawberry capillary hemangiomas, and capillary cavernous hemangiomas, are referred to as type 3 hemangiomas.[70] Juvenile hemangioma has also been called *strawberry nevus.*[172] Type 4 anomalies encompass arteriovenous fistulas, including arterial hemangioma.[70] Cirsoid angiomas, or arteriovenous malformations, are considered type 5 hemangiomas.[70,86] In addition to cavernous and capillary types, mixed lesions and hemangiolymphangiomatous lesions have been described.[172] Capillary hemangiomas are the most common type of hemangioma.[17,70] Intramuscular hemangiomas account for less than 1% of all hemangiomas.[19] Hemangiomas can also be classified as high-flow or low-flow lesions, which help determine the choice of therapy.[65] Other systems are based on the endothelial characteristics or diameter of the vascular structures that comprise the lesion.[150,174]

### Clinical presentation

Most hemangiomas are not evident at birth but present within the first month of life and grow until the second year of life.[17,208] The most common sites of occurrence in the head and neck are the scalp, neck, and face.[252] The skin is the most commonly involved organ.[244] A precursor lesion of pale skin sometimes surrounded by telangiectasia is often evident. After the second year, the size of the lesion stabilizes for approximately 1 year, after which involution may begin. The vast majority of these lesions undergo regression by the age of 5 years.[17]

On physical examination, these tumors are typically soft, painless, compressible, and indistinct. They can be located on the skin or mucosa, or within muscle, bone, or salivary gland tissue (Fig. 17–12). Audible bruits are detected if there is a significant AV malformation component.[172] Neonatal presentation consists of light pink staining over the forehead or back of neck.[70] Salmon patch is light pink to rust colored and is most common on the back of the neck, forehead, or eyelids. Spider angiomas consist of a small central arteriole with a stellate pattern of radiating capillaries. These often appear at the age of 3 or 4 years. Strawberry marks are pale halos of skin surrounded by telangiectasia.[70] Capillary hemangiomas are bright red or purple with well-defined borders showing varying degrees of lobulation and blanch with pressure.[17,70] Cavernous hemangiomas blanch with pressure as well and are generally raised and red to purple in color.[86] They are soft and indiscreet with a "bag of worms" texture. Increasing size can be noted with the valsalva maneuver. Pure cavernous forms are less common

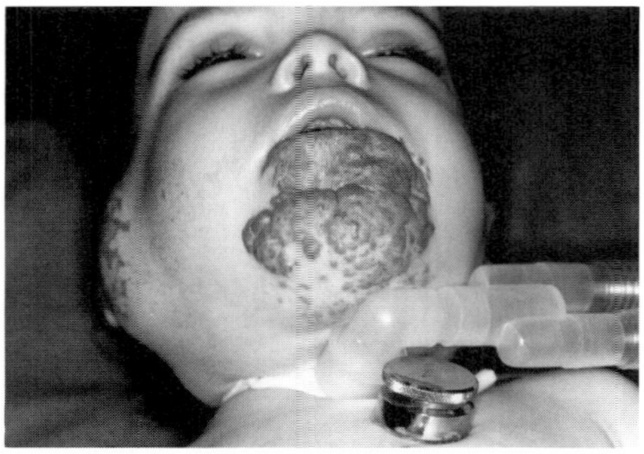

**Fig. 17–12.** Cervicofacial hemangioma of the neck in a child with airway obstruction who required a tracheotomy.

than the mixed variety.[17] In general, port wine stains do not blanch with pressure. They are usually pink to deep red in infancy and darken to a deep purple by middle age. Also, the surface of the lesion tends to become raised and nodular by that time. Hypertrophy of the soft tissue and bone underlying the port wine stain is common. Collagen degeneration may allow abnormal vessels to dilate.[8] The distribution of port wine stains may correspond to the sensory branches of the trigeminal nerve.[44,162]

The vast majority of childhood salivary gland hemangiomas occur in the parotid gland, although they can present within the submandibular triangle.[17,89,180,206]

Large hemangiomas in the neonatal period can be life-threatening. Heart failure presumably secondary to a large head and neck hemangioma has been reported. Changes in clinical parameters, such as rapid growth of the lesion, altered cry, stridor, dyspnea, cyanosis, changes in feeding, swallowing difficulties, tachycardia, or heart murmur should alert one to the possibility of heart failure.[59]

Hemangiomas may be associated with syndromes. These include Von Hippel disease, Maffucci syndrome, Sturge-Weber syndrome, and Kasabach-Merritt syndrome.[172]

### Diagnosis

Any patient with a hemangioma of the head and neck requires a comprehensive medical history and physical examination. Endoscopy of the upper aerodigestive tract should be performed when involvement of these structures is suspected. A barium esophagram is a complementary study in these instances. Plain radiographs should also be obtained during the initial radiographic evaluation. A pathognomonic finding is the presence of laminated smooth phleboliths within a large venous plexus on plain film. In addition, soap bubble appearance of multicystic bone resorption is typical.[17]

Doppler ultrasound is a noninvasive technique that can aid in the diagnosis of hemangiomas of the head and neck. CT with contrast is unable to determine high-flow from low-flow lesions or the presence of feeding vessels.[160] Ultrasound alone is unable to differentiate between hemangioma and lymphangioma.[17] Doppler ultrasound offers the ability to determine a high- vs. low-flow lesion and is useful in any case in which the diagnosis of a neck mass is unclear.[160] Ultrasound also can help predict outcome in cases of hemangioma. An increase in the number of fistulae detected within the lesion is associated with a decreased possibility of regression.[22]

CT should be obtained prior to any interventional therapy.[17] It can demonstrate bone erosion, involvement of major vessels, mediastinal or intracranial extension, or displacement of upper aerodigestive tract structures.[169] Angiography is another technique that is useful in the evaluation of hemangiomas of the head and neck. It is able to differentiate between hemangiomas and vascular malformations.[31] Direct puncture of vascular malformations and injection of contrast material can be performed if an arteriogram fails to demonstrate a vascular lesion.[25] A technique of radiolabeling autologous blood with technicium 99 to confirm vascular tumors from other soft tissue tumors in children has also been described. This is especially useful in hemangiomas that are deep in location and lack cutaneous involvement.[208] Valsalva maneuver in combination with scintigraphic evaluation can help to more accurately discern the actual size of the hemangioma. Postoperative scintigraphic evaluation can be helpful in determining the presence of residual hemangioma following surgical excision.[244]

#### Histology

Hemangiomas are found at different locations within the skin and subcutaneous tissues. They are typically nonencapsulated lesions.[70] Cutaneous capillary hemangiomas or nevus flammeus are located primarily in the superficial dermis.[166,197] Intradermal hemangiomas are located in the deep dermis.[70] Strawberry nevi are located in the subcutaneous tissues.[166] Port wine stains are found at various depths in the skin, either in the epidermis, dermis, or subdermis.[44,70]

Hemangiomas are divided histologically into categories based on the size of the vessels.[17] The most common categories include capillary, cavernous, or mixed types. The capillary form demonstrates a thin wall and small vessels lined by a single layer of flattened or plump endothelial cells. Cavernous hemangiomas contain larger dermal and subcutaneous vessels which are separated by scanty connective tissue stroma.[17] Additional categories include venous hemangioma (cirsoid angioma) and complex malformation.[20,70] Cirsoid angiomas are uncommon vascular lesions composed primarily of venous tributaries situated within a loose fibrous stroma.[8,20] Complex malformations often have mature bone and atrophic muscle fibers present on histologic examination.[20] Growth phases of hemangiomas are characterized by endothelial hyperplasia while, during regression, there is decreased cellularity present.[17] Indirect aminoperoxidase staining technique with factor 8–related protein will suggest the vascular nature of a hemangioma.[206] Malignant transformation most commonly follows radiation therapy and presents as a hemangiosarcoma.[70,220]

### Treatment

Cosmetic concerns are important in hemangiomas of the head and neck.[199] Children with port wine stains may suffer significant psychological sequelae as a result of their condition.[192] There is often pressure from the parents of a child with a hemangioma to initiate some form of treatment. Most lesions should be observed patiently for the expected regression which characterizes this congenital anomaly.[17] Spontaneous involution takes place in 85% of hemangiomas.[127,199] Most commonly, hemangiomas will begin to regress after 12 months of age.[199] Some authors suggest watching cavernous hemangiomas for 10 years before any treatment is initiated.[86] This conservative approach is also recommended for parotid hemangiomas.[180] Approximately 3%–5% of hemangiomas require aggressive therapy due to their size, involvement of vital structures, or life-threatening complications.[251] Other indications for therapy include easy excision, atypical growth or rapid growth, and failure of involution after a period of observation.[17,199] More aggressive therapy is also indicated if osseous deformity is the result of hemangioma.[31]

Nonsurgical treatment of hemangiomas includes electrodessication, compression therapy, embolization, cryotherapy, sclerosing therapy, radiation, steroids, and other chemotherapeutic agents.[17,199]

Zarem and Edgerton in 1967 were the first to recommend systemic steroid therapy for hemangiomas.[190,263] The mechanism of action is unclear.[17] Rates of response to systemic steroid therapy range from 29% to 100% and are more effective in younger patients.[17,40,207] Capillary hemangiomas show a greater response in infancy than cavernous hemangiomas.[172] Hemangiomas that are life threatening or cause dysfunction can be treated successfully by this modality.[17] Early use of steroids can prevent the need for tracheotomy in those patients with hemangiomas causing airway obstruction.[40] While systemic therapy has been shown to be effective in the treatment of hemangiomas, the potential of side effects remains a limiting factor.

Intralesional injection of steroids has been used with documented cases of regression.[17] Indications include ulceration, bleeding, rapid growth, or cosmetic deformity.[207] Various combinations have been used, including triamcinolone and betamethasone. Intralesional injection has been shown to inhibit further growth and promote regression. Response rates of 75% have been reported for those patients treated with intralesional injection.[207]

Several other chemotherapeutic agents have been used in the treatment of hemangiomas. Antifibrinolytic agents prevent clot degradation and can promote regression through local clot formation and fibrosis.[17] Aminocaproic acid and tranexamic acid have both been used. Cyclophosphamide and intra-arterial 5–fluorouracil have been used for large and inoperable lesions.[54,180,251] Antiestrogen therapy has been successful for intramuscular hemangiomas.[220]

The $CO_2$, argon, flash-pumped dye, and neodymium YAG lasers have all been used with success.[17,199] The advantage of the $CO_2$ laser is its ability to coagulate.[172] The argon laser, because of its selective absorption by hemoglobin and deep penetration while sparing overlying skin, has been used successfully to treat many cutaneous vascular lesions.[17,45,86,199] Many surgeons only treat port wine stains after puberty while others feel infants and children can undergo treatment successfully with little morbidity and a cosmetically more acceptable lesion as they grow older.[8,192] Port wine stains show significant improvement following treatment with the argon laser.[45] These treatments can be spaced a year apart. Although improvement is seen in 60%–75% of patients, hypertrophic scarring occurs in 9%–26% of patients treated with the argon laser.[8,192] A test spot on the skin is currently recommended to identify those patients who form hypertrophic scars or keloids.[17]

The YAG laser is also effective in the treatment of hemangiomas because of its ability to penetrate deeply into soft tissue, coagulate vessels up to 7 mm in diameter, and cause deep photocoagulation.[175,199] Local anesthesia has been found to alter the optical quality of the target and most patients undergo general anesthesia.[86] Thermal energy is dissipated quickly when used to treat high-flow vascular abnormalities.[175] For this reason, high-flow lesions such as AV malformations are not amenable to treatment by the YAG laser.[199]

The tuneable flashlamp pumped pulsed dye laser is a new technique that has demonstrated usefulness in the treatment of hemangiomas. Sedation or a general anesthetic is usually necessary for this procedure. The treatment area may result in a sunburn-like pain for several hours and can be followed by blistering of the skin. Purpura is usually produced for 10–14 days following therapy, which is replaced by a brownish discoloration the following week. Following re-evaluation in 6 weeks, additional portions of the port wine stain can be treated. This technique can be used in prepubescent children.[192]

Angiography with embolization has been used effectively as single therapy and in combination with surgery.[17,117,122,199,210] Embolization alone is indicated in the palliative treatment of inoperative lesions. Various embolization materials have been used.[17,86,169,220] Successful embolization makes resection of the hemangioma less difficult and decreases blood loss.[65] Resection specimens consist of a combination of hemangioma and fibrosis with necrosis.[72] It is essential that the interventional radiologist be knowledgable of the vascular anatomy and the important anastomoses between the extra- and intracerebral circulation.[169]

Opinion varies as to the most appropriate time for surgical excision following embolization. As a general rule, smaller lesions can undergo immediate resection, whereas larger lesions sometimes require a delay.[17] Preoperative embolization and surgical resection within 48–72 hours offers the best surgical opportunity for treatment.[199] Despite angiographic demonstration of primary blood supply, significant blood loss can occur during surgical excision.[170] Surgical resection of hemangiomas with ligation of feeding vessels has been described but recurrence is common.[14,17] Arterial ligation in combination with steroid therapy can be effective in large and complex hemangiomas.[254] Ligation of the feeding vessels promotes collateralization and eliminates these vessels as potential embolization routes in the future.[17,122,169] If collateralization occurs via the ophthalmic, ethmoidal, or meningeal arteries, postoperative embolization therapy is not recommended. Intramuscular hemangiomas are treated best by complete surgical excision.[172] Preoperative chemotherapy and radiation therapy followed by superficial parotidectomy with excision of the hemangioma and resolution of congestive heart failure has been described.[180] Cardiopulmonary bypass and deep hypothermia have been used in conjunction with surgical resection. Controlled intraoperative hypotension is an additional technique to limit blood loss during resection of hemangioma.[245] Free musculocutaneous flaps have been used following resection of extensive head and neck hemangioma for soft tissue replacement.[210]

Many authors advocate conservative therapy in the treatment of Kasabach-Merritt syndrome. Application of specially designed compression dressings have been utilized.[199] This condition has been treated by radiation, steroids, and splenectomy. Steroids are especially useful in this syndrome.[86] In addition, superselective embolization and intratumoral ligation have also been utilized.

### Complications

Complications of hemangiomas range from infection, hemorrhage, thrombocytopenia, ulceration, congestive heart failure and airway obstruction to cosmetic deformities. The most common complication of capillary hemangiomas is ulceration, usually due to infection.[17] Chondritis and cellulitis as a result of these lesions have been reported.[86] Recurrent bleeding episodes from a large head and neck hemangioma is not unusual.[210] Increasing friability with a greater tendency toward bleeding occurs as the child ages.[192] Scarring often results without altering the rate of resolution.[17]

Alteration in skeletal structures is not an uncommon complication of hemangiomas.[26] Vascular lesions can cause depression and demineralization of the outer cortex, hypoplasia, and distortion of the mandible. Malocclusion may result also. The mechanism of bone alteration remains unclear.[36] Facial nerve paralysis can occur from a large parotid hemangioma.[251] Congestive heart failure and airway obstruction are also much reported.[99,180]

## Cystic hygroma/lymphangioma

The term *hygroma* is taken from the Greek word meaning "watery tumor."[29,102] *Lymphangioma* is used interchangeably with *cystic hygroma*. These lesions are congenital anomalies of the lymphatic system and usually are diagnosed in infancy.[29] Lymphangiomas have also been classified as both neoplasms and hamartomas.[193] In 1828 Redenbacher provided one of the first descriptions of cystic hygromas, a lesion he referred to as a "ranula congenita."[29,215] Koester in 1872 was the first to suggest that these anomalies were lymphatic in origin.[215] Cystic hygromas comprise less than 5% of congenital neck masses.[29] More than 90% of cystic hygromas are reported in the cervical region.[111]

### Etiology

Although malformations, angiectasis, hematomas, and benign neoplasms all have been considered as the origin for cystic hygromas, the most widely accepted explanation for these lesions is that they arise from anomalous embryologic development of the lymphatic system.[29,159] Sabin showed that the lymphatic system develops from five primitive sacs derived from the venous system.[186] The paired jugular sacs, a single retroperitoneal sac, and the paired posterior sacs near the sciatic veins are evident by the seventh embryonic week.[29,158,186,193] The jugular lymphatic sacs exist next to the jugular veins, are the first to develop, and are usually the largest.[158,255] According to Sabin's centrifugal theory, endothelial sprouting from these sacs extends outward to form the peripheral lymphatic system.[29,186]

The centripetal theory, proposed by McClure and Huntington, states that the lymphatic system does not develop from the lymph sacs outward but from mesenchymal clefts which gradually extend from the periphery to connect to the venous circulation.[29,30,111]

In addition to the congenital variety, there are four types of acquired cystic hygromas. These include traumatic, infectious, iatrogenic, and neoplastic. The development of cystic hygromas following surgical procedures, minor trauma, or in response to chronic inflammation or infection has been reported. Moreover, Kennedy reports a case of a metastatic carcinoma causing obstruction to lymphatic drainage and a resultant cystic lymphangioma.[111]

### Classification

Capillary lymphangiomas are masses composed of capillary-size lymphatic channels which often invade the epidermis. Cavernous lymphangiomas contain larger, dilated sinuses which invade surrounding soft tissue. They are composed of one or more endothelial layers but can be without an adventitial layer. The largest of the cystic structures are cystic hygromas, which often surround neural and vascular structures.[29,179] They are frequently large, multiloculated cystic structures.[179,260] An additional category of hemangiolymphangioma was suggested by Saijo et al. in 1975.[187]

### Clinical presentation

There appears to be a bimodal distribution of patients presenting with cystic hygromas.[260] Forty percent of cystic hygromas appear in the newborn and 80%–90% present by the second year of life.[29,140,204,260] From birth to 2 years of age is the period of greatest lymphatic growth and may explain presentation of cystic hygromas in 90% of patients during this time.[234] A second group of lesions appears after the age of 20 years and occasionally into the fifth and sixth decade, although this is considered unusual.[29,116,140,144,260]

Between 45 and 75% of cystic hygromas occur in the head and neck region.[29,140] The neck is the single-most common structure involved by this tumor.[140] Both the posterior and anterior triangle have been reported as the most common sites of origin.[29] When cystic hygromas occur in the anterior cervical triangle, they usually extend into the submandibular and submental spaces and occasionally into the floor of mouth.[29,164] Only a few hygromas are found exclusively in the midline.[156]

Most patients present with a slowly growing, asymptomatic mass.[29,140] The mass tends to be soft and doughy to palpation and is usually not discrete (Fig. 17–13).[58,111,140] The skin overlying the mass can occasionally be thin secondary to stretching and atrophy of the subcutaneous tissues.[255] These masses are usually compressible and irregular, have a lobulated texture, and transilluminate.[140] Lymphangiomas can also present as small cystic cutaneous nodules.[193] They typically invade surrounding structures and fascial planes.[58]

A sudden increase in size indicates either hemorrhage from

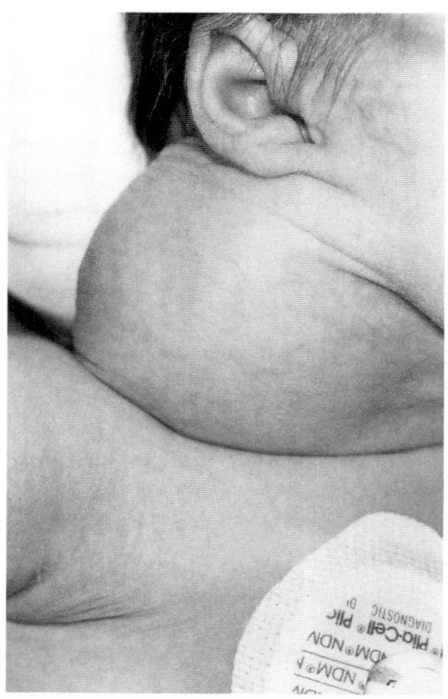

**Fig. 17–13.** Typical physical appearance of a large cervical cystic hygroma.

trauma or infection following an upper respiratory infection.[29,140,149] Rapid enlargement due to upper respiratory infection is thought to be due to excessive lymphatic filtration and lack of adequate drainage.[164] Repeat infection leads to increased sclerosis and further enlargement.[156] Sudden enlargement of cystic hygroma due to infection was associated with a high mortality rate in the preantibiotic era. These deaths were usually secondary to toxemia or respiratory obstruction.[248]

The size and site of lesion are the most common factors determining additional symptomatology.[58] Extension occurs to the floor of mouth, base of tongue, larynx, or mediastinum.[58] Difficulties in breathing and swallowing are common symptoms and indicate involvement of the upper aerodigestive tract.[140,260] Nearly 41% of children with cystic hygroma of the neck suffer upper airway and feeding problems and these patients can present with failure to thrive.[58,193] Macroglossia due to lymphangiomatous involvement of the tongue usually occurs in the anterior two-thirds.[193] Suprahyoid cystic hygroma causes feeding and airway difficulties in a much higher percentage of patients compared to infrahyoid cystic hygroma.[179]

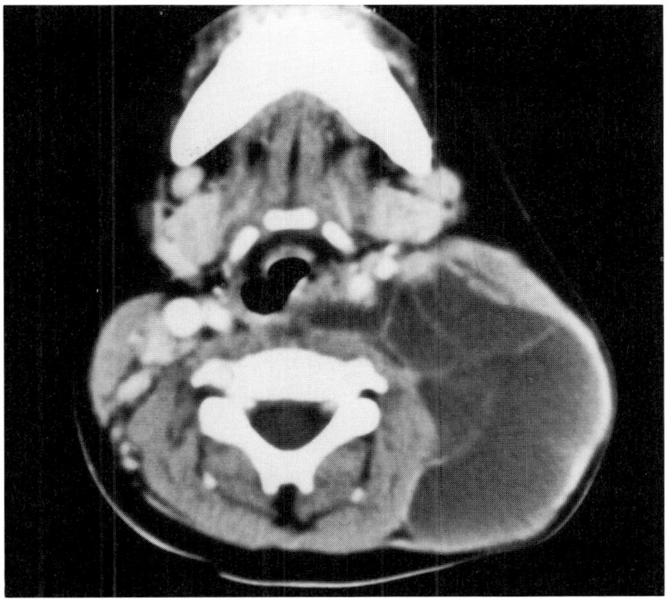

**Fig. 17–14.** Typical radiographic appearance of a cervical cystic hygroma consisting of a multiloculated cytic mass filled with low attenuation material with smooth septations and contrast enhancement with injection of contrast agent.

## Diagnosis

The evaluation of a patient with cervical cystic hygroma should include a careful history and physical examination. Endoscopic examination is recommended for those patients in whom hypopharyngeal or laryngeal involvement is suspected.[140] An elevated level of $\alpha$-fetoprotein has been noted with cystic hygroma in Turner syndrome, but the amount is normal in the majority of cases.[139,184] Inadvertent aspiration of the cystic hygroma may give elevated amniotic fluid $\alpha$-fetoprotein levels.[164]

Cystic hygroma is currently diagnosed more commonly on account of the technical advances in ultrasound.[47] In general, ultrasound demonstrates a cystic mass with linear septations and indistinct borders. There can be a focal area of thickening and increased echogenicity due to the presence of lymphatic tissue and organizing thrombus.[256] Cystic hygromas can demonstrate solid components relating to cyst walls or septae. Focal hemorrhage and calcification will show high echogenicity.[260] Cystic hygromas can simulate other lesions, such as an encephalocele.[154] The earliest ultrasound diagnosis of fetal cervical cystic hygroma can be made at 10 weeks gestational age.[47]

The initial radiographic evaluation should include anteroposterior and lateral neck films of the soft tissues of the neck.[193] A preoperative chest radiograph is essential to rule out mediastinal involvement.[30,50] Computed tomography is considered by many to be the method of choice for evaluating the cystic hygroma.[26,256] Typically, CT will show multiloculated cystic masses with smooth septations and contrast enhancement (Fig. 17–14).[51] Cystic hygromas appear as thin-walled masses with homogeneous density but can be single or multicystic.[256] The cyst wall can enhance without contrast.[260] Cystic hygromas are usually low-attenuation cystic masses filled with near-water density material and tend to be located posterior to the sternocleidomastoid muscle.[256,260] Many cystic hygromas originate in the posterior triangle and displace the sternocleidomastoid muscle laterally and often wrap around the muscle as well. Cystic hygromas that appear after the age of 2 years more commonly extend into the mediastinum and axilla.[256] Hemangiomas frequently infiltrate muscle and contain adipose tissue, but this is unusual for cystic hygromas.

MRI is a noninvasive technique that offers several advantages in the evaluation of cervical cystic hygromas. MRI is superior to CT in delineation of soft tissue structures.[260] It is better able to define the extent of the lesion, provides three-dimensional evaluation of the mass, and helps in more accurate preoperative surgical planning. There is no ionizing radiation and less need for contrast material.

### Histology

There are four histologic types of lymphangioma: cavernous lymphangioma, which is the most common, capillary lymphangioma, cystic hygroma, and hemangiolymphangioma. Often a combination of histologic types is found in the same patient.[140] Cystic hygroma consists of multiloculated cystic masses usually greater than 1 cm in diameter.[102] Hemangiolymphangiomas are suspected when there is excessive bleeding at the time of excision.[193] In addition, lymphangiomatous involvement of the skin is possible and demonstrates vesicle-like lesions within the papillary layer of the dermis. These lymphangiomatous lesions within the skin represent dilation of dermal lymphatics.[111]

Lymphangiomas are lined with a single layer of flattened endothelium and contain a protein-rich fluid.[132] The vessels lack smooth muscle.[178] The fluid contained within the cyst is usually serous, clear, or straw colored and often contains cholesterol crystals.[58,62] New vessel formation is commonly present.[178] Lymphangioma is differentiated from simple dilation of lymphatics or lymphangiectasis by invasion of surrounding tissue.[187]

## Treatment

Rapid enlargement of cystic hygromas can lead to acute airway obstruction.[179] Acute management is directed toward relief of airway obstruction or dysphagia.[193] Aspiration is an effective temporizing measure if there is compromise of the upper aerodigestive tract.[29] Initial needle aspiration and intubation should be followed by tracheotomy in most cases.[193] Complications of aspiration include infection and hemorrhage. This technique should be used for emergency decompression only.[140]

Some authors advocate careful observation, since some lesions undergo spontaneous resolution.[34] There are other reports of spontaneous regression followed by recurrence many years later. Regression usually leaves loose redundant skin at the site of the lesion.[156] One must consider the possibility of increased difficulty of surgical excision with enlargement of the hygroma or its recurrent infection when making the decision of close observation.[30,111]

Several nonsurgical techniques have been used in the treatment of cervical cystic hygromas. Diathermy has been used in the past but with limited success.[111,187] Radium seed implantation has been used as a primary mode of therapy.[111,140] Sclerosing agents such as ethemoline, boiling water, sodium morrhuate, quinine, urethane, hypotonic saline, tetracycline, cyclophosphamide, 25% glucose, and bleomycin have been introduced into lesions in an attempt to cause fibrosis.[29,51,99,140,248] These agents occasionally obliterate the cysts but can cause injury to the surrounding soft tissue.[90] Potential risks of the use of sclerosing agents include bacteremia, injury to the great vessels or brachial plexus, or the inadvertent injection of the sclerosing agent into the venous system. Steroids are not useful in the treatment of lymphangiomas.[140]

Some authors feel that premature infants with cervical cystic hygromas should be allowed to grow until normal birth weight is attained before recommending surgery.[30] Others recommend early resection to avoid the complications of infection. For lymphangiomas extending into the parotid gland, observation has been recommended until the age of 3 to 5 years, at which time parotidectomy can be performed. Surgical excision of a cystic hygroma should be delayed at least 3 months following acute infection.[111,156] In patients in whom respiratory tract involvement by these lesions is suspected, endoscopy and marsupialization can be used.[111] Unroofing the cyst is desirable in cases of small amounts of residual tumor.[140] Superficial capillary lymphangiomas of the skin can be treated with primary excision and closure or split-thickness skin grafting. According to some authors, operative removal of cervical cystic hygroma is only recommended if there is no regression by the age of 5 years.[193]

Considering the natural history of recurrence and enlargement, the most widely accepted treatment remains surgical removal.[29] In long-term follow-up, most cases that underwent complete excision were cured.[119,187]

### Complications

Complications of cystic hygroma include upper aerodigestive tract obstruction, aspiration, pneumonia due to upper airway obstruction, macroglossia, and recurrence.[255] Recurrence usually presents within 1 year of treatment and is associated with suppurative infections of the lymphangioma prior to surgery and delayed resection. Recurrence following complete excision is found in 6% of cases.[29] Incomplete excision is associated with up to 52% risk of recurrence.[29,58,161,187] Infrahyoid cystic hygromas demonstrate lower complication and recurrence rates with minimal potential for long-term impairment compared to suprahyoid lesions.[39,179] There are case reports of recurrences even after 21 years. High doses of steroids and antimicrobial agents can be useful in the treatment of recurrence. Tracheotomy must occasionally be performed to secure the airway, but the initial use of steroids and antimicrobials in high doses for presumed infection can be successful.[191]

Other surgical complications include muscle weakness, Horner syndrome, recurrent laryngeal nerve paralysis, postoperative infection, recurrent airway obstruction, and death.[154] Permanent nerve paralysis occurs in 12%–33% of cases of resection of cervical cystic hygromas.[58,111] The potential for intraoperative nerve injury is related to the size and the extent of the cystic hygroma rather than the age of the patient at operation.[58] Damage to the seventh, ninth, tenth, eleventh, and twelfth cranial nerves, as well as the cervical sympathetic chain and brachial plexus, is possible. Sepsis and fistula formation are additional complications of surgical excision. A mortality rate of between 2.5 and 5% is found in most large series.[111] Mortality rates approach 50% for massive infiltrating cystic hygroma of the neck in infants.[15]

## Sternocleidomastoid tumor of infancy

The sternocleidomastoid tumor of infancy (SCTI) is usually considered within the spectrum of conditions known as *congenital muscular torticollis* (CMT). Other terms used interchangeably include sternomastoid torticollis, fibromatosis colli, nodular fasciitis, or sternomastoid fibrosis.[231]

The most common cause of torticollis is congenital fibrosis within the sternocleidomastoid muscle seen with SCTI. This anomaly is not a true tumor but a fibrous swelling within the sternocleidomastoid muscle.[231,233] Estimates of incidence range from 4 per 1,000 births to 5 per 10,000 births.[28,126] It is the most common neck mass presenting in the immediate perinatal period.[231] By contrast, CMT is usually seen between the ages of 3 or 4 years and is not necessarily associated with SCTI. The majority of cases of CMT present after the age of 1 year.[126] Thirty-four percent of patients with CMT had no evidence of tumor.[105]

### Etiology

The pathophysiology of SCTI remains unclear and several hypotheses have been proposed.[231] Many authors feel that birth trauma with resultant injury of the sternocleidomastoid muscle and eventual fibrosis of the injury site is the most likely cause.[126,138,225,231] Cases of SCTI being present at birth lend less credence to this hypothesis.[225] The presence of SCTI following cesarean section has been attributed to injury to the sternocleidomastoid muscle during violent extraction from the uterus.[126,225]

### Clinical presentation

SCTI is more common in males, whereas CMT is more common in females.[126] Overall, there is no racial or sexual predisposition noted.[126,231] Both conditions have been found to be more common on the right and in children delivered with breech presentation.[135] However, others report no statistical difference between sides.[105,131,233] The majority of cases involve first-born children.[126,233] SCTI typically presents within the first 2 months of life.[231,233] It is usually firm and painless to palpation and has a fusiform shape.[233] The size varies from 1 to 3 cm in diameter. Between 2 and 3% are isolated.[105] The majority of tumors are found in the inferior and middle one-third of the sternocleidomastoid muscle.[231,233] The most superior one-third of the muscle is rarely affected. SCTI can involve either the sternal or clavicular heads of the muscle.

The natural history of SCTI is stabilized growth followed by spontaneous resolution. The mass will usually reach maximum size at 8 weeks and will remain unchanged for the next 8 to 12 weeks.[233] Resolution occurs over the next 6 to 8 months. Half of the patients with SCTI have normal muscle by the age of 6 months while 30% will have palpable fibrosis without torticollis.[105]

### Diagnosis

A complete history and physical examination is essential in the evaluation of this anomaly.[233] The most consistent physical finding is the presence of a mass and head tilt. Computed tomography is helpful in localizing the lesion to the sternocleidomastoid muscle and is recommended in those cases in which torticollis presents with neurologic deficit. An ultrasound examination may be a simple means of localizing the mass to the sternocleidomastoid muscle. Open biopsy should be reserved for those cases in which diagnosis is uncertain or the lesion fails to resolve spontaneously.[231]

The diagnosis of sternocleidomastoid tumor of infancy must be entertained in any infant presenting with a lateral neck mass. There have been no cases of malignancy associated with SCTI.[81] However, the lesion must be differentiated from other more aggressive processes such as desmoid tumors, neuroblastoma, rhabdomyoma or rhabdomyosarcoma, and fibrosarcoma.[13,231]

#### Histology

On gross examination, SCTI is usually glistening white with a whirled or lobulated appearance. Histologically, it appears to be composed of dense fibrous tissue without normal striated muscle. When muscle is present within the lesion, there is loss of striations, as well as edema, and vacuoles are present within the cells.[233] The degree of collagen deposition and fibroblast proliferation varies from case to case.[231] Electron microscopic evaluation reveals that the lesion is more similar to tendon and ligament than to muscle.[142]

### Treatment

While some authors recommend early excision to prevent the possibility of permanent deformity, most advocate conservative nonoperative treatment for this lesion due to the natural history of resolution in the majority of cases.[113,126,131] Therapy should be instituted prior to 1 year of age for the best long-term results. Physiotherapy with stretching of the sternocleidomastoid muscle along with heat and massage is beneficial.[231,233] Other exercise techniques include tilting the head away from the contracted side and rotating the chin towards the contracted side. Placement of toys and other objects in a position where stretching is necessary is also helpful.

Estimates of the success of conservative therapy range from 70% to 90%. In one series, the majority of patients having good results from conservative therapy were treated before the age of 1 year and had less than 30° limitation of rotation prior to treatment. Conservative therapy fails more commonly when it is initiated after 6 to 12 months of age.[34,126] Patients are reported to progress to torticollis despite physical therapy in 21% of cases.[126] Surgery is indicated when the mass or the torticollis is present for longer than 1 year, when craniofacial asymmetry develops, or when there is failure of an adequate trial of physiotherapy.[34,233]

The variety of surgical procedures recommended range from simple release of the fibrous band to partial and complete excision of the sternocleidomastoid muscle.[7] Historically, this lesion has been corrected surgically by sectioning both sternal and clavicular heads of the sternocleidomastoid muscle.[13,231] Both bipolar and unipolar releases and open tenotomy have been performed.[126]

Long-term follow-up is essential, due to the recurrence of some tumors and the development of delayed torticollis or craniofacial asymmetry. There are documented cases in which the mass has disappeared and reappeared during the growth spurts of childhood. This should be discussed with parents and followed closely.[233]

#### Complications

Approximately 10%–20% of patients will develop late torticollis and 25% will have some degree of persistent asymmetry or tightness of the sternocleidomastoid muscle. Children compensate for the torticollis by elevating the affected shoulder girdle laterally and shifting the head toward the affected side. This can lead to cervical scoliosis, lumbar scoliosis, and chronic pain. Plagiocephaly is found in almost one-third of patients with congenital muscular torticollis.[28] Plagiocephaly can become more pronounced in patients with sternocleidomastoid tumors because the infant tends to maintain his or her head in a fixed position while sleeping.[28,38] An additional complication of the sternocleidomastoid tumor of infancy and resultant torticollis is hypoplasia of the ipsilateral side of the face. Underdevelopment of the malar eminence and inferior displacement of the eye, ear, and corner of the mouth may result.[81,126]

## Dermoid

Dermoids cysts in the head and neck are unusual lesions.[123,176,240] Dermoids are often considered within the more general category of teratomas.[98,230] Teratomas are divided into epidermoid cysts, dermoid cysts, and true teratomas based on the number of germ cell derivatives present.[230] Dermoids are germ-cell-derived teratomas having an ectodermal dominance with the presence of both ectoderm and mesoderm.[18,230] Teratomas are distinguished by the addition of endodermally derived cells. Those are the most common form of teratoma.[98,230]

Approximately 6.9% of dermoid cysts affect the head and neck.[123,155,259] Over 80% arise primarily in the periorbital, nasal, and oral regions.[136,155,214] The periorbital area is the most common site in the head and neck, accounting for 47% of dermoids in this region.[136] Approximately 23% of these tumors in the head and neck are located in the floor of mouth.[123] Those of the neck account for 9–24% of dermoids of the head and neck, and up to 22% of midline neck lesions in most series.[136,155,214,216]

### Etiology

There are several theories attempting to explain the etiology of dermoids.[155] Embryologic rests of epithelial cells, traumatic implantation of dermal and epidermal elements, and variants of a thyroglossal duct cyst have all been offered as possible explanations.[49,73,98,136] The most widely accepted theory argues that cells from different germ-cell layers become trapped during embryologic development.[98,155,259] In the developing embryo, multipotential cells can become trapped at the time of closure of the anterior neuropore. These cells undergo differentiation based on germ-cell origin. Their typical location is along lines of embryologic fusion.[2,98,136,155,216] Congenital rests containing cells of both ectodermal and mesodermal origin eventually form dermoid cysts. These cysts have been further subdivided into four groups based on location.[136] Group 1 is located in the periorbital region, between the developing maxillary and mandibular processes of the naso-optic groove or pit. Group 2 is located on the dorsum of the nose as a result of inclusion during ossification of the frontonasal plate. Group 3 lesions are found in the midline of the submental region near the fusion of the first and second branchial arches.[136,259] They can be located in the submental, submandibular, or thyrohyoid region of the neck. Group 4 lesions are found in the suprasternal, thyroidal, or suboccipital regions and are the rarest type of dermoid cyst. Lesions from the latter two groups are most often confused with branchial and thyroglossal anomalies.[136]

### Classification

Sublingual dermoid cysts are divided into two groups based on their relation to the mylohyoid muscle.[2,123] They usually occur during the development of the anterior tongue and are located at the junction of the tuberculum impar and the medial aspect of the horizontal processes of the first branchial arch.[240] The genioglossus group rests on the mylohyoid muscle and bulges superiorly into the mouth, displacing the tongue and spreading the genioglossus muscle. These lesions also are called *floor-of-mouth dermoids*. The sublingual ones account for 1.4% of all dermoids and approximately 23% of those occurring in the head and neck.[2,55,176] The second type of sublingual dermoid cyst can enlarge inferiorly, spreading the geniohyoid muscle and producing a submental mass.[2,240] This is referred to as the *geniohyoid* or *submental dermoid cyst*.[142,240] There is often a sinus tract or fibrous connection from the cyst to the midline of the floor of mouth, mandible, or the hyoid bone.[123,240] This tract is considered evidence in support of the theory of epithelial rests trapped within lines of fusion during development.[123]

Although it has been stated that midline dermoids always appear above the mylohyoid muscle, a review of the literature shows that they can also present below the mylohyoid muscle.[2,123,216] When they occur below the mylohyoid muscle they can present as a submental or submandibular mass.[55] The latter lesions are called *lateral dermoid cysts*. The cysts can travel around the posterior border of the mylohyoid muscle or through small openings in which arterial branches of the submandibular artery travel.[2,155,240] Submental dermoids can pass through these openings to present as submental or submandibular masses as well, displacing the submandibular gland and its duct.[2,123,155]

Some authors argue that dermoid cysts located in the lateral neck have a separate embryologic origin and arise from the ventral aspect of the first pharyngeal pouch or first branchial cleft.[2,195,240]

### Clinical presentation

Sublingual dermoids are rarely found in infants and usually are diagnosed in the second or third decade of life.[123] They often grow slowly without secondary infection and become symptomatic when increased activity of the epithelial tissues fills the lumen with keratin debris. This generally occurs during adolescence and most of these lesions present between the ages of 15 and 35 years.[259] These patients present with a mass in the floor of the mouth or submental region, interfering with mastication, articulation, or swallowing.[123]

Dermoids of the neck can account for as many as 22% of midline or near-midline neck lesions.[49,107,214,219,240] Most are reported in children under 3 years of age.[214] They usually are found within the subcutaneous tissues (Fig. 17–15).[18] The mass is soft and doughy if it contains sebaceous material.[123] The cysts are usually smooth-walled, often have attachments to the hyoid bone, and may develop fistulas as a result of repeated infection.[123,219] Dermoid cysts have been reported to occur within the thyroid gland and to mimick a cold thyroid nodule, and in association with second branchial anomalies, TGDC, and midline cervical clefts.[43,84,136,223]

### Diagnosis

Any patient suspected of having a sublingual, submental, or midline neck dermoid must have a thorough documentation of history and physical examination. A mass in the neck may be the initial and only presentation of a sublingual dermoid.[73] If filled with sebaceous material, a dermoid cyst will not transilluminate.[176] Radiographic evaluation may include a lateral neck roentgenogram to determine the extent of the cyst and detect any airway compression.[216] Plain films and sialography are helpful but nondiagnostic.[240] Xeroradiography is considered more helpful than plain radiographs in determining the extent of the lesion, but is rarely used today.[73] Computed tomography of the neck is more specific and can help differentiate dermoid cysts from lipomas if there is evidence of fat density.[240,259]

On ultrasound, dermoids demonstrate a smooth border with clear demarcation. The internal contents are echogenic with both fine and coarse homogeneity. The cyst may appear solid if filled entirely with keratin debris. Internal echo is consistent with the presence of blood or inflammatory debris. They generally do not show posterior enhancement. These characteristics help differentiate these anomalies from other solid tumors in the neck that can appear similar on ultrasound, such as lipomas.[259] Because ultrasound is readily available, inexpensive, and able to differentiate solid from cystic lesions, it is often recommended as the initial procedure of choice to evaluate sublingual, submental, or midline neck masses.[230,240]

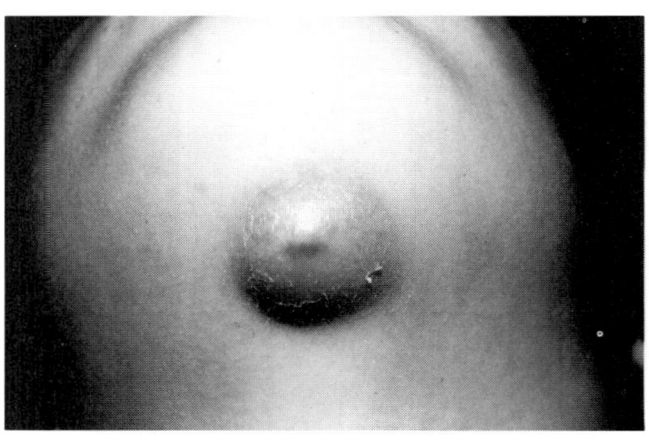

**Fig. 17–15.** Typical location of a dermoid cyst in the submental space.

Radiographic imaging in combination with fine needle aspiration to evaluate these lesions has also been recommended. Aspiration often produces a thick creamy fluid. Aspiration with injection of contrast material has been found to be less helpful.[73] Ultrasound can be used as well to localize the cyst cavity for aspiration.[240] A preoperative thyroid scan is suggested by some authors to eliminate the possibility of ectopic thyroid tissue as the substance of the mass.[73] Often the correct diagnosis can be based clinically on location, palpation, and history alone.[259]

### Histology

Epidermoid cysts are lined by stratified squamous epithelium but contain no additional skin appendages. Dermoid cysts are characterized by a fibrous wall containing skin structures and are lined by keratinizing stratified squamous epithelium, which accounts for its content of cheesy, keratinous debris. The presence of respiratory, gastrointestinal, or connective tissue derivatives within a midline neck cyst is consistent with the diagnosis of teratoma.[216,259] The essential histologic feature of the dermoid cyst, therefore, is the presence of additional skin appendages such as sebaceous and sweat glands.[49,136,259] Thyroglossal duct cysts may demonstrate inflammation with squamous metaplasia of the nonkeratinizing type, whereas dermoids generally do not.[217] There are no reported cases of malignant degeneration of dermoid cysts in the neck.[73,136]

### Treatment

The recommended treatment of dermoid cysts of the neck is surgical excision.[240] Indications for surgery are to prevent infection, obtain a diagnosis, avoid functional impairment, or remove a cosmetically unacceptable lesion.[136] Sublingual dermoids with no cervical extension can be approached through an intraoral incision.[2,240] Dissection of a large floor-of-mouth dermoid may be assisted by decompressing the cyst during the procedure. Excision of the epithelium-lined tract leading to the mandible is important to prevent recurrence.[73] Elective tracheotomy should be considered when the lesion is found deep within the tongue or floor of mouth.[123] Submental dermoids can be approached by a transverse submental skin incision. Lateral dermoids require a submandibular approach.[240] A cervical approach is also indicated when large lesions extend into the neck.[2] Removal of the submandibular gland is sometimes needed to gain access in cases of large dermoid cysts causing airway obstruction. Preoperative decompression is helpful in aiding endotracheal intubation in these situations.[240] Again, the sinus tract must be completely excised to avoid recurrence.[123]

While most authors consider simple excision as the treatment of choice for dermoids of the neck, others feel that this approach may be suboptimal.[49,217] They argue that the intraoperative differentiation of midline neck masses is important because it dictates the type of operative procedure to be utilized.[49] Dermoids have the capability of forming deep tracts with attachments to periosteum or hyoid bone.[49,136] Intraoperative aspiration or open examination of the cyst prior to excision is advocated by some to ensure accurate diagnosis and avoid the morbidity of a more extensive resection.[49] The Sistrunk procedure is recommended by others as the treatment of choice of any midline cyst with an attachment to the hyoid bone.[49,55] Recurrence is rare and is associated with incomplete removal.[240]

## Cervical teratoma

The term *teratoma* is derived from the Greek *teraton* or monster.[1] Unlike other congenital neck masses, teratomas are true tumors with neoplastic qualities.[91,250] They are divided into gonadal and extragonadal forms with the extragonadal types commonly arising in median or paramedian locations.[96,145,250] They are rare neoplasms in the head and neck.[83] Teratomas, including dermoids, occur in 1:4,000 births, but head and neck teratomas account for less than 3% of cases.[1,79] The most common sites in the head and neck region are the anterior lateral neck, followed by the face, oropharynx, nasopharynx, and orbit.[229] Cervical teratomas account for roughly half of extragonadal germ-cell tumors of the head and neck.[93] There are less than 150 cases of cervical teratoma reported in the world literature.[83] The majority of these lesions occur in the newborn or stillborn infant.[1,83] They often present with respiratory distress secondary to airway compression. Because they are rare, the diagnosis and need for immediate operative therapy may go unrecognized.[83] Unlike the overall category of teratomas, in which there is a female preponderence, there is no racial or sex predilection in case of cervical teratoma.[1,53]

### Etiology

The pathogenesis of teratomas is still unknown.[42] Theories include origin from primordial germ cells or primitive somatic cells that have escaped influence of organizers and inducers.[229] The usual distribution of teratomas points to a disturbance at the notocord and other adjacent structures which are derived by invagination of tissue at Henson's node early in embryonic development. This location in the embryo is considered one of the "primary organizers" of fetal development.[100] Embryologic experimentation has shown that removal of the primary organizer region can result in chaotic growth and differentiation without forming a defined organ.[1,100] The theory of congenital inclusion argues that teratomas form as a result of inclusion of germ-cell layers into deeper tissues secondary to failure of complete closure of fusion lines during embryogenesis.[96] These germ cells may migrate abnormally from the yolk sac to the genital ridge. It is these cells which escape the control of embryonic organizers during fetal life.[145]

An additional hypothesis states that teratomas represent an extreme form of incomplete twinning in which a small portion of cells separate at the blastula stage and form an incomplete embryo.[9,94,145] Teratomas of the neck in the form of a completely developed fetus have been described.[1,183]

### Classification

True teratomas are composed of all three germ-cell layers that are histologically identifiable. Those of the head and neck are divided into basal, cranial, and cervical forms.[1] Cervical teratomas have been classified based on the presence of and proximity to the thyroid gland because many of those reported in the literature are contained within or adjacent to the thyroid gland.[1,83,250]

### Clinical presentation

Cervical teratomas can present as early as the second trimester of fetal development and as late as adulthood.[96,250] They typically present within the first year of life and diagnosis is most common immediately following delivery unless a fetal ultrasound has been performed.[85,94,100] There is no evidence that sex, race, maternal age, or parity are associated with the development of cervical teratoma.[96] Congenital cervical teratomas present as soft, mobile masses which extend from the midline to the lateral aspect of the neck, adjacent to the thyroid gland.[183,221,239] The consistency varies from cystic to firm and the surface of the tumor mass is usually irregular.[1,250] The tumors are well defined and movable beneath the skin.[85] Often there is dilation of the veins overlying the mass.[183,250] There is usually fixation to the deep cervical fascia and occasionally to the platysma.[221] Tumors are equally distributed between each side of the neck and midline.[85] As a general rule, immature teratomas are more solid than mature teratomas and they can displace the larynx and trachea to one side.[100,229] An extension of the tumor superiorly may displace floor-of-mouth structures.[183]

Tumors presenting in the neonate and pediatric population are usually quite large, the largest ones ranging from 10 to 12 cm.[114,250] Tumors of this size can extend from the mandible to the clavicle.[250] Extension of a cervical teratoma into the mediastinum has been reported.[202] There may be compression of the vagus or recurrent laryngeal nerve.[183] Lateral displacement of the carotid artery to within 2 mm of the skin surface has been described.[93] Teratomas from other sites, such as the pharynx and sphenoid bone, can extend into the neck and present as a neck mass as well.[91,145]

Prenatal diagnosis of fetal cervical teratoma is unusual and occurs when ultrasound evaluation of maternal polyhydramnios reveals a rapidly growing fetal mass.[96,167,194] This can occur as early as the second trimester.[239] The size of the teratoma in the fetus has been correlated with the occurrence of polyhydramnios.[85] Fetuses with cervical teratoma also may have dystocia or difficult labor due to the presence of a mass. A neck mass may be the only presentation of a teratoma detected in the prenatal period. This usually occurs when a prenatal ultrasound is obtained for reasons other that polyhydramnios, such as twinning.[96]

In newborns with cervical teratoma, respiratory distress, dysphagia, and aspiration are the presenting symptoms and can be life threatening.[221] Respiratory distress can occur due to both intrauterine and postpartum tracheal compression.[83] Most infants with cervical teratomas have some degree of respiratory distress at or shortly after birth.[85,250] Newborns can also be asymptomatic at birth but, due to rapid tumor enlargement, may quickly experience respiratory embarrassment.[250] Upper airway obstruction by teratoma of the tonsil or nasopharynx is also possible.[1]

Older children will present with a neck mass requiring differentiation from other congenital neck masses.[221] Cervical teratoma can expand within the deeper layers of the neck and may not be obvious upon physical examination until a significant size is reached. These patients can develop dysphagia, aspiration, and velopharyngeal insufficiency.[91] Fibrous attachment to the pyramidal lobe of the thyroid is often confused with thyroglossal duct cyst. Mobility is most common in the horizontal planes since the tumor is attached to the hyoid bone or the thyroid gland.[221]

Stillbirth, prematurity, fetal malpresentation, and dystocia are associated with cervical teratoma.[1,250] Premature labor is thought to be due to the large bulk of the tumor.[79] Dystocia is noted in 58% of cases of cervical teratoma and is caused by intrauterine malposition such as face or brow presentation. Cervical teratomas should be considered in any case of dystocia of unknown etiology.[94] Maternal polyhydramnios is noted in approximately 18%–30% of neonates born with cervical teratomas.[1,185,239] This may be due to esophageal compression by the tumor with resultant dysphagia.[1,239] Imperforate anus, chondrodystrophy, pulmonary and cardiac hypoplasia are associated with cervical teratoma.[83,85] The simultaneous occurrence of liver and cervical teratomas has been reported.[53] To date, there are no familial cases of cervical teratoma in the literature.[85]

### Diagnosis

Ultrasound offers a noninvasive technique to evaluate any fetus suspected of having a cervical teratoma and is particularly useful in the evaluation of polyhydramnios.[167] Ultrasound can suggest the correct diagnosis by demonstrating a huge mass which approximates the size of the fetal head, contains areas of calcification, and is partially solid and partially cystic with well-defined borders.[239] These findings help to differentiate teratomas from cystic hygroma, which is multiloculated and cystic, and congenital thyroid goiter, which is a solid mass.[83] Polyhydramnios can occur when a teratoma reaches 5 cm in diameter.[85,185,232] The demonstration of the absence of a fluid-filled stomach has been used as a criterion for the diagnosis of upper gastrointestinal tract obstruction as the cause of polyhydramnios; however, this observation is unreliable since gastric secretions may partially fill an otherwise obstructed upper gastrointestinal tract.[167,232] The inability of the fetus to swallow amniotic fluid can be confirmed by contrast amniography.[167]

A thorough history and physical examination, including maternal obstetric history of polyhydramnios or dystocia, is mandatory in any newborn with respiratory distress and a large neck mass.[94,100,232,239] Elevated $\alpha$-fetoprotein levels are associated with sacrococcygeal and intracranial teratoma but have not been demonstrated with cervical teratomas.[92,232] Calcifications observed on chest radiographs or CT scans have been considered a pathognomonic radiographic finding, but this can be demonstrated in less than 50% of cases.[1,83,185,239] Half of the patients will also show compression or deviation of the trachea in addition to calcifications on chest radiographs.[83,250] Evidence of pulmonary involvement, such as atelectasis or lobar collapse, is a significant radiographic finding because it increases the urgency for surgery.[83] A barium esophagram will reveal mild displacement of the cervical esophagus by tumor.[221]

Radioisotope studies of the thyroid gland allow determination of the size of the thyroid gland and the presence or absence or ectopic thyroid tissue.[221] Fine needle aspiration biopsy of neck masses has been advocated.[1] The presence of both ectoderm and endoderm in the aspiration specimen should help in the diagnosis and prevent delay in surgical intervention.[1,83]

Cystic hygroma is often difficult to differentiate from teratoma and is the most common preoperative diagnosis in cases of histogically proven cervical teratoma.[1,83,93,185,250] These lesions are poorly defined and are soft in consistency when compared to teratomas that are well defined and freely mobile.[93] Congenital goiter can simulate cervical teratoma, both in location and on examination.[100] This type of neck mass typically demonstrates symmetrical enlargement and is rare outside of endemic areas.[250] It may cause tracheal compression, but does not contain areas of calcification.[100] Thyroid cysts can also mimic cervical teratomas, but they lack the mixture of germ-cell layers necessary for the diagnosis of teratoma.[250] Any large tumor presenting in a neonate with both solid and cystic components and located laterally in the neck suggests a teratoma.[232]

### Histology

The essential histologic feature of the cervical teratoma is the presence of three germ-cell layers not normally present in the region of the tumor.[1,53,250] The most mature differentiation of teratomas is represented by parasitic twinning.[183] Other examples of well-differentiated teratomas within the neck are well reported.[181,226]

Regardless of whether the tumor is thyroidal or extrathyroidal, the histologic features are always similar.[114] Thyroid tissue as part of the tumor or as a pseudocapsule is not uncommon.[83] On gross examination, the tumors are large and gray, semifirm, and contain neuroid-appearing tissue.[114] The cystic fluid in the tumor is usually amber with variable degrees of clarity.[183] Neuroglial elements predominate, with almost 70% of cervical teratomas containing neural tissue.[83,85] The neuroblastic tissue is typically arranged in a rosette pattern.[96] Teratomas often contain bronchial epithelium, ependymally-lined cysts, smooth muscle, liver, and cartilage and bone within the tumor mass.[96,250] These mesenchymal tissues are often at various stages of maturation.[250] According to some authors, the degree of immaturity of the tumor determines the malignant potential of the lesion.[114]

## Treatment

If the diagnosis of dystocia due to fetal teratoma is not made until after intrauterine death of the fetus, some form of destructive operation to reduce the volume of the tumor and allow vaginal delivery is recommended. If the fetus is alive, every attempt should be made for successful delivery as there can be excellent outcome with surgical therapy.[94] Elective cesarean section can be performed when lung maturity has been established. The presence of a neonatologist and a pediatric otolaryngologist to establish an airway, if there is airway obstruction, is recommended. In addition, a pediatric surgeon or neonatologist with expertise in extracorporeal membrane oxygenation (ECMO) can be a life-saving alternative if an airway cannot be established.

If acute airway obstruction occurs, decompression via aspiration with improvement of respiratory symptoms can be performed.[93,100] Laying the infant on the side of the tumor may relieve the tracheal compression.[12] Endotracheal intubation is preferred initially for securing an adequate airway.[1] This is usually possible, but emergent bronchoscopy may be necessary to maintain airway patency. Failure to improve the patient's condition with endotracheal intubation suggests pulmonary hypoplasia secondary to intrauterine tracheal obstruction.[83] Tracheal aspiration and oxygen administration in a patient with a teratoma in respiratory distress is an additional alternative.[85] Tracheotomy can often be avoided but has been necessary in cases in which the airway cannot be secured via endotracheal intubation.[83] It is a procedure of last resort because it is difficult and dangerous in a neonate with a large tumor blocking the trachea.[1,85]

If the airway is secured with an endotracheal tube, operative therapy should be offered as an urgent but not emergency procedure.[83,98] Large symptomatic tumors require early excision. These are most common in neonates.[250] It is usually performed successfully on account of the well-encapsulated and poorly vascularized nature of the tumor.[98]

### Complications

A mortality rate of 80% to 100% exists for those patients who do not undergo surgical resection in the neonatal period.[83,85,202,239] The most common cause of death is airway obstruction from tracheal compression by the large cervical mass.[185,221] Respiratory compromise is a significant component contributing to an increased mortality rate associated with delay in treatment, usually due to difficulty in diagnosis.[1,83] Respiratory distress in a infant with cervical teratoma is life threatening and prompt surgical intervention is recommended.[83,239]

Resection of cervical teratoma in the neonate is associated with a mortality rate of 9% to 17%.[83,85,202] Postoperative aspiration pneumonia contributes significantly to morbidity and mortality.[85] Delivery and surgical management may result in retention of secretions, atelectasis, pneumonia, and contribute to respiratory compromise.[93] Transient vocal cord paralysis is also a factor.[1,93] There have been no reported recurrences of cervical teratomas that were removed during the neonatal period. One case of an adult with a benign cervical teratoma is considered a recurrence of a childhood tumor by some authors.[83] Long-term follow-up in most studies of neonatal teratoma of the neck is lacking.[85,221,229] Unlike neonatal teratomas, however, recurrence is common in adults.[42,83] It can be treated with more radical therapy, but most adult patients die of local recurrence or diffuse metastatic disease.[42,114] The most important overall variable affecting long-term survival in teratomas is complete resection.

## Thymic anomalies

Thymic anomalies are among the rarest congenital masses in the neck.[130,189,247] These lesions are unusual because they often are asymptomatic and go unrecognized. Most are discovered incidentally.[219] The incidence of ectopic cervical thymic tissue in the general population has been reported as high as 21%.[74,247] The prevalence of cervical thymic anomalies in childhood may be related to the continued development of the thymus during this period.[104]

Several varieties of thymic tissue can be located in the neck.[82,189] Aberrant thymic rests are found commonly during autopsies in about 20% of patients and are usually of little clinical importance.[130,189,219,242] A second category is an undescended cervical thymus, which occurs when a solid lobe of thymus fails to descend with or without the parathyroid complex. It is different from the accessory cervical thymus in that only half of the normally bilobed thymus is present in the mediastinum, whereas in the accessory cervical thymus only a small portion is sequestered in the neck.[262] On occasion, the entire thymus can be located ectopically in the neck.[189,247] Thymoma is another category of thymic tissue found in the neck.[189,247] It has been found both at autopsy and at operation for a cervical mass.[104] Cervical extension of mediastinal thymus occurs when there is a low midline mass consisting of thymic tissue at the thoracic inlet due to incomplete mediastinal descent.[262]

Cervical thymic cysts are the most important variety of cervical thymic anomalies because of their clinical presentation.[104,189,247,262] Although it is the least common lateral cystic neck mass, it must be differentiated from other pediatric cystic neck masses, the majority of which are anomalies of the branchial system.[124,130] Cervical thymic cysts are probably more frequent than the number of cases reported.[66]

### Embryology and etiology

The thymus develops from sacculations from the ventral aspect of the third pharyngeal pouch during the sixth week of embryonic life.[37,130] By the sixth week, the third pharyngeal pouch has subdivided into a dorsal and ventral wing.[177] The dorsal wing corresponds to the inferior parathyroid glands and the ventral wing eventually becomes the thymus.[124,177,219] There are minor contributions from the fourth pharyngeal pouch to the primordial thymus.[121,219] The sacculations rapidly elongate caudally and medially into a tubular structure known as the *thymopharyngeal tract* which eventually becomes obliterated.[130,219]

Endodermal cells begin to proliferate by the middle of week 7 to become paired solid masses. By the end of the seventh week, the primordial thymus has undergone considerable elongation and usually remains associated with the parathyroid glands derived from the third pharyngeal pouch. The distal tips of the thymus begin to approach the midline. During week 8, the primordial thymus descends to the level of the aortic arch.[247] The proximal portion of the elongated thymic stalk usually atrophies and disappears. The descending thymic lobes do not unite until the beginning of the ninth week when they descend in front of the large vessels of the thorax. The thymus then fuses in the midline to descend posterior to the sternum into the superior mediastinum.[5,219,247] Here, the thymus is in contact with the pericardium, great vessels, and thoracic inlet.[5,219] It takes about 3 weeks for the entire process of thymic descent to occur.

Unlike a second branchial tract, which would pass from the pharyngeal tonsillar fossae between the internal and external carotids, the third pharyngeal pouch tract passes from the pyriform sinus through the thyrohyoid membrane between the common carotid artery and vagus, posterior and inferior to the glossopharyngeal nerve, and then lateral to the thyroid. The fourth pharyngeal pouch, which gives rise to parathyroid tissue, may contribute a small amount of thymic tissue that is thought to be incorporated in the main part of the gland. Occasionally, it can remain associated with the parathyroid gland, which may explain why thymic tissue can be found with parathyroid explorations. A fourth pharyngeal pouch tract would extend from the apex of the pyriform sinus inferior to the superior laryngeal nerve, external to the recurrent laryngeal nerve, and then pass inferiorly along the trachea and eventually between the arch of the aorta and subclavian artery.[262]

During the tenth week, the thymic anlage, which consists of cords of primitive pharyngeal endodermal epithelial cells, is invaded by mesenchymal cells from adjacent tissue. The mesenchymal tissue forms the reticular network and lymphoid follicles of the thymus, which eventually degenerate into Hassell's corpuscles. Squamous epithelium from the second cervical cleft or sinus can also invade the thymic anlage and form Hassell's corpuscles.[61] Therefore, Hassell's corpuscles can be of ectodermal or endodermal origin.[222]

By the third embryonic month, the migration has been completed and the bilobed thymus gland has developed.[130] The thymus has undergone differentiation and contains both a cortex and medulla.[254] Hassell's corpuscles are also evident by the third month. The thymus increases in size to approximately 30–40 gm at puberty. Its largest relative size is at age 4 where it is 12–15 gm. It achieves its greatest absolute size at puberty.[16] Following puberty, the lymphoid component disappears and is replaced by fat or connective tissue, but Hassell's corpuscles remain.[254]

The pathogenesis of solid cervical thymic tissue is divided into three possible mechanisms. The first possibility is a failure of the unilateral gland to descend.[262] This would present as a solid mass of thymic tissue within the neck. In an undescended thymus, only half of the normal amount of tissue is present in the mediastinum. The presence of an undescended parathyroid gland, which normally moves with the thymus, is also indicative of an undescended thymic parathyroid complex. This has been demonstrated by several authors.[219] A second explanation of solid thymic tissue in the neck is a sequestered focus of thymic tissue along its normal path of descent.[219,262] In this situation, a normal amount of tissue is present in the mediastinum.[219] The final possibility is a failure of the rostral fragments of the thymus to involute after the majority of the gland has descended into the mediastinum.

The pathogenesis of cystic cervical thymic tissue remains controversial.[262] Embryonal remnants of branchial anomalies or the thymopharyngeal duct is one possible explanation.[66,130,218,247] A persistent thymopharyngeal duct containing solid thymic tissue can have a cystic variant.[262] Sequestrated tissue produced during the involution of the thymus can undergo cystic degeneration, or a neoplastic process in the lymphocytoreticular or connective tissues of the neck may explain their existence.[66,218,219,247] They also could arise from lymphatic or connective tissue that has arrested in various stages of thymic development.[66,218,247]

Other authors feel that thymic cysts are acquired and not developmental. Acquired cysts can be inflammatory, traumatic, or neoplastic.[5,247] Cysts derived from the degeneration of Hassell's corpuscles are one type of acquired thymic cyst. This theory is based on histologic evidence of progressive cystic change within Hassell's corpuscles.[5,66,218,247] Inflammatory thymic cysts are associated with congenital syphilis and tuberculosis, or can be idiopathic.[12,198] Traumatic thymic cysts have been reported secondary to blunt trauma or prior thoracotomy and are found primarily in the mediastinum. Neoplastic thymic cysts are caused by cystic degeneration within a thymoma or lymphoma.[198] A thymic cyst of neoplastic origin is probably classified better as a thymoma with cystic degeneration.[35] Currently, the most popular theories are cystic degeneration of Hassell's corpuscles or cystic change within remnants of the thymopharyngeal duct.[196,219,228]

### Clinical presentation

Cervical thymic anomalies are usually not found at birth but appear later in life.[5] Two-thirds of these lesions occur in the first decade of life.[104,177,222] Almost 75% of patients with histologically proven cervical thymic cysts are less than 20 years of age at presentation.[104] Overall, the age at presentation ranges from 8 days to 74 years.[121,254] Males are affected twice as often as females.[82,222,247]

The most common complaint by an affected patient is the

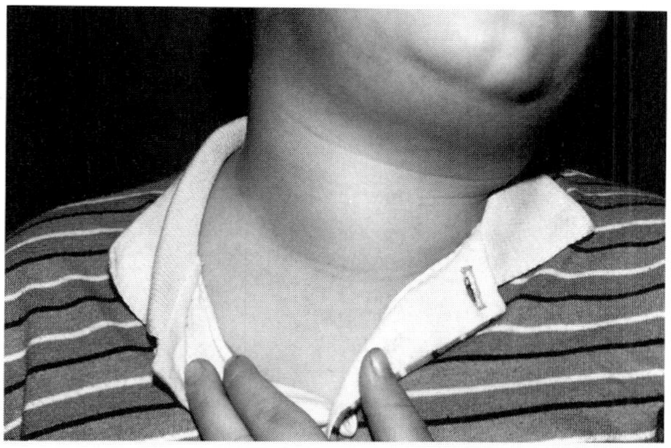

**Fig. 17–16.** Physical appearance of a thymic cyst which usually presents as a soft compressible suprasternal mass.

presence of the mass.[121,177] Almost 90% of patients have asymptomatic, painless swelling (Fig. 17–16).[5,130,247] Approximately 3% will note a post-traumatic mass.[3,130] The appearance of the mass may be sudden, due to infection, hemorrhage, venous engorgement, or cystic degeneration, or may be slowly progressive.[121,142,222,262] Fluctuation in size is common.[247] Upper respiratory infection (URI) often can be a prelude to the discovery of the mass.[247] Most patients present to the physician within 6 to 9 months of noticing the mass.[104,247] The size of the mass ranges from a small, unilocular swelling to large, multiloculated lesions.[177] They can vary from 1 to 17 cm in length and are consistently mobile.[196,247]

Thymic anomalies can result in compression and displacement of neighboring structures.[219] About 6%–10% of patients complain of dysphagia, dyspnea, cervical pain, or hoarseness.[23,177,247] Respiratory compromise may also occur.[247] Tracheal obstruction due to thymic masses within the trachea has been reported.[125] Neonates may suffer respiratory arrest due to a large, congenitally aberrant cervical thymus.[139,219]

Cervical thymic anomalies can be located anywhere from the mandibular angle to the superior mediastinum.[130,157,196] Thymic cysts are more common than solid lesions.[157,219,238] The majority of cysts are found in the lower third of the neck anterior to and extending beneath the sternocleidomastoid muscle.[130,177] Other locations of thymic anomalies include the thyroid gland, trachea, posterior pharynx, and pyriform sinus.[247,262]

Half of all cervical thymic cysts extend into the mediastinum.[124,247] This connection may consist of a solid cord remnant of thymic tissue or may be continuous with the cervical cyst.[222,247,262] The valsalva maneuver may produce a transient increase in size.[222] This may represent vascular engorgement or transmission of increased intrathoracic pressure.[222,262] Cervicomediastinal thymic cysts can present with vocal cord paralysis due to traction on the recurrent laryngeal nerve.[12] Pericardial tamponade secondary to a cervicomediastinal thymic cyst has also been reported.[4]

Cervical thymic cysts may have inclusions of other endocrine tissue. Most commonly, ectopic thyroid and parathyroid tissue are found.[104] Cervical thymic cysts may also be associated with myasthenia gravis.[200] While 15% of patients with myasthenia gravis have thymic neoplasms, this condition has been reported in association with only one case of cervical thymoma.[66,254] Other diseases associated with cervical thymic cysts include Hodgkin disease, thyrotoxicosis, aplastic anemia, neurofibromatosis, and Down syndrome. Unilateral cleft lip and alveolar cleft may be present in association with bilateral thymus in the skin of the neck.[37,104,189] These cases most likely represent coincidental findings.[189]

### Diagnosis

Initial evaluation includes a complete history and physical examination. The thymus is visible on chest radiographs until 2 years of age, after which it becomes increasingly difficult to identify.[37] A mediastinal shadow can be noted on a routine chest radiograph when there is extension into the chest.[124,200,222] Persistence of thymopharyngeal duct cysts, extending through the thyrohyoid membrane into the pyriform sinus, can be demonstrated on a barium esophagram or by water-soluble dye injected into the mass preoperatively. The ability to trace the duct back to the pharynx is helpful in determining the extent of surgical repair and its embryologic origin.[262] Fluoroscopy can help to differentiate laryngoceles from thymic anomalies.[222]

Computed tomography provides excellent visualization of the anomaly and helps to direct the surgical approach. Thymic cysts appear as large homogeneous water-density masses (Fig. 17–17). Computed tomography can demonstrate thymic origin by showing the mass contained within the carotid sheath and its connection to the thymus within the mediastinum.[124] It can also delineate mediastinal extension.[247] MRI may offer enhanced soft tissue contrast. Ultrasound examination of a neck mass can show both a homogeneous and nonhomogeneous solid mass, or even a cystic mass.[200,219] Some authors recommend ultrasound as an initial screening test and reserve computed tomography for those cases in which ultrasound is inconclusive or if further information is needed.[247]

Thyroid scans may be helpful in differentiating cervical thymic anomalies from thyroid masses.[222,254] Gallium and technetium are not stored selectively in the thymus.[254] However, in adults, thymic cysts may produce areas of decreased uptake on a thyroid scan and be confused with thyroid malignancy.[12,68] Fine needle aspiration is not a useful aid in diagnosis at this time.[130]

#### Histology

These lesions can be unilocular or multilocular.[247] Most are multilocular and contain clear or straw-colored fluid.[130,196] They can also contain semisolid material with necrotic debris and old blood.[196] Cholesterol can be found within the fluid and the walls of the cyst.[5,130,196] Hemosiderin deposition within some cysts suggests previous hemorrhage.[57,196] The epithelial lining may be ciliated or nonciliated, stratified or pseudostratified, cuboidal or columnar, and usually contains Hassell's corpuscles.[104,130,196,247] Ulceration of the epithelial wall is common.[130] The cysts can be lined by fibrous tissue due to the destruction of the epithelial lining from either infection or pressure necrosis.[5] Proliferation of the lining epithelium with pseudoepitheliomatous changes may be confused with malignancy.[224] The wall of the cyst can vary in thickness from a few mm to as much as 1 cm. Both the external capsule and internal septae of the cyst are composed of highly cellular and vascularized fibrous tissues.[104] Lymphocytes are present as aggregates and in a diffuse, scattered pattern.[104,196] The lymphoid

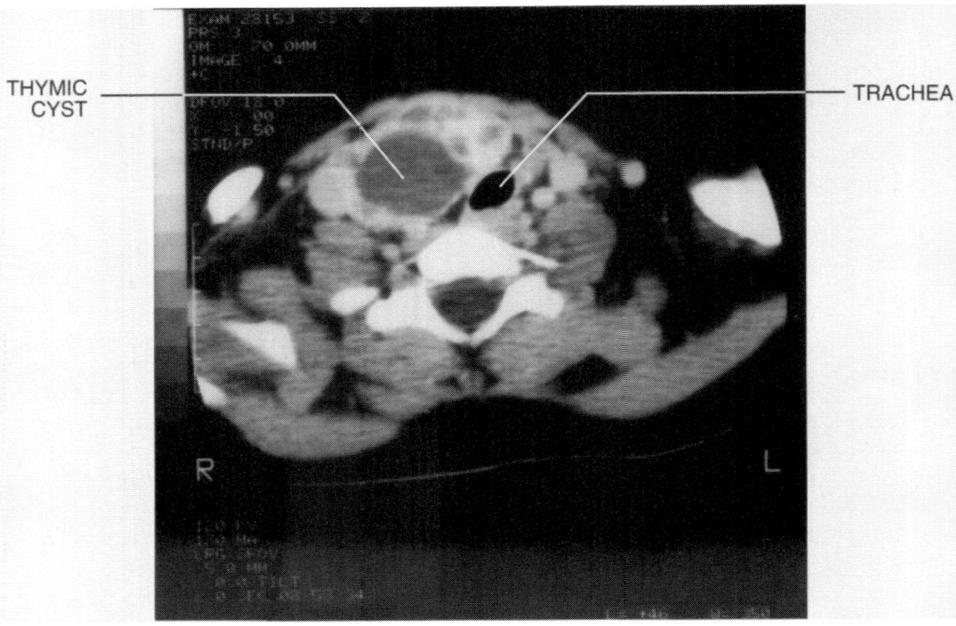


**Fig. 17–17.** Radiographic appearance of a thymic cyst as a large, homogeneous water-density mass with superior mediastinal extension and tracheal compression.

tissue within the wall of the thymic cyst has been demonstrated to be of thymic origin.[130] Parathyroid tissue may be found in the wall of some thymic cysts.[130,219,222]

Cervical thymic cysts are differentiated histologically from other cystic masses in the neck. A branchial anomaly is usually devoid of thymic tissue remnants within the cyst wall. Lymphoid tissue associated with branchial cysts demonstrates germinal centers which are not features of thymic cysts.[130] Thymic elements in contact with the cyst wall and giant cell reaction are distinguishing features of thymic cysts.[104,247] Thymic parenchyma within the cyst is a pathognomonic finding.[196] Frequently a thymic cyst is atrophic and may not reveal its true nature unless serial sections are made. For this reason, many cases of thymic cysts have been misdiagnosed as branchial cysts because of inadequate sampling of the resected tissue.[189]

The lateral cystic neck mass can encompass a wide variety of histological diagnoses.[196] Cervical cysts may contain salivary, gastric, and gastrointestinal tissue.[101,196] Thymic anomalies are often misdiagnosed as lymphadenitis, branchial cysts, thyroglossal duct cysts, cystic hygromas, thyroid adenomas, or parathyroid, dermoid, or epidermoid cysts.[66,196] In fact, there are very few cases of preoperative diagnosis of cervical thymic anomalies.[5] The two most frequent preoperative diagnoses are branchial cysts and cystic hygromas.[222] Branchial cysts present in a similar anatomic location. Thymic cysts are most common in the first decade of life, while branchial cysts are more common in the third decade.[130] Branchial and thyroglossal cysts normally do not enlarge with a valsalva maneuver, rarely extend to the clavicle, and more often present with signs and symptoms of recurrent infection or inflammation. Cystic hygromas tend to be more lateral and transilluminate brilliantly.[87] Cholesterol crystals within the cystic fluid and granulomas with lymphoid aggregates in the wall of the cervical cyst occur with many varieties of cervical cysts and do not aid in diagnosis.[3]

Malignant tumor can be confused with the thymic cervical cyst as well.[196] Thymomas located adjacent to and displacing the thyroid gland can mimic thyroid carcinoma.[219] Metastatic papillary thyroid cancer can present as a lateral cervical cyst.[196] Solid thymic tissue can be confused with metastatic squamous cell carcinoma if frozen section examination of thymic tissue obtained during parathyroid exploration is performed.[104]

### Treatment

Few thymic anomalies can be diagnosed correctly prior to surgical excision.[222,247] Once diagnosed intraoperatively, complete surgical excision is considered the treatment of choice.[121,130,219,247] Partial excision to relieve symptoms is recommended in a neonate, unless it is documented that mediastinal thymic tissue exists.[121,219,262] Removal of a normal thymic remnant is not advised.[222] Normal thymic tissue located within the skin of the neck should not be resected but excised from the skin and placed beneath the skin with an intact vascular pedicle.[37] Frozen section of the mass can aid in diagnosis and prevent removal of normal thymic tissue.[222]

Excision is accomplished through a transcervical approach. Parallel stepladder incisions will provide a cosmetically acceptable approach to large lesions.[222,254] Thymic cysts may adhere to the vagus nerve, carotid artery, jugular vein, phrenic nerve, or recurrent laryngeal nerve.[222,247] Cysts are commonly located within the carotid sheath.[222] Thymic cysts can arise from the thyroid gland.[67] In addition, fibrous tissue attachment to the base of skull behind the styloid process is also possible. The possibility of mediastinal extension must be entertained prior to surgical resection.[247] This may consist only of a solid fibrous cord extending into the mediastinum.[104,124] Cervical lesions with mediastinal extension can be removed through a supraclavicular approach with preparation for sternotomy, if necessary.[12,222] Other authors recommend a median sternotomy approach to the cervicomediastinal thymic cyst. This incision can be extended into the neck for greater exposure.[200]

### Complications

Tracheal compression noted preoperatively is important in guiding early postoperative respiratory care. Postoperative respiratory compromise is a common complication following excision of cervical thymic anomalies. Tracheotomy is rarely necessary. Prolonged intubation can be used to allow postoperative respiratory distress to resolve. It has been suggested that the tenseness of the cyst in combination with tracheal compression may result in a form of tracheomalacia that can resolve over time. Patients with respiratory compromise in the immediate perioperative period have no long-term sequelae.

There is a 2% incidence of recurrence of thymic cysts in adults. With complete excision, no recurrences in children have been reported. It is not known whether a second cyst can occur once a child has reached adulthood.[247] There are no reports of malignant degeneration in children or the development of myasthenia gravis or immunologic deficiencies following excision of a cervical thymic cyst.[121,247,254]

## Midline cervical cleft

The midline cervical cleft of the neck is an unusual congenital anomaly and can be considered within the larger group of craniofacial clefts which includes oblique clefts as well as transverse facial clefts.[67,223] The midline cervical cleft is not considered a true cleft because there is no gap between adjacent skin areas.[63] Congenital webbing of the neck was described by Kobrinski in 1893. An entity known as pterygium colli was described by Funke in 1902. Both pterygium colli and midline cervical cleft appear to be similar defects.[258]

The midline cervical cleft has been associated with a wide range of fusion defects, ranging from underdevelopment to absence of associated neck structures.[241] The usual lesion consists of a vertical midline defect of the skin and deeper neck tissues but sparing the chin.[67] It may extend from the lower lip to the manubrium and involve deeper structures as well. In addition, cysts and fistulae are also associated with this congenital anomaly. These other anomalies include thyroglossal duct cysts, dermoid cysts, and branchial anomalies.[67,223] The combination of midline cervical cleft and thyroglossal duct cyst has been described in several case reports.[6]

### Etiology

Multiple theories have been proposed to explain the presence of the midline cervical cleft. Some authors believe that alterations in the normal fusion of second and third branchial arches result in clefts of the lower neck structures, including the mandible, hyoid, manubrium, and superior aspect of the sternum.[223] It is possible that in uncomplicated cases of midline cervical cleft, mesodermal arches fuse normally in the midline but overlying ectoderm does not.[63,258] In more severe cases, the hyoid bone, thyroid cartilage, and other mesenchymal structures are absent from the defect area. While there are no branchial contributions to the sternum, the abnormalities in the surrounding region probably contribute to abnormalities in this area in severe cases.[149]

Although it is unusual for this anomaly to be associated with clefts of the lower lip and mandible, some authors have suggested that lack of closure of first arch structures leads to subsequent maldevelopment of second and third arch structures.[71,78,149] The term *anterior gnathoschisis* has been used to refer to midline defects of the lower lip and mandible.[149] Failure of the first arch to unite in the midline results in a spectrum of lower lip and mandibular clefts. Anomalies of the anterior two-thirds of the tongue can be included in this first arch category.[223] The mandibular processes fuse at approximately the fifth week of development while the anterior tongue and sternum fuse in the midline in the seventh and ninth weeks, respectively.[149] Both mechanical factors and vascular abnormalities have been proposed as causes of these fusion defects.[241]

Exteriorization of a thyroglossal remnant with exposure of the underlying mucosa is another hypothesis.[80] This theory fails to explain milder cases in which the hyoid bone is not involved and more severe cases involving more structures than that which is seen classically in a thyroglossal duct cyst.[63,78] An additional theory suggests that adherence between the pericardial roof and the pharynx during the fifth week of gestation causes abnormal fusion of the branchial arches. At approximately the fifth week, the embryo is 5 mm in length. At this stage, the cephalic end of the embryo is sharply flexed in the branchial region with the ventral surface of the pharynx immediately adjacent to the superior aspect of the primordial cardiac region.[149] Adherence between these two regions could explain a failure of normal development in the neck.[78,149]

### Clinical presentation

This anomaly usually is noted at birth.[6] In general, adequate tissue is present but there is a failure of midline fusion.[149] There has been no sex predilection noted in multiple reviews of this anomaly, although some authors report its occurrence almost exclusively in Caucasian females.[6,63] The midline cervical cleft usually extends from the inferior aspect of the mentum to the suprasternal notch. The area is often noted to be weeping serous fluid in the neonate with gradual resolution of the drainage over the next several months.[241] The cleft is reddened with atrophic and desquamated epithelium.[78] The superior aspect of the cleft has a nipple-like appearance (Fig. 17–18).[67,241] The

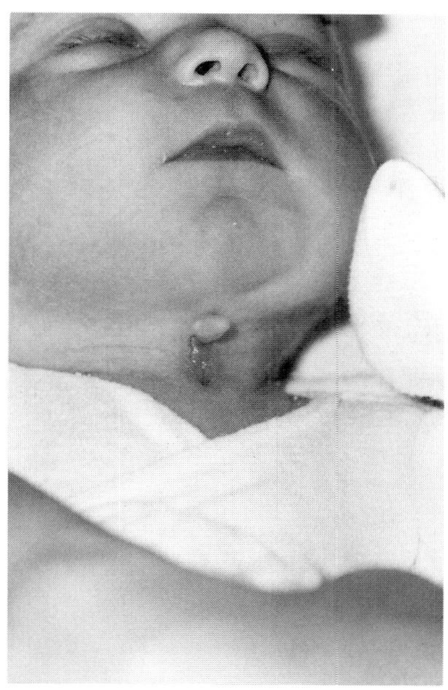

**Fig. 17–18.** Appearance of a midline cervical cleft with nipple-like protrusion at the superior aspect of the cleft.

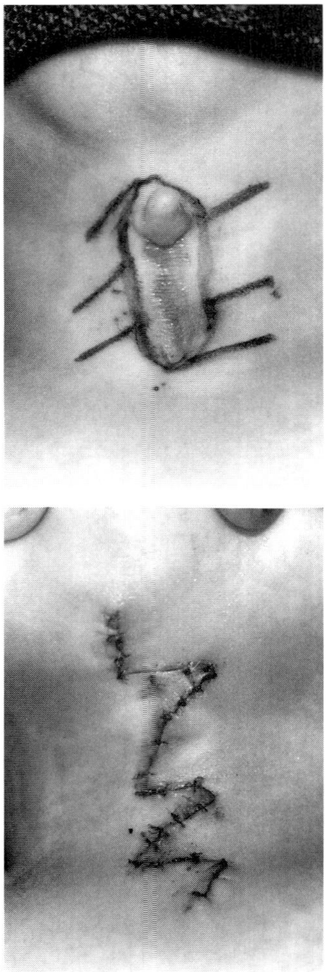

A

B

**Fig. 17–19.** Proposed surgical excision of a midline cervical cleft (A) and Z-plasty closure (B).

inferior aspect of the cleft may intermittently drain due to the presence of heterotopic salivary tissue.[241] Severe clefts may extend from the lower lip and through the midline of the mandible and often the anterior portion of the tongue is adherent to the defect of the mandibular symphysis.[223]

The area of the defect eventually heals as a widened scar and is often accompanied by a cord of subcutaneous tissue which forms a web.[63,67] The web can cause scar contracture of the neck, limiting range of motion.[241] In minor cases, these lesions can present in young children or young adults as a fibrous subcutaneous cord and it is noticed only when the neck is fully extended.[80,133] In such cases, the patient tends to become symptomatic as the fibrous band begins to limit movement of the neck. A bony spur in the submental portion of the mandible is radiologically evident in many patients.[78] This entity represents hypertrophic bone growth, secondary to traction on the fibrous cord.[241] The bony outgrowth is not present with minor lesions limited to the infrahyoid region.[78]

## Diagnosis

The relationship of any associated fistula to the cleft is important in differentiating midline cervical fistula of cleft origin from thyroglossal duct origin. The fistula from a midline cervical cleft, in general, is located caudally, while that due to thyroglossal duct anomalies is located cranially.[241] Bronchogenic cysts are usually located in the suprasternal notch area. They, too, have a fistulous opening that can drain mucoid material intermittently. This type of cyst has been found to extend into the superior mediastinum where it is continuous with the aortic arch.[146]

### Histology

Histologically, the excised subcutaneous cord is similar in appearance to specimens of fibromatosis colli.[243] Examination of the cleft shows a covering of stratified squamous epithelium with a mild disorganization of the deeper layers. Fibrosis is found primarily in the subcutaneous layers. Skin appendages are usually absent within the dermis layer of the cleft.[67,78] An absence of mesenchyme within the midline may explain their absence.[243]

A significant percentage of patients who present with a midline cervical cleft will have an associated cyst or sinus. A branchial cyst in association with a midline cervical cleft is considered when the cyst cavity contains skin epithelium and muscle bundles but lacks cartilage. The diagnosis of bronchogenic cyst is made when the cyst lacks muscular layers but contains cartilage.[67]

## Treatment

Treatment entails complete removal of the cleft and cord. Simple excision or transection of the fibrous band will lead to a recurrence of the contracted area.[63,78] The ribbed scar tissue resulting from healing of the cleft often can be removed by complete surgical excision followed by Z-plasty closure techniques (Fig. 17–19A, B).[63,67] The time of repair is based on the severity of the defect. Earlier repair is recommended for larger defects. Most authors suggest that only soft tissue be repaired in infants.[223] Repair of less severe cases of this anomaly can be deferred until the patient is 2 to 4 years of age.[78] Postoperative complications include recurrent scarring, which may be cosmetically unacceptable.[241]

## References

1. Abemayor E, Newman A, Bergstrom L, Dudley J, Magidson JG, Ljung BM: Teratomas of the head and neck in childhood. Laryngoscope 94:1489–1492, 1984.
2. Al-Chaayat M, Kenyon GS: Midline sublingual dermoid cyst. J Laryngol Otol 104:578–580, 1990.
3. Allard R: The thyroglossal cyst. Head Neck Surg 5:134–146, 1982.
4. Allee G, Logue B, Mansour K: Thymic cyst simulating multiple cardiovascular abnormalities and presenting with pericarditis and pericardial tamponade. Am J Cardiol 31:377–380, 1973.
5. Al-Shihabi BM, Jackson JM: Cervical thymic cyst. J Laryngol Otol 96:181–189, 1982.
6. Anderson BL, Svendsen EP: Midline cervical clefts. Scand J Plast Reconstr Surg 12:169–170, 1978.
7. Armstrong D, Pickerell K, Fetter B, Pitts W: Torticollis: an analysis of 271 cases. Plast Reconstr Surg 35:14–25, 1965.
8. Ashinoff R, Geronemus RG: Flashlamp-pumped pulsed dye laser for port-wine stains in infancy: earlier versus later treatment. J Am Acad Dermatol 24:467–472, 1991.
9. Ashley DJB: Origin of teratomas. Cancer 32:390–394, 1973.
10. Athow AC, Fagg M, Drake DP: Management of thyroglossal cyst in children. Br J Surg 76:811–814, 1989.
11. Bailey H: Thyroglossal cysts and fistulae. Br J Surg 12:579–589, 1925.

12. Bailey RL, Hilde RL, Smith TR, Thompson RJ: Cervicomediastinal thymic cyst with vocal cord paralysis. Cancer 39:347–349,1977.
13. Balkany TJ, Mishke RE: Mastoid release for congenital torticollis. Laryngoscope 90:337–338, 1980.
14. Bardach J, Panje W: Surgical management of the large cavernous hemangioma. Otolaryngol Head Neck Surg 89:792–796, 1981.
15. Barrand KG, Freeman NC: Massive infiltrating cystic hygroma of the neck in infancy. Arch Dis Child 48:523–531, 1973.
16. Barrick B, O'Kell RT: Thymic cysts and remnant cervical thymus. J Pediatr Surg 4:355–357, 1969.
17. Bartlett JA, Riding KH, Salkeld LJ: Management of hemangiomas of the head and neck in children. J Otolaryngol 17:111–120, 1988.
18. Batsakis JG: Nomenclature of developmental tumors. Ann Otol Rhinol Laryngol 93:98–99, 1984.
19. Beecham JE, Behrens HW: Intramuscular hemangioma of the head and neck: report of a case involving the prevertebral muscles. Head Neck Surg 10:402–405, 1988.
20. Beham A, Fletcher CDM: Intramuscular angioma: a clinicopathological analysis of 74 cases. Histopathology 18:53–59, 1991.
21. Bhaskar SN, Bernier JL: Histogenesis of branchial cysts: a report of 468 cases. Am J Pathol 35:407–423, 1959.
22. Bingham HG: Predicting the course of a congenital hemangioma. Plast Reconstr Surg 63:161–166, 1979.
23. Bistritzer T, Tamir A, Oland J, Varsano D,Manor A, Gall R, Aladjam, M: Severe dyspnea and dysphagia resulting from an aberrant cervical thymus. Eur J Pediat 144:86–87, 1985.
24. Bourjat P, Cartier J, Woerther JP: Thyroglossal duct cyst in hyoid bone: CT confirmation. J Comput Assist Tomogr 12:871–873, 1988.
25. Boxt L, Levin DC, Fellows KE: Direct puncture angiography in congenital venous malformations. AJR 140:135–136, 1983.
26. Boyd JB, Mulliken JB, Kaban LB, Upton J, Murray JE: Skeletal changes associated with vascular malformations. Plast Reconstr Surg 74:789–795, 1984.
27. Bradley PJ, Narula A, Maorgan DALM, Harvey L, MacLennan KA: Haemangiopericytoma of the larynx. J Laryngol Otol 103:234–238, 1989.
28. Brendenkamp JK, Hoover LA, Berke GS, Shaw A: Congenital muscular torticollis. Arch Otolaryngol Head Neck Surg 116:212–216, 1990.
29. Brock ME, Smith RJH, Parey S, Mobley DL: Lymphangioma. An otolaryngologic perspective. Int J Pediatr Otorhinolaryngol 14:133–140, 1987.
30. Brooks JE: Cystic hygroma of the head and neck. Laryngoscope 83:117–128, 1973.
31. Burrows PE, Lasjaunias PL, Ter Brugge KG, Flodmark O: Urgent and emergent embolization of lesions of the head and neck in children: indications and results. Pediatrics 80:386–394, 1987.
32. Byard RW, Bourne AJ, Silver MM: The association of lingual thyroglossal duct remnants with sudden death in infancy. Int J Pediatr Otorhinolaryngol 20:107–112, 1990.
33. Byrd SE, Richardson M, Gill G, Lee AM: Computer-tomographic appearance of branchial cleft and thyroglossal duct cysts of the neck. Diagn Imaging 52:301–312, 1983.
34. Canale ST, Griffin DW, Hubbard CN: Congenital muscular torticollis: a long term follow-up. J Bone Joint Surg 64:810–816, 1982.
35. Ceuppens H: Thymic cyst in an unusual site. Neth J Surg 36:17–18, 1984.
36. Chandrasoma P, Janssen M: A thyroglossal cyst lined by gastric epithelium [letter]. JAMA 247:1406, 1982.
37. Civi I, Kurtay M, Civi S: Bilateral thymus found in association with bilateral cleft lip and palate. Plast Reconstr Surg 83:143–147, 1989.
38. Clarren SK, Smith DW, Hanson JW: Helmet treatment for plagiocephaly and congenital muscular torticollis. J Pediatr 94:43–46, 1979.
39. Cohen SR, Thompson JW: Lymphangiomas of the larynx in infants and children: a survey of pediatric lymphangioma. Ann Otol Rhinol Laryngol 127:1–20, 1986.
40. Cohen SR, Wang CI: Steroid treatment of hemangioma of the head and neck in children. Ann Otol Rhinol Laryngol 81:584–590, 1972.
41. Coleman WR, Homer RS, Kaplan RP: Branchial cleft heterotopia of the lower neck. J Cutan Pathol 16:353–358, 1989.
42. Colton JJ, Batsakis JG, Work WP: Teratomas of the neck in adults. Arch Otolaryngol 104:271–273, 1978.
43. Comas AP: Dermoid cyst mimicking cold thyroid nodule [letter]. Lancet 2:421, 1979.
44. Conway H, McKinney P, Climo M: Permanent camouflage of vascular nevi of the face by intradermal injection of insoluable pigments (tattooing): experience through twenty years with 1022 cases. Plast Reconstr Surg 40:457–462, 1967.
45. Cosman B: Role of retreatment in minimal-power argon laser therapy for port-wine stains. Laser Surg Med 2:43–57, 1982.
46. Cox EF: Excision of branchial sinus and fistula tracts using arterial intimal strippers. Surg Gynecol Obstet 117:676–768, 1963.
47. Cullen MT, Gabrielli S, Green JJ, Rizzo N, Mahoney MJ, Salafia C, Bovicelli L, Hobbins JC: Diagnosis and significance of cystic hygroma in the first trimester. Prenat Diagn 10:643–651, 1990.
48. Cumberworth VL, Bradley PJ: Atypical thyroglossal duct cyst. J Laryngol Otol 103:700–703, 1989.
49. deMello DE, Lima JA, Liapis H: Midline cervical cyst in children. Arch Otolaryngol Head Neck Surg 113:418–420, 1987.
50. de Orbe Rueda A, Arellano CP, de Rojas FD, Mateo AA: Ultrasound diagnosis of mediastinal cystic hygroma. J Clin Ultrasound 12:180–182, 1984.
51. Dickerhoff R, Bode U: Cyclophosphamide in nonresectable cystic hygroma. Lancet 335:1474–1475, 1990.
52. Dilkes MG, Chapman J, Stafford ND: Per-oral excision of a branchial cyst. J Laryngol Otol 104:143–144, 1990.
53. Dische MR, Gardner HA: Mixed teratoid tumors of the liver and neck in trisomy 13. Am J Clin Pathol 69:631–637, 1978.
54. Donegan WL, Ridenhour CE: Treatment of cavernous hemangioma of the tongue by continuous intra-arterial infusion of 5 fluoro-uracil. Am J Surg 114:948–952, 1967.
55. Drucker C, Gerson CR: Sublingual contiguous thyroglossal and dermoid cysts in a neonate. Int J Pediatr Otorhinolaryngol 23:181–186, 1992.
56. Drumm AJ, Chow JM: Congenital neck masses. Am Fam Physician 39:159–163, 1989.
56a. Elahi MM, Dubé P, Manoukian JJ, Tewfik TL, Schloss MD: Partial thyroidectomy and selective neck dissection in the management of pyriform sinus fistulal. J Otolaryngol (in press).
57. Ellis HA: Cervical thymic cysts. Br J Surg 54:17–20, 1967.
58. Emery PJ, Bailey CM, Evans JNG: Cystic hygroma of the head and neck: a review of 37 cases. J Laryngol Otol 98:613–619, 1984.
59. Enjolras O, Riche MC, Merland JJ, Escande JP: Management of alarming hemangiomas in infancy: a review of 25 cases. Pediatrics 85:491–498, 1990.
60. Feldman JI, Kearns DB, Pransky SM, Seid AS: Catheterization of branchial sinus tracts: a new method. Int J Pediatr Otolaryngol 20:1–5, 1990.
61. Fielding JF, Farmer AW, Lindsay WK, Conen PE: Cystic degeneration in persistent cervical thymus: a report of four cases in children. Can J Surg 6:178–186, 1963.
62. Figi FA: Radium in the treatment of multilocular lymph cyst of the neck in children. AJR 21:473–480, 1929.
63. Fincher SG, Fincher GG: Congenital midline cervical cleft with subcutaneous fibrous cord. Otolaryngol Head Neck Surg 101:399–401, 1989.
64. Finn DG, Buchalter IH, Sarti E, Romo T, Chodosh P: First branchial cleft cysts: clinical update. Laryngoscope 97:136–140, 1987.
65. Fradis M, Podoshin L, Simon J, Lazarov N, Shagrawi I, Boss JH: Combined treatment of large head and neck capillaro-venous malformation by a fibrosing agent. J Laryngol Otol 103:390–398, 1989.
66. Freifeld S, Petti G Jr: Cervical thymic cyst. NY State J Med 75:2553–2554, 1975.
67. French WE, Bale GF: Midline cervical cleft of the neck with associated branchial cyst. Am J Surg 125:376–381, 1973.
68. Fukada T, Itami M, Sawa H, Furakawa T,Fukakusa S, Tsuchihashi N, Kakehi H, Takahashi Y, Fujimoto Y, Futonaka H, Takemura T: A case of thymoma arising from undescended thymus. High uptake of thallium-201 chloride. Eur J Nucl Med 5:465–468, 1980.
69. Gardner DJ: Unusual CT appearance of a thyroglossal duct cyst carcinoma. J Otolaryngol 18:258–259, 1989.
70. Garfinkle TJ, Handler SD: Hemangiomas of the head and neck in children: a guide to management. J Otolaryngol 9:439–450, 1980.
71. Gargan TJ, McKinnon M, Mulliken JB: Midline cervical cleft. Plast Reconstr Surg 76:225–229, 1985.
72. Gatot A, Tovi F, Fliss DM, Yanai-Inbar I: Branchial cleft cyst manifesting as hypoglossal nerve palsy. Head and Neck 3:249–250, 1991.
73. Gibson WS, Fenton NA: Congenital sublingual dermoid cyst. Arch Otolaryngol 108:745–748, 1982.
74. Gilmour JR: Some developmental abnormalities of the thymus and parathyroids. J Pathol 52:213–218, 1941.
75. Girard M, DeLuca SA: Thyroglossal duct cyst. Am Fam Physician 42:665–669, 1990.
76. Godin MS, Kearns DB, Pransky SM, Seid AB, Wilson DB: Fourth

branchial pouch sinus: principles of diagnosis and management. Laryngoscope 100:174–178, 1990.

77. Gosain AK, Wildes TO: Lateral cervical cyst containing gastric epithelium. Arch Pathol Lab Med 112:96–98, 1988.
78. Gottlieb E, Lewin ML: Congenital midline cervical clefts of neck. N Y State J Med 66:712–718, 1966.
79. Gray BN: Teratoma of the neck. Aust N Z J Surg 42:294–297, 1973.
80. Gross RE, Connerly ML: Thyroglossal cyst and sinuses: a study and report of 198 cases. N Engl J Med 223:616–624, 1940.
81. Gruhn J, Hurwitt ES: Fibrous sternomastoid tumor of infancy. Pediatrics 8:525–526, 1951.
82. Guba A, Adam AE, Jaques DA, Chambers RG: Cervical presentation of thymic cysts. Am J Surg 136:420–436, 1978.
83. Gundry SR, Wesley JR, Klein MD, Barr M, Coran AG: Cervical teratomas in the newborn. J Pediatr Surg 18:382–386, 1983.
84. Haar JG, Boulos EJ, Sadeghi MH, Sheffer J: Association of a thyroglossal duct cyst and a dermoid cyst in the neck A case report. Ann Otol Rhinol Laryngol 90:181–182, 1990.
85. Hadju SI, Faruqe AA, Hadju EO, Morgan WS: Teratoma of the neck in infants. Am J Dis Child 3:412–416, 1966.
86. Handley GH: Hemangiomas of the head and neck. Ear Nose Throat J 66:19–24, 1987.
87. Hanid TK, Johnson AG, Kay L: Cervical thymic cyst. J Pediatr Surg 10:141–142, 1975.
88. Hanzlick RL: Lingual thyroglossal duct cyst causing death in a four week old infant. J Forensic Sci 29:345–348, 1984.
89. Har-El G, Heffner DK, Ruffy M: Haemangioma in a cervical lymph node. J Laryngol Otol 104:513–515, 1990.
90. Har-El G, Sasaki CT, Prager D, Krespi J: Acute suppurative thyroiditis and the branchial apparatus. Am J Otolaryngol 12:6–11, 1991.
91. Hawkins DB, Park R: Teratoma of the pharynx and neck. Ann Otol Rhinol Laryngol 81:848–853, 1972.
92. Hecht F, Grix A, Hecht BK, Berger C, Bixenman H, Szucs S, O'Keefe D, Finberg HJ: Direct prenatal diagnosis of a malignancy. Cancer Genet Cytogenet 11:107–111, 1984.
93. Hester TO, Camnitz PS, Albernaz MS, Kodroff MB: Superficial carotid artery secondary to cervical teratoma. Ear Nose Throat J 70:524–526, 1991.
94. Heys RF, Murray CP, Kohler HG: Obstructed labour due to foetal tumours: cervical and coccygeal teratoma. Two case reports. *Gynaecologia* 164:43–54, 1967.
95. Hirota J, Maeda Y, Ueta E, Osaki T: Immunohistochemical and histologic study of cervical lymphoepithelial cysts. J Oral Pathol Med 18:202–205, 1989.
96. Hitchcock A, Sears RT, O'Neill T: Immature cervical teratoma arising in one fetus of a twin pregnancy. Acta Obstet Gynecol Scand 66:377–379, 1987.
97. Hoffman MA, Schuster SR: Thyroglossal duct remnants in infants and children: reevaluation of histopathology and methods for resection. Ann Otol Rhinol Laryngol 97:483–486, 1988.
98. Holt GR, Holt JE, Weaver RG: Dermoids and teratomas of the head and neck. Ear Nose Throat J 58:37–62, 1979.
99. Howell DM, Gumbiner CH, Martin GEO: Congestive heart failure due to a giant cutaneous hemangioma. Clin Pediatr 23:504–506, 1984.
100. Irvine DW: Cervical teratoma in the newborn. Arch Otolaryngol 82:546–549, 1965.
101. Ishwariah TD, Froome K: An unusual thyroglossal cyst. Br J Surg 49:597–600, 1962.
102. Jasper RD, Goldberg MH, Zborowski RG: Lymphangioma and cystic hygroma. J Oral Maxillofac Surg 18:152–154, 1989.
103. Johnson LA, Polga JP: Follicular adenocarcinoma arising in a thyroglossal duct remnant. Clin Nucl Med 13:378, 1988.
104. Johnsen NJ, Bretlau P: Cervical thymic cyst. Acta Otolaryngol 82:143–146, 1976.
105. Jones PG: Torticollis. In: Pediatric Surgery 4th ed, KJ Welch, JG Randolph, MM Ravitch, JA O'Neil, MI Rowe, eds. Yearbook Medical Publishers, Chicago, 1985, pp 552–556.
106. Judd ES: Thyroglossal duct cysts and sinuses. Surg Clin North 43:1023–1032, 1963.
107. Katz AD: Midline dermoid tumors of the head and neck. Arch Surg 109:822–823, 1974.
108. Katz AD, Hachigan M: Thyroglossal duct cyst: a thirty year experience with emphasis on occurrence in older patients. Am J Surg 155:741–743, 1988.
109. Katz R, Bar-Ziv J, Preminger-Shapiro R, Ben-Tovim R, Rechnic Y: Pyogenic thyroiditis due to branchial pouch sinus. Isr J Med Sci 25:641–644, 1989.
110. Kawamura S, Kishino B, Miyauchi A, Takai S, Tajima K, Mashita K, Tarui S: The differential diagnosis of cystic neck masses by the determination of thyroglobulin concentrations in the aspirates. Clin Endocrinol 20:261–267, 1984.
111. Kennedy TL: Cystic hygroma-lymphangioma: a rare and still unclear entity. Laryngoscope 99:79–86, 1989.
112. Khafif RA, Prichep R, Minkowitz S: Primary branchiogenic carcinoma. Head Neck 11:153–163, 1989.
113. Kiesewetter WB, Nelson PK, Palladino VS, Koop HR: The sternomastoid "tumor" of infancy. J Otolaryngol 5:523–529, 1955.
114. Kimler SC, Muth WF: Primary malignant teratoma of the thyroid. Cancer 42:311–317, 1978.
115. Knight RP, Hamoudi AB, Vassy LE: The diagnosis and treatment of midline neck masses in children. Surgery 93:603–611, 1983.
116. Kreller JS, Carr RF, Quinn JH: Cystic hygroma in a 17-year-old patient: report of a case. J Oral Surg 36:808–810, 1978.
117. Kuhne D, Helmke K: Embolization with "Ethibloc" of vascular tumors and arteriovenous malformations in the head and neck. Neuroradiology 23:253–258, 1982.
118. Landua A, Reese DJ, Blumenthal DR, Chin NW: Tophaceous neck mass presenting as a thyroglossal duct cyst. Arthritis Rheum 33:910–911, 1990.
119. Langer JC, Fitzgerald PG, Desa D, Filly RA, Golbus MS, Adzick NS, Harrison MR: Cervical cystic hygroma in the fetus: clinical spectrum and outcome. J Pediatr Surg 25:58–62, 1990.
120. LaRouere MJ, Drake AF, Baker SA, Richter HJ, Magielski E: Evaluation and management of a carcinoma arising in a thyroglossal duct cyst. Am J Otolaryngol 8:351–355, 1987.
121. Lau HT, Barlow BA, Gandhi RP: Ectopic thymus: presenting as neck mass. J Pediatr Surg 19:197, 1984.
122. Leikensohn JR, Epstein LI, Vasconez LO: Superselective embolization and surgery of noninvoluting hemangiomas and A-V malformations. Plast Reconstr Surg 68:143–151, 1981.
123. Levecue H, Saraceno CA, Tang C, Blanchard CL: Dermoid cysts of the floor of mouth and lateral neck. Laryngoscope 89:296–305, 1979.
124. Levine C: Cervical presentation of a large thymic cyst: CT appearance. J Comput Assist Tomogr 12:656–657, 1988.
125. Lewis MR: Persistence of the thymus in the cervical area. J Pediatr 61:887–893, 1962.
126. Ling CM, Low YS: Sternomastoid tumor and muscular torticollis. Clin Orthop 86:144–150, 1972.
127. Lister WA: Natural history of stawberry nevi. Lancet 1:1429–1434, 1938.
128. LiVolsi VA, Perzin KH, Savetsky L: Carcinoma arising in median ectopic thyroid (including thyroglossal duct tissue). Cancer 34:1303–1315, 1974.
129. Lustmann J, Benoliel R, Zeltser R: Squamous cell carcinoma arising in a thyroglossal duct cyst in the tongue. J Oral Maxillofac Surg 47:81–85, 1989.
130. Lyons TJ, Dickson JAS, Variend S: Cervical thymic cysts. J Pediatr Surg 24:241–243, 1989.
131. MacDonald D: Sternomastoid tumor and muscular torticollis. J Bone Joint Surg 51B:432–443, 1969.
132. Mahboubi S, Potsic WP: Computed tomography of cervical cystic hygroma in the neck. Int J Pediatr Otol 18:47–51, 1989.
133. Maneksha RJ: Congenital cervical cleft with a possible thyroglossal cyst. Br J Plast Surg 14:32, 1961.
134. Martin H, Moffit M, Ehlich H: The case for branchiogenic cancer (malignant branchioma). Ann Surg 132:867–887, 1950.
135. Matt BJ, Lusk RP: Delineation of a deep neck abscess with magnetic resonance imaging. Ann Otol Rhinol Laryngol 96:615–617, 1987.
136. McAvoy JM, Zuckerbraun L: Dermoid cysts of the head and neck in children. Arch Otolaryngol 102:529–531, 1976.
137. McGuirt WF: Pediatric Otolaryngology Case Studies. Medical Examination Publishing, Garden City, NY, 1980.
138. McGuirt WF: Neck mass: patient examination and differential diagnosis. In:Otolaryngology—Head and Neck Surgery, Vol 2, CW Cummings, JM Frederickson, LA Harker, CJ Krause, DE Schuller, eds. CV Mosby, St Louis, 1986, pp 1587–1595.
139. McLeod DM, Karandy EJ: Aberrant cervical thymus: a rare cause of acute respiratory distress. Arch Otolaryngol 107:179–180, 1981.
140. Mentz HA, Graham HD, Blair P: Lymphangioma of the head and neck in infants. J La State Med Soc 140:13–15, 1988.
141. Mickel RA, Calcaterra TC: Management of recurrent thyroglossal ducts cysts. Arch Otolaryngol 109:34–36, 1983.

142. Mickelson MR, Cooper RR, Ponseti IV: Ultrastructure of the sternocleidomastoid muscle in muscular torticollis. Clin Orthop 110:11–18, 1975.
143. Middleton DS: The pathology of congenital torticollis. Br J Surg 18:188–204, 1930.
144. Miller JM, Taboada JC: Cystic hygroma colli in an adult. Johns Hopkins Med J 134:233–236, 1974.
145. Mills RP, Hussain SSM: Teratomas of the head and neck in infancy and childhood. Int J Pediatr Otorhinolaryngol 8:177–180, 1984.
146. Minami RT, Pletcher J, Dakin RL: Midline cervical cleft. J Maxillofac Surg 8:65–68, 1980.
147. Morris MR, Woody EA: A closer look at the thyroglossal cyst. Ear Nose Throat J 66:40–45, 1987.
148. Morrish TN, Manning SC: Branchial anomaly in a newborn presenting as stridor. Int J Pediatr Otorhinolaryngol 21:259–262, 1991.
149. Morton CB, Jordan HE: Median cleft of the lower lip and mandible, cleft sternum and absence of basihyoid. Arch Surg 30:647–656, 1935.
150. Mulliken JB, Glowacki J: Haemangiomas and vascular malformations in infants and children, a classification based on endothelial characteristics. Plast Reconstr Surg 63:412–420, 1982.
151. Myer CM III: Congenital neck masses. In: Otolaryngology, Vol 3, MM Paparella, DA Shumrick, JL Gluckman, WL Meyerhoff, eds. WB Saunders, Philadelphia, 1991, pp 2535–2543.
152. Nachlas NE: Thyroglossal duct cysts. Ann Otol Rhinol Laryngol 59:381–389, 1950.
153. Narcy P, Aumont-Grosskopf C, Bobin S, Manach Y: Fistulae of the fourth endobranchial pouch. Int J Pediatr Otorhinolaryngol 16:157–165, 1988.
154. Nevin NC, Nevin J: Cystic hygroma simulating an encephalocele. Prenat Diagn 3:249–255, 1983.
155. New GB, Erich JB: Dermoid cysts of the head and neck. Surg Gynecol Obstet 65:48–55, 1937.
156. Ninh TN, Ninh TX: Cystic hygroma in children: a report of 126 cases. J Pediatr Surg 9:191–195, 1974.
157. Nowak PA, Zarbo RJ: Aberrant solid cervical thymus. Ear Nose Throat J 67:670–677, 1988
158. Numata M, Asato S, Hosoe S, Itoh N, Hayashi S: Two cases of cystic lymphangioma in the neck region in adults. Lymphology 15:100–105, 1982.
159. Nussbaum M, Buchwald RP: Adult cystic hygroma. Am J Otolaryngol 2:159–162, 1981.
160. Oates CP, Wilson AW, Ward-Booth RP, Williams ED: Combined use of Doppler and conventional ultrasound for the diagnosis of vascular and other lesions in the head and neck. Int J Oral Maxillofac Surg 19:235–239, 1990.
161. Ogita S, Tsuto T, Tokiwa K, Takashi T: Intracystic injection of OK-432: a new sclerosing therapy for cytic hygroma. Br J Surg 74:690–691, 1987.
162. Ohtsuka H: Port wine stain: distribution patterns on the face and neck. Ann Plast Surg 24:409–414, 1990.
163. Olumide F: Thyroglossal cyst presenting with severe laryngeal obstruction. Niger Med J 3:53–54, 1973.
164. Osborne TE, Levin LS, Tilghman DM, Haller JA: Surgical correction of mandibulofacial deformities secondary to large cervical cystic hygromas. J Oral Maxillofac Surg 45:1015–1021, 1987.
165. Ostfeld EJ, Wiesel JM, Rabinson S, Auslander L: Parapharyngeal (retrostyloid)–third branchial cleft cyst. J Laryngol Otol 105:790–792, 1991.
166. Overholt SL, Gado M, Sessions DG, Ogura JH: Angiography in the diagnosis and management of extracranial vascular lesions of the head and neck. Laryngoscope 88:1769–1783, 1978.
167. Patel RB, Gibson JY, Cruz CA, Burkhalter JL: Sonographic diagnosis of cervical teratoma in utero. AJR 139:1220–1222, 1982.
168. Pelausa EO, Forte V: Sistrunk revisited: a ten-year review of revision thyroglossal duct surgery at Toronto's Hospital for Sick Children. J Otolaryngol 18:325–333, 1989.
169. Persky MS, Berenstein A, Cohen NL: Combined treatment of head and neck vascular masses with preoperative embolization. Laryngoscope 94:20–27, 1984.
170. Pickleman JR, Lee J, Staus F, Paloyan E: Thyroid hemangioma. Am J Surg 129:331–333, 1975.
171. Podoshin L, Fradis M, Goldstein J, Misselevitch I, Boss JH: Intrahyoid thyroglossal cyst. J Laryngol Otol 103:539–542, 1989.
172. Poe R, Blair PA: Hemangioma of the head and neck. J La State Med Assoc 139:17–20, 1987.
173. Ramos-Gabatin A, Watzinger W: Fine needle aspiration and cytology in the preoperative diagnosis of branchial cysts. South Med J 77:1187–1189, 1984.
174. Rappaport I, Yim D: Congenital arteriovenous fistulas of the head and neck. Arch Otolaryngol 97:350–353, 1973.
175. Rebeiz E, April MM, Bohigian RK, Shapshay SM: Nd-Yag laser treatment of venous malformations of the head and neck: an update. Otolaryngol Head Neck Surg 105:655–661, 1991.
176. Reddy VA, Radhakrishna K, Rao PLNG: Lingual dermoid. J Pediatr Surg 26:1389–1390, 1991.
177. Reiner M Beck RA: Cervical thymic cysts in children. Am J Surg 139:704–707, 1980
178. Reiner SA, Medina JE, Min KW: Pathology quiz case. Arch Otolaryngol Head Neck Surg 117:110–113, 1991.
179. Ricciardelli EJ, Richardson MA: Cervicofacial cystic hygroma. Arch Otolaryngol Head Neck Surg 117:546–553, 1991.
180. Robertson JS, Weigand DA, Schaitkin BM: Life-threatening hemangioma arising from the parotid gland. Arch Otolaryngol Head Neck Surg 104:858–862, 1991.
181. Roediger WE, Spitz L, Schmaman: Histogenesis of benign cervical 2znteratoma. Teratology 10:111–118, 1974.
182. Rogers SN, Feldman MA: Thyroglossal duct cyst recurrence [letter]. Br J Surg 75:932, 1988.
183. Rosedale RS: Neck teratomas. Arch Otolaryngol 82:535–542, 1965.
184. Rosendorff J, Mayo JR, Reichman P, Pinto MR, Bernstein R: Elevated alpha fetoprotein levels in the 45 X (Turner syndrome) fetus with cystic hygroma. Case report. S Afr Med J 16:621–624, 1982.
185. Rosenfeld CR, Coln CD, Duenhoelter JH: Fetal cervical teratoma as a cause of polyhydramnios. Pediatrics 64:176–179, 1979.
186. Sabin FR: On the origin of the lymphatic system from the veins, and the development of the lymph heart and thoracic duct in the pig. Am J Anat 1:367–389, 1901–1902.
187. Saijo M, Munro IR, Mancer K: Lymphangioma. Rev Reconstr Surg 56:642–651, 1975.
188. Sanerkin NG, Edwards P: Birth injury to the sternomastoid muscle. J Bone Joint Surg 48:441–446, 1966.
189. Sanusi ID, Carrington PR, Adams DN: Cervical thymic cyst. Arch Dermatol 118:122–124, 1982.
190. Sasaki GH, Pang CY, Wittliff L: Pathogenesis and treatment of skin strawberry hemangiomas: clinical and in vitro studies of hormonal effects. Plast Reconstr Surg 73:359–368, 1984.
191. Scally CM, Black HA: Cystic hygroma: massive recurrence in adult life. J Laryngol Otol 104:908–910, 1990.
192. Scheibner A, Wheeland RG: Use of the Argon-pumped tunable dye laser for port-wine stains in children. J Dermatol Surg Oncol 17:735–739, 1991.
193. Schloss MD, Sweet RC, Blais C, Tewfik TL: Lymphangioma in children. J Otolaryngol 13:95–98, 1984.
194. Schoenfeld A, Edelstein T, Joel-Cohen SJ: Prenatal ultrasonic diagnosis of fetal teratoma of the neck. Br J Radiol 51:742–744, 1978.
195. Seward GR: Dermoid cyst of the floor of mouth. Br J Oral Surg 3:36–47, 1965.
196. Shajrawi I, Gertner R, Fradis M, Podoshin L, Boss JH: Lateral cervical thymic cyst. Otolaryngol Head Neck Surg 102:759–761, 1990.
197. Shamir R, Kohn G, Metzker A: Nevus flammeus. Discordance in monozygotic twins. Am J Dis Child 145:85–86, 1991.
198. Shapiro J, Gallant A, Wechsler RJ, Steiner RM: Thymic cyst secondary to cervical irradiation: a complication of treated laryngeal cancer. Comput Med Imaging Graph 15:319–322, 1991.
199. Shapshay SM, David LM, Zeitels S: Neodymium-yag laser photocoagulation of hemangiomas of the head and neck. Laryngoscope 97:323–330, 1987.
200. Shin CS, Levowitz BS: Cervicomediastinal thymic cyst. N Y State J Med 73:2695–2698, 1973.
201. Shugar MA, Healy GB: The fourth branchial cleft anomaly. Head Neck Surg 3:72–75, 1980.
202. Silberman R, Mendelson IR: Teratoma of the neck. Report of two cases and review of the literature. Arch Dis Child 35:159–170, 1960.
203. Silverman P, Degesys G, Ferguson B, Bierre AR: Papillary carcinoma arising in a thyroglossal duct cyst: CT findings. J Comput Assist Tomogr 9:806–808, 1985.
204. Silverman PM, Korobkin M, Moore AV: CT diagnosis of cystic hygroma of the neck. J Comput Assist Tomogr 7:519–520, 1983.
205. Sistrunk WE: The surgical treatment of cysts of the thyroglossal tract. Ann Surg 71:121–122, 1920.
206. Slack RWT, Parker A: Rare submandibular swelling (capillary hemangioma). J Laryngol Otol 103:623–633, 1989.

207. Sloan GM, Bolton LL, Miller JH, Reinisch JF, Nichter LS: Radionuclide-labelled red blood cell imaging of vascular malformations in children. Ann Plast Surg 21:236–241, 1988.
208. Sloan GM, Reinisch JF, Nichter LS, Saber WL, Lew K, Morwood DT: Intralesional corticosteroid therapy for infantile hemangiomas. Plast Reconstr Surg 83:459–456, 1989.
209. Slotnick D, Som PM, Geirbfried J, Biller H: Thyroglossal duct cysts that mimic laryngeal massses. Laryngoscope 97:742–745, 1987.
210. Smith AR, van Urk H, Vaandrager M, van der Meulen, JC: Treatment of a large hemangioma in the head and neck region. Head Neck Surg 5:263–267, 1983.
211. Smith JF, Kielmovitch I: Branchial cyst anomaly in a newborn. Otolaryngol Head Neck Surg 100:163–165, 1988.
212. Som PM: Clinical radiology quiz. Am J Otolaryngol 10:430–431, 1989.
213. Som PM: Clinical radiology quiz. Am J Otolaryngol 11:63–64, 1990.
214. Som PM, Sacher M, Lanzierei CF: Parenchymal cysts of the lower neck. Radiology 157:399–406, 1985.
215. Som PM, Zimmerman RA, Biller HF: Cystic hygroma and facial nerve paralysis: a rare association. J Comput Assist Tomogr 8:110–113, 1984.
216. Soni NK, Chatterji PA: Massive sublingual-cervical dermoid. J Laryngol Otol 92:1151–1159, 1978.
217. Soucy P, Penning J: The clinical relevance of certain observations on the histology of the thyroglossal tract. J Pediatr Surg 19:506–509, 1984.
218. Speer FD: Thymic cysts: report of a thymus presenting cysts of three types. NY Med Coll Flower Hosp Bull 1:142–150, 1938.
219. Spigland N, Bensoussan AL, Blanchard H, Russo P: Aberrant cervical thymus in children: three case reports and review of the literature. J Pediatr Surg 25:1196–1199, 1990.
220. Stofman GM, Reiter D, Feldman MD: Invasive hemangiomas of the head and neck. Ear Nose Throat J 68:612–616, 1989.
221. Stone HH, Henderson D, Guidio FA: Teratomas of the neck. J Dis Child 113:222–225, 1967.
222. Strome M, Eraklis A: Thymic cysts in the neck. Laryngoscope 87:1645–1649, 1977.
223. Surendran N, Varghese B: Midline cleft of lower lip with cleft of the mandible and midline dermoid of the neck. J Pediatr Surg 26:1387–1388, 1991.
224. Suster S, Rosai J: Cystic thymomas. Cancer 69:92–97, 1992.
225. Suzuki S, Yamamuro T, Fujita A: The etiological relationship between congenital torticollis and obstetrical paralysis. Int Orthop 8:175–181, 1984.
226. Tahilyani NDA, Singh KM Occipital teratoma bearing digits and nails. Br J Surg 63:493, 1976.
227. Takato T, Takeda H, Kamei M: First branchial cleft sinus in hemifacial microsomia. Br J Plast Surg 42:95–97, 1989.
228. Takimoto T, Akemoto Y, Umeda R: Pharyngeal cyst arising from second branchial cleft. J Laryngol Otol 103:964–965, 1989.
229. Tapper D, Lack EE: Teratomas in infancy and childhood. Ann Surg 198:398–410, 1983.
230. Thomas MR, Nofal F, Cave APD: Dermoid cyst in the mouth: value of ultrasound. J Laryngol Otol 104:141–142, 1990.
231. Thomsen JR, Koltai PJ: Sternomastoid tumor of infancy. Ann Otol Rhinol Laryngol 98:955–959, 1989.
232. Thurkow AL, Visser GHA, deVries JA: Ultrasound observations of a malignant cervical teratoma of the fetus in a case of polyhydramnios: case history and review. Obstet Gynecol Reprod Biol 14:375–384, 1983.
233. Tom LWC, Handler SD, Wetmore RF, Potsic WP: The sternocleidomastoid tumor of infancy. Int J Pediatr Otorhinolaryngol 13:245–255, 1987.
234. Tom LWC, Kenealy JFX, Torsiglieri AJ: First branchial cleft anomalies involving the tympanic membrane and middle ear. Otolaryngol Head Neck Surg 105:473–477, 1991.
235. Topf P, Fried MP, Strome M: Vagaries of thyroglossal duct cysts. Laryngoscope 98:740–743, 1988.
236. Tovi F, Barki Y, Maor E: Cartilage within a thyroglossal duct anomaly. Int J Pediatr Otorhinoarymgol 15:205–210, 1988.
237. Tovi F, Fliss DM, Inbar-Yanai I: Hurthle cell adenoma of the thyroglossal duct. Head Neck Surg 10:346–349, 1988.
238. Tovi F, Mares AJ: The aberrant cervical thymus: embryology and clinical applications. Am J Surg 136:631–637, 1978.
239. Trecet JC, Claramunt V, Larraz J, Ruiz E, Zuzuarregui M, Ugalde FJ: Prenatal ultrasound diagnosis of fetal teratoma of the neck. J Clin Ultrasound 12:509–511, 1984.
240. Tuffin JR, Theaker E: True lateral dermoid cyst of the neck. Int J Oral Maxillofac Surg 20:275–276, 1991.
241. van der Staak FHJ, Pruszczynski M, Severijnen RSVM, van de Kaa CA, Festen C: The midline cervical cleft. J Pediatr Surg 26:1391–1393, 1991.
242. van der Wal N, Wiener JD, Allard RHD, Henzen-Logmans C, Van der Waal I: Thyroglossal cysts in patients over 30 years of age. Int J Oral Maxillofac Surg 16:416–419, 1987.
243. Van Duyn J: Congenital midline cervical cord with report of a case and a note on the etiology of congenital torticollis. Plast Reconstr Surg 31:576–586, 1963.
244. Veluvolu P, Daniels DL, Collier BD, Isitman AT, Duncavage A, Patel N, Thakur S, Joestgen T: Scintigraphic demonstration of a soft tissue cavernous hemangioma with valsalva maneuver. Clin Nucl Med 15:865–869, 1990.
245. Viguera MC, Terry RN: Induced hypotension for extensive surgery in an infant. Anesthesiology 27:701–702, 1966.
246. Vincent SD, Synhorst JB: Adenocarcinoma arising in a thyroglossal duct cyst: report of a case and review of the literature. J Oral Maxillofac Surg 47:633–635, 1989.
247. Wagner CW, Vincur CD, Weintraub WH, Golladay ES: Respiratory complications in cervical thymic cysts. J Pediatr Surg 23:657–660, 1988.
248. Ward PH, Harris PF, Downey W: Surgical approach to cystic hygroma of the neck. Arch Otolaryngol 91:508–514, 1970.
249. Ward RF, Selfe RW, St. Louis L, Bowling D: Computed tomography and the thyroglossal duct cyst. Otolaryngol Head Neck Surg 95:93–98, 1986.
250. Watanatittan S, Othersen HB, Hughson MD: Cervical teratoma in children. Prog Pediatr Surg 14:225–239, 1981.
251. Weber T, Connors RH, Tracy TF, Bailey PV: Complex hemangiomas of infants and children. Arch Surg 125:1017–1021, 1990.
252. Weimert TA, Gilmore BB Jr: Multiple head and neck haemangiomas in the adult: a case report and review of the literature. J Laryngol Otol 92:937–941, 1978.
253. Weiss SD, Orlich CC: Primary papillary carcinoma of a thyroglossal duct cyst: report of a case and review of the literature. Br J Surg 78:87–89, 1991.
254. Welch KJ, Tapper D, Vawter GP: Surgical treatment of thymic cysts and neoplasms in children. J Pediatr Surg 14:691–697, 1979.
255. Woodring AJ: Cervical cystic hygroma: a review of the literature and report of an unusual case. Ann Otol Rhinol Laryngol 77:978–983, 1968.
256. Woods D, Young JEM, Filice R, Dobranowski J: Late-onset cystic hygromas: the role of CT. J Can Assoc Radiol 40:159–161, 1989.
257. Work WP: Newer concepts of first branchial cleft defects. Laryngoscope 82:1581–1593, 1972.
258. Wynn-Williams D: Congenital midline cervical cleft and web. Br J Plast Surg 5:87–93, 1953.
259. Yasumoto M, Shibuya H, Gomi N, Kasuga T: Ultrasonographic appearance of dermoid and epidermoid cysts in the head and neck. J Clin Ultrasound 19:455–461, 1991.
260. Yuh WTC, Buehner LS, Kao SCS, Robinson RA, Dolan, KD, Phillips JI: Magnetic resonance imaging of pediatric head and neck cystic hygromas. Ann Otol Rhinol Laryngol 100:737–742, 1991.
261. Zakrzewski J: Quick-hardening polymers in the surgical treatment of congenital neck fistulae. J Laryngol Otol 89:345–347, 1975.
262. Zarbo RJ, McClatchey KD, Areen RG, Baker SB: Thymopharyngeal duct cyst: a form of cervical thymus. Ann Otol Rhinol Laryngol 92:284–289, 1983.
263. Zarem HA, Edgerton MT: The treatment of hemangiomas. Ann Surg 183:517–532, 1976.
264. Zink A, Raue F, Hoffman R, Ziegler R: Papillary carcinoma in an ectopic thyroid. Horm Res 35:86–88, 1991.

# Appendix E

## Syndromes and Conditions Associated with Anomalies of the Neck

AHMAD S. TEEBI, TED L. TEWFIK, and VAZKEN M. DER KALOUSTIAN

| Syndrome or condition | MIM No. POSSUM No.[a] | Inheritance[b] | Neck anomalies | Other manifestations |
|---|---|---|---|---|
| Aase syndrome or Blackfan-Diamond anemia[37] | **205600** 3002 | AR | Webbed neck | Short stature, triphalangeal thumb, congenital hypoplastic anemia improves with age, cleft lip/palate, cardiac defects |
| Ablepharon and macrostomia[38] | **200110** 3919 | AR | Webbed neck with excess skin | Absent eyelids, eyebrows, and eyelashes; cryptophthalmos, ectropion, microcephaly, sparse scalp hair, macrostomia, low-set or dysplastic ears, flared nostrils, prognathism, small penis or ambiguous genitalia, (MR) mental retardation |
| Achondroplasia[86] | ***100800** 3006 | AD | Cervicomedullary compression, sudden death in infancy or childhood (relatively higher than for normal children) | Short stature, short limbs (predominantly rhizomelic), macrocephaly, brachycephaly, trident hand, acetabular bony spurs, metaphyseal lucency of proximal femur, narrowed interpedicular distance, hypotonia, (homozygotes are severely affected and die early); gene location 4p16.3 |
| Albright hereditary osteodystrophy or Pseudohypoparathyroidism[18] | ***103580** 3364 | AD | Short or webbed neck | Short stature, brachydactyly with short 4th, 5th metacarpals; advanced bone age, hypocalcemia or hyperphosphatemia, soft tissue calcification, fibrous dysplasia of the bone, seizures, MR, variable age of onset, proposed gene location 20q13.11 |
| Atelosteogenesis, type 1 or Spondylo-humero-femoral dysplasia[40] | **108720** 3552 | AD | Short neck, cervical malsegmentation defects or vertebral clefts | Short stature, short limbs, (rhizomelic), multiple joint dislocations, platyspondyly, distal tapering of humerus or femur, brachydactyly, macrocephaly, epiphyseal or diaphyseal abnormality |
| Beals auriculo-osteo-dysplasia[44] | ***109000** 3035 | AD | Short or webbed neck with excess skin | Short stature, attached ear lobes, long and high clavicle; elbow dislocation, hypoplasia of the capitulum, hip dislocation |
| Beals contractural arachnodactyly[9,85] | ***121050** 3027 | AD | Relatively short neck | Tall stature, long limbs, contractures (improve with time), lens dislocation, aortic root dilatation, aortic valve incompetence, scoliosis, pectus deformity, "crumpled" upper helix of ears, proposed gene location 5q23–31 |
| Burton syndrome[12] | **245160** 3839 | AR | Abnormal neck, cervical kyphosis | Short stature, short ribs, brachydactyly, bulky joints, bony restriction of joint movement, down- |

**Appendix E** Syndromes and conditions associated with anomalies of the neck *(Continued)*

| Syndrome or condition | MIM No. POSSUM No.[a] | Inheritance[b] | Neck anomalies | Other manifestations |
|---|---|---|---|---|
| | | | | ward lens dislocation, metaphyseal abnormality, platyspondyly, microsomia with pursed lips (resembles Kniest dysplasia) |
| Campomelic or camptomelic dysplasia or dwarfism[56] | ***211970** 3049 | AR | Short or webbed neck with excess skin | Short stature, short limbs (mesomelic), bowed legs and thighs, pretibial skin dimples, hypoplastic scapulae, rib anomalies, tracheal cartilage hypoplasia, flat face, hypertelorism, micrognathia, cleft soft/ hard palate, sex reversal in phenotypic females with XY karyotype (common), early death, proposed gene location 17q24.3–25.1 |
| Cardio-facio-cutaneous (CFC) syndrome[68] | **115150** 3627 | AD | Short or webbed neck with excess skin | Short stature, curly and sparse hair, high forehead, antimongoloid slant of palpebral fissures, ptosis, hypertelorism, depressed nasal bridge, small nose, abnormal dentition, folded or posteriorly angulated ears, pulmonary atresia, other cardiac defects, hyperkeratotic skin, eczema or dermatitis, hypotonia, spasticity, seizures, MR (very common) |
| Cephaloskeletal dysplasia or Taybi-Linder syndrome[75] | **247400** 3445 | AR | Atlantoaxial instability or odontoid hypoplasia | Intrauterine growth ratardation (IUGR), short stature, short limbs, microcephaly, prominent eyes, sloping forehead, holoprosencephaly or other CNS malformations, agenesis of the corpus callosum, broad hands and feet, osteoporosis, metaphyseal abnormality, early death |
| Cerebro-costo-mandibular syndrome[21] | **117650** 3056 | AD ?AR | Webbed neck with excess skin, multiple vertebral defects or hemivertebrae | Mental retardation, severe micrognathia, cleft palate, glossoptosis, narrow and asymmetric chest, short ribs, abnormal rib number and structure, triangular face, tracheal abnormality, dysplastic kidneys |
| Cerebro-hepato-renal syndrome or Zellweger syndrome[63] | ***214100** 3057 | AR | Webbed neck with excess skin | Severe hypotonia, macrocephaly, high and narrow forehead, large fontanelles, wide sutures, broad cheeks, telecanthus, epicanthic folds, corneal and retinal changes, cystic kidney changes, growth deficiency, peroxisomal disorder |
| CHARGE association (**C**oloboma, **H**eart defects, **A**tresia choanae, **R**etardation of growth and development, **G**enital hypoplasia, **E**ar anomalies)[51] | **214800** 3480 | Sporadic ?AR | Short neck | Short stature, iris and retinal colobomas, choanal atresia, facial asymmetry, low-set or anteverted ears, sensorineural and conductive deafness, heart defects, urogenital anomalies, CNS anomalies, hypogonadism, MR |
| Chromosome 3, partial dup 3q and del 3p[71] | 3068 | | Webbed neck with excess skin | Failure to thrive, hirsutism, upslanting palpebral fissures, synophrys, thick eyebrows, small nose, cleft lip/palate, small penis or cryptorchidism, syndactyly, camptodactyly, polydactyly of the feet, cardiovascular anomalies, early death |

| Syndrome or condition | MIM No. POSSUM No.[a] | Inheritance[b] | Neck anomalies | Other manifestations |
|---|---|---|---|---|
| Chromosome 4, partial dup 4p[90] | 3070 | | Short or webbed neck with excess skin | Coarse facial features, microcephaly, deep-set eyes, broad nasal bridge, bulbous nose, pointed chin, choanal atresia, cardiac defects, skeletal abnormalities, hypotonia, seizures, severe MR |
| Chromosome 5, partial dup 5p[29] | 4713 | | Short neck | Hydro or macrocephaly, high forehead, broad nasal bridge, microstomia, micrognathia, low-set or posteriorly angulated ears, iris coloboma, cardiac defects, agenesis or hypoplasia of kidneys, agenesis or hypoplasia of cerebellum/corpus callosum, hypotonia, MR |
| Chromosome 9, partial del 9p[30,77] | 3081 | | Short, webbed, and broad neck | Trigonocephaly or ridged metopic sutures, synophrys, short nose, micrognathia, long fingers with terminal broadening, cardiovascular anomalies, hypotonia, MR |
| Chromosome 9, dup 9q[53] | 3117 | | Torticollis | IUGR, dolichocephaly, microcephaly, beaked nose, deep-set eyes, retrognathia, large ears, sensorineural deafness, contractures, camptodactyly, slender limbs, arachnodactyly, cardiac defects, pyloric stenosis, urogenital anomalies, hypotonia, MR |
| Chromosome 13, trisomy 13, or Patau syndrome[92] | 3090 | | Webbed neck with excess skin, multiple vertebral segmentation defects | Microphthalmia, scalp defects, microcephaly, holoprosencephaly, cleft lip/palate, polydactyly, variable organ defects, severe MR, early death, pseudotrisomy 13 exists with a normal karyotype |
| Chromosome 13, del 13q (q12q14→q14 q31)[11] | 3125 | | Short or webbed neck | Growth retardation, microcephaly, high and broad nasal bridge, microphthalmia, cleft soft/hard palate, scoliosis, focal lumbar agenesis, cardiac defects, hypospadias, cryptorchidism, small or absent thumb, short great toe, retinoblastoma, MR |
| Chromosome 18, partial del 18p[84] | 3095 | | Short or webbed neck | Growth retardation, sparse scalp hair, decreased pigmentation, microcephaly, broad face, ptosis, prominent ears, irregular teeth, macrostomia (facial dysmorphism may be subtle), holoprosencephaly, urogenital and skeletal defects, MR |
| Chromosome 18, trisomy 18, or Edward syndrome[23] | 3094 | | Short or webbed neck with excess skin | IUGR, microcephaly, prominent occiput, small palpebral fissure, microstomia, overlapping fingers (clenched hands), rocker-bottom feet, short sternum diaphragmatic hernia, ectrodactyly or limb deficiency, cardiac defects, urogenital anomalies, spasticity, severe MR, early death |
| Chromosome 21, trisomy 21, or Down syndrome[5] | 3100 | | Short or webbed neck with excess skin, cystic hygroma, atlantoaxial instability, odontoid hypoplasia, cervical vertebral defects | Hypotonia, brachycephaly, distinctive round facies with upward slanting palpebral fissures, Brushfield spots, epicanthic folds, small nose, tongue thrusting, broad hands, single palmar crease, fifth finger clinodactyly, recurrent ear |

**Appendix E** Syndromes and conditions associated with anomalies of the neck *(Continued)*

| Syndrome or condition | MIM No. POSSUM No.[a] | Inheritance[b] | Neck anomalies | Other manifestations |
|---|---|---|---|---|
| | | | | and respiratory infections, cardiac defects, duodenal atresia, characteristic gait, MR (variable) |
| Chromosome 22, trisomy 22[74] | 3703 | | Short or webbed neck with excess skin (resembles Turner syndrome) | IUGR, body asymmetry, microcephaly or macrocephaly, eye coloboma, microphthalmia, absent or hypoplastic nails, brachydactyly, horseshoe kidney, cardiac defects, streak gonads, genital anomalies, anal stenosis or atresia, CNS malformations, MR; most cases are mosaics |
| Chromosome X; 45,X or Turner syndrome[15] | 3104 | | Short or webbed neck with excess skin (remarkable), low posterior hairline, cystic hygroma | Congenital lymphedema with residual puffiness, short stature, broad chest, wide space between nipples, cubitus valgus, brachydactyly, short 4th metacarpal, streak gonads, primary amenorrhea or infertility, coarctation of aorta, normal to borderline intelligence, occasional MR |
| Chromosome X; 48,XXXX or Tetrasomy X syndrome[69] | 3105 | | Webbed neck with excess skin | Normal growth, microcephaly, upward slanting palpebral fissures, epicanthic folds, depressed nasal bridge, MR (variable), abnormal behavior or psychosis |
| Chromosome X; 49,XXXXY[33] | 3111 | | Short or webbed neck with excess skin | IUGR, hydrops fetalis, short stature, microcephaly, upward slanting palpebral fissures, flattened nose, broad nasal bridge, micrognathia, radioulnar dysostosis, coxa valga, talipes deformity, cardiac defects, genital defects, hypogonadism, hypoplasia of corpus callosum, MR |
| Costello syndrome[19,78] | ***218040** 3475 | AR | Short or webbed neck | Macrocephaly, short stature, distinctive coarse facies, curly hair, loose skin, thick hyperkeratotic skin over the dorsum of hand, elbow, knees; hyperextensible joints, later onset of warty nasal and perioral papillomata, MR, outgoing personality |
| Craniofrontonasal dysplasia[46] | **304110** 3798 | XL AD | Short or webbed neck | Craniosynostosis (coronal), variable hypertelorism, broad nasal bridge, bifid nose, facial asymmetry, antimongoloid slant of palpebral fissures, brittle nails with prominent longitudinal grooves, syndactyly of fingers, hypotonia, intelligence may be normal |
| De Barsy syndrome or cutis laxa, corneal clouding, MR[47] | ***219150** 3680 | | Webbed neck with excess skin | Loose skin with excessive wrinkling, skin pigmentation problems, microcephaly, large fontanelle, sparse scalp hair, corneal clouding or opacification, cataract, small hands or feet, hypotonia, MR, behavior disorder |
| Diastrophic dysplasia or Diastrophic dwarfism[20,39] | ***222600** 3185 | AR | Atlantoaxial instability or odontoid hypoplasia | Short stature, short bowed limbs, short tubular bones, (especially first metacarpal), carpal fusion, joint limitations and contractures, talipes, "hitch-hicker" thumb, hy- |

| Syndrome or condition | MIM No. POSSUM No.[a] | Inheritance[b] | Neck anomalies | Other manifestations |
|---|---|---|---|---|
| | | | | pertrophic or calcified auricular cartilage (cauliflower ears), cleft palate, micrognathia, laryngotracheal stenosis, epiphyseal, metaphyseal, or diaphyseal abnormalities; abnormality of type IX collagen, gene location 5q31–q34 |
| Dyggve-Melchior-Clausen syndrome[10,73] | ***223800** 3188 | AR | Short or webbed neck with excess skin, atlantoaxial instability | Short stature, short trunk, microcephaly, abnormal sella turcica, prognathism, small scapula, barrel chest, thoracolumbar kyphosis, scoliosis, platyspondyly, cone-shaped epiphyses, restricted joint mobility, small ilia with irregular calcification of iliac crest (lacy appearance), MR |
| Elejalde syndrome[64] | **200995** 3565 | AR | Short or webbed neck with excess skin, cystic hygroma | Large baby, short limbs, hydrops fetalis, craniosynostosis, hypertelorism, small nose, long philtrum, posteriorly angulated or folded ears, preaxial or postaxial polydactyly of hands and feet, hypoplastic lungs, dysplastic kidneys |
| Fetal alcohol syndrome[27] | 3218 | Teratogenicity | Short or webbed neck, multiple vertebral segmentation defects | Variable manifestations, IUGR, microcephaly, short palpebral fissures, epicanthic folds, smooth long philtrum, thin upper lip, renal and cardiac defects, hirsutism, variable MR, features resemble pyruvate dehydrogenase complex deficiency |
| Fetal trimethadione or tridione syndrome[48] | 3980 | Teratogenicity | Webbed neck with excess skin | IUGR, postnatal growth deficiency, brachycephaly, V-shaped eyebrows, broad nasal bridge, folded or low-set ears, cardiac defects, tapering fingers, genital anomalies, possible early death |
| Fibrochondrogenesis[8] | ***228520** 3642 | AR | Short neck, cervical vertebral defects | Short limb dwarfism (rhizomelic), short ribs, marked nasal hypoplasia, platyspondyly, various vertebral defects, characteristic bone histology, early death |
| Freeman-Sheldon syndrome or whistling face syndrome[17] | ***193700** 3156 | AD ?AR | Short neck | Whistling appearance of the mouth, H-shaped chin creases, hypertonia and respiratory problems at birth with feeding difficulties in infancy, overlapping fingers or ulnar deviation, joint dislocations, short stature |
| Frontometaphyseal dysplasia[32] | ***305620** 3236 | XL | Wide foramen magnum, atlantoaxial instability, cervical vertebral defects | Coarse facies with wide nasal bridge and prominent supraorbital ridges (results from frontal hyperostosis), micrognathia, deafness (mixed), joint limitations and contractures, dislocated radial heads, splayed metaphyses, diaphyseal changes |
| Fryns syndrome[6] | ***229850** 3608 | AR | Short or webbed neck with excess skin, vertebral defects | Macrocephaly, coarse facies, macrostomia, low-set or posteriorly angulated ears, cleft lip/palate, micrognathia, hypoplastic lungs, diaphragmatic hernia, various intestinal, urogenital, and CNS anomalies; stillbirth or early death |

**Appendix E** Syndromes and conditions associated with anomalies of the neck *(Continued)*

| Syndrome or condition | MIM No. POSSUM No.[a] | Inheritance[b] | Neck anomalies | Other manifestations |
|---|---|---|---|---|
| Hunter syndrome or Mucopolysaccaridosis, type 2[14] | ***309900** 3309 | XLR | Short or webbed neck | Short stature, hirsutism, thick skin, dense and coarse scalp hair, macrocephaly, abnormal sella turcica, coarse facies (mild), dysostosis multiplex, osteoporosis, bony restriction of joint mobility, hepatosplenomegaly (storage), MR, urinary excretion of dermatan and heparan sulphate; iduronate sulphate sulphatase enzyme defect; proposed gene location Xq27–q28 |
| Hurler syndrome or Mucopolysaccharidosis type 1H[87] | ***252800** 3308 | AR | Short and broad neck | Short stature, hirsutism, coarse hair, macrocephaly, abnormal sella turcica, coarse facies, corneal clouding, thick and bushy eyebrows, thick lips, macroglossia, conductive deafness, dysostosis multiplex, osteoporosis, bony restriction of joint mobility, claw hands, aortic or mitral valve abnormalities, hepatosplenomegaly (storage), MR, urinary excretion of dermatan and heparan sulfate, $\alpha$-L-iduronidase enzyme defect |
| Hypochondrogenesis[57] | ***200610** 3940 | AR | Short or webbed neck with excess skin, cystic hygroma | Short stature, short trunk and limbs, hydrops fetalis, macrocephaly, frontal bossing, hypertelorism, midface hypoplasia, short ribs and rib cage, platyspondyly, delayed ossification of the spine, epiphyseal or metaphyseal abnormality, hypotonia, longer survival and milder radiological features than achondrogenesis type 2 |
| Jarco-Levin syndrome or spondylothoracic dysplasia[59] | ***277300** 3410 | AR | Short or webbed neck, low posterior hair line | Short stature, short trunk, prominent occiput, broad forehead, short thorax with malsegmentation of ribs and vertebrae, kyphoscoliosis, inguinal or umbilical hernia, long digits, camptodactyly, syndactyly, respiratory problems, neural tube defects |
| Klippel-Feil anomaly, absent vagina, deafness[7] | **148860** 4329 | AD | Short or webbed neck with excess skin, low posterior hairline, multiple vertebral segmentation, defects include fusion of cervical vertebrae, limited movement of the head | Short stature, absent vagina, agenesis or hypogenesis of the kidneys, ventricular septal defect, conductive deafness |
| Klippel-Feil sequence[31] | ***148900** 3274 | Heterogeneous ?AD | Short or webbed neck, low posterior hairline, limited movement of the head (cervical vertebrae are fused and other vertebral defects, e.g., hemivertebrae, may be found), torticollis | Various associations (may indicate heterogeneity); reported associations include deafness (conductive or sensorineural); renal and cardiac defects, cleft palate, Sprengel deformity, scoliosis, encephalocele, MR |
| Kniest dysplasia or metatropic dwarfism, type 2[24,65] | ***156550** 3272 | AD ?AR | Short neck, atlantoaxial instability or odontoid hypoplasia | Short stature, short trunk and limbs, macrocephaly, round and flat face, midface hypoplasia, cleft palate, high-degree myopia, enlarged joints, progressive limitation of joint mobility, kyphoscoli- |

| Syndrome or condition | MIM No. POSSUM No.[a] | Inheritance[b] | Neck anomalies | Other manifestations |
|---|---|---|---|---|
| | | | | osis, platyspondyly, epiphyseal or metaphyseal abnormality; distinctive "Swiss cheese" chondro-osseous morphology |
| LEOPARD syndrome or Multiple lentigines syndrome[45] | ***151100** 3277 | AD | Short or webbed neck | *LEOPARD* stands for **L**entigines and nevi; **E**CG abnormalities of prolonged PR and QRS and abnormal P waves; **O**cular hypertelorism; **P**ulmonic stenosis and other cardiovascular defects; **A**bnormalities of genitalia; and **D**eafness, sensorineural; mental deficiency is not common |
| Lethal cystic hygroma, cleft palate[22] | 4175 | AR | Webbed neck with excess skin, cystic hygroma | Cleft hard palate, hydrops fetalis |
| Lethal multiple pterygium syndrome[34,58] | **253290** 4255 | AR | Webbed neck with excess skin, neck edema and cystic hygroma | IUGR, hypertelorism, cleft palate, hypoplastic lungs, multiple pterygia (webbing), multiple joint contractures, camptodactyly, talipes deformity, diaphragmatic hernia, stillbirth or neonatal death |
| Limb, pelvis, uterus hypoplasia or aplasia syndrome, or Al-Awadi- Raas-Rothschild syndrome[2,76] | ***276820** 3651 | AR | Short neck | Short forearms with absent ulnae, variable ray deficiency of fingers, radiohumeral synostosis, carpal fusion, one long bone in the lower limbs, rudimentary feet with variable ray deficiency, absent or hypoplastic uterus, normal intelligence |
| Lymphedema-distichiasis syndrome[81] | ***153400** 3744 | AD | Webbed neck with excess skin, edema | Distichiasis (double row of eyelashes) may cause corneal irritation and ulceration, later onset of lymphedema, usually from knee downward; epidural spinal cyst, partial ectropion of the lower lid, cleft soft/hard palate |
| Mandibulofacial dysostosis, Toriello type[91] | ***301950** 4291 | XLR | Webbed neck | Short stature, microcephaly, triangular or asymmetric face, ptosis, midface hypoplasia, broad nasal bridge, micrognathia, preauricular tags or pits, sensorineural or conductive deafness, pulmonic stenosis, MR |
| Marden-Walker syndrome[66] | ***248700** 3284 | AR | Short neck, multiple vertebral segmentation defects including cervical spine | IUGR, short stature, microcephaly, expressionless face, blepharophimosis, microstomia, arthrogryposis, camptodactyly, kyphoscoliosis, cardiac defect, CNS anomalies, hypotonia, seizures, MR |
| Meckel-Grüber syndrome or Dysencephalia splanchnocystica[25,89] | ***249000** 3287 | AR | Short or webbed neck | Occipital encephalocele, cystic kidney, postaxial polydactyly, microcephaly, microphthalmia, micrognathia, liver cysts or fibrosis, early death |
| Metatropic dysplasia or metatropic dwarfism[42] | ***250600** 3300 | AR | Short neck, atlantoaxial instability | Intrauterine dwarfism, severe short stature, apparently short trunk, small thorax, thoracic kyphoscoliosis (may appear in infancy), prominent joints, restricted mobility at large joints, |

**Appendix E** Syndromes and conditions associated with anomalies of the neck *(Continued)*

| Syndrome or condition | MIM No. POSSUM No.[a] | Inheritance[b] | Neck anomalies | Other manifestations |
|---|---|---|---|---|
| | | | | hyperextensibility of finger joints, metaphyseal flaring (develops in childhood), platyspondyly, square iliac wings |
| Morquio syndrome or Mucopolysaccharidosis type 4[55] | ***253000** 3311 | AR | Short neck, ondontoid hypoplasia | Onset of manifestations in early childhood, severe limitation of growth, mild coarse facies, deafness, short trunk, severe kyphosis, pectus carinatum, marked platyspondyly, joint restriction, knock knees, progressive hip degeneration and dislocation, hepatomegaly (storage), normal intelligence, urinary excretion of keratan sulphate; type 4A: N-acetylgalactosamine-6–sulphatase enzyme defect, type 4B: β-galactosidase defect |
| Multiple pterygium syndrome or Escobar syndrome[35] | ***265000** 3472 | AR | Short or webbed neck with excess skin | Short stature, pterygia (webbing) of the neck, axillae, antecubital, popliteal, and intercrural areas; joint contractures, camptodactyly, syndactyly, talipes, deformity, facies with ptosis, antimongoloid slant of palpebral fissures, cleft palate and micrognathia, vertebral anomalies, cryptorchidism |
| Neurofibromatosis-Noonan syndrome[4] (including Watson syndrome) | ***193520** 4205 | AD | Short or webbed neck with excess skin, low posterior hairline | Features of neurofibromatosis (NF-l) such as café-au-lait spots, excessive axillary and inguinal freckling, neurofibromas, and scoliosis, and features of Noonan syndrome (see below); considered a distinct entity |
| Noonan syndrome or Turner-like syndrome[62] | ***163950** 3335 | AD | Short or webbed neck with excess skin, low posterior hairline | Short stature of prenatal onset, broad forehead, hypertelorism, ptosis, antimongoloid slant of palpebral fissures, down-turned mouth angles, posteriorly angulated ears, shield chest, cubitus valgus, vertebral anomalies, pulmonic stenosis, other cardiac defects, cryptorchidism |
| Optiz trigonocephaly syndrome or (C) syndrome[13,52] | ***211750** 3048 | AR | Short, webbed neck with excess skin | IUGR, short stature, trigonocephaly or prominent metopic ridge, upward slanting palpebral fissures, epicanthic folds, broad alveolar ridge, frenulae or small nose, macrostomia, posteriorly angulated ears, hypotonia, omphalocele, contractures, postaxial polydactyly of fingers, syndactyly, preaxial polydactyly of the great toe, cardiac defects, MR; C phenotype is reported with several chromosomal anomalies |
| Pallister-Killian syndrome or Killian-Teschler-Nicola syndrome[70] | 3800 | | Short or webbed neck with excess skin | Short stature, coarse facies, macrostomia, broad and high forehead, sparse scalp hair, pigmentary skin changes, accessory nipples, cardiac defect, diaphragmatic hernia, hypoplastic lungs, caudal appendage, imperforate |

| Syndrome or condition | MIM No. POSSUM No.[a] | Inheritance[b] | Neck anomalies | Other manifestations |
|---|---|---|---|---|
| | | | | anus, hypotonia, seizures, MR, mosaic tetrasomy 12p in fibroblasts |
| Potter sequence[3,61] | ***191830** 3368 | Unknown ?AD ?AR | Webbed neck with excess skin | Phenotype seen in association with renal agenesis or dysplasia and oligohydramnios; microcephaly, loose skin, hypertelorism, semilunar creases below the eyes, cleft lip/palate, low-set ears, ear cartilage deficiency, hypoplastic lungs, diaphragmatic hernia, anal atresia or stenosis, sacral dysgenesis, contractures of large joints, talipes deformity |
| Roberts syndrome or Roberts-SC phocomelia syndrome[83] | ***268300** 3378 | AR | Short neck | Severe growth deficiency, microcephaly, sparse hair, tetramelic or symmetrical limb reduction (more severe in the upper limbs), variable hypoplasia or aplasia of long bones, contractures, midfacial defects, including cleft lip/palate, hypertelorism, broad nasal bridge, and capillary hemangioma; microphthalmia or prominent eyes, malformed ears, cardiac, renal, and CNS anomalies; severe MR |
| SCARF syndrome[49] | **312830** 4739 | XL | Short or webbed neck with excess skin | Craniosynostosis, plagiocephaly, sparse scalp hair, loose skin with excessive wrinkling, sloping forehead with low anterior hairline, hypertelorism, ptosis, broad nasal bridge, deeply grooved philtrum, low-set or posteriorly angulated ears, short sternum, hypoplastic or abnormally placed nipples, ambiguous genitalia, brachydactyly, talipes deformity, borderline-mild MR |
| Schimke immuno-osseous dysplasia[36] | ***242900** 4822 | AR | Short neck, odontoid hypoplasia | IUGR, failure to thrive, short trunk, spondyloepiphyseal dysplasia, progressive renal failure, recurrent infections, lymphopenia and defective cellular immunity, café-au-lait spots, pigmented nevi or lentigines, broad face, broad nasal bridge and tip, hypertelorism |
| Schinzel-Giedion syndrome or Midface-retraction syndrome[50] | **269150** 3025 | AR | Short or webbed neck | Severe postnatal growth deficiency, wide fontanelles and sutures, high forehead, coarse facies, midface hypoplasia, hypertelorism, choanal stenosis, limb shortness (mesomelic), simian creases, hydronephrosis, hypospadias, hypertrichosis, hepatomegaly, CNS and renal abnormalities, skull radiology: steep and short base, wide occipital synchondrosis, wormian bones |
| Schwartz-Jampel syndrome or chondrodystrophia myotonica[26] | ***255800** 3403 | AR | Short or webbed neck | Short stature, myotonia with muscular build, poor facial expression, blepharophimosis, microstoma with inability to widely open the mouth, joint limitation |

**Appendix E** Syndromes and conditions associated with anomalies of the neck *(Continued)*

| Syndrome or condition | MIM No. POSSUM No.[a] | Inheritance[b] | Neck anomalies | Other manifestations |
|---|---|---|---|---|
| | | | | in the hips, wrists, fingers, and spine; platyspondyly, flattening of femoral epiphyses, malignant hyperthermia, normal intelligence |
| Seckel-like with short limbs or Osteodysplastic primordial dwarfism, type 2[72] | ***210720** 3345 | AR | Short or webbed neck | IUGR, short stature, short limbs (acromesomelic), microcephaly with receding forehead, prominent nose with high nasal bridge, micrognathia, epiphyseal, metaphyseal or diaphyseal abnormalities, MR |
| Smith-Lemli-Opitz syndrome, type 2[60] | ***268670** 3645 | AR | Short or webbed neck | IUGR, short limbs (mesomelic), microcephaly, cleft palate, microphthalmia, cataract, short philtrum, tented upper lip, broad alveolar ridge, small tongue, folded ears, contractures of large joints, overlapping fingers and toes, postaxial polydactyly of fingers and toes, syndactyly, cardiac, renal or CNS anomalies, unilobar lungs, ambiguous genitalia, hypotonia, MR, defect in 7–dehydrocholesterol reductase |
| Spondylocostal dysplasia, AD, or costovertebral segmentation anomalies[54] | ***122600** 3393 | AD | Short or webbed neck | Short stature, short trunk, prominent occiput, multiple structural defects of vertebrae and ribs, abnormal rib number, progressive restriction of spinal mobility, scoliosis, thoracolumbar kyphosis, back pain (milder than Jarcho-Levin syndrome) |
| Spondyloepiphyseal dysplasia congenita[67] | ***183900** 3394 | AD | Short neck, odontoid hypoplasia | Short stature, short trunk, and short limbs (striking at birth); flat face, cleft palate, myopia, barrel chest, platyspondyly, kyphoscoliosis, apparently normal hands and feet, lag in epiphyseal mineralization, hypotonia, abnormal gait, proposed gene location 12q13.11–q13.2 |
| Spondyloepiphyseal dysplasia tarda[43] | ***313400** 3395 | XL | Short neck | Onset of manifestation between 5–10 years of age, short stature, short spine with platyspondyly, kyphosis, scoliosis, back and hip pain, hip stiffness, short femoral neck and mild epiphyseal irregularity; often disabling by the age of 60 years; proposed gene location Xp22 |
| Teebi overgrowth syndrome[80] | **277590** 4738 | AR | Short neck with excess skin | Large birth weight, tall stature, sparse scalp hair, macrocephaly, long palpebral fissures, antimongoloid slant, posteriorly angulated ear, large ear lobule, loose skin, joint laxity, long fingers, 5th finger clinodactyly, long great toe, advanced bone age, mild MR |
| Teebi-Shaltout syndrome[28,79] | **272950** 4944 | AR | Hump on the back of the neck | Scaphocephaly, sparse and curly scalp hair, hypertelorism, absent primary teeth, limited opening of the mouth, camptodactyly, sacrococcygeal dimple, caudal appendage |

| Syndrome or condition | MIM No. POSSUM No.[a] | Inheritance[b] | Neck anomalies | Other manifestations |
|---|---|---|---|---|
| Toriello-Carey syndrome[41] | **217980** 4568 | AR | Short or webbed neck | IUGR, microcephaly, blepharophimosis, telecanthus, cleft soft/hard palate, glossoptosis, micrognathia, small hands, cardiac defect, laryngeal abnormality, sensorineural, deafness, CNS anomalies, including agenesis of corpus callosum, seizures, hypotonia |
| Weaver syndrome[16,82] | 3429 | Unknown | Atlantoaxial instability | Macrosomia, rapid growth, advanced skeletal maturation, macrocephaly, brachycephaly, hypertelorism, antimongoloid slant of palpebral fissures, large ears, hoarse cry and voice, camptodactyly, prominent fingertip pads, hypotonia, developmental lag |
| Winchester syndrome[88] | ***277950** 3428 | AR | Atlantoaxial instability or odontoid hypoplasia | Short stature, coarse facies, thickened gingivae, thick lips, osteoporosis, contractures, carpotarsal osteolysis, progressive rheumatoid-like small joint destruction, corneal opacities |
| Yunis-Varon syndrome[1] | ***216340** 3485 | AR | Webbed neck | IUGR, short stature, brachycephaly, absent clavicles, absent thumbs and big toes, hypoplastic distal phalanges, sparse scalp hair, high forehead, small face, short and bulbous nose, micrognathia, malformed ears, hypotonia, MR |

[a]MIM, *M*endelian *I*nheritance in *M*an. A Catalog of Human Genes and Genetic Disorders, by Victor A. McKusick, 11th ed, The Johns Hopkins University Press, Baltimore, 1994; POSSUM, *P*icture *O*f *S*tandard *S*yndromes and *U*ndiagnosed *M*alformations, by Agnes Bankier et al., Murdoch Institute, Royal Children's Hospital, Victoria, Australia.
[b]AD, autosomal dominant; AR, autosomal recessive; XLR, X-linked recessive; XLD, X-linked dominant.
*confirmed gene and inheritance
#phenotype that can be caused by mutation in any of 2 or more genes.

## References


1. Ades LC, Morris LL, Richardson M, Pearson C, Haan EA: Congenital heart malformation in Yunis Varon syndrome. J Med Genet 30:788–792, 1993.
2. Al-Awadi SA, Teebi AS, Farag TI, Naguib KK: Profound limb deficiency, thoracic dystrophy, unusual facies and normal intelligence: a new syndrome? J Med Genet 22:36–38, 1985.
3. Allanson JE, Hunter AGW, Mettler GS, Jimenez C: Renal tubular dysgenesis: a not uncommon autosomal recessive syndrome: a review. Am J Med Genet 43:811–814, 1992.
4. Allanson JE, Upadhyaya M, Watson GH, Partington M, MacKenzie A, Lahey D, MacLeod H, Safarazi M, Broadhead W, Harper PS, Huson SM: Watson syndrome: is it a subtype of type 1 neurofibromatosis? J Med Genet 28:752–756, 1991.
5. Antonarakis SE: Parental origin of the extra chromosome 21 as indicated by analysis of DNA polymorphism. Down syndrome collaborative group. N Engl J Med 324:872–876, 1991.
6. Aymé S, Julian C, Gambarelli D, Mariotti B, Luciani A, Sudan N, Maurin N, Philip N, Serville F, Carles D, Rolland M, Giraud F: Fryns syndrome: report of 8 new cases. Clin Genet 35:191–201, 1989.
7. Baird PA, Lowry RB: Absent vagina and Klippel-Feil anomaly. Am J Obstet Gynecol 118:290–291, 1974.
8. Bankier A, Fortune D, Duke J, Sillence DO: Fibrochondrogenesis in male twins at 24 weeks gestation. Am J Med Genet 38:95–98, 1991.
9. Bawle E, Quigg MH: Ectopia lentis and aortic dilatation in congenital contractural arachnodactyly. Am J Med Genet 42:19–21, 1992.
10. Beighton P: Dyggve-Melchior-Clausen syndrome. J Med Genet 27:512–515, 1990.
11. Blanquet V, Créau-Goldberg N, de Grouchy J, Turleau C: Molecular detection of constitutional deletions in patients with retinoblastoma. Am J Med Genet 39:355–361, 1991.
12. Burton BK, Sumner T, Lager LO Jr, Rimoin DL, Adomian GE, Lachman RS, Nicastro JF, Kelley DL, Weaver RG: A new skeletal dysplasia: clinical, radiologic and pathologic findings. J Pediatr 109:642–648, 1986.
13. Chu TW, Teebi AS, Gibson L, Breg WR, Yang-Feng TL: FISH diagnosis of partial trisomy 13 and tetrasomy 13 in a patient with severe trigonocephaly (C) phenotype. Am J Med Genet 52:92–96, 1994.
14. Clarke JTR, Willard HF, Teshima I, Chang PL, Skomorowski MA: Hunter disease (mucopolysaccharidosis type II) in a karyotypically normal girl. Clin Genet 37:355–362, 1990.
15. Cole H, Huang B, Salbert BA, Brown J, Howard-Peebles PN, Black SH, Dorfmann A, Febles OR, Stevens CA, Jackson-Cook C: Mental retardation and Ulrich-Turner syndrome in cases with 45,X/46X,+mar: additonal support for the loss of the X-inactivation center hypothesis. Am J Med Genet 52:136–145, 1994.
16. Cole TRP, Dennis NR, Hughes HE: Weaver syndrome. J Med Genet 29:332–337, 1992.
17. Dallapicola B, Giannoti A, Lembo A, Sagui L: Autosomal recessive form of whistling face syndrome in sibs. Am J Med Genet 33:542–544, 1989.
18. Davies SJ, Huges HE: Imprinting in Albright's hereditary osteoarthropathy. J Med Genet 30:101–103, 1993.
19. Der Kaloustian VM, Moroz B, McIntosh N, Watters AK, Blaichman S: Costello syndrome. Am J Med Genet 41:69–73, 1991.

20. Diab M, Wu J-J, Shapiro F, Eyre D: Abnormality of type IX collagen in a patient with diastrophic dysplasia. Am J Med Genet 49:402–409, 1994.
21. Drossou-Agakidou V, Andreou A, Soubassi-Griva V, Pandouraki M: Cerebrocostomandibular syndrome in four sibs, two pairs of twins. J Med Genet 28:704–707, 1991.
22. Elejalde BR, de Elejalde MM, Leno J: Nuchal cysts syndromes: etiology, pathogenesis, and prenatal diagnosis. Am J Med Genet 21:417–432, 1985.
23. Evans DGR, Evans ID, Donnai D, Lindenbaum RH: Ankyloblepharon filiform adnatum in trisomy 18 Edwards syndrome. J Med Genet 27:720–721, 1990.
24. Farag TI, Al-Awadi SA, Hunt MC, Satyanath S, Zahran M, Usha R, Uma R: A family with spondyloepimetaphyseal dwarfism: a "new" dysplasia or Kniest disease with autosomal recessive inheritance? J Med Genet 24:597–601, 1987.
25. Farag TI, Usha R, Uma R, Mady SA, Al-Nagdy K, El-Badramany MH: Phenotypic variability in Meckel-Grüber syndrome. Clin Genet 38:176–179, 1990.
26. Figuera LE, Jimenez-Gil J, García-Gruz O, Cantú JM: Schwartz-Jampel syndrome: an atypical form. Am J Med Genet 47:526–528, 1993.
27. Froster UG, Baird PA: Congenital defects of the limbs and alcohol exposure in pregnancy: data from population based study. Am J Med Genet 44:782–785, 1992.
28. Froster UG, Rehder H, Höhn W, Oberheuser F: Craniofacial anomalies, abnormal hair, camptodactyly and caudal appendage (Teebi-Shaltout syndrome): Clinical and autopsy findings. Am J Med Genet 47:717–722, 1993.
29. Fujita M, Flori E, Lemaire F, Casanova R, Astruc D: A new case of "complete" trisomy 5p with isochromosome 5p associated with a de novo translocation t(5;8) (q11;q23). Clin Genet 45:305–397, 1994.
30. Giltay JC, Gerssen-Schoorl KBJ, van der Wagen A: A case of de novo interstitial deletion of chromosome 9 (p12p13). Clin Genet 46:271–272, 1994.
31. Gorlin RJ, Cohen MM, Levin LS: Syndromes of the Head and Neck. 3rd ed, Oxford University Press, New York, 1990, pp 886–889.
32. Gorlin RJ, Winter RB: Frontometaphyseal dysplasia—evidence for X-linked inheritance. Am J Med Genet 5:81–84, 1980.
33. Haeusler G, Frisch H, Guchev Z, Hadziselimovic F, Neuhold A, Vormittag W: Hypoplasia of the corpus callosum and growth hormone deficiency in the XXXXY syndrome. Am J Med Genet 44:230–232, 1992.
34. Hall JG: Editorial comment: the lethal multiple pterygium syndrome. Am J Med Genet 17:803–807, 1984.
35. Hall JG, Reed SD, Rosenbaum KN, Gershanik J, Chen H, Wilson KM: Limb pterygium syndromes: a review and report of eleven patients. Am J Med Genet 12:377–409, 1982.
36. Hashimoto K, Takeuchi A, Ieshima A, Takada M, Kasagi M: Juvenile variant of Schimke immunoosseous dysplasia. Am J Med Genet 49:266–269, 1994.
37. Hing AV, Dowton SB: Aase syndrome: novel radiologic features. Am J Med Genet 45:413–415, 1993.
38. Hornblass A, Refler DM: Ablepharon macrostomia syndrome. Am J Ophthalmol 99:552–556, 1985.
39. Horton WA, Rimoin DL, Lachman RS, Skovby F, Hollister DW, Spranger J, Scott CI, Hall JG: The phenotypic variability of diastrophic dysplasia. J Pediatr 93:609–613, 1978.
40. Hunter AGW, Carpenter BF: Atelosteogenesis 1 and Boomerang dysplasia: a question of nosology. Clin Genet 39:471–480, 1991.
41. Jespers A, Buntinx I, Melis K, Vaerenberg M, Janssens G: Two siblings with midline field defects and Hirschprung disease: variable expression of Toriello-Carey or new syndrome? Am J Med Genet 47:299–302, 1993.
42. Jones KL: Smith's Recognizable Patterns of Human Malformation, 5th ed. WB Saunders, Philadelphia, 1996, p 368.
43. Jones KL: Smith's Recognizable Patterns of Human Malformation, 5th ed. WB Saunders, Philadelphia, 1996, pp 358–359.
44. Jones KL: Smith's Recognizable Patterns of Human Malformation, 5th ed. WB Saunders, Philadelphia, 1996, p 476.
45. Jones KL: Smith's Recognizable Patterns of Human Malformation, 5th ed. WB Saunders, Philadelphia, 1996, p 530.
46. Kapusta L, Brunner HG, Hamel BCJ: Craniofrontonasal dysplasia. Eur J Pediatr 151:837–841, 1992.
47. Karnes PS, Shamban AT, Oslen DR, Fazio MJ, Falk RE: De Barsy syndrome: report of case, literature review, and elastin gene expression studies of the skin. Am J Med Genet 42:29–34, 1992.
48. Kelly TE: Teratogenicity of anticonvulsant drugs: review of the literature. Am J Med Genet 19:413–434, 1984.
49. Koppe R, Kaplan P, Hunter A, MacMurray B: Ambiguous genitalia associated with skeletal abnormalities, cutis laxa, craniostenosis, psychomotor retardation and facial abnormalities (SCARF syndrome). Am J Med Genet 34:305–312, 1989.
50. Labrune P, Lyonnet S, Zupan V, Imbert M-C, Goutieres F, Hubert P, Le Merrer M: Three new cases of the Schinzel-Giedion syndrome and review of the literature. Am J Med Genet 50:90–93, 1994.
51. Lacombe D: Facial palsy and cranial nerve abnormalities in CHARGE association. Am J Med Genet 49:351–352, 1994.
52. Lalatta F, Clerici Bagozzi D, Salmoiraghi MG, Tagliabue P, Tischer C, Zollino M, Di Rocco C, Neri G, Opitz JM: "C" trigonocephaly syndrome: clinical variability and possibility of surgical treatment. Am J Med Genet 37:451–456, 1990.
53. Lindgren Y, Rosinsky B, Chin J, Berry-Kravis E: Two patients with overlapping de novo duplication of the long arm of chromosome 9, including one case with Di George sequence. Am J Med Genet 49:67–73, 1994.
54. Lorenz P, Pupprecht E: Spondylocostal dysostosis—dominant type. Am J Med Genet 35:219–221, 1990.
55. Lowry RB, Snyder FF, Wesenberg RL, Machin GA, Applegarth DA, Morgan K, Carter RJ, Toone JR, Holmes TM, Dewar RD: Morquio syndrome (MPS IV A) and hypophosphatasia in a Hutterite kindred. Am J Med Genet 22:463–475, 1985.
56. Maraia R, Saal HM, Wangsa D: A chromosome 17p de novo paracentric inversion in a patient with campomelic dysplasia; case report and etiologic hypothesis. Clin Genet 39:401–408, 1991.
57. Maroteaux P, Stanescu V, Stanescu R: Hypochondrogenesis. Eur J Pediatr 141:14–22, 1983.
58. Martin NJ, Hill JB, Cooper DH, O'Brien GD, Masel JP: Lethal multiple pterygium syndrome: three consecutive cases in one family. Am J Med Genet 24:295–304, 1986.
59. McCall CP, Hudgins L, Cloutier M, Greenstein RM, Cassidy SB: Jarcho-Levin syndrome: unusual survival in a classical case. Am J Med Genet 49:328–332, 1994.
60. McKeever PA, Young ID: Smith-Lemli-Opitz syndrome II: a disorder of the fetal adrenals? J Med Genet 27:465–466, 1990.
61. McPherson E, Carey J, Kramer A, Hall JG, Pauli RM, Schimke RN, Tasin MG: Dominantly inherited renal dysplasia. Am J Med Genet 26:863–872, 1987.
62. Mendez HM, Opitz JM: Noonan syndrome—a review. Am J Med Genet 21:493–506, 1985.
63. Moser HW: Peroxisomal diseases. Adv Pediatr 36:1–38, 1989.
64. Nevin NC, Herron B, Armstrong MJ: An 18 week fetus with Elejalde syndrome (acrocephalopolydactylous dysplasia). Clin Dysmorph 3:180–184, 1994.
65. Poole AR, Pidoux I, Reiner A, Rosenberg L, Hollister D, Murray L, Rimoin DL: Kniest dysplasia is characterized by an apparent abnormal processing of C-propeptide of type II cartilage collagen resulting in imperfect fibril assembly. J Clin Invest 81:579–589, 1988.
66. Ramer JC, Frankel CA, Ladda RL: Marden-Walker phenotype: spectrum of variability in three infants. J Med Genet 45:285–291, 1993.
67. Ramesar R, Beighton P: Spondyloepiphyseal dysplasia in a Cape Town family: linkage with the gene for type II collagen (COL2A1). Am J Med Genet 43:833–838, 1992.
68. Reynolds JF, Neri G, Herrmann JP, Blumberg B, Goldwell JG, Miles PV, Opitz JM: New multiple congenital anomalies/mental retardation syndrome with cardio-facio-cutaneous involvement—the CFC syndrome. Am J Med Genet 25:413–427, 1986.
69. Robinson WP, Binkert F, Schinzel AA, Basaran S, Mikelsaar R: Multiple R: Multiple origins of X chromosome tetrasomy. J Med Genet 31:424–425, 1994.
70. Schinzel A: Tetrasomy 12p (Pallister-Killian syndrome). J Med Genet 28:122–125, 1991.
71. Schinzel A: Catalogue of Unbalanced Chromosome Aberrations of Man, Walter de Gruyter, Berlin 1984, p 142.
72. Shebib S, Hugosson C, Sakati N, Nyhan WL: Osteodysplastic variant of primordial dwarfism. Am J Med Genet 40:146–150, 1991.
73. Spranger J, Maroteaux P, Der Kaloustian VM: The Dyggve-Melchior-Clausen syndrome. Radiology 114:415–421, 1975.
74. Stratton RF, DuPont R, Mattern VL, Young RS, McCourt JW, Moore CM: Trisomy 22 confirmed by fluorescent in situ hybridization. Am J Med Genet 46:109–112, 1993.
75. Taybi H: Cephalo-skeletal dysplasia and microcephalic osteodysplastic primordial dwarfism. Pediatr Radiol 22:476, 1992.

76. Teebi AS: Limb/pelvis/uterus—hypoplasia/aplasia syndrome. J Med Genet 30:397, 1993.
77. Teebi AS, Gibson L, McGrath J, Meyn MS, Berg WR, Yang-Feng TL: Molecular and cytogenetic characterization of 9p- anomalies. Am J Med Genet 46:288–292, 1993.
78. Teebi AS, Shaabani IS: Further delineation of Costello syndrome. Am J Med Genet 47:166–168, 1993.
79. Teebi AS, Shaltout AA: New syndrome: craniofacial anomalies, abnormal hair, camptodactyly, and caudal appendage. Am J Med Genet 33:58–60, 1989.
80. Teebi AS, Sunderashan TS, Hammouri MY, Al-Awadi SA, Al-Saleh QA: A new autosomal recessive disorder resembling Weaver syndrome. Am J Med Genet 33:479–482, 1989.
81. Temple IK, Collin JRO: Distichiasis—lymphoedema syndrome: a family report. Clin Dysmorph 3:139–142, 1994.
82. Thompson EM, Hill S, Leonard JV, Pembrey ME: A girl with the Weaver syndrome. J Med Genet 24:232–234, 1987.
83. Van Den Berg DJ, Francke U: Roberts syndrome: a review of 100 cases and a new rating system for severity. Am J Med Genet 47:1104–1123, 1993.
84. Voiculescu I, Toder R, Back E, Osswald P, Schempp W: A retrospective CISS hybridization analysis of a case with de novo translocation t(18;22) resulting in an 18p- syndrome. Clin Genet 43:318–320, 1993.
85. Viljoen D: Congenital contractural arachnodactyly (Beals syndrome). J Med Genet 31:640–643, 1994.
86. Wassman ER Jr, Rimoin DL: Cervicomedullary compression with achondroplasia. J Pediatr 113:411, 1988.
87. Watts RWE, Spellacy E, Adams JH: Neuropathological and clinical correlations in Hurler disease. J Inherit Metab Dis 9:261–272, 1986.
88. Winter RM: Winchester's syndrome. J Med Genet 26:772–775, 1989.
89. Wright C, Healicon R, English C, Burn J: Meckel syndrome: what are the minimum diagnostic criteria? J Med Genet 31:482–485, 1994.
90. Wyandt HE, Milunsky J, Lerner T, Gusella JE, Hou A, MacDonald M, Adekunle S, Milunsky A: Characterization of a duplication in the terminal band of 4p by molecular cytogenetics. Am J Med Genet 46:72–76, 1993.
91. Zelante L, Vigliaroli L, Mingarelli R, Dallapicola B: Confirmation of the mandibulofacial dysostosis, Toriello type. Am J Med Genet 45:534–535, 1993.
92. Zoll B, Wolf J, Lensing-Hebben D, Pruggmayer M, Thorpe B: Trisomy 13 (Patau syndrome) with an 11–year survival. Clin Genet 43:46–50, 1993.

# VII

# THE LARYNX

# 18

# Embryology of the Larynx

JOHN J. MANOUKIAN and ANDRÉ K. TAN

The study of the primordial tissues serves several important functions: (1) understanding of normal relationships of body (organ) structures, (2) understanding of physiological changes, (3) appreciation of the development of congenital anomalies, and (4) management of patients with these anomalies.

The incidence of congenital laryngeal anomalies varies from 1:10,000 to 1:50,000 births.[23] They present with a very wide spectrum of clinical manifestations, ranging from minimal morbidity, such as dysphonia, to mortality due to acute airway obstruction.

## Evolution of the human respiratory tract

Classical postmortem dissections[14,25] and radiographic and cineradiographic studies[7,9] have shown that the position of the larynx plays a major role in determining the mechanisms of breathing, swallowing, and vocalization.[14,25]

In most mammals, the position of the larynx is extremely high in the neck, corresponding to the first to third or fourth cervical vertebrae (1–4).[17] Such an observation is also noted in nonhuman primates. In humans infants, the upper respiratory tract is similar to that of primates with a larynx located high in the neck at cervical vertebral levels of C1–4. This infant larynx migrates to a lower position at the age of 1½ to 2 years. By adulthood, the larynx is positioned at the levels of C4–7.[6]

By studying the pharyngolaryngeal position in our fossil ancestors, pioneer work by J.T. Laitman and co-workers demonstrated the relationship between basicranium flexion and the location of upper respiratory tract structures by using extant (living) primate models.[11,12] Their work showed that a nonflexed basicranium corresponds to a superiorly positioned larynx, while a flexed basicranium suggests a larynx located inferiorly in the neck. They were able to demonstrate that early hominids, like australopithecines of 1½ to 4 millions years ago, had nonflexed basicrania similar to that of primates.[10] The first evidence of basicranial flexion is noted in specimens of *Homo erectus* (early member of our own genus *Homo*).[6]

A larynx located high in the neck means that the epiglottis is positioned behind the soft palate, thus allowing direct passage of air from the nasal cavity towards the larynx and subsequently into the trachea and lungs. At the same time, food can pass into the esophagus through the piriform sinuses via the lateral food channels.[4,14] This separation of the respiratory and digestive tracts allows the organism to breath and swallow simultaneously. However, such a larynx provides a rather small supralaryngeal portion of the pharynx. This significantly decreases the range of sounds that an organism can produce by limiting the area for sound modification in the supralaryngeal pharynx. By contrast, an inferiorly located larynx means a crossover of the respiratory and digestive tracts superior to the larynx. This provides the ability to produce a wider range of sounds in a larger supralaryngeal pharynx.[6]

Because of the high postition of the larynx, infants of modern humans resemble early humanoids and primates in breathing, swallowing, and vocalization, as demonstrated by Laitman and co-workers.[7,18] The ability for the human infant to separate the respiratory and digestive passages permits uninterrupted deglutition during breathing or crying and vocalization. From an evolutionary point of view, such an ability is traded off for a more advantageous facility: the capability to produce a wider range of sounds with an inferiorly positioned larynx and larger supralaryngeal pharynx. It is obvious that such an evolutionary and developmental gain is crucial to human speech development and communication.

## Staging of development

Human development is divided into prenatal and postnatal periods. The prenatal period is further subdivided into embryonic and fetal periods (Fig. 18–1).

The embryonic period of human development constitutes roughly the first 8 weeks after conception. The standard for staging human embryonic development is the Carnegie system. Mall, the first director of the Carnegie Institution of Washington's Department of Embryology, started the Carnegie collection of human embryos in 1887.[20] He was the first investigator to describe human embryonic development in stages. This system classifies the human embryonic development into 23 stages. Instead of using embryo size or supposed chronological age, each of the 23 stages is defined by specific morphological characteristics.

The fetal period of human development is not classified into stages. This is a period of organ maturation following the embryonic organogenesis. In addition, physiologic activity and integration of organ systems take place.[22]

After birth, the larynx migrates from a relatively high position in the neck at about 2 years of age into a more inferior position. This descent of the larynx determines the manner in which a child breathes, swallows, and vocalizes.

### Prenatal development

#### Embryonic development

The larynx develops from the endodermal lining of the laryngotracheal tube (pharyngeal groove) of the foregut and the surrounding mesenchyme. This takes place between the fourth and sixth branchial arches. From *stages 1 to 8* of the Carnegie sys-

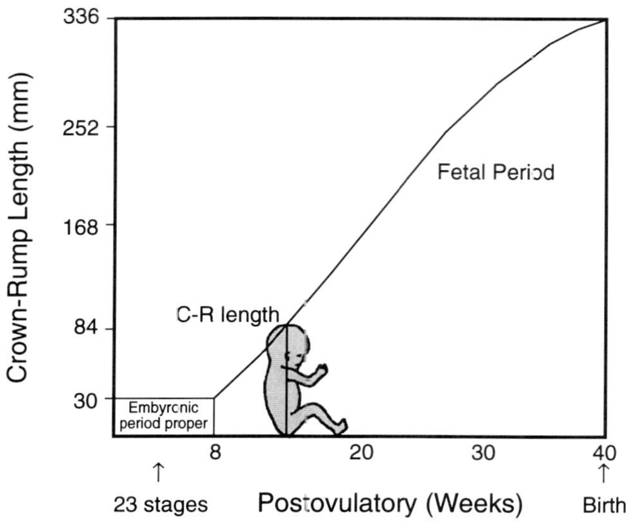


**Fig. 18–1.** The embryonic period proper, the first 8 weeks of development, is shown in relation to the fetal period. Crown-rump length of fetus is also shown. (With permission from JA Tucker and GF Tucker, Jr: Some aspects of fetal laryngeal development. Ann Otol Rhinol Laryngol 84:49–55, 1975.[21])

tem, the foregut is not identifiable and there is no evidence of development of the upper respiratory tract.

The foregut of the embryo first appears around the 20th day of age *(stage 9)*. A medially located pharyngeal groove can be identified. From this groove, the respiratory system develops.

At about 22 days of age *(stage 10),* with the continual growth of the pharyngeal groove, the primitive pharynx is evident with several pharyngeal arches and pouches.[15] The laryngeal sulcus and pulmonary primordium can also be identified.

Around 24 days of age *(stage 11),* the pulmonary primordium divides into the left and right lobes (lung buds).

On the 26th day of embryonic life *(stage 12),* the pulmonary primordium migrates caudally into the mesenchyme ventral to the foregut. This is the stage when the "respiratory tap" proposed by O'Rahilly and Müller[15] is turned on. According to this concept, the tracheoesophageal separation point remains fixed, while the tracheal bifurcation (lung buds) descends. This is an important stage because, from this stage onwards, the respiratory and digestive tracts develop separately. They can be distinguished from one another. The mesenchymal tissue separating the lung buds' and foregut's epithelia is termed the *tracheoesophageal septum* (Fig. 18–2).

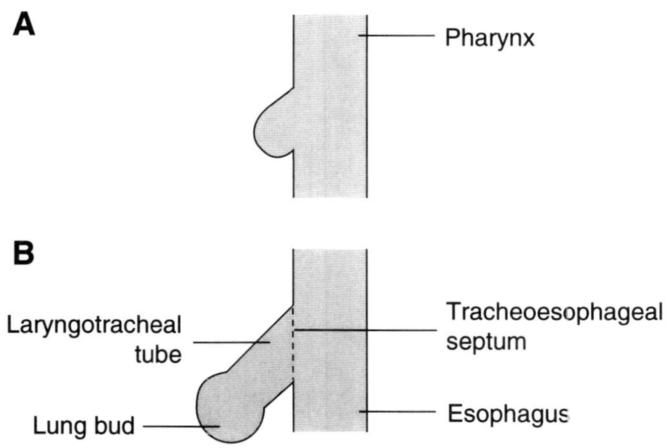


**Fig. 18–2.** Appearance of tracheoesophageal septum at stage 12 of embryonic development separating foregut into esophagus and laryngotracheal tube.

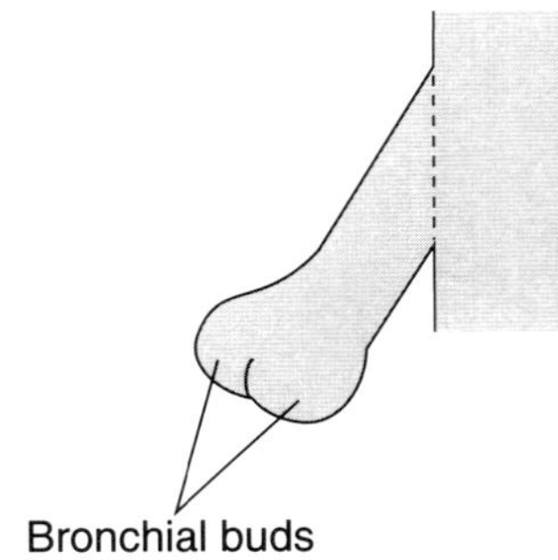


**Fig. 18–3.** Foregut at stage 13 of embryonic development showing appearance of left and right lung buds.

At *stage 13* the embryo is about 28 days old. At this point the left and right lung buds become more evident and the trachea can be identified with elongation of both the respiratory tract, esophagus, and the tracheoesophageal septum (Fig. 18–3).

At approximately 32 days of age *(stage 14),* on the floor of the pharynx, mesenchymal proliferation rapidly produces the hypopharyngeal eminence and arytenoid swelling. These swellings convert the vertically oriented laryngotracheal groove into a T-shaped primitive laryngeal aditus (Fig. 18–4). When the arytenoid swellings continue to grow and expand, median compression of the laryngeal groove causes the formation of the epithelial lamina by means of epithelial fusion (Fig. 18–5). Walander suggests, however, that according to a rat model, the epithelial lamina is a solid ventral outgrowth of the laryngeal groove.[24] While the origin of the epithelial lamina remains unsettled, it is important to realize that the development of the larynx depends on the initial formation, proliferation, and sequential cavitation of the lamina.[2,16]

At *stage 15* the embryo is about 33 days of age. Angiogenesis surrounding the primitive bronchi can now be identified. The capillary plexus distinguishes the esophagus and tracheobronchial tree. The laryngeal primordium as well as the superior laryngeal nerve become evident.

At about 37 days of age *(stage 16),* bilateral budding outgrowths within the epithelial lamina can be identified and become patent. They are the vestibulotracheal and pharyngotracheal canals. The recurrent laryngeal nerve is also seen.

At *stage 17* (40 days), the larynx and the epiglottis are clearly identifiable. Laryngeal cartilages (thyroid, cricoid, and epiglottis) and intrinsic musculature are seen as mesenchymal condensations. Tracheal condensation also becomes evident. The bronchopulmonary segments bud out peripherally from the tracheobronchial tree and invaginate the pleura.

At *stage 18* the embryo is about 44 days of age. Laryngeal cartilage condensation is most obvious ventrally and dorsally, with lateral thinning providing a slit-like appearance. The cricoid proliferates rapidly to a complete ring structure with a circular lumen.

At *stage 19,* the embryo is about 48 days of age. The epiglottis achieves its concave shape. Examination shows a well-

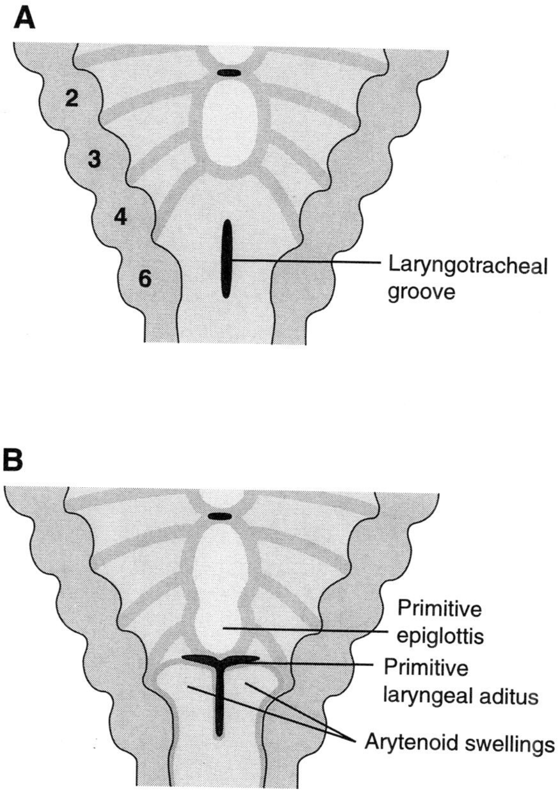


**Fig. 18–4.** Development of larynx at stage 14 showing the vertically oriented laryngotracheal groove (A) converting into a T-shaped primitive laryngeal aditus by arytenoid swellings (B).

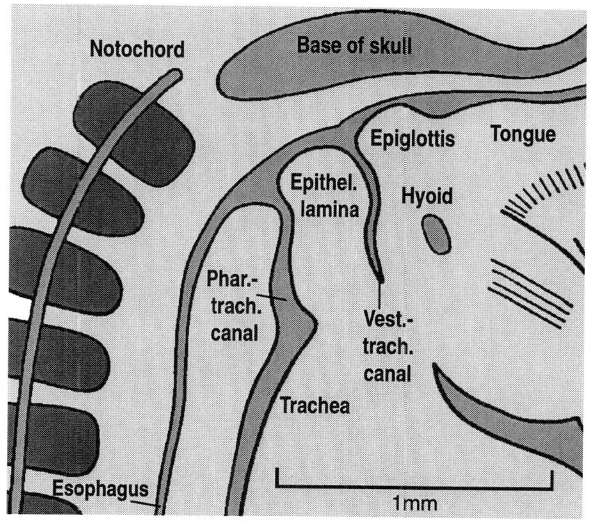


**Fig. 18–6.** Median section through the neck of a human embryo at stage 19. (With permission from JA Tucker and R O'Rahilly: Observations on the embryology of the human larynx. Ann Otol Rhinol Laryngol 81:520–523, 1972.[20])

differentiated striated musculature with innervation. The subsegmental bronchi of first generation are formed (Fig. 18–6).

At about 51 days of age *(stage 20),* the hyoid cartilage is evident. Second generation subsegmental bronchi are seen. (Fig. 18–7).

At about 52 days of age *(stage 21),* the thyroid gland can be identified at the location below and lateral to the cricoid cartilage. At this stage, all major bronchial buds are present.

*Stages 22–23* are reached at approximately 57 days of age. They mark the end of the embryonic development. The larynx can be identified clearly as an organ with supporting cartilages and musculature. The membrane of the vocal muscle can also be seen.[13] The epithelial lamina undergoes dissolution at this stage of cellular rearrangement and growth.[2] It should be noted that the respiratory tract epithelium resembles the pharynx while the esophagus is lined by pseudostratified columnar cells with a basement membrane.

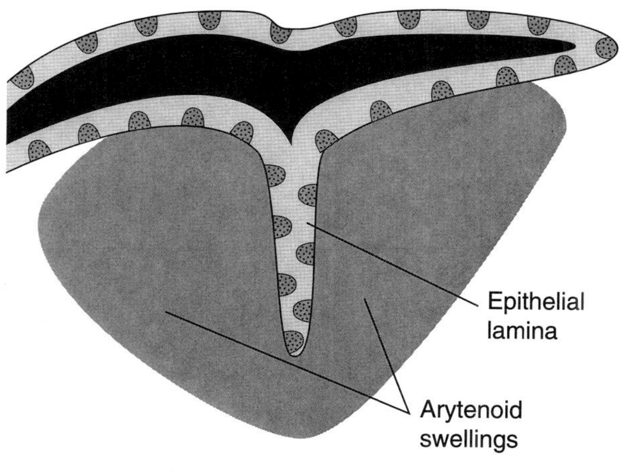


**Fig. 18–5.** Median compression of laryngeal groove (aditus) by arytenoid swellings causes formation of epithelial lamina.

### Fetal development

By the end of the embryonic developmental period, the fetus is approximately 9 weeks of age and about 30 mm in crown-rump (C-R) length. Fetal development is not described in stages. It covers the period from the age of 3 gestational months to full term. According to the Carnegie system, the fetal period begins with bone marrow formation in the humerus.[19,21]

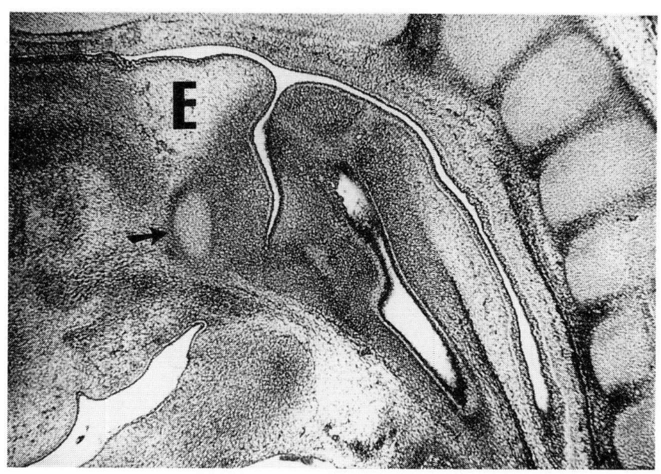


**Fig. 18–7.** Sagittal section through the neck of a human embryo at stage 20. The hyoid cartilage (arrow) is evident below the forming epiglottis (E). (With permission from JA Tucker, Carnegie Collection, 8226.)

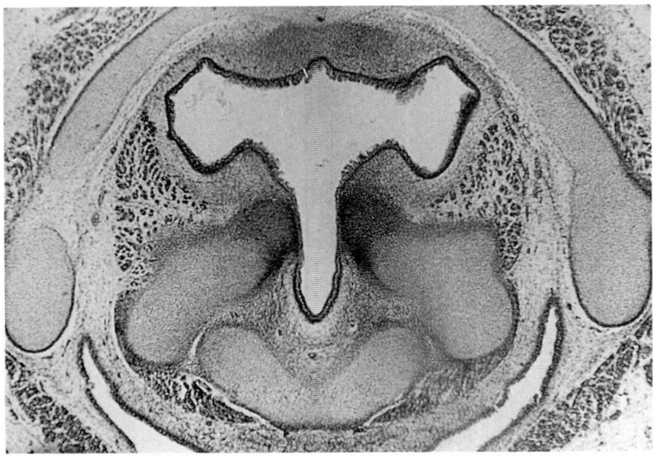

**Fig. 18–8.** Transverse section of larynx at weeks 9–12 of fetal period. (With permission from JA Tucker, Carnegie Collection, 3990.)

During the *third month,* or the 9th to the 12th week of gestation (Fig. 18–8), laryngeal growth includes the cartilaginous development of the vocal process of the arytenoids, ventral fusion of the thyroid cartilage laminae, and cricoid maturation. At about 10 weeks of age cartilage development is evident in the trachea and the primary bronchi. Ciliation of the esophagus occurs. The swallowing mechanism can be observed.[21]

In the *fourth month,* or the period between 13 and 16 weeks of gestation, laryngeal cartilaginous growth continues. Goblet cells and submucosal glands develop from the endoderm. During this period a different phase of tracheobronchial development, known as the *pseudoglandular phase,* begins. Dichotomous branching and multiplication of the bronchial tree occur.[5] The fetal breathing mechanism can be identified. Ciliation of the entire tracheobronchial tree is now complete.

During the *fifth to seventh months,* between 17 to 28 weeks gestational age, the epiglottis matures and fibroelastic cartilage appears. The cuneiform and corniculate cartilages can be identified (Fig. 18–9). The alveoli begin to produce surfactant between the 24th and 26th weeks.

The last fetal period covers the *8th month to term.* The fetus achieves a C-R length of about 300 mm by the end of 40 weeks of gestational age. The important event of this period is the change from interstitial growth to perichondrial growth of the cricoid cartilage. For more detailed description of the development of the cartilaginous tracheobronchial tree, the reader is referred to the study by Bucher and Reid.[1]

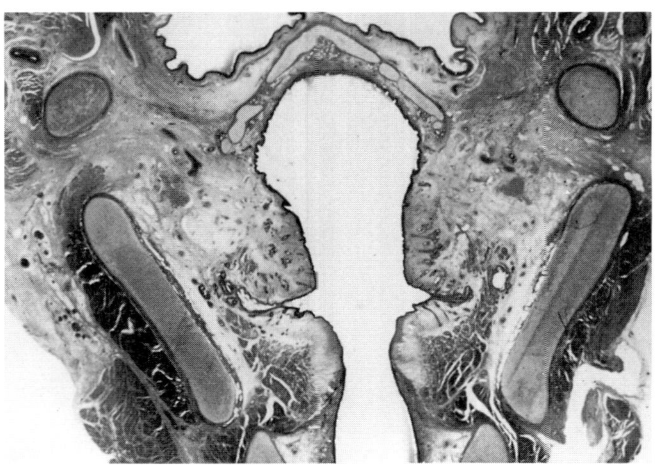

**Fig. 18–9.** Coronal section of larynx at weeks 17–28 of fetal period. (With permission from JA Tucker, Tucker Collection, 27.)

### Postnatal development

This period of human development is described neither by stages nor specific time periods. Rather, each organ system continues to grow and mature. Before it achieves its adult form and position, the infant larynx undergoes four basic maneuvers: (1) disproportional growth of laryngeal elements, (2) change in axis, (3) elongation, and (4) change of intralumenal shape.

During the *first 3 years* after birth, the larynx grows rapidly. The increase in size however, is not proportional for each element. The arytenoids remain relatively the same size while the rest of the larynx continues to grow. Thus, the arytenoids become smaller relative to the glottic chink. (Fig. 18–10).

The larynx, which is in a relatively high cervical position at birth, begins to assume a new position in the neck around the age of 18 months to 2 years. This migration is most noticeable at 2 years of age and continues until the age of approximately 6 years. During this period, the larynx and corresponding musculature descend from a relatively high cervical position of C1–4 to C4–7. This descent also allows a change in axis. In the infant, the vocal cords lie at an off-horizontal axis as they tend to slope inferiorly from posterior to anterior. In the adult, the vocal cords lie at a horizontal axis. The vertical axis of the infant's larynx also changes from an anteriorly curved position to a relatively straight vertical line.

Another important change in the infant's larynx is known as the *accordion effect.* The once overlapping hyoid and thyroid, as well as the thyroid and cricoid cartilages, become separated as the larynx grows and elongates vertically. This lengthening is best described as the elongation of the accordion.

Cricoid maturation continues well into the first decade[3] and occurs proportional to the glottic chink. In the pediatric larynx, the lumen is funnel-shaped with its apex at the subglottic area. In other words, the narrowest region of the pediatric larynx is at the subglottic area. In the adult, the subglottic region is wider than the glottic chink, and loses its funnel-shape appearance.

A thorough understanding of the embyrological, fetal, and postnatal development of the human larynx illuminates its anatomy and also helps the otolaryngologist and head and neck sur-

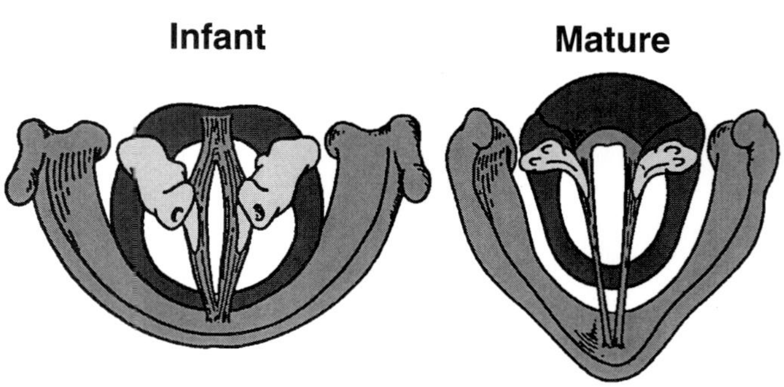


**Fig. 18–10.** Comparison of infant and adult larynx showing large arytenoids in infant in relation to glottic chink. The triangular-shaped thyroid of the mature larynx is also noted.

geon to appreciate the significance of specific congenital anomalies and to successfully manage the airway.

## References


1. Bucher U, Reid L: Development of the intrasegmental bronchial tree: the pattern of branching and development of cartilage at various stages of intra-uterine life. Thorax 16:207–218, 1961.
2. De Vries PA, De Vries CR: Embryology and development. In: The Pediatric Airway, H Bieman et al. eds. The Principles and Practice of the Pediatric Surgical Specialties, SL Gans, ed. WB Saunders, Philadelphia, 1991, pp 3–16.
3. Hawkins DB: Hyaline membrane disease of the neonate; prolonged intubation in management: effects on the larynx. Laryngoscope 88:201–224, 1978.
4. Humphrey T: The development of mouth opening and related reflexes involving oral area of human fetuses. Alabama J Med Sci 5:126–157, 1968.
5. Hutchins GM, Haupt HM, Moore GW: A proposed mechanism for the early development of the human tracheobronchial tree. Anat Rec 201:635–640, 1981.
6. Laitman JT: The Ontogenetic and Phylogenetic Development of the Upper Respiratory System and Basicranium in Man. Ph.D. dissertation, Yale University, New Haven, 1977.
7. Laitman JT, Crelin ES: Developmental change in the upper respiratory system of human infants. Perinatol/Neonatol 4:15–22, 1980.
8. Laitman JT, Crelin ES: Tantalum markers as an aid in identifying the upper respiratory structures of experimental animals. Lab Anim Sci 30:245–248, 1980.
9. Laitman JT, Crelin ES, Conlogue GJ: The function of the epiglottis in monkey and man. Yale J Biol Med 50:43–48, 1977.
10. Laitman JT, Heimbuch RC: The basicranium of Plio-Pleistocene hominids as an indicator of their upper respiratory systems. Am J Phys Anthropol 59:323–343, 1982.
11. Laitman JT, Heimbuch RC: Evolutionary biology and behavior. In: The Pygmy Chimpanzee, RL Susman, ed. Plenum, New York, 1984, pp 49–63.
12. Laitman JT, Heimbuch RC, Crelin ES: Developmental change in a basicranial line and its relationship to the upper respiratory system in living primates. Am J Anat 152:467–482, 1978.
13. Müller F, O'Rahilly R, Tucker J: The human larynx at the end of the embryonic period proper: the laryngeal and infrahyoid muscles and their innervation. Acta Otolaryngol 91:322–323, 1981.
14. Negus VE: The Biology of Respiration. E and S Livingstone, London, 1965.
15. O'Rahilly R, Müller F: Chevalier Jackson lecture. Respiratory and alimentary relations in staged human embryos. New embryological data and congenital anomalies. Ann Otol Rhinol Laryngol 93:421–429, 1984.
16. O'Rahilly R, Tucker JA: The early development of the larynx in staged human embryos. I. Embryos of the first five weeks (to stage 15). Ann Otol Rhinol Laryngol 82:1–27, 1973.
17. Reidenberg JS, Laitman JT: Position of the larynx in odontoceti (toothed whales). Anat Rec 218:98–106, 1987.
18. Sasaki CT, Levine PA, Laitman JT, Crelin ES: Postnatal descent of the epiglottis in man. A preliminary report. Arch Otolaryngol 103:169–171, 1977.
19. Smith EI: The early development of the trachea and esophagus in relation to atresia of the esophagus and tracheoesophageal fistula. Contrib Embryol Carnegie Inst 36:41–57, 1957.
20. Tucker JA, O'Rahilly R: Observations on the embryology of the human larynx. Ann Otol Rhinol Laryngol 81:520–523, 1972.
21. Tucker JA, Tucker GF: Some aspects of fetal laryngeal development. Ann Otol Rhinol Laryngol 84:49–55, 1975.
22. Tucker JA, Tucker GF: The Development of the Cricoid Cartilage in Staged Human Embryos and in Fetuses. Collegium, ORLAS, Munich, 1984.
23. Van den Broek P, Brinkman WFB: Congenital laryngeal defects. Int J Pediatr Otorhinolaryngol 1:71–78, 1979.
24. Walander A: Prenatal development of the epithelial primordium of the larynx in rat. Acta Anat 10 (Suppl 13):520–523, 1950.
25. Wind J: On the Phylogeny and Ontogeny of the Human Larynx: A Morphological and Functional Study. Walters-Noordhoff, Groningen, 1970.

# 19

# Congenital Anomalies of the Larynx

J. PAUL WILLGING and ROBIN T. COTTON

Abnormalities of the airway frequently present with stridor. Stridor is not a diagnosis, but rather a physical sign of turbulent airflow through a partial obstruction of the airway. Stridor may be inspiratory, expiratory, or biphasic, depending upon the location of the obstruction in the laryngotracheal airway. Severe airway obstruction need not be associated with stridor, however. The rate of airflow past an obstruction may be inadequate to generate audible turbulent airflow. Patients with stridor require immediate evaluation as significant respiratory compromise and death may occur if proper treatment is not initiated in a timely fashion.

Stridor in the infant is due to pathology of the larynx in 60% of cases.[16] Tracheal lesions account for 15% of cases, while bronchial lesions, infectious, and miscellaneous causes account for 25% of the cases of stridor. Congenital anomalies of the larynx not only impede the ventilatory function of the larynx, producing stridor, but also impair its ability to protect the lower respiratory tract. Feeding difficulties may result, presenting as frank dysphasia or subtle aspiration. The extent of laryngeal dysfunction is directly proportional to the degree of laryngeal disturbance. Symptoms of congenital laryngeal anomalies frequently present at birth but may be delayed. The common congenital laryngeal anomalies will be discussed with regard to their clinical presentation and management.

## Laryngomalacia

Laryngomalacia is the most common congenital laryngeal anomaly. It accounts for 60% of the laryngeal anomalies of the neonate.[16] Males are affected twice as often as females. It is generally a self-limiting condition, but may produce life-threatening obstructive apnea, cor pulmonale, and failure to thrive when severe.

Symptoms of laryngomalacia generally present within the first 2 weeks of life. Inspiratory stridor and noisy respiration are noted, and are more pronounced when the child is agitated. The airway noise is frequently related to position. A supine position is classically more aggravating to the condition than a prone position; a reclining position during feeding may also increase the degree of stridor. Neck extension will frequently decrease the intensity of airway noise. Symptoms increase over the first several months. Affected infants will maintain a normal cry without cyanosis. Dyspnea is rarely experienced and feeding difficulties are not uncommon. A gradual resolution of symptoms usually occurs by the age of 18 months.

The stridor of laryngomalacia develops from the partial obstruction of the supraglottic airway (Fig. 19–1). The epiglottis if frequently elongated and tightly curved upon itself, creating an omega shape to the cartilage. The epiglottis prolapses posteriorly on inspiration.[22] The epiglottis is derived from the third and fourth branchial arches. Overgrowth of the superior third arch derivative, elongates the epiglottis and causes lateral inward curling.[18] Prone positioning of the child allows the epiglottis to rest anteriorly, minimizing the obstruction.

The arytenoids in patients with laryngomalacia have a redundant mucosal covering. The bulky arytenoid masses prolapse anteriorly on inspiration.[22] It has been postulated that neurologic immaturity of the brain stem causes inadequate coordination of the laryngeal musculature, resulting in the paradoxical arytenoid movement on inspiration.[23]

The aryepiglottic folds of the larynx with laryngomalacia are foreshortened.[22] The supraglottic laryngeal structures are therefore tethered in a position partially obstructing the laryngeal inlet. The circumferential rimming of the supraglottic airway by the flaccid, redundant tissues of the epiglottis, arytenoids, and aryepiglottic folds produces the fluttering quality of the inspiratory noise associated with laryngomalacia. Expiration forces these tissues out of the airway and generally produces no noise.

While several explanations have been proposed for the development of laryngomalacia, none properly explain the distribution of the condition in the population. Most theories incorporate an element of immaturity, either of the cartilaginous elements or neuromuscular control, to account for the supraglottic structures being drawn into the supraglottic airway.[2] These theories would predict an increased representation of premature infants and infants with hypotonia. The premature infant does not appear to be at an increased risk for the development of laryngomalacia.[31] The hypotonic infant is difficult to evaluate, as hypopharyngeal collapse and glossoptosis seem to exert a much greater effect on the airway than the laryngomalacia that may be evident. Histologic studies of the larynx of laryngomalacia patients have failed to demonstrate any significant alterations of the cartilaginous or muscular elements to account for the clinical findings of laryngomalacia. Much work remains to be done to define the factors involved with the development of laryngomalacia.

Radiographic studies may suggest the diagnosis of laryngomalacia. There is frequently medial and inferior displacement of the arytenoids and epiglottis. Because this is a dynamic process, the film must be taken during inspiration to identify the abnormalities. Fluoroscopy is better able to illustrate the dynamic nature of the problem and demonstrate the collapse of the supraglottic structures with inspiration. Hypopharyngeal dilation is also seen on inspiration, accentuating the laryngeal obstruction. Chest radiographs should also be obtained to rule out associated anomalies of the lower respiratory tract, such as innominate artery compression, tracheomalacia, and vascular rings.

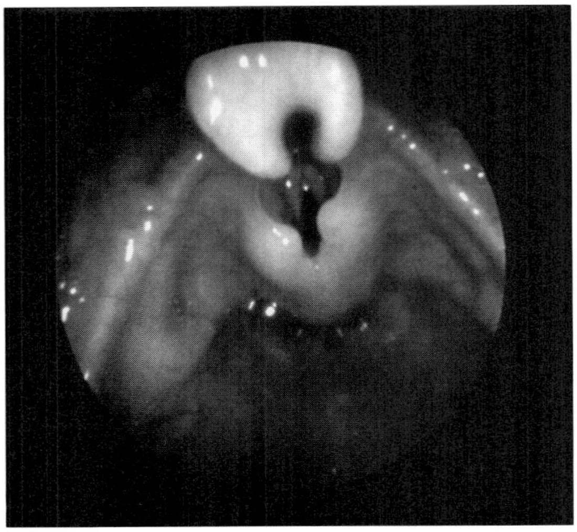

**Fig. 19–1.** Laryngomalacia is characterized by a long epiglottis, redundant mucosa covering the arytenoid cartilages, and short aryepiglottic folds.

The mainstay of diagnosis for laryngomalacia is flexible laryngoscopy. A long, omega-shaped epiglottis is visualized anteriorly, with large, bulky arytenoids posteriorly. Upon inspiration, the supraglottic structures collapse, creating a small, slit-like channel leading to the glottis. A determination can often be made as to the relative obstruction caused by the epiglottis and by the arytenoids. Prone positioning is more effective in improving the airway obstructed by a retrodisplacing epiglottis. In contrast, airway obstruction caused by the anterior prolapse of the arytenoids is improved by a supine positioning of the patient. The vocal cords in laryngomalacia are mobile. With increasing severity of the laryngomalacia, the ability to visualize the vocal cords, however, decreases. In severe cases of laryngomalacia, the vocal cords cannot be seen due to the supraglottic collapse.

The majority of patients with laryngomalacia require no intervention. Continued vigilance on the part of the otolaryngologist is required to ensure adequate feeding abilities, continued growth, and that the child is not developing significant breathing difficulties. In patients with obstructive apnea, failure to thrive, or other complications related to airway compromise, surgical intervention may be required.

Tracheotomy has in the past been the preferred surgical procedure for severe laryngomalacia. The area of obstruction was bypassed until the supraglottic pathology spontaneously resolved. Epiglottoplasty is an alternative method that has proven successful in the correction of the supraglottic obstruction and that has avoided the need for tracheotomy. Direct laryngoscopy and bronchoscopy must be performed prior to the epiglottoplasty to rule out concomitant pathology contributing to the obstruction of the airway. The larynx is then suspended, and the lateral edges of the epiglottis are trimmed, as well as the redundant arytenoid mucosa. A wedge is removed from the aryepiglottic folds allowing the epiglottis to spring anteriorly, increasing the dimension of the laryngeal inlet (Fig. 19–2). The patients are usually left intubated overnight with extubation the following morning.[31] Antibiotic coverage is maintained for 5 days to prevent supraglottic infection. Gastroesophageal reflux is associated with laryngomalacia. Perioperative use of antireflux measures (positioning and medications) is recommended to minimize the effect of gastric secretions on raw mucosal surfaces. Cautious excision of mucosa must be exercised to prevent the possibility of supraglottic stenosis.

## Vocal cord paralysis

Vocal cord paralysis is the second-most common congenital laryngeal anomaly. It accounts for 15% of congenital anomalies of the larynx.[16] The paralysis may be unilateral or bilateral.

The symptoms of unilateral vocal cord paralysis may be

A

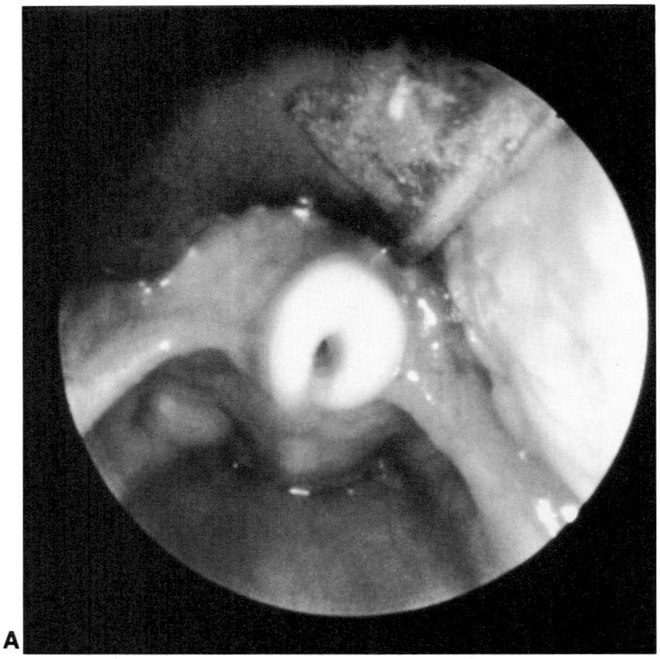

B

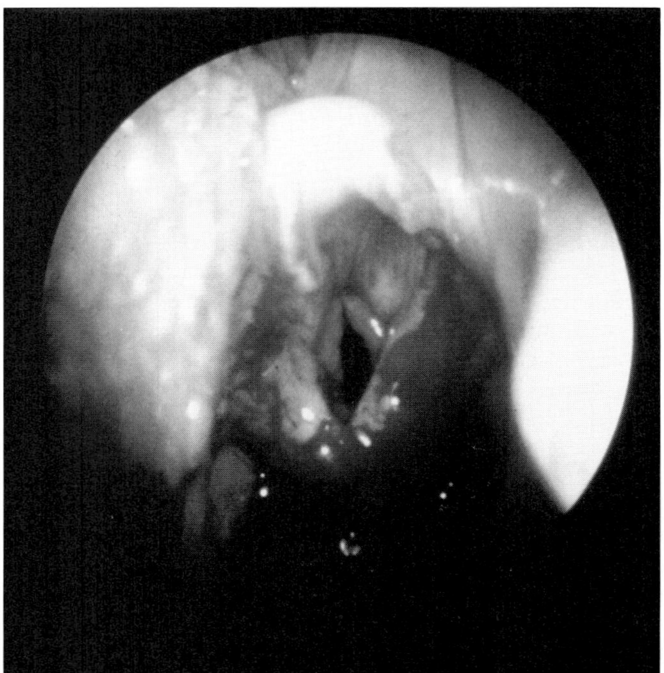

**Fig. 19–2.** A: A severe laryngomalacia with obstructive apnea and oxygen desaturation. B: Larynx immediately after epiglottoplasty showing redundant mucosa removed from arytenoid cartilages, trimming of the lateral edges of the epiglottic cartilage, and division of the aryepiglottic folds.

present at birth or may develop over the first several weeks of life. Unilateral paralysis is often well tolerated by the neonate and delayed diagnosis is not uncommon. Airway obstruction is minimal, and stridor is apparent only with periods of aggravation or stress. A weak or hoarse, breathy cry is commonly present with unilateral paralysis. Feeding difficulties, such as aspiration, may be present but are generally manageable without surgical intervention. Positioning the patient with the paralyzed vocal cord superior during feeding, combined with thickening agents when necessary, allow adequate nutritional intake in the majority of patients. Positioning the patient with the paralyzed vocal cord down will often improve the airway during periods of quiet respiration.

Bilateral vocal cord paralysis presents with acute airway distress. The cry is normal and there is a characteristic high-pitched inspiratory stridor that is present at rest and markedly exacerbated with agitation. Bilateral vocal cord paralysis is poorly tolerated in the neonate. Emergent intubation is frequently required to stabilize the airway, followed by tracheotomy.

The diagnosis of vocal cord paralysis is made by flexible laryngoscopy. Direct laryngoscopy and bronchoscopy are generally reserved for cases of bilateral vocal cord paralysis and cases of unilateral paralysis which demonstrate significant airway distress, where concomitant pathology of the airway may exist.

The etiology of congenital vocal cord paralysis is secondary to a neurologic abnormality. In general, bilateral paralysis is secondary to a central problem, while unilateral paralysis is caused by injury to the peripheral nervous system.[13] The entire course of the recurrent laryngeal nerve must be evaluated in cases of unilateral vocal cord paralysis. A chest X-ray may demonstrate cardiac or great vessel anomalies that impinge on the recurrent laryngeal nerve. The left recurrent laryngeal nerve is more prone to injury than the right, due to the longer course that the nerve takes through the neck and mediastinum.[13] The birth history may elicit a clue as to the etiology of the paralysis. A difficult delivery may result in stretching of the neck, with traction on the recurrent laryngeal nerve that may cause a unilateral paralysis.

Bilateral vocal cord paralysis is usually due to a central disorder. Head ultrasound or computed tomography is necessary to diagnose intracerebral hemorrhage, cerebral agenesis, hydrocephalus, or Arnold-Chiari malformation of the brain stem with herniation. Multiple cranial nerve deficits are common in cases of bilateral vocal cord paralysis. As a result, the incidence of chronic aspiration and dysphasia is increased in these patients. The majority of cases of vocal cord paralysis will have no identifiable cause.

Treatment of patients with vocal cord paralysis is generally supportive. Unilateral cases rarely require surgical intervention. Patients with bilateral vocal cord paralysis frequently require tracheotomy to bypass the glottic obstruction and to also provide access to aspirated materials in the airway. Observation for a minimum of 1 to 2 years is advised to allow for a spontaneous recovery. Should vocal cord function fail to return after this time, lateralization procedures, arytenoidectomy, or partial cordectomy procedures may be considered.[26]

## Congenital subglottic stenosis

Congenital subglottic stenosis is the third-most common laryngeal anomaly, accounting for 15% of cases. The etiology of congenital subglottic stenosis is felt to be failure of the laryngeal lumen to recanalize after it was obliterated during the eighth week of gestation. This mesenchyme condensation within the laryngeal lumen is recanalized beginning during the tenth week of gestation, to re-establish the laryngeal lumen.[28] Complete arrest of the process of recanalization will lead to complete laryngeal atresia. Incomplete recanalization will result in various degrees of subglottic stenosis with symptoms ranging from mild to severe. Children with mild to moderate congenital subglottic stenosis will have no symptoms until the airway is further narrowed by processes such as an upper respiratory tract infection. Recurrent croup may be the only clue to the diagnosis of a congenitally small subglottis. When the subglottic airway is narrowed to the point of generating symptoms, the voice will remain normal, but progressive respiratory difficulty will ensue with biphasic stridor, dyspnea, and marked suprasternal and intercostal retractions.

A complete physical examination should be performed to rule out any associated anomalies. Flexible laryngoscopy is essential to document vocal cord mobility. The telescope should not be passed below the level of the true vocal cords in order to avoid the severe vasovagal reflexes that are stimulated when the subglottis is irritated. Radiographs contribute information as to the location and extent of the subglottic stenosis.[11] High kilovoltage anteroposterior (AP) projections of the neck demonstrate lateral obstruction of the airway. The mainstay of diagnosis for subglottic stenosis, however, is rigid endoscopy. Under general anesthesia, the entire laryngeal–tracheal airway can be directly examined. The length of the stenosis as well as its thickness can be determined. An objective measurement of the residual laryngeal lumen can also be obtained by passing an endotracheal tube of known outside diameter through the stenosis.[24]

Subglottic stenosis is present when the airway lumen of the cricoid region of the airway measures less than 4 mm in a full-term infant, or 3 mm in a premature infant. It is difficult to determine the true incidence of congenital subglottic stenosis, as many patients are intubated in the neonatal period, and therefore by definition would be considered as having an acquired subglottic stenosis.

Congenital subglottic stenosis can be divided histopathologically into membranous and cartilaginous types. The membranous form of congenital subglottic stenosis is generally circumferential and soft to palpation with an instrument. The mucosa lining the subglottis is thickened secondarily due to an increase in the fibrous connective tissue layer of the submucosa. Hyperplasia and dilation of the mucous glands may also add to the thickness of the obstruction.

The cartilaginous variety of congenital subglottic stenosis is variable in its appearance. Mild cases have a normal-shaped subglottic lumen, but the caliber of the lumen is diminished. More commonly, the cricoid cartilage is abnormally shaped, having prominent lateral shelves. This creates a subglottic lumen with an elliptical appearance (Fig. 19–3).

The condition of most patients with congenital subglottic stenosis improves with age. Less than half of the patients with congenital subglottic stenosis will require a tracheotomy for maintenance of their airway.[19] There are cases that will require laryngeal reconstruction. In general, the reconstructive procedures required for congenital lesions are less radical than those required for the acquired subglottic lesions.[7]

Congenital subglottic stenosis may arise as an isolated anomaly or may be associated with other congenital lesions or syndromes. Down syndrome, for example, is well recognized as

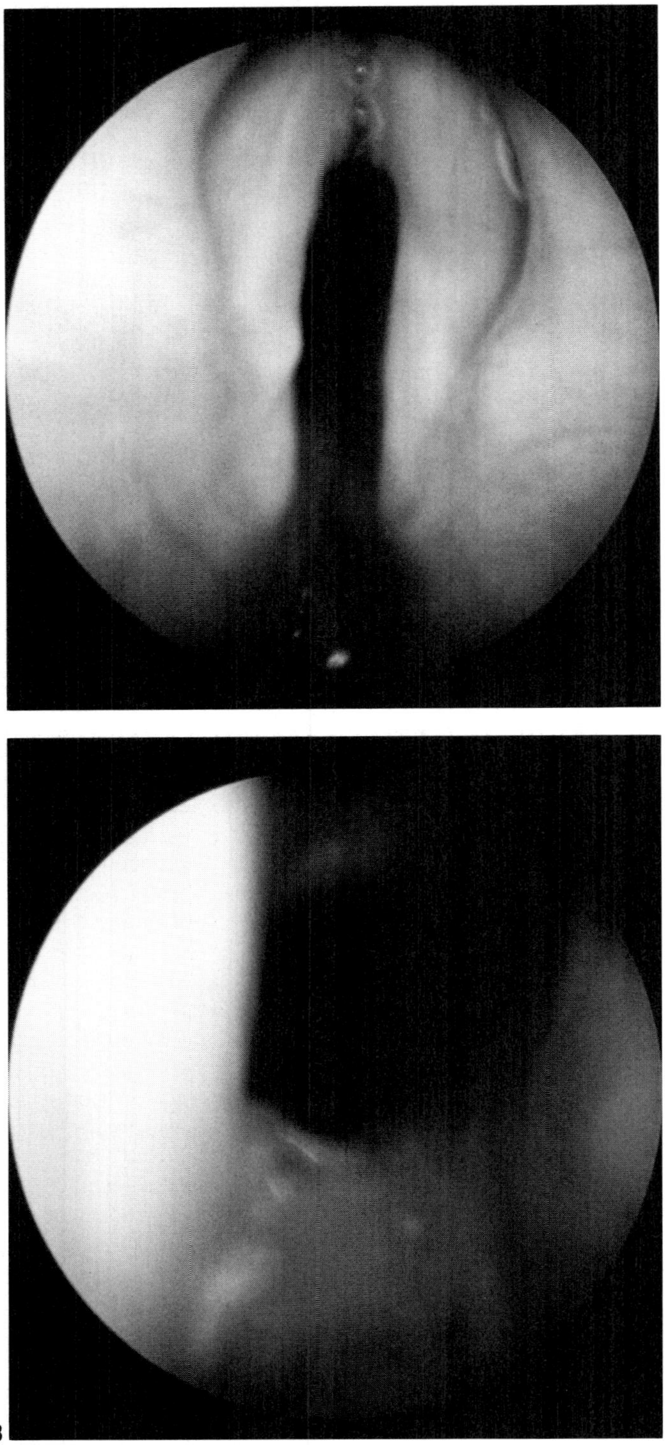

A

B

**Fig. 19–3.** A: Defective recanalization of the laryngeal lumen in the first trimester of gestation leads to diminished subglottic dimensions at delivery. B: An elliptical lumen results because of the prominent lateral cartilaginous shelves.

having a subglottis that is smaller than normal by one-half an endotracheal tube size. Routine intubation for all children must be approached with caution, as a congenitally small larynx can be significantly injured by an inappropriately-sized endotracheal tube.

## Laryngeal web

Part of the constellation of anomalies arising from defects in the recanalization of the larynx during the first trimester of gestation, the laryngeal web is a membrane of varying thickness that occludes the glottic lumen. Symptoms range from complete airway obstruction when the web completely obstructs the glottis to varying degrees of dysphonia. Intervention, therefore, ranges from observation to emergent tracheotomy in the delivery room.

Laryngeal webs should be evaluated endoscopically under general anesthesia to determine the extent of the defect at the glottic level, as well as its inferior extent into the subglottis. The web is generally located anteriorly, with a persistent posterior glottic opening. The thickness of the web is variable. Some webs are thin and transparent, involving only the vocal cords. Other webs are thick fibrous structures that fix the vocal cords and extend interiorly to obstruct the subglottic lumen.[5] A lateral, high-kilovoltage X-ray of the neck will demonstrate the extent of the lesion. The majority of laryngeal webs will demonstrate a "sail sign" on the X-ray, showing the anterior subglottic obstruction that is the remnant of the embryonic intraluminal laryngeal plug (Fig. 19–4).

Treatment of laryngeal webs must be modified according to the thickness of the membrane. Very thin, translucent webs will respond to endoscopic division with a knife or laser. More commonly, the web is thick anteriorly and will require an open repair with placement of a keel and temporary tracheotomy (Fig. 19–5). The keel is removed after 10 days. Follow-up endoscopy is necessary to monitor the final healing process. Additional dilations or laser procedures may be required to maximize voice quality postoperatively.[26]

## Laryngeal atresia

Laryngeal atresia is considered the rarest of all congenital laryngeal anomalies.[14] Laryngeal atresia is not compatible with life without emergent establishment of an airway. The airway must be established in the delivery room based on the clinical presentation of the neonate. The infant's color is good at birth but rapidly deteriorates with clamping of the umbilical cord. Active respiratory efforts are seen with intercostal and suprasternal retractions, but no airway is generated. The infant has no cry. Intubation attempts are unsuccessful. Tracheotomy is necessary to establish an alternative airway.

The diagnosis of laryngeal atresia is made endoscopically, after establishment of the alternative airway (Fig. 19–6). A persistent pharyngotracheal duct may be found posteriorly in the postcricoid area. This duct is not of adequate caliber to maintain ventilation. A tracheoesophageal fistula may be present, which at times may be of adequate size to permit mask ventilation, increasing the time available for the performance of the tracheotomy.

Laryngeal atresia is associated with maternal polyhydramnios. Maternal ultrasound allows the potential for prenatal diagnosis of the atresia.[30] With advanced knowledge of a potential airway problem at birth, a select team can be assembled in the delivery room to manage the infant's airway. The umbilical cord can be left intact to assist in oxygenation of the child while the tracheotomy is being performed.

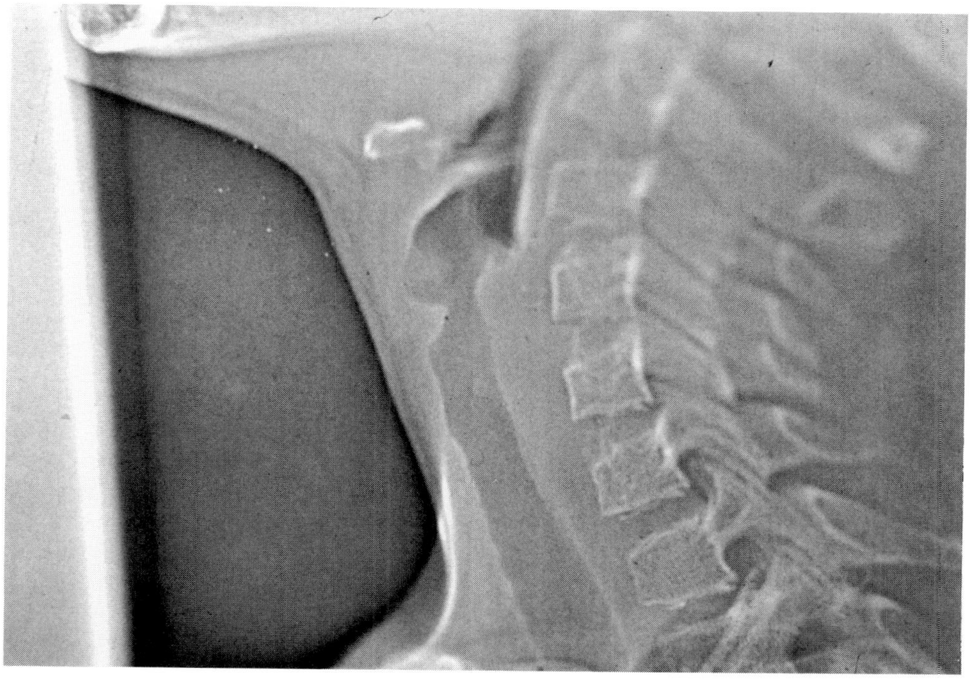

**Fig. 19–4.** Laryngeal webs generally have significant subglottic extension. This lateral neck X-ray demonstrates the involvement of the anterior subglottis. It is this subglottic extension that is responsible for the failure of many endoscopic repairs of laryngeal webs.

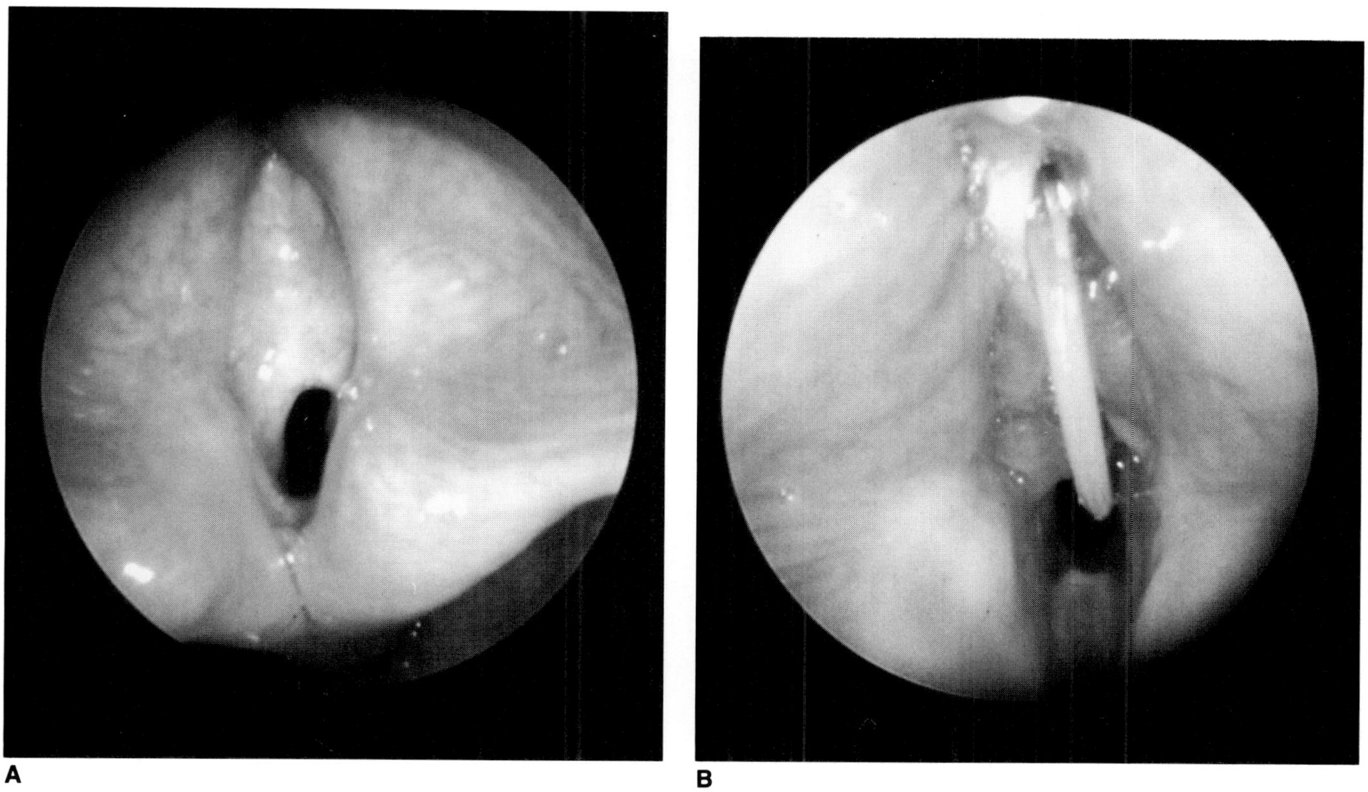

A B

**Fig. 19–5.** A: Congenital glottic web with residual posterior lumen. B: Thick anterior extension into the subglottis necessitates laryngofissure with keel placement for adequate repair.

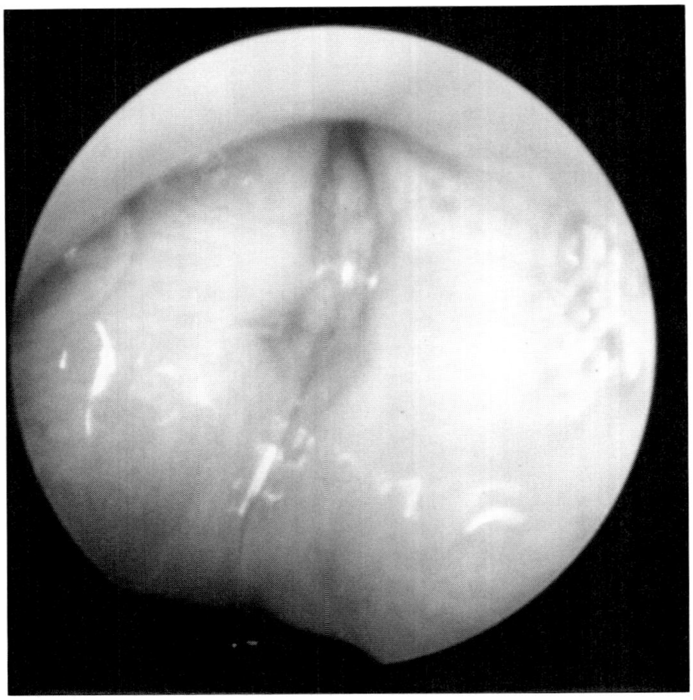

**Fig. 19–6.** Tracheotomy has been previously established to bypass this complete laryngeal atresia.

## Laryngeal cleft

The trachea and esophagus share a common lumen during embryogenesis. The tracheoesophageal septum separates these two structures by the 35th day of gestation.[21] Failure of the interarytenoid tissue or the cricoid cartilage to fuse in the posterior midline will result in a laryngeal cleft.[20] Incomplete formation of the tracheoesophageal septum produces a tracheoesophageal fistula. A high mortality rate is associated with laryngeal clefts, approaching 50%.[12] The mortality is a consequence of the delay in diagnosis and respiratory distress secondary to repeated episodes of aspiration. Multiple associated anomalies may exist concurrently with a laryngeal cleft (Table 19–1) which contribute to the overall mortality of this condition.[12]

Patients with laryngeal clefts present with aspiration and cyanosis during feeding. Increased tracheal secretions with occasional stridor may be noted. Voice abnormalities are present in many patients. Gastroesophageal reflux is a major contributor to the overall pulmonary embarrassment that develops with a laryngeal cleft. The severity of symptoms is related to the extent of the laryngeal cleft. Approximately 20% of patients with a laryngeal cleft will have a tracheoesophageal fistula, further increasing the risk of aspiration and respiratory failure.

Several classification systems exist for laryngeal clefts. The Evans classification system has four types.[3] The type I cleft extends into the interarytenoid notch but does not extend below the vocal cords or into the posterior cricoid lamina. Type II is a partial cleft through the cricoid cartilage, extending below the vocal cords but not completely through the posterior cricoid plate. Type III is a total cricoid cleft extending into the cervical trachea. Type IV is a laryngotracheoesophageal cleft, extending into the mediastinum.

**Table 19–1.** Anomalies associated with laryngeal cleft

| |
|---|
| Tracheoesophageal fistula |
| Laryngomalacia |
| Cleft lip and palate |
| Subglottic stenosis |
| Pulmonary anomalies: tracheal shortening, hypoplastic lungs |
| Cardiovascular defects: transposition of great vessels |
| Hamartomas |
| Gastrointestinal abnormalities: imperforate anus, rectal stenosis, mesenteric malrotation, Meckel's diverticulum |
| Genitourinary abnormalities: hypospadias, hypoplastic kidneys |

From Eriksen et al.[12]

Patients suspected of having a laryngeal cleft require radiographic evaluation. Chest radiographs may demonstrate nonspecific infiltrates suggestive of aspiration pneumonia. Contrast esophagrams may show spillover of the barium into the larynx or trachea. Laryngeal clefts are difficult to visualize radiographically. Frequently, multiple studies must be performed prior to demonstrating the defect.

Endoscopy is required to definitively make the diagnosis of a laryngeal cleft (Fig. 19–7). A high index of suspicion is required to identify type I and type II defects. Placement of an anterior commissure scope into the larynx will splay the posterior larynx and demonstrate the inferior extent of the cleft. Great care must be taken to document the relationship of the cleft to the level of the vocal cords.

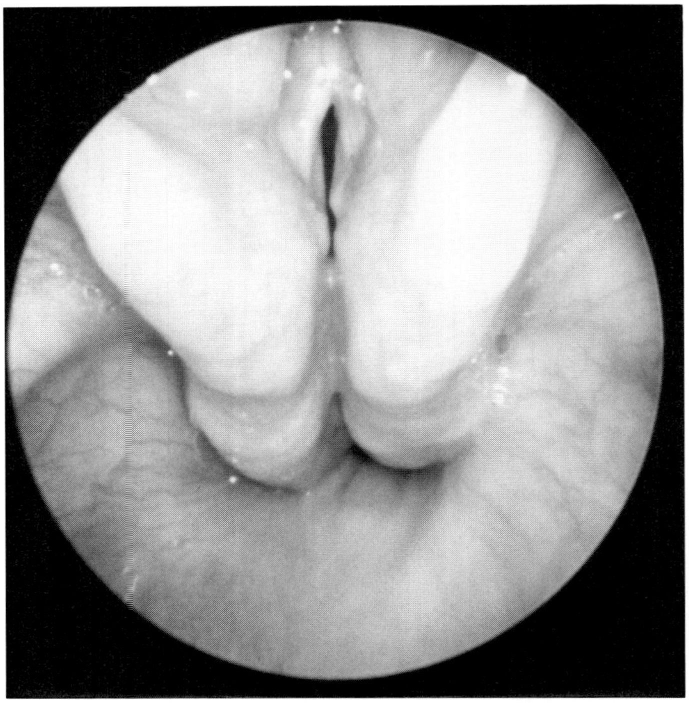

**Fig. 19–7.** Example of an Evans type III laryngeal cleft. Deep interarytenoid notching is evident. Placement of an anterior commissure scope splays the posterior larynx, allowing visualization of the inferior extent of the cleft.

Management of patients with a laryngeal cleft begins with protection of the airway from aspiration and maintenance of respiratory support. Nearly all patients will require tracheotomy, but endotracheal intubation can temporize the situation until the child is medically stable to undergo the procedure. Gastroesophageal reflux is commonly associated with laryngeal cleft and must be managed aggressively. Reverse Trendelenburg positioning and antireflux medications should be implemented. Gastrostomy and Nissen fundoplication must be considered in cases of refractory reflux.

The surgical approach for repair of the laryngeal cleft is dictated by the extent of the defect. Extensive clefts require a lateral pharyngotomy with creation of laterally-based flaps to allow multilayer closure of the cleft. The anterior laryngofissure generally provides adequate exposure for clefts as extensive as type III defects.[8] Complications include recurrent laryngeal nerve injury, breakdown of the repair site, excessive granulation tissue formation at the repair site, continued aspiration, and posterior glottic stenosis.[8]

## Laryngeal cysts

Congenital laryngeal saccular cysts are usually found within the aryepiglottic folds or between the true and false vocal cords (Fig. 19–8).[17] They differ from laryngoceles in that saccular cysts have no communication with the endolaryngeal lumen and are filled with mucous. When the 1 mm saccular orifice is obstructed, the saccule dilates with retained secretions.[10] They account for one-fourth of all laryngeal cysts. Laryngoceles are air-containing dilations of the saccule, which maintain a patent saccule orifice connecting to the laryngeal ventricle.

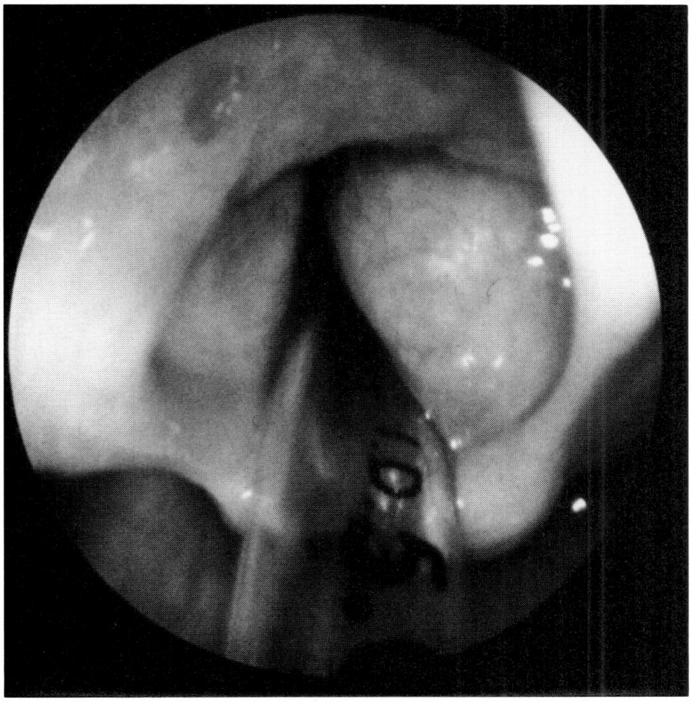

**Fig. 19–8.** Saccular cysts frequently present as a fullness within the aryepiglottic folds or within the false vocal cords, causing compromise.

Patients present with stridor and varying degrees of airway obstructions. Emergent intervention is occasionally required in the newborn. Endotracheal intubation is generally possible, as the cyst is compressible. Needle aspiration of the cyst may be used to temporize a critical airway but will generally lead to reaccumulation of fluid within the cyst.

Definitive treatment requires unroofing of the cyst and removal of the cyst lining. This can be done mechanically or by destroying the lining with a $CO_2$ laser.[29] Postoperative intubation until the laryngeal edema resolves obviates the need for tracheotomy in most cases. Recurrent lesions require an external approach for adequate exposure and excision of the cyst.

## Subglottic hemangioma

Subglottic hemangiomas are uncommon lesions accounting for 1.5% of all congenital laryngeal anomalies.[18] There is a 2:1 female predominance. Fifty percent of children with subglottic hemangioma will have cutaneous hemangioma. The lesion is a benign congenital vascular malformation derived from mesodermal rests.[1] The lesions demonstrate two distinct growth forms. The infantile hemangioma is composed of capillary-sized vessels, while the adult hemangioma develops large cavernous dilations. The lesion generally develops within the first 2 months of life. Subglottic hemangiomas are characterized by a rapid growth phase, which generally subsides by 1 year of age. A slow resolution phase ensues, leading in many instances to complete resolution of the lesion by 5 years of age.[25]

Patients with subglottic hemangioma are asymptomatic at birth. During the first few months of life the lesion increases in size, causing intermittent airway obstruction. There are no voice changes. With continued growth of the lesion, biphasic stridor develops and acute respiratory distress is not uncommon.

Neck X-rays will demonstrate an asymmetric narrowing of the subglottis on the A-P view and a posterior subglottic mass on the lateral film. Flexible laryngoscopy will demonstrate a normal supraglottic larynx with mobile vocal cords. Occasionally, a subglottic fullness can be seen. The definitive diagnosis requires direct laryngoscopy under general anesthesia. The lesion will have a pink or blue hue and appear as a smooth submucosal mass. The lesion is easily compressible. Hemangiomas classically arise from the posterolateral aspect of the subglottis (Fig. 19–9). The endoscopic appearance of the lesion is generally diagnostic, and biopsy is rarely required. Procurement of a biopsy is controversial, due to the risk of hemorrhage.[27]

Treatment of subglottic hemangioma must be tailored to the degree of airway obstruction. Observation may be appropriate for very small lesions, but most lesions require surgical intervention to manage the airway obstruction resulting from the mass. As the natural history of the lesion is one of complete resolution, retaining complete and normal laryngeal function, all interventions must leave the larynx in normal condition. Overly aggressive surgical intervention may result in severe complications, such as subglottic stenosis.[9] In many instances, tracheotomy is the best treatment modality, which allows the obstruction to be bypassed while giving the lesion time to spontaneously regress.

The $CO_2$ laser has the ability to decrease the size of the lesion while causing minimal edema and adjacent tissue injury.

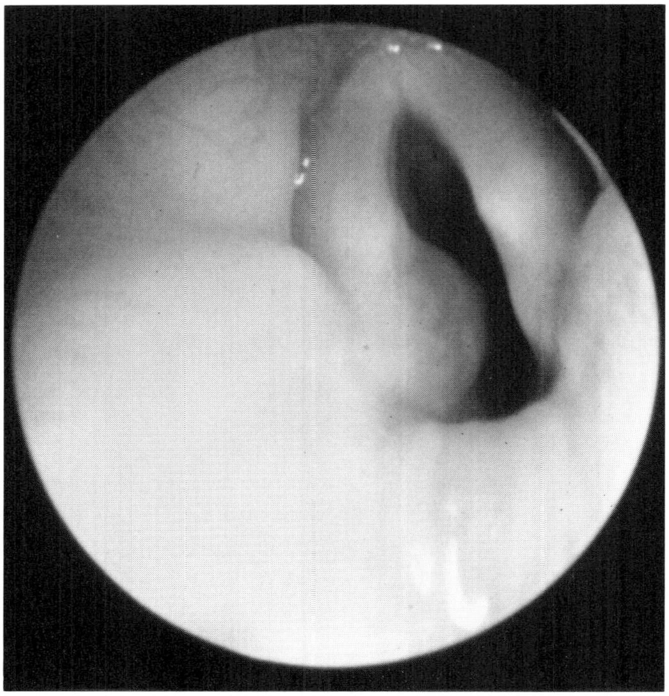

**Fig. 19–9.** Subglottic hemangioma generally present as a submucosal mass with a pink or blue hue. They often arise from the postero-lateral aspect of the subglottis.

The laser is most effective on capillary hemangioma, as the vessel size is such that hemorrhage is minimal. Vessels of cavernous hemangioma are generally beyond the ability of the $CO_2$ laser to adequately coagulate.

Steroids may be used as an adjunctive treatment for subglottic hemangioma. Steroids occupy estradiol sites and are felt to inhibit any supportive functions estradiol exhibits on hemangioma growth.[15] Steroids may also sensitize the microvasculature of the hemangioma to circulating endogenous vasoconstrictors that may lead to spontaneous involution.

Subglottic hemangiomas generally require surgical management. Tracheotomy alone should be considered for the majority of patients to ensure preservation of normal laryngeal structure and function. Judicious use of the laser may be appropriate for moderately sized lesions in an attempt to avoid tracheotomy.

## Lymphangioma

Lymphangiomas are uncommon malformations of the lymphatic system. They are derived from the same endodermal elements as those found in the developing venous system. Primary involvement of the larynx is rare, while secondary involvement by compressive effects of the mass is more common.[6] The lesion presents within the neonatal period in 50% of cases and 75% of cases are diagnosed within the first year of life.

Lymphangiomas are divided into three morphologic groups. Lymphangioma simplex is a lesion of capillary-size lymphatics. The cavernous lymphangioma is composed of dilated lymphatic channels. The cystic hygroma contains discrete cystic spaces. Lymphangiomas have no malignant potential but the invasive growth pattern decreases the likelihood of complete excision.[4]

Presenting symptoms of laryngeal lymphangioma relate to airway obstruction and voice alteration. Indirect laryngeal involvement from compressive effects of the lesions located in the floor of the mouth or tongue cause dysphagia and aspiration difficulties. Lymphangiomas have unpredictable growth potential and tremendous increases in the size of the lesion are possible when associated with upper respiratory tract infections (Fig. 19–10).

Treatment of laryngeal lymphangiomas is discouraging. The majority of patients will require tracheotomy to bypass the obstruction. These lesions tend to increase in size over time; thus surgical intervention is recommended when the patient's size and condition permit resection. Complete excision is rarely possible, so extirpation of the lesion should be temporized by the need to prevent long-term complications and maintain normal structures. The $CO_2$ laser has proven to be the most efficacious treatment modality for laryngeal lymphangiomas. The laser is used to open the cyst, after which the entire cyst wall is vaporized. Simple unroofing of the cyst will offer no long-term effect on the lesion. Staged procedures are commonly required in the treatment of lymphangioma. Radiation has been ineffective and the risk of inducing secondary malignancies has made this treatment modality unacceptable. Sclerosing agents have been advocated in the past, but long-term success with this treatment modality has been discouraging.

### References


1. Batsakis JG: Tumors of the Head and Neck—Clinical and Pathological Considerations, 2nd ed. Williams and Wilkins, Baltimore, 1979, pp 220–221.
2. Belmont JR, Grundfast K: Congenital laryngeal stridor (laryngomalacia): etiologic factors and associated disorders. Ann Otol Rhinol Laryngol 93:430–437, 1984.


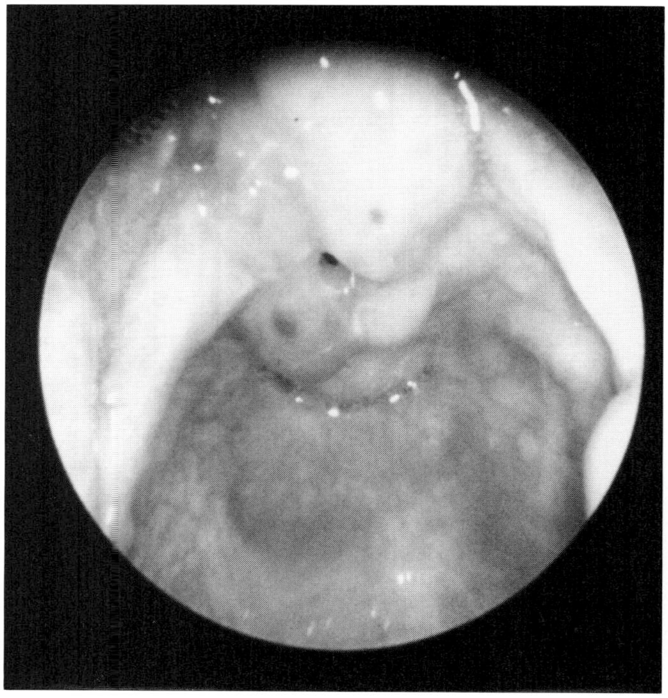

**Fig. 19–10.** Laryngeal lymphangiomas are rare. Complete excision is frequently not possible. Staged procedures are necessary to maintain function.

3. Benjamin B, Inglis A: Minor congenital laryngeal clefts: diagnosis and classification. Ann Otol Rhinol Laryngol 98:417–420, 1989.
4. Choa DI, Smith MC, Evans JN, Bailey CM: Subglottic hemangioma in children. J Laryngol Otol 100:447–454, 1986.
5. Cohen SR: Congenital glottic webs in children. A retrospective review of 51 patients. Ann Otol Rhinol Laryngol (Suppl) 121:2–16, 1985.
6. Cohen SR, Thompson JW: Lymphangiomas of the larynx in infants and children. A survey of pediatric lymphangioma. Ann Otol Rhinol Laryngol (Suppl) 127:1–20, 1986.
7. Cotton RT: The problem of pediatric laryngotracheal stenosis: a clinical and experimental study on the efficacy of autogenous cartilage grafts placed between the vertically divided halves of the posterior lamina of the cricoid cartilage. Laryngoscope 101 (Suppl 56):1–34, 1991.
8. Cotton RT, Schreiber JT: Management of laryngotracheoesophageal cleft. Ann Otol Rhinol Laryngol 90:401–405, 1981.
9. Cotton RT, Tewfik TL: Laryngeal stenosis following carbon dioxide laser in subglottic hemangioma. Report of three cases. Ann Otol Rhinol Laryngol 94:494–497, 1985.
10. DeSanto LW: Laryngocele, laryngeal mucocele, large saccules and laryngeal saccular cysts: a developmental spectrum. Laryngoscope 84:1291–1296, 1974.
11. Dunbar JS: Upper respiratory tract obstruction in infants and children. Am J Roentgen 109:227–246, 1970.
12. Eriksen C, Zwillenberg D, Robinson N: Diagnosis and management of cleft larynx. Literature reviewed and case report. Ann Otol Rhinol Laryngol 99:703–708, 1990.
13. Ferguson CF: Congenital abnormalities of the infant larynx. Otolaryngol Clin North Am 3:185–200, 1970.
14. Gatti WM, MacDonald E, Orfei E: Congenital laryngeal atresia. Laryngoscope 97:966–969, 1987.
15. Hawkins DB, Crockett DM, Kahlstrom EJ, MacLaughlin EF: Corticosteroid management of airway hemangiomas: long-term follow-up. Laryngoscope 94:633–637, 1984.
16. Holinger LD: Etiology of stridor in the neonate, infant and child. Ann Otol Rhinol Laryngol 89:397–400, 1980.
17. Holinger LD, Barnes DR, Smid LJ, Holinger PH: Laryngocele and saccular cysts. Ann Otol Rhinol Laryngol 87:675–685, 1978.
18. Holinger PH, Brown WT: Congenital webs, cysts, laryngoceles, and other anomalies of the larynx. Ann Otol Rhinol Laryngol 76:744–752,1967.
19. Holinger PH, Kutnick SL, Schild JA, Holinger LD: Subglottic stenosis in infants and children. Ann Otol Rhinol Laryngol 85:591–599, 1976.
20. Holinger LD, Tansek KM, Tucker GF: Cleft larynx with airway obstruction. Ann Otol Rhinol Laryngol 94:622–626, 1985.
21. Lim TA, Spanier SS, Kohut RI: Laryngeal clefts: a histopathologic study and review. Ann Otol Rhinol Laryngol 88:837–845, 1979.
22. McSwiney PF, Cavanagh NP, Languth P: Outcome in congenital stridor (laryngomalacia). Arch Dis Child 52:215–218, 1977.
23. Martin JA: Congenital laryngeal stridor. J Laryngol 77:290–294, 1963.
24. Myer CM 3rd, O'Connor DM, Cotton RT: Proposed grading system for subglottic stenosis based on endotracheal tube sizes. Ann Otol Rhinol Laryngol 103:319–323, 1994.
25. Pitanguy I, Caldeira AM, Calixto CA, Alexandrino A: Clinical evaluation and surgical treatment of hemangiomata. Head Neck Surg 7:47–59, 1984.
26. Richardson MA, Cotton RT: Anatomic abnormalities of the pediatric airway. Pediatr Clin North Am 31:821–834, 1984.
27. Shikhani AH, Jones MM, Marsh BR, Holliday MJ: Infantile subglottic hemangiomas. An update. Ann Otol Rhinol Laryngol 95:336–347, 1986.
28. Tucker JA, O'Rahilly R: Observations on the embryology of the human larynx. Ann Otol Rhinol Laryngol 81:520–523, 1972.
29. Vaughn CW: Use of the carbon dioxide laser in the endoscopic management of organic laryngeal disease. Otolaryngol Clinic North Am 16:849–864, 1983.
30. Watson WJ, Thorp JM Jr, Miller RC, Chescheir NC, Katz VL, Seeds JW: Prenatal diagnosis of laryngeal atresia. Ann J Obstet Gynecol 163:1456–1457, 1990.
31. Zalzal GH, Anon JB, Cotton RT: Epiglottoplasty for the treatment of laryngomalacia. Ann Otol Rhinol Laryngol 96:72–76, 1987.

# Appendix F

## Syndromes and Conditions Associated with Congenital Anomalies of the Larynx and Trachea

TED L. TEWFIK, AHMAD S. TEEBI, and VAZKEN M. DER KALOUSTIAN

| Syndrome or condition | MIM No. POSSUM No.[a] | Inheritance[b] | Ear, nose, and throat manifestations | Other manifestations |
|---|---|---|---|---|
| Adducted thumb syndrome, Christian syndrome or craniosynostosis, arthrogryposis, cleft palate[30] | ***201550** 3591 | AR | Myopathic face, micrognathia, cleft palate, low-set ears, abnormal shape of ears, torticollis, laryngomalacia, dysphagia | Craniosynostosis, microcephaly, downward slanting palpebral fissures, telecanthus, ophthalmoplegia, pectus excavatum, adducted thumbs, contractures, mental retardation, seizures, hypotonia, early death |
| Agnathia, synotia, microstoma or otocephaly syndrome[37] | **202650** 3478 | Sporadic | Absence of mandible, micrognathia, small nostrils, choanal atresia, microstomia, aglossia, blind mouth, cleft palate, low-set ears, ears fused in the midline, middle ear anomalies, bilobed epiglottis, rudimentary vocal cords, webbed neck | Epicanthal folds, epibulbar dermoids, abnormal rib number, vertebral anomalies, dextrocardia, situs inversus, hypoplastic lungs, renal agenesis, cardiac defects, holoprosencephaly, lethal |
| Atelosteogenesis, type 3[53] | 4761 | | Midface hypoplasia, microstomia, micrognathia, cleft palate, flat nasal bridge, anteverted nostrils, low-set ears, helix hypoplasia, stenosis of the external auditory canal, laryngomalacia | Prominent forehead, hypertelorism, long clavicles, atlantoaxial instability, scoliosis, cleft of vertebral bodies, multiple joint dislocations, rhizomelic short/bowed limbs |
| Bilateral ptosis, vocal cord paralysis[57] | 4792 | AD | Vocal cord paralysis, abnormal cry | Failure to thrive, normal intelligence, ptosis |
| Campomelic dysplasia or Campomelic dwarfism[17,32] | ***211970** 3049 | AR | Flat face and nose, anteverted nostrils, cleft palate, micrognathia, low-set ears, short neck, tracheal cartilage hypoplasia | Short/bowed limbs, pretibial skin dimples, macrocephaly, rib abnormalities, small scapulae, pectus excavatum, brachydactyly, sex reversal |
| Charcot-Marie-Tooth disease with other defects[10,48] | ***118200** 4384 | XLR<br>AD<br>AR | Micrognathia, high and narrow palate, sensorineural deafness, short neck | Kyphosis, abnormal gait, peroneal muscular atrophy, talipes deformity, pes cavus (hereditary motor/sensory neuropathy) |
| Chondrodysplasia punctata, Conradi-Hunermann type[23,26] | ***118650** 3063 | AD | Flat face, midface hypoplasia, depressed nasal bridge, tracheal abnormality | Short stature, short limbs, ichthyosis, increased skin pigmentation, scoliosis, contractures of large joints, epiphyseal stippling (X-rays), mild mental retardation |
| Chondrodysplasia punctata, rhizomelic type[44] | ***215100** 3064 | AR | Flat face, depressed nasal bridge, tracheal abnormality, dysphagia | Metaphyseal, epiphyseal or diaphyseal abnormality, spasticity, seizures, rhizomelic shortness of limbs, severe growth retardation, widespread punctate stippling (X-rays), mental retardation (MR) |
| Chondrodysplasia punctata, X-linked recessive[60] | ***302950** 3737 | XLR | Small nose, broad nasal bridge, anteverted nostrils, deafness, short neck, laryngeal abnormality | Cicatricial alopecia, ichthyosis, coarse hair, frontal bossing, short stature, MR (del Xp22) |
| Chromosome 5, partial del 5p or | 3073 | | High, shrill mewing cry, broad | Microcephaly, round face, hyper- |

**Appendix F** Syndromes and conditions associated with congenital anomalies of the larynx and trachea *(Continued)*

| Syndrome or condition | MIM No. POSSUM No.[a] | Inheritance[b] | Ear, nose, and throat manifestations | Other manifestations |
|---|---|---|---|---|
| Cri du chat syndrome[31,41] | | | cheeks, cleft lip/palate, micrognathia, broad nasal bridge, small posteriorly angulated ears, preauricular tags, laryngeal abnormality | telorism, hypotonia, heart defects, cryptorchidism, epicanthic folds, moderate to severe MR |
| Chromosome 7, partial dup 7q[47] | 3076 | | Micrognathia, beaked nose, everted lips, cleft palate, macroglossia, anteverted or bat ears, short neck, hearing abnormality, laryngeal abnormality | Short stature, macrocephaly or hydrocephalus, frontal bossing, hypertelorism, cryptorchidism, single palmar creases, MR |
| Craniofacial digital genital anomalies[21] | 4163 | | Narrow face, pointed chin, microstomia, micrognathia, anteverted ears, abnormal cry, laryngeal abnormality | Hypotelorism, syndactyly, arachnodactyly, pectus deformity, small penis, hypospadias, pyloric stenosis, MR |
| Cryptophthalmos, multiple congenital anomalies (MCA) syndrome, or Fraser syndrome[38,45] | ***219000** 3179 | AR | Asymmetric face, coloboma of nostrils, choanal atresia, cleft lip/palate, low-set ears, atresia of the external auditory canal, conductive deafness, laryngeal stenosis | Hypertelorism, cryptophthalmos (not obligatory), ambiguous genitalia, hypospadias, cryptorchidism, anal stenosis or atresia, thymic aplasia, hypotonia, MR |
| De la Chapelle dysplasia or Atelosteogenesis type 2, or Neonatal osseous dysplasia[52] | ***256050** 3847 | AR | Cleft palate, folded-down ears, abnormal neck, laryngeal stenosis, bronchomalacia | Short ribs, scoliosis, severely hypoplastic ulna and fibula, bowed limbs, bifid humeral metaphysis, lethal |
| Diastrophic dysplasia[18] | ***222600** 3185 | AR | Cauliflower ears, calcified ear cartilage, cleft palate, micrognathia, conductive deafness, tracheal and laryngeal abnormality, abnormal cry | Short stature, short/bowed limbs, hitch-hiker thumbs, contractures, cryptorchidism, epiphyseal or metaphyseal abnormality, brachydactyly, dislocated hips, kyphoscoliosis, respiratory obstruction |
| Distal muscular atrophy, deafness[6] | **158580** 4621 | AD | Sensorineural deafness, vocal cord paralysis, abnormal cry | Scoliosis, distal muscular atrophy, muscle weakness, abnormal gait |
| Facio-auriculo-vertebral dysplasia. Oculo-auriculo-vertebral dysphasia, or Goldenhar syndrome[9,46] | **164210** 3339 | AD AR | Facial asymmetry, triangular face, macrostoma, micrognathia, cleft palate, deafness, epibulbar dermoids, preauricular pits or tags, microtia or anotia, tracheoesophageal fistula, laryngeal abnormality | Intrauterine growth retardation (IUGR), microcephaly, microphthalmos, coloboma of eyelid, iris, and retina, oligodontia, hypoplastic lungs, dysplastic kidney, vertebral defects, agenesis of corpus callosum, hydrocephalus, MR |
| Farber lipogranulomatosis, generalized lipogranulomatosis, or acid ceramidase deficiency[39] | ***228000** 3436 | AR | Hoarseness of voice due to vocal cord thickening, macroglossia, thickened gingiva, hamartoma of mouth | Painful/swollen joints and subcutaneous nodules, cloudy corneal lymphadenopathy, hepatosplenomegaly, diffuse osteoporosis, nephropathy, seizures, MR |
| Flannery syndrome[12] | 4625 | | Imperforate oropharynx, mandibulofacial dysostosis, low-set and malformed ears, micrognathia, broad nasal bridge, abnormal esophagus | Hemivertebrae, abnormal rib number, arachnodactyly, clinodactyly of 5th finger |
| Fraser-Jéquier-Chen syndrome[13] | 4306 | | Laryngeal cleft, beaked nose, high narrow palate, low-set ears, preauricular tags | Pancreatic and renal dysplasia, short limbs, genital anomalies, imperforate anus, brachydactyly, polydactyly |
| Hydrolethalus syndrome[2] | ***236680** 3567 | AR | Micrognathia, flattened or cleft nose, glossoptosis, low-set ears, tracheal/laryngeal abnormality | Hydrocephalus, micropolygyria, polydactyly, segmental lung defect, heart defect |
| Hypothalamic-hamartoblastoma syndrome, or Ano-cerebro-digital syndrome, or Pallister-Hall syndrome[43] | ***146510** 3471 | | Flat face, glossoptosis, cleft palate, anteverted nostrils, micrognathia, prominent and low-set ears, ear cartilage deficiency, laryngeal cleft, tracheal abnormality | IUGR, macrocephaly, prominent occiput, abnormal sella turcica, hypothalamic hamartomas, agenesis of corpus collosum, hypopituitarism, scoliosis, genital anomalies, heart defects, imperforate anus, postaxial polydactyly or syndactyly, lethal |

| Syndrome or condition | MIM No. POSSUM No.[a] | Inheritance[b] | Ear, nose, and throat manifestations | Other manifestations |
|---|---|---|---|---|
| Hypothyroidism, spiky hair, deafness[3] | **241850** 4622 | XLR | Choanal atresia, cleft palate, micrognathia, bifid epiglottis | Spiky hair, scalp alopecia, borderline mental retardation, spasticity, hypothyroidism |
| Infantile type sialuria[15] | ***269920** 4308 | AR | Coarse facies, speech deficit, laryngeal abnormality | Neonatal ascites, short stature, hepatic fibrosis, hepatomegaly, ataxia/athetosis, moderate to severe MR (storage disorder) |
| Kaufman-McKusick syndrome, or hydrometrocolpos, polydactyly, congenital heart defect[58] | ***236700** 3510 | AR | Choanal atresia, cleft palate, congenital tracheal stenosis | Vaginal atresia, imperforate hymen, hydrometrocolpos, polydactyly, small penis, hydronephrosis, heart defect, imperforate anus |
| Keutel syndrome, or Pulmonary stenosis, brachydactyly, deafness, cartilage defect[14] | ***245150** 3675 | AR | Sensorineural deafness, midface hypoplasia, short philtrum, calcified ears, laryngeal/tracheal abnormality | Brachydactyly, soft tissue calcification, abnormal ossification, syndactyly, carpal fusion, peripheral pulmonary stenosis, heart defects, immune or hematological abnormalities, MR |
| Killian-Teschler-Nicola syndrome, or Pallister mosaic syndrome, or Chromosome 12, mosaic tetrasomy 12p[49] | 3800 | Sporadic | Coarse facies, broad nasal bridge, anteverted nostrils, long philtrum, large and low-set ears, thickened helix, cleft palate, short neck, laryngeal abnormality | Sparse hair, irregular skin pigmentation, accessory nipples, puffy eyelids, cataracts, optic nerve abnormality, inguinal/umbilical hernia, diaphragmatic hernia, genital anomalies, imperforate anus, caudal appendage, seizures, hypotonia, moderate to severe MR |
| Laryngeal abductor paralysis, MR, or Plott syndrome[40] | **308850** 4008 | XLR | Bilateral vocal cord paralysis, myopathic face, abnormal cry, dysphagia | Failure to thrive, MR, optic nerve abnormality, hypotonia |
| Laryngeal hypoplasia, encephalocele[34] | 4672 | | Laryngeal atresia, low-set and abnormal ears | Stillbirth, abnormal placenta, hydrops fetalis, contractures of large joints, other elbow and wrist deformities, horseshoe kidney, hydrocephalus, encephalocele |
| Laryngeal web, congenital heart disease[42] | 4156 | AD | Laryngeal web, subglottic stenosis, abormal cry | Short stature, heart defect |
| Laryngotracheoesophageal cleft, unilateral pulmonary hypoplasia[39a] | 4341 | | Laryngotracheoesophageal cleft, tracheoesophageal fistula, partial tracheal agenesis, micrognathia, microstomia, low-set ears | Abnormal rib structures, vertebral anomalies, heart defect, hypoplastic lung, pancreas/spleen abnormality |
| Lethal chondrodysplasia, Blomstrand type, or lethal dwarfism, advanced bone age[5] | 3815 | AR | Macroglossia, micrognathia, depressed nasal bridge, anteverted nostrils | Short-limb dwarf with normal-sized hands and feet, advanced skeletal maturation, hydrops fetalis, tarsal fusion, coarctation of aorta, lethal |
| MR, hypopituitarism, distal arthrogryposis[8] | **208080** 4799 | AR | Square face, midface hypoplasia, short nose, depressed bridge, anteverted nostrils, micrognathia, prominent ears, laryngeal abnormality | Failure to thrive, frontal bossing, ridged metopic sutures, delayed skeletal maturation, ulnar deviation of fingers, contractures, hypopituitarism, hydrocephalus, severe MR |
| Metaphyseal chondrodysplasia, Kaitila type[27] | **250230** 4064 | AR | Tracheobronchomalacia, thickened gingivae, broad alveolar ridge | Thoracolumbar kyphosis, scoliosis, hypermobile joints, cone-shaped epiphyses, brachydactyly, pectus deformity (progressive) |
| Metaphyseal chondrodystrophy, Sussman type[55] | 4197 | AR | Midface hypoplasia, laryngeal/tracheal abnormality | Short stature, short limbs, blue sclerae, cardiomyopathy, vertebral segmentation defects, spindle-shaped fingers |
| Multiple congenital anomalies, Hood-Hartwell type[22] | 4797 | | Laryngeal atresia, micrognathia, beaked nose, short philtrum, abnormal helix | Hypertelorism, delayed skeletal maturation, hypoplastic lungs, hypoplastic kidneys, ureteric reflux |

**Appendix F** Syndromes and conditions associated with congenital anomalies of the larynx and trachea *(Continued)*

| Syndrome or condition | MIM No. POSSUM No.[a] | Inheritance[b] | Ear, nose, and throat manifestations | Other manifestations |
|---|---|---|---|---|
| Multiple sulphatase deficiency, or juvenile sulfatidosis, Austin type[29] | ***272200** 4228 | AR | Flat and coarse face, depressed nasal bridge, anteverted nostrils, thick lips, deafness, short neck, abnormal esophagus | Puffy eyelids, epiphyseal abnormalities, hepatomegaly, hypotonia, cerebral cortex atrophy, dysostosis multiplex, MR (storage disorder) |
| Omphalocele, larynx/pharynx hypoplasia[51] | **182210** 4022 | AR | Broad nasal bridge, abnormal columella, down-turned mouth angles, thin lips, abnormal cry, pharyngeal and laryngeal hypoplasia | High-arched eyebrows, hypertelorism, scoliosis, omphalocele, hypotonia, MR |
| Opitz-Frias syndrome, G syndrome, or Opitz oculo-genital-laryngeal syndrome, type 2[1,59] | ***145410** 3239 | AD XLD | Broad nasal bridge, anteverted nostrils, cleft palate, posteriorly angulated ears, micrognathia, dysphagia, laryngeal abnormality | Hypertelorism, hypospadias, scrotal/anal anomalies (in the spectrum of BBBG syndrome) |
| Oral-digital-facial syndrome, type 4, or, Mohr/Majewski syndrome[16,36] | **258860** 3147 | AR | Midline cleft lip, cleft palate, fissured or lobulated tongue | Short stature, mesomelic shortness of limbs, multiple joint dislocations, tibial dysplasia, polydactyly, syndactyly, heart defects, irregular respiration, imperforate anus, MR |
| Pachyonychia congenita or Jadassohn-Lewandowsky syndrome[19a,54] | ***167200** 4181 | AD AR | Dysphonia secondary to thickening of the posterior commissure of the larynx, deafness (conductive), oral leukoplakia, natal teeth | Onycholysis, thickened nails, palmoplantar hyperkeratosis, cutaneous cysts, corneal leukokeratosis |
| Schwartz-Jampel syndrome, or myopathy, dwarfism, chondrodystrophy, or Osteochondromuscular dystrophy[24] | ***255800** 3403 | AR | Flat face, poor facial expression, micrognathia, microstomia, trismus, low-set ears | Blepharophimosis, pectus deformity, platyspondyly, inguinal hernia, small penis, dislocated hips, myotonia, electromyographic abnormality, muscle wasting, slow growth but normal mental development |
| Short-rib polydactyly syndrome, Majewski type, or polydactyly with neonatal chondrodystrophy type 2[4] | ***263520** 3389 | AR | Flattened short nose, anteverted nostrils, cleft lip/palate, low-set ears | Short ribs, short limbs, brachydactyly, syndactyly, polydactyly, heart defects, polycystic kidneys, abnormal pancreas, genital anomalies, short bowel (lethal) |
| Shy-Drager syndrome[33] | **146500** 4664 | AR | Vocal cord paralysis, speech defect | Decreased sweating, irregular respiration, hypotension, bowel and bladder incontinence, psychosis, tremor with no intellectual deterioration |
| Smith-Lemli-Opitz syndrome, type 2[28,35] | ***268670** 3645 | | Micrognathia, tented upper lip, short philtrum, cleft or high-arched palate, glossoptosis, low-set ears, short webbed neck, dysphagia, laryngeal abnormality | Short limbs, polydactyly, syndactyly, overlapping fingers, dislocated hip, heart defects, ambiguous genitalia, dysplastic kidneys, unilobular lungs, abnormal pancreas, agenesis of corpus callosum, MR |
| Thoraco-laryngo-pelvic dysplasia or thoracopelvic dysostosis[7] | **187770** 3606 | AD | Laryngeal hypoplasia | Respiratory distress, short stature, pectus deformity, short ribs, short round ilium, shallow sciatic notch, hypoplastic lungs |
| Toriello-Carey syndrome or Pallister syndrome[56] | **217980** 4568 | AR | Short nose, anteverted nostrils, cleft palate, glossoptosis, low-set ears, posteriorly angulated ears, sensorineural deafness, short neck, laryngeal abnormality | Microcephaly, agenesis of corpus callosum, short palpebral fissures, telecanthus, inguinal hernia, hypospadias, cryptorchidism, small hands, clinodactyly of 5th finger, heart defect, hypotonia (early death) |
| Tracheal agenesis association[11,61] | 2849 | | Laryngeal atresia, abnormal esophagus, tracheal agenesis | Limb deficiencies, wide carrying angle of elbow, abnormal palmar |

| Syndrome or condition | MIM No. POSSUM No.[a] | Inheritance[b] | Ear, nose, and throat manifestations | Other manifestations |
|---|---|---|---|---|
| | | | | dermatoglyphics, hypoplastic thumbs, lung segmental defects, duodenal atresia, imperforate anus |
| Ulnar-mammary syndrome of Pallister[50] | ***181450** 3420 | AD | Facial asymmetry, jaw abnormality, cleft soft palate, laryngeal abnormality | Asymmetric hypoplasia of ulnar rays, breast hypoplasia, scoliosis, small penis, cryptorchidism, apparent absence of sweat glands, imperforate hymen, pyloric stenosis |
| Urbach-Wiethe syndrome, lipoid proteinosis, or hyalinosis cutis et mucosae[20] | ***247100** 4830 | AR | Macroglossia, yellow infiltration of larynx, hoarseness of voice, tracheal abnormality | Subcutaneous yellow nodules, increased skin pigmentation, intracranial calcification, seizures, hyperlipidemia |
| Velo-cardio-facial syndrome or Shprintzen syndrome[25] | **#192430** 3132 | AD | High nasal bridge, cleft palate (often submucous), micrognathia, microtia, conductive deafness, nasal speech, laryngeal abnormality | Short stature, microcephaly, heart defects, ocular abnormalities, thymic aplasia, MR |
| White forelock with malformations or Goodman-Yahav-Frand syndrome[19] | **277740** 3505 | AD | High-arched palate, posterior angulation of ears, tracheal abnormality, bronchomalacia | Decreased hair pigmentation, white forelock, blue sclera, hypertelorism, myopia, paralysis of ocular muscles, winged scapulae, syndactyly, cardiac conduction defects |

[a]MIM, *M*endelian *I*nheritance in *M*an. A Catalog of Human Genes and Genetic Disorders, by Victor A. McKusick, 11th ed, The Johns Hopkins University Press, Baltimore, 1994; POSSUM, *P*icture *O*f *S*tandard *S*yndromes and *U*ndiagnosed *M*alformations, by Agnes Bankier et al., Murdoch Institute, Royal Children's Hospital, Victoria, Australia.
[b]AD, autosomal dominant; AR, autosomal recessive; XLR, X-linked recessive; XLD, X-linked dominant.
*confirmed gene and inheritance
#phenotype that can be caused by mutation in any of 2 or more genes.

## References


1. Allanson JE: G syndrome: an unusual family. Am J Med Genet 31:637–642, 1988.
2. Aughton DJ, Cassidy, SB: Hydrolethalus syndrome: report of an apparent mild case, literature review, and differential diagnosis. Am J Med Genet 27:935–942, 1987.
3. Bamforth JS, Hughes IA, Lazarus JH, Weaver CM, Harper PS: Congenital hypothyroidism, spiky hair, and cleft palate. J Med Genet 26:49–51, 1989.
4. Bernstein R, Isdale J, Pinto M, Du Toit Zaaijman J, Jenkins T: Short rib-polydactyly syndrome: a single or heterogeneous entity? A reevaluation prompted by four new cases. J Med Genet 22:46–53, 1985.
5. Blomstrand S, Claesson T, Save-Soderbergh J: A case of lethal congenital dwarfism with accelerated skeletal maturation. Pediatr Radiol 15:141–143, 1985.
6. Boltshauser E, Lang W, Spillman T, Hof E: Hereditary distal muscular atrophy with vocal cord paralysis and sensorineural hearing loss: a dominant form of spinal muscular atrophy? J Med Genet 26:105–108, 1989.
7. Burn J, Hall C, Marsden D, Matthew DJ: Autosomal dominant thoracolaryngopelvic dysplasia: Barnes syndrome. J Med Genet 23:345–349, 1986.
8. Chitayat D, Hall JG, Couch RM, Phang MS, Baldwin VJ: Syndrome of mental retardation, facial anomalies, hypopituitarism, and distal arthrogryposis in sibs. Am J Med Genet 37:65–70, 1990.
9. Cohen MM Jr, Rollnick BR, Kaye CI: Oculoauriculovertebral spectrum: an updated critique. Cleft Palate J 26:276–286, 1989.
10. Davis CJS, Bradley WG, Madrid R: The peroneal muscular atrophy syndrome: clinical, genetic, electrophysiological and nerve biopsy studies. I. Clinical, genetic and electrophysiological findings and classification. J Genet Hum 26:311–349, 1978.
11. Evans JA, Reggin J, Greenberg C: Tracheal agenesis and associated malformations: a comparison with tracheoesophageal fistula and the VACTERL association. Am J Med Genet 21:21–38, 1985.
12. Flannery DB: Syndrome of imperforate oropharynx with costovertebral and auricular anomalies. Am J Med Genet 32:189–191, 1989.
13. Fraser FC, Jéquier S, Chen MF: Chondrodysplasia, situs inversus totalis, cleft epiglottis and larynx, hexadactyly of hands and feet, pancreatic cystic dysplasia, renal dysplasia/absence, micropenis and ambiguous genitalia imperforate anus. Am J Med Genet 34:401–405, 1989.
14. Fryns JP, van Fleteren A, Mattelaer P, van den Berghe H: Calcification of cartilages, brachytelephalangy and peripheral pulmonary stenosis. Confirmation of the Keutel syndrome. Eur J Pediatr 142:201–203, 1984.
15. Gahl WA, Schneider JA, Aula PP: Lysosomal transport disorders: cystinosis and sialic acid storage disorders. In: The Metabolic and Molecular Bases of Inherited Disease, CR Scriver, AL Beaudet, WS Sly, D Valle (eds) 7th ed. McGraw-Hill, New York, 1995, pp 3763–3797.
16. Gillerot Y, Koulischer L: Oro-facial-digital syndrome II. Clin Genet 33:141–142, 1988.
17. Gillerot Y, Vanheck CA, Foulon M, Podevain A, Koulischer L: Campomelic syndrome: manifestations in a 20 week fetus and case history of a 5 year old child. Am J Med Gen 34:589–592, 1989.
18. Gollop TR, Eigier A: Prenatal ultrasound diagnosis of diastrophic dysplasia at 16 weeks. Am J Med Genet 27:321–324, 1987.
19. Goodman RM, Yahav Y, Frand M, Barzilay Z, Nissan E, Hertz M: A new white forelock (poliosis) syndrome with multiple congenital malformations in two sibs. Clin Genet 17:437–442, 1980.
19a. Gorlin RJ, Cohen MM Jr. Levin LS: Syndromes of the Head and Neck, 3rd ed. Oxford University Press, New York, 1990, pp 445–448.
20. Gorlin RJ, Cohen MM Jr, Levin LS: Syndromes of the Head and Neck, 3rd ed. Oxford University Press, New York, 1990, pp 507–511.
21. Harrod MJ, Keele DR, Howard J Sr: A syndrome of craniofacial, digital, and genital anomalies. Birth Defects 13:111–115, 1977.
22. Hood OJ, Hartwell EA, Shattuck KE, Rosenberg HS: Multiple congenital anomalies associated with a 47,XXX chromosome constitution. Am J Med Genet 36:73–75, 1990.
23. Hosenfeld D, Wiedemann HR: Chondrodysplasia punctata in an adult recognized as vitamin K antagonist embryopathy. Clin Genet 35:376–381, 1989.

24. Jones KL: Smith's Recognizable Patterns of Human Malformation, 5th ed. WB Saunders, 1996, p 218.
25. Jones KL, Smith's Recognizable Patterns of Human Malformation, 5th ed. WB Saunders, 1996, p 266.
26. Jones KL: Smith's Recognizable Patterns of Human Malformation, 5th ed. WB Saunders, 1996, p 390.
27. Kaitila II, Halttunen P, Snellman O, Takkunen O: A new form of metaphyseal chondrodysplasia in two sibs: surgical treatment of tracheobronchial malacia and scoliosis. Am J Med Genet 11:415–424, 1982.
28. Kohler HG: Brief clinical report: familial neonatally lethal syndrome of hypoplastic left heart, absent pulmonary lobation, polydactyly, and talipes, probably Smith-Lemli-Opitz (RSH) syndrome. Am J Med Genet 14:423–428, 1983.
29. Kolodny EH, Fluharty AL: Metachromatic leukodystrophy and multiple sulfatase deficiency: sulfatide lipidosis. In: The Metabolic and Molecular Bases of Inherited Disease, 7th ed. CR Scriver, AL Beaudet, WS Sly, D Valle, eds. McGraw-Hill, New York, 1995, pp 2693–2739.
30. Kunze J, Park W, Hansen KH, Hanafeld F: Adducted thumb syndrome. Report of a new case and a diagnostic approach. Eur J Pediatr 141:122–126, 1983.
31. Kushnick T, Kao KW, Lamb AN: Familial 5p-syndrome. Clin Genet 26:472–476, 1984.
32. Lee FA, Isaacs H Jr, Strauss J: The "campomelic" syndrome. Short life-span dwarfism with respiratory distress, hypotonia, peculiar facies, and multiple skeletal and cartilaginous deformities. Am J Dis Child 124:485–496, 1972.
33. Lee S, Chen CN: Clinical diversity of the Shy-Drager syndrome: a case in Hong Kong. Soc Med 82:225–226, 1989.
34. Machin GA, Popkin JS, Zachs D, Newbigging J, Walther G, Bell D: Fetus with asymmetric parietal encephalocele, and hydrops secondary to laryngeal atresia. Am J Med Genet (Suppl) 3:311–321, 1987.
35. McKeever PA, Young ID: Smith-Lemli-Opitz syndrome II: a disorder of the fetal adrenals? J Med Genet 27:465–466, 1990.
36. Meinecke P, Hayek H: Orofaciodigital syndrome type IV (Mohr-Majewski syndrome) with severe expression expanding the known spectrum of anomalies. J Med Genet 27:200–202, 1990.
37. Meinecke P, Padberg B, Laas R: Agnathia, holoprosencephaly, and situs inversus: a third report. Am J Med Genet 37:286–287, 1990.
38. Mortimer G, McEwan MP, Yates JR: Fraser syndrome presenting as monozygotic twins with bilateral renal agenesis. J Med Genet 22:76–78, 1985.
39. Moser HW: Ceramidase deficiency: Farber lipogranulomatosis. In: The Metabolic and Molecular Bases of Inherited Disease, CR Scriver, AL Beaudet, WS Sly, D Valle, eds, 7th ed. McGraw-Hill, New York, 1995, pp 2589–2599.
39a. Novak RM: Laryngotracheoesophageal cleft and unilateral pulmonary hypoplasia in twins. Pediatrics 67:732–734, 1982.
40. Opitz JM, Kaveggia EG, Durkin-Stamm MV, Pendleton E: Diagnostic/genetic studies in severe mental retardation. Birth Defects 14:1–38, 1978.
41. Overhauser J, McMahon J, Oberlender S, Carlin ME, Niebuhr E, Wasmuth JJ, Lee-Chen J: Parental origin of chromosome 5 deletions in the cri-du-chat syndrome. Am J Med Genet 37:83–86, 1990.
42. Paes BA, De Sa DJ, Hitch DA: Fatal malformations of the larynx and upper trachea. Laryngoscope 94:1477–1481, 1984.
43. Pallister PD, Hecht F, Herrman J: Three additional cases of the congenital hypothalamic "hamartoblastoma" (Pallister-Hall) syndrome. Am J Med Genet 33:500–501, 1989.
44. Poulos A Sheffield L, Sharp P, Sherwood G, Johnson D, Beckman K, Fellenberg AJ, Wraith JE, Chow CW, Usher S, et al: Rhizomelic chondrodysplasia punctata: clinical, pathologic, and biochemical findings in two patients. J Pediatr 113:685–690, 1989.
45. Ramsing M, Rehder H, Holzgreve W, Meinecke P, Lenz W: Fraser syndrome (cryptophthalmos with syndactyly) in the fetus and newborn. Clin Genet 37:84–96, 1990.
46. Rollnick BR, Kaye C, Nagatoshi R, Hauok W, Martin AU: Oculoauriculovertebral dysplasia and variants: phenotypic characteristics of 294 patients. Am J Med Genet 26:361–375, 1987.
47. Romain DR, Cairney A, Stewart D, Colombano-Green LM, Garry M, Parslow MI, Parfitt R, Smythe RH, Chapman CJ: Three cases of partial trisomy 7q owing to rare structural rearrangements of chromosome 7. J Med Genet 27:109–113, 1990.
48. Ruiz C, Rivas F, Ramirez-Casillar G, Vazquez-Santana, R, Mendoza-Chalita B Feria-Velasco A, Tapia-Arizmendi G, Cantu JM: A distinct congenital motor and sensory neuropathy (neuronal type) with dysmorphic features in a father and two sons. A variant of Charcot-Marie-Tooth disease. Clin Genet 31:109–113, 1987.
49. Schinzel A: Tetrasomy 12p (Pallister-Killian syndrome). J Med Genet 28:122–125, 1991.
50. Schinzel A: Ulnar-mammary syndrome, J Med Genet 24:778–781, 1987.
51. Shprintzen RJ, Goldberg RB: Dysmorphic facies, omphalocele, laryngeal and pharyngeal hypoplasia, spinal anomalies, and learning disabilities in a new dominant malformation syndrome. Birth Defects 15:347–353, 1979.
52. Sillence DO, Kozlowski K, Rogers JG, Sprague PL, Cullity GJ, Osborn RA: Atelosteogenesis: evidence for heterogeneity. Pediatr Radiol 17:112–118, 1987.
53. Stern HJ, Graham JM Jr, Lachman RS, Horton W, Bernini PM, Spiegel PK, Bodurtha J, Ives EJ, Bocian M, Rimoin DL: Atelosteogenesis type III: a distinct skeletal dysplasia with features overlapping atelosteogenesis and oto-palato-digital syndrome type II . Am J Med Genet 36:183–195, 1990.
54. Su WP, Chun WI, Hammond DE, Gordon H: Pachyonychia congenita: a clinical study of 12 cases and review of the literature. Pediatr Dermatol 7:33–38, 1990.
55. Sussman MD, Kelly T, Rosenbaum KN, Balian G: Abnormality of cartilage collagen in a patient with unclassified chondrodystrophy. J Orthop Res 2:339–345, 1984.
56. Toriello HV, Carey JC: Corpus callosum agenesis, facial anomalies, Robin sequence, and other anomalies: a new autosomal recessive syndrome? Am J Med Genet 31:17–23, 1988.
57. Tucker HM: Congenital bilateral recurrent nerve paralysis and ptosis: a new syndrome? Laryngoscope 93:1405–1407, 1983.
58. Vince JD, Martin NJ: McKusick-Kaufman syndrome: report of an instructive family. Am J Med Genet 32:174–177, 1989.
59. Wilson GN, Oliver WJ: Further delineation of the G syndrome: a manageable genetic cause of infantile dysphagia. J Med Genet 25:157–163, 1988.
60. Wohrle D Barbi G, Schulz W, Steinbach P: Heterozygous expression of X-linked chondrodysplasia punctata. Complex chromosome aberration including deletion of MIC2 and STS. Hum Genet 86:215–218, 1990.
61. Woo P, Karmody CS: Congenital laryngeal atresia. Histopathologic study of two cases. Ann Otol Rhinol Laryngol 92:391–395, 1983.

# VIII

## THE ESOPHAGUS

# 20

# Embryology of the Esophagus

JEAN-MARTIN LABERGE

Embryology of the human foregut has given rise to several hypotheses and much controversy. We will discuss esophageal development in the light of recent studies.

## Embryonic period

The embryonic period extends from conception to the ninth week. The entoblast first appears as a distinct layer 8 days after fecundation, and mesoblastic cells appear 1 week later. The entoblast lines the vitelline cavity at the end of the second week of development; with the craniocaudal plication of the embryo during the third and fourth weeks, part of the vitelline cavity becomes incorporated in the embryo. In the anterior part of the embryo this gives rise to the foregut (Fig. 20–1).

Towards the end of the third week of development, a ventral diverticulum appears in the primitive foregut, just caudal to the fourth and fifth pharyngeal pouches, and cranial to the hepatic primordium. This diverticulum grows caudally and divides to form the trachea, bronchi, and lungs. It was previously thought that the differentiation of the foregut into trachea and esophagus occurred through a process of septation: lateral folds were to fuse in the midline in a caudocranial direction to form a septum dividing the primitive foregut into the trachea ventrally and the esophagus dorsally. This theory, first proposed by His in 1885[5] and slightly modified by Smith in 1957,[14] continues to be illustrated in several recent embryology textbooks.[4,7,11,13]

Recent studies of human embryos by Zaw-Tun[16] and O'Rahilly,[12] and of chick embryos by Kluth et al.,[8] disagree with the former theory (Fig. 20–2). In the former theory, the diverticulum was thought to represent the lung bud or pulmonary primordium, while the trachea was to develop from the foregut, cephalad to this. The more current theory[8,12,15,16] can be summarized as follows: soon after its appearance the respiratory diverticulum develops bronchopulmonary buds; the trachea appears only after further caudal growth of the respiratory diverticulum.

Table 20–1 details relevant events in the development of the foregut and esophagus; the relation between age, length, stage, and actual events is only relative, since development may vary between embryos of the same size or same somite number.

During the fourth and fifth weeks of development, the heart and liver enlarge rapidly. Stretched by these structures, the esophagus, now a distinct tube between the respiratory diverticulum and the recognizable stomach, becomes elongated and narrow to near-complete obliteration at the level of the carina.[6,12,16] This narrowing appears to be caused by stretching rather than by cellular proliferation, since the columnar epithelium remains 1 to 3 cells thick; in fact, the walls are thinner as the lumen narrows.[16] Although some authors continue to say that epithelial proliferation may completely obliterate the lumen at this stage,[4,11] such "proliferation" or obliteration does not seem to occur in normal circumstances.[6,12,16] Vacuoles can be noted within the epithelium, but the esophageal lumen itself remains intact.[6] The esophageal length increases from 200–300 $\mu$m to 2.5 mm during those 2 weeks. It should be noted that the bronchial primordia curve dorsally and "embrace" the esophagus, possibly because of the growing pericardium anteriorly. This results in the tracheal bifurcation being very close to the front wall of the esophagus, at a point where the latter is so narrow that its lumen becomes barely visible microscopically.[16] It is interesting to relate these observations with congenital anomalies of the esophagus, the most frequent of which is esophageal atresia with a distal tracheoesophageal fistula. The fistula is usually with the distal trachea or carina. One theory is that epithelial division may be unable to keep pace with the rapid elongation, resulting in interruption; the lower end could remain blind (resulting in a pure atresia) or reattach itself to the nearest epithelial structure, the distal trachea. Other theories include a defect or failure of the mesenchyme between the two structures or an anomaly in the relative position of each within the embryo.[7] A purely mechanical theory would not explain the frequency of associated anomalies such as anorectal, cardiac, vertebral, renal, and limb malformations.

Between the sixth and eighth weeks of gestation, the esophageal epithelium remains stratified columnar and becomes 2 to 5 cells thick. It is surrounded by a layer of undifferentiated mesenchyme and a circular layer of myoblasts. As the circular muscle layer becomes well developed, some elements of the longitudinal layer appear in the lower esophagus.[3] Branches of the vagus nerves with terminal groups of cells are visible along the esophagus at this point;[4] myenteric ganglia are distinguishable at the end of this period.[3] Blood vessels from the aorta can be seen entering the submucosa.[4] It is also during this period that cartilage appears in the tracheobronchial tree. At the end of the embryonic period, the esophagus is 8 to 10 mm long. From its first appearance in the fourth week until the seventh week, the primitive pharyngeal floor (between the respiratory primordium and the esophagus) remains at a constant level in relation to the somites.[12] Therefore, the growth of the esophagus and tracheobronchial tree is mostly caudal until now, and not in both directions as was thought previously when the tracheal bifurcation was taken as the point of reference, and the trachea and esophagus were presumed to be divided from each other by an ascending septum and lateral infoldings of the foregut (Fig. 20–2).

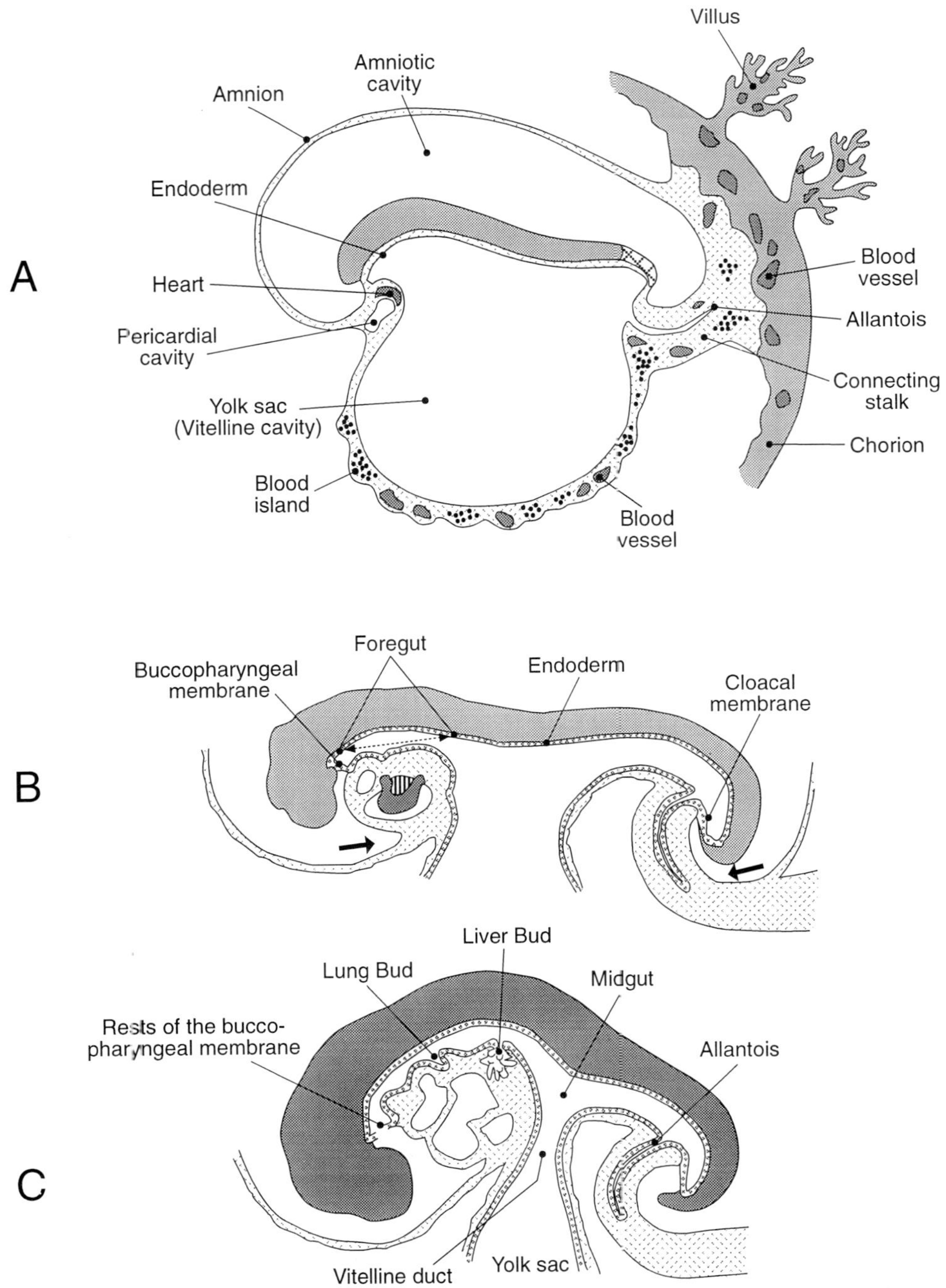


**Fig. 20–1.** Development of the foregut in the embryo: A: 19 days; B: 25 days; C: 28 days. (Modified from Sadler, 1985.[13])

## Fetal period

The fetal period of esophageal development covers the time from the ninth week until birth (Table 20–2).

The stratified columnar epithelium becomes ciliated during the tenth week, first in the middle third.[2,6] Mesenchymal ridges also lead to well-defined longitudinal folds of the mucosa at this time,[4] although these have been noted even earlier by others.[6] Arsenault and Ménard[2] studied the human fetal esophagus between the 10th and 16th week of gestation using organ culture. By autoradiography they showed proliferation of all layers of epithelial cells except ciliated cells. Mesenchymal cells in the submucosa and muscular cells in the muscularis propria were also proliferating to a lesser degree. The epithelial and mesenchymal proliferation appeared to decrease gradually from the tenth to the fifteenth week, while the muscular proliferation peaked at 11 to 12 weeks and then slowly decreased. Between the tenth and twelfth weeks the longitudinal muscle layer becomes well defined and ganglion cells appear in the myenteric plexuses. The muscularis mucosa also becomes apparent in the lower esophagus.[3]

At 12 weeks, the epithelium is completely ciliated and proliferation occurs only in basal cell layers. Epidermal growth factor (EGF) binding sites were found by Ménard et al[10] to correlate with cellular proliferation: while EGF binding sites are present in all undifferentiated cells of the stratified epithelium at 8–10 weeks, they are concentrated in the basal layers once the epithelium is ciliated.

**Table 20–1.** Esophageal development in the embryo (0–8 weeks)

| Age (days) | Length (mm) | Pairs of somites | Carnegie stage | Events |
|---|---|---|---|---|
| 20 | 1.5–2.5 | 1–3 | 9 | Foregut appears |
| 22 | 2.0–3.5 | 4–12 | 10 | Oropharyngeal membrane appears, hepatic primordium appears |
| 24 | 2.5–4.5 | 13–20 | 11 | Respiratory primordium (RP) appears, oropharyngeal membrane ruptures |
| 26 | 3.0–5.0 | 21–29 | 12 | Endoderm thickens ventrally (4–6 cells thick) while it is thin dorsally (1–3 cells). RP dilates into a diverticulum (RD) and develops bronchopulmonary buds (BrP). Mesoderm compresses the lateral walls of the primitive pharynx (PPh) between the 4th pharyngeal pouches and the RD. Primitive pharyngeal floor (PPhF) is a saddle-shaped wall between RP and esophagus. Stretching of foregut by rapid heart enlargement occurs. |
| 28 | 4.0–6.0 | 30 | 13 | Stomach is recognizable; esophagus elongates and narrows (to near-complete obliteration at the level of the carina) with unchanged wall thickness. RD elongates caudally, trachea and carina appear. |
| 32 | 5.0–7.0 | — | 14 | Mesoderm continues to indent lateral walls of PPh. BrP curve dorsally and embrace esophagus. Tracheal bifurcation is very close to front wall of esophagus. |
| 4th and 5th week | 2–10 | — | 10–15 | Septum transversum forms. Esophagus length increases from 200–300 $\mu$m to 2.5 mm. Esophageal epithelium is 1–3 cells thick. PPhF remains at a constant level (up to stage 19–7th wk) |
| 6th to 8th week | 10–30 | — | 16–23 | Esophageal epithelium is 2–5 cells thick (i.e., stratified columnar), surrounded by a layer of undifferentiated mesenchyme and a circular layer of myoblasts. Branches of vagus nerves develop with terminal groups of cells just outside. Scattered elements of longitudinal muscle layer are in lower esophagus. Cartilage appears in the tracheobronchial tree. Blood vessels from aorta enter submucosa. Esophageal length is 8–10 mm at end of embryonic period. |

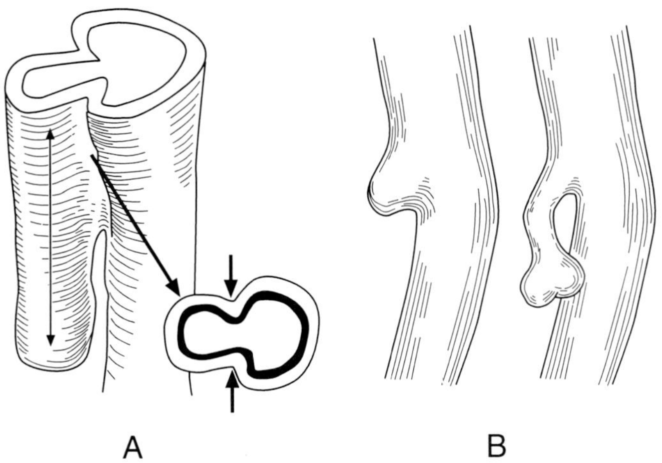


**Fig. 20–2.** Differentiation of the foregut into trachea and esophagus. A: In the former theory, lateral folds were to fuse in the midline in a caudocranial direction (process of septation). B: In the current theory, the tracheobronchial tree develops caudally from a ventral outpouching of the foregut. (Modified from Kluth et al., 1987.[8])

From 12 to 15 weeks, striated muscle appears in the upper esophagus and extends for a variable length. The muscularis mucosa becomes well defined[3] and the longitudinal mesenchymal ridges now give the typical mucosal folds.[4]

At some point during the fourth and fifth months of gestation, the ciliated columnar epithelium is replaced by stratified squamous epithelium. This starts in the midesophagus, then extends to the lower and finally upper parts.[6] The process by which the epithelium is replaced remained unclear, until studies by Ménard and Arsenault.[9] They used 12 to 16 weeks gestation human esophageal explants maintained in organ culture for up to 28 days. After 5 days of culture, the epithelium became thicker and a vacuolization process was noted in the upper half of the epithelium. The ciliated cells lifted off completely and the subjacent cells flattened (Fig. 20–3). Subsequently, even if the explants were maintained in culture, the epithelium remained stratified squamous, with the development of occasional islands of ciliated cells resting on the basal cell layers. The ultrastructure of the new epithelium was comparable to that of adult esophageal epithelium except for the presence of glycogen in the basal cells in the fetal esophageal explants. These

**Table 20–2.** Esophageal development in the fetus (9–40 weeks)

| Age (weeks) | Length (mm) | Events |
|---|---|---|
| 10 | 40–50 | Stratified columnar ciliated epithelium appears in the middle third. Proliferation of all layers of epithelial cells (except ciliated cells) as well as mesenchymal (submucosa) and muscular cells occurs. Mesenchymal ridges lead to longitudinal folds of the mucosa. |
| 10–12 | 40–80 | Intense epithelial proliferation occurs. Simple columnar epithelium (Mucin+) alternates with stratified ciliated.[6] Longitudinal muscle layer is well defined. Ganglion cells in myenteric plexuses appear. Muscularis mucosa appears in lower esophagus. |
| 12–15 | 80–120 | Stratified columnar ciliated epithelium is complete; proliferation is in basal cell layers only. Muscularis mucosa is well defined. Striated muscle appears in upper esophagus and extends for variable length. |
| 4th–6th month | 130+ | Stratified squamous epithelium starts in the middle esophagus, then in the lower and upper esophagus. Superficial glands develop from tall, simple, columnar epithelium. Ciliated cells may be present at birth in the upper esophagus. |

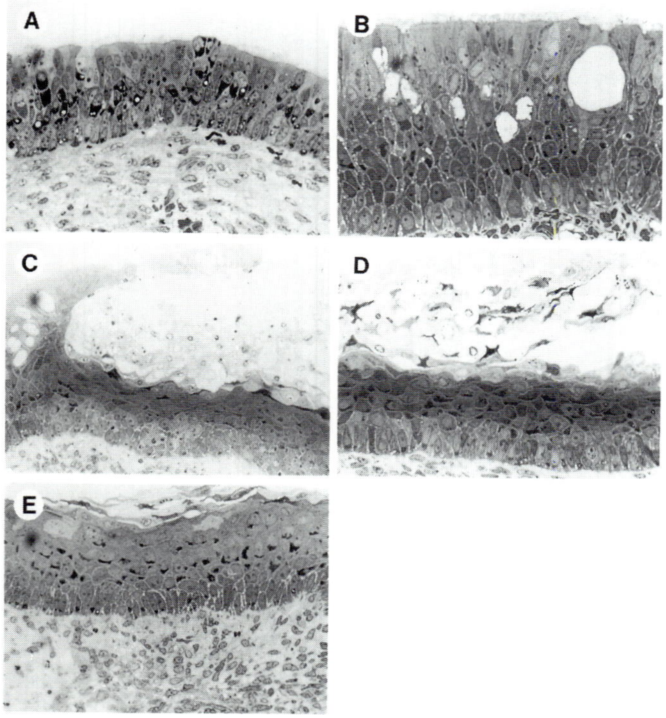

**Fig. 20–3.** Light microscopy of human fetal esophageal explants obtained at 14 weeks gestation and maintained in organ culture (sections stained with 1% methylene blue, 1% azur 11, and 1% borax). A: At the beginning of the culture a stratified ciliated epithelium with aggregates of glycogen is observed. × 110. B: After 5 days of culture the epithelium has increased in thickness and some vacuoles are present in the upper half of the epithelium. × 110. C: After 9 days of culture the upper half of the epithelium is being lifted off and the subjacent cells are flattened and some are desquamating. × 70. D: After 15 days of culture, the surface epithelium is stratified squamous. × 100. E: The general morphology remains unchanged after 21 days. × 100. (Reprinted from Ménard and Arsenault[9] by permission of John Wiley & Sons, Inc.)

well-done experiments help explain previous observations and invite speculations about the causes of the accelerated maturation seen in organ culture.

While most of the epithelium is being replaced, superficial glands form in the upper and lower esophagus. These seem to originate from tall, simple, columnar cells that first appear in the third month.[6] The deep esophageal glands are thought to appear late in gestation, most of their development being postnatal.

With completion of the morphological changes, growth continues at a slower pace, and the esophagus measures about 10 cm at term. In terms of function, swallowing begins at 14 weeks and is well established by the end of the fourth month. The physiology of the swallowing process and the anatomical relationships of the esophagus being outside the scope of this chapter, readers are referred to an excellent review of the subject.[1]

## References


1. Amoury RA: Structure and function of the esophagus in infancy and early childhood. In: Pediatric Esophageal Surgery, KW Ashcraft, TM Holder, eds. Grune and Stratton, Orlando, 1986, pp 1–28.
2. Arsenault P, Ménard D: Autoradiographic localization of [$^3$H]-thymidine incorporation in developing human esophagus. Anat Rec 220:313–317, 1988.
3. Gemonov VV, Kolesnikov LL: Development of oesophageal tissue structures in human embryogenesis. Anat Anz 171:13–15, 1990.
4. Gray SW, Skandalakis JE: Embryology for Surgeons: The Embryological Basis for the Treatment of Congenital Defects. WB Saunders, Philadelphia, 1972.
5. His W: Anatomie menschlicher Embryonen. III. Zur Geschichte der Organe. Vogel, Leipzig, 1885.
6. Johns BAE: Developmental changes in the oesophageal epithelium in man. J Anat 86:431–442, 1952.
7. Kluth D, Habenicht R: The embryology of usual and unusual types of esophageal atresia. Pediatr Surg Int 2:223–227, 1987.
8. Kluth D, Steding G, Seidi W: The embryology of foregut malformations. J Pediatr Surg 22:389–393, 1987.

9. Ménard D, Arsenault P: Maturation of human fetal esophagus maintained in organ culture. Anat Rec 217:348–354, 1987.
10. Ménard D, Renaud J, Beaulieu J-F: Distribution of EGF receptors during the development of the human esophagus. Gastroenterology 100:124, 1991.
11. Moore KL: The Developing Human, 4th ed. WB Saunders, Philadelphia, 1988.
12. O'Rahilly R, Müller F: Respiratory and alimentary relations in staged human embryos. Ann Otol Rhinol Laryngol 93:421–429, 1984.
13. Sadler TW: Langman's Medical Embryology, 5th ed. Williams & Wilkins, Baltimore, 1985.
14. Smith EI: The early development of the trachea and the esophagus in relation to atresia of the esophagus and tracheoesophageal fistula. Contrib Embryol Carnegie Inst 36:41–57, 1957.
15. Stovin PGI: Early lung development. Thorax 40:401–404, 1985.
16. Zaw-Tun HA: The tracheo-esophageal septum—Fact or Fantasy? Origin and development of the respiratory primordium and esophagus. Acta Anat 114:1–21, 1982.

# 21

# Congenital Anomalies of the Esophagus

LUONG T. NGUYEN and JEAN-MARTIN LABERGE

The embryonic foregut gives rise to the esophagus and trachea. Its development is the source of some important malformations that may be life threatening if there is any delay in diagnosis.

The major categories of esophageal anomalies are: atresia and tracheoesophageal fistula; stenosis and webs; cystic and tubular duplications, including dorsal enteric remnants (split notochord); laryngotracheoesophageal clefts; diverticula of esophagus; congenital bronchopulmonary foregut malformations; congenital short esophagus; and vascular malformations (discussed in Chapter 22).

## Esophageal atresia and tracheoesophageal fistula

### History

Esophageal atresia with or without fistula was first described in the seventeenth century.[58] Mortality was 100% before 1939 when Ladd and Leven,[45,46] working independently, succeeded in saving the first babies with this malformation. In 1941, Cameron Haight performed the first successful primary repair and this became the method of choice.[32] Since then, each decade has seen dramatic improvement in the results of treatment, thanks to tremendous progress in pediatric anesthesia and neonatal care, especially mechanical ventilation and total parenteral nutrition.

### Incidence

The reported incidence of esophageal atresia varies from 1 in 3,000 to 1 in 4,500 live births.[20] This anomaly has been described in twins and children of adults who had this malformation.[7,10,14,21,41,42,83] In a 1984 review, Van Staey et al. found 76 familial cases in the literature and added 2 cases.[80] In addition to genetic factors, developmental events related to infectious agents or other teratogenic substances may play a role.[13,64]

### Classification

The various types of esophageal atresia and/or tracheoesophageal fistula are usually regrouped as in Figure 21–1, although many anatomic variations have been described.[44]

In terms of prognosis, the classification proposed by Waterston in 1962 has been widely used.[81] This classification, which took into account the birth weight, the presence and severity of associated anomalies, and pneumonia has become obsolete with advances in neonatal care. At The Montreal Children's Hospital, we found that only severe pulmonary dysfunction (i.e., preoperative ventilator dependence) and the presence of major or life-threatening associated anomalies had a prognostic influence. Birth weight was not found to independently influence mortality. Therefore, we formulated a new classification to include only significant factors (Table 21–1).[66] Most patients fit into class I and have an excellent prognosis (>90% survival) while the few patients in Class II have a mortality rate in excess of 50%.

### Associated anomalies

Nearly 50% of all babies with esophageal atresia have other major malformations, and multiple malformations are the most common cause of postoperative complications and death.[9,24,51,72] Table 21–2 demonstrates the anomalies found in 95 patients at The Montreal Children's Hospital.

#### Cardiovascular malformations

The incidence of these malformations with esophageal atresia is variable (up to 28% in some series). The most common anomalies are patent ductus arteriosus, ventricular septal defect, atrial septal defect, and right aortic arch. More complex cardiac defects may be seen, especially when gastrointestinal or skeletal malformations are present.

#### Gastrointestinal malformations

The most frequent of these malformations in babies with esophageal atresia is imperforate anus (10%). The imperforate anus is usually discovered first. Therefore, any infant born with an imperforate anus must have a radio-opaque catheter passed into the stomach to rule out an esophageal atresia. Associated duodenal atresia can be missed if the initial radiographic study does not include the abdomen.

#### Musculoskeletal anomalies

Anomalies of this nature associated with esophageal atresia include hemivertebrae, rib malformations, and limb anomalies.

#### VATER (or VACTERL) association

The multiple malformations that characterize this association include the following: **V**ertebral anomalies; **A**nal malformations (imperforate anus); **C**ardiac malformations; **T**racheo-**E**sophageal anomalies (atresia, fistula); **R**enal anomalies; and **L**imb malformations (especially radial ray anomalies). This association is seen in approximately 10% of esophageal atresia patients.[55]

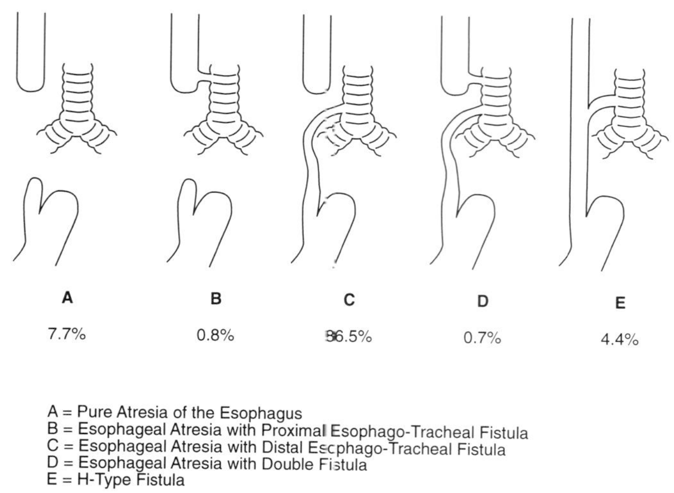


**Fig. 21–1.** Common types of esophageal atresia and/or tracheoesophageal (TE) fistula: A: pure atresia of the esophagus; B: esophageal atresia with proximal TE fistula; C: esophageal atresia with distal TE fistula; D: esophageal atresia with double fistula; E: H-type fistula. Percentages are rates of incidence.

### Other anomalies

Other anomalies associated with esophageal atresia have been described, including pulmonary hypoplasia, pulmonary sequestration, congenital diaphragmatic hernia, and tracheal atresia.[15,36,79]

### Diagnosis and preoperative care—clinical findings

The malformation can often be suspected in the fetus using ultrasound. Polyhydramios is present in nearly all cases of pure esophageal atresia and in up to 60% of esophageal atresia with tracheoesophageal fistula.

After birth, the first symptom is often excessive drooling. The first attempt to feed the baby will result in choking, cyanosis, and regurgitation. Respiratory distress is progressive and the breathing is noisy because of overflow of pharyngeal secretions into the trachea. Atelectasis of the right upper lobe is not a rare finding.

When mechanical ventilation is required, abdominal distension may be massive because of the free passage of air through the fistula into the stomach. Gastric rupture may occur. If an esophageal atresia without tracheoesophageal fistula is present, the abdomen remains flat, since no air can pass into the stomach.

Inability to pass a firm oral tube (at least #10 French) into the stomach confirms the diagnosis. The tube will stop at 10 to 12 cm. A soft and flexible tube should not be used since it may curl in the upper pouch, giving the illusion that it has passed into the stomach. A radiograph of the chest must be obtained to confirm the position of the tube.

Through a "head-to-toe" physical examination, the physician should assess the cardiopulmonary status and look for other anomalies, especially an imperforate anus.

**Table 21–1.** Montreal Children's Hospital Classification of esophageal atresia and tracheoesophageal fistula

| | Ventilation dependent | Associated anomalies |
|---|---|---|
| Class 1 | All patients who do not fulfill criteria for Class 2 | |
| Class 2 | Yes | Major |
| Class 2 | No | Life threatening |

**Table 21–2.** Associated anomalies in 95 patients at The Montreal Children's Hospital

| | |
|---|---|
| Cardiovascular | 20/95 |
| Gastrointestinal | 17/95 |
| Musculoskeletal | 17/95 |
| Craniofacial | 13/95 |
| Genitourinary | 10/95 |
| Respiratory | 9/95 |
| Central nervous system | 5/95 |
| Chromosomal | 3/95 |
| Miscellaneous | 1/95 |

### Investigation

The best radiographic examination is the *babygram,* a radiograph of the whole body which includes the neck, chest, abdomen, and pelvis (Fig. 21–2). Immediately before the X-ray is taken, the mucus should be aspirated and air insufflated through the catheter which is left in place. The upper pouch is sometimes best visualized on a lateral chest radiograph, which should also be done. The presence of gas in the abdomen is an important finding. In nearly all cases, a gas-free abdomen designates an atresia without distal fistula. A "double bubble" indicates an associated duodenal atresia.

The plain film is also examined for the presence of vertebral anomalies or a right-sided aortic arch. In 5–10% of cases, a right aortic arch may interfere with the standard operative approach.[33] Echocardiography can be used to determine the position of the aorta and especially to detect cardiac anomalies.[53]

Contrast studies of the upper pouch are not essential in all cases but may be useful in some patients.[37] When insertion of the oral or nasal tube has been traumatic or when the tube blocks at an unusually high or low level, a false passage may have occurred in a baby who does not have esophageal atresia. Other preoperative studies include a complete blood count, assessment of serum electrolytes, glucose, blood urea nitrogen (BUN), and creatinine, and a cross-matching of blood.

A sagittal computerized tomography (CT) scan can help determine the length of the gap between the upper pouch and the lower esophagus,[78] but this is rarely used clinically.

During the investigation, Replogle sump tube suction should be continued and antibiotics should be started. Intubation and mechanical ventilation may be required, according to the respiratory status.

In the operating room, prior to thoracotomy, bronchoscopy using a fiberoptic rigid bronchoscope is useful. It may identify a proximal fistula, show the exact location of the distal fistula, and help to confirm the side of the aortic arch.

### Operative strategy and technique

After a complete work-up, a decision is then made as to which approach will give the baby the best chance to survive, while restoring esophageal continuity as soon as possible.

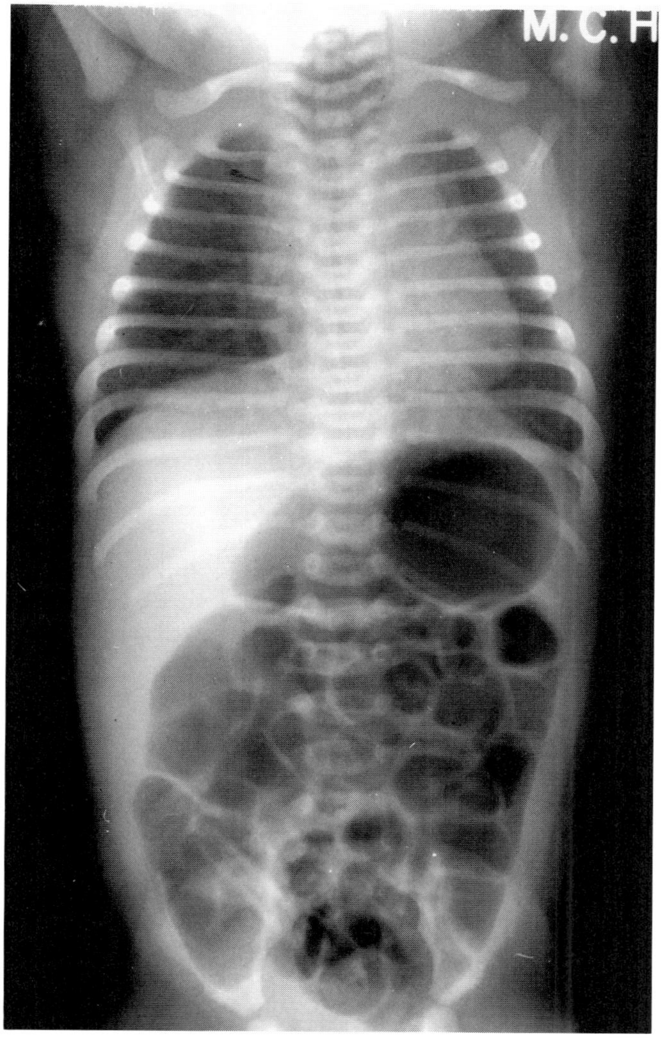

**Fig. 21–2.** A babygram shows a dilated proximal esophageal pouch and gas in the stomach and distal bowel.

### No immediate operation

Surgery can be delayed from several hours up to a few days if the respiratory status is not adequate or if the baby still requires other special studies (echocardiography, chromosome study).

### Gastrostomy and division of fistula

This can improve the respiratory status, decompress the abdomen, and save the baby's life, especially in cases of small prematures with respiratory distress syndrome. We believe that gastrostomy alone is inadequate in these patients because of their noncompliant lungs; the ventilation will go through the fistula into the more compliant stomach.

### Primary repair

This is the treatment of choice and can be accomplished in most patients.

Before surgery, we often establish a percutaneous central venous line to facilitate intraoperative monitoring and postoperative care. Various approaches can be used to gain access to the esophagus. We prefer a limited posterolateral thoracotomy without division of the serratus anterior, and an extrapleural approach (Fig. 21–3).

The lower esophagus is identified just distal to the azygos vein, under the vagus nerve. It is dissected only superiorly up to the junction with the trachea. The lower esophagus and its surrounding tissue should be left intact to preserve the blood vessels that arise directly from the aorta. The fistula is divided close to the trachea to avoid the formation of a blind pouch on the trachea. The trachea is closed with several fine sutures. The upper esophageal pouch is identified by having the anesthetist push a firm catheter into the blind pouch. Traction sutures are placed through all layers of the tip of the upper pouch. The pouch can be mobilized well up to the neck without fear of compromising its blood supply, which arises from the inferior thyroid arteries. The most difficult part of the surgery is the separation of the esophagus from the trachea. Sharp dissection is necessary because the esophagus is contiguous with the trachea at the distal end of the pouch. An upper pouch fistula may be encountered and should be divided and closed. The tip of the esophagus is then opened and the two ends are approximated.

The anastomosis may be carried out by several techniques. We prefer a single layer of interrupted synthetic resorbable 5–0 suture. Corner sutures are placed in the full thickness of either ends, with knots being tied outside the lumen. The posterior row of 3 or 4 sutures is placed with the knots inside the lumen. The Replogle tube is then gently pushed down further through the anastomosis into the stomach. The stomach is aspirated. With completion of the anastomosis, the tube is withdrawn to just above the anastomosis. A small chest tube (10F) is placed close to, but not in contact with, the anastomosis.

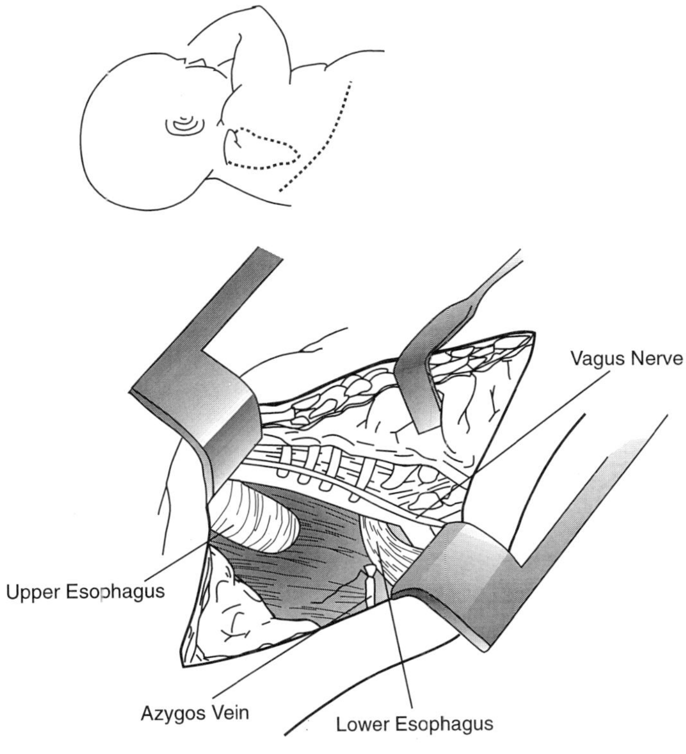


**Fig. 21–3.** Left posterolateral thoracotomy. Divided azygous vein, proximal pouch, and distal tracheoesophageal fistula. Vagus nerve is situated close to the fistula.

The tube is connected to underwater seal drainage to avoid an extrapleural pneumothorax.

### The long gap problem

When faced intraoperatively with a long gap after maximal mobilization, the surgeon has several options:

1. Attempt to repair despite tension. This option is not our preferred technique because of adverse results such as stenosis, leakage, or total dehiscence.[30]
2. Circular myotomy as described by Livaditis. This usually allows elongation of the upper pouch by 1 to 1.5 cm.[50] If necessary, a second or third myotomy can be done.[34] Functional results have been satisfactory.[48,76]
3. Creating a flap from the large upper pouch.
This elongates the upper pouch by about 1.5 cm.[2]
4. Simple closure of the esophagus is a safe method. However, it requires a repeat thoracotomy. The gap will decrease after a waiting period of 8 to 12 weeks.
5. "Suture-fistula" technique.[68,71] The two ends are tied by heavy, nonabsorbable suture. A fistula will be formed between the two ends and establish the continuity. The tract can then be dilated.

### Postoperative care

Neonatal critical care is managed by a team approach.[57] Parenteral nutrition is started when the baby is stable. Continuous suction on the Replogle tube is maintained. Care is taken not to insert the tube past the mark made by the anesthetist in the operating room.

About 1 week postoperatively, a contrast esophagram is carried out under fluoroscopy. This allows assessment of the anastomosis (leak, stenosis), the swallowing reflex, and the motility of the esophagus. The anastomosis always appears narrow. If the study doesn't show a leak, oral feeding should be started slowly because of poor sucking reflex. The child may be discharged when feeding well and gaining weight. It is very important to explain to the parents that there is some permanent scarring at the site of the anastomosis, which prevents normal distensibility, and that the esophagus will always have some degree of dysmotility. We therefore recommend pureed food up to 2 years and then minced food until 5 years of age when the child has learned to chew well before swallowing. Parents should also be well informed about other complications such as gastroesophageal reflux, recurrent fistula, and their consequences.

### Complications

Complications may be related to associated anomalies and prematurity. We will concentrate only on complications related to the tracheoesophageal defect and its treatment. These may be divided into the following:

1. Early complications: anastomotic leak, dehiscence, recurrent fistula, and stenosis[18,35,37,75]
2. Intermediate complications: gastroesophageal reflux, and tracheomalacia[25,28,29,59]
3. Long-term complications: dysphagia, scoliosis, and chest wall deformities.[17]

Fortunately, most anastomotic leaks are minor and seal spontaneously, especially with an extrapleural approach in which the risk of empyema is extremely low. A leak is suspected when drainage from the chest tube is saliva. A small amount of saliva indicates a small leak, which will be shown on the contrast esophagram. Oral feedings are delayed, and most of these leaks will seal spontaneously. A small leak may result in a stenosis of the anastomotic site which will require postoperative dilatation. A major leak or dehiscence of the suture line is indicated by copious drainage associated with major air leaks. This requires urgent thoracotomy to prevent mediastinitis and empyema.

A recurrent tracheoesophageal fistula is a serious complication. The classic approach is a repeat right thoracotomy, transpleural division of the fistula, and interposition of healthy tissue such as pericardial flap or intercostal muscle flap. Endoscopic obliteration has been described, but recurrences are high.[67,70]

Gastroesophageal reflux may present with vomiting, recurrent pneumonia, failure to thrive, and stenosis of the anastomotic site. Evaluation should include repeat contrast radiographs, 24–hour esophageal pH monitoring, and nuclear "milk scan."

Medical treatment is often effective. Esophageal stenosis in this context may respond well to dilatation and medical treatment. Surgery is required in 5% to 20% of patients after esophageal atresia repair. Its indications are repeat pneumonia or failure to thrive, despite optimal medical treatment, and stenosis, despite medical treatment and dilatations.

Severe tracheomalacia, most often at the level of the upper pouch, can often be suspected when the child experiences episodes of "dying spells." Tracheal compression between the aortic arch and the distended upper esophagus can often be seen on the lateral view of the chest X-ray. Bronchoscopy demonstrates tracheal collapse on expiration. The incidence of severe tracheomalacia requiring aortopexy varies from 2.5% to more than 25% of patients.[29,73]

### Long-term results

The overall survival rate is over 90%. Mortality is usually related to the associated anomalies rather than to the esophageal malformation. Despite an esophagus with dysmotility, long-term results are good and most patients live comfortably.[4,16,51] The pulmonary symptoms, esophageal dysmotility, and nutritional status improve with time;[37] however, there is a risk of persistent gastroesophageal reflux and Barrett's esophagus, which could give rise to esophageal cancer.[1,49]

## Esophageal atresia without fistula

Esophageal atresia without fistulous connection to the trachea accounts for approximately 5% to 8% of esophageal anomalies.[37] The gap between the upper pouch and the lower esophagus is long, which precludes any surgical attempt to bring the two ends together in the first days of life.[38]

### Symptomatology and clinical findings

The malformation can be suspected by ultrasonography during intrauterine life. Polyhydramnios is present in nearly all cases.

When the baby is born, excessive drooling combined with a scaphoid abdomen are the most important findings. The "babygram" findings of dilated upper pouch, coupled with an absence of air below the diaphragm are pathognomonic of pure atresia without fistula.

A type C malformation with tracheoesophageal fistula blocked by thick mucus at birth can mimic a pure atresia without fistula and present a gas-free abdomen. If the baby develops episodes of respiratory distress after birth, a proximal fistula should be suspected and an endoscopic examination should be done as soon as possible.[13,37]

### Surgical treatment

In the past, an immediate cervical esophagostomy was performed to drain the saliva away from the trachea. The baby would be fed via a gastrostomy. When the infant was a year old or older, the reconstruction of the missing esophagus would be done, using a gastric tube or a segment of colon or small bowel.[37]

Several attempts have been made by other authors to bring the two ends as close as possible. The two ends of the esophagus were stretched by variable techniques, such as bouginage, using mercury-filled bougie,[39,52] and stretching by electromagnetic current.[58] It has become clear, however, that the esophagus can grow in the first months of life, as demonstrated by Puri et al.,[66a] and Bensoussan and others,[8] making mechanical stretching unnecessary. Maximal growth appeared to be between 8 and 12 weeks.

Currently, we perform a feeding gastrostomy soon after the diagnosis is made. Surgical technique is more delicate than a routine gastrostomy because the stomach is very small, just bigger than the size of a thumb. We prefer to place the gastrostomy near the lesser curvature, keeping the greater curvature intact. Therefore, if the baby needs a reversed gastric tube, the construction of a tube from the intact greater curvature would be much easier. The baby is then kept in the neonatal intensive care unit (NICU), with continuous suction of the upper pouch and feeding via gastrostomy.

Radiographs are obtained at intervals with contrast material in the stomach and a radio-opaque tube in the esophagus. The contrast material will outline the lower esophagus by gastroesophageal reflux, which is usually present in those babies. Therefore, the gap will be appreciated. Primary repair may become feasible at 2 to 3 months of age.

According to Bensoussan et al.,[8] a gap which measures less than two verteral bodies can be brought together without excessive tension on the anastomosis. In some cases when the gap is still excessive after 3 months, a gastric or colon bypass technique may be required for reconstruction of the esophagus.

Kimura et al. have proposed a staged technique using extrathoracic stretching of the upper pouch brought out as a cutaneous esophagostomy.[43] Each time, the cutaneous esophagostomy is dissected free from subcutaneous tissues and then placed under traction further down on the chest wall. The esophageal continuity can be re-established when the upper esophagus can reach the lower esophagus.

### Complications

Complications are similar to those found in esophageal atresia with tracheoesophageal fistula. Oral feeding can be a problem, because these babies may lose the suction reflex.

## Tracheoesophageal fistula without atresia

Congenital tracheoesophageal fistula without atresia (H type or N type TEF) was first described at autopsy by Lamb[56] in 1873. Its incidence varies between 1 and 11% of esophageal malformations.[81] The first successful surgical repair was carried out on a 6-year-old boy via a transtracheal approach.[31]

### Symptomatology

Patients with H-type tracheoesophageal fistula become symptomatic at a later date than patients with esophageal atresia and tracheoesophageal fistula, but most of them present in the newborn period.[5] There are no significant features in the antenatal period; polyhydramnios is rare. There are three major presenting symptoms:

1. Coughing and choking precipitated by feeding. This is a classic mode of presentation and may or may not be associated with cyanosis. It occurs in 80% of patients.[5]
2. Abdominal distension caused by the passage of air through the fistula. The catheter test can be done at bedside; with the tip of the catheter in the esophagus and the other end under water, one can expect to see vigorous bubbling if a fistula is present. Distension of the abdomen is described in over 30% of patients
3. The third mode of presentation is recurrent, often severe pneumonia, which is usually of chemical origin and unresponsive to antibiotics. It can be found in over 70% of patients.[5]

### Diagnostic methods

H-type tracheoesophageal fistula may be suspected on the grounds of clinical symptoms. Investigation is required in order to confirm it and demonstrate its location.

#### Radiologic studies (Fig. 21–4)

The initial barium swallow with videofluoroscopy, although rarely diagnostic, may establish an alternative diagnosis, such as incoordination of the oropharynx, gastroesophageal reflux, or esophageal dysmotility. However, it may also lead to confusion if the infant aspirates the contrast material.

Many techniques have been described, including the use of a radio-opaque catheter, where the tip is inserted in the distal esophagus and the contrast material injected with sufficient pressure to dilate the esophagus.[54] According to Shandling et al.,[5] the fistula can be visualized by contrast studies in approximately 70% of patients. They stressed the importance of repeated contrast examination. Rigid bronchoscopy using a Hopkins' rod lens telescope is very helpful in diagnosis and treatment.[7] The fistula can be catheterized and the catheter left in place; this will facilitate the identification of the fistula at the time of surgery.[7,26]

### Operative technique

Most H-type fistulas are above or at the level of the clavicle and can be reached through a cervical incision. In some cases, partial division of sternocleidomastoid muscle or omohyoid muscle is helpful. A thoracotomy is required in the 10–20% of H-type tracheoesophageal fistulas[5] that are intrathoracic.

In most cases, we prefer to use a right cervical approach to avoid injury to the thoracic duct. With the child supine and the neck hyperextended and turned partially to the left, a transverse incision is made in the lower skin-fold. The carotid sheet and the median portion of the sternocleidomastoid muscle are retracted laterally. The tracheoesophageal groove is bluntly dissected paying attention to hemostasis. The right recurrent nerve, in its position behind the inferior thyroid artery and along the tracheoesophageal groove, must be carefully visualized and preserved. The anterior surface of the esophagus and the posterior surface of the trachea must be also carefully and gently dissected. The presence of a catheter in the fistula,

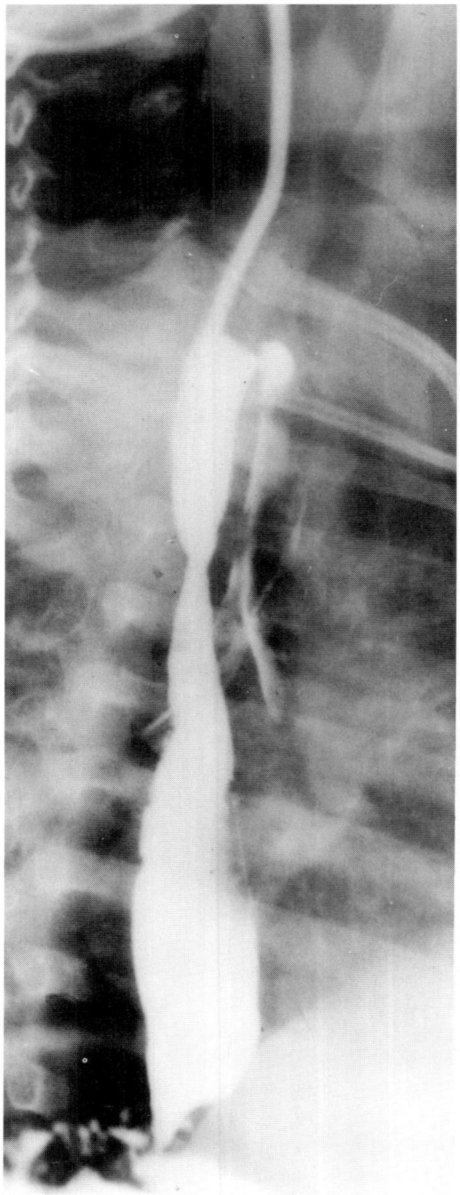

Fig. 21–4. H-Type tracheoesophageal fistula visualized by contrast study.

placed by bronchoscopy at the beginning of the procedure, will greatly facilitate the visualization of the fistula, and will prevent excessive dissection and traction on the recurrent laryngeal nerve (Fig. 21–5). The fistula is then divided and oversewn with 5–0 synthetic suture. A muscle flap from the omohyoid muscle can be interposed at the site of the fistula between the trachea and the esophagus.

### Complications

A recurrent fistula may become apparent after surgery. Its incidence is between 10% and 15%. This requires reoperation with tissue flap interposition.[5] Endoscopic obliteration has been reported.[70] A recurrent laryngeal nerve palsy can be temporary or permanent. Shandling reported a 10% incidence of temporary recurrent laryngeal nerve palsy.[5] Myers and Egami, in their series between 1950 and 1985, recorded an incidence of 30% of recurrent nerve injury.[60] Yazbeck and Dubuc recorded no recurrent nerve palsy in their series of 16 infants.[84] This is a better reflection of current results with this malformation.

## Congenital esophageal stenosis and webs

Esophageal atresia may be complicated by postoperative stenosis, most frequently at the site of anastomosis or in the distal esophagus secondary to gastroesophageal reflux. However, congenital stenosis can also occur in the distal esophagus, away from the site of the anastomosis.

The first case of congenital esophageal stenosis with an esophageal atresia was reported by Dunbar in 1958 from The Montreal Children's Hospital.[23] Up until 1990, 46 cases had been reported, including 6 cases from The Montreal Children's Hospital.[61] Distal esophageal diaphragms or webs or membranous atresia have also been described.[44]

### Histology

Histology was available in 13 of 46 cases reported.[61] The majority (11/13) had tracheobronchial rests and three had fibromuscular stenosis (Fig. 21–6 to 21–8). Nihoul-Fékété et al.[63] in their experience with 20 patients found 6 cases of steno-

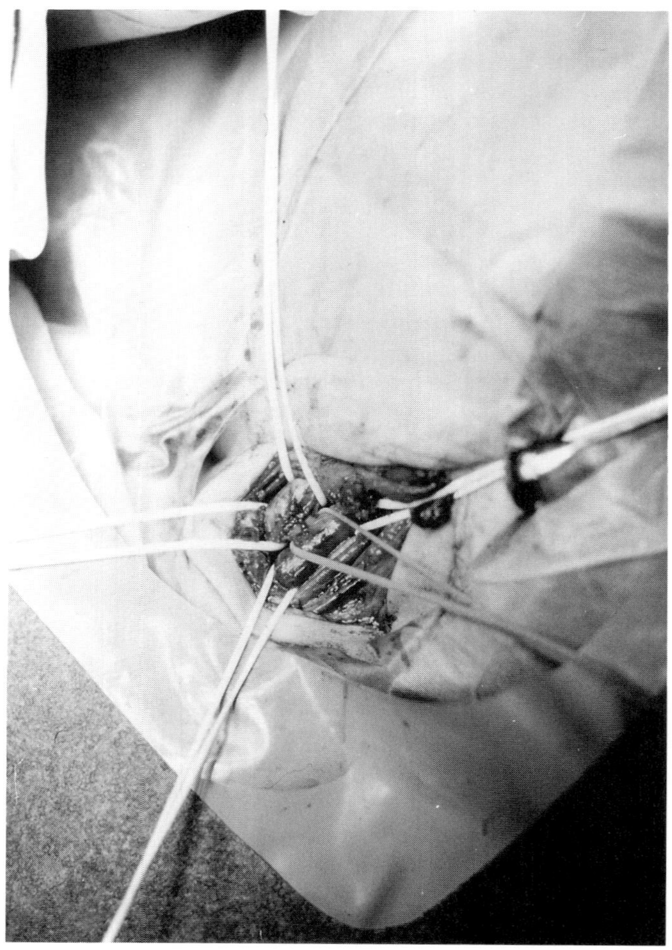

Fig. 21–5. Both trachea and esophagus are dissected and isolated above and below the fistula by umbilical tapes. The fistula is encircled by a vessel loop.

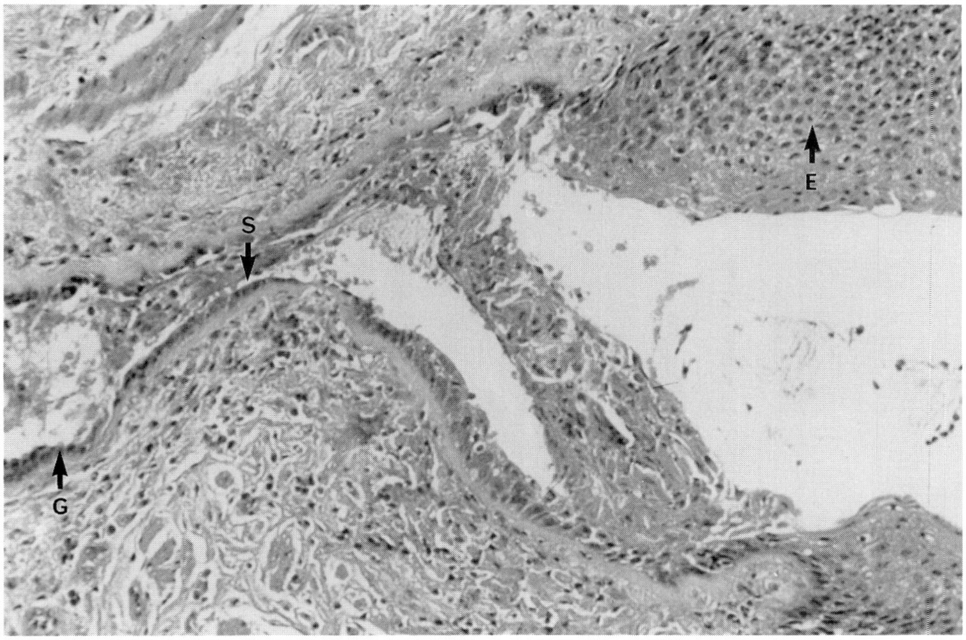


**Fig. 21–6.** Note area of fibromuscular stenosis (S) with different types of lining: glandular (G) and epidermoid (E).

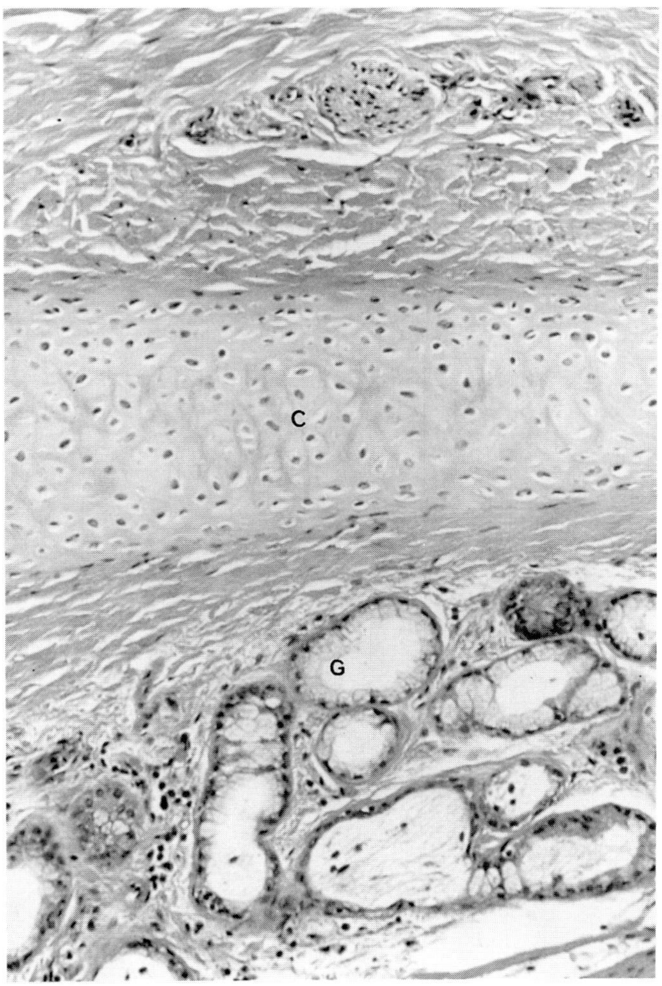


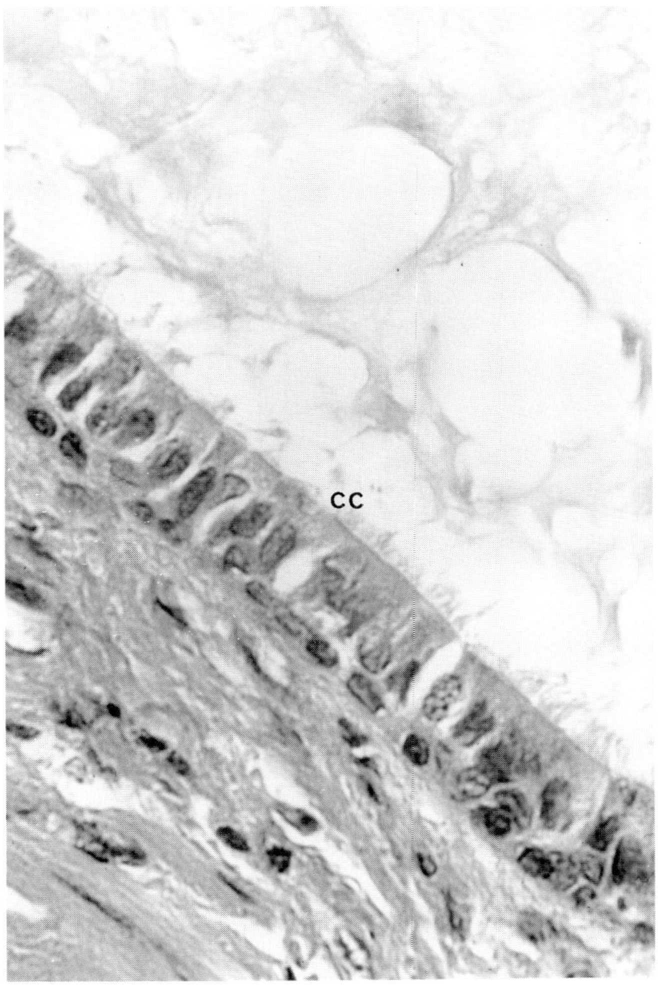


**Figs. 21–7,8.** Fibromuscular stenosis of the distal esophagus under microscopic examination. Cartilage rests (C) and glandular formation (G) are found. The lining is made of ciliated cells (CC).

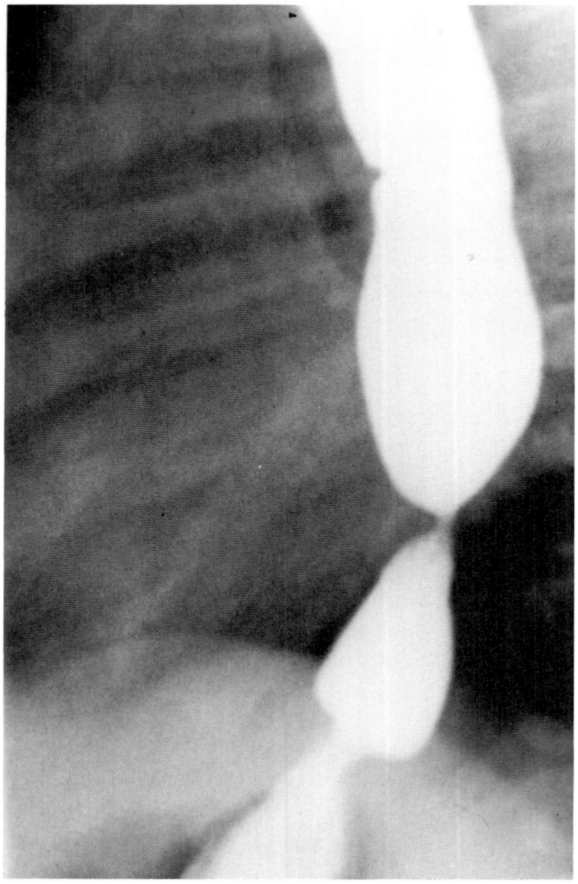

**Fig. 21–9.** Esophagram shows stenosis of the distal esophagus.

sis caused by membranous diaphragm and 10 cases of fibromuscular stenosis. In their series, 18/20 patients had esophageal stenosis alone, without atresia or tracheoesophageal fistula.

### Classification

Nihoul-Fékété et al.[63] classify congenital esophageal stenosis according to histology into group I: tracheobronchial rests (cartilage, respiratory mucus glands, ciliated epithelium); group II: membranous diaphragm; and group III: fibromuscular stenosis.

### Diagnosis

The diagnosis of congenital esophageal stenosis begins with a high index of suspicion. Early symptoms include aspiration with recurrent pneumonia mimicking a recurrence of tracheoesophageal fistula. Dysphagia may become apparent after introduction of solid foods at 4–6 months of age.[63] Because many children after esophageal atresia repair have gastroesophageal reflux, the diagnosis of congenital stenosis may be delayed.

The investigation should include a review of the feeding history and of the initial and repeat cineesophagrams (Fig. 21–9). Endoscopy with biopsy and pH monitoring of the esophagus may also be useful. Even with these investigations, it may be difficult to distinguish congenital esophageal stenosis from strictures due to gastroesophageal reflux.

### Treatment

After investigation, we recommend a single bouginage, which can be combined with the first esophagoscopy. For those caused by fibromuscular stenosis, dilatation may be the only treatment required. If the esophagram shows persistence of the stenosis, a series of hydrostatic balloon dilatations to one atmosphere pressure should be undertaken. If there is a failure of improvement after 2 or 3 dilatations, surgery is recommended. Because the stenosis is short—1–2 cm in length—a limited resection is all that is required.

The long-term prognosis is excellent in most cases, although a high incidence of postoperative gastroesophageal reflux has led some authors to recommend an antireflux procedure at the time of esophageal resection.[63]

## Foregut duplications

Esophageal cystic or tubular duplications are foregut derivatives. They can be associated, therefore, with an extralobar sequestration or a stenosis or atresia of the esophagus.[19] Because of their common origin, bronchogenic cysts and esophageal duplications may be difficult to differentiate histologically.

Cysts, round or tubular, are usually located in the posterior mediastinum, usually on the right side (Fig. 21–10). They may be separated from the esophagus or share a commom wall with

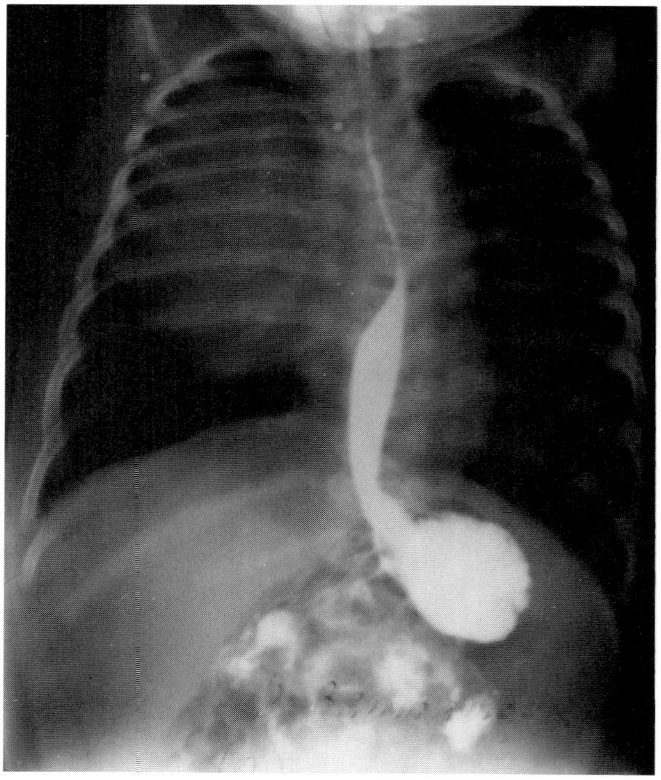

**Fig. 21–10.** Duplication of esophagus: cystic mass displacing the mediastinum and compressing the upper esophagus.

it. They rarely communicate with the esophagus. They may contain gastric mucosa.[19]

### Dorsal enteric remnants

Esophageal duplications may be associated with vertebral anomalies and intraspinal cysts.[77] These are often associated with intra-abdominal intestinal duplications. These anomalies are believed to arise from the failure of the notochord to detach itself from the endoderm, with persistence of a neurenteric canal, i.e., the split notochord theory.[77] A long tubular duplication of the esophagus can also be contiguous with an intestinal duplication, and the extension passes through the esophageal hiatus behind the stomach and pancreas to join the duodenum or jejunum. These duplications are commonly lined partly by gastric mucosa and cause severe hemorrhage.[3]

### Symptoms and clinical findings

Large cystic or tubular duplications can cause cardiac or respiratory problems. When vertebral anomalies are associated, neurological symptoms often predominate.

The chest X-ray may show a soft tissue mass with displacement of the mediastinum. Ultrasonography will differentiate solid from cystic masses while a barium study will confirm extrinsic pressure on the esophagus. Computed tomography may help to plan for surgical removal and nuclear medicine (technetium scan) may identify ectopic gastric mucosa. In the past, myelography with or without computed tomography was used to detect intraspinal cysts when vertebral anomalies were present. Magnetic resonnance imaging (MRI) should now be the examination of choice.

The surgical treatment consists of careful removal of the duplication cyst. On the common wall with the esophagus, a mucosectomy removing the lining would be appropriate. If the duplication cyst extends through the diaphragm, even by a small fistulous tract, a subsequent laparotomy will be required to remove the intra-abdominal duplication.[3] Complete removal gives excellent results. In the presence of an intraspinal cyst, this should be approached first, unless the mediastinal part is symptomatic.[77]

## Diverticulum of esophagus

True congenital diverticula are extremely rare. In the literature, Borrie and Wilson[11] reported a congenital diverticulum of the midesophagus associated with an H-type tracheoesophageal fistula in an 11-year-old boy. Nelson[62] reported a case of true diverticulum originating at the level of $T_1$ and compressing the trachea. The pulsion diverticulum has also been reported.[27] It is the herniation of the mucosa through defects in the muscular wall. Symptoms are similar to those seen in adults, i.e., vomiting, regurgitation, and recurrent lung infections. Some authors believe that this lesion is very likely an incomplete form of duplication.[19]

## Laryngotracheoesophageal cleft (LTEC)

Laryngotracheoesophageal cleft is a rare malformation characterized by a midline defect of variable length between the posterior larynx and trachea and the anterior wall of the esophagus.[22] Its severe forms are usually lethal.

### Classification

LTEC has been classified into three types[82] (Fig. 21–11): type 1 (31%) is a cleft limited to the larynx involving part or all of the cricoid plate; type 2 cleft (47%) extends into the trachea as far as the proximal six rings; and the type 3 (22%) defect extends to the carina.

### Associated anomalies

Associated anomalies include cardiovascular anomalies in 16% to 33% of patients, and genitourinary tract anomalies, including undescended testis, hypospadias, renal agenesis, and multicystic kidney, are found in 14% to 44% of patients. LTEC may also be associated with esophageal atresia or tracheoesophageal fistula.[22]

### Symptomatology

The severity of the symptoms vary with the length of the cleft. Clinical manifestations may be life threatening at birth, but a small lesion of type 1 can remain unsuspected for several years.[22] Symptoms are respiratory distress, cyanosis, and choking and coughing during feeding.

### Diagnosis

Laryngotracheoesophageal clefts may be difficult to diagnose. There are many reports of failure to recognize this lesion after multiple diagnostic attempts.[6,65] A high index of suspicion may

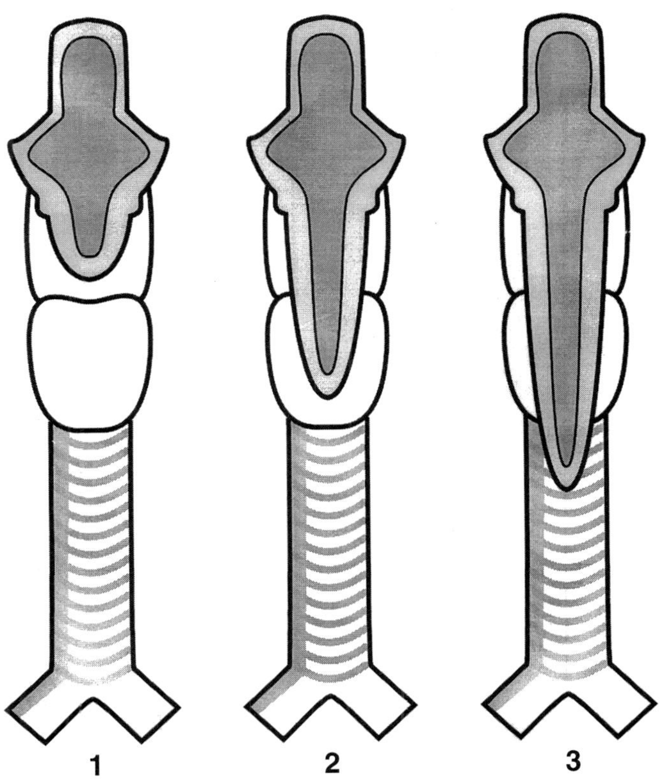


**Fig. 21–11.** Classification of laryngotracheoesophageal clefts. Type 1: cleft limited to the larynx, involving part or all of the cricoid plate. Type 2: cleft extends into the proximal tracheal rings. Type 3: defect extends to the carina.

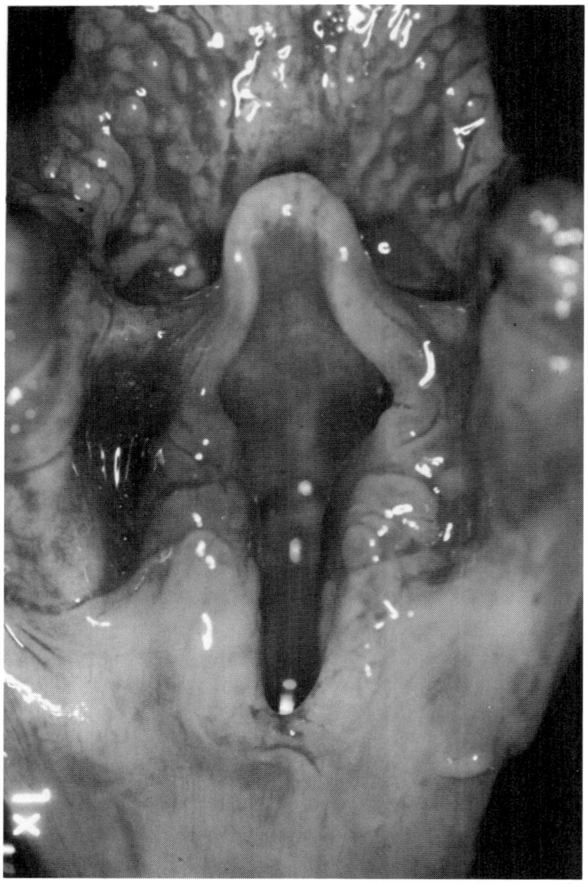

**Fig. 21–12.** Autopsy finding in a patient. A laryngotracheoesophageal cleft, type 2.

make us think about the possibility of a laryngotracheoesophageal cleft, especially when the endotracheal tube is dislodged in the esophagus.[82] Endoscopy remains the definitive method of diagnosis, but the redundancy of the esophageal mucosa may make the endoscopic visualization difficult[82](Fig. 21–12).

### Treatment

For small clefts, treatment may not be necessary. The condition of infants with clefts confined to the larynx (type 1) tends to improve with growth and the majority have not required repair. We agree with Lim and associates[47] that if the infant is symptomatic only when fed, a trial of nasogastric or gastrostomy tube feedings should be employed and definitive repair performed only if thickened oral feedings cannot be tolerated after several months.

Emergency endotracheal intubation or tracheostomy may be required for respiratory distress in more severe cases. Gastric decompression is necessary to prevent aspiration. In large laryngotracheoesophageal clefts, we prefer a gastrostomy to a nasogastric tube, because the tube may become displaced anteriorly obstructing the trachea.

### Surgical repair

A tracheostomy is always required at the time of operation. Three operative approaches have been employed. The anterior approach involves the division of the cricoid and upper trachea in the midline. This approach allows adequate visualization. The edges of the cleft are incised bilaterally from within. The esophagus and the trachea are each approximated in turn.

The lateral laryngopharyngotomy approach is most widely used. Esophageal tissue should be left on the tracheal side to avoid compromising the airway.

In the posterior approach the esophagus is entered from behind to minimize the danger of possible injury to the recurrent and superior laryngeal nerves. Interposition of strap muscle as recommended by Donahoe and Hendren is effective.[21a] Extensive clefts require a combined cervical and thoracic approach.

Postoperatively, the patient is fed by gastrostomy or nasogastric tube. The tracheostomy is left in place.

### Results

Recurrence is reported in about 10% of patients.[65] The survival rate in recent years has improved dramatically. Before 1970, only 18% of patients survived, as compared with a 75% survival rate since that time.[82] Nevertheless, laryngotracheoesophageal clefts remain a great challenge. Gastroesophageal reflux, tracheomalacia, tracheostomy dependence, and feeding difficulties contribute to long-term morbidity.

## Congenital bronchopulmonary foregut malformations

Congenital bronchopulmonary foregut malformations (CBPFM) are rare congenital anomalies characterized by a communication between the esophagus and an isolated portion of the respiratory system (a lung, lobe, or segment).[40,69] Srikanth et al.[74] found 51 cases in the literature and added six of their own. Symptoms may be respiratory distress, cough while feeding, and recurrent pneumonia.

In most cases, radiologic studies confirm the diagnosis. Surgery gives excellent results in over 80% of patients.

## Congenital short esophagus

Congenital short esophagus is extremely rare.[12] It does not allow the stomach to be placed in the abdomen. Therefore, it is usually associated with a hiatus hernia. The child may present with vomiting or failure to thrive in the first month of life. Surgical intervention is the treatment of choice and consists of an antireflux Collis-Nissen type procedure.

### References

1. Adzick NS, Fisher JH, Winter HS, Saandler RH, Hendren H: Esophageal adenocarcinoma 20 years after esophageal atresia repair. J Pediatr Surg 24:741–744, 1989.
2. Bar-Maor JA, Shoshany G, Sweed Y: Wide gap esophageal atresia: a new method to elongate the upper pouch. J Pediatr Surg 24:882–883, 1989.
3. Beardmore HE, Wiglesworth FW: Vertebral anomalies and alimentary tract duplications. Pediatr Clin North Am 5:457–474, 1958.
4. Beasley SW, Myers NA: Trends in mortality in esophageal atresia. Pediatr Surg Int 7:86–89, 1992.
5. Bedard D, Girvan DP, Shandling B: Congenital H-type tracheoesophageal fistula. J Pediatr Surg 9:663–668, 1974.
6. Bell DW, Christiansen TA, Smith TE Jr, Stucker FJ: Laryngotracheoesophageal cleft: the anterior approach. Ann Otol Rhinol Laryngol 86:616–622, 1977.

7. Benjamin B, Pham T: Diagnosis of H-type tracheoesophageal fistula. J Pediatr Surg 26:667–671, 1991.
8. Bensoussan AL, Letourneau JN, Blanchard H: Cure de l'atrésie de l'oesophage de type I et II: Anastomose primaire différée. Chir Pediatr 24:109–112, 1983.
9. Besser AS, Roberts CC, Ashcroft KW: Esophagus, atresia. In: Birth Defects Encyclopedia, M-L Buyse, ed. Blackwell Scientific Publications, Cambridge, 1990, p 641.
10. Blank RH, Prillaman PE Jr, Miron GR: Congenital esophageal atresia with tracheoesophageal fistula occurring in identical twins. J Thorac Cardiovasc Surg 53:192–196, 1967.
11. Borrie J, Wilson RLK: Oesophageal diverticula: principle of management and appraisal of classification. Thorax 35:759–767, 1980.
12. Brown RE, Madge GE, Howell TR: Congenital short esophagus in the newborn. Dig Dis 15:863–868, 1976.
13. Cass D, Auldist A: Oesophageal atresia with proximal tracheo-oesophageal fistula. Pediatr Surg Int 2:212–215, 1987.
14. Chen H, Goei GS, Hertzler JH: Family studies on congenital esophageal atresia with or without tracheoesophageal fistula. Birth Defects 15:117–144, 1979.
15. Chen JM, Schloss MD, Laberge J-M: Extensive upper aerodigestive tract anomalies in "VACTERL" association. Arch Otolaryngol Head Neck Surg 117:1407–1410, 1991.
16. Chetcuti P, Myers NA, Phelan PD, Beasley SW: Adults who survived repair of congenital oesophageal atresia and tracheo-oesophageal fistula. Br Med J 297:344–346, 1988.
17. Chetcuti P, Myers NA, Phelan PD, Beasley SW, Dickens DR: Chest wall deformity in patient with repaired esophageal atresia. J Pediatr Surg 24:244–247, 1989.
18. Chittmittrapap S, Spitz L, Kiely EM, Brereton RJ: Anastomotic leakage following surgery for esophageal atresia. J Pediatr Surg 27:29–32, 1992.
19. Dehner LP: Pediatric Surgical Pathology, 2nd ed. Williams & Wilkins, Baltimore, 1987, pp 334–336.
20. de Lorimier AA, Harrisson MR: Esophageal atresia: embryogenesis and management. World J Surg 9:250–257, 1985.
21. Dennis NR, Nicholas JL, Kovar I: Oesophageal atresia: 3 cases in 2 generations. Arch Dis Child 48:980–983, 1983.
21a. Donahoe PK, Hendren WH: The surgical management of laryngotracheoesophageal cleft with tracheoesophageal fistula and esophageal atresia. Surgery 71:636–368, 1972.
22. Dubois JJ, Pokorny WJ, Harberg FJ, Smith RJ: Current management of laryngeal and laryngotracheoesophageal clefts. J Pediatr Surg 25:855–860, 1990.
23. Dunbar, JS: Congenital oesophageal stenosis. Pediatr Clin North Am 5:433–455, 1958.
24. Ein SH, Shandling B, Wesson D, Filler RM: Esophageal atresia with distal tracheoesophageal fistula: associated anomalies and prognosis in the 1980's. J Pediatr Surg 24:1055–1059, 1989.
25. Filler RM, Messineo A, Vinograd I: Severe tracheomalacia associated with esophageal atresia: results of surgical treatment. J Pediatr Surg 27:1136–1140, 1992.
26. Filston HC, Rankin JS, Kirks DR: The diagnosis of primary and recurrent tracheoesophageal fistulas: value of selective catheterization. J Pediatr Surg 17:144–148, 1982.
27. Fiser WP, Euler AR, Golladay ES: Pharyngoesophageal pulsion diverticulum (Zenker) in a ten-year-old boy. J Pediatr Surg 16:727–729, 1981.
28. Garabedian EN, Aubert P, Cotin G, Belas M, Gruner M: Sténoses post-anastomotiques dans les atrésies de l'oesophage: Etude à propos de 23 cas. Ann Otolaryngol Chir Cervicofac 104:157–161, 1987.
29. Guy JM, Triglia JM, Louis C, Panuel M, Carcassonne M: Esophageal atresia, tracheomalacia and arterial compression: role of aortopexy. Eur J Pediatr Surg 1:261–265, 1991.
30. Hagberg S, Rubenson A, Sillen U, Werkmäster K: Management of long gap esophagus: experience with end-to-end anastomosis under maximal tension. Prog Pediatr Surg 19:88–92, 1986.
31. Haight C: Some observations on esophageal atresia and tracheoesophageal fistulas of congenital origin. J Thorac Cardiovasc Surg 34:147–172, 1957.
32. Haight C, Towsley HA: Congenital atresia of the esophagus with tracheoesophageal fistula. Extrapleural ligation of fistula and end-to-end anastomosis of esophageal segments. Surg Gynecol Obstet 76:672–688, 1943.
33. Harrisson MR, Hanson BA, Mahour GH, Takahashi M, Weitzmann JJ: The significance of right aortic arch in repair of esophageal atresia and tracheoesophageal fistula. J Pediatr Surg 12:861–869, 1977.
34. Hoffman DG, Moazam F: Transcervical myotomy for wide-gap esophageal atresia. J Pediatr Surg 19:680–682, 1984.
35. Hoffer FA, Winter HS, Fellows KE, Folman J: The treatment of postoperative and peptic esophageal strictures after esophageal atresia repair. Pediatr Radiol 17:454–458, 1987.
36. Hoffman MA, Superina R, Wesson DE: Unilateral pulmonary agenesis with esophageal atresia and distal tracheoesophageal fistula: report of two cases. J Pediatr Surg 24:1084–1085, 1989.
37. Holder TM: Esophageal atresia and tracheoesophageal malformation. In: Pediatric Surgery, 2nd ed, KW Ashcraft, TM Holder, eds. WB Saunders, Philadelphia, 1993, pp 249–269.
38. Holder TML, Ashcraft KW: Esophageal atresia and tracheoesophageal malformations. In: Pediatric Surgery, TM Holder, KW Ashcraft, eds. WB Saunders, Philadelphia, 1980, pp 266–283.
39. Howard R, Myers NA: Esophageal atresia: a technique for elongation of the upper pouch. Surgery 58:725–727, 1965.
40. Johnson F, Lain T: Radionuclide evaluation of a communicating bronchopulmonary foregut malformation. Pediatr Radiol 7:175–177, 1978.
41. Kashuk JL, Lilly JR: Esophageal atresia in father and son. J Pediatr Surg 18:621–622, 1983.
42. Kiesewetter WB, Bower RJ: Tracheoesophageal fistula in parent and offspring: a rare occurrence. Am J Dis Child 134:896, 1980.
43. Kimura K, Nishijima E, Tsugawa C, Matsumoto Y: A new approach for the salvage of unsuccessful esophageal atresia repair: a spiral myotomy and delayed definitive operation. J Pediatr Surg 22:981–983, 1987.
44. Kluth D: Atlas of esophageal atresia. J Pediatr Surg 11:901–919, 1976.
45. Ladd WE: The surgical treatment of esophageal atresia and tracheoesophageal fistulas. New Engl J Med 230:625–637, 1944.
46. Leven NL: Congenital atresia of esophagus with tracheoesophageal fistula: report of successful extrapleural ligation of fistulous communication and cervical esophagostomy. J Thoracic Surg 10:648–657, 1941.
47. Lim TA, Spanier SS, Kohut RI: Laryngeal clefts: a histopathology study and review. Ann Otol Rhinol Laryngol 88:837–845, 1979.
48. Lindahl H, Louhimo I: Livaditis myotomy in long-gap esophageal atresia. J Pediatr Surg 22:109–112, 1987.
49. Lindahl H, Rintala R, Sariola H: Chronic esophagitis and gastric metaplasia are frequent complications of esophageal atresia. J Pediatr Surg 28:1178–1180, 1993.
50. Livaditis A: Esophageal atresia: A method of overbridging large segmental gaps. Z Kinder Chir 13:298–306, 1973.
51. Louhimo I, Lindahl H: Esophageal atresia: primary results of 500 consecutively treated patients. J Pediatr Surg 18:217–229, 1983.
52. Mahour GH, Woolley MM, Gwin JL: Elongation of the upper pouch and delayed anastomotic reconstruction in esophageal atresia. J Pediatr Surg 9:373–383, 1974.
53. Mee RBB, Beasley SW, Auldist AW, Myers NA: Influence of congenital heart disease on management of oesophageal atresia. Pediatr Surg Int 7:90–93, 1992.
54. Moncrief JA, Randolph JG: Congenital tracheoesophageal fistula without atresia of the esophagus. A method for diagnosis and surgical correction. J Thorac Cardiovasc Surg 51:434–442, 1966.
55. Muraji T, Mahour GH: Surgical problems in patients with VATER-associated anomalies. J Pediatr Surg 27:550–554, 1984.
56. Murray M, Kappelman M, Dorst AMJ, Haller A, Stambler A: H-type tracheoesophageal fistula. J Dis Child 118:568–575, 1969.
57. Myers NA: Oesophageal atresia. Editorial comments. Pediatr Surg Int 7:83–85, 1992.
58. Myers NA, Aberdeen GH: Congenital esophageal atresia and tracheoesophageal fistula. In: Pediatric Surgery, 3rd ed, MM Ravitch, KJ Welch, CD Benson, E Aberdeen, JG Randolph, eds.Year Book Medical Publishers, Chicago, 1979, pp 446–469.
59. Myers NA, Beasley SW, Auldist AW: Secondary esophageal surgery following repair of esophageal atresia with distal tracheoesophageal fistula. J Pediatr Surg 25:773–777, 1990.
60. Myers NA, Egami K: Congenital tracheoesophageal fistula. "H" or "N" fistula. Pediatr Surg Int 2:198–211, 1987.
61. Neilson IR, Croitoru DP, Guttman FM, Youssef S, Laberge J-M: Distal congenital esophageal stenosis associated with esophageal atresia. J Pediatr Surg 26:478–481, 1991.
62. Nelson AR: Congenital true esophageal diverticulum. Report of a case unassociated with other esophago–tracheal anomalies. Ann Surg 145:258–264, 1957.
63. Nihoul-Fékété C, De Backer A, Lortat-Jacob S, Pellerin D: Congenital esophageal stenosis. A review of 20 cases. Pediatr Surg Int 2:86–92, 1987.

64. Ozimek CD, Grimson RC, Aylsworth AS: An epidemiologic study of tracheoesophageal fistula and esophageal atresia in North Carolina. Teratology 25:53–59, 1982.
65. Pillsbury HC, Fischer ND: Laryngotracheoesophageal cleft. Diagnosis, management, and presentation of a new diagnostic device. Arch Otolaryngol 103:735–737, 1977.
66. Poenaru D, Laberge JM, Neilson IR, Guttman FM: A new prognositic classification for esophageal atresia. Surgery 113:426–432, 1993.
66a. Puri P, Blake N, O'Donnell B, Guiney EJ: Delayed primary anastomosis following spontaneous growth of esophageal segments in esophageal atresia. J Pediatr Surg 16:180–183, 1981.
67. Rangecroft L, Bush GH, Lister J, Irving IM: Endoscopic diathermy obliteration of recurrent tracheoesophageal fistulae. J Pediatr Surg 19:41–43, 1984.
68. Rehbein F, Schweder N: Reconstruction of the esophagus without colon transposition in cases of atresia. J Pediatr Surg 6:746–752, 1971.
69. Rodgers BM, Harman PK, Johnson AM: Bronchopulmonary foregut malformations: The spectrum of anomalies. Ann Surg 203:517–524, 1986.
70. Schmittenbecher PP, Mantel K, Hoffman U, Berlien H-P: Treatment of congenital tracheoesophageal fistula by endoscopic laser coagulation: preliminary report of three cases. J Pediatr Surg 27:26–28, 1992.
71. Shafer AD, David TE: Suture fistula as a means of connecting upper and lower segments in esophageal atresia. J Pediatr Surg 9:669–673, 1974.
72. Sillen U, Hagberg S, Rubenson A, Werkmaster K: Management of esophageal atresia: review of 16 years' experience. J Pediatr Surg 23:805–809, 1988.
73. Spitz L, Kiely EM, Brereton RJ: Esophageal atresia: five year experience with 148 cases. J Pediatr Surg 22:103–108, 1987.
74. Srikanth MS, Ford EG, Stanley P, Mahour GH: Communicating broncho-pulmonary foregut malformations: classification and embryogenesis. J Pediatr Surg 27:732–736, 1992.
75. Stringer DA, Ein SH: Recurrent tracheo-esophageal fistula: a protocol for investigation. Radiology 151:637–641, 1984.
76. Sumitomo K, Ideda K, Nagasaki A: Esophageal manometrical assessment after esophageal circular myotomy for wide-gap esophageal atresia. Jpn J Surg 18:218–223, 1988.
77. Superina RA, Ein SH, Humphreys RP: Cystic duplications of the esophagus and neurenteric cysts. J Pediatr Surg 19:527–530, 1984.
78. Tam PK, Chan FL, Saing H: Direct sagittal CT scan: a new diagnostic approach for surgical neonates. J Pediatr Surg 22:397–400, 1987.
79. Udassin R, Zamir O, Peleg O, Lernau OZ: Coexisting left diaphragmatic hernia and esophageal atresia. Pediatr Surg Int 2:301–303, 1987.
80. Van Staey M, De Bie S, Matton MT, De Roose J: Familial congenital esophageal atresia. Hum Genet 66:260–266, 1984.
81. Waterston DJ, Bonham Carter RE, Aberdeen E: Oesophageal atresia: tracheo–esophageal fistula: a study of survival of 218 infants. Lancet 1:819–822, 1962.
82. Wolfson PJ, Schloss M, Guttman FM, Nguyen L: Laryngotracheoesophageal cleft. Arch Surg 119:228–230, 1984.
83. Woolley MM, Chinnock RF, Paul RH: Premature twins with esophageal atresia and tracheo-esophageal fistula. Acta Paediatr 50:423–430, 1961.
84. Yazbeck S, Dubuc M: Congenital tracheoesophageal fistula without esophageal atresia. Can J Surg 26:239–241, 1983.

# 22

# Vascular Anomalies Involving the Trachea and Esophagus

ROBERT L. WILLIAMS

Mediastinal vascular anomalies have been found at autopsy during the last 300 years and their clinical and radiographic features were described in the first half of this century. The identification and management became clinically important in 1945 when Gross reported the first successful surgical division of a double aortic arch.[24]

Congenital malformations of the major mediastinal arteries may displace or encircle the trachea and esophagus as isolated lesions, in association with congenital heart disease, or as a component of a multisystem syndrome. The clinical features range from incidental asymptomatic findings to life threatening airway obstruction. This chapter will concentrate on the major vascular rings (Table 22–1). The pathogenesis is fascinating, the clinical features are variable, and the modalities available for investigation are diverse. The treatment is specific and the prognosis is almost always excellent.

## Incidence

The true incidence of vascular anomalies is difficult to determine for many are asymptomatic and found only at autopsy. The incidence of anomalous right subclavian artery with a left aortic arch is well established at about 0.5% of the general population from contrast examinations of the upper gastrointestinal tract. The incidence of vascular rings in children with cardiac problems is reasonably well known. One to two percent of 17,271 children referred to the cardiac clinics of the Boston Children's Hospital and the Toronto Sick Children's Hospital from 1950 to 1970 had a vascular ring.[36] This, of course, is an underestimate of the incidence in the general population for, as will be shown, most patients with rings do not have congenital heart disease and many are asymptomatic. The right aortic arch with anomalous left subclavian artery and ligamentum arteriosum is the most common vascular ring. Most of these patients are asymptomatic, however, and double aortic arch is the most common surgical lesion.

## Etiology

Information on the etiology of vascular anomalies in humans can only be surmised from clinical associations. For example, there is a high incidence of abnormalities of the aortic arch and conotruncus in patients with the DiGeorge syndrome, which is a defect of structures derived from the third and fourth pharyngeal pouches. Experimental embryologists have produced cardiac and aortic anomalies by applying topical catecholamines or ionizing radiation to chick embryos at critical stages of development. Neural crest cells that migrate from specific rostral somites have been shown to influence cardiac conotruncal development and the mesenchymal components of the pharyngeal pouches. Aortic arch and cardiac defects can be produced by extirpation of precise portions of the neural crest of the chick embryo before this migration occurs.[29] All these mechanisms, probably acting by changing local embryonic hemodynamics for altered patterns of flow, can lead to abnormal cardiovascular development even in the late-gestation fetal lamb.[40]

## Functional embryology

A knowledge of current concepts of normal human embryology is useful in understanding the pathological anatomy. The following brief summary is from Barry[3] and Edwards.[14]

In very early embryonic life there are two paired aortae emerging from the rostral cardiac sac. These turn dorsally and elongate caudally to persist as the two paired dorsal aortae. The proximal aortae fuse to form the aortic sac in continuity with the primitive heart. The distal dorsal aortae fuse to form the midline descending aorta. The ventral and dorsal portion of the paired aortae are joined by six pairs of interconnecting arteries. These come to be associated with each of the classical pharyngeal pouches of Rathke. Intersegmental arteries also arise from the dorsal aorta to supply the body somites.

The arch system is bilaterally symmetrical at this stage of development. The regression of certain segments and the differential growth of other vessels leads to the normal left-sided aortic arch (Fig. 22–1). The fourth and sixth arch and the first seven dorsal intersegmental arteries are of particular interest. The left fourth arch persists as that part of the left arch between the left common carotid and left subclavian arteries. The right fourth arch becomes the proximal right subclavian artery. The proximal sixth arch forms the proximal right and left pulmonary arteries. Both distal sixth arches form a ductus arteriosus but the right almost always regresses at an early stage. The more distal branches of the pulmonary arteries arise from the post branchial plexus. The left subclavian artery forms from the seventh dorsal intersegmental artery and that portion of the left dorsal arch distal to the left sixth arch. It migrates relatively cranially by differential growth and normally originates from the arch proximal to the left sixth arch (the ductus arteriosus). The third arch contributes to the carotid circulation and the fifth arch is transient and thought to form no part of the normal mature aortic system.

In this chapter, the term *ductus arteriosus* will be used in the fetus and ligamentum arteriosum after birth; however, it must be realized that it takes several weeks after birth for a true ligamentum to form and the ductus may remain patent abnor-

**Table 22–1.** Congenital vascular anomalies that may encircle or displace the trachea and/or esophagus

| |
|---|
| Double aortic arch* |
| Both arches patent |
| One arch partially atretic |
| Right aortic arch |
| Mirror image branching |
| Usual branching |
| Retroesophageal left ductus |
| Anomalous left subclavian artery* |
| Left retroesophageal descending aorta |
| Normal branching |
| Anomalous left subclavian artery |
| Right cervical aorta |
| Left aortic arch |
| Anomalous right subclavian artery |
| Right retroesophageal descending aorta |
| Normal branching |
| Anomalous right subclavian artery |
| "Anomalous innominate artery"* |
| Left cervical aorta |
| Severe cardiac malposition |
| Anomalous left pulmonary artery "sling"* |

*Major clinical lesions—see text for details.

mally particularly when associated with congenital heart disease.

Edwards modified the Barry schematic diagram into a clinically useful hypothetical double aortic arch with bilateral ducti arteriosi (Fig. 22–2).[45] Notice that the heart and lungs have been removed, the descending aorta is in the midline, and the distal dorsal aortic roots have been elongated. The relationship of the major vessels to the trachea and esophagus, however, is clearly appreciated. The final left or right aortic arch and most of the vascular rings can be explained by persistence or failure of regression of structures indicated in this diagram.

The *normal left arch* with a left descending aorta and left ligamentum arteriosum results from regression of the right ductus and the eighth segment of the right dorsal aorta (area 1 in Fig. 22–2).

A *double aortic arch* of the usual type results from regression of the right ductus and failure of regression of the eighth segment of the right dorsal aorta (area 1 in Fig. 22–2).

A *right aortic arch with anomalous left subclavian artery* and ligamentum arteriosum results from regression of that segment of the left aortic arch between the carotid and subclavian arteries which is derived from the left fourth aortic arch (area 4 in Fig. 22–2). There is also regression of the right ductus.

## Clinical manifestations

The clinical manifestations are almost exclusively respiratory with the severity and age of onset related to the degree of airway compression. The severely symptomatic neonates usually have a double aortic arch or, less frequently, a pulmonary artery sling. In a surgical series of 51 vascular lesions, 39 were symptomatic neonates and 25 of these were symptomatic from the time of birth.[39]

Respiratory stridor with an inspiratory and expiratory component may be associated with a harsh cry, tachypnea, and wheezing. All these features are accentuated by any activity, including feeding. The amount of respiratory distress may be exquisitely sensitive to head position and the baby may extend the neck presumably to improve the airway narrowing. There may be episodes of cyanosis leading to a cardiorespiratory arrest which requires resuscitation, intubation, and emergency surgery. There may be a barking cough and recurrent episodes of lower respiratory tract infections.

The findings on physical examination may include intermittent cyanosis, increased effort of breathing, indrawing, abnormal head position, audible wheezing, barking cough, and coarse upper airway sounds and wheezing on auscultation.

True dysphagia is difficult to assess because feeding difficulties may be related to respiratory distress and many of the lesions are corrected before the introduction of solid foods. Most of the information is from older patients with milder rings. Many parents will volunteer the information that the child who previously had only mild respiratory symptoms feeds more easily after an operation. Foreign bodies may obstruct the esophagus above the ring and lead to its recognition.[10] Dysphagia from an anomalous right subclavian artery (dysphagia lusorum) is difficult to document in the modern literature. The difficulty in swallowing solid foods and the abnormal increase in midesophageal pressure were relieved in three children aged 2 to 4 years by the division of an anomalous right subclavian artery.[31]

Life-threatening aortoesophageal fistula associated with prolonged nasogastric intubation has been reported in 6 patients ranging in age from 3 months to 80 years. There were two children with a double aortic arch and four adults with an anomalous right subclavian artery.[34]

## Differential diagnosis

The differential diagnosis of chronic intrathoracic airway obstruction will vary with the age of presentation. Since most symptomatic vascular lesions occur in the first 2 years of life, this discussion will be confined to diseases of this age-group. It must be remembered that the inflammatory edema and exudate of an acute upper or lower respiratory tract infection may accentuate or uncover the clinical features of a vascular lesion.

The differential diagnosis is somewhat different in neonates than in later infancy. A tight double aortic arch or pulmonary artery sling can be symptomatic from birth and must be distinguished from other congenital lesions narrowing the airway. Intraluminal lesions such as congenital tracheal stenosis or subglottic hemangioma will all ultimately require endoscopy for their precise diagnosis. Examples of congenital masses which compromise the intrathoracic airway from without are cystic hygroma, foregut duplication cyst, neurenteric cyst, teratoma, bronchogenic cyst, or neurogenic tumors such as neuroblastoma. The presence of these lesions is usually obvious on chest radiographs and this leads to the appropriate investigation.

The differential diagnosis changes somewhat after the neonatal period, although milder forms of the above lesions may not come to medical attention until later when masses have enlarged or cysts grown because of secretion or hemorrhage into

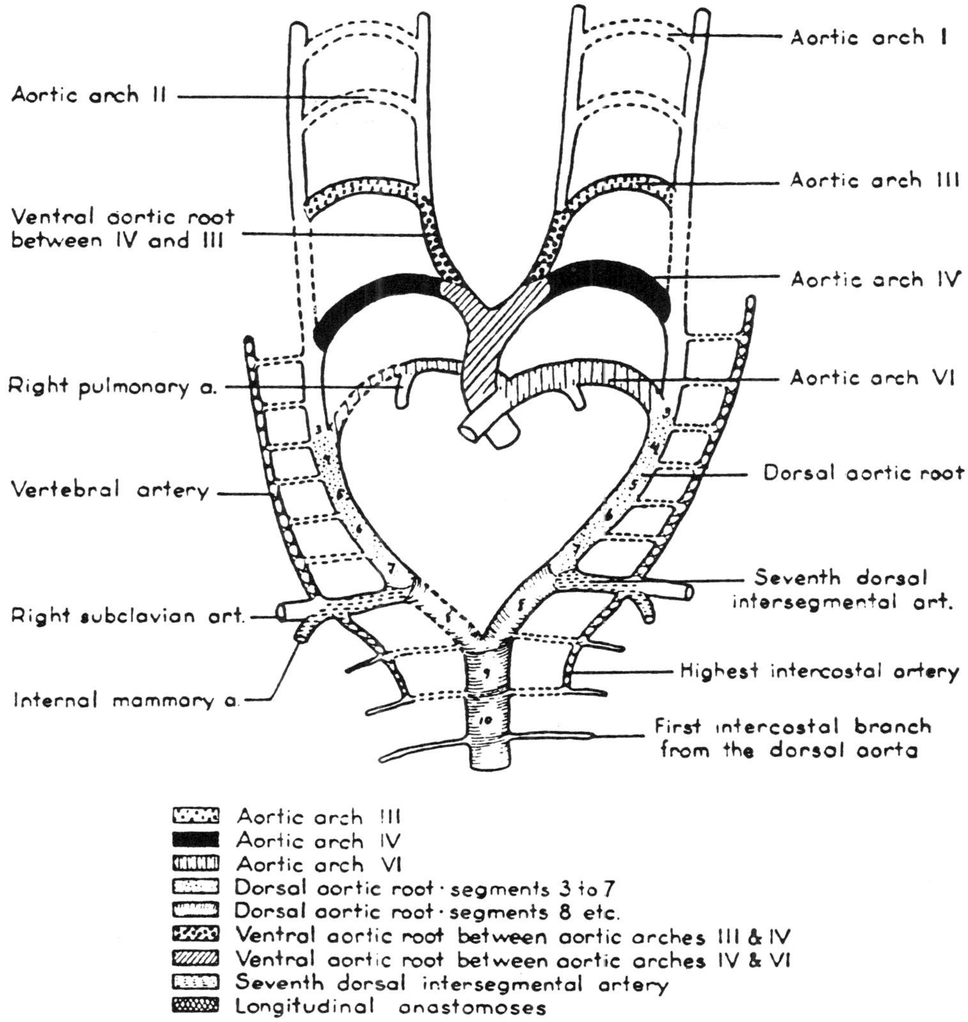


**Fig. 22–1.** Schematic diagram of the embryonic paired aortic arches (I–VI) and the somitic intersegmental branches of the dorsal aorta (3–10). Components that normally regress in the human embryo are indicated by dashed lines. (From Barry, 1951,[3] with permission.)

their lumen. Intraluminal lesions in older children include foreign bodies in the airway or esophagus, hemangioma, papilloma, and adenoma. True primary tracheomalacia is a diagnosis of exclusion. In older children, lymphadenopathy secondary to infection or lymphoma-leukemia may compress the airway from without.

A vascular lesion should not be considered as a cause of true dysphagia in an older child until achalasia, a foreign body, or esophageal stricture (from caustic ingestion, reflux peptic esophagitis, or previous esophageal surgery) have all been excluded by contrast esophagograms, endoscopy, and/or manometry.

## Investigation

The plain chest radiograph and the barium esophagogram with fluoroscopy are the basis of investigation of the child with clinical features of intrathoracic airway obstruction. Most common vascular lesions can be identified by these methods and further imaging is reserved for lesions with atypical features or those requiring operation depending on the preference of the surgeon.

### Chest radiograph

Most children with vascular rings have generous lung volumes because of air trapping. When there is an inequality of aeration between the two lungs, a vascular sling should be suspected. The side of the aortic arch is obvious in older patients and may be inferred by the contralateral deflection of the trachea in young children. This, however, is not an infallible method.[47] The arch may be displaced cephalad (cervical aorta) or may be large from cardiac (tetralogy of Fallot) or aortic (Marfan syndrome) disease. If the arch or trachea is poorly visualized because of a large thymus, the filtered-beam, high-kV technique may be useful. The side of the descending aorta may be ipsilateral or contralateral to the aortic arch. Tracheal stenosis, a tracheobronchial hemangioma, or a foreign body may be visible.

### Barium esophagogram

This should be performed under fluoroscopy for visualization of pulsating vessels. The common lesions have been grouped by the appearance of the lateral esophagogram (Fig. 22–3).[4] The side of the descending aorta is confirmed in the frontal

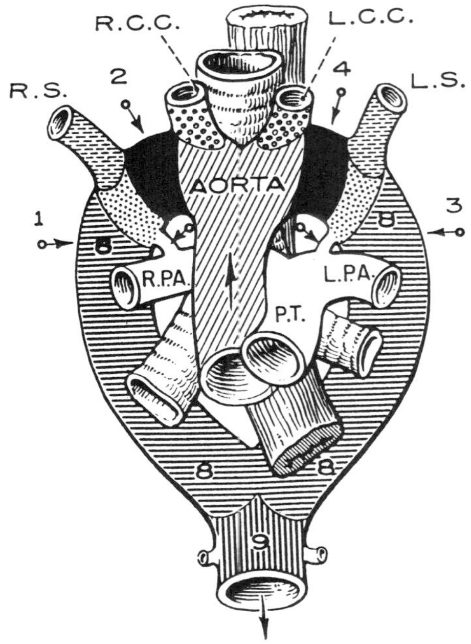


**Fig. 22–2.** Schematic ventral view of Edward's hypothetic double aortic arch with bilateral ductus arteriosi and midline ascending and descending aorta. The shading is similar to that in Fig. 21–1. Arrows point to the four key locations where regression occurs; they are numbered 1–4. P.T. = pulmonary trunk; L.P.A. = left pulmonary artery; R.P.A. = right pulmonary artery; L.S. = left subclavian artery; L.C.C. = left common carotid artery; R.C.C. = right common carotid artery; R.S. = right subclavian artery. (From Stewart et al., 1964,[45] with permission.)

view and an anomalous subclavian artery may be seen coursing obliquely toward the right shoulder.

If the chest radiograph shows a normal left aortic arch and descending aorta and the barium esophagogram is normal, a surgical vascular ring can be confidently excluded. Further studies are indicated to delineate milder vascular lesions with unusual features or to search for other causes of intrathoracic airway obstruction.

## Sonography

Two-dimensional sonography with color Doppler sampling can characterize the anatomy in most lesions.[27] This technique is very operator dependent and a knowledge of the anatomy combined with an ordered logical approach is essential.

The suprasternal notch approach is used to determine the sequence of branching of the arch vessels and a right innominate artery characterizes a normal left aortic arch. An anomalous right subclavian artery can usually be identified. In double aortic arch the side of the dominant arch can be determined. The branching of the main pulmonary artery can be identified and in pulmonary artery sling, the left pulmonary artery can be seen arising from the right pulmonary artery and followed around the posterior trachea toward the left lung.

Sagittal scanning in the high left parasternal position will identify the side of the descending aorta with respect to the trachea and the esophagus. These relationships can also be confirmed using a subcostal window.

The patency and direction of flow in vessels can be determined with color Doppler sampling.

## Angiography

This has traditionally been reserved for atypical or complex lesions, especially if surgery is planned. It has the advantage of showing excellent aortic and great vessel anatomy and can be combined with the investigation of any concomitant heart disease. It requires ionizing radiation, the injection of contrast medium, and often an arterial puncture. A double aortic arch with atresia between the left carotid and left subclavian artery cannot be confidently differentiated from a right aortic arch with anomalous left subclavian artery and ligamentum arteriosum by this technique.

The transfemoral retrograde arterial or venous transseptal approach may be utilized. Optimal anatomy is obtained with biplane oblique views with cranial angulation.

## Computerized tomography (CT)

Considerable information can be obtained with dynamic, fast CT scanning during bolus central venous infusion of contrast. This technique is gradually being replaced by magnetic resonance and should be reserved for babies who are too sick to undergo this long procedure.

## Magnetic resonance (MR)

MR has the advantage of not requiring ionizing radiation, the injection of contrast medium, or vascular puncture. The images may be collected in the axial, coronal, sagittal, or angled planes.[28] There is simultaneous display of the cardiovascular and tracheobronchial anatomy. The disadvantages are related to the time and cost of the examination and the necessity for intravenous sedation. In centers with facilities and experience, this is the procedure of choice for displaying the anatomy.

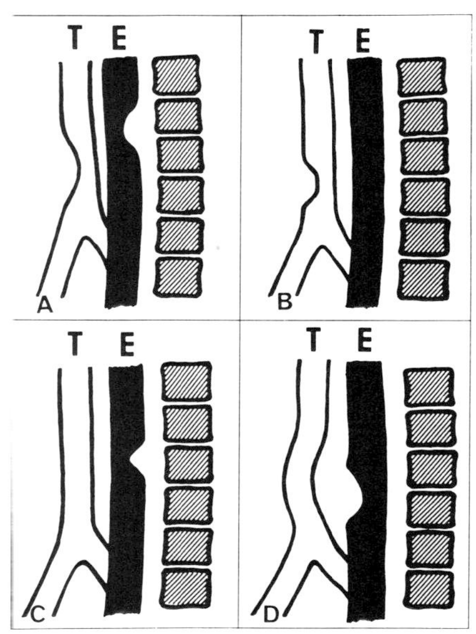


**Fig. 22–3.** Four patterns of vascular compression anomalies on the trachea (T) and esophagus (E), lateral projection. Pattern A is found in the double aortic arch or right aortic arch with anomalous left subclavian artery and ligamentum arteriosum. Pattern B is found in the innominate artery syndrome. Pattern C is found in the anomalous right subclavian artery. Pattern D is found in the anomalous left pulmonary artery or pulmonary artery sling. (From Berdon and Baker, 1972,[4] with permission.)

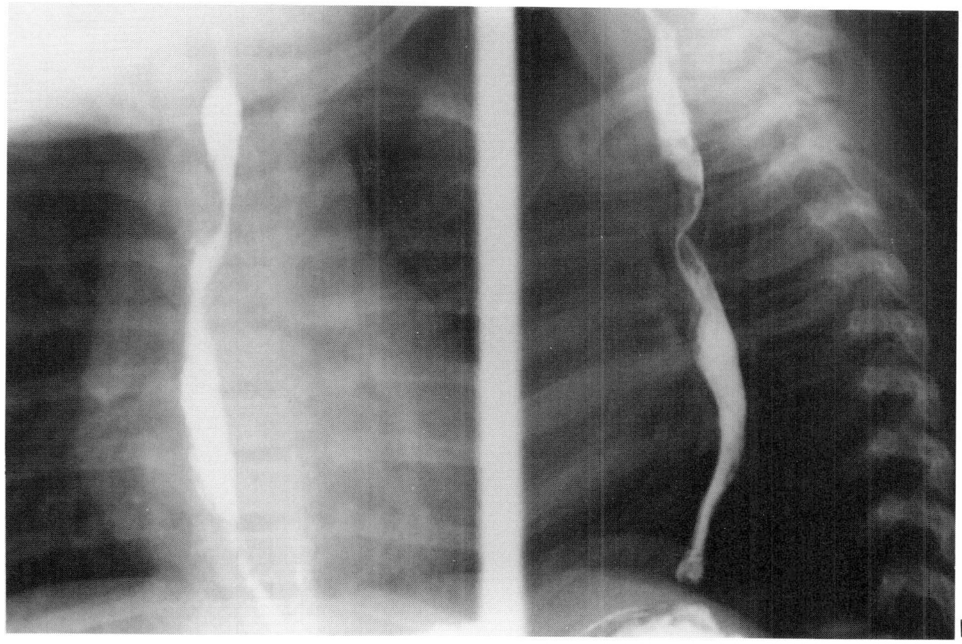
A B

**Fig. 22–4.** Barium esophagogram in double aortic arch. Frontal view (A) demonstrates large right cephalad indentation and smaller left caudal indentation. Lateral view (B) shows large posterior indentation and anterior indentation of tracheal air column.

## Endoscopy

Although the site and severity of vascular indentations and pulsations on the major airways can be visualized directly by this technique, it is usually not necessary. Endoscopy requires some form of general anesthesia in often very sick children. It is used mainly to identify intrinsic lesions or to assess the degree of tracheomalacia or the deformities of the tracheobronchial tree in the ring-sling complex (see below).

## Double aortic arch

A double aortic arch is the most important vascular ring and will be discussed in some detail. It accounts for at least 50% of the lesions in most large (greater than 20) surgical series.[7,30,39,51] The lesion may also be asymptomatic and found only at autopsy. The incidence of congenital heart disease, usually tetralogy of Fallot, was as high as 8% in the above series.

Embryologically, this can be thought of as a failure of regression of the eighth segment of the right dorsal aorta. This leads to persistence of all components of the hypothetic double aortic arch (Fig. 22–2), further modified by regression of the right ductus arteriosus and inclination of the descending aorta to the left of the midline. There can be no innominate artery. Both the right and the left arch are usually patent and the right is usually the larger and more cranial. As a general rule, the descending aorta is on the side opposite the larger arch, but exceptions occur. Atresia can occur at any segment, but it is very rare in the right arch. The most common site is distal to the left subclavian artery where the arch is completed by a fibrous band which preserves the completeness of the vascular ring. Although a left (and rarely right) ligamentum arteriosum is usually present, it does not contribute to the ring but may influence the severity of symptoms.

A double aortic arch is usually a disease of infancy and most babies are symptomatic in the neonatal period. There may be a delay in the diagnosis; surgical series contain examples of babies who were intubated or tracheostomized for many days before recognition. The spectrum of clinical features ranges from severe respiratory distress in the neonate to an asymptomatic adult. Most infants have stridor, harsh cry, repeated respiratory infections, and indrawing and wheezing (see Clinical manifestations and Differential diagnosis). The typical frontal chest radiograph has large lung volumes with a midline trachea and left descending aorta. There is an anterior indentation on the tracheal air column in the lateral view and a large posterior esophageal indentation at T3–T4 on the well-filled barium esophagogram (Fig. 22–4). The frontal esophagogram shows bilateral indentations with the right usually larger and more cephalad than the caudal and smaller left indentation. Sonography, especially from the suprasternal notch, will show four separate head and neck vessels and the two arches, and determine the side of the larger arch and the descending aorta (Fig. 22–5).

At this point, with typical clinical and simple imaging findings, most surgeons proceed to a left thoracotomy, realizing that there is a possibility that part of the left arch may be atretic or that the defect may conceivably be a right aortic arch with anomalous left subclavian artery and left ligamentum arteriosum. The anatomy is defined and the left arch is test-occluded while the carotid, subclavian, and femoral pulses are palpated. The arch is divided at its narrowest portion (usually distal to the left subclavian artery) and the stumps are ligated and oversewn. The arch is dissected free of mediastinal structures and the ligamentum is divided. The mortality and morbidity are low if the operation is performed semielectively. The perioperative course is determined by the tightness of the ring and the severity of secondary focal tracheomalacia. Most patients are extubated on the day of the operation but this may be delayed. Parents should be informed before the operation that the breathing may remain noisy for several weeks or months after the operation. The long-term prognosis is excellent.[39]

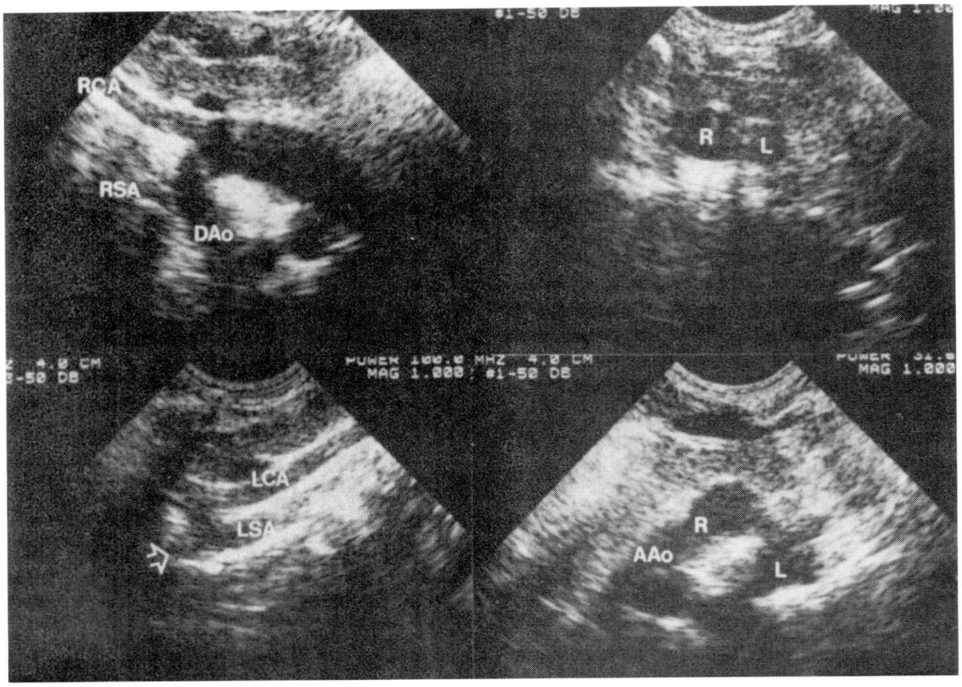


**Fig. 22–5.** Echocardiographic appearance of double aortic arch from the suprasternal notch. In the sagittal plane, the right aortic arch (upper left) and the left aortic arch (lower left) are demonstrated with separate origin of the carotid and subclavian arteries on each side. Scanning anterior in the coronal plane (upper right) reveals the characteristic bilateral echolucencies of double aortic arch. The right aortic arch (R) appears larger than the left aortic arch (L) in both the sagittal and coronal views. Scanning in the sagittal plane from right to left (lower right) reveals a complete vascular ring encircling the trachea and the esophagus. RCA = right carotid artery; RSA = right subclavian artery; DAo = descending aorta; LCA = left carotid artery; LSA = left subclavian artery; AAo = ascending aorta. (From Morrow and Huhta, 1972,[35] with permission.)

If the clinical and simple imaging features are atypical or the surgeon wishes more precise delineation of the anatomy, further investigations may be performed. Angiography was formerly the "gold standard" (Fig. 22–6); however, if the patient is suitable, axial and coronal MR images (Fig. 22–7) give superior delineation of the anatomy and clearly visualize the central airways. Bronchoscopy should rarely be necessary. The surgeon may prefer to perform a right thoracotomy when the left aortic arch component is larger.[33]

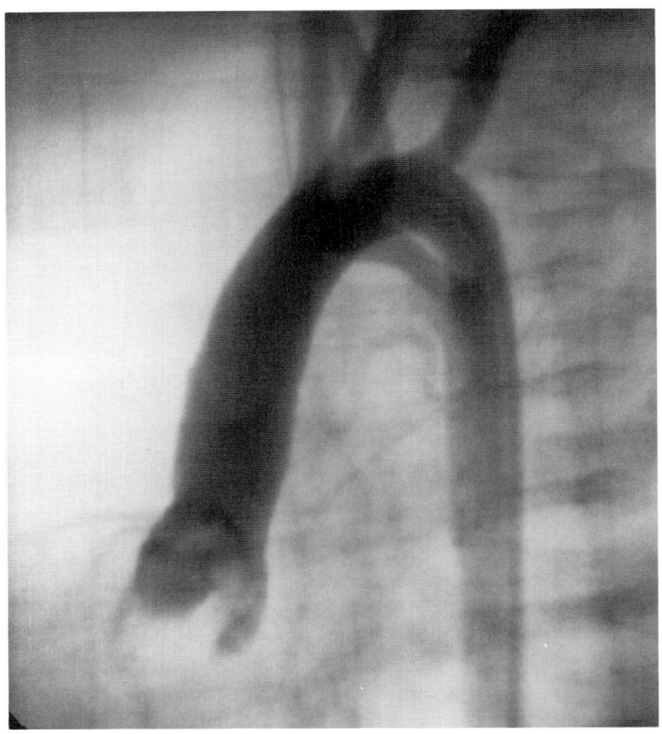

**Fig. 22–6.** Double aortic arch. Retrograde ascending aortogram. Left anterior oblique projection with mild cranial angulation. Retrograde arterial catheter has passed around the larger and more cephalad of the two arches. The four great arteries are seen arising separately from each arch.

## Right aortic arch

A vascular ring should be strongly suspected when a right aortic arch is identified, particularly in the absence of congenital heart disease. Shuford and Sybers[43] have classified the types of right aortic arch (Fig. 22–8) on the basis of site of interruption of the embryonic left arch in the hypothetic double arch diagram of Edwards.

### Mirror image branching (type 1 in Fig. 22–8)

This is the opposite of the normal arch and is thought to result from resorption of the eighth segment of the left dorsal aorta (area 3 in Fig. 22–2). The ligamentum usually arises from the base of the left-sided innominate artery (the first branch of the arch) and there is no vascular ring. The arch passes to the right of the trachea above the right bronchus and displaces the trachea to the left. There is a very high (up to 98%) association with cyanotic congenital heart disease, particularly tetralogy of

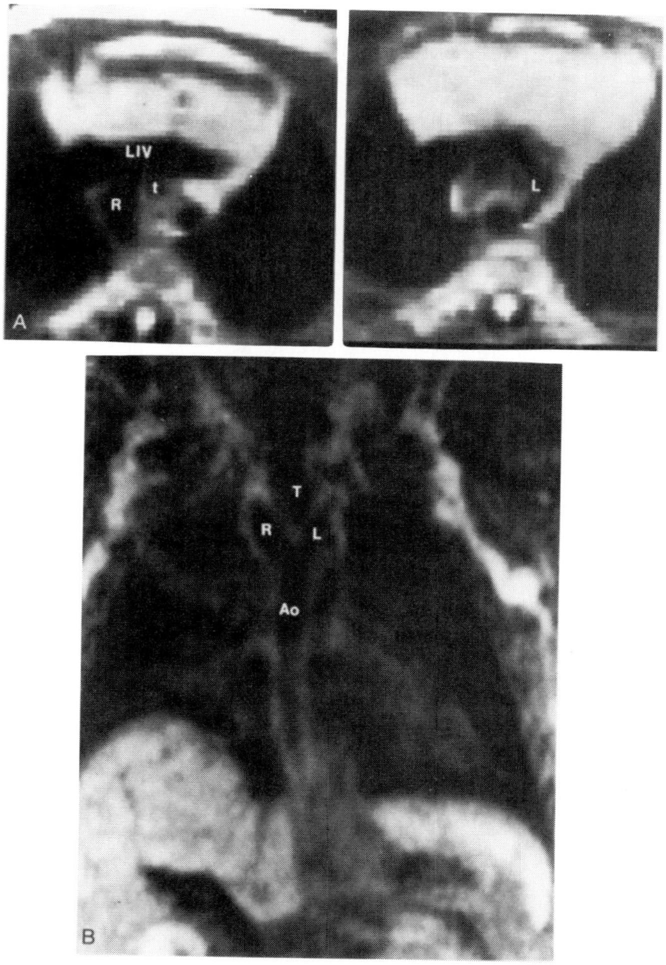


**Fig. 22–7.** Double aortic arch. Magnetic resonance (MR) axial images (A) showing the larger and more cranial right arch and the smaller left arch (L) 5mm. more caudal. Coronal MR scan (B) through the posterior aspect of the double arch encircling the trachea (T) in another patient. R = right sided arch; L = left arch; Ao = descending aorta. (From Bank and Hernandez, 1988,[2] with permission.)

Fallot and truncus arteriosus—conditions associated with a large aortic arch. This may cause symptomatic compression of the right bronchus without a vascular ring.[20]

Rarely, the ligamentum may originate from the right-sided proximal descending aorta or from a retroesophageal diverticulum thought to be a remnant of the distal left aortic arch (type 2 in Fig. 22–8). The left ligamentum then passes to the left pulmonary artery and produces a vascular ring.

### Anomalous left subclavian artery with ligamentum arteriosum (type 3 in Fig. 22–8)

This is the most common vascular ring and should be strongly suspected in a patient with a right-sided aortic arch and symptoms of airway obstruction with no evidence of congenital heart disease. It is the second (after double aortic arch) most frequent surgical lesion.

It is thought to result from regression of that segment of the left aortic arch between the carotid and subclavian arteries which is derived from the left fourth aortic arch (area 4 in Fig. 22–2). There is a large retroesophageal diverticulum of Kommerell which represents the distal left arch. A left ligamentum passes from the diverticulum to the left pulmonary artery to complete the vascular ring. There can be no innominate artery. The descending aorta is usually on the right. Rarely, the origin of the left subclavian artery is narrow and the distal segments are filled from retrograde flow in the ipsilateral vertebral artery (vertebral-subclavian artery steal).

Although this is the most common vascular ring, it is rarely symptomatic. In the minority of patients there are symptoms of mild airway obstruction or dysphagia, but this is unusual before the age of 2 years. There is a large posterior indentation in the barium esophagogram. Sonography is usually diagnostic and shows a right aortic arch with absence of an innominate artery and a retroesophageal left subclavian artery. At times, the lesion cannot be confidently differentiated from a double aortic arch with atresia of the left arch between the left carotid and subclavian arteries. The surgical approach (left thoracotomy) is similar, however, and angiography or MR is usually not necessary.

### Anomalous left innominate artery (with left ligamentum) (type 4 in Fig. 22–8)

This is exceedingly rare and is thought to result from regression of the arch between the ascending aorta and the left carotid artery. The left innominate artery would then arise as the last branch of the right arch, pass behind the esophagus, and give rise to the left subclavian and carotid arteries. The left ligamentum completes the ring.[23]

### Circumflex retroesophageal right aortic arch

In this rare lesion, there is a right aortic arch, usually with normal mirror-image branching, and the aorta passes behind the esophagus to descend on the left. A ring may be formed by a left ligamentum passing from the descending aorta to the left pulmonary artery. The ring is usually loose; dysphagia is more prominent than respiratory symptoms; and there is a high (33%)

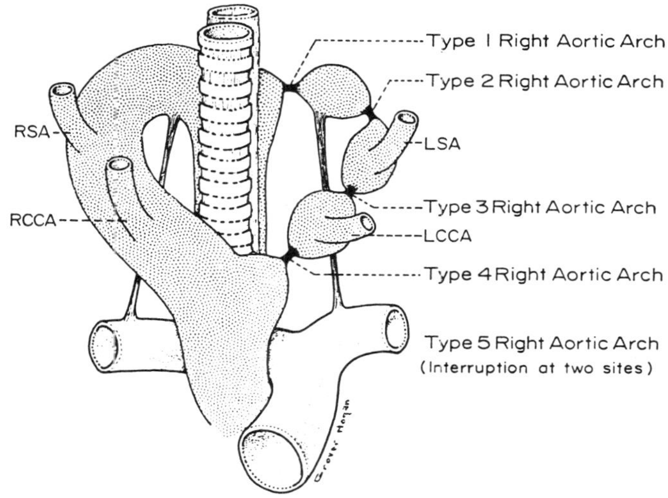


**Fig. 22–8.** Diagram showing sites in the embryonic left arch in the hypothetic double aortic arch where interruption results in the different types of right aortic arch. RCCA = right common carotid artery; RSA = right subclavian artery; LSA = left subclavian artery; LCCA = left common carotid artery. (From Shuford and Sybers, 1974,[43] with permission.)

association with tetralogy of Fallot.[42] Some patients will also have an aberrant left subclavian artery which makes the lesion difficult to distinguish between double aortic arch and left arch atresia.

### Right cervical aorta

In this rare lesion, the aortic arch rises above the clavicle and may be as high as the second cervical vertebra. The descending aorta crosses behind the esophagus at the fourth thoracic vertebra and usually descends on the contralateral side to the arch. There is almost always no innominate artery. The internal and external carotid arteries usually arise separately from the arch. The left subclavian artery is often anomalous. There may be a vascular ring if the ligamentum is contralateral to the arch and arises from the descending aorta. Congenital heart disease is rare.

The embryology is unclear. Clinical evidence has been found to support either persistence of the third aortic arch or failure of descent of the aortic arches from the normal embryonic cervical position.[26]

The patient may be asymptomatic or may present with dysphagia or respiratory manifestations in the presence of a ring. There is always a pulsatile mass in the neck, and when it is compressed, the femoral pulses will decrease in amplitude.

The cervical aortic arch can usually be diagnosed clinically. The frontal chest radiograph shows a right superior mediastinal mass with leftward displacement of the trachea and usually a left-sided descending aorta. There is no aortic knob. There is anterior displacement of the trachea in the lateral view. Although considerable information on the course and branching of the aorta can be obtained by a barium esophagogram, CT, and sonography, those symptomatic patients being considered for surgery should have high-quality MR and/or angiography.

## Left aortic arch

### Anomalous right subclavian artery

The right subclavian artery may arise as the last branch of the normal aortic arch and pursue a retroesophageal course obliquely upward into the right arm. It is thought to result from regression of the right fourth aortic arch between the right carotid artery and the right subclavian artery (area 2 in Fig. 22–2). Occasionally, the origin may be dilated and is called the *diverticulum of Kommerell,* which is thought to be a remnant of the right distal aortic arch. As the ligamentum is almost always on the left, there is no vascular ring.

This branching is so common (0.5% of the population) that it may be considered a normal variation. It is frequently found in Down syndrome and in tetralogy of Fallot.

The vessel may sometimes be seen on the well-penetrated frontal chest radiograph either as a density on the superior margin of the aortic arch (where it may simulate a mediastinal mass) or coursing obliquely upward to the right, superimposed on the tracheal air column. There is a small posterior indentation on the barium esophagogram. The vessel may be demonstrated by sonography, CT, angiography, or MR; however, this is rarely necessary.

This is almost always a benign lesion. There are no respiratory manifestations and, if the vessel is found during the investigation of dysphagia, a vigorous search must be carried out for other causes before reimplantation of the artery is considered. Rare clinical problems attributed to this vessel include: a site of lodgement of an esophageal foreign body;[10] aorticoesophageal fistula during prolonged nasogastric intubation;[34] and true dysphagia if the diverticulum is large or becomes aneurysmal with age.

### Anomalous innominate artery or *innominate artery syndrome*

The clinical significance of innominate artery syndrome is controversial. The original description[25] was of a group of infants with stridor, cyanosis, and apnea who improved when an "anomalous" innominate artery was sutured to the sternum. The symptoms were thought to be related to tracheal compression by an innominate artery arising more distally than usual from the arch and crossing in front of the trachea. Crowding of structures in the infant's superior mediastinum was considered by some to be a contributing factor.

The reported incidence has varied considerably in the past 45 years. Some centers have reported large surgical series[1,16] and most reports of operations for relief of airway compression by vascular anomalies describe some cases of this syndrome. Nevertheless, it was recognized early that symptoms ascribed to this condition often improved with time and many adopted a conservative approach to management. Some babies have no relief of symptoms after operation.[32]

There is a group of infants with stridor, apnea, cyanosis, and recurrent pneumonia in various combinations of severity who have normal barium esophagograms. These infants may have (1) an anterior indentation of the trachea just below the thoracic inlet while the head is in a neutral position (Fig. 22–9); (2) a strong pulsation of the anterior trachea noted during bronchoscopy with diminution of the right carotid and brachial pulses during gentle compression by the endoscopist; or (3) angiographic[5] or MR[18] demonstration of the innominate artery anterior to the trachea and narrowing the lumen. These observations have been used to support this diagnosis and each requires critical evaluation.

Anterior tracheal narrowing on a lateral chest radiograph may be seen in many babies with no symptoms of airway compression.[49] An indentation was found in 30% of 156 random radiographs of children under 2 years of age.[46] This indentation was also found in a high proportion of children with no stridor who underwent angiography during the investigation of congenital heart disease. The innominate artery arose partially (51%) or completely (44%) to the left of the trachea in 172 children, almost all of whom were under 2 years of age. Thus, moderate anterior tracheal indentation and the demonstration of an innominate artery crossing in front of the trachea do not confirm the diagnosis for, in fact, the anterior innominate artery is not anomalous but is following its normal course in almost all children.

The concept of upper mediastinal "crowding" was examined with MR in 16 infants with stridor.[18] Pulsating anterior tracheal indentation was observed at endoscopy in 8 babies. The position of the innominate artery and the transverse and sagittal upper mediastinal measurements were similar in both groups. There was no relation to the size and position of the thymus. It seems unlikely that the mediastinal "crowding" in the young infant is a significant culprit. An exception is the neonate with

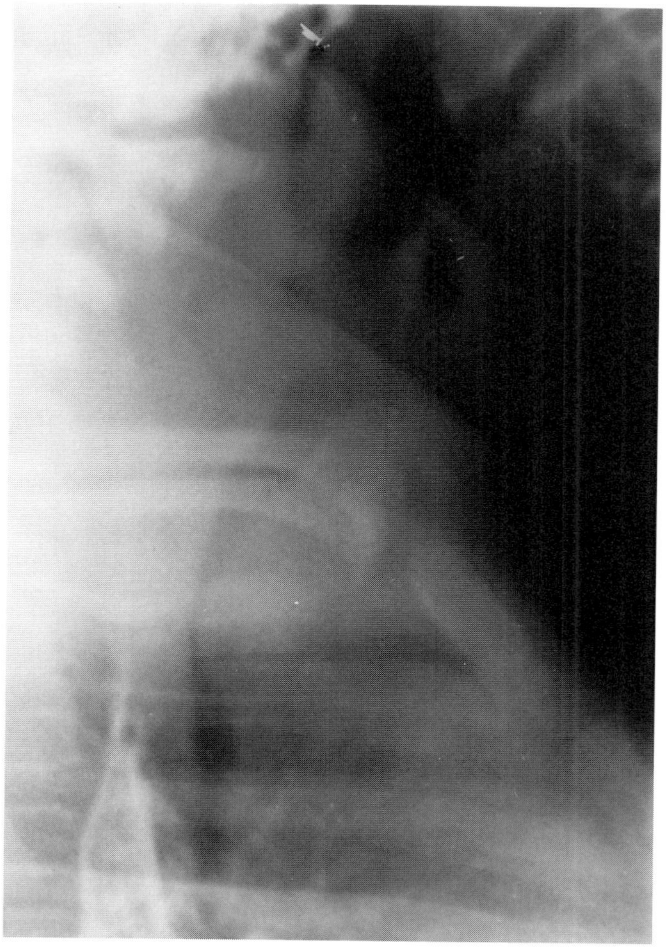

**Fig. 22–9.** Innominate artery syndrome. Lateral barium esophagogram in a 5-month-old infant after repair of a tracheoesophageal fistula. Note severe anterior indentation of the trachea just below the thoracic inlet.

esophageal atresia with a distal fistula and a dilated upper esophageal pouch. Partial thymectomy and aortopexy are advocated in these babies.

What then is the innominate artery syndrome? It clearly is not associated with an innominate artery arising too distally on the aortic arch, for this is the normal infant anatomy. It is not related to crowding of the trachea in the infant's superior mediastinum, for measurements are similar in infants with other reasons for stridor. We are left with the strong suspicion that there are some infants with an intrinsic localized softening of tracheal cartilage—primary tracheomalacia. This is supported by the tendency toward gradual spontaneous regression of symptoms in unoperated children and the improvement after an operation similar to that used for tracheomalacia in patients with very severe symptoms.[9]

The diagnosis is made by a combination of exclusion of other causes of airway compression by methods previously described, the findings of severe, localized airway narrowing on lateral chest radiograph, and definite, prominent anterior tracheal pulsation at endoscopy. Operation should be reserved for those few infants with the above findings and life-threatening apnea. Unpublished observations on many babies over several years strongly support conservative management.

#### Circumflex retroesophageal left aortic arch

This uncommon lesion may be recognized on the frontal chest radiograph by a normal left aortic arch (with the tracheal air column to the right of the midline) plus a right-sided descending aorta. The barium esophagogram shows a large posterior indentation from the transverse distal arch. The anomaly is usually asymptomatic and the general clinical features are similar to a circumflex retroesophageal right aortic arch. There is a high incidence of congenital heart disease. A vascular ring may occur if there is an anomalous right subclavian artery and a right ligamentum arteriosum to the right pulmonary artery. This may compress the right bronchus and lead to hyperinflation of the right lung.[12] The precise anatomy can be determined with sonography, MR, or angiography, and a symptomatic ring is usually divided through a right thoracotomy.

#### Left cervical aorta

A cervical aorta is less common on the left and is associated with a pulsatile mass in the left supraclavicular region. Usually, the aorta descends on the right. The variability of vessel branching, theories of embryogenesis, clinical features, and approach to imaging and management are similar in both types of cervical aorta.

#### Severe cardiac malposition

A baby with abdominal situs solitus, complex intracardiac lesions, a left-sided aorta, a large main pulmonary artery, and a left patent ductus arteriosus has been described in whom there was severe stridor associated with tracheal compression. There was anterior indentation of the trachea by a large main pulmonary artery which had been rotated forward and to the right in association with the dextrocardia.[41] "Pseudovascular rings" can also be associated with dextrocardia secondary to right lung agenesis.

### Anomalous left pulmonary artery (pulmonary vascular sling)

A pulmonary artery sling is an airway compression syndrome in which the left pulmonary artery arises anomalously as a branch of the right pulmonary artery. It passes posteriorly along the right lateral wall of the trachea above the right bronchus and then turns to the left between the trachea and esophagus to enter the left hilum where it may compress the left main stem bronchus (Fig. 22–10). It is thought to result from a failure of development of the left sixth proximal arch and the excessive development of the left postbranchial pulmonary plexus occurring between the trachea and the esophagus. This then connects the postductal branch pulmonary artery to the right pulmonary artery. A left ligamentum arteriosum may accentuate the compression.

There is a high incidence of associated congenital anomalies, which often determines the prognosis. The incidence of major congenital heart disease, especially ventricular septal defects, was 27% in 130 patients collected by Gikonyo et al.[21] Sixty-eight patients died and most had important abnormalities of the tracheobronchial tree. There was a hypoplastic distal trachea in almost 50% of patients. This was usually associated with an

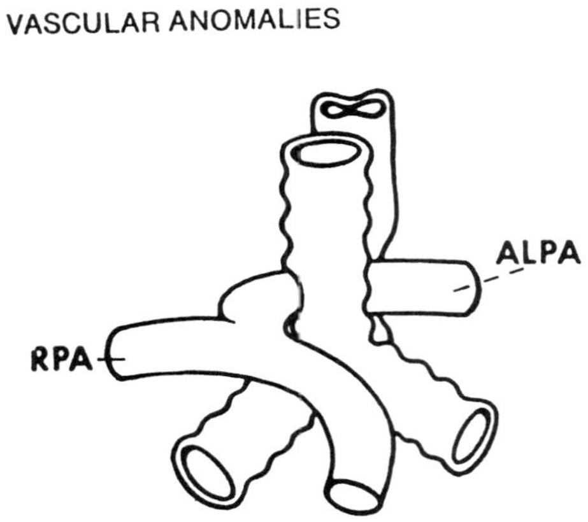


**Fig 22–10.** Representation of pulmonary sling with left pulmonary artery having anomalous origin from the right pulmonary artery. RPA = right pulmonary artery; ALPA = anomalous left pulmonary artery.[4] (From Berdon and Baker, 1972,[4] with permission.)

absent pars membranacea producing complete tracheal rings. Other findings included stenosis of a main stem bronchus and epiarterial bronchus (bronchus suis). Often, more than one tracheobronchial anomaly was present.

The clinical manifestations are usually determined by the associated anomalies. Although a vascular sling has been discovered as a hilar mass in an asymptomatic adult, most cases present in early infancy and many neonatal fatalities have been reported. These severely affected babies are almost all examples of the "ring-sling complex"[6] with tracheal stenosis associated with complete rings of tracheal cartilage. The clinical features are those of severe intrathoracic airway obstruction. Often the infants require intubation and the position of the endotracheal tube is critical.

The lesion may be investigated by an array of modalities, the choice of which will depend on the equipment and skill available (Table 22–2). Ideally, the complex will be suspected by clinical features, a chest radiograph, and a barium esophagogram with fluoroscopy. The diagnosis can be confirmed by sonography, and the tracheal anomalies determined by careful endoscopy. Associated nonrespiratory anomalies will modify the approach. The differential diagnosis of a soft tissue density between the anterior esophagus and the lower trachea includes lymphadenopathy, central bronchogenic cyst, and the very rare ductal sling.[8]

The management will depend on the severity of symptoms and on the associated anomalies of the tracheobronchial tree. The technique for the relief of the sling is well established and has a low mortality. When severe tracheal narrowing is present, the mortality approaches 50% in some series and some airway obstruction may persist in up to 45% of the survivors, in spite of attempts to resect localized areas of tracheal stenosis or incise the complete tracheal rings and insert a pericardial patch.

## Large proximal aorta and pulmonary arteries

When the great arteries become very large, they may displace and then compress the central airways leading, especially in infants, to poor drainage of secretions with increased lower respiratory tract infections and/or peripheral atelectasis. This is particularly true when the aortic arch is large, because of its normal contact with the lower trachea and left bronchus. Stanger et al.[44] have demonstrated that children with congenital cardiac defects associated with large left-to-right shunts (usually ventricular septal defect and complete AV canal) often have large main and branch pulmonary arteries which compress central airways.

The usual diseases associated with the large proximal aorta at all ages are classified in Table 22–3. Airway compression becomes more important when the aorta is aneurysmal. Marfan syndrome is an important example.

Marfan syndrome is an autosomal dominant connective tissue disorder resulting from a defect of the fibrillin 1 gene on chromosome 15.[11] The major phenotypic expression is in the musculoskeletal, ocular, and cardiovascular systems.[37] The patients are tall with little subcutaneous fat. The limbs and fingers are long and the arm span exceeds the height. There is kyphoscoliosis and pectus excavatum. The joints are hypermobile and easily dislocatable. The lens is frequently dislocated. There is myopia and a risk of retinal detachment.

The major cardiovascular abnormality is cystic medial necrosis of the thoracic aorta, which may progress to a fatal dissecting aneurysm. Less important lesions are mitral valve insufficiency, dilated main pulmonary artery, and aneurysm of the ductus arteriosus. Aortic root dilatation may begin as early as the first and as late as the fifth decade of life. It starts in the

**Table 22–2.** Modalities for investigation of pulmonary artery sling

| | |
|---|---|
| Chest radiography: frontal view with high kV filtered beam | Hyperinflation<br>Unilateral right obstructive emphysema<br>Unilateral left obstructive emphysema<br>Mediastinal mass<br>Low left hilum<br>Indentation of right lower trachea<br>Displacement of lower trachea to the left<br>Short trachea with increased carinal angle |
| Barium esophagogram (with fluoroscopy) | Pulsating anterior indentation at the level of carina |
| Sonography (coronal plane from the suprasternal notch; parasternal short axis view) | Absence of normal bifurcation of the main pulmonary artery (MPA); origin of LPA from RPA; posterior and left lateral course of LPA<br>Rule out associated congenital heart disease |
| Pulmonary angiography with 60° of cranial angulation in the frontal plane | Demonstrate precise pulmonary arterial anatomy |
| Computed tomography (CT) (dynamic axial images with bolus infusion of contrast) | LPA arising from posterior proximal RPA and passing between trachea and esophagus |
| Magnetic resonance (MR) (axial and coronal images) | As with CT<br>Assess tracheal diameter and length |
| Endoscopy | Assess tracheal diameter, tracheomalacia, complete tracheal rings, and proximal bronchial abnormalities |

**Table 22–3.** Airway displacement by large central great arteries

| |
|---|
| *LARGE AORTA* |
| Congenital heart disease |
| Tetralogy of Fallot (especially with pulmonary atresia) |
| Truncus arteriosus |
| Severe valvular aortic stenosis or insufficiency |
| Atherosclerotic aneurysm |
| Traumatic aneurysm |
| Cystic medial necrosis |
| Marfan syndrome |
| Ehlers-Danlos syndrome |
| Pseudoxanthoma elasticum |
| Turner syndrome |
| Idiopathic |
| Infectious aortitis |
| Staphylococcus, salmonella, and treponema pallidum |
| Inflammatory aortitis |
| Takayasu's arteritis |
| Rheumatoid and psoriatic arthritis |
| Spondyloarthropathies |
| Systemic lupus erythematosus and scleroderma |
| Iatrogenic aneurysm |
| Post-arch reconstruction for hypoplastic left heart syndrome (Norwood procedure) |
| Post-repair of coarctation of the aorta |
| *LARGE MAIN AND BRANCH PULMONARY ARTERIES* |
| Congenital heart disease |
| Absent pulmonic valve (usually with tetralogy) |
| Large left-to-right shunt lesions (VSD, PDA, AV canal) |

aortic sinuses and quickly leads to aortic insufficiency. As the aorta dilates, the trachea and left bronchus become displaced and compressed. Because of the catastrophic nature of an acute dissecting aneurysm, it has recently been recommended that these patients have yearly sonographic measurements of the aortic root diameter and that the aneurysm be electively repaired when the measurement exceeds 6 cm.[22]

## Intraluminal hemangioma

Infantile hemangiomas usually occur in the subglottic cervical trachea but can be found throughout the trachea and even occasionally in the proximal bronchi. There is a proliferation of capillary endothelium with multilamination of the basement membrane with the accumulation of mast cells, fibroblasts, and macrophages.[15] It is the most common subglottic soft tissue mass in children[13] and occurs twice as frequently in females.[17,38] A knowledge of the natural history of the true capillary hemangioma is very important for guiding management. They are present at birth, enter a proliferative phase, and enlarge for 6 to 9 months. They then usually regress and involute over 1 to 3 years.[52] Chemical mediators, perhaps involving the pericyte, have been implicated in this evolution.

Classically, this is a disease of early infancy and most series confirm the observation of Teft[50] who reported that 27 of 28 children presented before the age of 3 months. About 50% will have associated cutaneous hemangiomas. The clinical features are stridor, retractions, wheezing, and even cyanosis, all made worse by feeding, crying, or respiratory infections. Most infants are initially thought to have viral croup; however, cough is rarely a feature and true croup is unusual in the first few months of life.[48]

The diagnosis can almost always be made by high-quality soft tissue radiographs of the trachea in frontal and lateral projection during inspiration and expiration. An asymmetrical subglottic endotracheal lesion is usually clearly visible (Fig. 22–11). If endoscopy is performed, a bluish submucosal, asymmetric, compressible, posterolateral mass is clearly visible. Biopsy is rarely indicated. The differential diagnosis includes a subglottic granuloma secondary to prolonged neonatal intubation, congenital subglottic tracheal stenosis, including the complete tracheal ring complex, and the very rare papilloma.

Treatment should be as conservative as possible because of the usual natural history. Nevertheless, there are infants with life-threatening upper airway obstruction who require oral prednisone often combined with laser therapy. Tracheostomy and surgical excision should be avoided unless the above regime has failed after 2 years. Franks[19] has recently reported the resection of a steroid resistant hemangioma located in the lower trachea and left main bronchus using cardiopulmonary bypass to maintain oxygenation. Although these hemangiomas are radiosensitive, radiotherapy is contraindicated because of the well-documented increased incidence of late thyroid malignancy.

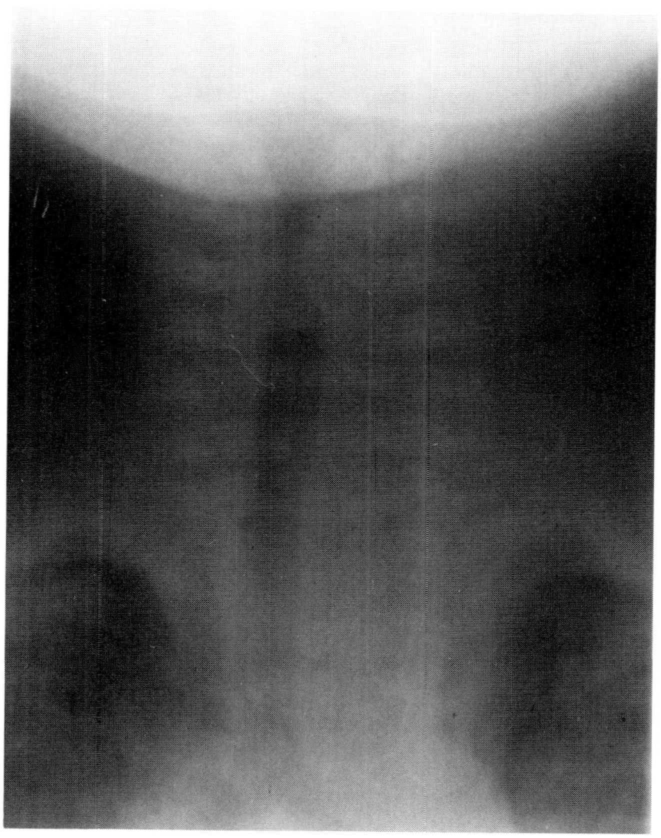

**Fig. 22–11.** Subglottic hemangioma. Frontal radiograph with soft tissue technique (130 kVp and 1 mm copper filtration) shows asymmetric subglottic soft tissue density narrowing the tracheal air column.

Occasionally the trachea is displaced and even invaded by large, complex cavernous hemangiomas of the neck and mediastinum. These may trap platelets (Kasabach-Merritt syndrome), hemorrhage, or become infected. The diagnosis and extent of the lesion can be assessed by contrast-infused CT, MR and, occasionally, angiography. The treatment is more difficult, as involution is unpredictable. Steroid therapy may need to be complemented with embolization and surgical excision. Cyclophosphamide, tranexaminic acid, and interferon $\alpha$-2A have been used with some effect in a small number of intractable patients.[15]

## Summary

The clinically important vascular lesions of the trachea and esophagus are double aortic arch, right aortic arch with anomalous left subclavian artery and ligamentum arteriosum, and the pulmonary artery sling. They have a wide clinical spectrum, but their prompt recognition and treatment in the infant with severe airway obstruction can be lifesaving. Recent advances have been made in noninvasive diagnosis. Other lesions involving the airway have been discussed; however, in most of these, the presentation is less dramatic.

### References

1. Backer CL, Ilbawi MN, Idriss FS, DeLeon SY: Vascular anomalies causing tracheoesophageal compression. Review of experience in children. J Thorac Cardiovasc Surg 97:725–731, 1989.
2. Bank ER, Hernandez RJ: CT and MR of congenital heart disease. Radiol Clin North Am 26:241–262, 1988.
3. Barry A: The aortic arch derivatives in the human adult. Anat Rec 111:221–238, 1951.
4. Berdon WE, Baker DH: Vascular anomalies and the infant lung: rings, slings and other things. Semin Roentgenol 7:39–64, 1972.
5. Berdon WE, Baker DH, Bordiuk J, Mellins R: Innominate artery compression of the trachea in infants with stridor and apnea. Radiology 92:272–278, 1969.
6. Berdon, WE, Baker DH, Wung JT, Chrispin J, Kozlowski K, de Silva M, Bales P, Alford B: Complete cartilage-ring tracheal stenosis associated with anomalous left pulmonary artery: the ring-sling complex. Radiology 152:57–64, 1984.
7. Bertolini A, Pelizza A, Panizzon G, Moretti R, Bava CL, Calza G, Tacchino A: Vascular rings and slings. Diagnosis and surgical treatment of 49 patients. J Cardiovasc Surg 28:301–312, 1987.
8. Binet JP, Conso JF, Losay J, Narcy P, Raynaud EJ, Beaufils F, Dor C, Bruniaux J: Ductus arteriosus sling: report of a newly recognized anomaly and its surgical correction. Thorax 33:72–75, 1978.
9. Cohen D: Tracheopexy: aorto-tracheal suspension for severe tracheomalacia. Aust Pediatr J 17:117–121, 1981.
10. Currarino G, Nikaidoh H: Esophageal foreign bodies in children with vascular ring or aberrant right subclavian artery: coincidence or causation? Pediatr Radiol 21:406–408, 1991.
11. Dietz HC, Cutting GR, Pyeritz RE, Maslen CL, Sakai LY, Corson GM, Puffenberger EG, Hamosh A, Nanthakumar EJ, Curristin SM, et al: Marfan syndrome caused by a recurrent de novo missense mutation in the fibrillin gene. Nature 353:337–339, 1991.
12. Dominguez R, Oh KS, Dorst JP, Young LW: Left aortic arch with right descending aorta. Am J Roentgenol 130:917–920, 1978.
13. Dunbar JS: Upper respiratory tract obstruction in infants and children. Am J Roentgenol 109:227–246, 1970.
14. Edwards JE: Anomalies of the derivatives of the aortic arch system. Med Clin North Am 32:925–949, 1948.
15. Ezekowitz RA, Mulliken JB, Folkman J: Interferon alfa-2a therapy for life-threatening hemangiomas of infancy. N Engl J Med 326:1456–1463, 1991.
16. Fearon B, Shortreed R: Tracheobronchial compression by congenital cardiovascular anomalies in children. Syndrome of apnea. Ann Otol Rhinol Laryngol 72:949–969, 1963.
17. Finn MC, Glowacki J, Mulliken JB: Congenital vascular lesions: clinical application of a new classification. J Pediatr Surg 18:894–900, 1983.
18. Fletcher BD, Cohn RC: Tracheal compression and the innominate artery: MR evaluation in infants. Radiology 170:103–107, 1989.
19. Franks R, Rothera M: Cadiopulmonary bypass for resection of low tracheal haemangioma. Arch Dis Child 65:630–632, 1990.
20. Gidding SS, Beekman RH, Lebowitz E, Wesley J, Coran A, Behrendt D, Rosenthal A: Airway compression by a right aortic arch in the absence of a vascular ring. Chest 85:703–705, 1984.
21. Gikonyo BM, Jue KL, Edwards JE: Pulmonary vascular sling: report of 7 cases and review of the literature. Pediatr Cardiol 10:81–89, 1989.
22. Gott VL, Pyeritz RE, Magovern GJ Jr, Cameron DE, McKusick VA: Surgical treatment of aneurysms of the ascending aorta in the Marfan syndrome. Results of composite-graft repair in 50 patients. N Engl J Med 314:1070–1074, 1986.
23. Grollman JH Jr, Bedynek JL, Henderson HS, Hall RJ: Right aortic arch with an aberrant retroesophageal innominate artery: angiographic diagnosis. Radiology 90:782–783, 1968.
24. Gross RE: Surgical relief for tracheal obstruction from a vascular ring. N Engl J Med 233:586–590, 1945.
25. Gross RE, Neuhauser EBD: Compression of the trachea by an anomalous innominate artery. An operation for its relief. Am J Dis Child 75:570–574, 1948.
26. Haughton VM, Fellows KE, Rosenbaum AE: The cervical aortic arches. Radiology 114:675–681, 1975.
27. Huhta JC: Pediatric Imaging/Doppler Ultrasound in the Chest: Extra Cardiac Diagnosis. Lea & Febiger, Philadelphia, 1986.
28. Jaffe RB: Magnetic resonance imaging of vascular rings. Semin Ultrasound CT MR 11:206–220, 1990.
29. Kirby ML: Cardiac morphogenesis—recent research advances. Pediatr Res 21:219–224, 1987.
30. Lowe GM, Donaldson JS, Backer CL: Vascular rings: 10–year review of imaging. Radiographics 11:637–646, 1991.
31. Martin GR, Rudolph C, Hillemeier C, Heyman MB: Dysphagia lusorum in children. Am J Dis Child 140:815–816, 1986.
32. Maurseth K: Sténoses trachéales par compression du tronc innominé. Ann Radiol 9:287–294, 1966.
33. McFaul R, Millard P, Nowicki E: Vascular rings necessitating right thoracotomy. J Thorac Cardiovasc Surg 82:306–309, 1981.
34. McKeating J, Smith S, Kochanck P, Perper J, Orenstein S, Nakayama D: Fatal aortoesophageal fistula due to double aortic arch: an unusual complication of prolonged nasogastric intubation. J Pediatr Surg 25:1298–1300, 1990.
35. Morrow WR, Huhta JC: Aortic arch and pulmonary artery anomalies In: The Science and Practice of Pediatric Cardiology, vol II A Garson, JT Bricker, DG McNamara, eds. Lea & Febiger, Philadelphia, 1990, pp. 1421–1452.
36. Nadas AS, Fyler DC: Pediatric Cardiology, 3rd ed. WB Saunders, Philadelphia, 1972, pp 683.
37. Pyeritz RE, McKusick VA: The Marfan syndrome: diagnosis and management N Engl J Med 300:772–777, 1979.
38. Richardson MA, Cotton RT: Anatomic abnormalities of the pediatric airway. Pediatr Clin North Am 31:821–834, 1984.
39. Roesler M, De Leval M, Chrispin A, Stark J: Surgical management of vascular ring. Ann Surg 197:139–146, 1983.
40. Rudolph AM, Heymann MA, Spitznas U: Hemodynamic considerations in the development of narrowing of the aorta. Am J Cardiol 30:514–525, 1972.
41. Scherer D, Westcott JL: Dextrocardia, left aortic arch, and tracheal compression. An unusual type of vascular ring. Radiology 103:383–384, 1972.
42. Schneeweiss A, Blieden L, Shem-Tov A, Deutsch V, Neufeld HN: Retroesophageal right aortic arch. Pediatr Cardiol 5:191–195, 1984.
43. Shuford WH, Sybers RG: The Aortic Arch and its Malformations with Emphasis on the Angiographic Features. Charles C Thomas, Springfield, IL 1974.
44. Stanger P, Lucas RV Jr, Edwards JE: Anatomical factors causing respiratory distress in acyanotic congenital heart disease. Special reference to bronchial obstruction. Pediatrics 43:760–769, 1969.
45. Stewart JR, Kincaid OW, Edwards JE: An Atlas of Vascular Rings and Related Malformations of the Aortic Arch System. Charles C. Thomas, Springfield, IL, 1964.
46. Strife JL, Baumel AS, Dunbar JS: Tracheal compression by the innominate artery in infancy and childhood. Radiology 139:73–75, 1981.

47. Strife, JL, Matsumoto J, Bisset GS 3rd, Martin R: The position of the trachea in infants and children with right aortic arch. Pediatr Radiol 19:226–229, 1989.
48. Sutton TJ, Nogrady MB: Radiologic diagnosis of subglottic hemangioma in infants. Pediatr Radiol 1:211–216, 1973.
49. Swischuk LE: Anterior tracheal indentation in infancy and early childhood: normal or abnormal? Am J Roentgenol 112:12–17, 1971.
50. Teft M: The radiotherapeutic managment of subglottic hemangioma in children. Radiology 86:207–214, 1966.
51. Tucker BL, Meyer BW, Lindesmith GG, Stiles QR, Jones JJ: Congenital aortic vascular ring. Arch Surg 99:521–523, 1969.
52. Weber TR, Connors RH, Tracy TF Jr, Bailey PV: Complex hemangiomas of infants and children. Individualized management in 22 cases. Arch Surg 125:1017–1021, 1990.

# Appendix G

## Syndromes and Conditions Associated with Tracheoesophageal Fistula or Abnormal Esophagus

TED L. TEWFIK, AHMAD S. TEEBI, and VAZKEN M. DER KALOUSTIAN

| Syndrome or condition | MIM No. POSSUM No.[a] | Inheritance[b] | Ear, nose, and throat manifestations | Other manifestations |
|---|---|---|---|---|
| Achalasia-adrenal-alacrima syndrome or 3A syndrome[6] | ***231550**<br>4241 | AR | Neurosensory deafness, esophageal achalasia | Short stature, increased skin pigmentation, lack of lacrimation, optic nerve atrophy, polyneuropathy, dementia, ataxia, hypotonia, adrenal malfunction |
| Achalasia-microcephaly syndrome[20] | **200450**<br>4243 | AR | Dysphagia, esophageal achalasia | Microcephaly, mental retardation (MR), abnormal palmar dermatoglyphics, recurrent lung inflammatory disease |
| Acrorenal syndrome[33] | **102520**<br>3672 | AD | Abnormal esophagus | Short stature, carpal and tarsal fusion, brachydactyly, polydactyly, cleft hand and foot, ureteric abnormality, renal failure, MR |
| Alport syndrome[24] | ***104200**<br>**203780**<br>***301050**<br>4509 | XLR<br>AR<br>AD | Sensorineural deafness, esophageal and tracheal leiomyomatosis | Nephritis with hematuria, cataract, keratoconus, macular pigmentary abnormality |
| Arthrogryposis, CNS calcifications[14] | **208110**<br>4650 | AR | Myopathic facies, trismus, long philtrum, abnormal esophagus | Contractures of large joints, ulnar deviation of fingers, calcified blood vessels, intracranial calcifications, hypotonia |
| Brachmann-de Lange syndrome or Cornelia de Lange syndrome[9,23] | **122470**<br>3183 | Usually sporadic<br>AD<br>AR | Micrognathia, short nose, depressed nasal bridge, flared nostrils, down-turned mouth angles, cleft palate, thin lips, low-set ears, abnormal cry, abnormal esophagus, dysphagia | Short stature, cutis marmorata, microcephaly, synophrys, long eyelashes, hypogonadism, diffuse osteoporosis, brachydactyly, syndactyly, missing toes, hallux valgus, hypotonia, severe mental retardation |
| CHARGE association (**C**oloboma, **H**eart defect, **R**etardation of growth and development, **G**enital hypoplasia, **E**ar anomalies)[31,34] | **214800**<br>3480 | Sporadic<br>AR | Structural asymmetry of face, facial palsy, midface hypoplasia, micrognathia, choanal atresia, cleft lip/palate, abnormal helix, deafness—conductive or sensorineural—early feeding problems | Short stature or stunted growth, eye colobomas, omphalocele, hypogonadism, heart defects, agenesis of kidneys, ureteric abnormalities, MR |
| Chromosome 8, trisomy 8 mosaicism, or Warkany syndrome[15,25] | 3077 | | Coarse and myopathic face, micrognathia, flattened nose, broad nasal bridge, thick lips, low-set or anteverted ears, prominent antihelix, conductive deafness, short neck, abnormal esophagus | Large birth weight, tall stature, deep palmar and plantar creases (cat paw), absent nails, deep-set eyes, pectus deformity, scoliosis, kyphosis (thoracolumbar), multiple vertebral malsegmentation, renal anomalies |
| Chromosome 13, del 13q (q22 or 31qter)[21] | 3091 | | High nasal bridge, small nose, microstomia, abnormal location of ears, micrognathia, short neck, webbed neck, abnormal esophagus | Small for gestational age, sloping forehead, epicanthic folds, upward slanting palpebral fissures, colobomatous microphthalmia, hypospadias, cryptorchidism, abnormal female genitalia, single palmar creases, talipes, defor- |

**Appendix G** Syndromes and conditions associated with tracheoesophageal fistula or abnormal esophagus (*Continued*)

| Syndrome or condition | MIM No. POSSUM No.[a] | Inheritance[b] | Ear, nose, and throat manifestations | Other manifestations |
|---|---|---|---|---|
| | | | | mity, neural tube and brain defects, heart defects, severe MR, early death |
| Chromosome 18, trisomy 18 or Edward syndrome[7,28] | 3094 | | Triangular face, micrognathia, small nose, choanal atresia, microstoma, cleft palate, low-set ears, absent helix, short neck, TEF | Small for gestational age, prominent occiput, increased body hair, cutis marmorata, small palpebral fissures, short sternum, delayed skeletal maturation, overlapping fingers, rocker-bottom feet, diaphragmatic hernia, severe MR |
| Chromosome 21, trisomy 21, or Down syndrome[40,42] | 3100 | | Small nose, depressed nasal bridge, protruding tongue, small folded ear, open mouth, narrow palate, short neck, deafness—conductive or sensorineural—TEF | Microcephaly, flat occiput, upward eye slant, epicanthus, Brushfield spots, pectus deformity, atlantoaxial instability, umbilical hernia, cryptorchidism, clinodactyly of 5th finger, single palmar creases, flat foot, heart defects, duodenal atresia, characteristic gait, hypothyroidism |
| Chromosome X, triploidy 69XXX/XXY, or triploidy[35] | 3114 | | Micrognathia, broad nasal bridge, choanal atresia, down-turned mouth angles, cleft lip/palate, macroglossia, dysplastic micrognathia, low-set ears, short neck | Premature or small for gestational age, corneal opacities, retinal coloboma, microphthalmia, ambiguous genitalia, hypospadias, syndactyly of fingers, talipes valgus, hypoplastic lungs, diaphragmatic hernia, malrotation of gut, Arnold Chiari malformation, neural tube defects, moderate to severe MR |
| Coach syndrome or MR, ataxia, hepatic fibrosis[44] | 4624 | Unknown | Flat face, esophageal varices | Hypertelorism, choroidal coloboma, hepatic fibrosis, splenomegaly, cerebellar vermis hypoplasia/aplasia, ataxia, hypotonia, MR |
| Colobomata, TEF, heart defects[26] | 4359 | Unknown | Structural asymmetry of face, facial palsy, low-set ears, abnormal voice, TEF | Microphthalmia, dislocated lens, coloboma of iris, heart defects |
| Deafness, vitiligo, achalasia[22] | ***221350**<br>3855 | AR | Sensorineural deafness, achalasia of the esophagus | Short stature, vitiligo, muscle weakness or wasting |
| DiGeorge sequence or, thymic aplasia syndrome, or third and fourth pharyngeal pouch syndrome[11,19] | ***188400**<br>3186 | Mostly sporadic AD | Anteverted nostrils, choanal atresia, short philtrum, cleft palate, bifid uvula, posteriorly angulated ears, middle ear abnormalities, esophageal atresia | Hypertelorism, short palpebral fissure, epicanthic folds, aortic arch abnormality, thymic aplasia, frequent infections, lymphocyte dysfunction, hypoparathyroidism, hypocalcemia, MR; may be associated with chromosome deletion of 22q11 |
| Dyserkeratosis congenita syndrome or Zinsser-Engman-Cole syndrome[5,41] | **127550**<br>**224230**<br>***305000**<br>3191 | AD<br>AR<br>XLR | Oral mucosal abnormalities (leukoplakia), thinning of ear drum, sensorineural deafness, dysphagia with esophageal strictures and diverticulae | Usually normal at birth; increased skin pigmentation, leukoplakia, telangiectasia, premature graying of hair, nail changes, defects of the lacrimal system; hyperkeratosis or hyperhidrosis of palms and soles (in the first decade), multiple fractures, and progressive marrow failure; malignancy, death in adult life; proposed gene location Xq28. |
| Epidermolysis bullosa dystrophica or Epidermolysis bullosa, Hallopeau-Siemens type[10,36] | ***#226600***<br>3216 | AR | Anomalies of tongue, enamel defects, discoloration of teeth, diminished mouth opening, prognathism, feeding difficulties | Dermolytic blisters after minor trauma, thin skin, dysplastic nails, syndactyly of fingers, claw hand, contractures (due to scarring) |

| Syndrome or condition | MIM No. POSSUM No.[a] | Inheritance[b] | Ear, nose, and throat manifestations | Other manifestations |
|---|---|---|---|---|
| Esophageal atresia, coloboma, talipes[30] | 3914 | Unknown | Esophageal atresia | Coloboma of iris or retina, talipes deformities |
| Esophageal leiomyomata, nephritis, deafness[4] | 4422 | AD | Sensorineural deafness, esophageal leiomyomatosis | Congenital cataract, nephritis with hematuria, renal failure, visceral leiomyomata (variant of Alport syndrome) |
| Female pseudohermaphroditism, Müllerian/urinary/anal dysplasia[45] | 4482 | Unknown | Abnormal esophagus | Ambiguous genitalia, uterine abnormality, urogenital sinus, limb defect (ray), dysplastic kidneys, ureteric or urethral abnormality, imperforate anus |
| Femoral hypoplasia, unusual facies[16] | **134780**<br>3232 | AD<br>Multifactorial | Short nose, hypoplastic alae nasi, broad nasal bridge, thin lips, long philtrum, cleft palate, micrognathia, prominent ears, abnormal pinnae, abnormal esophagus | Short stature, short limbs, scoliosis, hypoplastic femur/fibula, dislocated hips, polydactyly of feet, dysplastic kidneys, genital abnormalities, heart defects |
| Focal dermal hypoplasia or Goltz-Gorlin syndrome[27] | ***305600**<br>*3204 | XLD | Oral papillomas, cleft palate, oligodontia, cleft tongue, mixed deafness, broad nasal tip, coloboma of nostrils, outstanding simple pinnae, narrow auditory canals, esophageal papillomas | Short stature, atrophic skin macules, areas of fat herniation, linear or reticular hyperpigmentation or hypopigmentation, absent nails, sparse scalp hair, eye colobomas, hypoplastic clavicles, diffuse osteoporosis, polydactyly, oligodactyly, syndactyly, MR |
| Infantile myofibromatosis with MCA[32] | 4798 | Unknown | Esophageal atresia | Subcutaneous nodules, annular pancreas, sacral, vertebral, and kidney defects |
| Maternal (PKU) syndrome or phenylketonuria PKU embryopathy[18,29] | ***261600**<br>3533 | Teratogenicity | Depressed nasal bridge, long philtrum, cleft palate | Microcephaly, epicanthal folds, heart defects, MR, behavior disorders, seizures |
| Microcephaly, TEF, hand defect[8] | 4063 | AD | Low-set ears, abnormal esophagus, TEF | Microcephaly, missing fingers, overlapping fingers, rocker-bottom foot, syndactyly, duodenal atresia, MR |
| MR, chest asymmetry, muscle hypoplasia[1] | 4043 | Unknown<br>XL<br>AR | High nasal bridge, high-arched palate, abnormal cry, abnormal esophagus | Failure to thrive, poor musculature, macrocephaly, pectus deformity, dolichocephaly, arachnodactyly, absence of subcutaneous tissue, contractures of large joints, severe MR |
| Multiple odontoma, esophageal stenosis[39] | 4426 | AD | General enlargement of the jaw, maxillary and mandibular cysts, esophageal stenosis, leiomyomatosis | Aortic and pulmonic stenosis, cardiomyopathy, hepatocellular liver disease, fibrosis |
| Potter sequence or oligohydramnios sequence[17,46] | ***191830**<br>3368 | Heterogenous | Micrognathia, flattened nose, cleft lip/palate, low-set ears, webbed neck, esophageal atresia | Ambiguous genitalia, cryptorchidism, uterine-vaginal abnormality, contracture of large joints, hypoplastic lungs, dysplastic kidneys, ureteric and bladder abnormalities, imperforate anus |
| Pulmonary agenesis and microphthalmia[43] | 3577 | Unknown | Depressed nasal bridge, abnormal columella, deeply grooved philtrum, prominent antihelix, esophageal atresia | Bilateral pulmonary agenesis, heart defects, microphthalmia, eventration of diaphragm |
| Schisis association[12] | 4137 | Unknown | Cleft lip/palate, encephalocele, abnormal esophagus, TEF | Omphalocele, inguinal hernia, diaphragmatic hernia, neural tube defects |
| Sirenomelia sequence, or caudal regression syndrome[38] | 3399 | Multifactorial (higher frequency in infants of diabetic mothers) | Micrognathia, depressed nasal bridge, low-set ears, abnormal esophagus | Hemivertebrae, sacral agenesis, ambiguous genitalia, urogenital sinus, variable fusion or hypoplasia of lower limbs, horseshoe kidney, imperforate/stenotic anus, MR |

**Appendix G** Syndromes and conditions associated with tracheoesophageal fistula or abnormal esophagus (*Continued*)

| Syndrome or condition | MIM No. POSSUM No.[a] | Inheritance[b] | Ear, nose, and throat manifestations | Other manifestations |
|---|---|---|---|---|
| Tetraamelia with pulmonary hypoplasia or aplasia[37] | ***273395** 4849 | AR | Lateral cleft lip, low-set ears, abnormal esophagus | Absence of 4 limbs, hydrocephalus, hypoplastic lungs and pulmonary vessels |
| TEF, bat ears, symphalangism of the 5th finger, or Blaichman syndrome[2] | 3554 | Unknown | Facial palsy, limited opening of the mouth, broad nasal bridge, bat ears, TEF | Upward slanting palpebral fissures, epicanthal folds, vertebral abnormality, symphalangism of the 5th finger/clinodactyly, irregular-shaped toes, abnormal palmar dermatoglyphics |
| VACTERL association with hydrocephalus[13] | 4843 | AR XLR | Micrognathia, low-set ears, atresia of the external auditory canal, TEF | Hydrocephalus, agenesis of corpus callosum, MR; in addition to the spectrum of VACTERL or VATER association (see below) |
| VATER Association or VACTERL association: **V**ertebral, **A**nal, **C**ardiac, **T**racheo-**E**sophageal, **R**enal, and **L**imb defects [3] | **192350** 3425 | Sporadic Unknown AD (some cases) | TEF | Vertebral defects, anal stenosis or atresia, radial ray-renal abnormalities, cardiac defects, limb defects, pulmonary abnormalities |

The following syndromes also may have an abnormal esophagus: (1)facio-auriculo-vertebral dysplasia (Goldenhar syndrome); (2) Flannery syndrome; (3) laryngotracheoesophageal cleft, unilateral pulmonary hypoplasia; (4) multiple sulphatase deficiency; (5) Opitz-Frias syndrome; and (6) tracheal agenesis association.

## References


1. Benthem LH, van Driessen O, Haneveld GT: Cryptorchidism, chest deformities, and other congenital anomalies in three brothers. Arch Dis Child 45:590–592, 1970.
2. Blaichman S: Tracheoesophageal fistula, protruding pinnae, proximal interphalangeal symphalangism of fifth finger. A new syndrome? Am J Med Genet 13:233–234, 1982.
3. Chetcuti P, Dickens DR, Phelan PD: Spinal deformity in patients borh with oesophageal atresia and tracheo-oesophageal fistula. Arch Dis Child 64:1427–1430, 1989.
4. Cochat P, Guibaud P, Garcia Torres R, Roussel B, Guarner V, Larbre F: Diffuse leiomyomatosis in Alport syndrome. J Pediatr 113:339–343, 1988.
5. Davidson HR, Connor JM: Dyskeratosis congenita. J Med Genet 25:843–846, 1988.
6. Ehrich E, Aranoff G, Johnson WG: Familial achalasia associated with adrenocortical insufficiency, alacrima, and neurological abnormalities. Am J Med Genet, 26:637–644, 1987.
7. Evans DG, Evans ID, Donnai D, Lindenbaum, RH: Ankyloblepharon filiforme adnatum in trisomy 18 Edwards syndrome. J Med Genet 27:720–721, 1990.
8. Feingold M: Familial microcephaly with skeletal abnormality. Case report. Synd Ident 3:16–17, 1975.
9. Filippi G: The de Lange syndrome. Report of 15 cases. Clin Genet 35:343–363, 1989.
10. Gorlin RJ, Cohen MM, Levin LS: Syndromes of the Head and Neck, 3rd ed. Oxford University Press, New York, 1990, pp 501–506.
11. Greenberg F, Courtney KB, Wessels RA, Huhta J, Carpenter RJ, Rich DC, Ledbetter DH: Prenatal diagnosis of deletion 17p13 associated with DiGeorge anomaly. Am J Med Genet 31:1–4, 1988.
12. Hershey DW, Haesslein HC, Marr CC, Adkins JC: Familial abdominal wall defects. Am J Med Genet 34:174–176, 1989.
13. Iafolla AK, McConkie-Rosell A, Chen YT: VATER and hydrocephalus: distinct syndrome? Am J Med Genet 34:174–176, 1989.
14. Illum N, Reske-Nielsen E, Skovby F, Askjaer SA, Bernsen A: Lethal autosomal recessive arthrogryposis multiplex congenita and whistling face and calcifications of the nervous svstem. Neuropediatrics 19:186–192, 1988.
15. Jones KL: Smith's Recognizable Patterns of Human Malformation, 5th ed. WB Saunders, Philadelphia, 1996, p 24.
16. Jones KL: Smith's Recognizable Patterns of Human Malformation, 5th ed. WB Saunders, Philadelphia, 1996, p 310.
17. Jones KL: Smith's Recognizable Patterns of Human Malformation, 5th ed. WB Saunders, Philadelphia, 1996, p 570.
18. Jones KL: Smith's Recognizable Patterns of Human Malformation, 5th ed. WB Saunders, Philadelphia, 1996, p 580.
19. Jones KL: Smith's Recognizable Patterns of Human Malformation, 5th ed. WB Saunders, Philadelphia, 1996, p 616.
20. Khalifa MD: Familial achalasia, microcephaly, and mental retardation. Case report and review of literature. Clin Pediatr 27:509–512, 1988.
21. Kiss P, Osztovics M: Association of 13q deletion and Hirschprung's disease. J Med Genet 26:100–104, 1989.
22. Konigsmark BW, Gorlin RJ: Genetic and Metabolic Deafness. WB Saunders, Philadelphia, 1976, p 246.
23. Kumar D, Blank CE, Griffiths BL: Cornelia de Lange syndrome in several members of the same family. J Med Genet 22:296–300, 1985.
24. Legius E, Proesmans W, Van Damme B, Geboes K, Lerut T, Eggermont E: Muscular hypertrophy of the oesophagus and "Alport-like" glomerular lesions in a boy. Eur J Pediatr 149:623–627, 1990.
25. Lessick M, Israel J, Szego K, Wong P: Leiomyosarcoma in a patient with trisomy 8 mosaicism. Med Genet 7:643–644, 1990.
26. Lilliquist KJ, Warburg M, Andersen SR, Hagerstrand I: Colobomata of the iris, ciliary body and choroid in an infant with oesophago-tracheal fistula and congenital heart defects. An unknown malformation complex. Acta Paediatr Scan 69:427–430, 1990.
27. Mann M, Weintraub R, Hashimoto K: Focal dermal hypoplasia with an initial inflammatory phase. Pediatr Dermatol 7:278–282, 1990.
28. Marion RW, Wiznia, AA, Hutcheon RG, Rubinstein A: Craniofacial dysmorphism in children with human immunodeficiency virus infection. J Pediatr 113:784–785, 1988.
29. Matalon R, Michals K, Blau N, Rouse B: Hyperphenylalaninemia due to inherited deficiencies of tetrahydrobiopterin. Adv Pediatr 36:67–89, 1989.
30. Mehes K: Esophageal atresia, coloboma, and clubfood in two unrelated infants. Hum Genet 67:354, 1985.
31. Meinecke P, Polke A, Schmiegelow P: Limb anomalies in the CHARGE association. J Med Genet 26:202–203, 1989.
32. Michel M, Ninane J, Claus D, Gosseye S, Wese FX, Moulin D: Major malformations in a case of infantile myofibromatosis. Eur J Pediatr 149:251–252, 1990.
33. Miltenyi M, Balogh L, Schmidt L, Detre Z, Hernady T, Czeizel A: A new varient of the acrorenal syndrome associated with bilateral oligomeganephronic hypoplasia. Eur J Pediatr 142:40–43, 1984.
34. Oley CA, Baraitser M, Grant DB: A reappraisal of the CHARGE association. J Med Genet 25:147–156, 1983.
35. Pettenati MJ, Mirkin LD, Goldstein DJ: Diploid-triploid mosaicism: report of necropsy findings. Am J Med Genet 24:23–28, 1986.
36. Price T, Katz VL: Obstetrical concerns of epidermolysis bullosa. Obstet Gynecol Surv 43:445–449, 1988.

37. Rosenak D, Ariel I, Arnon J, Diamant YZ, Ben Chetrit A, Nadjari M, Zilbnerman R, Yaffe H, Cohen T, Ornoy A: Recurrent tetraamelia and pulmonary hypoplasia with multiple malformations in sibs. Am J Med Genet 38:25–28, 1991.
38. Rudd NL, Klimek ML: Familial caudal dysgenesis: evidence for a major dominant gene. Clin Genet 38:170–175, 1990.
39. Schmidseder R, Hausamen JE: Multiple odontogenic tumors and other anomalies. An autosomal dominantly inherited syndrome. Oral Surg Oral Med Oral Pathol 39:249–258, 1975.
40. Serra A, Neri G: Trisomy 21: conference report and 1990 update. Am J Med Genet (Suppl) 7:11–19, 1990.
41. Shahidi NT: Fanconi anemia, dyskeratosis congenita, and WT syndrome. Am J Med Genet (Suppl) 3:263–278, 1987.
42. Sheridan R, Lierena J JR, Matkins S, Debenham P, Cawood A, Bobrow M: Fertility in a male with trisomy 21. J Med Genet 26:294–298, 1989.
43. Spear GS, Yetur P, Beyerlein RA: Bilateral pulmonary agenesis and microphthalmia. Am J Med Genet (Suppl) 3:379–382, 1987.
44. Verloes A, Lambotte C: Further delineation of a syndrome of cerebellar vermis hypo/aplasia, oligophrenia, congenital ataxia, coloboma, and hepatic fibrosis. Am J Med Genet 32:227–232, 1989.
45. Wenstrup RJ, Pagon RA: Female pseudohermaphroditism with anorectal, mullerian duct, and urinary tract malformations: report of four cases. J Pediatr 107:751–754, 1985.
46. Wilson RD, Baird PA: Renal agenesis in British Columbia. Am J Med Genet 21:153–169, 1985.

# IX

## Selected Syndromes and Conditions

# Selected Syndromes and Conditions

TED L. TEWFIK, AHMAD S. TEEBI, and VAZKEN M. DER KALOUSTIAN

## Aarskog syndrome

### Facio-digito-genital syndrome

(MIM Nos. 100050, *305400; POSSUM No. 3001)

#### General manifestations

Short stature and normal intelligence is seen in 90% of patients. Bone age is retarded. The hands are short and broad (80%); mild cutaneous syndactyly is observed in 60% with marked hyperextensibility of the proximal interphalangeal joints in 70% of cases. The feet are also broad, with bulbous toes (70%). Mild pectus excavatum is common.

The most peculiar genital finding is the shawl scrotum where a scrotal fold extends dorsally to surround the penile shaft (80%). Cryptorchidism and inguinal hernia are common (60%–75%).

Ocular findings include large cornea, amblyopia, deficient ocular elevation, blue sclerae, posterior embryotoxon, and a variety of refractive errors.[3]

Other occasional malformations include growth hormone deficiency and single palmar crease.[2,6,8,10,11]

#### Otolaryngological manifestations

The majority of patients (90%) have hypertelorism, with a broad nasal bridge and anteverted nostrils. Fifty to sixty percent of patients have a widow's peak. The eyelids are ptosed, and there is an antimongoloid slant of the palpebral fissures. The philtrum is long and the maxilla is hypoplastic. The external ears are thickened. Latent nystagmus may occur. Delayed dental eruptions and missing teeth have been reported. Cleft lip/palate may also be seen.[2,3,4,6,7]

#### Etiology

Aarskog syndrome is of X-linked recessive inheritance.[1,5] The locus is at Xp11.21.[10]

The faciogenital dysplasia *(FGD1)* gene responsible for Aarskog syndrome has been cloned. It encodes a putative Rha/Rac guanine nucleotide exchange factor involved in mammalian morphogenesis. An intragenic Taq I polymorphism facilitates the accurate carrier detection of individuals at risk.[9]

#### Differential diagnosis

Similar syndromes include autosomal recessive facio-digito-genital syndrome (Kuwait type), Robinow syndrome, Opitz syndrome, Naguib-Richieri-Costa syndrome, Teebi hypertelorism syndrome, and cranio-fronto-nasal dysplasia.[12]

#### References

1. Bawle E, Tyrkus M, Lipman S, Bozimowski D: Aarskog syndrome: full male and female expression associated with an X-autosome translocation. Am J Med Genet 17:595–602, 1984.
2. Berry C, Cree J, Mann T: Aarskog syndrome. Arch Dis Child 55:706–710, 1980.
3. Brodsky MC, Keppen LD, Rice CD, Ranels JD: Ocular and systemic findings in the Aarskog (facial-digital-genital) syndrome. Am J Ophthalmol 109:450–456, 1990.
4. DeSaxe M, Kromberg JG, Jenkins T: The Aarskog (facio-digital-genital) syndrome in South Africa. A report of three families. S Afr Med J 65:299–303, 1984.
5. Escobar V, Weaver DD: Aarskog syndrome, new findings and genetic analysis. JAMA 240:2638–2641, 1978.
6. Grier RE, Farrington FH, Kendig R, Mamunes P: Autosomal dominant inheritance of the Aarskog syndrome. Am J Med Genet 15:39–46, 1983.
7. Hoo JJ: The Aarskog (Facio-digito-genital) syndrome. Clin Genet 16:269–276, 1979.
8. Kodama M, Fujimoto S, Namikawa T, Matsuda I: Aarskog syndrome with isolated growth hormone deficiency. Eur J Ped 135:273–276, 1981.
9. Pasteris NG, Gorski JL: An intragenic Taq I polymorphism in the faciogenital dysplasia (FGD1) locus, the gene responsible for Aarskog syndrome. Hum Genet 96:494, 1995.
10. Porteous MEM, Curtis A, Lindsay S, Williams O, Goudie D, Kamakari S, Bhattacharya SS: The gene for Aarskog syndrome is located between DXS255 and DXS566 (Xq11.2–Xq13). Genomics 14:298–301, 1992.
11. Porteous ME, Goudie DR: Aarskog syndrome. J Med Genet 28:44–47, 1991.
12. Teebi AS, Rucquoi JK, Meyn MS. Aarskog syndrome: report of a family with review and discussion of nosology. Am J Med Genet 46:501–509, 1993.

## Achondroplasia

(MIM No. *100800; POSSUM No. 3006)

#### General manifestations

Achondroplasia is the most common chondrodysplasia with a frequency of 1:26,000 live births.[6] It presents with a large head, frontal bossing, and a small foramen magnum. The cranial base is short with early closure of the spheno-occipital suture. The vertebral bodies are cuboid with small interpedicular distances. Partial occipitization of the atlas occurs in most cases. Kyphoscoliosis is present. The sacrum is narrow and horizontally oriented. The thoracic cage is small and the legs are frequently bowed. The limb bones are shortened, especially the humerus and the femur (rhizomelic). The metacarpals and phalanges are short but disproportionately large in relation to the radius, ulna, and humerus.[2,3,7,10] A "trident" hand is common.

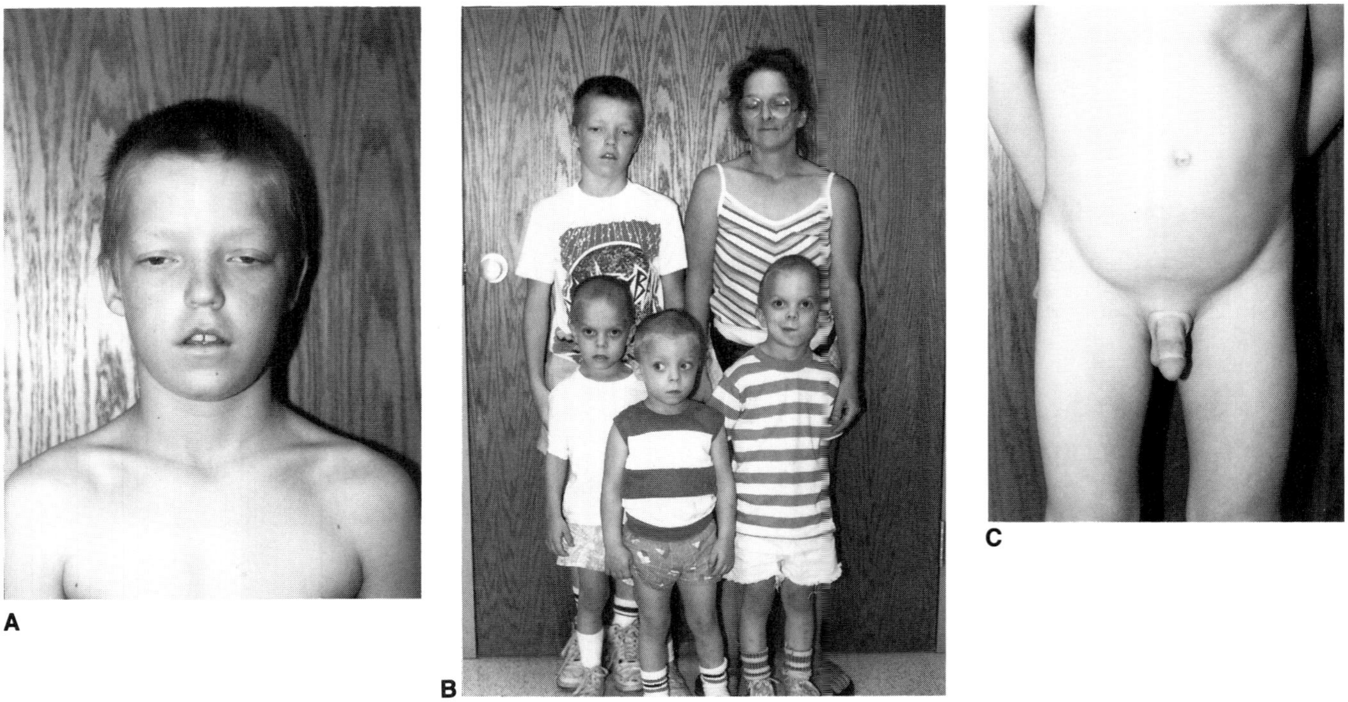

**Fig. 1.** Aarskog syndrome. A: Note broad forehead, hypertelorism, ptosis, and low-set ears. B: Family of patient in A. C: Note shawl scrotum.

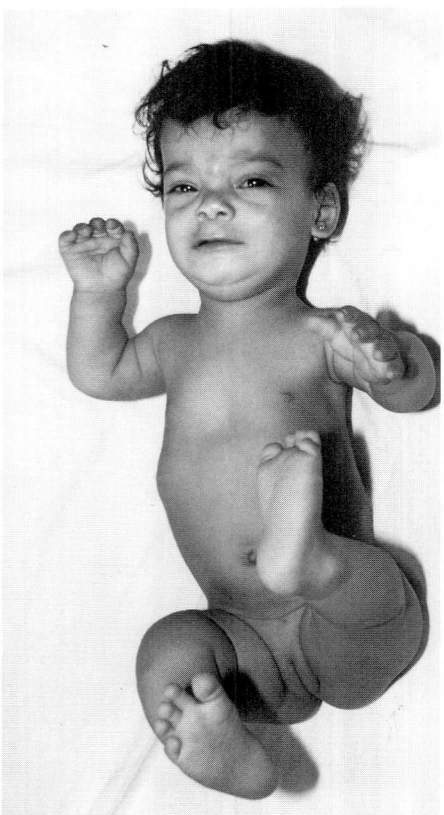

**Fig. 2.** Achondroplasia. Note the enlarged calvarium, frontal bossing, midfacial hypoplasia, low nasal bridge, and short limbs.

Intelligence is normal. The progressive narrowing of the spinal canal in the craniocaudal direction predisposes patients, with age, to neurological sequalae. Cervicomedullary compression may result in unexpected death in childhood.[2,6,8]

### Otolaryngological manifestations

Hypoplasia of the midface, low nasal bridge, and repeated ear infections with sensorineural or conductive hearing loss may occur. Dysfunction of the eustachian tube has been documented. Acoustic neuroma and progressive otosclerosis has also been described.[2–4]

### Etiology

Inheritance is autosomal dominant with complete penetrance. The great majority of cases represent fresh mutations. Advanced paternal age is a contributing factor. The condition is due to mutations in fibroblast growth factor receptor 3 (FGFR3).[5,9] Achondroplasia, the milder disorder of hypochondroplasia and the more severe disorder of thanatophoric dysplasia are allelic.[1,5,7a]

### Differential diagnosis

Achondroplasia should be differentiated from hypochondroplasia, pseudoachondroplasia, and thanatophoric dwarfism.

## References

1. Bellus GA McIntosh I, Smith EA, Aylsworth AS, Kaitila I, Horton WA, Greenhaw GA, Hecht JT, Francomano CA: A recurrent mutation in the tyrosine kinase domain of fibroblast growth factor receptor 3 causes hypochondroplasia. Nat Genet 10:357–359, 1995.

2. Brinkmann G, Schlitt H, Zorowka P, Spranger J: Cognitive skills in achondroplasia. Am J Med Genet 47:800–804, 1993.
3. Hall JG: The natural history of achondroplasia. Basic Life Sci 48:3–9, 1988.
4. Langer LO Jr, Baumann PA, Gorlin RJ: Achondroplasia. Am J Roentgenol 100:12–26, 1967.
5. Le Merrer M, Rousseau F, Legeai-Mallet L, Landais JC, Pelet A, Bonaventure J, Sanak M, Weissenbach J, Stoll C, Munnich A, Maroteaux P: A gene for achondroplasia—hypochondroplasia maps to chromosome 4p. Nat Genet 6:318–321, 1994.
6. Maroteaux P, Lamy M: Achondroplasia in man and animals. Clin Orthop 33:91–103, 1964.
7. Murdoch JL, Walker BA, Hall JG, abbey H, Smith KK, McKusick VA: Achondroplasia—genetic and statistical survey. Ann Hum Genet 33:227–244, 1970.
7a. Naski MC, Wang Q, Xu J, Ornitz DM: Graded activation of fibroblast growth factor receptor 3 by mutations causing achondroplasia and thanatophoric dysplasia. Nat Genet 13:233–237, 1996.
8. Pauli RM, Scott CI, Wassman ER Jr, Gilbert EF, Leavitt LA, Ver Hoeve J, Hall JG, Partington MW, Jones KL, Sommer A, et al: Apnea and sudden unexpected death in infants with achondroplasia. J Pediatr 104:342–348, 1984.
9. Shiang R, Thompson LM, Zhu YZ, Church DM, Fielder TJ, Bocian M, Winokur ST, Wasmuth JJ: Mutations in the transmembrane domain of FGFR3 cause the most common genetic form of dwarfism, achondroplasia. Cell 78:335–342, 1994.
10. Siebens AA, Hungerford DS, Kirby NA: Curves of the achondroplastic spine: a new hypothesis. Johns Hopkins Med J 142:205–210, 1978.

## Alport syndrome

### Hereditary nephropathy and deafness

(MIM No. *104200, 203780, #301050; POSSUM No. 4509)

This syndrome was described by Alport in 1927[1] as an inherited kidney disease characterized by hematuria, proteinuria, and progressive "perceptive deafness."[20]

#### General manifestations

Alport syndrome (AS) comprises a group of hereditary diseases characterized by progressive defects of capillaries and the glomerular basement membranes of the kidneys (glomerulonephritis). Other features include progressive sensorineural hearing loss (SNHL), ocular problems, and defects of blood platelets.[20]

Alport syndrome is classified into 6 types:[20]

Type I. Autosomal dominant inheritance. Juvenile onset of end-stage renal disease (ESRD) with SNHL.

Type II. X-linked dominant inheritance. Juvenile onset of ESRD and SNHL.

Type III. X-linked dominant inheritance. Adult onset of ESRD and SNHL.

Type IV. X-linked dominant inheritance. Adult onset of ESRD; normal hearing.

Type VA. Autosomal dominant inheritance with nephritis, SNHL, macrothrombocytopathy, and leucocyte inclusions (MIM No.153640). Also known as Fechtner syndrome.

Type VB. Autosomal dominant inheritance with nephritis, SNHL, and macrothrombocytopathy (MIM No.153650). Also known as Epstein syndrome.[4]

Type VI. Autosomal dominant inheritance with juvenile nephritis and SNHL (MIM No. 203780).

Recurrent gross or microscopic hematuria is usually seen more in males than females. Histologically, the glomerular basement membrane is thickened.[2] "Basket weave" alteration of the lamina densa of the capillary basement membrane is described as pathognomonic on electron microscopy.[22] Ophthalmologic anomalies occur in 10% of patients. Lenticonus, anterior polar cataracts, and spherophakia are described.[13,16,18]

Treatment includes the use of hearing aids, renal dialysis, and possible kidney transplantation in end-stage renal failure patients.

#### Otolaryngological manifestations

Approximately 45% of AS females and 55% of males are reported to experience a slowly progressive, symmetrical, mild to moderately severe, mid- and high-frequency SNHL.[20] The hearing loss is more severe in males. It can occur as early as 10 years of age and has been described as socially nonsignificant until the second decade of life; generally, the high frequencies are affected.[5,7,10] It is important to screen family members, as 30–50% of relatives may show SNHL. However,

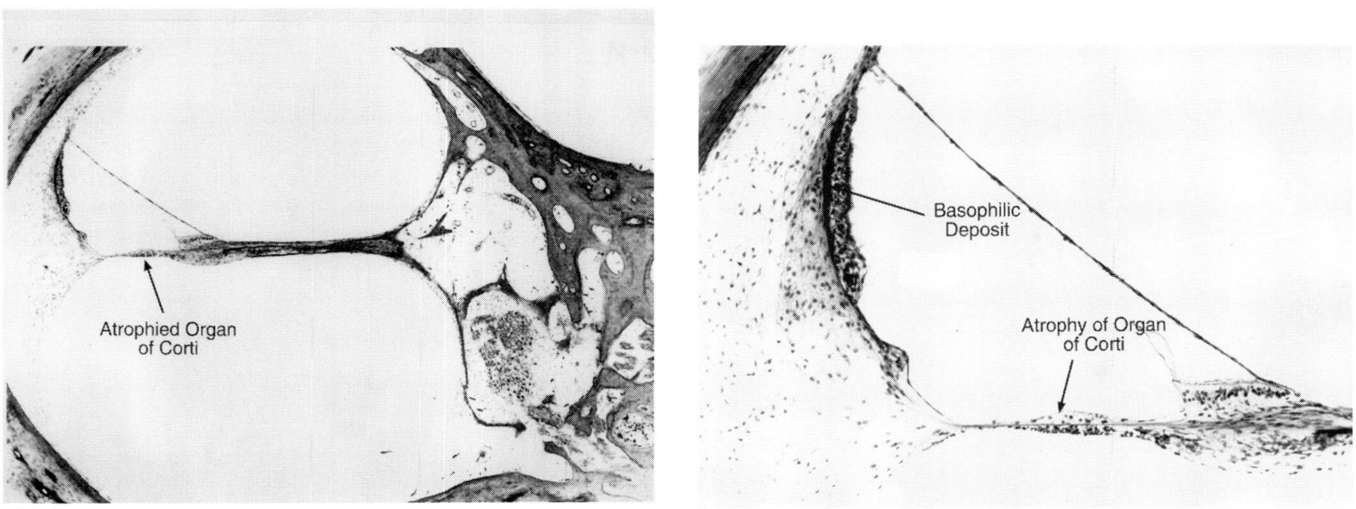


**Fig. 3.** Alport syndrome. A,B: Photomicrographs of the temporal bone showing atrophic organ of Corti at the basal end of the cochlea. In B, note mounds of cells without pillar cells (arrow directed toward the atrophic organ of Corti). There is patch atrophy of the striae vasculares and scattered homogeneous basophilic deposits at the interface between striae and the spiral ligaments. (From H Schuknecht, *Pathology of the Ear,* 2nd ed., Lea & Febiger, Philadelphia, 1993, p. 125, with permission.)

there may be no correlation between the hearing loss and kidney function.

Various publications describe the histological structure of the inner ear in AS.[8,11,12,15,21] The basal turns of the organ of Corti show degeneration of the hair cells and the striae vascularis. Reduction of the spiral ganglion neurons has been reported.[6] Very few systematic assessments of oculovestibular function have been reported with AS. Histologic sections have shown cyst-like vesicle formations under each utricular macule. Nystagmus was not consistently confirmed as an ocular symptom.[20]

### Etiology

Alport syndrome may follow the autosomal dominant, autosomal recessive, and X-linked dominant patterns of inheritance (see above). AS can show tremendous clinical variability between kindreds (phenotype heterogeneity).[20]

Genetic linkage studies using restriction fragment length polymorphism (RFLP) technology and clinical tests of renal function to define the phenotype have mapped type III AS to Xq22, with little evidence for genetic heterogeneity.[3] A missense transition (362G→A) in exon 3 of the COL4A5 gene has been identified in a male patient with late-onset AS.[19] Major COL4A5 gene rearrangements were found in patients with juvenile-type AS.[17] Mutations in the COL4A3 or COL4A4 genes (2q37) were demonstrated in parents with autosomal recessive AS.[14a] Splice-mediated insertion of an Alu sequence in the COL4A3 mRNA was identified.[14]

### Differential diagnosis

AS should be differentiated from glomerulonephritis associated with hematuria, and hereditary nephritis without deafness that is probably a separate entity (MIM No.161900).[9]

### References


1. Alport AC: Hereditary familial congenital hemorrhagic nephritis. Br Med J 1:504–506, 1927.
2. Antignac C: Molecular genetics of basement membranes: the paradigm of Alport syndrome. Kidney Int (Suppl) 49:S29–S33, 1995.
3. Atkin CL, Hasstedt SJ, Menlove L, Cannon L, Kirschner N, Schwartz C, Nguyen K, Skolnick M: Mapping of Alport syndrome to the long arm of the X chromosome. Am J Hum Genet 42:249–255, 1988.
4. Brodie HA, Chole RA, Griffin GC, White JG: Macrothrombocytopenia and progressive deafness: a new genetic syndrome. Am J Otol 13:507–511, 1992.
5. Cassidy G, Brown K, Cohen M, Demaria W: Hereditary renal dysfunction and deafness. Pediatrics 35:967–979, 1965.
6. Celes-Blaubach A, Garcia-Zozaya J, Pérez-Requejo J, Brass K: Vestibular disorders in Alport's syndrome. J Laryngol Otol 88:663–674, 1974.
7. Chiricosta A, Jindal SL, Metuzals J, Koch G: Nephropathy with hematuria (Alport's syndrome). Am Med Assoc J 102:396–401, 1970.
8. Crawfurd MD, Toghill PJ: Alport's syndrome of hereditary nephritis and deafness. Quart J Med 37:563–576, 1968.
9. Dockborn RJ: Hereditary nephropathy without deafness. Am J Dis Child 114:135–138, 1967.
10. Ferguson AC, Rance CP: Hereditary nephropathy with nerve deafness (Alport's syndrome). Am J Dis Child 124:84–88, 1972.
11. Fujita S, Hayden RC: Alport's syndrome. Arch Otolaryngol 90:453–466, 1969.
12. Gregg JB, Becker SF: Concomitant progressive deafness, chronic nephritis and ocular lens disease. Arch Ophthalmol 69:293–299, 1963.
13. Hauser J: Nephropathie chronique héréditaire avec surdité et atteinte oculaire. Schweiz Med Wochenschr 104:724–728, 1974.
14. Knebelmann B, Forestier L, Drouot L, Quinones S, Chuet C, Benessy F, Saus J, Antignac C: Splice-mediated insertion of an Alu sequence in the COL4A3 mRNA causing autosomal recessive Alport syndrome. Hum Mol Genet 4:675–679, 1995.

14a. Lemmink HH, Mochizuki T, van den Heuvel LP, Schroder CH, Barrientos A, Monnens LAH, van Oost BA, Brunner HG, Reeders ST, Smeets HJM: Mutations in the type IV collagen $\alpha3$ (COL4A3) gene in autosomal recessive Alport syndrome. Hum Mol Genet 3:1269–1273, 1994.

15. Myers GJ, Tyler HR: The etiology of deafness in Alport's syndrome. Arch Otolaryngol 96:333–340, 1972.
16. Nielsen CE: Lenticonus anterior and Alport's syndrome. Acta Ophthalmol 56:518–530, 1978.
17. Renieri A, Galli L, Grillo A, Bruttini M, Neri T, Zanelli P, Rizzoni G, Massella L, Sersa A, Meroni M, et al: Major COL4A5 gene rearrangements in patients with juvenile type Alport syndrome. Am J Med Genet 59:380–385, 1995.
18. Streeter BW, Robinson MR, Wallace R, Jones DB: Lens capsule abnormalities in Alport's syndrome. Arch Ophthalmol 105:1693–1697, 1987.
19. Turco AE, Rossetti S, Biasi MO, Rizzoni G, Massella L, Saarinen NH, Renieri A, Pignatti PF, Demarchi M: A novel missense mutation in exon 3 of the COL4A5 gene associated with late-onset Alport syndrome. Clin Genet 48:261–263, 1995.
20. Wester DC, Atkin CL, Gregory MC: Alport syndrome: clinical update. J Am Acad Audiol 6:73–79, 1995.
21. Winter LE, Cram BM, Banovetz JD: Hearing loss in hereditary renal disease. Arch Otolaryngol 88:238–241, 1968.
22. Yoshikawa N, White RHR, Amerson AH: Familial hematuria: clinicopathological correlations. Clin Nephrol 17:172–182, 1982.


## Alström syndrome

### (MIM No. *203800; POSSUM No. 3020)

Alström et al.[1] described this syndrome in a Swedish kindred in 1959. It is characterized by retinitis pigmentosa, hearing loss, and diabetes mellitus.

### General manifestations

Blindness occurs by the second decade. Retinal degeneration causes nystagmus and loss of central vision initially, then spreads to the periphery of the retina.[1] Other ocular changes include glaucoma, dislocated lens, vitreous fibrosis and optic atrophy. Diabetes mellitus starts in early adulthood and is the result of resistance to the action of insulin. Moderate obesity is a part of this syndrome and usually responds to diet. Intelligence is normal. Chronic nephropathy may result in renal failure. Secondary sexual characteristics may be normal, despite small testes and elevated serum gonadotropins.[4] Cardiomyopathy due to myocardial fibrosis was reported by Warren et al.,[3] although they also stated that it may not be a feature of the syndrome. Other manifestations include acanthosis nigricans[2] and aminoaciduria.

### Otolaryngological manifestations

Deafness is progressive, sensorineural, starts in the first decade (ages 7–10), and becomes moderately severe by the third decade. Audiological investigations indicate cochlear involvement.[2]

### Etiology

Alström syndrome follows the autosomal recessive pattern of inheritance. It is frequent among French Acadians in Nova Scotia and Louisiana.

### Differential diagnosis

Bardet-Biedl syndrome differs from it by having polydactyly, mental retardation, and hypogonadism.

### References

1. Alström C, Hallgren B, Nilsson L, Asander H: Retinal degeneration combined with obesity, diabetes mellitus, and neurogenic deafness. Acta Psychiatr Neurol Scand 34:1–35, 1959.
2. Goldstein JL, Fialkow PJ: The Alström syndrome. Medicine 52:53–71, 1973.
3. Warren SE, Schmitt SJ, Bauman AJ, Gianelly RE, Landsberg L, Baim DS: Late onset dilated cardiomyopathy in a unique familial syndrome of hypogonadism and metabolic abnormalities. Am Heart J 114:1522–1524, 1987.
4. Weinstein RL, Klinan B, Scully RE: Familial syndrome of primary testicular insufficiency with normal virilization, blindness deafness and metabolic abnormalities. N Engl J Med 281:989–977, 1969.

## Antley-Bixler syndrome

(MIM No. *207410; POSSUM No. 3570)

The syndrome is characterized by craniosynostosis, hypoplasia of the midface, proptosis, dysplastic ears, radiohumeral synostosis, femoral bowing and/or fractures.

### General manifestations

Radiohumeral synostosis, multiple joint contractures, and inability to extend the fingers are common. The range of movement is decreased in the hips, knees, wrists, and ankles. The femora are bowed and the interphalangeal joints are enlarged. Fingers may be elongated with narrow nails. The chest and pelvis are narrow (20%). Camptodactyly (80%), rocker-bottom feet (60%), and syndactyly (20%) are observed. Ocular proptosis is very common.

Urogenital abnormalities, including hypoplastic labia minora, enlarged clitoris, duplicated kidneys, and vaginal atresia, are documented.[5,6]

Other defects may be seen, including cardiovascular malformations, hydrocephalus, imperforate anus, and lumbar meningomyelocele.[3]

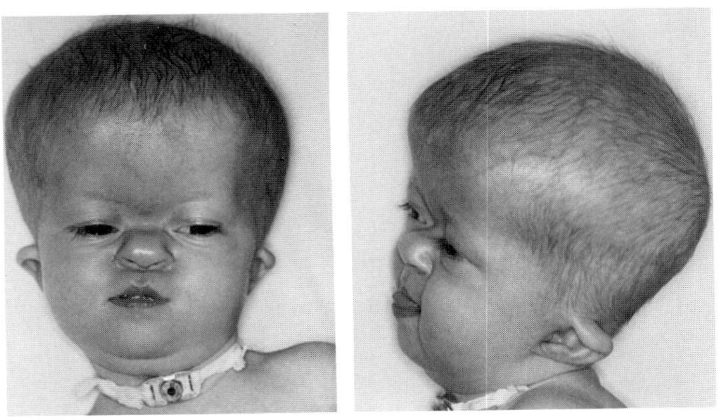

A B

**Fig. 4.** Antley-Bixler syndrome. A,B: Note the biparietal bossing, brachycephaly, malformed ears, and low nasal bridge. (From RJ Gorlin et al., *Syndromes of the Head and Neck,* 3rd ed. Oxford University Press, New York, 1990, p. 533.)

### Otolaryngological manifestations

The skull is brachycephalic with frontal and biparietal bossing due to craniosynostosis of the coronal and lambdoid sutures. The anterior fontanel is large. The nose is large and pear-shaped, and the nasal bridge is low. There is severe hypoplasia of the midface. Atresia or stenosis of the choanae occurs in 80% of the cases. The ears are abnormal (100%), often low set and protruding. The external auditory canals are stenotic (50%). Preauricular tags are seen occasionally. Respiratory depression is the main cause of death early in infancy.[1,2,4,7]

### Etiology

Antley-Bixler syndrome follows the autosomal recessive pattern of inheritance.

### Differential diagnosis

This disorder should be differentiated from campomelic syndrome and syndromes with radiohumeral synostosis.

### References

1. Delozier CD, Antley Rm, Williams R, Green N, Hiller RM, Bixler D, Engel E: The syndrome of multisynostotic osteodysgenesis with long bone fracture. Am J Med Genet 7:391–403, 1980.
2. Delozier-Blanchet CD: Antley-Bixter syndrome from a prognostic perspective. Am J Med Genet 32:262–263, 1989.
3. Escobar LF, Bixler D, Sadore M, Bull MJ: Antley-Bixler syndrome from a prognostic perspective: Am J Med Genet 32:262–263, 1989.
4. Pincus RL, Urbina MC, Gallo RA, DeFrietas J: The otolaryngological manifestations of Antley-Bixler syndrome. Otolaryngol Head Neck Surg 104:276–278, 1991.
5. Robert E, Bethenod M, Bourgeois J: Le syndrome d'Antley-Bixler. J Genet Hum 32:291–298, 1984.
6. Robinson LK, Powers NG, Dunklee P, Sherman S, Jones KL: The Antley-Bixler syndrome. J Pediatr 101:201–205, 1982.
7. Schinzel A, Savoldelli G, Bruier J, Sigg P, Massina C: Antley-Bixler syndrome in sisters: a term newborn, a prenatally diagnosed fetus. Am J Med Genet 14:139–147, 1983.

## Apert syndrome

**Acrocephalosyndactyly type I**
(MIM No. *101200; POSSUM No. 3007)

Apert is credited with the first description of this syndrome in 1906.[1] However, Wheaton had reported it earlier.[13] Recent extensive reviews are available.[5,6,8]

### General manifestations

The major diagnostic criteria are craniosynostosis and syndactyly of the hands and feet.

The skull is acrocephalic with a shortened anteroposterior (AP) diameter and flat occiput. The craniosynostosis involves the coronal suture. The forehead is prominent. The fontanelles are large and close at a later age. The palpebral fissures slant downward. The corners of the mouth are down-turned and it is sometimes described as *trapezoid mouth.* Dental anomalies include delayed and ectopic eruptions and shovel-shaped incisors.[9] Malocclusion with mesial molar occlusion and severe crowding of the teeth are also frequently noted.

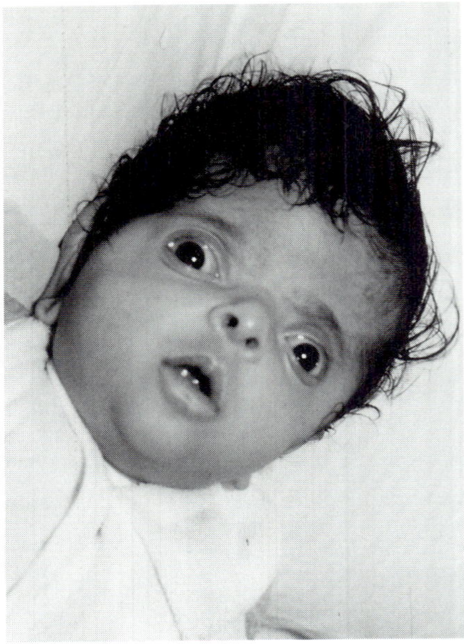

A

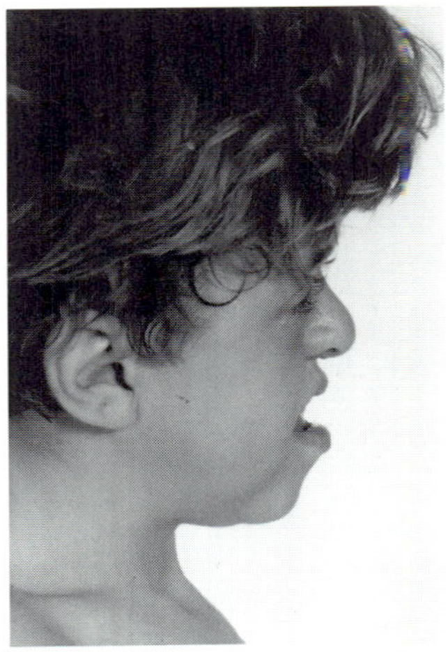

B

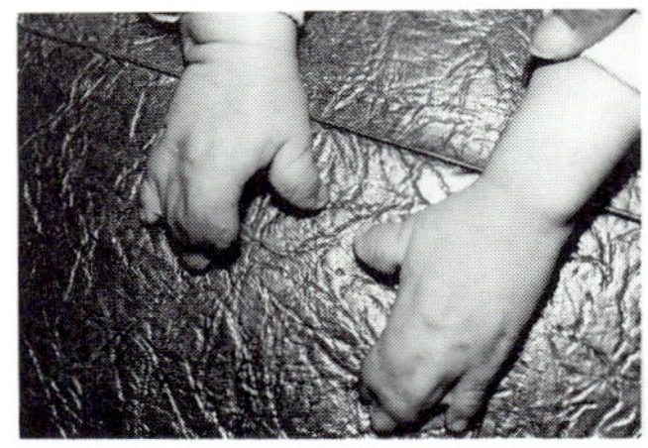

C

**Fig. 5.** Apert syndrome. Note the depressed nasal bridge and the downward slanting palpebral fissures (A), the parrot-like nose (B), and syndactyly of the fingers (C).

A significant number of Apert syndrome patients are mentally retarded. Malformations of the corpus callosum and/or the limbic structures do occur. Other findings include gyral abnormalities, megalencephaly, hypoplasia of the white matter, and heterotropic gray matter.[4,5] Patton et al. found that half of their patients had an IQ of 70.[12] Normal intelligence has been observed by others.[3] The pituitary fossa and the basiocciput are significantly larger than normal in Apert patients.[13]

Anomalies of the hands include syndactyly of the second, third, and fourth fingers that form a mid-digital mass. The first and fifth fingers may join the hand mass or be separate from it. The distal phalanx of the thumb is often broad. Syndactyly is also noted in the feet and involves the second, third, and fourth toes. Fusion of the tarsal bones and an extra metatarsal have been noted.[14,16] Other anomalies include abnormalities of the cervical vertebrae (single fusion 37%, multiple fusion 31%). C5 and C6 are often involved.[8]

Moderate to severe acne at adolescence occurs in 70% of patients. Synostosis of the radioulnar complex, pyloric stenosis, ventricular septal defects, and polycystic kidneys are rare occurrences.

## Otolaryngological manifestations

The nasal bridge is depressed, and the midface is typically hypoplastic. The palate is narrow and is described as *byzantine-arch-shaped*. Cleft palate may also occur (30%). Anomalies of the ears include otitis media, conductive hearing loss, fixation of the stapedial foot plate, and wide cochlear aqueduct. Temporal bone studies revealed absence of the internal auditory canals in one patient[2] and enlarged subarcuate fossa in another report.[10] Anomalies of the airway have also been reported, as well as tracheal stenosis, obstructive sleep apnea, and cor pulmonale with resultant early death.[6]

## Etiology

Apert syndrome follows the autosomal dominant pattern of inheritance. An increased paternal age is a factor in most of sporadic cases, which account for the majority. Exclusive paternal origin of new mutations in Apert syndrome has been reported.[10a] The incidence of Apert syndrome is estimated to be 15.5 per million and it represents 4.5% of all cases of craniosynostosis.[7]

Mutations have been found in fibroblast growth factor receptor 2 (FGFR2).[11] These consist of specific missense substitutions involving adjacent amino acids (Ser252Trp or Pro253Arg) in the linker between the second and third extracellular immunoglobulin domains of FGFR2. It has been found that cleft palate is significantly more common in Ser252Trp patients, whereas the syndactyly is more severe with the Pro253Arg mutation. It is concluded that there may be subtle differences in the phenotype resulting from the different mutations. These may relate to varying patterns of temporal and tissue-specific expression of different fibroblast growth factors which are the ligands for FGFR2.[15]

## Differential diagnosis

Apert syndrome should be differentiated from Crouzon syndrome, Pfeiffer syndrome and Saethre-Chotzen syndrome.

## References

1. Apert E: De l'acrocéphalosyndactylie. Bull Soc Med Paris 23:1310–1330, 1906.
2. Bergström LV, Neblett LM, Hemenway WG: Otologic manifestations of acrocephalosyndactyly. Arch Otolaryngol 96:117–123, 1972.
3. Cohen MM Jr: Craniosynostosis: Evaluation and Management. Raven Press, New York, 1986.
4. Cohen MM Jr, Kreiborg S: Agenesis of the corpus collosum. Its associated anomalies and syndromes with special reference to the Apert syndrome. Neurosurg Clin N Am 32:565–568, 1991.
5. Cohen MM Jr, Kreiborg S: The central nervous system in the Apert syndrome. Am J Med Genet 35:36–45, 1990.
6. Cohen MM Jr, Kreiborg S: Upper and lower airway compromise in the Apert syndrome. Am J Med Genet 44:90–93, 1992.
7. Cohen MM Jr, Kreiborg S, Lammer EJ, Cordero JF, Mastroiacovo P, Erickson JD, Roeper P, Martinez-Frias ML: Birth prevalence study of the Apert syndrome. Am J Med Genet 42:655–659, 1992.
8. Kreiborg S, Barr M Jr, Cohen MM Jr: Cervical spine in the Apert syndrome. Am J Med Genet 43:704–708, 1992.
9. Kreiborg S, Cohen MM Jr: The oral manifestations of Apert sydrome. J Craniofac Genet Dev Biol 12:41–48, 1992.
10. Lindsay JR, Black FO, Donnelly WN Jr: Acrocephalosyndactyly

(Apert's syndrome). Temporal bone findings. Ann Otol Rhinol Laryngol 84:174–178, 1975.
10a. Moloney DM, Slaney SF, Oldridge M, Wall SA, Sahlin P, Stenman G, Wilkie AOM: Exclusive paternal origin of new mutations in Apert syndrome. Nat Genet 13: 48–53, 1996.
11. Park W-J, Belus GA, Jabs EW: Mutations in fibroblast growth factor receptors: phenotypic consequences during eukaryotic development. Am J Hum Genet 57:748–754, 1995.
12. Patton MA, Goodship J, Hayward R, Landsown R: Intellectual development in Apert's syndrome: a long-term follow-up of 29 patients. J Med Genet 25:164–167, 1988.
13. Richtsmeier JT: Comparative study of normal, Crouzon, and Apert craniofacial morphology using finite element scaling analysis. Am J Phys Anthropol 74:473–493, 1987.
14. Schauerte EW, St-Aubin PM: Progressive synostosis in Apert's syndrome (acrocephalosyndactyly) with a description of roentgenographic changes in the feet. Am J Roentgenol 97:67–73, 1966.
15. Slaney SF, Oldridge M, Hurst JA, Morriss-Kay GM, Hall CM, Poole MD, Wilkie AOM: Differential effects of FGFR2 mutations on syndactyly and cleft palate in Apert syndrome. Am J Hum Genet 58:923–932, 1996.
16. Wheaton SW: Two specimens of congenital cranial deformity in infants associated with fusion of fingers and toes. Trans Pathol Soc London 45:238–241, 1894.

## Beals syndrome

### Contractural arachnodactyly
(MIM No. *121050; POSSUM No. 3027)

#### General manifestations

This syndrome is characterized by congenital joint contractures of the knees, elbows, fingers, and ankles in addition to adducted thumbs and narrow, long fingers with flexion of proximal interphalangeal joints (camptodactyly). Toes are also long and curve in, which is associated with occasional metatarsus adductus or talipes equinovarus deformities. The joint contractures improve spontaneously with time or respond to physiotherapy. Hypoplasia of the muscles, particularly those of the lower legs, is a frequent finding.

Most patients are taller than average and exhibit kyphoscoliosis. The scoliosis is usually progressive.[3,4] Intelligence is normal.

Cardiovascular findings include mitral valve prolapse, aortic root dilatation, congenital heart defects (ASD, VSD, or hypoplastic aorta).[1,3,8] Intraocular colobomata, microphthalmia, ectopia lentis, myopia, and keratoconus have also been reported.[2,3,8]

#### Otolaryngological manifestations

These include "crumpled" ears with ill-defined conchae, flattened anti-helix, prominent crura, micrognathia, a high-arched palate, and a relatively short neck.

#### Etiology

Beals syndrome is caused by a mutation of the fibrillin 2 *(FBN 2)* gene on the long arm of chromosome 5.[5,7] Inheritance is autosomal dominant with variable expressivity.[4,5,6,8]

#### Differential diagnosis

Beals syndrome should be differentiated from Marfan syndrome.[4,7]

#### References

1. Anderson RA, Koch S, Camerini-Otero RD: Cardiovascular findings in congenital contractural arachnodactyly: report of an affected kindred. Am J Med Genet 18:265–271, 1984.
2. Bass HN, Sparkes RS, Crandall BF, Marcy SM: Congenital contractural arachnodactyly, keratoconus and probable Marfan syndrome in the same pedigree. J Pediatr 98:591–593, 1981.
3. Bawle E, Quigg MH: Ectopia lentis and aortic root dilatation in congenital contractural arachnodactyly. Am J Med Genet 42:19–21, 1992.
4. Beals RK, Hecht F: Congenital contractural arachnodactyly. A heritable disorder of connective tissue. J Bone Joint Surg 53:987–993, 1971.
5. Putnam EA, Zhang H, Ramirez F, Milewicz DM: Fibrillin-2 *(FBN2)* mutations result in the Marfan-like disorder, congenital contractural arachnodactyly. Nat Genet 11:456–458, 1995.
6. Ramos Arroyo MA, Weaver DD, Beals RK: Congenital contractural arachnodactyly. Report of four additional families and review of literature. Clin Genet 27:570–581, 1985.
7. Tsipouras P, Del Mastro R, Sarfarazi M, Lee B, Vitale E, Child AH,

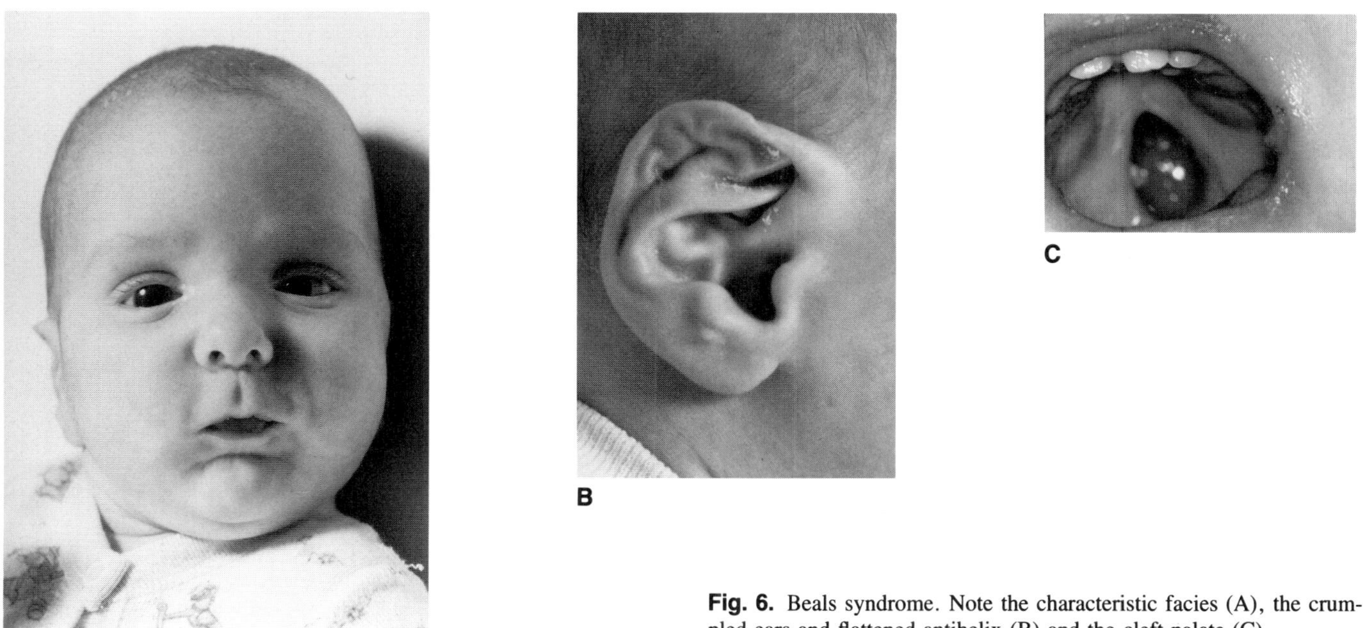

A B C

**Fig. 6.** Beals syndrome. Note the characteristic facies (A), the crumpled ears and flattened antihelix (B) and the cleft palate (C).

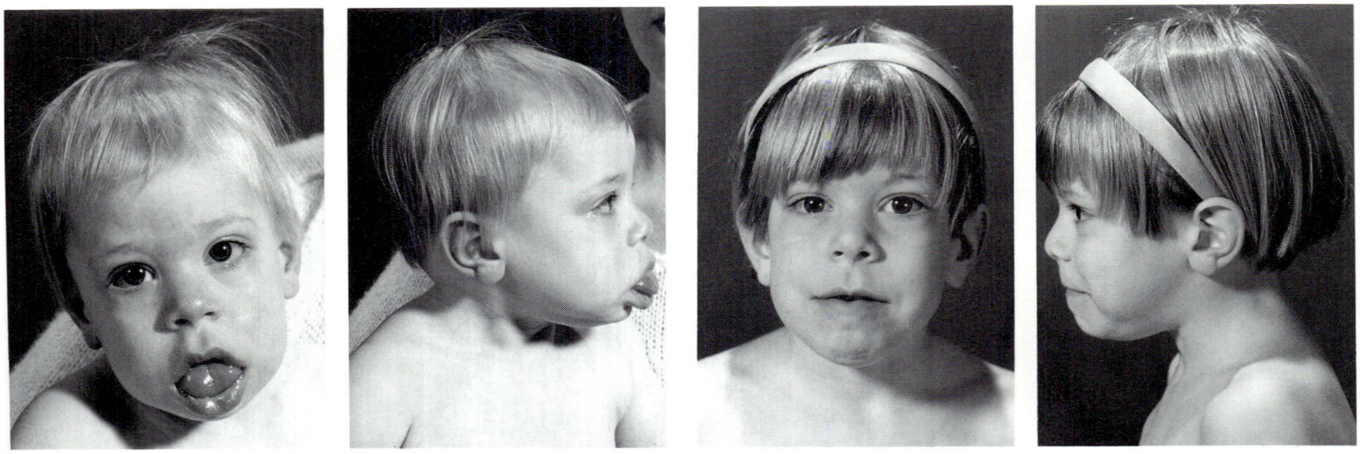

A B C D

**Fig. 7.** Beckwith-Wiedemann syndrome. A,B: note the macroglossia, prognathism, infraorbital hypoplasia, and linear crease of the ear lobule. C,D: The same patient, a few years later (after surgical correction of the macroglossia).

Godfrey M, Devereux RB, Hewett D, Steinmann, et al: Genetic linkage of the Marfan syndrome, ectopia lentis, and congenital contractural arachnodactyly to the fibrillin gene on chromosome 15 and 5. The International Marfan Syndrome Collaborative Study. N Engl J Med 326:905–909, 1992.

8. Viljoen D: Syndrome of the month: Congenital contractural arachnodactyly (Beals syndrome). J Med Genet 31:1640–1643, 1994.

## Beckwith-Wiedemann syndrome

(MIM No. *130650; POSSUM No. 3036)

### General manifestations

Macrosomia is a constant feature. Visceromegaly involving the kidneys, spleen, and liver is seen in the majority of cases. Neonatal hypoglycemia is common. The infant death rate of 20% is due to congestive heart failure or severe malformations.[2]

Advanced bone age is common and there may be widening of the metaphyses and cortical thickening of the long bones. The growth curve remains above the 90th percentile for the first 5 years of life. Intelligence is normal in most patients. Mild to moderate mental retardation is occasionally seen. Seizures, hydrocephaly, and subdural hematomas have been reported. Cardiovascular anomalies include ASD, PDA, VSD, Fallot's tetralogy and, occasionally, coarctation of the aorta and pulmonary stenosis.[1–4] Other manifestations include hemihyperplasia, omphalocele, polydactyly, diaphragmatic eventration, imperforate anus, bicornuate uterus, hypospadias, and cryptorchidism. Immunodeficiency and cardiomyopathy have been reported.

There is an increased possibility (7.5%) of developing neoplasms, especially embryonal tumors. Wilms tumor, adrenocortical carcinoma, and hepatoblastoma are among the most common neoplasms.

### Otolaryngological manifestations

Macroglossia is evident from birth on. Prognathism, infraorbital hypoplasia, and capillary nevus flammeus of the face become more obvious in the first year of life. The ears display indentations on the posterior rim of the helix and concha and unusual linear creases of the lobule. Cleft palate, submucous cleft, as well as preauricular pits and conductive hearing loss have been reported.[2,5,8,9]

### Etiology

Most cases are sporadic. Approximately 15% of cases have positive family history. Familial cases are inherited in an autosomal dominant manner with incomplete penetrance. Maternally imprinted genes at chromosome 11p15 have been implicated in familial and sporadic cases. A small number of patients have cytogenetic abnormalities at 11p15.[2] Paternally inherited duplications or isodisomies of 11p15 are associated with this condition. It is proposed that a double dose of the active paternal gene of insulin-like growth factor 2 (IGF2) is responsible for the pathogenesis. Normally, the maternal IGF2 is imprinted and not transcribed. However, in certain cases, there is disruption of IGF2 imprinting in Beckwith-Wiedemann syndrome and both maternally and paternally inherited genes are active.[6,7,10,12]

### Differential diagnosis

Beckwith-Wiedemann syndrome should be differentiated from infants of diabetic mothers, Perlman syndrome and Simpson-Golabi-Behmel syndrome.[11]

### References

1. Combs JT, Grunt JA, Brandt IK: New syndrome of neonatal hypoglycemia. N Engl J Med 275:236–243, 1966.
2. Elliott M, Maher ER: Beckwith-Wiedemann syndrome. J Med Genet 31:560–564, 1994.
3. Irving IM: Exomphalos with macroglossia: a study of 11 cases. J Pediatr Surg 2:499–507, 1967.
4. Kosseff AL, Herrmann J, Opitz JM: The Wiedemann-Beckwith syndrome: genetic considerations and a diagnostic sign. Lancet 1:844, 1972.
5. Niikawa N, Ishikiriyama S, Takahashi S, Inagawa A, Tonoki H, Ohta Y, Hase N, Kamei T, Kajii T: The Wiedemann-Beckwith syndrome: pedigree studies on five families with evidence for autosmal dominant inheritance with variable expressivity. Am J Med Genet 24:41–55, 1986.
6. Ohlsson R, Nyström A, Pfeifer-Ohlsson S, Töhönen V, Hedborg F, Schofield P, Flam F, Ekström TJ: *IGF2* is parentally imprinted during human embryogenesis and in the Beckwith-Wiedemann syndrome. Nat Genet 4:94–97, 1993.

7. Reik W, Brown KW, Schneid H, Le Bouc Y, Bickmore W, Maher ER: Imprinting mutations in the Beckwith-Wiedemann syndrome suggested by an altered imprinting pattern in the *IGF2-H19* domain. Hum Mol Genet 4:2379–2385, 1995.
8. Shafer AD: Primary macroglossia. Clin Pediatr 7:357–363, 1968.
9. Takato T, Kamei M, Kato K, Kitano I: Cleft palate in the Beckwith-Wiedemann syndrome. Ann Plast Surg 22:347–349, 1989.
10. Weksberg R, Shen DR, Fei YL, Song QL, Squire J: Disruption of insulin-like growth factor 2 imprinting in Beckwith-Wiedemann syndrome. Nat Genet 5:143–150, 1993.
11. Weksberg R, Squire JA, Templeton DM: Glypicans: A growing trend. Nat Genet 12:225–227, 1996.
12. Weksberg R, Teshima I, Williams BRG, Greenberg CR, Pueschel SM, Chernos JE, Fowlow SB, Hoyme E, Anderson IJ, Whiteman DAH, Fisher N, Squire J: Molecular characterization of cytogenetic alterations associated with the Beckwith-Wiedemann syndrome (BWS) phenotype refines the localization and suggests the gene for BWS is imprinted. Hum Mol Genet 2:549–556, 1993.

## Binder syndrome

(MIM No. 155050; POSSUM No. 3330)

Binder syndrome is also known as Maxillonasal dysplasia, Binder type, or Maxillonasal dysostosis, or congenitally flat nose syndrome.

This condition was first described by Binder in 1962.[1] It is regarded by some authors[11] as a nonspecific anomaly of the nasomaxillary complex.

### General manifestations

Various anomalies of the first two cervical vertebrae are described in 15 to 50% of cases. The association of megaesophagus, dysautonomia, and Binder syndrome led some authors to classify it as a neurocristopathy.[7] Ocular findings include juvenile glaucoma and goniodysgenesis.[2] Cardiac anomalies, mild mental retardation,[5,11] achalasia,[7] diaphragmatic hernia, and genital anomalies are considered uncommon manifestations.[11]

### Otolaryngological manifestations

The nose is flat and hypoplastic, the nasofrontal angle is absent, the nasolabial angle is acute, the nasal septum is atrophied, and the columella is shortened. The sense of smell is preserved, despite atrophy of the nasal mucosa. X-ray findings include absence of the anterior nasal spine, retrognathia of the maxilla, and increased gonial angle.[9] Class III malocclusion develops due to the short maxilla and relative prognathism of the mandible. The frontal sinuses are poorly pneumatized.[1,3] The upper lip contour is convex and the philtrum is poorly developed. Labiomaxillary clefts are occasionally seen.[5,8] Hearing loss has been documented in 5% of patients.[4,6]

### Etiology

Most cases are sporadic. A hereditary basis has been suggested.[5,10]

### Differential diagnosis

Binder syndrome should be differentiated from Stickler syndrome and pseudohypoparathyroidism.

#### References

1. Binder KH: Dysostosis maxillo-nasalis ein arhinencephaler Missbildungkomplex. Dtsch Zahnarzt Z 17:438–444, 1962.
2. Bron A, Bertrand AM, Chabod C, Royer J: Syndrome de Binder et goniodysgénésies. A propos d'un cas. Ophtalmologie 4:242–245, 1990.
3. Delaire J, Tessier P, Tulasne JF, Resche F: Clinical and radiologic aspects of maxillonasal dysostosis (Binder's syndrome). Head Neck Surg 3:105–22, 1980.
4. Ferguson JW, Thompson RPJ: Maxillonasal dysostosis (Binder syndrome). A review of the literature and case reports. Eur J Orthodont 7:145–148, 1985.
5. Holmstrom H: Clinical and pathologic features of maxillonasal dysplasia (Binder's syndrome). Significance of the prenasal fossa on etiology. Plast Reconstr Surg 78:559–567, 1986.
6. Horswell BB, Holmes AD, Barnett JS, Levant BA: Maxillonasal dysplasia (Binder's syndrome). A critical review and case study. J Oral Maxillofac Surg 45:114–122, 1987.
7. Narcy C, Foucaud P, Cargill G, Sablier G, LeGuillou C, Contencin P, Navarro J: Association méga-oesophage, syndrome de Binder et dysautonomie: une nouvelle neurocristopathie? Arch Fr Pediatr 44:119–121, 1987.
8. Olow-Nordenram MAK, Radberg CT: Maxillo-nasal dysplasia (Binder syndrome) and associated malformations of the cervical spine. Acta Radiol 25:353–360, 1984.
9. Olow-Nordenram MAK, Thilander B: The craniofacial morphology in persons with maxillonasal dysplasia (Binder syndrome). Am J Orthodont 95:148–158, 1989.
10. Olow-Nordenram MAK, Valentin J: An etiologic study of maxillo-

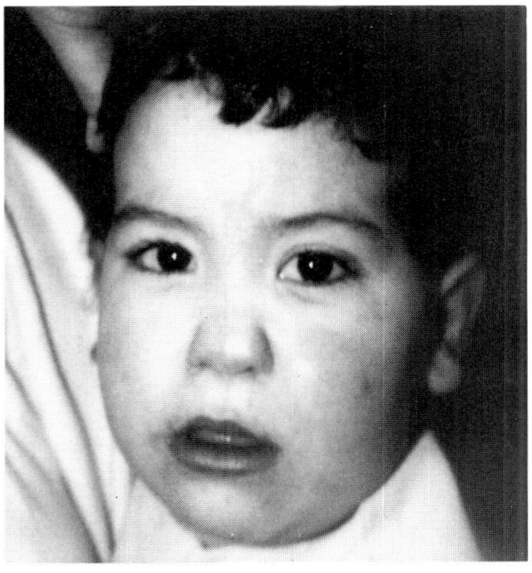

A

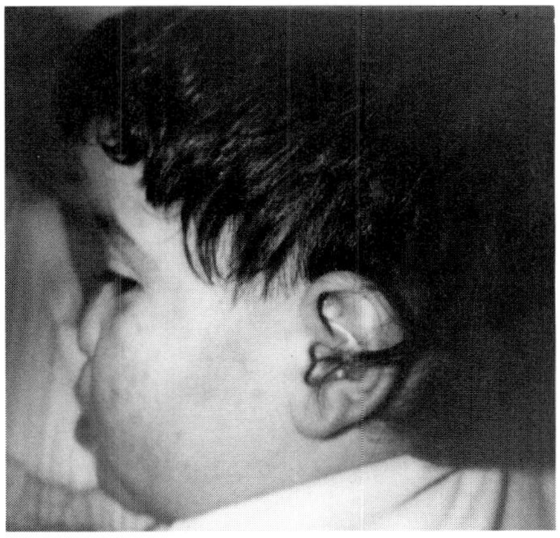

B

**Fig. 8.** Binder syndrome. A,B: Note the flat nose and absent nasofrontal angle.

nasal dysplasia—Binder's syndrome. Scand J Dent Res 96:74, 1988.
11. Toriello HV: Is Binder syndrome really a syndrome? Presented at David W. Smith Workshop on Malformations and Morphogenesis, Greenwood, South Carolina August 15–19, 1989.

## Branchio-oto-renal syndrome (BOR syndrome)

### Melnick-Fraser syndrome
(MIM No. *113650; POSSUM No. 3133)

The association of auricular malformations, branchial fistulae, deafness, and renal anomalities was first described in 1975.[13] Later, Fraser et al. further delineated the syndrome.[8] The prevalence is estimated to be 1:40,000 in the general population.

#### General manifestations

Renal dysplasia is reported in over two-thirds of patients and varies from tapered superior poles (duplication of the collecting system) to marked agenesis of the kidney.[1,7] This syndrome may include Potter sequence.[18]

#### Otolaryngological manifestations

The preauricular pits are blind, pin head–sized depressions in the superior part of the pinna of the ear. They are seen in 75 to 85% of patients. Other external ear malformations (40%–60%) may include preauricular tags, lop or bat ears, and microtia. The external auditory canals may be atretic.[4,8]

Anomalies of the middle ear include anomalies of the ossicles, facial nerve, and fallopian canals. Computerized tomography of the temporal bones may demonstrate a hypoplastic cochlea and absent or hypoplastic semicircular canals. Mondini dysplasia has also been reported. Hearing loss (75%–90%) is usually stable and may be conductive, sensorineural, or mixed.[2,4,9,16]

It is estimated that 2% of profoundly deaf children have BOR syndrome.

The branchial fistulae (63%) are usually bilateral in the lower part of the neck and the external openings are on the medial border of the sternomastoid muscle.[5,8] Other associated manifestations include aplasia or stenosis of the lacrimal ducts (8%–9%), a high-arched or cleft palate, deep overbite,[3] and facial nerve anomalies. Hemifacial microsomia is considered to be a severe form by some authors.[10,17]

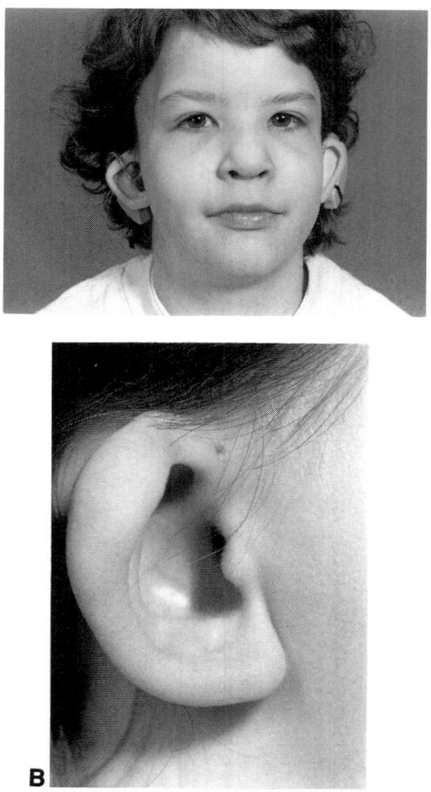

**Fig. 9.** Branchio-oto-renal syndrome. Note the prominent lop ears, hearing aids (A) and preauricular pit (B).

#### Etiology and pathogenesis

Inheritance is autosomal dominant with high penetrance and variable expression.

Pathogenesis is presumed to be due to a deficiency in differentiation of the first and second branchial arches. The anomalies of the renal system are the result of abnormal interaction between the ureteric bud and the metanephric blastema. It is interesting to note that the inner ear (stria vascularis) and the renal glomeruli share a common antigen, and more than one group have described histopathologic changes on temporal bone examinations.[6,14,18]

The gene for this condition is mapped to chromosome 8q12.2–q21.2.[12,15,20]

#### Differential diagnosis

BOR syndrome should be differentiated from other ear and renal anomalies, e.g., autosomal dominant dysmorphic pinna–polycystic kidney syndrome,[11] cat eye syndrome,[19] and ear-pits deafness syndrome (MIM No.125100).

Renal investigations should be considered in any deaf child with preauricular pit or branchial cleft fistula or cyst.

#### References

1. Carmi R, Binshtock M, Abeliovich D, Bar-Ziv J: The branchio-oto-renal (BOR) syndrome. Report of bilateral renal agenesis in three sibs. Am J Med Genet 14:625–627, 1983.
2. Chitayat D, Hodgkinson KA, Chen MF, Haber GD, Nikishima S, Sanda I: Branchio-oto-renal syndrome: further delineation of an under-diagnosed syndrome. Am J Med Genet 43:970–975, 1992.
3. Côté A, O Regan S: The branchio-oto-renal syndrome. Am J Nephrol 2:144–146 1982.
4. Cremers CWRJ, Fikkers-von Noord M: The ear pits-deafness syndrome. Clinical and genetic aspects. Int J Pediatr Otorhinolaryngol 2:309–322 1980.
5. Cremers CW, Thijssen HO, Fischer AJ, Marres EH: Otological aspects of the ear pit-deafness syndrome. ORL J Otorhinolaryngol Relat Spec 43:223–239, 1981.
6. Fitch N, Lindsay JR, Srolovitz H: The temporal bone in the preauricular pit, cervical fistula, hearing loss syndrome. Ann Otol Rhinol Laryngol 85:268–275, 1976.
7. Fraser FC: Autosomal dominant duplication of the renal collecting system, hearing loss, and external ear anomalies: a new syndrome? Am J Med Genet 14:473–478, 1983.
8. Fraser FC, Link D, Clogg D, Nogrady B: Genetic aspects of the BOR syndrome-branchial fistulas, ear pits, hearing loss and renal anomalies. Am J Med Genet 2:241–252, 1978.
9. Gimsing S, Dyrmose J: Branchio-oto-renal dysplasia in three families. Ann Otol Rhinol Laryngol 95:421–426, 1986.
10. Heimler A Lieber E: Branchio-oto-renal syndrome: reduced penetrance and variable expressivitiy in four generations of a large kindred. Am J Med Genet 25:15–27, 1986.

11. Hilson D: Malformation of ear as sign of malformation of genito-urinary tract. Br Med J 2:785–9, 1957.
12. Kumar S, Kimberling WJ, Connolly CJ, Tinley S, Marres HA, Cremers CW: Refining the region of branchio-oto-renal syndrome and defining the flanking markers on chromosome 8q by genetic mapping. Am J Hum Genet 55:1188–1194, 1994.
13. Melnick M, Bixler D, Silk K, Yune H, Nance WE: Autosomal dominant branchio-oto-renal dysplasia. Birth Defects 11:121–128, 1975.
14. Melnick M, Hodes ME, Nance WE, Yune H, Sweeney A: Branchio-oto-renal dysplasia and bronchio-oto-dysplasia: two distinct autosomal dominant disorders. Clin Genet 13:425–442, 1978.
15. Ni L, Wagner MJ, Kimberling WJ, Pembrey ME, Grundfast KM, Kumar S, Daiger SP, Wells De, Johnson K, Smith RJ: Refined localization of the branchiootorenal syndrome gene by linkage and haplotype analysis. Am J Med Genet 51:176–184, 1994.
16. Ostri B, Johnsen T, Bergmann I: Temporal bone findings in a family with branchio-oto-renal syndrome (BOR). Clin Otolaryngol 16:163–167, 1991.
17. Rollnick BR, Kaye CI: Hemifacial microsomia and the branchio-oto-renal syndrome. J Craniofac Genet Develop Biol. 1 (Suppl):287–295, 1985.
18. Saito R: Anomalies of the auditory organ in Potter's syndrome. Histopathological findings in the temporal bone. Arch Otolaryngol 1208:484–488, 1982.
19. Schinzel A, Schmid W, Fraccaro M, Tiepolo L, Zuffardi O, Opitz JM, Lindsten J, Zetterqvist P, Snell H, Baccichetti C, Tenconi R, Pagon RA: The "Cat eye syndrome": dicentric small marker chromosome probably derived from a No. 22 (tetrasomy 22pter-q11) associated with a characteristic phenotype. Hum Genet 57:148–158, 1981.
20. Vincent C, Kalatzis V, Compain S, Levilliers J, Slim R, Graia F, Pereira ML, Nivelon A, Croquette MF, Lacombe D, et al: A proposed new contiguous gene syndrome on 8q consists of Branchio-Oto-Renal (BOR) syndrome, Duane syndrome, a dominant form of hydrocephalus and trapeze aplasia; implications for the mapping of the BOR gene. Hum Mol Genet 3:1859–1866, 1994.

## Campomelic syndrome

### Campomelic or camptomelic dysplasia
(MIM No. *211970; POSSUM No. 3049)

Spranger et al[15] and later Maroteaux et al[11] are credited for recognizing this syndrome in 1970 and 1971, respectively.

#### General manifestations

The lower limb bones are bowed anteriorly, and the arm bones may demonstrate the same abnormalities.[12] The pretibial skin dimples associated with bowing of the legs and thighs are characteristic. The scapulae are hypoplastic, the sterum is demineralized, and there is generalized kyphoscoliosis. Talipes equinovarus is a common manifestation. Dislocated hips and increased acetabular angle are frequent. Cardiovascular abnormalities, renal malformations, ambiguous genitalia, and ano-

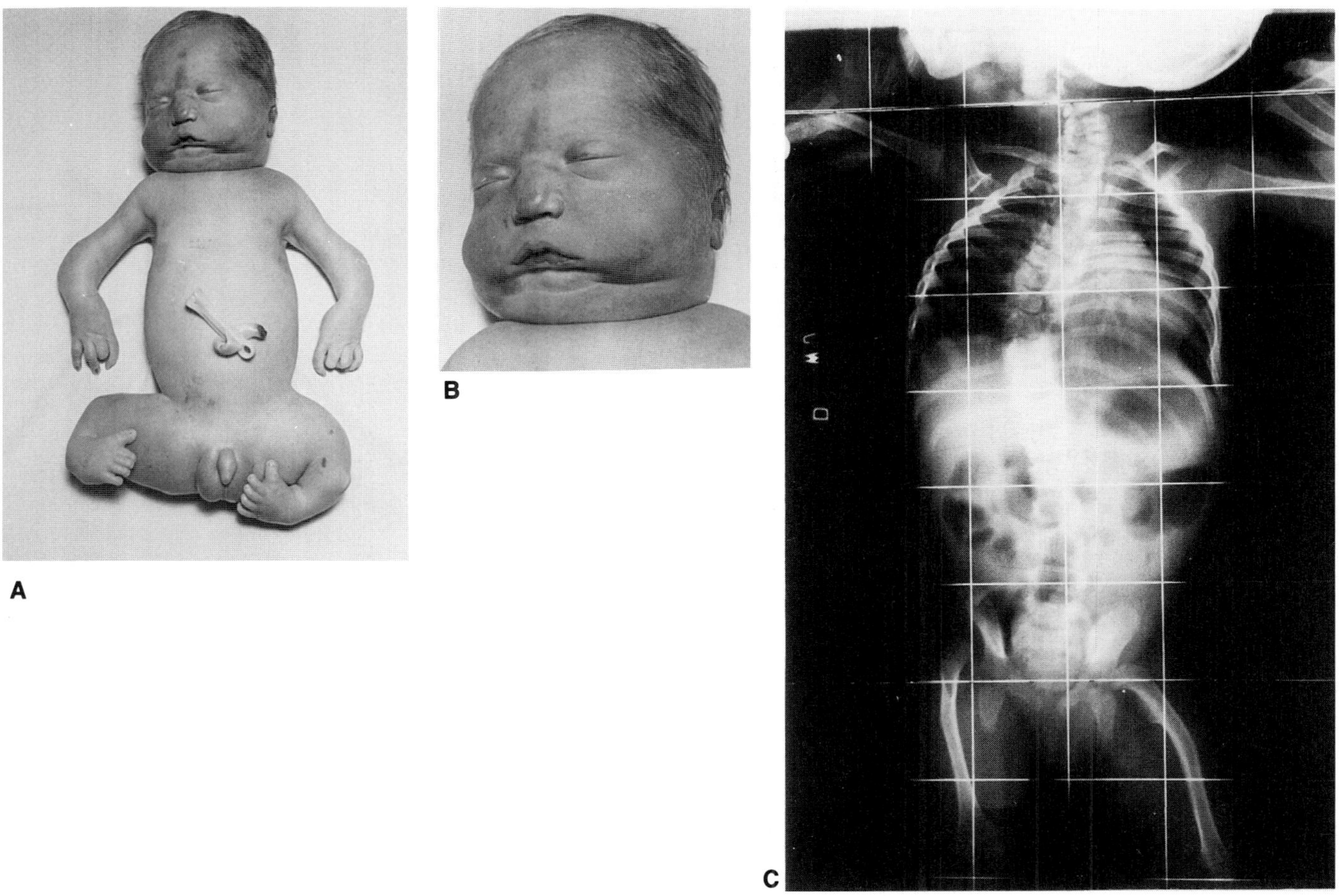

**Fig. 10.** Campomelic syndrome. Note the micrognathia and bent lower extremities (A), the short palpebral fissures, flat nasal bridge, and short neck with redundant skin (B). C: Radiogram demonstrating severe scoliosis and dislocated right hip. (A,B from RJ Gorlin et al., *Syndromes of the Head and Neck,* Oxford University Press, New York, 1990, p. 183, courtesy of Dr. RE Stevenson. C from Y. Gillerot et al., Am J Med Genet 34:589, 1989, with permission.)

rectal atresia[13] have been described. Sex reversal was observed in about half of females with 46,XY karyotypes. These sex-reversed females are H-Y antigen negative.[5,6,12]

This syndrome is characterized by early death in the neonatal period from respiratory failure and failure to thrive. Very few patients survive beyond the first year.[7] Craniofacial anomalies include hydrocephalus, and gross cellular disorganization of the cortex, caudate nucleus, and thalamus. Acampomelic campomelic dysplasia[3,9] has also been reported. Prenatal diagnosis by ultrasonography is described.[2]

### Otolaryngological manifestations

The face is small, the fontanelles are large, and the nose is usually small with a flat nasal bridge and anteverted nostrils. Cleft palate is present in most cases.[1] The ears are usually low set. Takahashi et al.[16] have described specific temporal bone changes. These include deformities of the vestibule and the semicircular canals, abnormal cartilagenous and osseous tissues, hypoplastic cochlea, aberrant course of the facial nerve, and hypoplasia of the middle ear ossicles. The vertebrae of the neck are usually flat and short. Tracheobronchomalacia has been described.[14]

### Etiology

Campomelic dysplasia is an autosoml recessive disorder. The observed female:male ratio is 3:1. The site of campomelic dysplasia locus (17q) was demonstrated by Young et al.[18] and Maraia et al.[10]

It has been established that autosomal sex reversal and campomelic dysplasia are caused by mutations in and around the SRY-related gene *SOX9*.[4,17]

### Differential diagnosis

Campomelic syndrome should be differentiated from syndromes with congenital bowing of long bones[8] and kyphomelic dysplasia.

### References


1. Beluffi G, Fraccaro M: Congenital and clinical aspects of campomelic dysplasia. Prog Clin Biol Res 104:53–65, 1982.
2. Cordone M, Lituania M, Zampatti C, Passamonti U, Magnano GM, Toma P: In utero ultrasonographic features of campomelic dysplasia. Prenat Diagn 9:745–750, 1989.
3. Decsi T, Botykai A: Campomelic dysplasia without campomelia. Päediatr und Padol 27:29–30, 1992.
4. Foster JW, Dominguez-Steglich MA, Guioli S, Kowk G, Weller PA, Stevanovic M, Weissenbach J, Mansour S, Young ID, Goodfellow PN, et al: Campomelic dysplasia and autosomal sex reversal caused by mutations in an SRY-related gene. Nature 372:525–530, 1994.
5. Gorlin RJ, Cohen MM, Levin LS: Syndromes of the Head and Neck, 3rd ed. Oxford University Press, New York, 1990, pp 181–184.
6. Hall D, Spranger JW: Congenital bowing of the long bones. A review and phenotype analysis of 13 diagnosed cases. Eur J Pediatr 133:131–138, 1980.
7. Houston CS, Opitz JM, Spranger JW, MacPherson RI, Reed M, Gilbert H, Herrmann J, Schinzel A: The campomelic syndrome. A review, report of 17 cases and follow up on the currently 17 year old boy first reported by Maroteaux et al. in 1971. Am J Med Genet 15:3–28, 1983.
8. Kozlowski K, Butler HO, Galatius-Jensen F, Tullock A: Syndromes of congenital bowing of the long bones. Pediatr Radiol 7:40–48, 1978.
9. MacPherson RI, Skinner SA, Donnenfeld AE: Acampomelic campomelic dysplasia. Pediatr Radiol 20:90–93, 1989.
10. Maraia R, Saal HM, Wangson D: A chromosome 17q de novo paracentric inversion in a patient with campomelic dysplasia; case report and etiologic hypothesis. Clin Genet 39:401–408, 1991.
11. Maroteaux P, Spranger JW, Opitz JM, Kucera J, Lowry RB, Schimke RN, Kagan SM. Le syndrome campomélique. Presse Med 22:1157–1162, 1971.
12. Pazzaglia UE, Beluffi G: Radiology and histopathology of the bent limbs in campomelic dysplasia. Implications in the aetiology of the disease and review of theories. Pediatr Radiol 17:50–55, 1987.
13. Rebage Moises V, Arnal Alonso JM, Perez Gascon M, Baldellow Vasquez A, Anton Jimenez R, Used Aznar MM, Romo Montejo A, Marco Tello A: Campomelic dysplasia associated with anorectal atresia. An Esp Pediatr 31:483–485, 1989.
14. Shinwell ES, Hengerer AS, Kendig JW: A third case of bronchoscopic diagnosis of tracheobronchomalacia in campomelic dysplasia. Pediatr Pulmonol 4:192, 1988.
15. Spranger J, Langer L, Maroteaux P: Increasing frequency of a syndrome of multiple osseous defects. Lancet 21:716, 1970.
16. Takahashi H, Sando I, Masutani H: Temporal bone histopathological findings in campomelic dysplasia. J Laryngol Otol 106:361–365, 1992.
17. Wagner T, Wirth J, Meyer J, Zabel B, Held M, Zimmer J, Pasantes J, Bricarelli FD, Keutel J, Hustert E, et al: Autosomal sex reversal and campomelic dysplasia are caused by mutations in and around the SRY-related gene SOX9. Cell 79:1111–1120, 1994.
18. Young ID, Zuccolo JM, Maltby EL, Broderick NJ: Campomelic dysplasia associated with a de novo 2q;17q reciprocal translocation. J Med Genet 29: 251–252, 1992.


## CHARGE association

### (MIM No. 214800; POSSUM No. 3480)

The acronym *CHARGE association* was coined by Pagon et al[13] in 1981. Components are **C**oloboma of the eye, **H**eart disease, **A**tresia of the choanae, **R**etarded development and growth, **G**enital anomalies, and **E**ar anomalies and/or deafness.[13]

### General manifestations

Choanal atresia is associated with over 65% of cases. It is bilateral in over two-thirds of patients.[2] In unilateral cases, it is more common on the left side.

Colobomatous malformations are seen in 80% of cases. They range from iris coloboma with intact vision to anophthalmia and retinal colobomas. Microphthalmia and nystagmus may also occur.

Cardiac anomalies may include tetrology of Fallot, PDA, VSD, ASD, coarctation of the aorta, or right-sided aortic arch.

Mental deficiency is reported in the majority of cases ranging from mild to severe. Central nervous system malformations have also been described, such as arhinencephaly and/or holoprosencephaly.[4,5,10]

Minor kidney anomalies, cryptorchidism, microphallus, congenital hypothyroidism,[11] imperforate anus, and pectus carinatum have also been reported.[9,14]

### Otolaryngological manifestations

Anomalies of the external ear include a low-set ear and posteriorly angulated, asymmetric, or cup-shaped pinnae. Anomalies of the inner ear, termed by Guyot et al. as "charge dysplasia of the temporal bone," include Mondini dysplasia of the pars inferior and complete absence of the pars superior.[1,6,7] Hearing loss is conductive or sensorineural and often asymmetrical.[3,8]

Other anomalies include Robin or DiGeorge sequence, facial asymmetry, micrognathia, feeding difficulties, tracheoesopha-

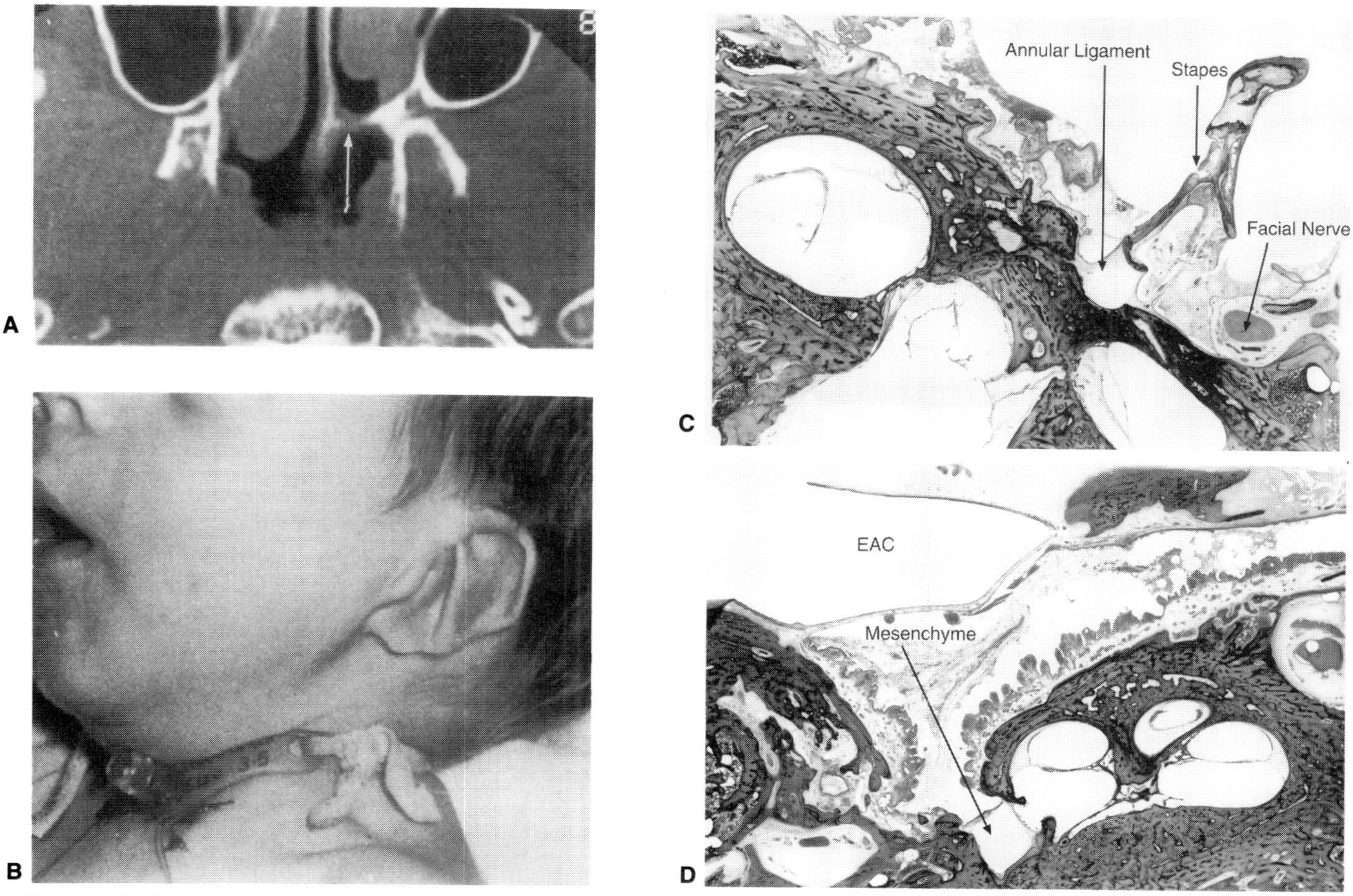


**Fig. 11.** CHARGE association. A: CT scan demonstrating choanal atresia. B: Note the low-set ear and tracheotomy. C,D: Temporal bone of a 7½-month-old-female showing severe dysplasia of the stapes, absent oval window, and mesenchyme obliterating round window niche. External auditory canal, tympanic membrane, malleus, and incus are all normal. (A,B from D Morgan et al., Arch Otolaryngol Head Neck Surg 119:49, 1993; C,D from HF Schuknecht, *Pathology of the Ear,* 2nd ed., Lea & Febiger, Philadelphia, 1993, p. 142, with permission.)

geal fistula, esophageal atresia,[9] cleft lip/palate, and upper airway abnormalities.

### Etiology and pathogenesis

In most cases the syndrome is sporadic. Autosomal dominant or recessive mutations have been suggested as the cause of this syndrome. Translocations involving chromosome 6 and 8 have been reported.[15] Other chromosomal abnormalities have also been suggested.[16] The CHARGE association is most probably due to abnormality in the migration and/or development of the cephalic neural crest cells.[16,17] A locus or loci for a gene or genes causing some of the anomalies of CHARGE association may reside in the region of 14q22–q24.3.[12]

### Differential diagnosis

CHARGE association should be considered in all cases with ocular colobomas, mental retardation, vertebral anomalies, and cleft palate/lip.

### References

1. Asher BF, McGill TJ, Kaplan L, Friedman EM, Healy GB: Airway complications in CHARGE association. Arch Otolaryngol Head Neck Surg 116:594–595, 1990.
2. Bergström L, Owens O: Posterior choanal atresia: a syndromal disorder. Laryngoscope 94:1273–1276, 1984.
3. Brown DP, Israel SM: Audiologic findings in a set of fraternal twins with CHARGE association. J Am Acad Audiol 2:183–188, 1991.
4. Chittmittrapap S, Spitz L, Kiely EM, Brereton RJ: Oesophageal atresia and associated anomalies. Arch Dis Child 64:364–368, 1989.
5. Clementi M, Tenconi R, Turolla L, Silvan C, Bortotto L, Artifoni L: Apparent CHARGE association and chromosome anomaly, chance or contiguous gene syndrome. Am J Med Genet 41:246–250, 1991.
6. Guyot JP, Gacek RR, DiRaddo P: The temporal bone anomaly in CHARGE association. Arch Otolaryngol Head Neck Surg 113:321–324, 1987.
7. Harvey AS, Leaper PM, Bankier A: CHARGE association: clinical manifestations and developmental outcome. Am J Med Genet 39:48–55, 1991.
8. Hurst JA, Meinecke P, Baraitser M: Balanced t(6;8) (6p8p;6q8q) and the CHARGE association. J Med Genet 28:54–55, 1991.
9. Kutiyanawala M, Wyse RK, Brereton RJ, Spitz L, Kiely EM, Drake D, Blake K: CHARGE and esophageal atresia. J Pediatr Surg 27:558–560, 1992.
10. Lin AE, Siebert JR, Graham JM Jr: Central nervous system malformations in the CHARGE association. Am J Med Genet 37:304–310, 1990.
11. Marin JF, Garcia B, Quintana A, Barrio R, Sordo MT, Lozano C: The CHARGE association and athyreosis. J Med Genet 28:207–208, 1991.
12. North KN, Wu BL, Cao BN, Whiteman DA, Korf BR: CHARGE association in a child with de novo inverted duplication (14)(q22→q24.3). Am J Med Genet 57:610–614, 1995.
13. Pagon RA, Graham JM Jr, Zonana J, Yong SI: Coloboma, congenital heart disease, and choanal atresia with multiple anomalies. CHARGE association. J Pediatr 99:223–227, 1981.

14. Paparella MM: Mondini's deafness—review of the histopathology. Ann Otol Rhinol Laryngol 89 (Suppl):1–10, 1980.
15. Russel-Eggitt M, Blake KD, Taylor DC, Wyse RK: The eye in the CHARGE association. Br J Ophthalmol 74:421–426, 1990.
16. Siebert JR, Graham JM Jr, MacDonald C: Pathologic features of the CHARGE association: support for involvement of the neural crest. Teratology 31:331–336, 1985.
17. Stack CG, Wyse RK: Incidence and management of airway problems in the CHARGE associaton. Anaesthesia 46:582–585 1991.

## Cockayne syndrome

(MIM No. *216400, 216411, *133540; POSSUM No. 3149)

This syndrome was reported by Cockayne in 1936 as proportionate dwarfism with retinal atrophy and deafness.[1] It is characterized by senile-like changes beginning in infancy, retinal degeneration, impaired hearing, and photosensitivity of the skin.[6]

### General manifestations

In Cockayne syndrome (CS), growth retardation is evident in the second year of life. There is usually kyphosis of the dorsal region and biconvex flattening of the vertebrae. The limbs display joint limitations and sometimes cyanosis. The hands are disproportionately large.[10] Radiographically, the skull base is often thickened. Photosensitive dermatitis is manifested on the face and sun-exposed areas.[14]

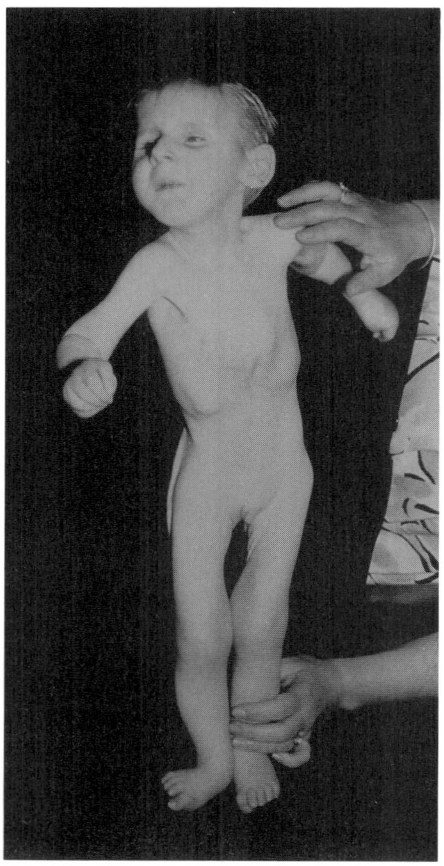

**Fig. 12.** Cockayne syndrome. Early onset of Cockayne syndrome. Note the lack of subcutaneous fat, the prominent facial bones, and sunken eyes. (With permission from MA Patton et al., J Med Genet 26:154, 1989.)

Ocular findings are enophthalmos, retinal pigmentary degeneration (salt-and-pepper type), optic atrophy, cataracts, corneal opacities, photophobia, and nystagmus. Moderate to severe mental deficiency becomes evident after the first year. Other neurological findings include microcephaly, choreoathetosis, peripheral neuropathy, progressive cerebellar ataxia, and intracranial calcifications.[10,11]

Prenatal diagnosis of Cockayne syndrome has also been reported by Lehmann et al.[7]

The name *CAMFAK syndrome* or *Cockayne syndrome type II* has been proposed for the condition that manifests with pre- or perinatal onset instead of at the age of 2 years.[8,13] Cockayne syndrome type III with high intelligence has also been described.[2]

### Otolaryngological manifestations

The lack of subcutaneous fat, prominence of the facial bones, slender nose, and sunken eyes give these patients a senile-looking or bird-like facies. Sensorineural deafness and large ears are additional manifestations.

### Etiology

Cockayne syndrome is due to autosomal recessive inheritance. Interstitial 10q21.1 deletion was reported in a patient with clinical and neurologic manifestations consistent with late-onset Cockayne syndrome.[3]

CS is one of the syndromes associated with DNA repair defects.[5,9,14] Following ultraviolet (UV) irradiation, cultured CS cells are unable to restore RNA synthesis rates to normal levels. This has been attributed to a specific deficiency in the ability to repair damage in actively transcribed regions of DNA. This failure of RNA synthesis to recover following UV irradiation has been used in a complementation test. Restoration of normal RNA synthesis rates in UV-irradiated heterokaryons was to indicate donors of different complementation groups. With this method, two complementation groups (CS-A and CS-B) have been found, with no obvious racial, clinical, or cellular distinctions.[12] The CSA and CSB genes have been cloned.[4]

### Differential diagnosis

Cockayne syndrome should be differentiated from other photosensitivity syndromes (Bloom syndrome, xeroderma pigmentosum, erythropoietic porphyria).

### References

1. Cockayne EA: Dwarfism with retinal atrophy and deafness. Arch Dis Child 11:1–8, 1936.
2. Czeizel AE, Marchalko M: Cockayne syndrome type III with high intelligence. Clin Genet 48:331–333, 1995.
3. Fryns JP, Bulcke J, Verdu P, Carton H, Kleczkowska A, Van den Berghe H: Apparent late-onset Cockayne syndrome and interstitial deletion of the long arm of chromosome 10 del(10)(q11.23q21.2). Am J Med Genet 40:343–344, 1991.
4. Henning KA, Li L, Iyer N, McDaniel LD, Reagan MS, Legerski R, Schultz RA, Stefanini M, Lehmann AR, Mayne LV, et al: The Cockayne syndrome group A gene encodes a WD repeat protein that interacts with CSB protein and a subunit of RNA polymerase II TFIIH. Cell 82:555–564, 1995.
5. Itoh T, Cleaver JE, Yamaizumi M: Cockayne syndrome complementation group B associated with xeroderma pigmentosum phenotype. Hum Genet 97:176–179, 1996.

6. Jones KL: Smith's Recognizable Patterns of Human Malformation, 5th ed. WB Saunders, Philadelphia, 1996, pp 144–145.
7. Lehmann AR, Francis AJ, Giannelli F: Prenatal diagnosis of Cockayne's syndrome. Lancet 1:486–488, 1985.
8. Lowry RB: Early onset of Cockayne syndrome. Am J Med Genet 13:209–210, 1982.
9. Rainbow RB, Howes MA: A deficiency in the repair of UV and gamma-ray damaged DNA in fibroblasts from Cockayne's syndrome. Mutat Res 93:235–247, 1982.
10. Scott-Emuakpor AB: A syndrome of microcephaly and cataract in four siblings: a new genetic syndrome. Am J Dis Child 131:67–69, 1977.
11. Smits MG, Gabreels FJ, Froeling PG, de Abreu RA, Thijssen HD, Renier WO: Calcium-phosphate metabolism in autosomal recessive idiopathic strio-pallido-dentate calcinosis and Cockayne's syndrome. Clin Neurol Neurosurg 85:145–153, 1983.
12. Stefanini M, Fawcett H, Botta E, Nardo T, Lehmann AR: Genetic analysis of twenty-two patients with Cockayne syndrome. Hum Genet 97:418–423, 1996.
13. Talwer D, Smith SA: CAMFAK syndrome: a demyelinating inherited disease similar to Cockayne syndrome. Am J Med Genet 34:194–198, 1989.
14. Windmiller J, Whalley PJ, Fink CW: Cockayne syndrome with chromosomal analysis. Am J Dis Child 105:204–208, 1963.

## Coffin-Lowry syndrome

(MIM No. *303600; POSSUM No. 3150)

### General manifestations

All males and approximately two-thirds of females with this syndrome show mental retardation. IQ varies between 5 and 60. Mild to moderate growth deficiency occurs after birth. The hands are soft and the fingers are wide proximally and tapered distally. The nails are short and broad, the finger joints are hyperextensible. The sternum is short and bifid. Pectus carinatum or excavatum is common. Thoracolumbar kyphoscoliosis and anterior superior marginal vertebral defects are often seen. Distal muscle atrophy and hypotonia are not uncommon. Microcephaly, thick calvarium, dilated lateral ventricles, inguinal herniae, and rectal prolapse are occasional findings.[3,4,7]

### Otolaryngological manifestations

The forehead is square with prominent eyebrows. Hypertelorism and downward slanting palpebral fissures are observed. The nose is short and bulbous with a thick septum and flared alae. The midface is mildly hypoplastic. The lips are thick and full and the philtrum is elongated. The tongue may have a midline furrow. The ears are prominent. Sensorineural hearing loss is documented. Coarseness of the facies increases with age. Hypodontia, malocclusion, and premature tooth loss is common.[2] Speech is severely retarded. The paranasal sinues and mastoids may be hypoplastic.

### Etiology and pathogenesis

Coffin-Lowry syndrome is of X-linked semidominant inheritance, with many sporadic cases. Possible pathogenesis may be related to an underlying lysosomal storage disease and alteration in glycosaminoglycan metabolism.[5,8] The gene is at Xp22.1–p22.2.[1,5,6]

### Differential diagnosis

The coarse facies resemble the mucopolysaccharidoses.

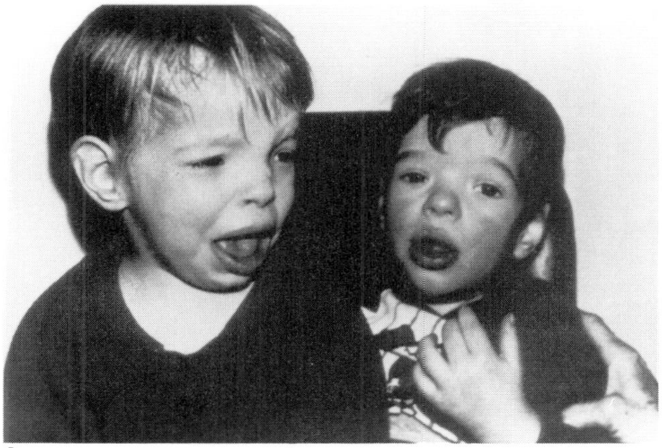

A

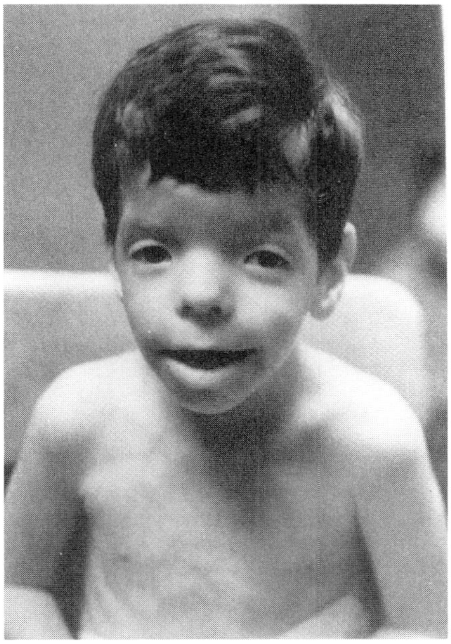

B

**Fig. 13.** Coffin-Lowry syndrome. Note the hypertelorism and midfacial hypoplasia (A), and the elongated philtrum, downward slanting palpebral fissures, and short nose (B). (From JK Hartsfield, Jr, et al., Am J Med Genet 45:552, 1993, with permission.)

### References

1. Biancalana V, Trivier E, Weber C, Weissenbach J, Rowe PS, O'Riordan JL, Partington MW, Heyberger S, Oudet C, Hanauer A: Construction of a high-resolution linkage map for Xp22.1–p22.2 and refinement of the genetic localization of the Coffin-Lowry syndrome gene. Genomics 22:617–625, 1994.
2. Hartsfield JK Jr, Hall BD, Grix AW, Kousseff BG, Salazar JF, Haufe SM: Pleiotropy in Coffin-Lowry syndrome: sensorineural hearing deficit and premature tooth loss as early manifestations. Am J Med Genet 34:552–557, 1993.
3. Haspeshagh M, Fryns JP, Beusen L, Van Dessel F, Vinken L, Moens E, Van den Berghe H: The Coffin-Lowry syndrome. Eur J Pediatr 143:82–86, 1984.
4. Hunter AG, Partington MW, Evans JA: The Coffin-Lowry syndrome: experience from four centres. Clin Genet 21:321–335, 1982.
5. Miyazaki K, Yamanaka T, Ishida Y, Oohira A: Calcified ligamenta flava in a patient with Coffin-Lowry syndrome: biochemical analysis of glycosaminoglycans. Jpn J Hum Genet 35:215–221, 1990.
6. Partington MW, Mulley JC, Sutherland GR, Thode A, Turner G: A family with the Coffin-Lowry syndrome revisited: localization of CLS to Xp21–pter. Am J Med Genet 30:509–521, 1988.
7. Temtamy SA, Miller JD, Hussels-Maumenee I: The Coffin-Lowry syndrome: an inherited faciodigital mental retardation syndrome. J Pediatr 86:724–731, 1975.

8. Vine DT, Gold JT, Grand AD: Etiology of the weakness in Coffin-Lowry syndrome. Am J Hum Genet 39:A85, 1986.

## Coffin-Siris syndrome

(MIM No. *135900; POSSUM No. 3151)

### General manifestations

Mental retardation is seen in all patients. The fifth finger and toe nails are hypoplastic or absent. Other digits may be hypoplastic. Hypotonia and lumbosacral hirsutism are seen in all patients. The bone age is retarded in 80% of patients.

The joints are lax, and radial dislocation at the elbow is common. Coxa vara and small patellae are frequent occurrences. Occasional abnormalities include ptosis, hypertelorism, patent ductus arteriosus, ventricular septal defects, and Fallot's tetralogy. Gastric and duodenal ulcers, neonatal intussusception, malrotation and Dandy Walker malformations may be seen.[2,5,6]

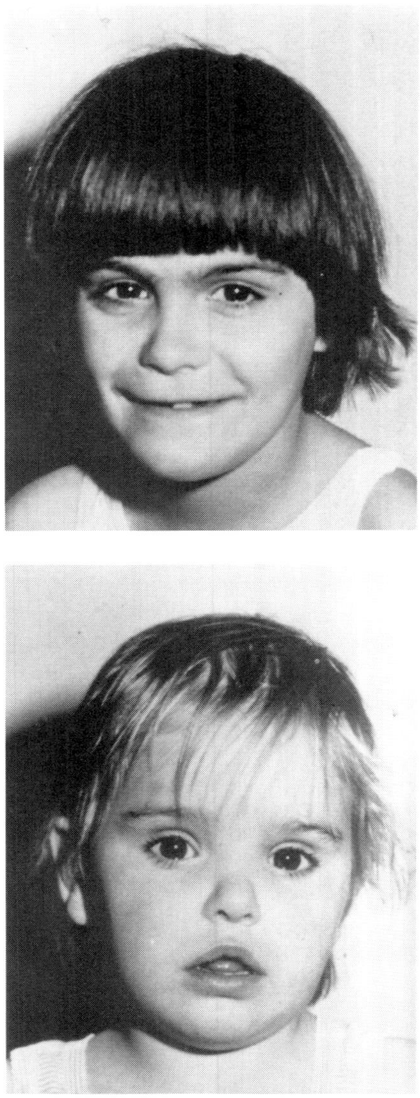

**Fig. 14.** Coffin-Siris syndrome. A,B: Note the mild coarseness of the facies, with bushy eyebrows and characteristic upturned nose. (From M Haspeslagh et al., Clin Genet 26:374, 1984, with permission; courtesy of Dr. JP Fryns.)

### Otolaryngological manifestations

Mild microcephaly (65%) occurs frequently in this syndrome. The facies are coarse and the eyebrows are thick and bushy. The nasal bridge is low and the tip is bulbous and upturned. Preauricular tags may occur. Scalp hair may be scarce. Choanal atresia has been reported. Sucking and feeding difficulties are common.[3,6]

### Etiology

Autosomal dominant and autosomal recessive inheritance have been suggested. Partial biotinidase deficiency was found in association with the syndrome. The ratio of female to male is 4:1.[1,4,7]

#### References

1. Burlina AB, Sherwood WG, Zacchello F: Partial biotinidase deficiency associated with Coffin-Siris syndrome. Eur J Pediatr 149:628–629, 1990.
2. De Bassio WA, Kemper TL, Knoefel JE: Coffin-Siris syndrome: neuropathologic findings. Arch Neurol 42:350–353, 1985.
3. de Jong G, Nelson M: Choanal atresia in two unrelated patients with the Coffin-Siris syndrome. Clin Genet 42:320–322, 1992.
4. Haspeslagh M, Fryns JP, Van den Berghe H: The Coffin-Siris syndrome: report of a family and further delineation. Clin Genet 26:374–378, 1984
5. Levy P, Baraitser M: Coffin-Siris syndrome. J Med Genet 28:338–341, 1991.
6. Qazi QH, Heckman LS, Markouizos D, Verma RS: The Coffin-Siris syndrome. J Med Genet 27:333–336, 1990.
7. Richieri-Costa A, Monteleone-Neto R, Gonzales ML: Coffin-Siris syndrome in a Brazilian child with consanguineous parents. Rev Bras Genet 9:169–177, 1986.

## Cohen syndrome

(MIM No. *216550; POSSUM No. 3152)

This syndrome is characterized by hypotonia, obesity, prominent incisors, mental retardation, short philtrum, micrognathia, narrow hands and feet, and a high-arched palate.

### General manifestations

Most individuals are short, obese, hypotonic, and mentally retarded. The IQ ranges from 30 to 70.[1,2] Other features of the syndrome include delayed puberty, downward slanting palpebral fissures, decreased visual acuity, constricted visual fields, chorioretinal dystrophy, and optic atrophy.[6] A mottled retina has been described in some patients.[4]

Cubitus valgus and hyperextensible joints are present in half of the cases. Heart defects may occasionally be observed and include mitral valve prolapse, pseudotruncus with ventricular septal defect, or isolated VSD. Rare anomalies include microphthalmia, mild cutaneous syndactyly, seizures, and ureteropelvic obstruction.[3,5,7,9]

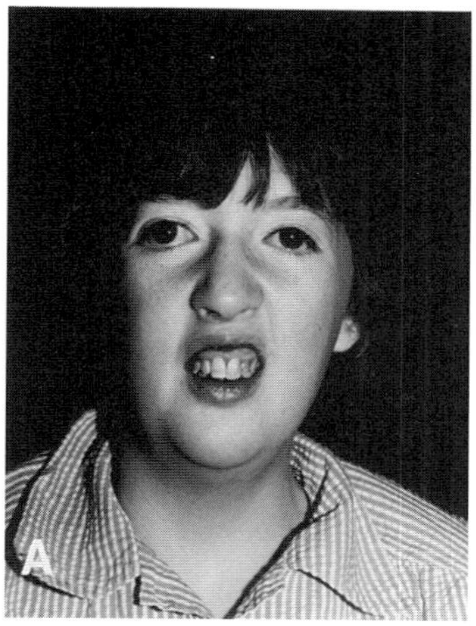


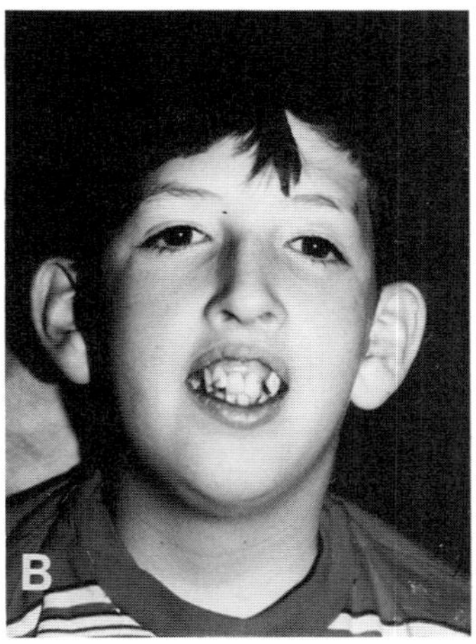


**Fig. 15.** Cohen syndrome. A,B: Patients with mild microcephaly, downward-slanting palpebral fissures, open mouth, and short philtrum. (With permission from MM Cohen, Jr et al., J Pediatr 83:280, 1973.)

### Otolaryngological and dental manifestations

Such manifestations commonly include an open mouth, a short philtrum, exposed upper gingivae, and prominent upper central incisors. Maxillary hypoplasia, mild micrognathia, a high nasal bridge, and a high and narrow palate are also noted.[3,5,7,9]

### Etiology

Cohen syndrome is of autosomal recessive inheritance. Probably there are multiple causative alleles. The gene was mapped to chromosome 8.[8]

### Differential diagnosis

Cohen syndrome should be distinguished from Prader-Willi syndrome.

#### References


1. Carey JC, Hall BD: Confirmation of the Cohen syndrome. J Pediatr 93:239–244, 1978.
2. Cohen MM Jr, Hall BD, Smith DW, Graham CB, Lampert KJ: A new syndrome with hypotonia, obesity, mental deficiency and facial, oral, ocular and limb anomalies. J Pediatr 83:280–284, 1973.
3. Grise A Jr, Nelson S: New obesity, mental retardation syndrome resembling Cohen syndrome. Proc Greenwood Ctr 6:123, 1987.
4. Kondo I, Negataki S, Miyagi N: The Cohen syndrome: does mottled retina separate a Finnish and a Jewish type? Am J Med Genet 37:109–113, 1990.
5. Kousseff BG: Cohen syndrome: further delineation and inheritance. Am J Med Genet 17:317–319, 1980.
6. Norio R, Raitta C, Lindahl E: Further delineation of the Cohen syndrome; report on chorioretinal dystrophy, leukopenia and consanguinity. Clin Genet 25:1–14, 1984.
7. North C, Palton MA, Baraitser M, Winter RM: The clinical features of the Cohen syndrome: further case reports. J Med Genet 22:131–134, 1985.
8. Tahvanainen E, Norio R, Karila E, Ranta S, Weissenback J, Sistonen P, de la Chapelle A: Cohen syndrome gene assigned to the long arm of chromosome 8 by linkage analysis. Nat Genet 7:201–204, 1994.
9. Zeller WP, Rademaker D, Kent D, Hasiakos P, Wong P: A consideration in evaluation of short stature. Cohen syndrome. Ill Med J 171:31–33, 1987.


## Cornelia de Lange syndrome

### De Lange syndrome
(MIM No. 122470; POSSUM No. 3183)

This syndrome is characterized by thin lips with down-turned angles, synophyrs, anomalies of extremities, primordial growth deficiency, and mental retardation.

### General manifestations

Short stature of prenatal onset is characteristic (100%). Osseous maturation is retarded (50%). Microbrachycephaly is common (50%–90%). Mental retardation, which is often severe, occurs in 75%–100% of cases. Hirsutism is seen in 97% of patients. The nipples and umbilicus are hypoplastic. Micromelia occurs two-thirds of the time, while phocomelia and/or oligodactyly occur in one-third of the cases and limb involvement may be uni- or bilateral.[4] The eyelashes are curly and long and synophrys is characteristic. Genitourinary anomalies such as hypoplastic kidneys, cryptorchidism, bicornuate uterus, and dysplasic ovaries are documented.[5,8] Gastrointestinal and cardiovascular anomalies are not rare.

### Otolaryngological manifestations

The nose is small with anteverted nostrils and a flat nasal bridge (100%). The philtrum is long. The lips are thin with a small "beak" on the upper lip and a corresponding notch in the lower lip. The mouth has characteristic down-turned angles. Micrognathia and a prominent meatal spur are common. The

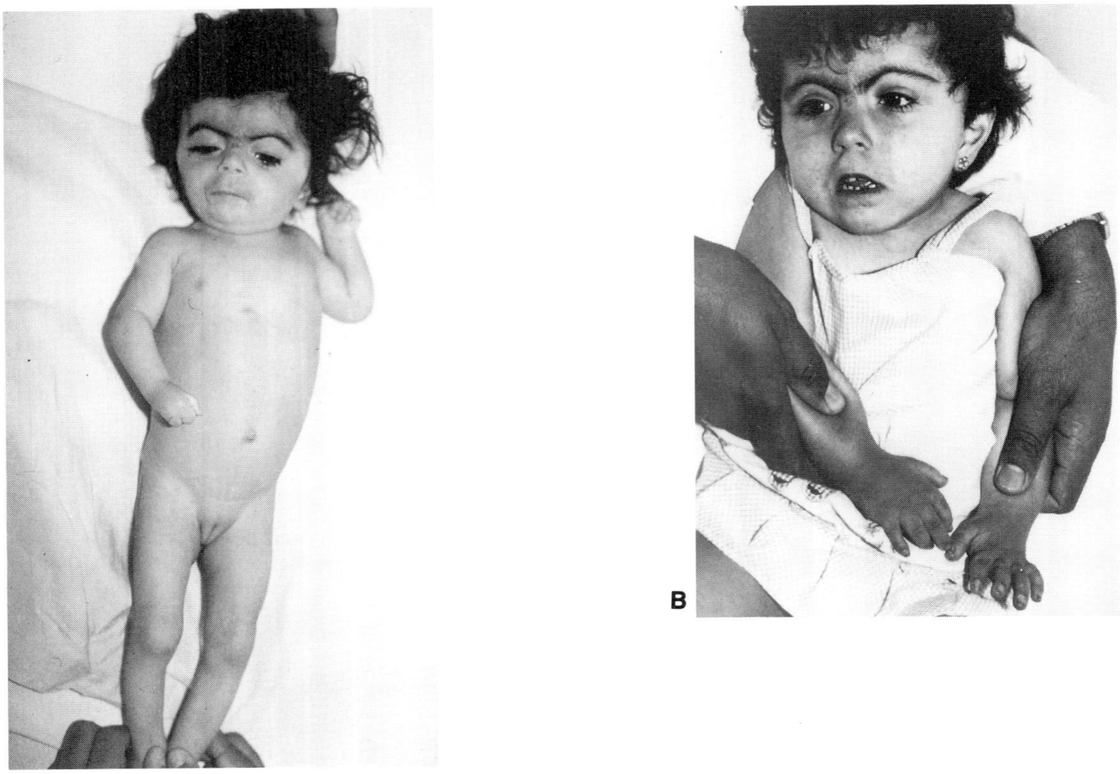


**Fig. 16.** Cornelia de Lange syndrome. A,B: Note the characteristic bushy eyebrows with synophrys, thin and down-turned lips, flat nasal bridge, and abnormalities of the limbs.

ears may be small or malformed and hirsute. Hearing loss is sensorineural and is documented in approximately one-fourth of the cases.[1,2,6]

The palate may be high arched (50%), the neck is thick and short. Dental anomalies, late tooth eruption, and widely spaced teeth are common (93%). A weak, low-pitched cry is common in infancy and speech delay occurs in over 75% of cases.

### Etiology

Causation is unknown. Most cases are sporadic. Autosomal dominant inheritance is suggested in some cases. Autosomal recessive inheritance has been proposed in other cases.[3,7]

### Differential diagnosis

Cornelia De Lange syndrome should be differentiated from dup (3q) syndrome and fetal alcohol syndrome.

### References

1. Falek A, Scmidt R, Jervis G: Familial de Lange syndrome with chromosome abnormalities. Pediatrics 37:92–101, 1966.
2. Filippi G: The de Lange syndrome; report of 15 cases. Clin Genet 35:343–363, 1989.
3. Fryns J, Dereymaeker AM, Hoefnagels M, D'Hondt F, Mertens G, van den Berghe H: The Brachman de Lange syndrome in two siblings of normal parents. Clin Genet 31: 413–415, 1987.
4. Halal F, Preus M: The hand profile in de Lange syndrome: diagnostic criteria. Am J Med Genet 3:317–312, 1979.
5. Hawley PP, Jackson LG, Kurnit DM: Sixty four patients with Brachmann de Lange syndrome: a survey. Am J Med Genet 20:453–459, 1985.
6. Marres HA, Cremers CW, Jongbloet PH: Hearing levels in the Cornelia de Lange syndrome. A report of seven cases. Int J Pediatr Otorhinolaryngol 18:31–37, 1989.
7. Naguib KK, Teebi AS, Al-Awadi SA, Marafie MJ: Brachmann de Lange syndrome in sibs. J Med Genet 24:627–629, 1987.
8. Vischer D: Typus degenerativus amstelodamensis (Cornelia de Lange syndrome) Helv Paediatr Acta 20:415–445, 1965.

## Craniometaphyseal dysplasia

(MIM No. *123000, 218400; POSSUM No. 3162)

### General manifestations

Most changes are the result of increasing bony sclerosis of the skull and metaphyseal ends of the long bones. Intelligence is usually normal.[1–7] However, a few patients have shown mental retardation.[5]

### Otolaryngological manifestations

During infancy the root of the nose begins to broaden and an elevated wing of bone gradually extends bilaterally over the nasal bridge to the zygomas. Other features include narrowing of the nasal lumen leading to obstruction and mouth breathing, choanal stenosis, progressive mixed hearing loss that manifests in childhood, peripheral facial nerve paralysis, headache, and optic atrophy as a result of bony encroachment on the optic foramina. Occasionally there is delayed eruption of the permanent teeth and supernumerary teeth.[1–7] Osteoclast-like cells are 40% of the normal in number.[8]

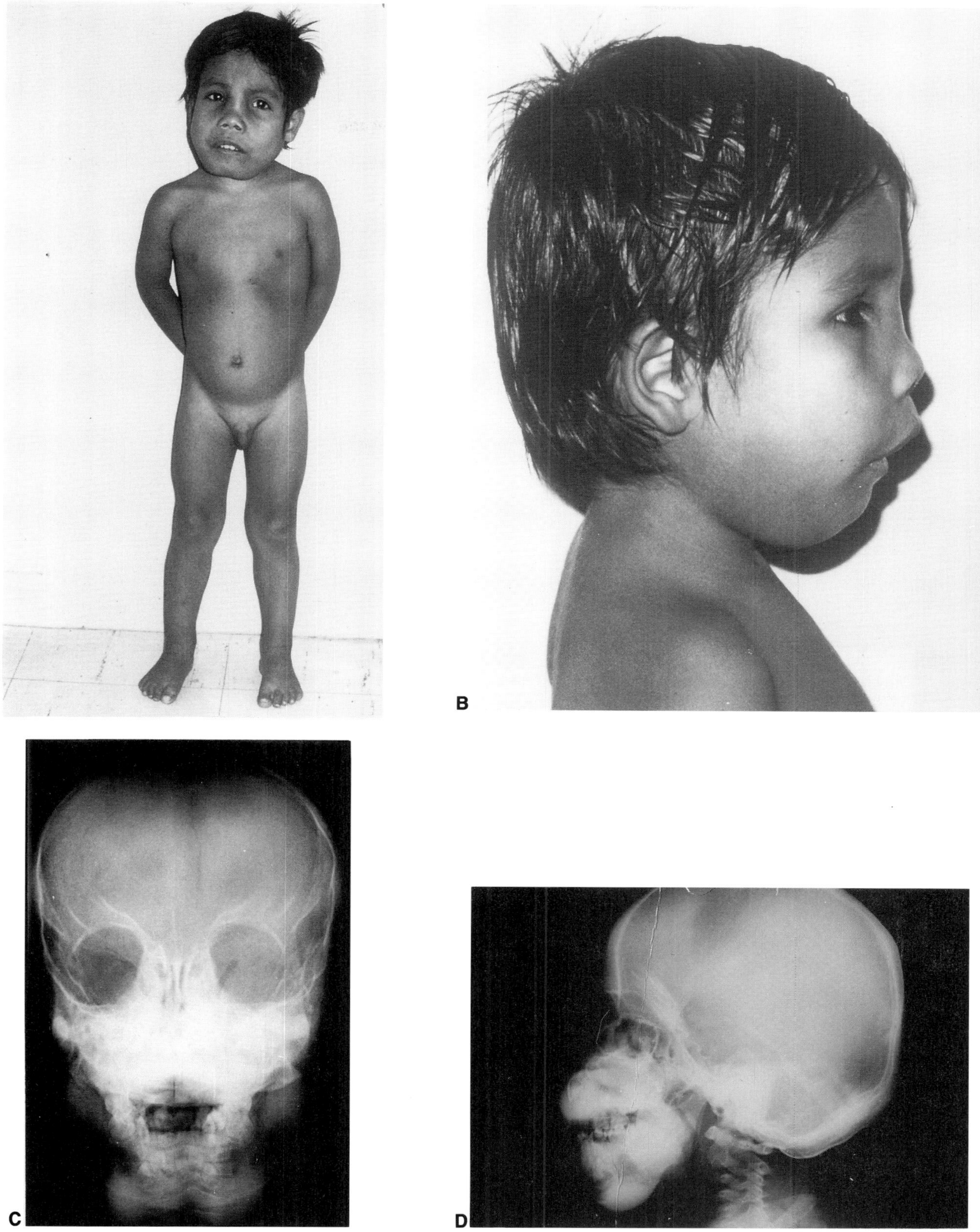

**Fig. 17.** Craniometaphyseal dysplasia. A,B: Note the broad nasal bridge and open mouth. C,D: Skull X-rays demonstrating hyperostosis and sclerosis of the calvarium, base of the skull, and mandible. (With permission from A Carnevale et al., Clin Genet 23:17, 1983.)

Radiographically, hyperostosis and sclerosis of the calvarium, base of the skull, and mandible are present. Underpneumatization of the mastoid bones is evident. Frontonasal hyperostosis also occurs.

### Etiology

Both autosomal recessive and autosomal dominant forms exist.[4,7] The extreme variability of expression of the dominant form makes it difficult to differentiate it from the recessive form.

### Differential diagnosis

Craniometaphyseal dysplasia should be differentiated from craniodiaphyseal dysplasia and Pyle disease.

### References

1. Beighton P, Hamersma H, Horan F: Craniometaphyseal dysplasia—variability of expression within a large family. Clin Genet 15:252–258, 1979.
2. Cooper JC: Craniometaphyseal dysplasia: a case report and review of the literature. Br J Oral Surg 12:196–204, 1974.
3. Kietzer G, Paparella MM: Otolaryngological disorders in craniometaphyseal dysplasia. Laryngoscope 79:921–941, 1969.
4. Penchaszadeh VB, Gutierrez ER, Figueroa E: Autosomal recessive craniometaphyseal dysplasia. Am J Med Genet 5:43–55, 1980.
5. Reardon W, Hall CM, Dillon MJ, Baraitser M: Sibs with mental retardation, supraorbital sclerosis, and metaphyseal dysplasia: frontometaphyseal dysplasia, craniometaphyseal dysplasia, or a new syndrome? J Med Genet 28:622–626, 1991.
6. Stool SE, Caruso VG: Cranial metaphyseal dysplasia. Otolaryngologic aspects. Arch Otolaryngol 97:410–412, 1973.
7. Taylor DB, Sprague P: Dominant craniometaphyseal dysplasia—a family study over five generations. Australas Radiol 33:84–89, 1989.
8. Yamamoto T, Kurihara N, Yamaoka K, Ozono K, Okada M, Yamamoto K, Matsumoto S, Michigami T, Ono J, Okada S: Bone marrow-derived osteoclast-like cells from a patient with craniometaphyseal dysplasia lack expression of osteoclast-reactive vacuolar proton pump. J Clin Invest 91:362–367, 1993.

## Cri du chat syndrome

POSSUM No. 3073

### General manifestations

Affected individuals exhibit microcephaly, hypotonia, and severe developmental retardation. Cardiovascular defects are common, the most frequent being the patent ductus arteriosus. Musculoskeletal abnormalities include diastasis recti, inguinal hernia, talipes, dislocated hips, and partial syndactyly. Single palmar creases and short metacarpals are frequent. Bowel rotation and cryptorchidism may also occur.[1,4,7]

Respiratory and feeding difficulties are known complications. Ocular findings include epicanthal folds, strabismus, deficient tearing, and tortuous retinal vessels in adulthood.

### Otolaryngological manifestations

The characteristic mewy cry (cat cry) is present only during infancy. The high shrill disappears with age in 98% of patients. The origin of the cry is thought to be central rather than due to laryngeal abnormality. The facies are round with hypertelorism and a broad nasal root. Malocclusion and a high-arched palate are seen in most cases. Cleft palate/lip is seen occasionally. The frontal sinuses are large in adult patients. The ears are posteriorly angulated and preauricular tags may exist.[1,3,5] The neck is short and the hair is gray in adulthood.

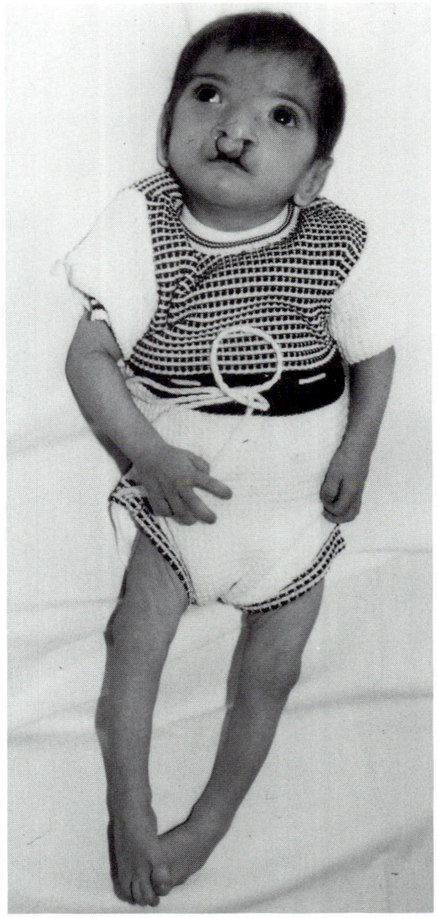

**Fig. 18.** Cri du chat syndrome. Note the cleft lip/palate and microcephaly.

### Etiology

This syndrome is associated with partial deletion of the short arm of chromosome 5. This could be either a de novo deletion (85%) or an unbalanced translocation inherited from a carrier parent (15%). Cri-du-chat syndrome as such is a contiguous gene syndrome with all the additional features mentioned above under general manifestations. The isolated cat-like cry feature is associated with the specific critical region of 5p15.2.[2] The frequency of this syndrome is 1:50,000 births.[6] Approximately 1% of profoundly retarded patients are diagnosed with cri-du-chat syndrome.

### References

1. Breg WR, Steele MW, Miller OJ, Warburton D, DeCaproa A, Allderdice PW: The cri-du-chat syndrome in adolescents and adults: clinical findings in 13 older patients with partial deletion of the short arm of chromosome No 5(5p-). J Pediatr 77:782–791, 1970.
2. Gersh M, Goodart SA, Pasztor LM, Harris DJ, Weiss L, Overhauser J: Evidence for a distinct region causing a cat-like cry in patients with 5p deletions. Am J Hum Genet 56:1404–1410, 1995.

3. Hashimoto T, Tsukino R, Chiyo H, Furuyama J: Reciprocal translocation t(5;6)(p13q27) through three generations: case report of cri-du-chat syndrome. Hum Genet 53:145–147, 1980.
4. Howard RO: Ocular abnormalities in the cri-du-chat syndrome. Am J Ophthalmol 73:949–954, 1972.
5. Manning KP: The larynx in the cri-du-chat syndrome. J Laryngol Otol 91:887–892, 1977.
6. Niebuhr E: The cri-du-chat syndrome. Hum Genet 44:227–275, 1978.
7. Wilkins LE, Brown JA, Nance WE, Wolfe B: Clinical heterogeneity in 80 home-reared children with cri-du-chat syndrome. J Pediatr 102:528–533, 1983.

## Crouzon syndrome

### Craniofacial dysostosis
(MIM No. *123500; POSSUM No. 3158)

Crouzon syndrome was originally described in 1912.[5] It is characterized by cranial deformity due to premature craniosynostosis, hypoplastic midface, exophthalmos, hypertelorism, and mandibular prognathism. This syndrome is estimated to occur in 16.5 per 1 million.[4]

### General manifestations

Craniosynostosis of the coronal, sagittal, and lambdoid sutures may occur, giving the skull a brachycephalic shape. Occasionally, scaphocephaly or clover-leaf deformity may occur.[12] Crouzon syndrome constitutes approximately 4.8% of cases with craniosynostosis.[4]

Proptosis occurs in most cases secondary to the shallow orbits. It may result in exposure keratitis. Optic nerve involvement is usually evident in half of the cases. Other ocular findings include megalocornea, nystagmus, keratoconus, ectopia lentis, or colobomas of the iris.[3,7]

Frequent headaches, seizures, and mental deficiency may also occur. Acanthosis nigricans has been described in associa-

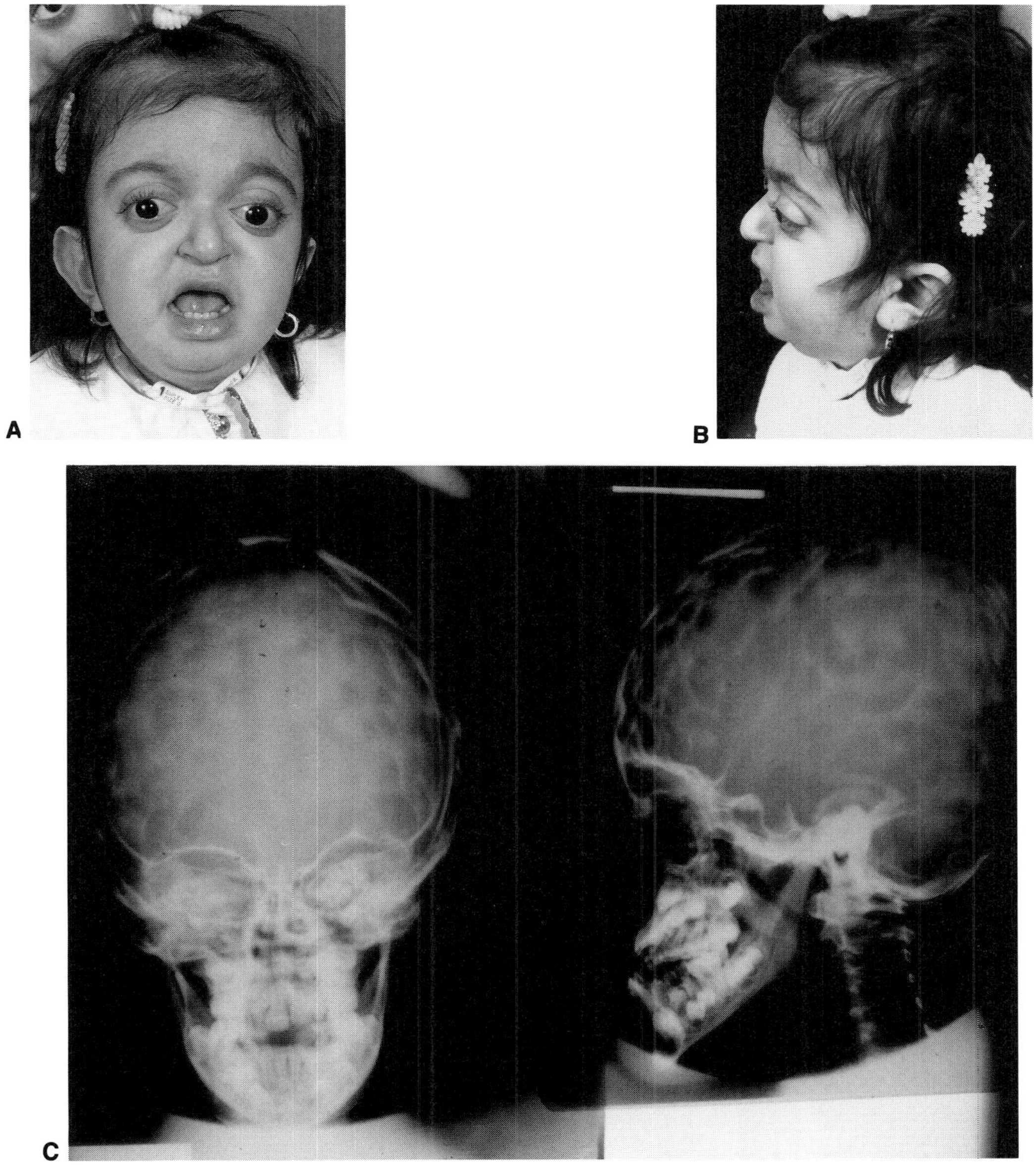

**Fig. 19.** Crouzon syndrome. A,B: Note the shallow orbits, proptosis, and parrot-like nose. C: Skull X-ray showing copper-beaten appearence.

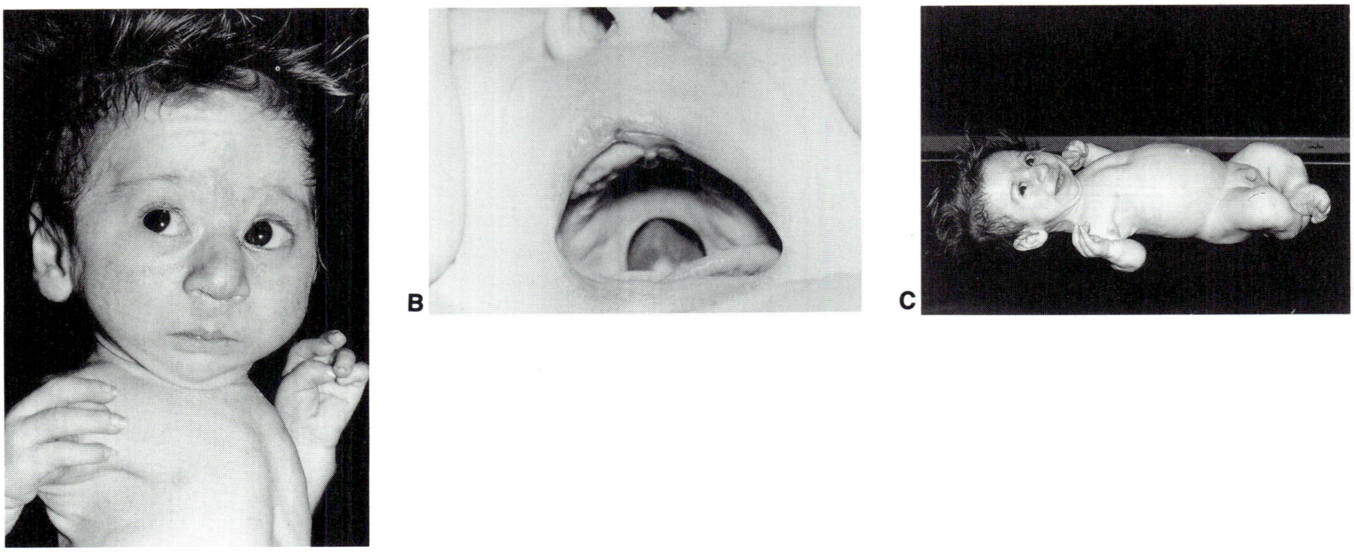

**Fig. 20.** Diastrophic dysplasia. Note the abnormal nose and flared nostrils (A); the cleft palate (B); and short and characteristic lower extremities (C).

tion with Crouzon syndrome.[2,6] Surgical treatment is usually directed toward correcting the craniosynostosis. Facial abnormalities may be corrected using the Tessier procedure.[13]

### Otolaryngological manifestations

It is estimated that 30 to 55% of Crouzon patients have hearing loss. The hearing loss is usually conductive. The external auditory canals may be atretic. Ossicular fixation and deformities have been described as well.[1,7]

Anomalies of the palate include lateral palatal swellings in 50% of cases but cleft lip/palate is not common.[7,11] The maxillary teeth are often crowded and there is usually an anterior open bite. The nose is frequently parrot-like. Calcification of the stylohyoid ligament occurs most of the time. Anomalies of the cervical vertebrae involve mostly C2 and C3.[8]

### Etiology

This syndrome is inherited as an autosomal dominant trait with complete penetrance. Expressivity is variable. Increased paternal age is a factor in sporadic cases. Many mutations have been described in the *FGFR2* gene.[10] Crouzon syndrome with acanthosis nigricans is due to a mutation in the *FGFR3* gene.[9]

### Differential diagnosis

Crouzon syndrome should be differentiated from nonsyndromic craniosynostosis, Apert syndrome, Pfeiffer syndrome, and Saethre-Chotzen syndrome.

#### References

1. Boedts D: La surdité dans la dysostose craniofaciale ou maladie de Crouzon. Acta Otorhinolaryngol Belg 21:143–155, 1967.
2. Breitbart AS, Eaton C, McCarthy JGH: Crouzon's syndrome associated with acanthosis nigricans. Ramifications for the craniofacial surgeon. Am Plast Surg 22:310–315, 1989.
3. Cohen MM Jr: Craniosynostosis: Diagnosis, Evaluation, and Management. Raven Press, New York, 1986.
4. Cohen MM Jr, Kreiborg JS: Birth prevalence studies of the Crouzon syndrome: comparison of direct and indirect methods. Clin Genet 41:12–15, 1992.
5. Crouzon O: Dysostose cranio-faciale héréditaire. Bull Mem Soc Med Hôp (Paris), 33:545–555, 1912.
6. Koizumi H, Tomoyori T, Sato KC, Ohkaware A: An association of acanthosis nigricans and Crouzon Syndrome. J Dermatol 19:122–126, 1992.
7. Kreiborg S: Crouzon syndrome. Scand J Plast Reconstr Surg (Suppl) 18:1–198, 1981.
8. Kreiborg S, Barr M Jr, Cohen MM Jr: Cervical spine in the Apert syndrome. Am J Med Genet 43:704–708, 1992.
9. Meyers GA, Orlow SJ, Munro IR, Przylepa KA, Jabs EW: Fibroblast growth factor receptor 3 (FGFR3) transmembrane mutation in Crouzon syndrome with acanthosis nigricans. Nat Genet 11:462–464, 1995.
10. Park W-J, Bellus GA, Jabs EW: Mutations in fibroblast growth factor receptors: phenotypic consequences during eukaryotic development. Am J Hum Genet 57:748–754, 1995.
11. Peterson-Falzone SJ, Pruzansky S, Parris PJ, Laffer JL: Nasopharyngeal dysmorphology in the syndromes of Apert and Crouzon. Cleft Palate J 18:237–250, 1981.
12. Rohatgi M: Cloverleaf skull a severe form of Crouzon's syndrome: a new concept in a etiology. Acta Neurochir 108:45–52, 1991.
13. Tessier P: The definitive plastic surgical treatment of the severe facial deformities of craniofacial dysostosis. Crouzon's and Apert's diseases. Plast Reconstr Surg 48:419–442, 1971.

## Diastrophic dysplasia

### Diastrophic dwarfism
(MIM No. *222600; POSSUM No. 3185)

### General manifestations

In addition to hyperplastic auricular cartilage (cauliflower ears), this syndrome is characterized by short tubular bones (especially first metacarpal) and joint limitations with talipes.

The short stature is prenatal. Talipes varus progresses with age and is resistant to treatment. The proximal phalangeal joints have limited flexion, and the thumbs are hypermobile and laterally displaced (hitchhiker's thumb). Scoliosis is progressive, kyphosis may be seen as well. Symphalangism occurs in the proximal interphalangeal joints and radiologically all tubular bones are short and thick. Hip dislocation and patellar subluxation may occur. Early calcification of the ribs, intracranial calcification, and facial hemangiomas are documented.[1,3,7,9,10]

### Otolaryngological manifestations

The facies include circumoral fullness. The nose is broad with flared nostrils and a narrow nasal bridge. Acute swelling of the pinnae develop in the first few weeks of life. The ears feel cystic and may be fluctuant. The swelling resolves after approximately 4 weeks, leaving the cartilage thickened, hard, and calcified (85%). The external auditory canals are narrow. Deafness of the conductive type may occur due to ossicular abnormalities or fusion. Abnormalities of the tracheal, laryngeal, and bronchial cartilages have resulted in collapse of the airway and death. Cleft palate occurs in one-third of patients. Glossoptosis occurs in 10% of cases.[4,5,8,10]

### Etiology

Inheritance is autosomal recessive. The responsible gene is located at 5q32–q33.1.[6,6a,6b,9a] An abnormality of type IX collagen has been reported.[2] The diastrophic dysplasia gene encodes a novel sulfate transporter (DTDST).[6a]

### Differential diagnosis

Arthrogryposis, achondroplasia, and cartilage-hair hypoplasia may be confused with this condition. Pseudodiastrophic dysplasia bears a remarkable resemblance to diastrophic dysplasia, but the former has the additional presence of platyspondyly.

### References


1. Butler MG, Gale DD, Meaney FJ: Metacarpophalangeal pattern profile analysis in diastrophic dysplasia. Am J Med Genet 28:685–689, 1987.
2. Diab M, Wu JJ, Shapiro F, Eyre D: Abnormality of type IX collagen in a patient with diastrophic dysplasia. Am J Med Genet 49:402–409, 1994.
3. Dorn U, Rosenkranz U, Bosch: Der diastrophische Zwergwuchs. Z Orthop Ihre Grenzgeb 118:359–366, 1980.
4. Friedman SI, Taber P, Hillister DW, Rimoin DL: A lethal form of diastrophic dwarfism. In: Skeletal Dysplasia, D Bergsma, ed. Excerpta Medica, Amsterdam, 1974, pp 43–49.
5. Godbersen GS, Hosenfeld D, Pankau R: Diastrophic dysplasia. A congenital syndrome with remarkable changes of the external ear and stridor. HNO 38:256–258, 1990.
6. Hästbacka J, Kaitila I, Sistonen P, de la Chapelle A: Diastrophic dysplasia gene maps to the distal long arm of chromosome 5. Proc Natl Acad Sci USA 87:8056–8059, 1990.

6a. Hästbacka J, de la Chapelle A, Mahtani MM, Clines G, Reeve-Daly MP, Daly M, Hamilton BA, Kusumi K, Trivedi B, Weaver A et al.: The diastrophic dysplasia gene encodes a novel sulfate transporter: postional cloning by fine-structure linkage disequilibrium mapping. Cell 78:1073–1087, 1994.

6b. Kaplan NL, Hill WG, Weir BS: Likelihood methods for locating disease genes in nonequilibrium population. Am J Hum Genet 56:18–32, 1995.

7. Krecak J, Starshak RJ: Cervical kyphosis in diastrophic dwarfism: CT and MR findings. Pediatr Radiol 17:321–322, 1987.
8. Naselli A, Di Battista E, Vignolo M, de Toni T, Toma P: La displasia diastrophica. Minerva Pediatr 35:8912–8917, 1983.
9. Richards BS: Atlanto-axial instability in diastrophic dysplasia. A case report. J Bone Joint Surg 73:614–616, 1991.

9a. Saltman DL, Dolganov GM, Warrington JA, Wasmuth JJ, Lovett M: A physical map of 15 loci on human chromosome 5q23–q33 by two-color fluorescence in situ hybridisation. Genomics 16:726–732, 1993.

10. Walker BA, Scott CI Jr, Hall JG, Murdoch JL, McKusick VA: Diastrophic dwarfism. Medicine 51:41–60, 1972.


## DiGeorge sequence

(MIM No. *188400; POSSUM No. 3186)

### General manifestations

This sequence may present with severe cardiovascular and craniofacial features that may be associated with abnormalities originating from the third and fourth pharyngeal pouches, and with hypoplasia or aplasia of the thymus and/or the parathyroid glands.

Thymic hypoplasia or aplasia results in defective cell-mediated immunity and frequent infections early in life. Infants who survive with milder manifestations of DiGeorge sequence are moderately to severely retarded. The parathyroid hypoplasia or aplasia results in hypocalcemic tetany and seizures in infancy.[9,11]

Cardiovascular anomalies include conotruncal defects such

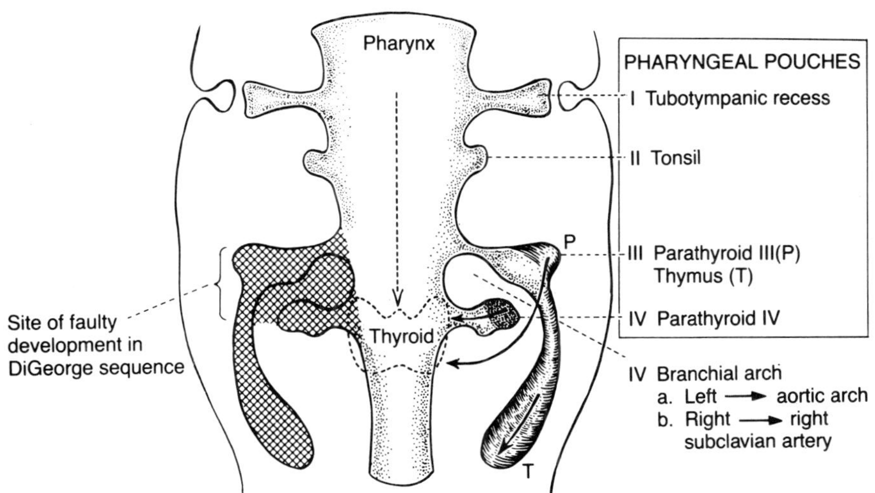


**Fig. 21.** DiGeorge sequence. Schematic appearance of anterior foregut and its derivatives, fifth week of development. (With permission from KL Jones, *Smith's Recognizable Patterns of Human Malformation,* 4th ed., WB Saunders, Philadelphia, 1988.)

as right aortic arch, interrupted aorta, PDA, VSD, and tetralogy of Fallot.[12]

The incidence is 1:20,000 births.

### Otolaryngological manifestations

Craniofacial anomalies include hypertelorism, epicanthic folds, downward slanting palpebral fissures, a short philtrum, cleft lip/palate, and choanal atresia. Abnormalities of the ears include low-set, posteriorly-angulated ears with pointed pinnae and middle ear defects. Other defects include esophageal atresia and anomalies of the speech muscles.[3,10,11,12]

**Table 1.** Conditions with DiGeorge sequence*

| |
|---|
| *CHROMOSOMAL* |
| dup(1q) |
| del(5p) |
| dup(8q) |
| del(10p) |
| del(22q) |
| *MONOGENIC* |
| Isolated autosomal dominant |
| Isolated autosomal recessive |
| Velo-cardio-facial syndrome |
| Zellweger syndrome |
| *TERATOGENIC* |
| Diabetic embroypathy |
| Fetal alcohol syndrome |
| Retinoid embryopathy |
| *ASSOCIATIONAL* |
| Arhinencephalia/DiGeorge |
| CHARGE/DiGeorge |
| Cardiofacial/DiGeorge |

*Modified from Gorlin et al. 1990.[6b]

### Etiology

Partial monosomy of the long arm of chromosome 22 (22q11.2) is present in most patients with DiGeorge sequence. Patients with velo-cardio-facial syndrome (Shprintzen syndrome) have been shown to have deletions in the same region.[3] Microdeletions were detected in 83% of the DiGeorge sequence patients and 68% of the velo-cardio-facial syndrome patients.[3] Deletions of the 22q11.2 region have been associated with a wide range of developmental defects (DiGeorge syndrome, velo-cardio-facial syndrome, and isolated conotruncal cardiac defects) that have been classified under the controversial acronym *CATCH 22*.[6,13] DiGeorge sequence has also been reported in infants of diabetic mothers and as a part of the teratogenic effects of maternal intake of alcohol and vitamin A.[5,8,10] It is also associated with other conditions (see Table 1). Most cases are sporadic. However, autosomal dominant or recessive inheritance has been suggested in certain instances.[14]

A zinc finger gene *(ZNF74)* is consistently deleted in DiGeorge syndrome.[1] Also, the human mitochondrial citrate transporter protein gene is localized in the region of chromosome 22q11 which is critical to DiGeorge syndrome.[7] Moreover, a candidate gene, which becomes disrupted as a result of a balanced translocation, has been cloned.[2,4] A transcription map of the DiGeorge and velo-cardio-facial syndrome minimal critical region on 22q11 has been established.[6a]

### References


1. Aubry M, Demczuk S, Desmaze C, Aikem M, Aurias A, Julien J-P, Rouleau GA: Isolation of a zinc finger gene consistently deleted in DiGeorge syndrome. Hum Mol Genet 2:1583–1587, 1993.
2. Budarf ML, Collins J, Gong W, Roe B, Wang Z, Bailey LC, Sellinger B, Michaud D, Driscoll DA, Emanuel BS: Cloning a balanced translocation associated with DiGeorge syndrome and identification of a disrupted candidate gene. Nat Genet 10:269–277, 1995.
3. Conley ME, Beckwith JB, Mancer JF, Tenckhoff L: The spectrum of the DiGeorge syndrome. J Pediatr 94:883–890, 1979.
4. Demczuk S, Aledo R, Zucman J, Delattre O, Desmaze C, Dauphinot L, Jalbert P, Rouleau GA, Thomas G, Aurias A: Cloning of a balanced translocation breakpoint in the DiGeorge syndrome critical region and isolation of a novel potential adhesion receptor gene in its vicinity. Hum Mol Genet 4:551–558, 1995.
5. Driscoll DA, Salvin J, Sellinger B, Budarf ML, McDonald-McGinn DM, Zackai EH, Emanuel BS: Prevalence of 22q11 microdeletions in DiGeorge and velocardiofacial syndromes: implications for genetic counselling and prenatal diagnosis. J Med Genet 30:813–817, 1993.
6. Glover TW: CATCHing a break on 22. Nat Genet 10:257–258, 1995.

6a. Gong W, Emanuel BS, Collins J, Kim DH, Wang Z, Chen F, Zhang G, Roe B, Budarf ML: A transcription map of the DiGeorge and velo-cardio-facial syndrome minimal critical region on 22q11. Hum Mol Genet 5:789–800, 1996.

6b. Gorlin RJ, Cohen MMJr, Levin LS: Syndromes of the Head and Neck, 3rd ed. Oxford University Press, New York, 1990, p 665.

7. Heisterkamp N, Mulder MP, Langeveld A, Tenhoeve J, Wang Z, Roe BA, Groffen J: Localization of the human mitochondial citrate transporter protein gene to chromosome 22q11 in the DiGeorge syndrome critical region. Genomics 29:451–456, 1995.
8. Lammer EJ, Opitz JM: The DiGeorge anomaly as a developmental field defect. Am J Med Genet 2:113–127, 1986.
9. Müller W, Peter HH, Wilken M, Juppner H, Kallfelz HC, Krohn HP, Miller K, Rieger CH: The DiGeorge syndrome I. Clinical evaluation and course of partial and complete forms of the syndrome. Eur J Pediatr 147:496–502, 1988.
10. Novak RW, Robinson HB: Coincident DiGeorge anomaly and renal agenesis and its relation to maternal diabetes. Am J Med Genet 50:311–312, 1994.
11. Steele RW, Limas C, Thurman GB, Schuelein M, Bauer H, Bellanti JA: Familial thymic aplasia. Attempted reconstitution with fetal thymus in a Millipore diffusion chamber. N Engl J Med 287:787–791, 1972.
12. Van Mierop LHD, Kutsche LM: Cardiovascular anomalies in DiGeorge syndrome and importance of neural crest as a possible pathogenic factor. Am J Cardiol 58:133–137, 1986.
13. Wilson DI, Burn J, Scambler P, Goodship J: DiGeorge syndrome: part of CATCH 22. J Med Genet 30:852–856, 1993.
14. Winter WE, Silverstein JH, Barrett DJ, Kiel E: Familial DiGeorge syndrome with tetralogy of Fallot and prolonged survival. Eur J Pediatr 141:171–172, 1984.


## Down syndrome

### Trisomy 21
(MIM #190685; POSSUM No. 3100)

This syndrome is the most common of the chromosomal abnormality syndromes. L. Down[7] report of 1866 set forth the clinical manifestations of the syndrome that bears his name. Later, Lejeune,[13] Polani et al.,[15] and Clarke et al.[4] reported on the extra chromosome, the translocation type, and the mosaicism, respectively.

### General manifestations

The diagnosis of Down syndrome can be made during the early newborn period. Four out of ten signs are needed to make a clinical diagnosis (see Table 1). However, a final diagnosis

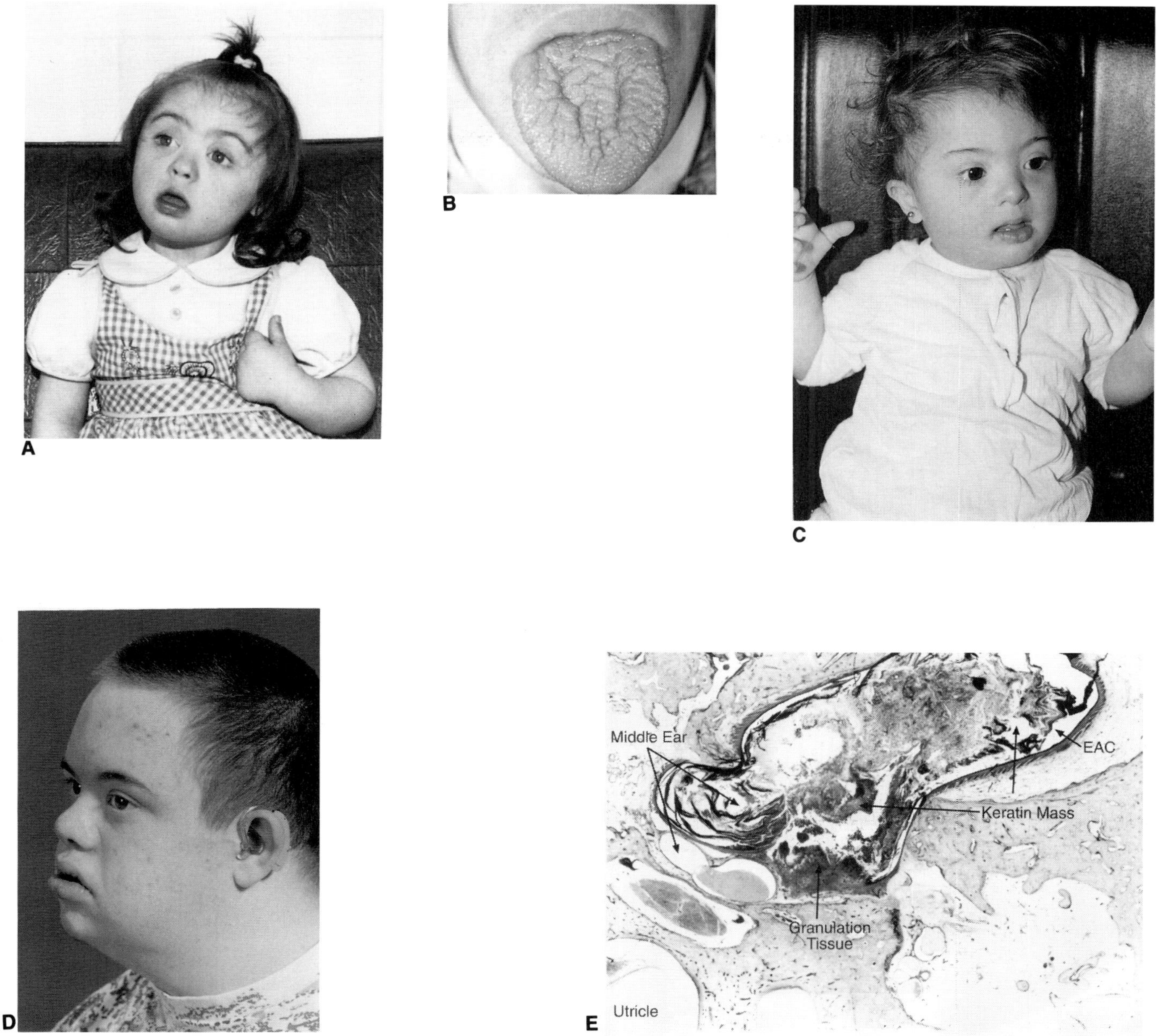


**Fig. 22.** Down syndrome. Note the flat facial features, flat nasal bridge, and epicanthal folds (A); and the fissured tongue (B). C: Patient with mild expression of the syndrome. D: Patient with hearing loss—note hearing aid. E: Middle ear section showing cholesteatoma of the external auditory canal and middle ear. The ossicles are partially resorbed. Granulation tissue is seen on the promontory and a massive keratin plug fills the external auditory canal and middle ear. (E from HF Schuknecht, *Pathology of the Ear,* 2nd ed., Lea & Febiger, Philadelphia, 1993, p. 187, with permission.)

may be made only after having the results of the chromosomal pattern.

The eyes have speckled irises (Brushfield spots) and fine opacities are seen in the lens on slit lamp examination. Mental deficiency is a hallmark of the syndrome. The IQ varies between 30 and 50. Various brain lesions have been described, including abnormalities of the cerebellar peduncles and fibrous gliosis of the white matter. The frequency of epilepsy is estimated to be 5%. Older patients develop changes characteristic of Alzheimer's disease.[14,17,19]

Cardiac anomalies are seen in approximately 40% of patients; atrioventricular communis or ventricular septal defects, Fallot's tetralogy, and patent ductus arteriosus occur in decreasing order of frequency.[8] Atlantoaxial instability is seen in 10%–20% of cases. The hands have short metacarpals and phalanges with clinodactyly and hypoplastic midphalanx of the fifth finger. Single palmar creases and ulnar loop dermal ridge patterns are seen in a high percentage of cases. There is a wide gap between the first and second toes. Male patients have a small penis and low testosterone production and are almost all infertile. The hair is often sparse, and cutis marmorata and dry hyperkeratotic skin are not uncommon.

Other uncommon anomalies include tracheoesophageal (TE) fistula, incomplete fusion of the vertebrae, cryptorchidism, syndactyly, and keratoconus. The main cause of death is cardiovascular malformation and is highest in the first 2 years of life. Leukemia occurs in 1% of patients. Lymphomas, testicular carcinoma, and CNS tumors have also been reported.

### Otolaryngological manifestations

Flat facial features, small or absent paranasal sinuses, hypertelorism, small nasal bridge, and oblique palpebral (upward slanting) fissures occur in over 80% of patients.[11,16,18] The tongue is relatively large and protrudes from the mouth. It may be furrowed or fissured. Occasionally, true macroglossia is present.

The ears are small with overfolding of the superior part of the helix. The external auditory canals are stenotic, especially at the isthmus (bony-cartilagenous junction). Conductive hearing loss occurs in 60% of patients, with a high incidence of serous otitis. Sensorineural hearing loss occurs in 10% of patients. The cochlea is sometimes shorter than usual. Ossicular chain anomalies, especially the stapes, may be seen.[1,2,6]

The lips are broad and dry, and rhagade furrows around the mouth are seen. The tonsils are often hypertrophied and not recessed in the fossae. The palate is narrow. Cleft lip/palate is occasionally seen.[3,9] Gingivitis, periodontal disease, and dental caries exist in certain patients. Microdontia, hypoplasia of the enamel, posterior crossbite, and widely-spaced teeth are frequent occurrences. Articulation defects and dysrhythmic or explosive speech are associated with a low-pitched, hoarse voice.[5,12]

### Etiology

95% of cases are due to 21 trisomy with 47 chromosomes. Mosaicism is observed in 1%–2% of patients. Translocations account for 3 to 4% of patients involving chromosome 14, 21 or 22 (i.e., 14/21, 21/21 or 22/21). A sub-region of chromosome 21 (21q22.3) has been associated with mental retardation and several characteristic morphological features. This is the Down syndrome critical region.[6a]

Incidence of the syndrome increases with advanced maternal age, being 1 per 1,500 for mothers aged 15 to 29 and 1:50 for those over 40. The general incidence is 1 in 600 of all live births.

**Table 1** Ten cardinal features of Down syndrome in the newborn

| Feature | Percent of occurrence |
|---|---|
| Flat facial profile | 90% |
| Poor Moro reflex | 85% |
| Hypotonia | 80% |
| Hyperflexibility of joints | 80% |
| Excess skin on back of neck | 80% |
| Slanted palpebral fissures | 80% |
| Dysplastic pelvis | 70% |
| Anomalous auricles | 60% |
| Dysplasia of midphalanx of fifth finger | 60% |
| Simian crease | 45% |

From Hall B: Mongolism in newborns. A clinical and cytogenic study. Acta Paediatr Scand 154:1–95, 1964,[10] with permission.

### References


1. Aase JM, Wilson AC, Smith DW: Small ears in Down's syndrome: a helpful diagnostic aid. J Pediatr 82:845–847, 1973.
2. Balkany TJ, Downs MP, Jafek BW Krajicek MJ: Hearing loss in Down's Syndrome. Clin Pediatr 18:116–118, 1979.
3. Butterworth T, Leoni EP, Beerman H, Wood MG, Strean LP: Cheilitis of mongolism. J Invest Dermatol 35:347–352, 1960.
4. Clarke CM, Edwards JH, Smallpeice V: 21 trisomy/normal mosaicism in an intelligent child with some mongoloid features. Lancet 1:1028–1030, 1961.
5. Cohen MM Sr, Cohen MM Jr: The oral manifestations of trisomy G (Down's syndrome). Birth Defects 7:241–251, 1971.
6. Cunningham C, McArthur K: Hearing loss and treatment in young Down's syndrome children. Childcare Health Dev 7:357–374, 1981.

6a. Delabar JM, Theophile D, Rahmani Z, Chettouh Z, Blouin JL, Prieur M, Noel B, Sinet PM: Molecular mapping of twenty-four features of Down syndrome on chromosome 21. Europ J Hum Genet 1:114–124, 1993.

7. Down JLH: Observations on an ethnic classification of idiots. Clinical Lecture Reports, London Hospital, 3:259, 1866.
8. Fabia J, Drolette M: Life tables up to age 10 for mongols with and without congenital heart defects. J Ment Defic Res 14:235–242, 1970.
9. Gorlin RJ, Cervenka J, Pruzansky S: Facial clefting and its syndromes. Birth Defects 7:3–49, 1971.
10. Hall B: Mongolism in newborns. A clinical and cytogenetic study. Acta Paediatr Scand 154:1–95, 1964.
11. Jensen GM: Dentoalveolar morphology and developmental changes in Down's syndrome. Am J Orthodont 64:607–618, 1973.
12. Le Clech G, Journel H, Roussey M, Lemarec B: La première dentition du trisomique 21, à propos de 114 enfants suivis régulièrement. Ann Pediatr 33:795–798, 1986.
13. Lejeune J: Le Mongolisme. Premier exemple d'aberration autosomique humaine. Ann Genet 1:41–49, 1959.
14. Melyn M, White D: Mental and developmental milestones of non-institutionalized Down's syndrome children. Pediatrics 52:542–545, 1973.
15. Polani P, Briggs JH, Ford CE, Clarke CM, Berg JM: A mongol girl with 46 chromosomes. Lancet 1:721–724, 1960.
16. Roche AF, Seward FS, Sunderland S:: Nonmetrical observations on cranial roentgenograms in mongolism. Am J Roentgenol 85:659–662, 1961.
17. Solitare GB, Lamarche JB: Brain weight in the adult mongol. J Ment Defic Res 11:79–84, 1967.
18. Spitzer R, Rabinowitch JY, Wybar KC: A study of the abnormalities of the skull, teeth and lenses in mongolism. Can Med Assoc J 84:567–572, 1961.
19. Urioste M, Valcarcel E, Gomez MA, Pinel I, Garcia de Leon R, Diaz de Bustamante A, Tebar R, Martinez-Grias ML: Holoprosencephaly and trisomy 21 in a child born to a non-diabetic mother. Am J Med Genet 30:925–928, 1988.


## EEC syndrome

### Ectrodactyly-ectodermal dysplasia-clefting syndrome
(MIM No. *129900; POSSUM No. 3211)

Reports associating ectrodactyly (lobster-claw anomaly) of the hands and feet with cleft lip and ectodermal dysplasia date back to the early 1800s.[4,10] In 1970, Rüdiger et al.[16] suggested the designation *EEC* association.

### General manifestations

The majority of patients show absent lacrimal puncti, diminished tearing, dacryocystitis, and blepharophimosis leading to photophobia, corneal ulcers, keratoconjunctivitis, and loss of vision.[5,7,9] Ectrodactyly usually involves all the extremities. Syndactyly may occasionally be seen. Decreased sweating, mild dystrophy of the nails, light-colored sparse hair and pigmented nevi are described.[5,10,16] Mental retardation, renal anomalies, and cryptorchidism are occasionally reported.[2,5,9,11] Growth hormone deficiency has also been reported.[8]

### Otolaryngological manifestations

Cleft lip/palate is seen in the majority of patients. It is often bilateral. The maxilla is hypoplastic. Other anomalies include

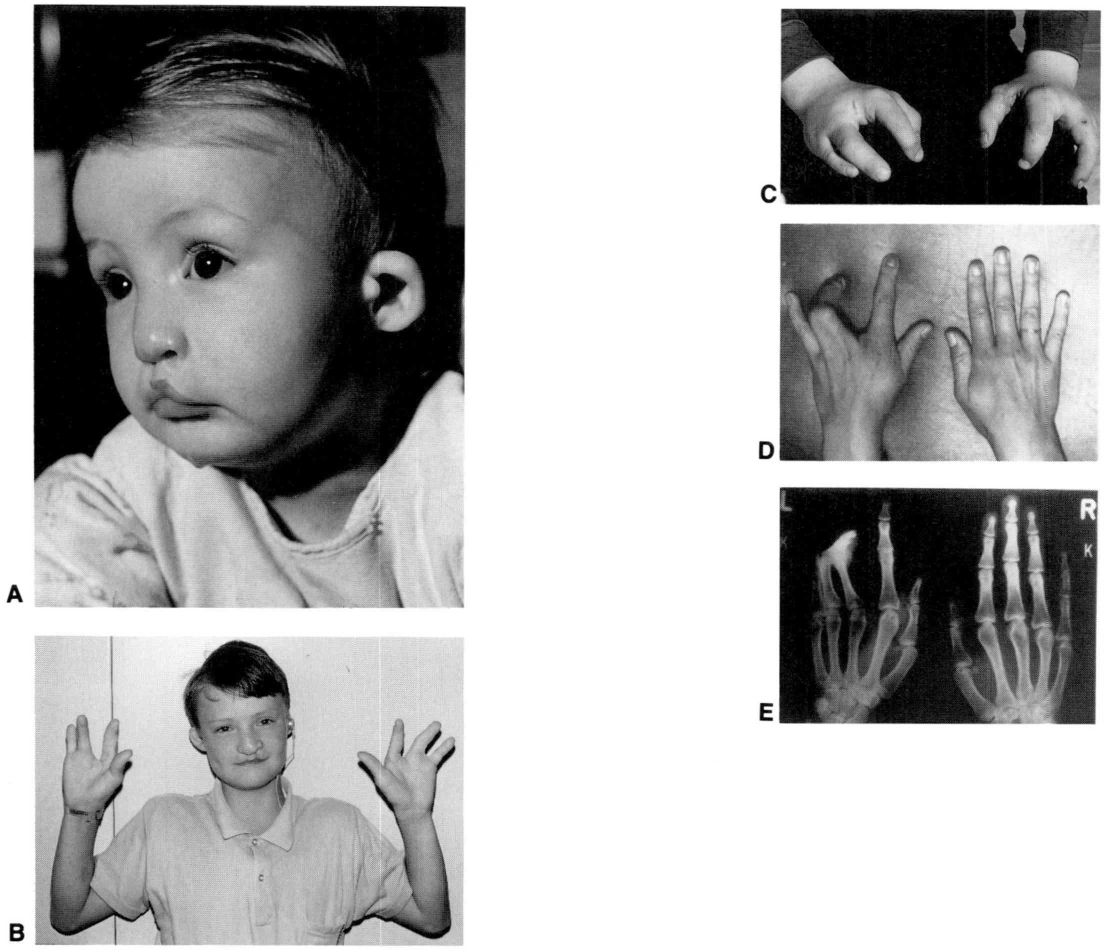

**Fig. 23.** EEC syndrome. A: Note abnormal pinna and repaired cleft lip. B: Note abnormal pinnae, hearing aid, repaired cleft lip and bilateral ectrodactyly. C: Ectrodactyly. D,E: Note ectrodactyly of the left hand with the corresponding roentgenogram. (D,E from W Kuster et al., Clin Genet 28:130, 1985, with permission.)

missing teeth, dysplasia of enamel, and dental caries. Furrowed tongue, xerostomia, and atresia of Stenson's ducts are reported. Thirty percent of patients have conductive hearing loss. Dysphonia due to dry mucous membranes was also reported. Malformed auricles and absent stapes are occasionally seen.[3,10,12,13,14,17,19]

### Etiology

Causation of this syndrome is associated with autosomal dominant inheritance. Low penetrance and variable expressivity have been observed.[7,9,18]

EEC syndrome is associated with chromosome 7 anomalies and it has been suggested that the responsible gene is in the region of 7p11.2–q21.3.[15] The finding of a reciprocal translocation between chromosomes 7 and 9 followed by fluorescence in situ hybridization studies suggests that the site of this condition is at 7p11.21.[6] A paracentric inversion (7) (q22.1;q36.3) was also reported.[1]

### Differential diagnosis

EEC syndrome should be differentiated from Rapp-Hodgkin syndrome, fetal alcohol syndrome, and odontotrichomelic syndrome.

## References


1. Akita S, Kuratomi H, Abe K, Harada N, Mukae N, Niikawa N: EC syndrome in a girl with paracentric inversion (7) (q22.1;q36.3). Clin Dysmorphol 2:62–67, 1993.
2. Aldenhoff P, von Muhlendahl KE, Waldenmaier C: Das EEC-Syndrom. Monatschrift Kinderheilkd 126:575–578, 1978.
3. Chiang TP, Robinson GC: Ectrodactyly, ectodermal dysplasia, and cleft lip/palate syndrome. The importance of dental anomalies. J Dent Child 41:38–42, 1974.
4. Cruveillier J: Anatomie pathologique du corps humain. In: Maladie des extrémités, Vol II, part 38. S. Baillière, Paris, 1829–1842.
5. Fried K: Ectrodactyly-ectodermal dysplasia-clefting (EEC) syndrome. Clin Genet 3:396–400, 1972.
6. Fukushima Y, Ohashi H, Hasegawa T: The breakpoints of the EEC syndrome (ectrodactyly, ectodermal dysplasia and cleft lip/palate) confirmed to 7q11.21 and 9p12 by fluorescence in situ hybridization [Letter]. Clin Genet 44:50, 1993.
7. Jaworska M, Popiolek J: Genetic counseling in lobster-claw anomaly: discussion of variability of genetic influence in different families. Clin Pediatr 7:396–399, 1968.
8. Knudtzon J, Aarskog D: Growth hormone deficiency associated with the ectrodactyly-ectodermal dysplasia-clefting syndrome and isolated absent septum pellucidum. Pediatrics 79:410–412,1987.
9. Kuster W, Majewski F, Meinecke P: EEC syndrome without ectrodactyly? Report of 8 cases. Clin Genet 28:130–135, 1985.
10. Leibowitz MR, Jenkins T: A newly recognized feature of ectrodactyly, ectodermal dysplasia, clefting (EEC) syndrome: Comedone naevus. Dermatologica 169:80–85, 1984.

11. London R, Heredia RM, Israel J: Urinary tract involvement in EEC syndrome. Am J Dis Child 139:1191–1193, 1985.
12. Parkash H, Sidhu SS, Dhannani N, Grewal MS: Ectrodactyly, ectodermal dysplasia, cleft lip and palate (EEC)—a rare syndrome. Indian J Pediatr 50:337–340, 1983.
13. Peterson-Falzone SJ, Caldarelli DD, Landahl KL: Abnormal laryngeal vocal quality in ectodermal dysplasia. Arch Otolaryngol 107:300–304, 1981.
14. Pries C, Pittleman D, Miller M, Solomon LM, Pashayan HM, Pruzansky S: The EEC syndrome. Am J Dis Child 127:840–844, 1974.
15. Qumsiyeh MB: EEC syndrome (ectrodactyly, ectodermal dysplasia and cleft lip/palate) is on 7p11.2–q21.3 [Letter] Clin Genet 42:101, 1992.
16. Rüdiger RA, Haase W, Passarge E: Assocation of ectrodactyly, ectodermal dysplasia and cleft lip/palate. Am J Dis Child 120:160–163, 1970.
17. Temtamy S, McKusick VA: The genetics of hand malformations. Birth Defects 14:157–172, 1978.
18. Walker JC, Clodius L: The syndromes of cleft lip, cleft palate and lobster claw deformities of hands and feet. Plast Reconstr Surg 32:627–636, 1963.
19. Wiedemann HR, Dibbern H: EEC-Syndrom. Med Welt 31:1862–1863, 1980.

A

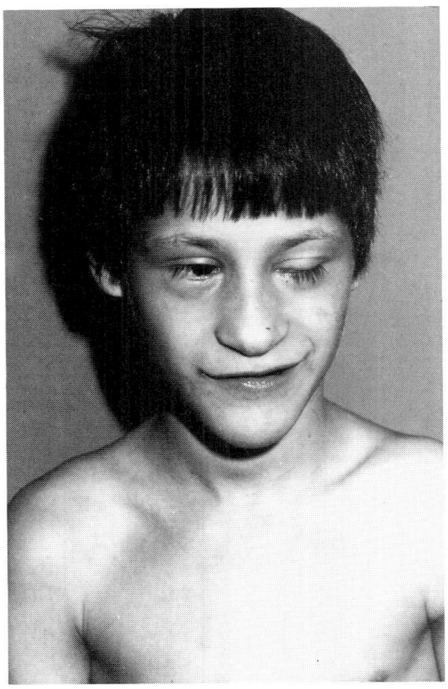

B

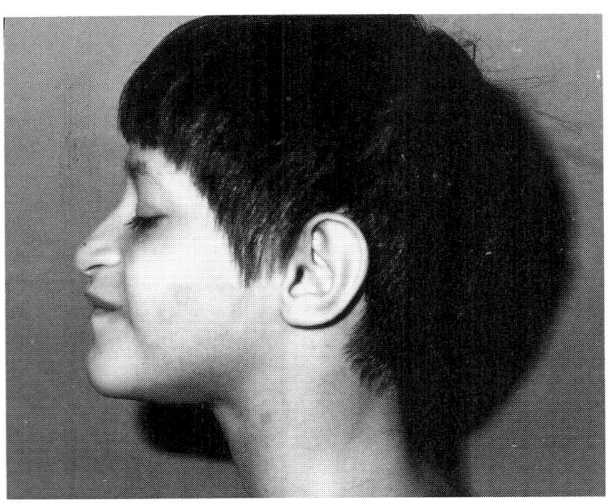

**Fig. 24.** Fetal alcohol syndrome. A,B: Note the narrow forehead, ptosis of the left eyelid, midfacial hypoplasia, and thin upper lip.

## Fetal alcohol syndrome

(POSSUM No. 3218)

In 1968, P. Lemoine of Nantes, France, recognized that intake of alcohol by a pregnant mother can have serious effects on the developing fetus. The more severe end of the spectrum of these effects is recognized as the *fetal alcohol syndrome*.[4,6]

### General manifestations

Characteristic features include prenatal and postnatal growth deficiency and microcephaly, with an average IQ of 63. Irritability and hyperactivity are common. Seizures disorders have been identified in 10%–20% of patients. Neural tube defects may be present.[1,6,7]

Other than the otolaryngological anomalies, patients may have hypoplasia of the optic nerve, increased tortuosity of the retinal vessels, and severe microphthalmia and colobomas.

Cardiac,[9] renal,[5] and skeletal anomalies may be present. Malignant neoplasms of embryonal origin have also been reported.[2]

### Otolaryngological manifestations

Facial dysmorphic features include a narrow forehead, short palpebral fissures, epicanthal folds, ptosis of the eyelids, midface hypoplasia, a short nose, a smooth philtrum, a thin upper lip, and a hypoplastic mandible.[10] Cleft palate or cleft lip may be present. Both conductive and sensorineural hearing loss are frequent.[3]

### Etiology

Alcohol[8] and its major metabolite, acetaldehyde,[8a] may be teratogenic. Alcohol-related developmental abnormalities can be due to restriction of cell growth during critical periods. The amount of alcohol intake needed to cause fetal alcohol syndrome is not clearly established.

### Differential diagnosis

Fetal alcohol syndrome should be differentiated from Dubowitz syndrome, de Lange syndrome, familial blepharophimosis syndrome, and fetal phenylketonuria (PKU) effect.

### References

1. Castro-Gago M, Rodriguez-Cervilla J, Ugarte J, Novo I, Pombo M: Maternal alcohol ingestion and neural tube defects. J Pediatr 104:796–797, 1984.
2. Cavdar AO: Fetal alcohol syndrome, malignancies and zinc deficiency. J Pediatr 105:335, 1984.
3. Church MW, Gerkin KP: Hearing disorders with fetal alcohol syndrome. Pediatrics 82:147–154, 1988.
4. Clarren SK, Smith DW: The fetal alcohol syndrome. N Engl J Med 298:1063–1067, 1978.
5. Debeukelaer MM, Randall CL, Stroud DR: Renal anomalies in the fetal alcohol syndrome. J Pediatr 91:759–760, 1977.
6. Graham JM Jr, Hanson JW, Darby BL, Barr HM, Streissguth AP: Independent dysmorphology evaluation at birth and 4 years of age for children exposed to varying amounts of alcohol in utero. Pediatrics 81:772–778, 1988.

7. Kennedy LA: The pathogenesis of brain abnormalities in the fetal alcohol syndrome: an integrating hypothesis. Teratology 29:363–368, 1984.
8. Larsson G, Bohlin AB, Tunell R: Prospective study of children exposed to variable amounts of alcohol in utero. Arch Dis Child 60:316–321, 1985.
8a. Ryle PR, Thomson AD: Acetaldehyde and fetal alcohol syndrome. Lancet 2:219–220, 1983.
9. Sardor GG, Smith DF, MacLeod PM: Cardiac malformations in the fetal alcohol syndrome. J Pediatr 98:771–773, 1981.
10. Wood RE: Fetal alcohol syndrome: Its implications for dentistry. J Am Dent Assoc 95:596–599, 1977.

## Fetal rubella syndrome

(POSSUM No. 3222)

The effects of rubella virus on the fetus were first described by Gregg in 1941.[3]

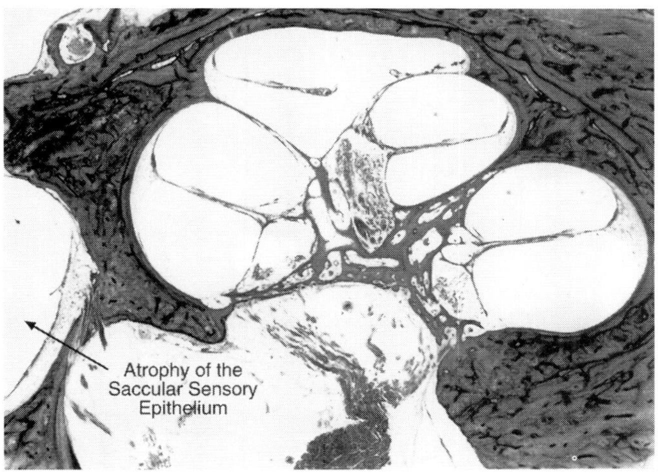


A

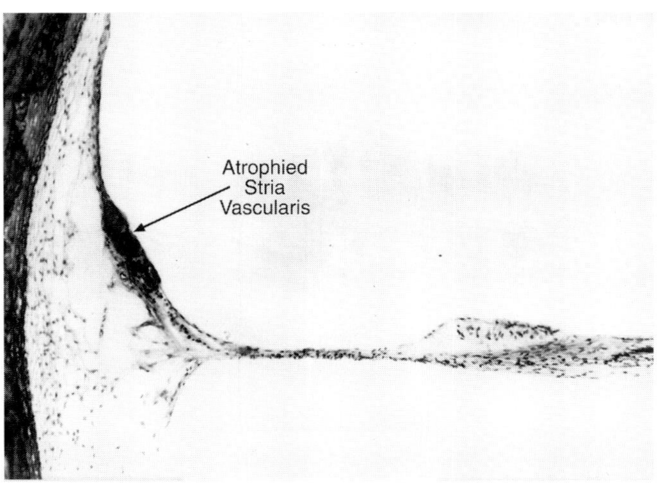


B

**Fig. 25.** Fetal rubella syndrome. A: The walls of the saccule are partially collapsed on the atrophied otolithic membrane. B: The organ of Corti consists of a thin layer of flattened cells. The stria vascularis is composed of a small layer of compact cells associated with scattered basophilic cystic structures. (With permission from HF Schuknecht, *Pathology of the Ear,* 2nd ed., Lea & Febiger, Philadelphia, 1993, p. 146).

### General manifestations

Fetal death may occur or the infant may be born with low birth weight, hepatosplenomegaly, large anterior fontanel, cataract, glaucoma, corneal opacities, chorioretinitis, microphthalmia, myocardial disease, septal heart defect, and patent ductus arteriosus. In addition, anemia, thrombocytopenia, purpura, jaundice, and interstitial pneumonia may occur. Pleocytosis, elevated cerebrospinal fluid (CSF) protein levels, and elevated serum IgM are documented.[4–7] Mental deficiency is common and 80% have an IQ below 80.

Endocrine anomalies include insulin-dependent diabetes mellitus, parathyroid gland problems, and hypopituitarism. Diabetes mellitus may develop later in life. Other findings include renal disease, hypospadias, cryptorchidism, and CNS anomalies.

Patients who survive infancy may have a normal life span. Early intensive treatment, special education, and a multidisciplinary approach are essential for the care of patients with multiple handicaps.[4–7]

### Etiology

This syndrome results from intrauterine rubella virus infection. The effects depend on the time of pregnancy when exposure occurs and may range from no effect to deafness only, to the full spectrum of the syndrome. Major effects occur when a nonimmune mother acquires the infection during the first trimester of the pregnancy.[1,3,6] However, cases of rubella embryopathy have also been recorded after previous maternal immunity.[2]

The virus remains in the tissues and infants with congenital rubella shed it in saliva, urine, and stools for months after birth. Shedding of virus is uncommon after the age of 1 year.

#### References

1. Cooper LZ, Krugman S: Diagnosis and management: congenital rubella. Pediatrics 37:335–338, 1966.
2. Das BD, Lakhani P, Kurtz JB, Hunter N, Watson BE, Cartwright KA, Caul EO, Roome APCH: Congenital rubella after previous maternal immunity. Arch Dis Child 65:545–546, 1990.
3. Gregg NM: Congenital cataract following German measles in the mother. Trans Ophthalmol Soc Aust 3:35, 1941.
4. Hardy JB: Clinical and development aspects of congenital rubella. Arch Otolaryngol 98:230–236, 1973.
5. Menser MA, Dods L, Harley JD: A twenty-five-year follow-up of congenital rubella. Lancet 2:1347–1350, 1967.
6. Miller E, Cradock-Watson JE, Pollock TM: Consequences of confirmed maternal rubella at successive stages of pregnancy. Lancet 2:781–784, 1982.
7. Ueda K, Nishida Y, Oshima K, Shepard TH: Congenital rubella syndrome: correlation of gestation age at time of maternal rubella with type of defect. J Pediatr 94:763–765, 1979.

## Fragile X syndrome

(MIM No. *309550; POSSUM No. 3324)

Lubs documented in 1969 the presence of a fragile site on the long arm of the X chromosome in affected males and some female carriers in one family.[4] The syndrome represents 50% of cases of X-linked mental retardation. The incidence is 1 in 1,250 males.

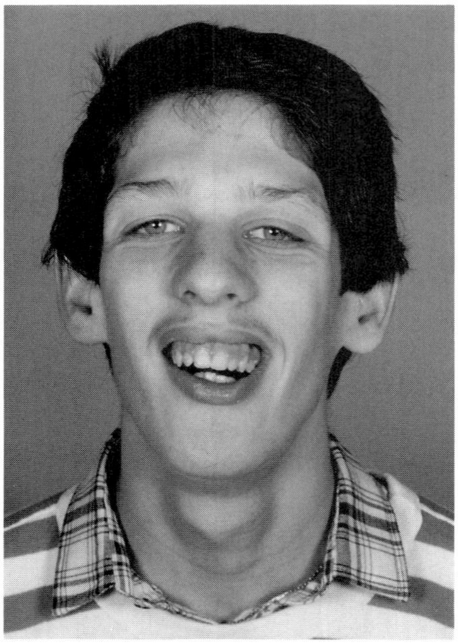

**Fig. 26.** Fragile X syndrome. Note the characteristic facies, downward slanting palpebral fissures, and prominent mandible. (Courtesy of Dr. B Lemieux.)

### General manifestations

Mental deficiency is present in 80% of affected males and 35% of carrier females. I.Q. varies in males between 30 and 55. When present in females, mental retardation is usually mild or borderline.[5,6,10] The life span is normal.

Retarded motor development, clumsiness, hyperactivity, hypotonia, automutilation, autistic or aggressive behavior, and seizures may also be present.[10] Macroorchidism, soft testes, hyperpigmented scrotum, and penile enlargement are noted in half of the affected individuals. Joint laxity in the fingers, knees, and ankles as well as flat feet, soft velvety skin, and mitral valve prolapse with mild aortic dilatation may be associated with this condition.[1,2,6,8,10]

### Otolaryngological manifestations

Increased head circumference, a prominent forehead, a broad-based nose, prognathism, large ears with everted pinnae, and absent lobules are characteristic of this syndrome. Speech is delayed and repetitive phrases are often expressed. The palate is high arched, occasionally cleft, with prominent palatine ridges, crossbite and open bite.[3,6,9]

### Etiology

Fragile X syndrome is of X-linked inheritance. The X chromosome shows a light-staining site at Xq27.3 in 40%–60% of cells.[8] The *FMR-1* gene has been identified at this site, containing an unstable region of DNA, segregating with the phenotype. This region involves CGG repeat sequences. The normal number of repeats is around 60 and the phenotype becomes manifest when the threshhold of 200 repeats is passed. A pedigree may have male carriers of the premutation (CGG repeats of 60–200). The CGG repeat number is increased when the gene passes through a female. The reliable diagnosis of this condition is presently done by molecular analysis.[5,7]

### References


1. Chudley AE, Hagerman RJ: Fragile X syndrome. J Pediatr 110:821–831, 1987.
2. Fryns JP: The Fragile X syndrome. A study of 83 families. Clin Genet 26:497–528, 1984.
3. Loehr JP, Synhorst DP, Wolfe RR, Hagerman RJ: Aortic root dilatation and mitral valve prolapse in the fragile X syndrome. Am J Med Genet 23:189–194, 1986.
4. Lubs HA: A marker X chromosome. Am J Hum Genet 21:231–244, 1969.
5. Oostra BA, Jacky PB, Brown WT, Rousseau F: Guidelines for the diagnosis of fragile X syndrome. J Med Genet 30:410–413, 1993.
6. Opitz JM, Sutherland GR: International workshop on the fragile X and X-linked mental retardation. Am J Med Genet 17:5–94, 1984.
7. Rousseau F: The fragile X syndrome: implications of molecular genetics for the clinical syndrome. Eur J Clin Invest 24:1–10, 1994.
8. Schmidt A: Fragile site Xq27 and mental retardation. Clinical and cytogenetic manifestation in heterozygotes and hemizygotes of five kindreds. Hum Genet 60:322–327, 1982.
9. Shellhart WC, Casamassimo PS, Hagerman RJ, Belanger GK: Oral findings in fragile X syndrome. Am J Med Genet 23:179–187, 1986.
10. Veenema H, Veenema T, Geraedts JP: The fragile X syndrome in a large family. II. Psychological investigations. J Med Genet 24:32–38, 1987.


## Fraser syndrome

### Cryptophthalmos syndrome, Fraser type
(MIM No.'s *219000; POSSUM No. 3179)

### General manifestations

Mental retardation occurs in more than 80% of cases. Soft tissue syndactyly has been observed in 70% of patients. It may affect the fingers and toes. Abnormalities of the genitals occur in 50%–80% of cases; these include cryptorchidism, hypoplastic penis, large clitoris/labia majora, rudimentary uterus, and atresia of the vagina. Renal agenesis has been reported in 80% of cases. Gonadoblastoma may be found. Occasional anomalies

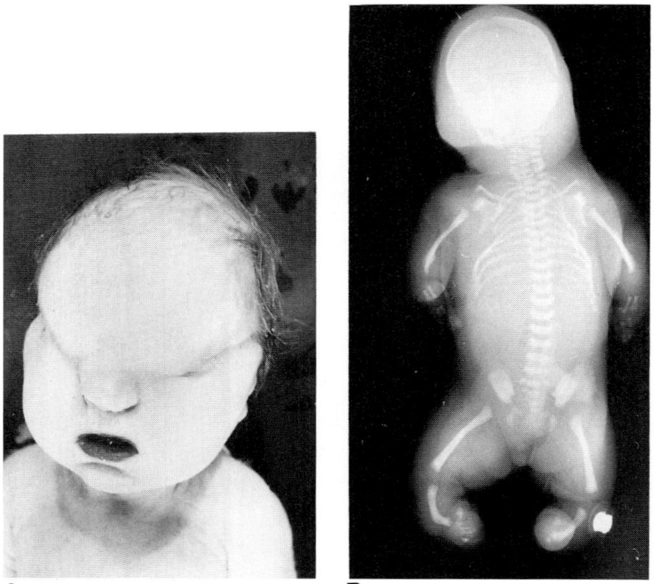

A B

**Fig. 27.** Fraser syndrome. A: Note bilateral cryptophthalmos. B: Skeletal X-ray showing micromelia of all limbs, with marked bowing of the tibiae. (With permission from PA Boyd et al., Am J Med Genet 31:159–168, 1988, courtesy of Dr. JW Keeling.)

include calcified falx cerebri, encephalocele, omphalocele, pulmonary hyperplasia, and congenital heart lesions.[4–6,8]

### Otolaryngological manifestations

Cryptophthalmos is present in 89% of cases. It is mostly bilateral. Upper lid colobomas, microphthalmia, symblepharon, and epibulbar dermoids may be present. Anomalies of the ears are described in 60%–80% of patients. They include microtia, low-set ears, absent pinnae, and atresia of the external auditory canals. Ossicular anomalies may occur. No inner ear anomalies are described. Anomalies of the nose include beaked nose, notched or pinpoint nostrils, choanal atresia, and alar colobomas. Laryngeal atresia, stenosis, fusion of the vocal cords, and laryngeal webs are documented. Cleft lip/palate and tongue-tie occur in 10% of patients. Malocclusion and hypoplastic teeth are also known to occur.[1–3,7,9,10]

### Etiology

Fraser syndrome is of autosomal recessive inheritance.

### References


1. Ford FR, Irving RM, Jones NS, Bailey CM: ENT manifestations of Fraser syndrome. J Laryngol Otol 106:1–4, 1992.
2. Goldhammer Y, Smith J: Cryptophthalmos syndrome with basal encephaloceles. Am J Ophthalmol 80:146–149, 1975.
3. Karas DE, Respler DS: Fraser syndrome: a case report and review of the otolaryngologic manifestations. Int J Pediatr Otolaryngol 31:85–90, 1995.
4. Labbe A, Dechelotte P, Lemery D, Malpuech G: Pulmonary hyperplasia in Fraser Syndrome. Ped Pulmonology 14:131–134, 1992.
5. Levine RS, Powers T, Rosenberg HK, Siegel CA, Bilaniuk LT: The cryptophthalmos syndrome. Am J Roentgenol 143:375–376, 1984.
6. Lurie IW, Cherstvoy ED: Renal agenesis as a diagnostic feature of the cryptophthalmos-syndactyly syndrome. Clin Genet 25:528–532, 1984.
7. Mina MM, Greenberg C, Levin B: ENT abnormalities associated with Fraser syndrome: case report and literature review. J Otolaryngol 127:233–236, 1988.
8. Mortimer C, McEwan HP, Yates JRW: Fraser syndrome presenting as monozygotic twins with bilateral renal agenesis. J Med Genet 22:76–78, 1985.
9. Thomas IT, Frias JL, Felix V, Sanchez de Leon L, Hernandez RA, Jone MC: Isolated and syndromic cryptophthalmos. Am J Med Genet 25:85–98, 1986.
10. Waring GO, Shields JA: Partial unilateral cryptophthalmos with syndactyly, brachycephaly and renal anomalies. Am J Ophthalmol 79:437–440, 1975.


## Fryns syndrome

### (MIM No. *229850; POSSUM No. 3608)

Fryns et al.[3] reported this multiple congenital anomaly syndrome in 1979. The main features include cleft palate, diaphragmatic hernia, coarse facies, and acral hypoplasia. It is estimated that the prevalence of the syndrome is 0.7 to 1 in 10,000 births.[1]

### General manifestations

Diaphragmatic hernia is the constant feature of this syndrome. It is usually unilateral and commonly on the left side. Pulmonary hypoplasia and the absence of lung lobulations may contribute to the pathogenesis. Other anomalies include gastrointestinal malrotations, atresia of the duodenum or esophagus, omphalocele, and aganglionosis of the gut and anal anomalies. Cardiac defects (ASD, VSD), cystic kidneys, bicornuate uterus, hypoplastic vagina, cryptorchidism, distal limb hypoplasia, and extranumerary vertebrae may occur.[1,3–5] Hydramnios in the second trimester and intrauterine death in the third trimester occur frequently.

### Otolaryngological manifestations

The face is coarse and hirsute. Macrostoma, cleft lip or palate, flat nasal bridge, large nose with anteverted nostrils, and narrow palpebral fissures occur. The auricles are poorly shaped and the attached ear lobes are hypoplastic. The neck is short and broad. Olfactory bulb agenesis is reported.[3,4,6]

### Etiology

Fryns syndrome is of autosomal recessive inheritance.[2]

### Differential diagnosis

Fryns syndrome should be differentiated from Brachman de Lange syndrome, trisomy 18 syndrome, Rüdiger syndrome, and Zellweger syndrome.

### References


1. Aymé S, Julian C, Gambarelli D, Mariotti B, Luciani A, Sudan N, Maurin N, Philip N, Serville F, Carles D, et al: Fryns syndrome. Report on 8 new cases. Clin Genet 35:191–201, 1989.
2. Bamforth JS, Leonard CO, Chodirker BN, Chitayat D, Gritter HL, Evans JA, Keena B, Pantzar R, Friedman JM, Hall JG: Congenital diaphragmatic hernia, coarse facies and acral hypoplasia: Fryns syndrome. Am J Med Genet 32:93–99, 1989.
3. Fryns JP, Moerman F, Goddeeris P, Bosuyt C, Van den Berghe H: A new lethal syndrome with cloudy corneae, diaphragmatic defects and distal limb deformities. Hum Genet 50:65–70, 1979.
4. Goddeeris P, Fryns JP, van den Berghe H: Diaphragmatic defects, cranial dysmorphism, cleft palate and distal limb deformities: a new lethal syndrome. J Genet Hum 28:57–60, 1980.
5. Meinecke P, Fryns JP: The Fryns syndrome: diaphragmatic defects, craniofacial dysmorphism, and distal digital hypoplasia: further evidence for autosomal recessive inheritance. Clin Genet 28:516–520, 1985.
6. Moerman P, Fryns J, Van den Berghe H, Cevleiger H, Lauveryns JM: The syndrome of diaphragmatic hernia, abnormal face and distal limb anomalies (Fryns syndrome): report of two sibs with further delineation of the multiple congenital anomaly (MCA) syndrome. Am J Med Genet 31:805–814, 1988.


## Gardner syndrome

### (MIM No. *175100; POSSUM No. 3766)

### General manifestations

The main findings of this syndrome are polyposis of the colon and rectum with a tendency toward malignant degeneration, multiple osteomas of the facial bones, cutaneous epidermoid cysts, and fibrous hyperplasia of the skin and mesentery. Other sites of polyposis include the stomach and small intestine. Carcinoma of the ampulla of Vater has also been described.[5,8,12]

Desmoid tumors occur in a high percentage of patients with

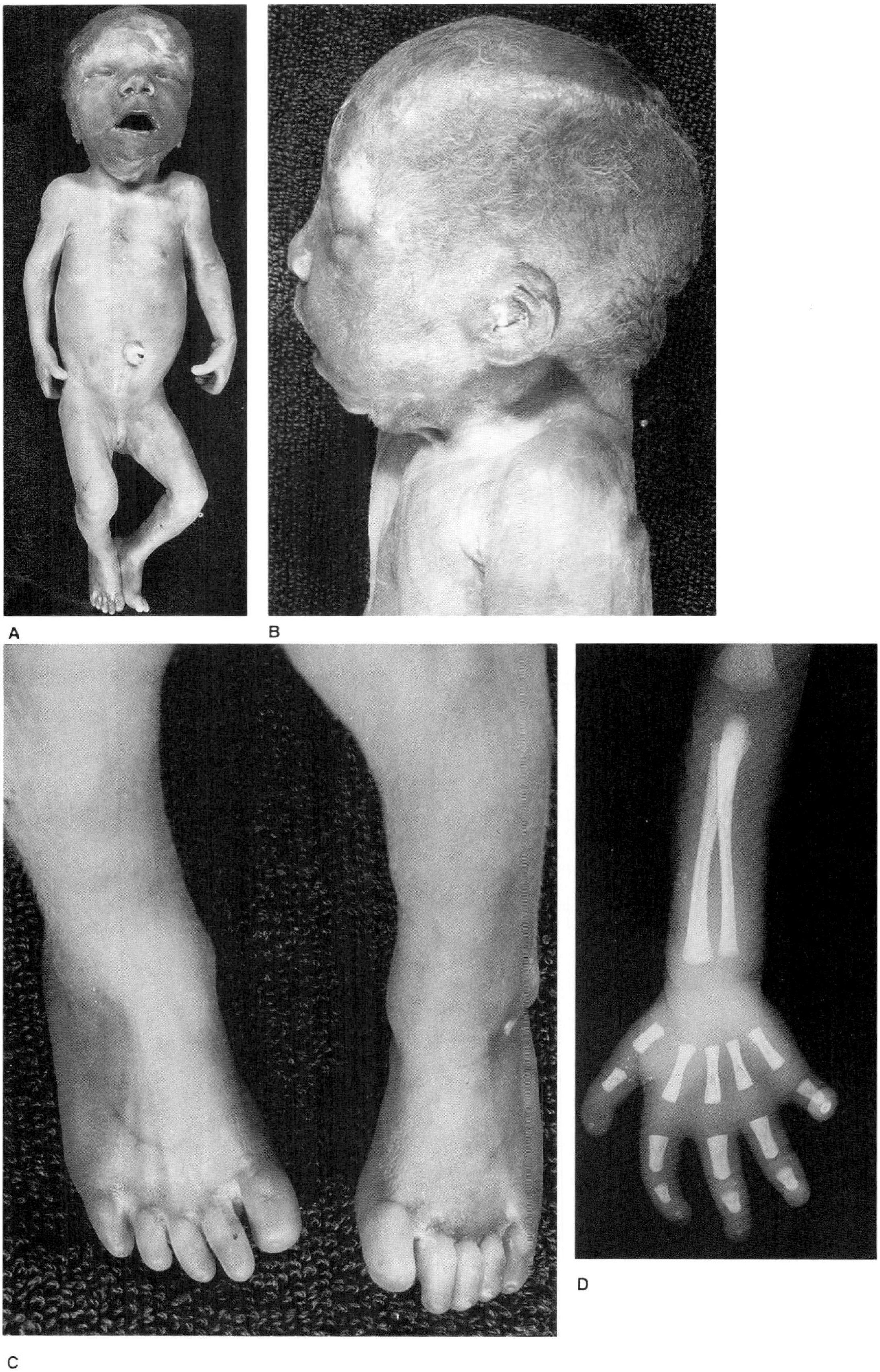

**Fig. 28.** Fryns syndrome. Note the flat, upturned nose, macrostoma, and short philtrum (A); low-set ears with posterior angulation (B); and hypoplastic terminal digits (C). D: X-ray showing agenesis of terminal phalanges. (With permission from JP Fryns et al., Hum Genet 50:65, 1979.)

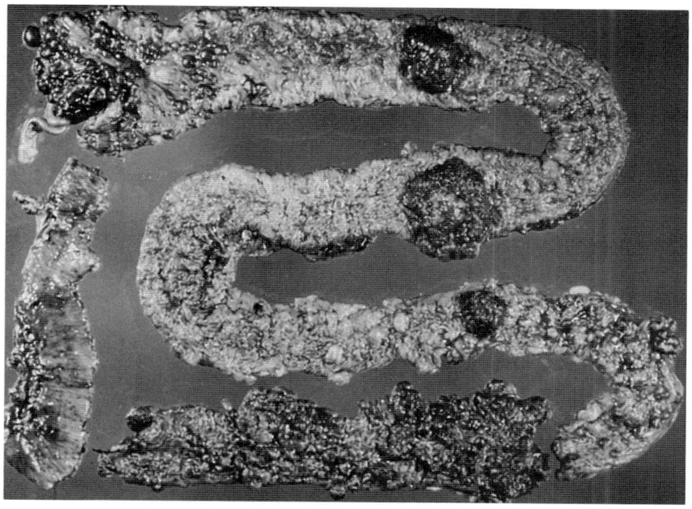

**Fig. 29.** Gardner syndrome. Note multiple polyps of the colon. (From RJ Gorlin et al.: *Syndromes of the Head and Neck,* 3rd ed., Oxford University Press, 1990, p. 368.)

Gardner syndrome. They may be seen a few years after surgery in the abdominal wall or may occur in the different musculoaponeurotic structures. Mesenteric fibrosis is also frequent.[7,9]

Epidermoid cysts of the skin occur in approximately 50% of cases. They occur on the extremities and scalp. The cysts appear usually in the fourth decade and precede the occurrence of the intestinal polyps. Histologically, a high number of the cysts resemble pilomatrixomas.[3,8,12]

Other manifestations include bilateral congenital hypertrophy of the retinal epithelium in some pedigrees. Various CNS tumors, papillary cancer of the thyroid, adrenal adenoma, neurofibroma, and basal cell carcinoma have been reported.[2,10,11]

### Otolaryngological manifestations

Osteomas of the calvaria, paranasal sinuses and the jaws are commonly seen. The rest of the skeletal systems (e.g., radius, ulna, metacarpals) may also be involved, but this is usually minimal compared to the face.[6,13] Supernumerary teeth have also been described.

### Etiology

Gardner syndrome is of autosomal dominant inheritance with markedly variable expressivity.[11] The gene has been mapped to the long arm of chromosome 5 (5q21–q22).[1,12] The syndrome is caused by germ-line mutations of the adenomatous polypsis coli gene (APC).[4]

### Differential diagnosis

Gardner syndrome should be differentiated from other syndromes with intestinal polyposis and, in particular, Turcot syndrome with CNS tumors.

#### References


1. Burn J, Chapman PD, Eastham EJ: Annotation: familial adenomatous polyposis. Arch Dis Child 71:103–107, 1994.
2. Cohen SB: Familial polyposis coli and its extracolonic manifestations. J Med Genet 19:193–203, 1982.
3. Cooper PH, Fechner RE: Pilomatrixoma-like changes in the epidermal cysts of Gardner's syndrome. J Am Acad Dermatol 8:639–644, 1983.
4. Davies DR, Armstrong JG, Thakker N, Horner K, Guy SP, Clancy T, Sloan P, Blavi V, Dodd C, Warnes TW, Harris R, Evans DGR: Severe Gardner syndrome in families with mutations restricted to a specific region of the APC gene. Am J Hum Genet 57:1151–1158, 1995.
5. Hamilton SR, Bussey HJR: Ilial adenomas after colostomy in nine patients with adenomatous polyposis coli/Gardner's syndrome. Gastroenterology 77:1252–1257, 1979.
6. Ida M, Nakamura T, Utsunomiya J: Osteomatosis changes and tooth abnormalities found in the jaws of patients with adenomatosis coli. Oral Surg Oral Med Oral Path 52:2–11, 1981.
7. Kratzer GL, Kasumi A, Krash AJ: Gardner syndrome: a study and follow-up of a family. Am J Med Genet 41:393–397, 1991.
8. Leppard B, Bussey HJR: Epidermoid cysts, polyposis coli and Gardner's syndrome. Br J Surg 62:387–393, 1975.
9. McAdam WAF, Goligher JC: The occurrence of desmoids in patients with familial polyposis coli. Br J Surg 57:618–631, 1970.
10. Michels VV, Stevens JC: Basal cell carcinoma in a patient with intestinal polyposis. Clin Genet 22:80–82, 1982.
11. Naylor EW, Gardner EJ: Penetrance and expressivity of the gene responsible for the Gardner syndrome. Clin Genet 11:381–393, 1977.
12. Rasheed S, Rhim JS, Gardner EJ; Inherited susceptibility to retrovirus-induced transformation of Gardner syndrome cells. Am J Med Genet 35:919–931, 1983.
13. Watne AL: Syndromes of polyposis coli and cancer. Curr Prob Cancer 7:3–31, 1982.


## Goldenhar syndrome

### Oculo-auriculo-vertebral dysplasia spectrum or Facio-auriculo-vertebral sequence
(MIM No. 164210; POSSUM No. 3339)

Gorlin et al.[8] proposed the term *oculo-auriculo-vertebral dysplasia* for the spectrum of anomalies ranging from hemifacial microsomia, which denotes unilateral microtia, mandibular hypoplasia, and microstoma, to Goldenhar syndrome, which also includes epibulbar dermoids and vertebral anomalies.

### General manifestations

Blepharoptosis, microphthalmia, epibulbar tumors, as well as retinal abnormalities have been documented. Visual acuity is usually reduced.

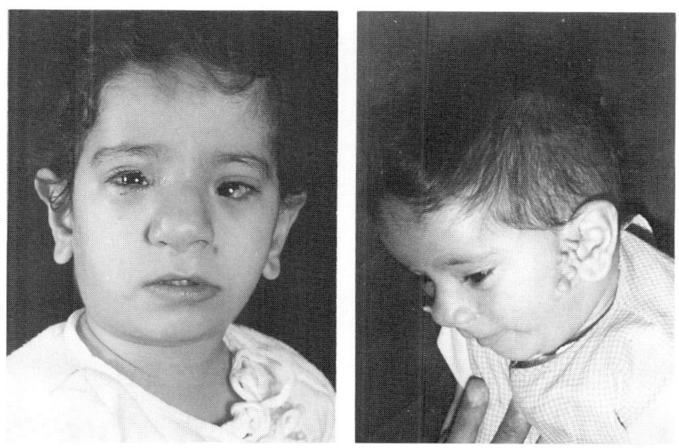

A B

**Fig. 30.** Goldenhar syndrome. Note the epibulbar dermoid of the left eye, coloboma of the right upper eyelid, and the left hemifacial hypoplasia (A), as well as the preauricular appendages and abnormal pinna (B). (With permission from VM Der Kaloustian, AK Kurban, *Genetic Diseases of the Skin,* Springer-Verlag, Berlin, 1979, p. 103.)

Mental retardation varies in the reported series between 5 and 15%.[17] Children with anophthalmia/microphthalmia and cleft lip/palate seem to be at increased risk for cerebral malformation and mental retardation.[16] Various cardiac anomalies are described, ranging from ventricular septal defect, patent ductus arteriosus, and Fallot's tetralogy to coarctation of the aorta.[6,13] Renal ectopia and hydronephrosis are less common. Talipes equinovarus deformities and other limb anomalies are rare occurrences.

### Otolaryngological manifestations

The mandibular ramus and condyles are hypoplastic. The maxilla, malar, and temporal bone are smaller on one side.[14] The mastoid is also poorly pneumatized. Approximately one-third of the cases show bilateral involvement.

The right side is involved in 60% of cases.[13] Macrostoma or pseudomacrostoma (lateral cleft-like extension of the corner of the mouth) is a usual occurrence.

The parotid gland is also affected (agenesis or displaced salivary tissue).[7] Cleft palate/lip occurs approximately 10% of the time. Delayed dental development occurs on the hypoplastic side,[4] as do lingual and palatal malformations.[15,18] Microtia or occasional anotia, and preauricular tags occur between the tragus and the corner of the mouth. The middle ear demonstrates ossicular anomalies and an abnormal course of the facial nerve. Hearing loss is more commonly conductive than sensorineural.[1,2,19] Cervical vertebral anomalies occur in 30% of cases.[5] Hemivertebrae and fused vertebrae have been described. Tracheal and pulmonary anomalies and tracheoespophageal fistula are less common.[3,10]

### Etiology and pathogenesis

Sporadic occurrence in the majority of cases. One to two percent of reported cases occur in families suggesting autosomal dominant transmission.[12] Animal models have shown that vascular disruption and hematoma formation affect the developing structures of the jaw and ear regions in utero. Other hypotheses suggest that disturbance of the population of the neural crest cells occurs between days 30 and 45 of gestation. The frequency of the condition ranges between 1:3,500 and 1:25,000 births.[9,11]

### Differential diagnosis

Goldenhar syndrome should be differentiated from Townes-Brooks syndrome, Nager syndrome, VATER, and CHARGE associations.

### References


1. Aleksic S, Budzilovich G, Greco MA, McCarthy J, Reuben R, Margolis S, Epstein F, Feigin I, Pearson J: Intracranial lipomas, hydrocephalus and other CNS anomalies in oculoauriculo-vertebral dysplasia (Goldenhar-Gorlin syndrome). Childs Brain 11:285–297, 1984.
2. Bassila MK, Goldberg R: The association of facial and/or sensorineural hearing loss in patients with hemifacial microsomia. Am J Med Genet 26:287–291, 1989.
3. Bowen AD, Parry WH: Bronchopulmonary foregut malformation in the Goldenhar anomalad. Am J Roentgenol 134:186–188, 1980.
4. Farias M, Vagervik K: Dental development in hemifacial microsomia. Eruption and agenesis. Pediatr Dent 10:140–143, 1988.
5. Figueroa AA, Friede H: Craniovertebral malformations in hemifacial microsomia. J Craniofac Genet Dev Biol Suppl 1:167–178, 1985.
6. Friedman S, Savador M: The high frequency of congenital heart disease in oculo-auriculo-vertebral dysplasia (Goldenhar's syndrome). J Pediatr 85:873–874, 1974.
7. Gorlin RJ, Cohen MM Jr, Levin SL: Syndromes of the Head and Neck, 3rd ed. Oxford University Press, New York, 1990, p 646.
8. Gorlin RJ, Jue KL, Jacobson U, Goldschmidt E: Oculoauriculovertebral dysplasia. J Pediatr 63:991–999, 1963.
9. Grobb WC: The first and second branchial arch syndrome. Plast Reconstr Surg 36:485–508, 1965.
10. Inglis AF Jr, Kokesh J, Siebert J, Richardson HA: Vertically fused tracheal cartilage. An underrecognized anomaly. Arch Otolaryngol Head Neck Surg 118:436–438, 1992.
11. Poswillo D: Otomandibular deformity: pathogenesis as a guide to reconstruction. J Maxillofac Surg 2:64–72, 1974.
12. Regenbogen L, Godel V, Goya V, Goodman RM: Further evidence for an autosomal dominant form of oculo-auriculo-vertebral dysplasia. Clin Genet 21:161–167, 1982.
13. Rollnick BR, Kaye CI, Nagatoshi K, Hauck W, Martin AO. Oculoauriculovertebral dysplasia and variants. Phenotype characteristics of 294 patients. Am J Med Genet 26:361–375, 1987.
14. Rune B, Selvik G, Sarnos KV, Jacobson S: Growth in hemifacial microsomia studies with the aid of roentgen stereophotogrammetry and metallic implants. Cleft Palate J 1:128–146, 1981.
15. Samuels L, Lawson LI, Rowe LO: Characteristics of patients with hemifacial microsomia at the craniofacial center. In: Treatment of Hemifacial Microsomia, EP Harvold, ed. Alan R. Liss, New York, 1983, pp 51–55.
16. Schrander-Stumpel CT, de Die-Smulders CE, Hennekam RC, Fryns JP, Bouckaert PX, Brouwer OF, da Costa JJ, Lommen EJ, Maaswinkel-Mooy PD: Oculoauriculovertebral spectrum and cerebral anomalies. J Med Genet 29:326–331, 1992.
17. Shokeir MHK: The Goldenhar syndrome: a natural history. Birth Defects 13:67–83, 1977.
18. Shprintzen RJ, Croft CB, Berkman MD, Rakoff SJ: Velopharyngeal insufficiency in the facio-auriculo-vertebral malformation complex. Cleft Palate J 17:132–137, 1980.
19. Wells MD, Phelps PD, Michaels L: Oculo-auriculo-vertebral dysplasia: a temporal bone study of a case of Goldenhar syndrome. J Laryngol Otol 97:689–696, 1983.


## Gorlin syndrome

### Basal cell nevus syndrome
(MIM No. *109400; POSSUM No. 3527)

Gorlin and Goltz are credited with recognizing the full extent of this syndrome in 1960.[7] It is characterized by marfanoid habitus and skeletal anomalies, odontogenic dyskeratotic cysts, intracranial calcifications, and a predisposition toward basal cell carcinoma of the skin (BCC), medulloblastoma, ovarian fibromas, and a variety of other tumors.[6]

### General manifestations

Calcification of the falx cerebri and cerebelli, lumbarization of the sacrum, vertebral anomalies, spina bifida occulta, and pectus excavatum or carinatum occur in approximately one-third of patients. The palms and soles may show characteristic pits. They provide a diagnostic clue in patients before age 30. Other findings include meningiomas, mesenteric cysts, iris and optic colobomas, cataracts, glaucoma, nystagmus, strabismus, hypogonadism, and anosmia.[1,2,8,10,11] Calcified ovarian fibromas, ovarian carcinomas, cardiac fibroma, fetal rhabdomyoma, subcutaneous calcifications of skin, agenesis of corpus callosum, and mental retardation have also been reported.[12] Mental deficiency occurs in less than 10% of cases.

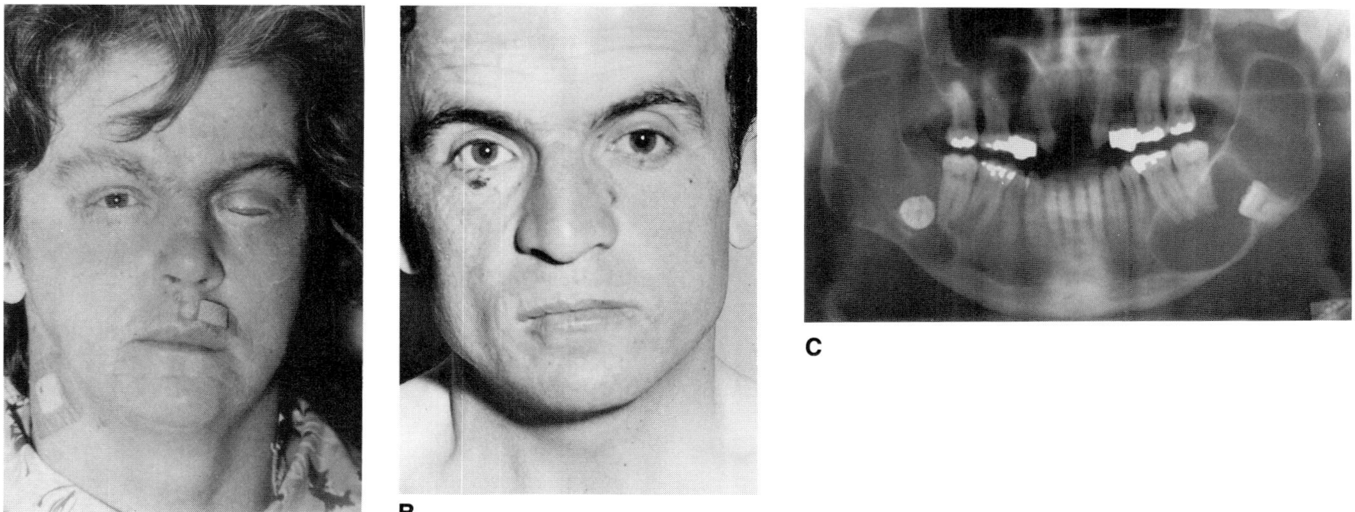

A B C

**Fig. 31.** Gorlin syndrome. A,B: Patients with numerous basal cell carcinomas. C: Panorex showing multiple keratocysts of the jaws. (A and B from VM Der Kaloustian, AK Kurban, *Genetic Diseases of the Skin,* Springer-Verlag, Berlin, 1979, p. 214; C from RJ Gorlin et al., *Syndromes of the Head and Neck,* 3rd ed., Oxford University Press, 1990, p. 373.)

### Otolaryngological manifestations

The frontoparietal bossing and increased size of the skull give these patients a characteristic facies in over two-thirds of cases.

The nose is broad, especially at the root, with mild hypertelorism and mild prognathism. Odontogenic keratocysts of the jaws and multiple basal cell nevi prone to carcinomatous changes occur over the neck, trunk, face, and upper limbs in over 50% of cases.[6] The nevi increase significantly in number around the age of puberty. Cleft lip and/or palate occurs in about 5% of patients.[12]

### Etiology

Inheritance is autosomal dominant. Paternal age is a factor in fresh mutational cases which represent 40% of patients.[8] This syndrome is an example of developmental defects and neoplasia related to a tumor-suppressor gene showing tight linkage to 9q22.3.[3–5] A two-hit model for the developmental defects has been suggested.[9] Mutation analysis revealed alterations of the human PTC gene in nevoid basal cell carcinoma syndrome (NBCCS) patients.[6a,6b]

### Differential diagnosis

Gorlin syndrome should be differentiated from Gardner syndrome. Jaw cysts, if few in number, may be mistaken for usual dental cysts or isolated keratocysts. The calcification of several organs may suggest pseudohypoparathyroidism.

### References


1. Berlin NI, Van Scott EJ, Clendenning WE, Archard HO, Block JB, Witkop C, Haynes HA: Basal cell nevus syndrome. Ann Intern Med 64:403–421, 1966.
2. Esser R, B Bohwert B: Neurologic symptoms of basal cell nevus syndrome. Eur Neurol 19:335–338, 1980.
3. Farndon PA, Del Mastro RG, Evans DG, Kilpatrick MW: Location of gene for Gorlin syndrome. Lancet 339:581–582, 1992.
4. Farndon PA, Morris DJ, Hardy C, McConville CM, Weissenbach J, Kilpatrick MW, Reis A: Analysis of 133 meioses places the genes for nevoid basal cell carcinoma (Gorlin) syndrome and Fanconi anemia group C in a 2–6 cM interval and contributes to the fine map of 9q22.3. Genomics 23:486–489, 1994.
5. Gailani MR, Bale SJ, Leffel DJ, DiGiovanna JJ, Peck GL, Poliak S, Drum MA, Pastakia B, McBride OW, Kase R, Green M, Mulvihill JJ, Bale AE: Developmental defects in Gorlin syndrome related to putative tumor suppressor gene in chromosome 9. Cell 69:111–117, 1992.
6. Gorlin RJ: Nevoid basal cell carcinoma syndrome. Medicine 66: 96–113, 1987.

6a. Hahn H, Wicking C, Zaphiropoulos PG, Gailani MR, Shanley S, Chidambaram A, Vorechovsky I, Holmberg E, Unden AB, Gillies S et al.: Mutations of the human homolog of drosophila *patched* in the nevoid basal cell carcinoma syndrome. Cell 85:841–851, 1996.

6b. Johnson RL, Rothman AL, Xie J, Goodrich LV, Bare JW, Bonifas JM, Quinn AG, Myers RM, Cox DR, Epstein EHJr, Scott MP: Human homolog of *patched,* a candidate gene for the basal cell nevus syndrome. Science 272:1668–1671, 1996.

7. Gorlin RJ; Goltz RW: Multiple nevoid basal-cell epithelioma, jaw cysts and rib syndromes. N Engl J Med 262:908–912, 1960.
8. Jones KL, Smith DW, Harvey MA, Hall BD, Quan L: Older paternal age and fresh gene mutation: data on additional disorders. J Pediatr 86:84–88, 1975.
9. Levanat S, Gorlin RJ, Fallet S, Johnson DR, Fantasia JE, Bale AE: A two-hit model for developmental defects in Gorlin syndrome. Nat Genet 12:85–87, 1996.
10. Rayner CR, Towers JF, Wilson JS: What is Gorlin syndrome? The diagnosis and management of basal cell nevus sydrome, based on a study of thirty-seven patients. Br J Plast Surg 30:62–67, 1977.
11. Southwick GJ, Schwartz RA: The basal cell nevus sydrome. Disasters occurring among a series of 36 patients. Cancer 44:2294–2305, 1979.
12. Van Dijk E, Neering H: The association of cleft lip and palate with basal cell nevus syndrome. Oral Surg 50:214–217, 1980.


## Hallermann-Streiff syndrome

### Oculo-mandibulo-facial or François dyscephalic syndrome

(MIM No. 234100; POSSUM No. 3342)

A hypoplastic mandible, pinched nose, proportionate dwarfism, hypotrichosis, microphthalmia, and congenital cataract characterize this syndrome.

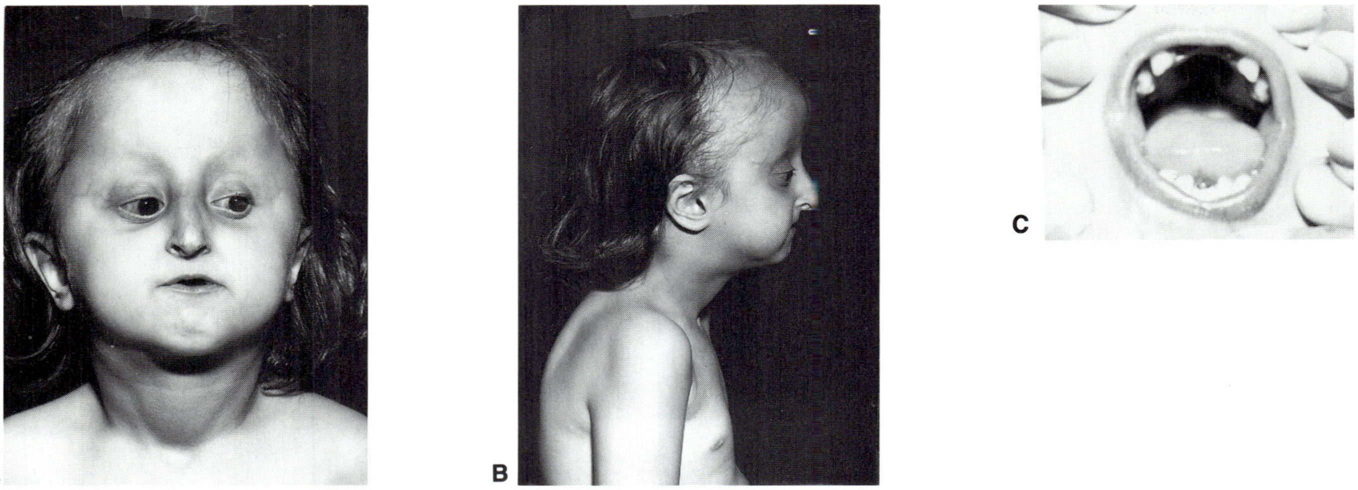

**Fig. 32.** Hallermann-Streiff syndrome Note sparse hair over the anterior part of the skull, absent eyebrows, scanty eyelashes and dilated nasal veins (A); the parrot-like profile (B); and partial anodontia (C). (With permission from VM Der Kaloustian, AK Kurban, *Genetic Diseases of the Skin,* Springer-Verlag, Berlin, 1979, p. 99.)

### General manifestations

Abnormal shape of the skull, with frontal and parietal bossing and brachycephaly, is present in almost all cases. Proportionate short stature occurs in approximately two-thirds of patients. Hypotrichosis and skin atrophy are also common (over 80%). Ocular manifestations are very common and include congenital cataract (80%–90%), microphthalmia (80%), nystagmus, strabismus (35%–40%), blue sclera (25%), iris atrophy, and fundus abnormalities.[11,12] Mental deficiency is present in 15%–30% of cases. Hypogenitalism (10%), enlarged clitoris, hypospadias, and cryptorchidism may be seen. Syndactyly, winged scapulae, cardiac anomalies, hypoparathyroidism, and deficient humoral immunity have been documented.[2,3,6]

### Otolaryngological manifestations

Characteristic features include malar and mandibular hypoplasia with micrognathia. The chin often shows central clefting or dimpling. There is also characteristic anterior displacement of the temporomandibular joint on X-rays. The nose is small, thin, and pointed. It tends to become parrot-shaped with advanced age. The cartilagenous tip is hypoplastic and the septum is often deviated. The palate is high arched. Teeth may be present at birth. Enamel dysplasia and malocclusion are common. The sinuses are hypoplastic. The skin is atrophied mostly over the nose and scalp. Scalp veins are prominent. Tracheomalacia has been reported. Respiratory obstruction may result in cor pulmonale.[1,4,5,7–10]

### Etiology

Most cases are sporadic. However, autosomal recessive inheritance is a possibility.

### Differential diagnosis

Hallermann-Streiff syndrome should be differentiated from Progeria and Treacher Collins syndrome.

### References

1. Barrucand D, Benradi C, Schmitt J: Le syndrome de François. A propos de deux cas. Rev Otoneuroophtalmol 50:305–326, 1978.
2. Chandra RK, Joglekar S, Antonio A: Deficiency of humoral immunity and hypoparathyroidism associated with the Hallermann-Streiff syndrome. J Pediatr 93:892–893, 1978.
3. Dinwiddie R, Gewitz M, Taylor JF: Cardiac defects in the Hallermann-Streiff syndrome. J Pediatr 92:77–78, 1978.
4. François J: François dyscephalic syndrome. Birth Defects 18:595–619, 1982.
5. Honda E, Inone T, Domon M, Sasaki T, Uchida T: Dental radiographic signs characteristic to Hallermann-Streiff syndrome. Oral Surg Oral Med Oral Path 70:121–125, 1990.
6. Imamura S, Ikeda E, Yoshida H: Hallermann-Streiff syndrome: case report. Dermatologica 160:3654–357, 1980.
7. Ponte F: Further contributions to the study of the syndrome of Hallermann and Streiff. Ophthalmologica 143:399–402, 1962.
8. Robinson M: Respiratory obstruction and cor pulmonale in the Hallermann-Streiff syndrome. Am J Med Genet 41:515–516, 1991.
9. Salbert BA, Stevens CA, Spence JE: Tracheomalacia in Hallermann-Streiff syndrome. Am J Med Genet 41:521–523, 1991.
10. Sclaroff A, Eppely BL: Evaluation and surgical correction of the facial skeletal deformity in Hallermann-Streiff syndrome. Int J Oral Maxillofac Surg 16:738–733, 1987.
11. Van Balen AT: Dyscephaly with microphthalmos, cataract and hypoplasia of the mandible. Ophthalmologica 141:53–63, 1961.
12. Walter JR, Jones DH: Spontaneous cataract absorption in Hallermann-Streiff syndrome. Ophthalmologica 150:401–408, 1965.

## Inner ear dysplasias

The dysplasias of the inner ear may be sporadic or hereditary. They may occur uni- or bilaterally. There are various types,[1,2,5,6,9,12,16,17] including the following:

1. Mondini dysplasia (incomplete development of the bony and membranous labyrinth)
2. Scheibe dysplasia (cochleo-saccular aplasia)
3. Trisomal dysplasias (which include trisomy 13,18,21, or 22). Other chromosomal dysplasias are seen in deletion syndromes, e.g., Cri du chat syndrome (or 5p-) and triploidy (XXX or XXY).
4. Large vestibular aqueduct syndrome
5. Michel aplasia or complete absence of the inner ear
6. Alexander type (membranous cochlear aplasia)

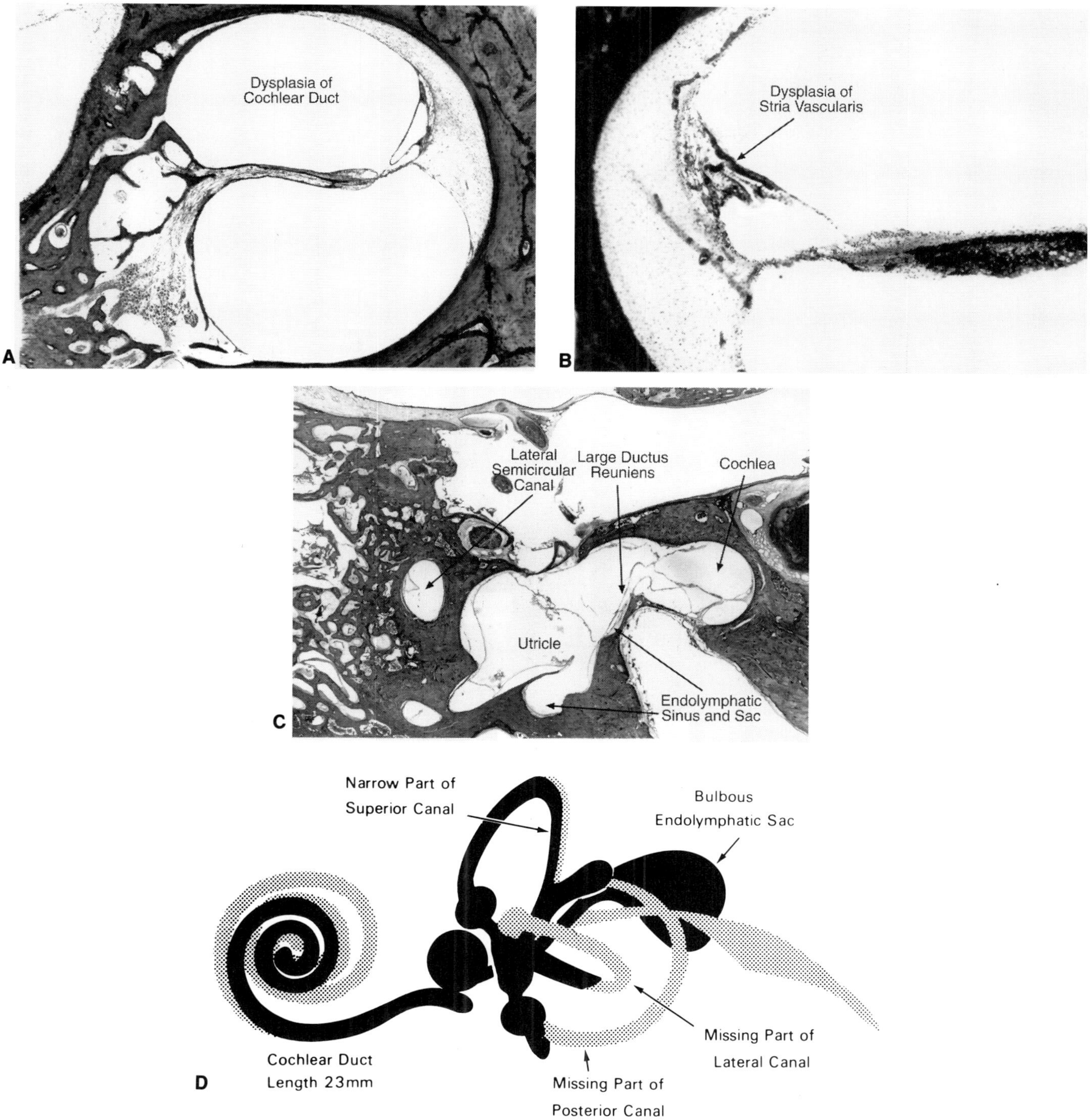


**Fig. 33.** Inner ear dysplasias. A: Scheibe dysplasia. Temporal bone of a male aged 10 years with profound hearing loss from birth. The organ of Corti consists of a flattened mound of cells containing remnants of pillars and undifferentiated cells. Reissner's membrane is depressed onto the striae vasculares and organ of Corti obliterates the endolymphatic space. In some areas, the striae vasculares are atrophied, and in others they are hyperplastic. B: Scheibe dysplasia. Temporal bone of a newborn male who survived 10 hours. In the basal turn, the striae vasculares form multiple layers between spiral ligament and partly collapsed Reissner's membrane. C: Mondini dysplasia. The cochlear compartment is round and has a vestigial modiolus and hypoplastic organ of Corti. The cochlea communicates widely with the vestibule. The utricle is enlarged. The maculae and cristae are hypoplastic. The population of cochlear and vestibular neurons is severely diminished. The endolymphatic sac is bulbous. D: Mondini dysplasia. Diagram showing the dysmorphic features of the right membraneous labyrinth (black area) superimposed on the normal configuration (gray area). The cochlea has two-and-one-half turns but is only 20 mm in length. Parts of the semicircular canals are missing and the endolymphatic sac is bulbous. (All figures with permission from HF Schuknecht, *Pathology of the Ear,* 2nd ed., Lea & Febiger, Philadelphia, 1993. A and B from p. 178, courtesy of Dr. L Ruedi, University of Zurich, Switzerland; C from p. 181; D from p. 183, courtesy of Drs. Peron and Schuknecht.)

7. Bing-Siebenmann type (underdevelopment of the membranous labyrinth, particularly of the sense organ, with a well-formed bony labyrinth)

Schuknecht[16] disagrees about including types 6 and 7, because of the lack of clinical and histological documentation, as well as type 5, or Michel aplasia, because of its extreme rarity.

### Mondini dysplasia

The first description of this anomaly dates back to 1791.[10] The dysmorphic features include a dwarf cochlea (of one-and-a-half turns approximately instead of the usual two-and-a-half turns).[14] The modiolus is vestigial and the organ of Corti is deformed and may be reduced to a mound of undifferentiated cells. The stria vascularis is also hypoplastic and Reissner's membrane may be collapsed. The utricle and saccule are usually enlarged and the macula and cristae are also hypoplastic. The endolymphatic sac may appear bulbous.[13,15,16]

Mondini dysplasia is easily diagnosed radiologically.[13,18] It may occur in association with DiGeorge, Klippel-Feil, Pendred, or trisomy syndromes.[7,18]

Periplymphatic fistulae and recurrent meningitis may occur with Mondini dysplasia. Nonsyndromal familial Mondini dysplasia has been described.[3]

### Scheibe malformation

This anomaly[4,8,11,16] involves the cochlea and saccule that are considered as the newer (phylogenetically) part of the inner ear. The semicircular canals and utricle are normal.

The organ of Corti is usually reduced and consists of undifferentiated cells with remnants of pillars. Reissner's membrane may be depressed on the stria vascularis and limbus. As a result, the endolymphatic space may be obliterated. The stria vascularis may be replaced by fibrous tissue and may show cystic spaces and PAS-positive deposits.

Saccular changes include collapse of the wall on the macula, atrophy of the sensory epithelium, and deformed otolithic membrane.

For further details regarding the anomalies seen in chromosomal disorders, the reader is referred to reference 16, which gives an excellent overview of the subject.

### References


1. Arcand P, Desrosiers M, Dubé J, Abela A: The large vestibular aqueduct syndrome and sensorineural hearing loss in a pediatric population. J Otolaryngol 20:247–250, 1991.
2. Cawthorne TE, Hinchcliffe R: Familial perceptive deafness. Pract Otorhinolaryngol 19:69–83, 1957.
3. Chan KH, Eelkema EA, Furman JMR, Kamerer DB: Familial sensorineural hearing loss: a correlative study of audiologic, radiographic and vestibular findings. Ann Otol Rhinol Laryngol 100:620–625, 1991.
4. Fisch L: Deafness as part of a hereditary syndrome. J Laryngol Otol 73:355–382, 1959.
5. Hirsch BE, Weissman JL, Curtin HD, Kamerer DB: Magnetic resonance imaging of the large vestibular aqueduct. Otolaryngol Head Neck Surg 118:1124–1127, 1992.
6. Jackler RK, De La Cruz A: The large vestibular aqueduct syndrome. Laryngoscope 99:1238–1243, 1989.
7. Jackler RK, Luxford WM: Congenital malformations of the inner ear. Laryngoscope (Suppl 40) 97:1–24, 1987.
8. Lindsay JR: Histopathology of deafness due to postnatal viral disease. Arch Otolaryngol 98:258–264, 1973.
9. Michel EM: Mémoires sur les anomalies congénitales de l'oreille interne, avec la première authentique d'absence complète d'oreilles internes et de nerfs auditifs, et de l'absence partielle de l'oreille moyenne chez un sourd et muet, mort à l'âge de douze ans. Gazette Médicale Strasbourg 23:55–58, 1863.
10. Mondini C: Anatomia surdi nati sectio. De Bononiensi Scientiarum et Artium Instituto atque Academia Commentarii, Bononiae 7:28–29, 419–431, 1791.
11. Nomura Y, Kawabata I: Scheibe dysgenesis of the inner ear. J Laryngol Otol 94:1345–1352, 1980.
12. Ormerod FC: The pathology of congenital deafness. J Laryngol Otol 74:919–950, 1960.
13. Paparella MM: Mondini deafness. A review of histopathology. Ann Otol Rhinol Laryngol (Suppl) 89:1–10, 1980.
14. Paparella MM, Schachern PA: Sensorineural hearing loss in children-genetic. In: Otolaryngology, 3rd ed, MM Paparella, ed. WB Saunders, Philadelphia, 1994, p 1580.
15. Schuknecht HF: Mondini dysplasia. A clinical and pathological study. Ann Otol Rhinol Laryngol (Suppl) 89:1–23, 1980.
16. Schuknecht HF: Pathology of the Ear, 2nd ed. Lea & Febiger, Baltimore, 1993, pp 177–189.
17. Suehiro S, Sando I: Congenital anomalies of the inner ear. Ann Otol Rhinol Laryngol (Suppl) 88:1–23, 1979.
18. Valvassori GE, Naunton RF, Lindsay JR: Inner ear anomalies: clinical and histological considerations. Ann Otol Rhinol Laryngol 78:929–938, 1969.


## Kartagener syndrome

### Dextrocardia, bronchiectasis and sinusitis
(MIM No. *244400; POSSUM No. 3763)

#### General and otolaryngological manifestations

Pansinusitis during childhood, absence of the frontal sinuses, and thick nasal rhinorrhea are characteristic presenting symptoms. The mastoid air cells are poorly developed. Otitis media due to eustachian tube dysfunction results in deafness, usually of the conductive type. Anosmia and nasal polyps are frequent complications. Recurrent pneumonia and chronic cough are common. It is estimated that one-tenth of the cases of bronchiectasis are due to Kartagener syndrome.

Situs inversus with gross defects in cardiac septation may occur. One-sixth of situs inversus cases have this syndrome. Myringotomy and insertion of bilateral pressure equalization tubes (PET) are required for the serous middle ear effusion. Early treatment of respiratory infection may help in preventing bronchiectasis. Removal of affected lobes of the lung may be needed later to treat the bronchiectasis. In vitro fertilization may be used in the management of sterility. Associated anomalies include polysplenia or asplenia syndrome, rheumatoid arthritis, thyrotoxicosis, biliary atresia, abnormal subclavian artery, and glomerulonephritis.[2,3,6,7,10,11]

#### Etiology and pathogenesis

Kartagener syndrome is of autosomal recessive inheritance. Autosomal dominant or X-linked inheritance has also been suggested.[8,9] The primary defect is abnormality of the cilia of the respiratory tract. This leads to blockage of the paranasal sinuses, eustachian tubes, and the lungs. Immobility of the sperm produces sterility in males; affected females may have decreased fertility. The lack of dynein arms is the most common structural abnormality in the respiratory and fallopian cilia and sperm tails.[1,4,5,12]

#### Differential diagnosis

Young syndrome (MIM No. 279000) patients have bronchiectasis, sinusitis, and azoospermia but not situs inversus or abnormal cilia.

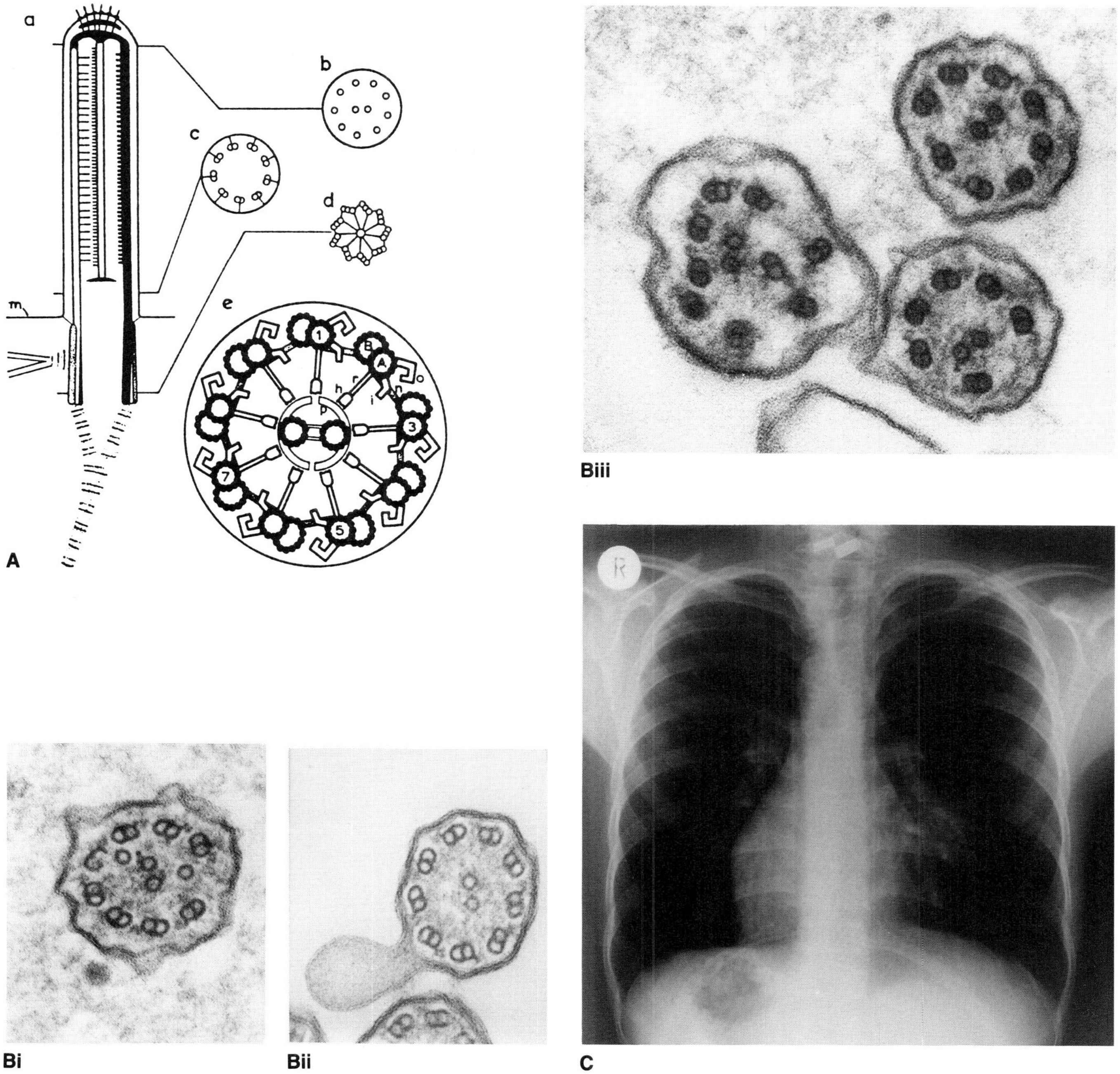


**Fig. 34.** Kartagener syndrome. A: Diagram of a normal celium. Note the outer microtubular doublets and two central microtubules in e. Details of structures are seen in different cross sections b, c, and d. a, ciliary shaft; n, nexin; r; radial spokes; h; dilated heads, p, projections, o, outer and i, inner dynein arms. (From MA Sleigh et al., Am Rev Resp Dis 137:727, 1988, courtesy of Dr. JR Blake.) B: Electron micrograph of abnormal cilia. i: Disruption of outer doublet organization and number with internalization of doublets. ii: Disruption of outer doublet organization and number with fragmentation of a doublet. iii: Absence of inner dynein arms and radial spokes. (Courtesy of Drs. D Gaskin and M Corriveau.) C: Situs inversus. (Courtesy of Drs. M Davis and A Coates.)

## References


1. Afzelius BA: Immotile cilia. Thorax 35:401–404, 1980.
2. Aitken RJ, Ross A, Lees MM: Analysis of sperm function in Kartagener's syndrome. Fertil Steril 40:696–698, 1983.
3. Bhugra D: Kartagener's syndrome. Br J Clin Pract 39:38–39, 1985.
4. Corbeel L, Cornillie F, Lauweryns J, Boel M, van den Berghe G: Ultrastructural abnormalities of bronchial cilia in children with recurrent airway infections and bronchiectasis. Arch Dis Child 56:929–933, 1981.
5. Eavey RD, Nadol JB Jr, Holmes LB, Lairs NM, Lapey A, Joseph MP, Strome M: Kartagener's syndrome: a blinded controlled study of cilia ultrastructure. Arch Otolaryngol Head Neck Surg 112:646–650, 1986.
6. Gershoni-Baruch R, Gottfried E, Pery M, Sahiu A, Etzioni A: Immotile cilia syndrome including polysplenia, situs inversus and extrahepatic biliary atresia. Am J Med Genet 33:330–333, 1989.
7. Johrdoerfer R, Feldman PS, Rubel EW, Guerrant JL, Eggleston P, Selden RF: Otitis media and the immobile cilia syndrome. Laryngoscope 89:769–778, 1979.
8. Moreno A, Murphy EA: Inheritance of Kartagener syndrome. Am J Med Genet 8:305–313, 1981.
9. Narayan D, Kirshnan SN, Upender M, Ravikumar TS, Mahoney MJ, Dolan F Jr, Teebi AS, Haddad GG: Unusual inheritance of primary ciliary dyskinesia (Kartagener's syndrome). J Med Genet 31:493–496, 1994.
10. Rossmann CM, Forrest JB, Rubbin RE, Newhouse MT: Immotile cilia

syndrome in persons with and without Kartagener's syndrome. Am Rev Respir Dis 121:1011–1016, 1980.
11. Schidlow DV, Katz SM, Turtz MG, Donner RM, Capasso S: Polysplenia and Kartagener syndromes in a sibship: association with abnormal respiratory cilia. J Pediatr 100:401–404, 1982.
12. Sturgess JM, Thompson NW: Genetic aspects of immotile cilia syndromes. Am J Med Genet 25:149–160, 1986.

## Keutel syndrome

### (MIM No. *245150; POSSUM No. 3675)

This syndrome is characterized by brachytelephalangy, peripheral pulmonary stenosis, deafness, and calcification of the auricular cartilages.

### General and otolaryngological manifestations

The striking features of this syndrome are widespread diffuse calcifications of the nose, pinnae, larynx, epiglottis, trachea, and ribs. These changes are seen as early as 3 years of age . Hearing loss may be conductive or mixed. The ossicle of the middle ear may have malformations. Hearing loss is greater in the higher frequencies and deafness ranges from 30 to 75 dB. Middle ear infections contribute to the hearing loss. Speech is nasal, due to a relatively short palate.[1–7] The face is flat. The nose is small with a depressed bridge and small nares.

The hands and feet have short, malformed terminal phalanges, short nails, and interphalangeal webbing. Peripheral pulmonary artery stenosis (at the bifurcation of the pulmonary arteries) occurs in most cases.[3,6,7]

### Etiology

Keutel syndrome is of autosomal recessive inheritance.

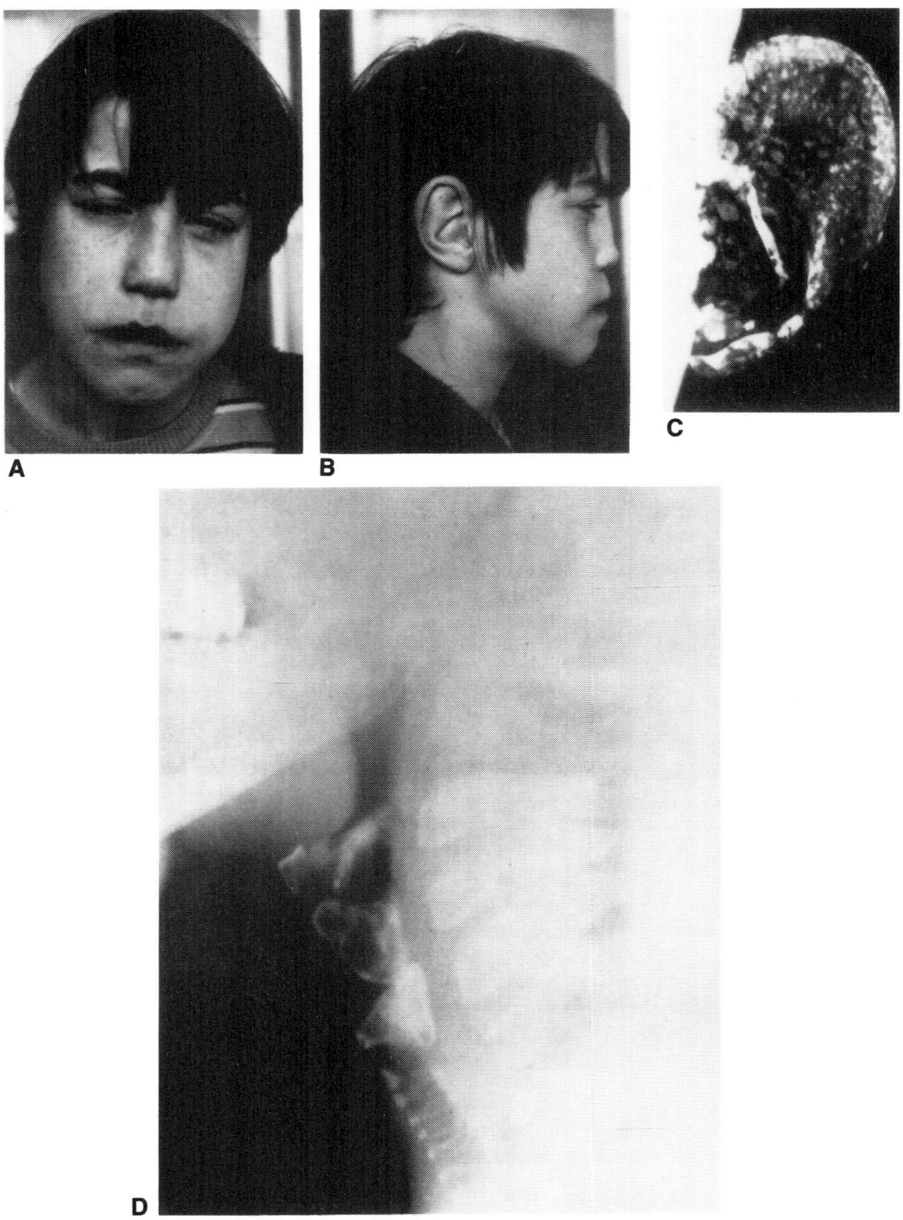

**Fig. 35.** Keutel syndrome. A,B: Midfacial hypoplasia and depressed nose. C: Calcified pinna on X-ray. D: Radiograph of the neck showing calcified thyroid cartilage. (From JP Fryns et al., Eur J Pediatr 142:201, 1984, with permission.)

### References


1. Cormode EJ, Dawson M, Lowry RB: Keutel syndrome: clinical report and literature review. Am J Med Genet 24:289–294, 1986.
2. Dibartolomeo JR: The petrified auricle: comments on ossification, calcification and exostoses of the external ear. Laryngoscope 95:566–576, 1985.
3. Fryns JP, van Fleteren A, Mattelaer P, van den Berghe H: Calcification of cartilages, brachytelephalangy and peripheral pulmonary stenosis. Confirmation of the Keutel syndrome. Eur J Pediatr 142:201–203, 1984.
4. Keutel J, Jorgensen G, Gabriel P: A new autosomal recessive syndrome with peripheral pulmonary stenosis, brachytelephalangism, neural hearing loss and abnormal cartilage calcifications/ossifications. Birth Defects 8:60–68, 1972.
5. Khosroshahi HE, Uluoglu O, Olgunturk R, Basaklar C: Keutel syndrome: a report of four cases. Eur J Pediatr 149:188–191, 1989.
6. Primrose DA: A slowly progressive degenerative condition characterized by mental deficiency, wasting of limb musculature and bone abnormalities, including ossification of the pinnae. J Ment Def Res 26:101–106, 1982.
7. Ziereisen F, De Munter C, Perlmutter N: The Keutel syndrome. Report of a case and review of the literature. Pediatr Radiol 23:314–315, 1993.


## Klippel-Feil anomaly

(MIM No. *148900; POSSUM No. 3274)

Anomalies of the cervical vertebrae were originally described by Klippel and Feil.[14] The only constant characteristic of the

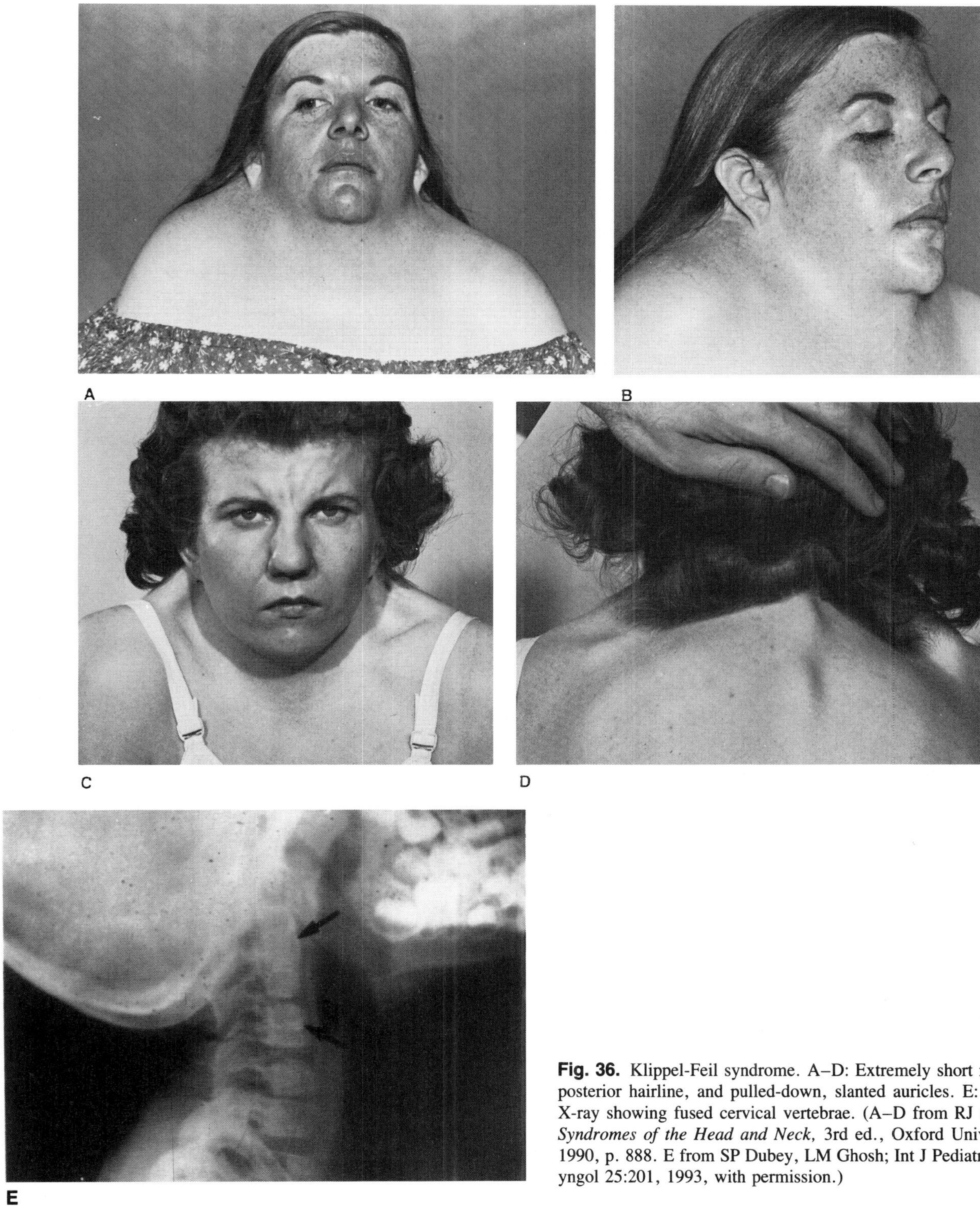

**Fig. 36.** Klippel-Feil syndrome. A–D: Extremely short neck, low-set posterior hairline, and pulled-down, slanted auricles. E: Lateral neck X-ray showing fused cervical vertebrae. (A–D from RJ Gorlin et al., *Syndromes of the Head and Neck,* 3rd ed., Oxford University Press, 1990, p. 888. E from SP Dubey, LM Ghosh; Int J Pediatr Otorhinolaryngol 25:201, 1993, with permission.)

syndrome is fusion of the cervical vertebrae due to failure of segmentation of the somites in utero.[19]

### General manifestations

These include convergent squint, nystagmus, and atrophy of the choroid plexus.[12] Scoliosis with or without kyphosis occurs in most patients. Other common findings include spina bifida occulta and urinary tract anomalies (agenesis of the kidneys, horseshoe kidney, or ectopic renal malformations).

Hypospadias and cryptorchidism may occur. The neurological complications should be kept in mind after minor cervical trauma. They usually occur in the first decade of life. Intracranial tumors, pulmonary and cardiovascular anomalies have also been reported.[2,6,17]

### Otolaryngological manifestations

Hearing loss is described as mixed, conductive, or sensorineural. It occurs in 25%–50% of patients.[4,8,18] Inner ear anomalies, vestibular involvement, bifid tongue, cleft palate, velopharyngeal insufficiency and laryngeal anomalies have also been reported.[5,7,20,21]

### Clinical types, etiology, and pathogenesis

Feil[9] classified the anomalies of this syndrome as three clinical types:

1. Type I is characterized by extensive fusion of the cervical and upper thoracic vertebrae. It is more common in females (1.3/1.0). Most cases are sporadic.[11]
2. In type II fusion occurs between one or two intervertebral spaces (C2–C3 and C5–C6). It is inherited as an autosomal dominant trait and atlantoaxial fusion is often described. Some cases appear to have an autosomal recessive inheritance.[11,13]
3. Type III involves fusion of the cervical and lower dorsal or lumbar vertebrae. Autosomal recessive inheritance has been suggested.[11]
4. Type IV was proposed by Raass-Rothchild et al.[16] and encompasses different fusions of the cervical, upper and lower thoracic, and lumbar segments. Most cases are sporadic.

The possibility of teratogenic etiology has been raised.[19] Others believe that this syndrome is due to subclavian disruption sequence.[3] Of all these types, type II is the less severe and most common form, the characteristics being a short-webbed neck, limited cervical movements, and a low hairline. One of the genes responsible for Klippel-Feil anomaly may be located at 5q11.2 or 17q23, two sites involved in a de novo, apparently balanced, reciprocal translocation.[10]

### Differential diagnosis

Others syndromes that are associated with Klippel-Feil anomalies include Wildervanck syndrome, which is characterized by abducens paralysis and retracted eye globe (Duane anomaly), severe hearing loss (congenital sensorineural or conductive), occasional cleft palate, and/or torticollis. It is more common in females.[8] MURCS association (**M**üllerian duct aplasia, **R**enal aplasia, and **C**ervicothoracic **S**omatic dysplasia), is also associated with Klippel-Feil syndrome. Occasionally hypoplastic uterus and absent vagina are reported.[1,15]

### References


1. Baird PA, Lowry RB: Absent vagina and the Klippel-Feil anomaly. Am J Obstet Gynecol 188:290–291, 1974.
2. Bhagat R, Paul K, Singh VK, Paut C, Gupta A, Jaggi OP: Pulmonary developmental anomaly associated with Klippel-Feil syndrome and anomalous atrioventricular conduction. Chest 101:1157–1158, 1992.
3. Brill CB, Peyster RG, Keller MS, Galtman L: Isolation of the right subclavian artery with subclavian steal in a child with Klippel-Feil anomaly: an example of the subclavian artery supply disruption sequence. Am J Med Genet 26:933–940, 1987.
4. Daniilidis J, Maganaris T, Dimitriadis A, Iliades T, Manolidis L: Stapes gusher and Klippel-Feil syndrome. Laryngoscope 88:1178–1183, 1978.
5. Derkay CS, Grundfast KM, McCullough DC: Sudden onset of velopharyngeal insufficiency in Klippel-Feil syndrome. Ear Nose Throat J 69:548–552, 1990.
6. Dickman-Guiroy B, Huang PS: Klippel-Feil syndrome in association with a craniocervical dermoid cyst presenting as aseptic meningitis in an adult: case report. Neurosurgery 25:652–655, 1989.
7. Ene F, Fikcas G, Cioflea O, Ene E: Peripheral-type acute cochleovestibular involvement in the Klippel-Feil syndrome. Comments on 2 clinical cases. Rev Chir Otolaryngol 34:45–56, 1989.
8. Everberg G, Ratjen E, Sorensen H: Wildervank's syndrome: Klippel Feil syndrome associated with deafness and retraction of the eyeball. Br J Radiol 36:562–567, 1963.
9. Feil A: L'absence et la diminution des vertèbres cervicales. Thèses, Librairie Littéraire et Médicale, Paris, 1919.
10. Fukushima Y, Ohashi H, Wakui K, Nishimoto H, Sato M, Aihara T: De novo apparently balanced reciprocal translocation between 5q11.2 and 17q23 associated with Klippel-Feil anomaly and type A1 brachydactyly. Am J Med Genet 57:447–449, 1995.
11. Gunderson CH, Greenspan RH, Glazer GH, Lubs HA: The Klippel-Feil syndrome: genetic and clinical re-evaluation of cervical fusion. Medicine 46:491–512, 1967.
12. Helmi C, Pruzansky S: Craniofacial and extracranial malformations in the Klippel-Feil syndrome. Cleft Palate J 17:65–88, 1980.
13. Juberg RC, Gershank JJ: Cervical vertebral fusion (Klippel-Feil) syndrome with consanguineous parents. J Med Genet 13:246–249, 1976.
14. Klippel M, Feil A: Un cas d'absence des vertèbres cervicales. Nouvelle Iconogr Salpet 25:223–250, 1912.
15. Mecklenburg RS, Krueger PM: Extensive genitourinary anomalies associated with the Klippel-Feil syndrome. Am J Dis Child 128:92–93, 1974.
16. Raas-Rothschild A, Goodman RM, Grunbaumm, Berger I, Minouni M: Klippel-Feil anomaly with sacral agenesis: an additional subtype, type IV. J Craniofac Genet Dev Biol 9:399–400, 1989.
17. Smith BA, Griffin C: Klippel-Feil syndrome. Ann Emerg Med 21:876–879, 1992.
18. Stewart EJ, O'Reilly BF: Klippel-Feil syndrome and conductive deafness. J Laryngol Otol 103:947–949, 1989.
19. Warkany J: Congenital Malformations: Notes and Comments. Yearbook Medical Publishers, Chicago, 1971.
20. Widgersow AD: Klippel-Feil anomaly, cleft palate and bifid tongue. Ann Plast Surg 25:216–277, 1990.
21. Windle-Taylor PC, Emery PJ, Phelps PD: Ear deformities associated with the Klippel-Feil syndrome. Ann Otol Rhinol Laryngol 90:210–216, 1981.


## Larsen syndrome

### (MIM Nos. *150250, *245600; POSSUM No. 3275)

This syndrome was first described by Larsen, Schottstaedt, and Bost in 1950.[6] It is characterized by flat facies, multiple congenital dislocations, club foot deformities, short fingernails, and a cleft palate.

### General manifestations

Bilateral joint dislocations involving the knee, hips, and elbows occur in 70 to 80% of patients. Pseudoclubbing of the fingers, which are cylindrical and have extra creases, occurs in 75% of cases.[3] Radiologically, multiple carpal ossification cen-

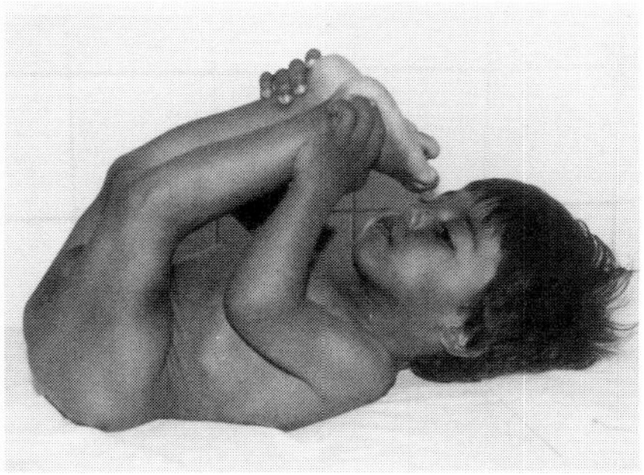

**Fig. 37.** Larsen syndrome. Note the hyperflexed hips and hyperextended knees due to joint dislocation.

ters are recognized. The eyes are wide set and the cervical vertebrae may show kyphosis that could lead to quadriplegia or death.

Other findings include congenital heart disease such as ASD, VSD, aortic dilatation, and valvular anomalies.[5] Mental retardation is seen in 15% of cases.

### Otolaryngological manifestations

The nose is flat with hypertelorism and a depressed nasal bridge, the forehead is prominent, and the palate high arched and often cleft. Micrognathia is usually seen.[3,4,7] Anomalies of the upper airway include laryngomalacia or laryngotracheal stenosis.[2,9] Hearing loss can be sensorineural or mixed.[10,11] The temporal bone findings are well described[4] and include dislocation of the incudomalleal joint, abnormal foot plate, poorly developed mastoid system, and mesenchymal remnants in the attic and mesotympanum.

### Etiology

Larsen syndrome is of autosomal dominant inheritance. An autosomal recessive form is also reported and is usually more severe.[1,8] The pathogenesis is unknown. However, it is considered by some authors[10] as a generalized mesenchymal disorder. The gene for the autosomal dominant type is localized to chromosome region 3p21.1–p14.1 in the proximity of, but distinct from, the COL7A1 locus.[12]

### Differential diagnosis

Diagnosis is often confused with otopalatodigital syndrome which is characterized by pugilistic facies, hearing loss, and paddle-shaped metatarsal bones. Arthrogryposis, cerebro-oculofacial syndrome (COFS), and Ehler-Danlos syndrome are also in the differential diagnosis. A lethal, Larsen-like multiple joint dislocation syndrome should be considered when dealing with neonatal cases.[1]

### References


1. Chan H, Chang C-H, Perrin E, Perrin J: A lethal, Larsen-like multiple joint dislocation syndrome. Am J Med Genet 13:149–161, 1981.
2. Crowe AV, Kearns DB, Mitchell DB: Tracheal stenosis in Larsen's syndrome. Arch Otolaryngol Head Neck Surg 155:626, 1989.
3. Gorlin RJ, Cohen MM Jr, Levin LS: Syndromes of the Head and Neck, 3rd ed, Oxford University Press, New York, 1990, pp 722–724.
4. Kaga K, Suzuki J, Kimizuka M: Temporal bone pathology of two infants with Larsen's syndrome. Int J Pediatr Otolaryngol 22:257–267, 1991.
5. Kiel EA, Frias JL, Victorica BE: Cardiovascular manifestations in the Larsen syndrome. Pediatrics 71:942–946, 1983.
6. Larsen LJ, Schottstaedt ER, Bost F: Multiple congenital dislocations associated with characteristic facial abnormality. J Pediatr 37:574–581, 1950.
7. Latta RJ, Graham CB, Aase J, Scham SM, Smith DW: Larsen's syndrome: a skeletal dysplasia with multiple joint dislocations and unusual facies. J Pediatr 78:291–298, 1971.
8. Myers TL: Larsen syndrome. In: Birth Defects Encyclopedia, ML Buyse, ed. Blackwell Scientific Publications, Cambridge, 1990, p 1029.
9. Ronningen H, Bjerkrein I: Larsen syndrome. Acta Orthop Scand 49:138–142, 1978.
10. Samuel AW, Davies DR: The Larsen syndrome with multiple congenital dislocations and a normal facies. Int Orthop 5:229–232, 1981.
11. Stanley CS, Thelin JW, Miles JH: Mixed hearing loss in Larsen syndrome. Clin Genet 33:395–398, 1988.
12. Vujic M, Hallstensson K, Wahlstrom J, Lundberg A, Langmaack C, Martison I: Localization of a gene for autosomal dominant Larsen syndrome to chromosome region 3p21.1–14.1 in the proximity of, but distinct from, the COL7A1 locus. Am J Hum Genet 57:1104–1113, 1995.


## Lenz-Majewski syndrome

### (MIM No. 151050; POSSUM No. 3045)

This syndrome is characterized by a large head, a particular facies, choanal atresia, dysplastic enamel, loose skin, skeletal anomalies, and mental retardation.[4]

### General manifestations

Characteristic features include a large head, with a prominent forehead and widely separated sutures. All affected children are mentally retarded. Cutis laxa is present during infancy. Later, the skin becomes atrophic and prominent veins as well as cutis marmorata become evident.[2] The skull shows progressive sclerosis. The long bones demonstrate cortical thickening and skeletal maturation is retarded.[1] The fingers are short, the clavicles and ribs are broad. Hypotonia and inguinal hernias are common. Cryptorchidism, hypospadias, and an anteriorly placed anus are documented.

### Otolaryngological manifestations

Sensorineural hearing loss is frequent. The ears are large and floppy. Hypertelorism, nasolacrimal stenosis, and enamel dysplasia are also frequent findings.[1–4]

### Etiology

The occurrence is sporadic. Lenz-Majewski syndrome is possibly due to de novo autosomal dominant mutations. Advanced paternal age may be a predisposing factor.

### Differential diagnosis

This syndrome should be differentiated from craniometaphyseal dysplasia and craniodiaphyseal dysplasia.

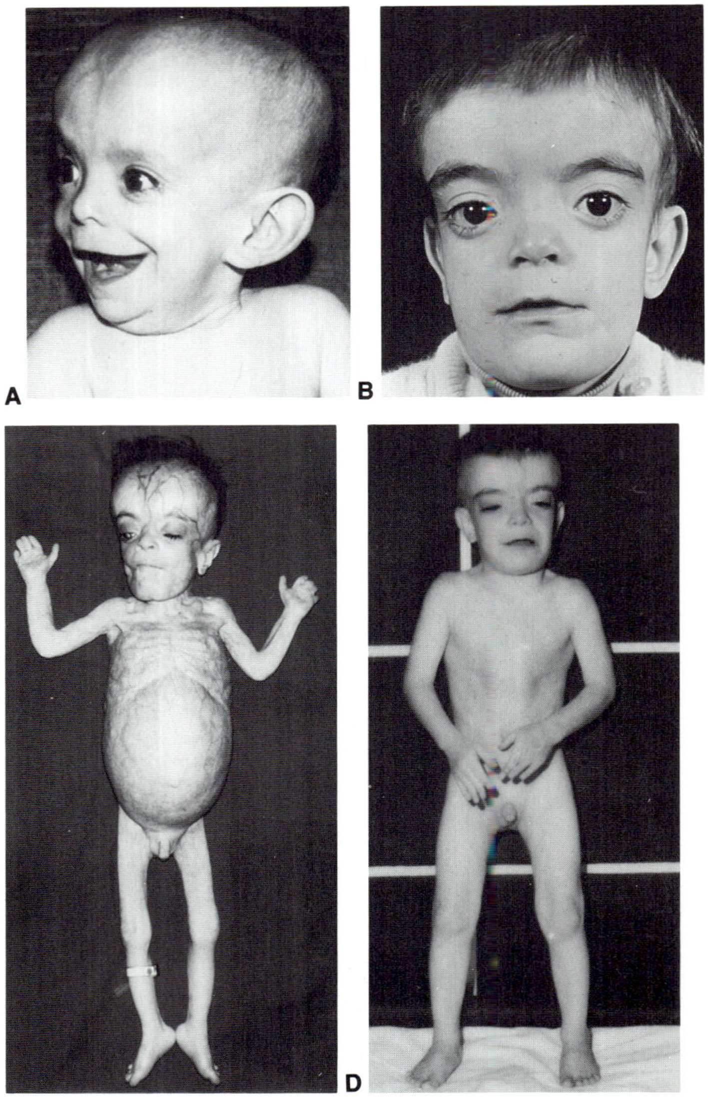

**Fig. 38.** Lenz-Majewski syndrome. A,B: Note the prominent veins, atrophic skin, and hypertelorism. C,D: Relatively large head contrasts with relatively small torso and extremities. (From M Robinow et al.: J Pediatr 91:417, 1977, with permission.)

### References


1. Gorlin RJ, Whitley CB: Lenz-Majewski syndrome. Radiology 149:129–131, 1983.
2. Kaye CJ, Fisher DE, Esterly NB: Cutis laxa, skeletal anomalies, and ambiguous genitalia. Am J Dis Child 127:115–117, 1974.
3. Macpherson RI: Craniodiaphyseal dysplasia, a disease or group of diseases? J Can Assoc Radiol 25:22–33, 1974.
4. Robinow M, Johanson AJ, Smith TH: The Lenz-Majewski hyperostotic dwarfism. A syndrome of multiple congenital anomalies, mental retardation, and progressive skeletal sclerosis. J Pediatr 91:417–421, 1977.


## LEOPARD syndrome

(MIM No. *151100; POSSUM No. 3277)

The acronym *LEOPARD* was developed by Gorlin, Anderson, and Blaw in 1969.[1] It is derived from **L**entigines, **E**lectrocardiographic anomalies, **O**cular hypertelorism, **P**ulmonary stenosis, **A**bnormal genitalia, **R**etardation of growth, and **D**eafness (sensorineural), which are the main features of the syndrome.

### General manifestations

Lentigines differ from freckles in being darker in color and having more melanocytes per unit of skin area. They are not related to sunlight exposure. The size of the lentigines varies between 1 and 5 mm and may only spare the mucosal surfaces. Occasionally they may form café-au-lait spots (1–5 cm).[11] The lentigines usually increase with age.[5]

Electrocardiographic changes occur in approximately half of the subjects and are described as prolonged PR interval, QRS, and P wave abnormalities. Complete bundle branch block has also been reported.[8,9]

Pulmonary stenosis, the most common cardiac anomaly (40%), is usually mild. Other lesions like hypertrophic cardiomyopathy and right or left ventricular hypertrophy may occur.[4,11]

Hypospadias and cryptorchidism are frequently present.[3] Growth retardation occurs in most patients (85%). Mild mental retardation occurs in over 25% of patients.[2,7]

Death from respiratory insufficiency has also been documented.[6] The association of LEOPARD syndrome and Marfan syndrome has been reported in three patients.[10]

### Otolaryngological manifestations

Early onset of deafness, which is sensorineural in 25% of cases, often occurs. The face is triangular with hypertelorism, mild prognathism, low-set ears, and mild pterygium colli. Anosmia or hyposmia may occur.

### Etiology

This syndrome is inherited as autosomal dominant with high penetrance and varying phenotypic expression.

### Differential diagnosis

LEOPARD syndrome should be differentiated from Noonan Syndrome, Aarskog syndrome, rubella embryopathy, and Turner syndrome.

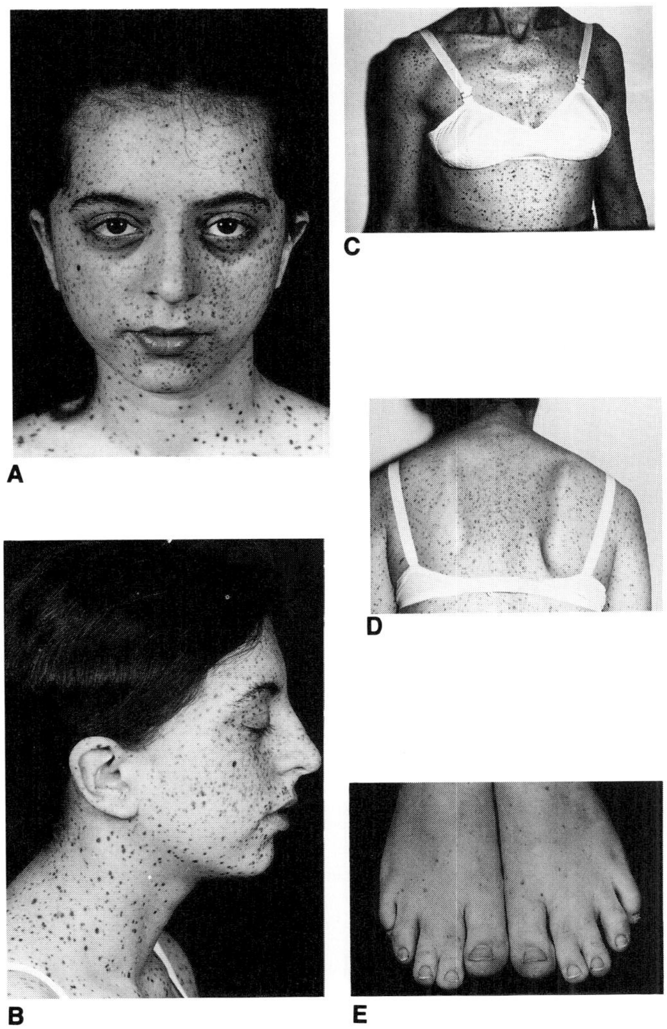

**Fig. 39.** Leopard syndrome. A–E: Note the numerous lentigenes of the face, neck, chest, back, and feet. (From chapter by F Char in *Clinical Delineation of Birth Defects,* D Bergsma ed., vol. 7, no. 8, pt. 12, 234–235, Balitmore, Williams & Wilkins, 1971, with permission; courtesy of Dr. V McKusick.)

### References


1. Gorlin RJ, Anderson RC, Blaw M: Multiple lentigines syndrome. Am J Dis Child 117:558–563, 1969.
2. Gorlin RJ, Anderson RC, Moller JH: The Leopard (multiple lentigines) syndrome revisited. Laryngoscope 81:1674–1681, 1971.
3. Moynahan EJ: Multiple symmetrical moles with "psychic" and somatic infantilism and genital hypoplasia. First male case of a new syndrome. Proc R Soc Med 55:959–960, 1962.
4. Moynahan EJ: Progressive cardiomyopathic lentiginosis. First report of autopsy findings in a recently recognized inheritable disorder (autosomal dominant). Proc R Soc Med 63:445–451, 1970.
5. Nordlund JJ, Lerner AB, Braverman IM, McGuire JS: The multiple lentigines syndrome. Arch Dermatol 107:259–261, 1973.
6. Peter JR, Kemp JS: Leopard syndrome: death because of chronic respiratory insufficiency. Am J Med Genet 57:340–341, 1990.
7. Pickering D, Laski B, MacMillan DC, Rose V: 'Little leopard' syndrome. Description of three cases and review of 24. Arch Dis Child 46:85–90, 1971.
8. Seuanez H, Mane-Garzon F, Kolski R: Cardio-cutaneous syndrome (The "LEOPARD" syndrome). Review of the literature and a new family. Clin Genet 9:266–276, 1976.
9. Smith RF, Pulicicchio LU, Holmes AV: Generalized lentigo, electrocardiographic abnormalities, conduction disorders and arrhythmias in three cases. Am J Cardiol 25:501–506, 1970.
10. Torok L, Szentendrei L, Szili M, Budai S: Progressive cardiomyopathic lentiginosis (Leopard syndrome) in 3 patients combined with Marfan syndrome. Z Hautkr 65:197–201, 1990.
11. Voron DA, Hatfield HH, Kalkhoff RK: Multiple lentigines syndrome: case report and review of the literature. Am J Med 60:447–56, 1976.


## Marfan syndrome

### (MIM No. #154700; POSSUM No. 3285)

Marfan described this syndrome in 1896.[9] The cardinal features occur in three systems: the skeletal, ocular, and cardiovascular systems. It is inherited as an autosomal dominant trait with high penetrance and variable expressitivity. The majority of patients have relatives with the syndrome.

### General manifestations

Ocular findings include ectopia lentis (50%–80%), myopia, and flat cornea. Glaucoma and retinal detachment may occur, but these are usually seen after cataract removal. Eighty percent of patients have good vision.[10] The ascending aorta is progressively dilated due to the cystic necrosis of the media. Mitral valve prolapse is noted in most cases. Other cardiovascular anomalies include aneurysm of the descending aorta and pulmonary artery.[1,2,13] Musculoskeletal anomalies are characteristic. These include arachnodactyly (88%), dolichostenomelia, pectus excavatum or carinatum (68%), and scoliosis. It is presumed that the growth is due to a defect in a fibrous element of the periosteum. Joints may be hypermobile (56%) or congenitally contracted. Recurrent dislocation of the big joints is not uncommon. Pulmonary capacity is reduced in Marfan's syndrome and patients may develop pneumothorax. Occasional features are inguinal herniae and neuropsychological problems. Sacral meningocele was also reported.[6,7,14]

### Otolaryngological manifestations

The palate is narrow and highly arched. Cleft palate may occur. The teeth are crowded and malocclusion is frequent. Frontal bossing and prominent supraorbital ridges are also noted. The paranasal sinuses are enlarged. Hearing loss may occur and it

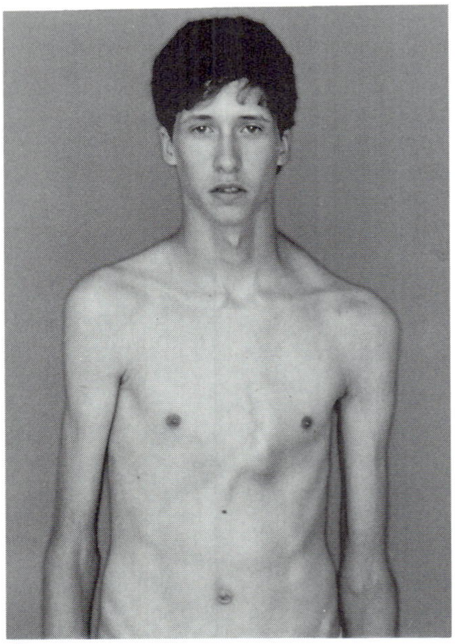

A

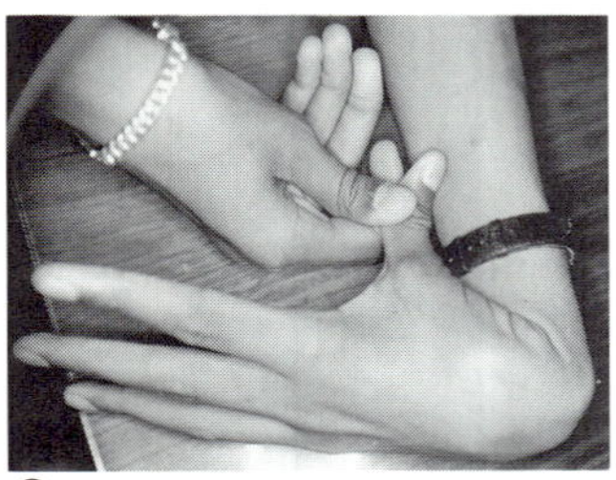

C

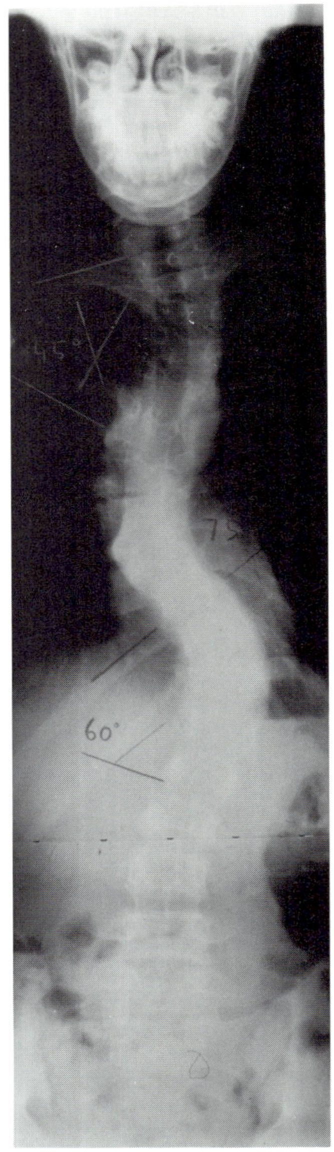


B

**Fig. 40.** Marfan syndrome A: Patient with pectus carinatum. B: Roentgenogram showing kyphoscoliosis. C: Arachnodactyly and hyperextensible joints. (Courtesy of Dr. V Arlet.)

is usually due to recurrent otitis. Temporal bone changes include narrowing of the vestibular aqueduct, bulging round window, dilatation of the endolymphatic duct and utriculoampullary space.[3,8,12]

### Etiology

This syndrome appears to be due to a mutation of the fibrillin 1 *(FBN1)* gene located on chromosome 15.[4,11] This makes prenatal and presymptomatic diagnosis possible by molecular methods.[5,15]

### Differential diagnosis

Marfan syndrome should be differentiated from other conditions with marfanoid habitus such as Klinefelter syndrome and congenital contractural arachnodactyly. Patients with homocystinuria may have marfanoid habitus and ectopia lentis usually associated with mental retardation.

### References


1. Chen S, Fagan LF, Nouri S, Donahoe JL: Ventricular dysrhythmias in children with Marfan's syndrome. Am J Dis Child 139:273–276, 1985.
2. Come PC: Echocardiographic assessment of cardiovascular abnormalities in the Marfan syndrome: comparison with clinical findings and with roentgenographic estimation of aortic root size. Am J Med 74:465–474, 1983.
3. Gauthier R: Ein Beitrag zur Arachnodaktylie. Z Kinderheilkunde 43:724–736, 1927.
4. Godfrey M, Menashe V, Weleber RG, Koler RD, Bigley RH, Lovrien E, Zonana J, Hollister DW: Cosegregation of elastin-associated microfibrillar abnormalities with the Marfan phenotype in families. Am J Hum Genet 46:652–660, 1990.
5. Godfrey M, Vandemark N, Wang M, Velinov M, Wargowski D, Tsipouras P, Han J, Becker J, Robertson W, Droste S, et al: Prenatal diagnosis and a donor splice site mutation in fibrillin in a family with Marfan syndrome. Am J Hum Genet 53:472–480, 1993.
6. Hall JR, Pyeritz RE, Dudgeon DL, Haller JA Jr: Pneumothorax in the Marfan syndrome: prevalence and therapy. Ann Thorac Surg 37:500–504, 1984.
7. Hollister DW: Marfan syndrome: Neuropsychological aspects. Am J Med Genet 31:331–338, 1988.

8. Kelemen G: Marfan's syndrome and hearing organ. Acta Otolaryngol 59:23–32, 1965.
9. Marfan M: Un cas de déformation congénitale des quatres membres, plus prononcée aux extrémités, caracterisée par l'allongement des os avec un certain degré d'amincissement. Bull Mem Soc Med Hopital, Paris 13:220–226, 1896.
10. Maumenee IH: The eye in Marfan syndrome. Birth Defects 18:515–524, 1982.
11. McKusick VA: Mendelian Inheritance in Man, A Catalog of Human Genes and Genetic Disorders, 11th ed., The Johns Hopkins University Press, Baltimore, 1994.
12. Nelson LB, Maumenee IH: Ectopia lentis. Surv Ophthalmol 27:143–160, 1982.
13. Pyeritz RE, Wappel MA: Mitral valve dysfunction in Marfan syndrome: clinical and echocardiographic study of prevalence and natural history. Am J Med 74:797–807, 1983.
14. Raftopoulos C, Delechese F, Graude P, Rodesh C, Brotchi J: Anterior sacral meningocele and Marfan syndrome: a review. Acta Chir Belg 93:1–7, 1993.
15. Wang M, Mata J, Price CE, Iversen PL, Godfrey M: Prenatal and presymptomatic diagnosis of the Marfan syndrome using fluorescence PCR and an automated sequencer. Prenat Diagn 15:499–507, 1995.

## Melkersson-Rosenthal syndrome

### Cheilitis granulomatosa

(MIM No. *155900; POSSUM No. 3491)

This syndrome is characterized by recurrent or persistent lip swelling, facial swelling, facial palsy, and furrowed tongue.

#### General manifestations

Characteristic features include auditory and visual disturbances, swelling in the hands and chest, blepharospasm, epiphora and megacolon.

#### Otolaryngological manifestations

The swelling of the lips is usually of sudden onset and is unilateral or bilateral. The upper lip is affected in most cases and may remain swollen permanently. This occurs in 75% of patients. Facial palsy occurs after the lip swelling and sometimes precedes it. Facial swelling usually involves the eyelids, chin, and forehead in 50% of cases.[10] The oral mucosa and the gingiva may show swelling.[9] Histologically, the swollen tissues exhibit chronic granulomatous changes similar to sarcoidosis or tuberculosis.

Lingual fissures occur in 40% of cases. Defects of taste along the anterior two-thirds of the tongue, lip fissuring, and exposure keratitis are seen in long-standing cases.[2,5]

Surgical excision and reconstruction is recommended for the swollen orofacial tissues.[1] Total facial nerve decompression for recurrent facial palsy is also advocated.[3]

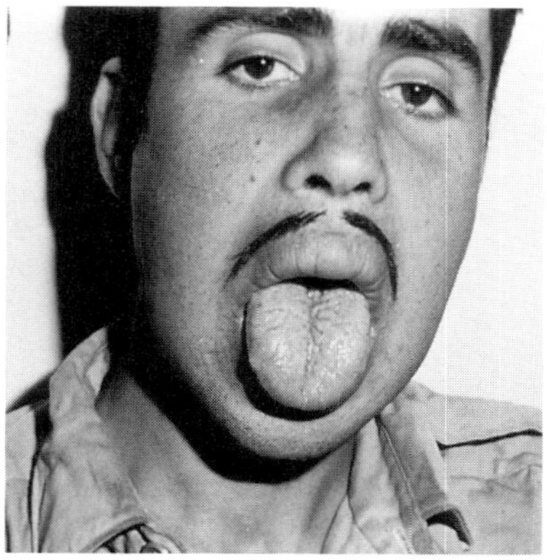

**Fig. 41.** Melkersson-Rosenthal syndrome. Patient with edema of the lip and scrotal tongue. (From VM Der Kaloustian, AK Kurban, *Genetic Diseases of the Skin,* Springer-Verlag, Berlin, 1979, p. 207, with permission.)

#### Etiology and pathogenesis

Most cases are sporadic.[7] Familial occurrences suggest an autosomal dominant transmission.[8] This syndrome is remarkably variable in its expression. The disease begins in childhood or early adulthood.[6] It is considered a local immune response and vasomotor disturbance affecting the vasa vasorum of the vessels supplying the facial nerve and neighboring structures.[4]

#### Differential diagnosis

Melkersson-Rosenthal syndrome should be differentiated from Hughes thick lips and oral mucosa syndrome.

#### References

1. Glickman LT, Gruss JS, Birt BD, Kohli-Dang N: The surgical management of Melkersson-Rosenthal syndrome. Plast Reconstr Surg 89:815–821, 1992.
2. Graaf-Radford SB: Melkersson-Rosenthal: a review of the literature and a case report. S Afr Med J 60:71–74, 1981.
3. Graham MD, Kartush JM: Total facial nerve decompression for recurrent facial paralysis: an update. Otolaryngol Head Neck Surg 101:442–444, 1989.
4. Hernandez G, Hernandez F, Lucas M: Meischer's granulomatous cheilitis. J Oral Maxillofac Surg 44:474–478, 1986.
5. Hornstein O, Schwermann H: Das sogenannte Melkersson-Rosenthal-Syndrome (ein schliesslich "cheilitis granulomatosa" Miescher). Ergebnisse Int Med Kinderheilkunde 17:190–263, 1962.
6. Kunstadter RH: Melkersson syndrome. A case report of multiple recurrences of Bell's palsy and episodic facial edema. Am J Dis Child 110:559–561, 1965.
7. Langevitz P, Engelberg JS, Tsur H, Cabili S: Melkersson-Rosenthal syndrome: an oligo-symptomatic form. South Med J 79:1159–1160, 1986.
8. Lygidakis C, Tsankanikas C, Ilias A, Vassilopoulos D: Melkersson-Rosenthal's syndrome in four generations. Clin Genet 15:189–192, 1979.
9. Worsaae N, Puidborg JJ: Granulomatous gingival manifestations in Melkersson-Rosenthal syndrome. Oral Surg 49:131–138, 1980.
10. Zimmer VM, Rogers RS, Reeve CM, Sheridan PJ: Orofacial manifestations of Melkersson-Rosenthal syndrome. A study of 42 patients and review of 220 cases from the literature. Oral Surg Oral Med Oral Pathol 74:610–619, 1992.

## Miller syndrome

(MIM No. *263750; POSSUM No. 3487)

#### General manifestations

The major manifestations include first branchial arch anomalies combined with defects of the extremities, variable degrees of mandibulofacial dysostosis with lower lid colobomas, vertebral and rib defects, accessory nipples, and postaxial limb defects.

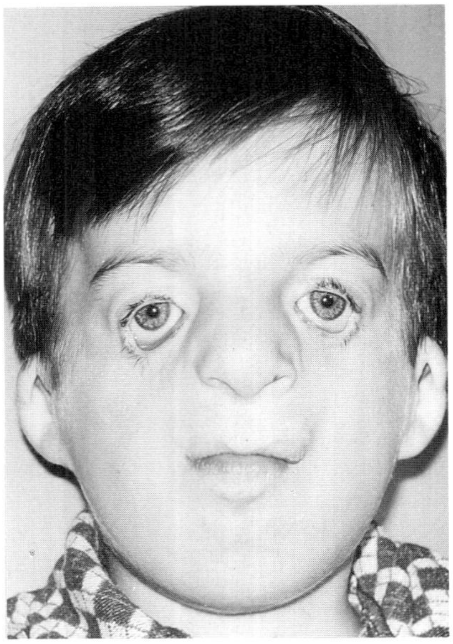

A

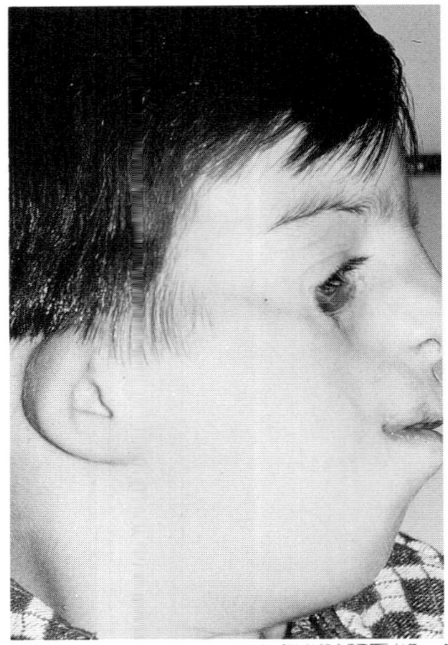

B

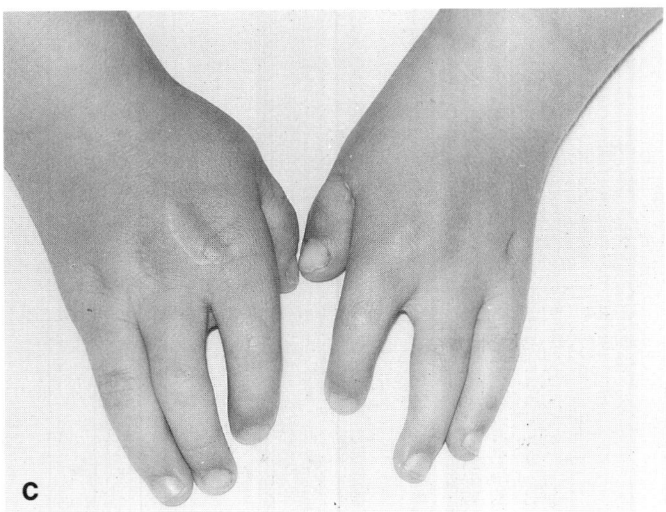

C

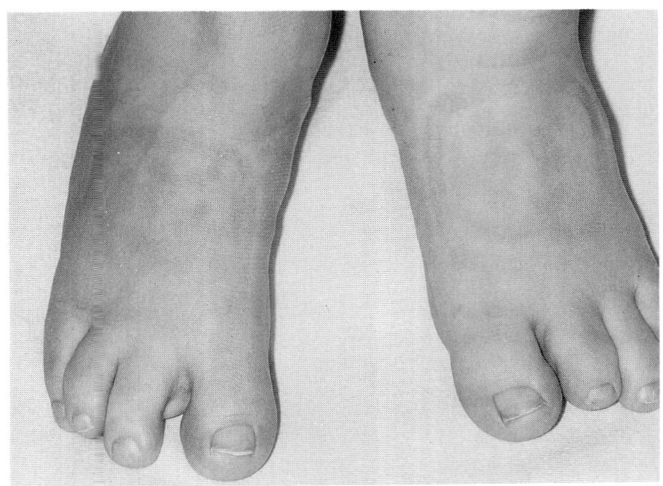

D

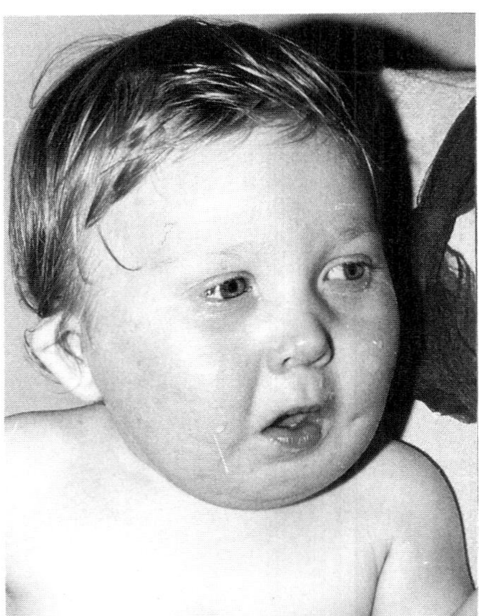

E

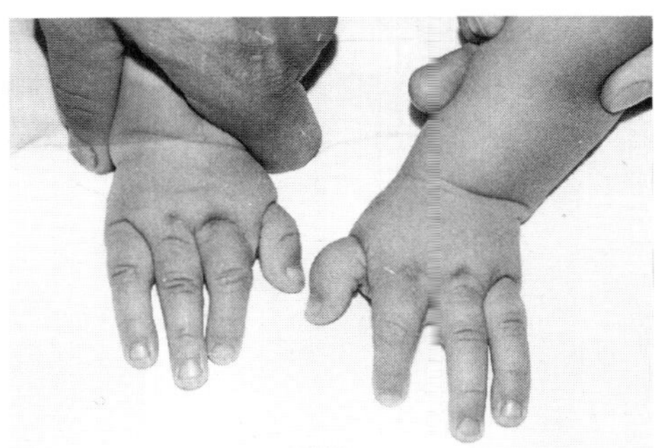

F

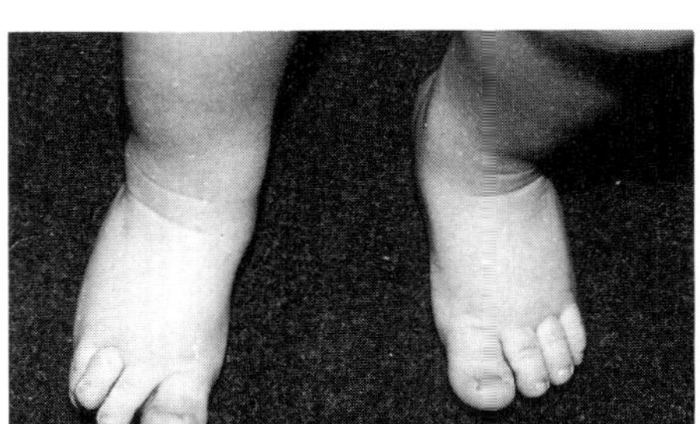

G

**Fig. 42.** Miller syndrome. Note the downward slanting palpebral fissures, ectropion of the lower lids, malformed ears, and repaired cleft lip (A,B), and postaxial agenesis of the fingers and toes (C,D). E–G: Affected patient with classical anomalies of the hands and feet. (A–D from MM Cohen Jr, Dysmorphic syndromes with craniofacial manifestations, in *Oral Facial Genetics,* RE Stewart, GH Prescott, eds., CV Mosby, St. Louis, 1976; E–G from KH Chrzanowska et al., Clin Genet 35:157, 1989, with permission.)

Oligodactyly and hypoplastic thumbs are the hallmarks of the syndrome.[3,4,7,8] Abnormal thumbs occur in half of the cases. Radioulnar synostosis and a short ulna and radius have been reported. Patent ductus arteriosus, ventricular septal defect with endocardial cushion defects, and genitourinary abnormalities have been described.[2–8]

### Otolaryngological manifestations

These include hypoplastic malar bones with downward slanting palpebral fissures, lower lid colobomas, micrognathia, and cleft palate.[1,6,7] The ears are hypoplastic and cup shaped. The facies resembles that of patients with Treacher Collins syndrome.

### Etiology

Miller syndrome is probably of autosomal recessive inheritance.[2,5] Autosomal dominant transmission with variable expressivity was documented in a large kindred.[1]

### Differential diagnosis

Miller syndrome should be differentiated from Nager syndrome.

#### References

1. Allanson JE, McGillivray BC: Familial clefting syndrome with ectropion and dental anomaly without limb anomalies. Clin Genet 27:426–429, 1985.
2. Fineman RM: Recurrence of the postaxial acrofacial dysostosis syndrome in a sibship: implications for genetic counselling. J Pediatr 98:87–88, 1981.
3. Fryns JP, van den Berghe H: Brief clinical report: acrofacial dysostosis with postaxial limb deficiency. Am J Med Genet 29:205–209, 1988.
4. Genée E: Une forme extensive de dysostose mandibulofaciale. J Genet Hum 17:45–52, 1969.
5. Giannotti A, Digilio MC, Virgili Q, Obregon MG, Guadagni AM, Ventura T, Dallapiccola B: Familial postaxial acrofacial dysostosis syndrome. J Med Genet 29:752, 1992.
6. Jackson IT, Bauer B, Salch J, Sullivan C, Argenta LC: A significant feature of Nager's syndrome: palatal agenesis. Plast Reconstr Surg 84:219–226, 1989.
7. Meinecke P, Wiedemann HR: Robin sequence and oligodactyly in mother and son—probably a further example of the postaxial acrofacial dysostosis syndrome. Am J Med Genet 27:953–956, 1987.
8. Smith DW, Jones KL: Case report 28. Syndrome Ident 3:7–8, 1975.

## Möbius syndrome

(MIM No. 157900; POSSUM No. 3217)

This syndrome was first described by Möbius in 1888.[9] Many authors consider this syndrome to be one of the oromandibular limb hypogenesis spectrum conditions.[5]

### General manifestations

Along with cranial nerve palsies, defects of the limbs (adactyly, syndactyly) may be seen, as well as hypoplasia or aplasia of the pectoral musculature. Poland anomaly is seen in 15% of cases.[13]

Mild mental retardation has been reported. Cardiovascular and urogenital anomalies are rare.[6,10,13]

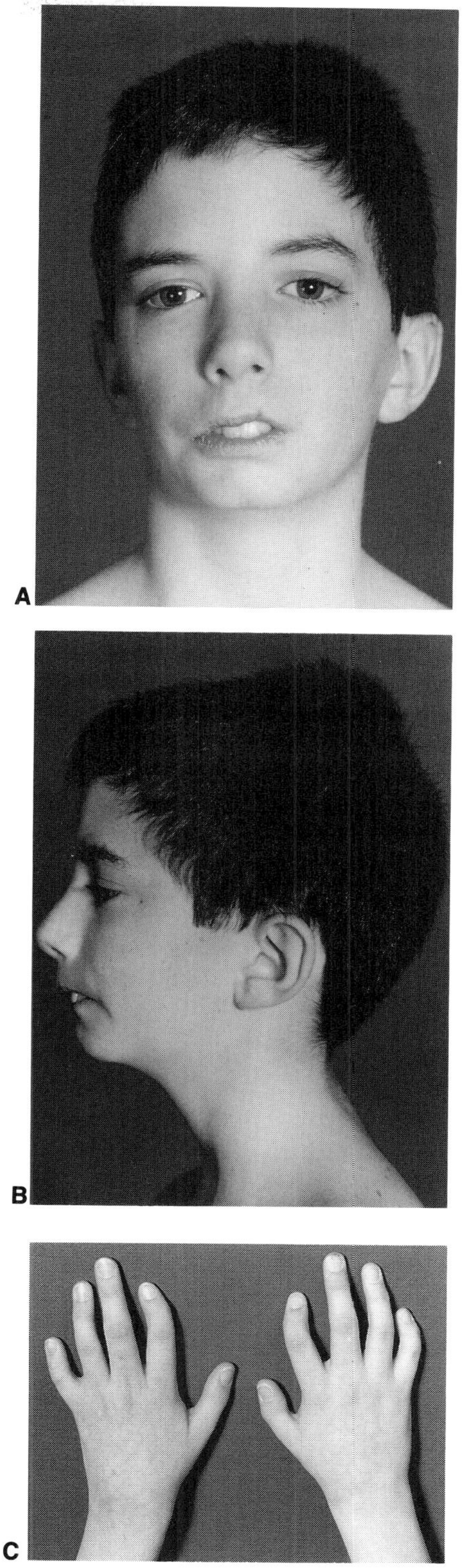

**Fig. 43.** Möbius syndrome. Note the bilateral facial paresis and mask-like facies (A,B) and abnormal digits (C).

### Otolaryngological manifestations

These include cranial nerve palsies, mostly of the sixth and seventh cranial nerves. This gives rise to a mask-like facies if the palsy is bilateral.[4] Paralysis of the abducens nerve is the most common ocular finding. Unilateral palsy may occur.[3] The mouth is small with drooping angles. The other cranial nerves may be affected as well (XII, IX, V, and III), resulting in lingual hypoplasia, dysfunction of the palate, and ocular ophthalmoplegia with conjunctivitis and/or keratitis.[3,12] The nose is broad, the mandible is hypoplastic, and the ears frequently lack cartilage. Hearing loss is infrequent.

### Etiology and pathogenesis

The etiology is unknown. Although most cases have been sporadic, familial recurrence is not rare.[7a,9] Autosomal dominant inheritance has been suggested in some cases.[2] The theory of subclavian artery disruption was proposed by Baviuck and Weaver.[1] Other theories include delayed formation of blood vessels, early uterine compression, and blood vessel edema.[14] Vascular disruption of the basilar artery and ischemia of the brain stem has also been proposed.[7,8] Deletion of chromosome 13 (q12.2) was reported in 1991.[11] In a Dutch family, the gene for Möbius syndrome was localized to chromosome 3q, indicating genetic heterogeneity.[7a] This heterogeneity was further proven by the exclusion of both loci in another family with Möbius syndrome.[7a]

### Differential diagnosis

Möbius syndrome should be differentiated from congenital myopathies and oromandibular-limb hypogenesis or aglossia-adactylia syndrome.

### References


1. Baviuck JNB, Weaver DD: Subclavian artery supply disruption sequence: hypothesis of a vascular etiology for Poland, Klippel-Feil, and Möbius anomalies. Am J Med Genet 23:903–918, 1986.
2. Dotti MT, Federico A, Palmeri S, Guazzi GC: Congenital oculo-facial paralysis (Moebius syndrome): evidence of dominant inheritance in two families. Acta Neurol 11:434–438, 1989.
3. Evans PR: Nuclear agenesis. Möbius syndrome: The congenital facial diplegia syndrome. Arch Dis Childh 30:237–243, 1955.
4. Gutman D, Sharon A, Laufer D: Moebius' syndrome. Br J Oral Surg 11:20–24, 1973.
5. Hall BD: Aglossia-adactylia. Birth Defects 7:233–236, 1971.
6. Hanissian AS, Fusk F, Hayes WT, Duncan JM: Möbius syndrome in twins. Am J Dis Child 120:472–475, 1970.
7. Harbord MG, Finn JP, Hall-Craggs MA, Brett EM, Baraitser M: Moebius' syndrome with unilateral cerebellar hypoplasia. J Med Genet 26:579–582, 1989.

7a. Kremer H, Kuyt LP, van den Helm B, van Reen M, Leunissen JAM, Hamel BCJ, Jansen C, Mariman ECM, Frants RR, Padberg GW: Localization of a gene for Möbius syndrome to chromosome 3q by linkage analysis in a Dutch family. Hum Mol Genet 9:1367–1371, 1996.

8. Lipson AH, Webster WS, Brown-Woodman PD, Osborn RA: Moebius syndrome: animal model-human correlations and evidence for a brainstem vascular etiology. Teratology 40:339–350, 1989.
9. Möbius RJ: Über angeborene doppelseitige Abducens-Facialis Lahmung. München Med Wochenschr 35:91–94, 108–111, 1888.
10. Olson WH, Bardin CW, Walsh GO, Engel WK: Möbius syndrome: lower motor neuron involvement and hypogonadotrophic hypogonadism. Neurology 20:1002–1008, 1970.
11. Slee JJ, Smart RD, Viljoen DL: Deletion of chromosome 13 in Moebius syndrome. J Med Genet 28:413–414, 1991.
12. Steigner M, Steward RE, Setoguchi Y: Combined limb deficiencies and cranial nerve dysfunction: report of six cases. Birth Defects 11:133–141, 1975.
13. Sugarman GI, Stark HH: Möbius syndrome with Poland's anomaly. J Med Genet 10:192–196, 1973.
14. Van Allen MI: Fetal vascular disruptions: mechanisms and some resulting birth defects. Pediatr Ann 10:219–233, 1981.


## The mucopolysaccharidoses

The mucopolysaccharidoses (MPS) are inherited storage disorders caused by a deficiency in lysosomal enzymes necessary for the degradation of mucopolysaccharides (glycosaminoglycans). Accumulation of mucopolysaccharide molecules results in cell, tissue, and organ dysfunction. There are several enzyme deficiencies that give rise to six distinct types of MPS. These types share many clinical manifestations to varying degrees. The manifestations include abnormal facies, skeletal changes (dysostosis multiplex), organomegaly, and a chronic and progressive course.[10,24] Mental retardation, hearing impairment, vision problems, joint limitation, and cardiovascular dysfunction may be additional features. All MPS are inherited in an autosomal recessive manner with the exception of MPS-2 (Hunter syndrome), which is an X-linked recessive disorder.[24]

## MPS-I (Hurler, Scheie, and Hurler-Scheie syndromes)

(MIM No. *252800; POSSUM Nos. 3308, 3312)

### General manifestations

An MPS-IH (Hurler syndrome) infant appears normal at birth but may have umbilical or inguinal hernias. Clinical diagnosis is usually made in the first or second year of life. Macrocephaly, coarse facial features, a prominent forehead, macroglossia, joint stiffness including claw hands and other skeletal deformities, and hepatosplenomegaly with protuberant abdomen are usually the presenting features.[10,24] Patients may be large in infancy but growth failure occurs afterwards. Communicating hydrocephalus appears to be common. Developmental delay is apparent in the second year of life and severe mental retardation is usually the rule. Cardiac complications include valvular changes, coronary artery disease and endocardial fibroelastosis.[8,29,34] Progressive corneal clouding begins in infancy and glaucoma can be an early complication. The skin is dry, the hair is coarse, and the teeth are widely spaced. Most children have recurrent upper respiratory infections, ear infections, noisy breathing, and chronic nasal discharge due to marked lymphoid tissue hypertrophy. Obstructive airway disease, pneumonias, and cardiac failure are the common causes of death, which usually occurs by the age of 10 years.[24,33]

Radiologic changes include a large skull with thickened calvarium, premature closure of lambdoid and saggital sutures, J-shaped sella turcica, a thick skull base with calcified stylohyoid ligaments, dysplastic cervical vertebrae with subluxation of C1–C2, anterior hypoplasia of lumbar vertebrae with kyphosis, enlarged diaphyses of long bones, irregular metaphyses, abnormal development of epiphyseal centers, short and thickened clavicles, and a poorly formed pelvis with small femoral heads and coxa valga.[10,24] The ribs are oar shaped and the phalanges have short and widened epiphyses.

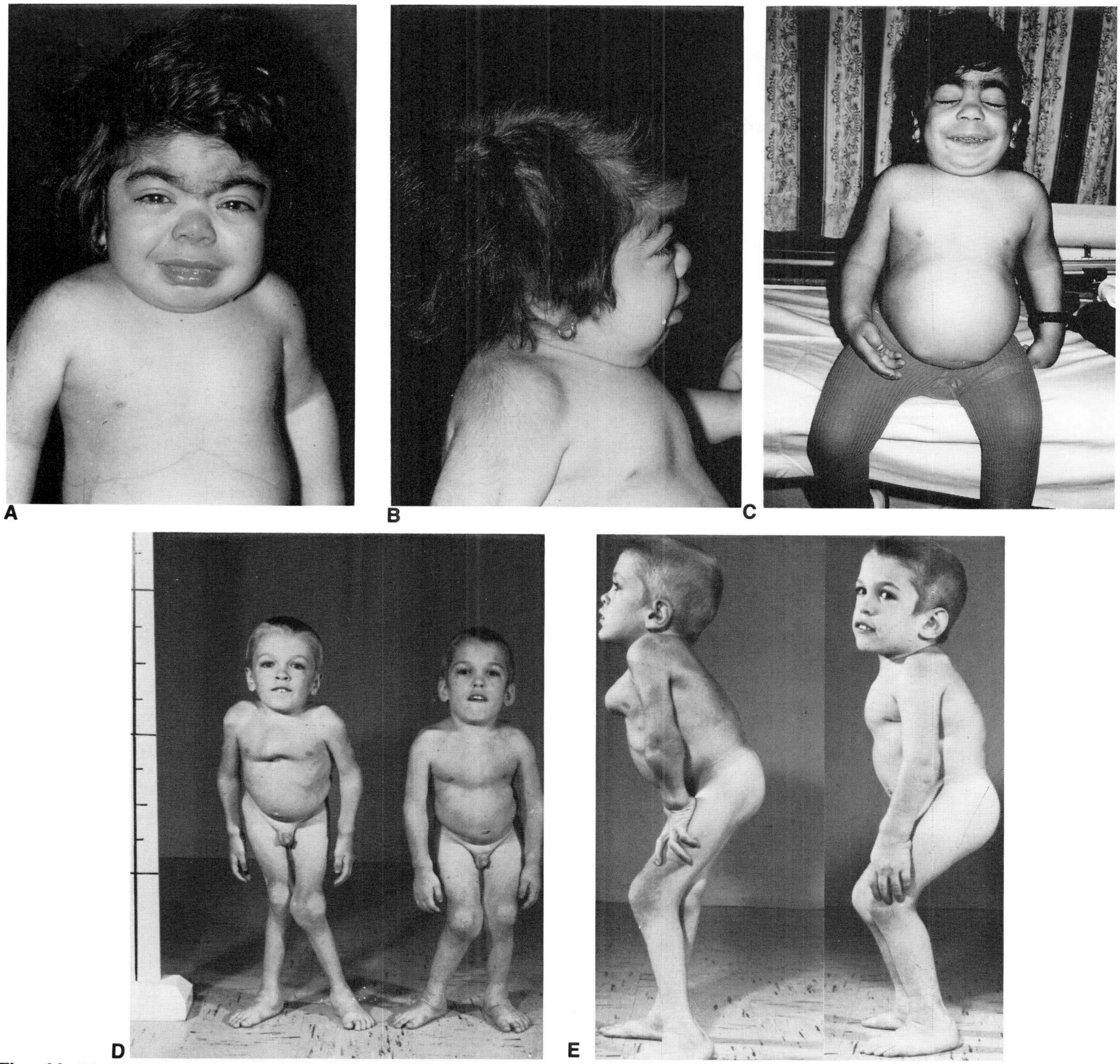

**Fig. 44.** Mucopolysaccharidoses. A–C: Patients with Hurler syndrome. Note the characteristic coarse facies and hepatosplenomegaly. D,E: Morquio syndrome. Note the dwarfism, kyphosis, flexed knees, short neck, and protruding sternum. (D,E from H Zellweger et al., J Pediatr 59:549, 1961, with permission.)

MPS-IH/S (Hurler-Scheie syndrome) is characterized by a less progressive course as compared with MPS-IH, as there is little or no intellectual dysfunction.[10,24] Corneal clouding, deafness, joint stiffness and valvular heart disease develop usually in the beginning of the second decade of life and cause significant impairment. Coarse facial features with micrognathia and dysostosis multiplex are observed. Cervical cord compression due to mucopolysaccharide accumulation in the dura occurs. Survival to adulthood is common. Cardiac and respiratory complications are the most common cause of death.

MPS-IS (Scheie syndrome) is characterized by corneal clouding, aortic valve disease, coarse facies, joint stiffness, and normal stature and intelligence.[10,24] The joint involvement is most prominent in the hands due to claw-hand deformity. Carpal-tunnel syndrome is common. Aortic valve disease with regurgitation or stenosis occurs due to deposition of mucopolysaccharides on the valve and cordae tendinae.[6] Cervical cord compression occurs, but less commonly than in MPS-IH/S patients. Deafness is not very common. Glaucoma and pigmentary retinopathy may develop. Diagnosis is often made in the second decade of life. Life expectancy is probably normal.

### Otolaryngological manifestations

In MPS-IH, otolaryngological manifestations include a depressed nasal bridge and broad nose with anteverted nostrils.

The lips are patulous and the mouth is held open.[7] Middle ear infection is common due to eustachian tube obstruction.[10,11] Some degree of hearing loss is very common and is usually a combination of conductive and sensorineural elements. Dentigenous cysts occur because of the pooling of dermatan sulfate in the hyperplastic dental follicles.[7,10] Enlargement of the gingiva results from mouth breathing and lack of oral hygiene. Sleep apnea results from airway obstruction and a small mandible.

### Etiology

The deficiency in $\alpha$-L-iduronidase results in a wide spectrum of clinical manifestations. Hurler syndrome is the most severe, Scheie syndrome is the mild form, and Hurler-Scheie syndrome is the intermediate form.[24] All are characterized by excessive urinary excretion of dermatan and heparan sulfate and the absence of $\alpha$-L-iduronidase activity.

The gene encoding MPS-I has been localized to chromosome 4p16.3 by in situ hybridization and has been confirmed by other methods.[31] It has been cloned and mutation analysis revealed a number of mutant alleles, two of which are common.[24,32] The milder forms of MPS are likely to have at least one mutant allele that permits some residual activity.

## MPS-II (Hunter syndrome)

(MIM No. *309900; POSSUM No. 3309)

### General manifestations

Two forms are recognized: mild and severe. They are separated on clinical grounds since iduronate sulfatase enzyme activity appears to be equally deficient in both forms. The severe form of Hunter syndrome is reminiscent of Hurler syndrome except for the absence of corneal clouding and a slower progression of somatic and CNS involvement.[33,38,43,44] The occurrence of pebbly, ivory-colored skin lesions over the back, upper arms, and thighs is distinctive to MPS-II and has no correlation with the severity of the disease.[24] Death occurs in the early teens due to cardiopulmonary disease.

The mild form of Hunter syndrome is somewhat similar to MPS-IS, with normal intelligence.[42] Visual impairment is common and is usually due to retinal dysfunction and chronic papilledema.[2] Carpal-tunnel syndrome and joint stiffness are common. Patients with mild MPS-II may survive into the sixth and seventh decades of life.[42] Death may occur earlier due to cardiopulmonary complications.

### Otolaryngological manifestations

Some degree of deafness is universal.[27]

### Etiology

The gene for MPS-II has been mapped to Xq28 by several methods including in situ hybridization with cloned cDNA.[21,37] About one-fifth of patients have deletions or rearrangements detectable on Southern blots.[24] The majority of MPS-II patients appear to have point mutations and minor rearrangements.[15,18]

## MPS-III (Sanfilippo syndrome)

(MIM Nos. *252900, *252920, *252930, *252940; POSSUM No. 3310)

### General manifestations

MPS-III is characterized by mild somatic disease and severe progressive CNS involvement.[25] The infant with Sanfilippo syndrome appears normal at birth. Presentation occurs after the second year of life and features can include delayed development, hyperactivity, poor attention span and aggressive behavior, coarse hair, sleep disturbances, and mild hepatosplenomegaly.[10,24,25,39] Coarse facies and macroglossia are not prominent features as compared with other MPS and skeletal involvement including joint stiffness is usually minimal. Height is usually normal. Corneal clouding is absent. Severe neurologic deterioration and seizures occur in most patients, accompanied by rapid social and adaptive regression.[25] Progression to severe cortical atrophy occurs late in the disease.

MPS-III type A is the most severe, with earlier onset and more rapid progression of disease and reduced lifespan. Type B is clinically heterogeneous as well as type D, which is very rare.[20] Type C is an intermediate form of MPS-III between type A and mild forms of type B.

### Otolaryngological manifestations

Severe hearing loss is common and poor speech is the rule.

### Etiology

Patients with this syndrome are classified into four clinically similar types which are biochemically diverse. Each is characterized by a deficiency in an enzyme necessary for the degradation of heparan sulfate. The four enzymes are heparan N-sulfatase (type A); $\alpha$-N-acetylglucosaminidase (type B); acetyl CoA:$\alpha$-glucosaminide acetyltransferase (type C); and N-acetyl glucosamine 6-sulfatase (type D).[24]

The gene for MPS-IIID has been localized to 12q14 by in situ hybridization.[30]

## MPS-IV (Morquio syndrome)

(MIM Nos. *253000, #253010; POSSUM No. 3311)

### General manifestations

Clinical manifestations in the two types of MPS-IV are widely variable and include short trunk dwarfism, spondyloepiphyseal dysplasia, fine corneal deposits, and normal intelligence.[14,24,40] Patients are apparently normal at birth. First symptoms of Morquio syndrome appear between 1 and 4 years of age and include genu valgus, kyphosis, growth failure with short trunk and neck, and waddling gait with a tendency to fall.[3,13,26] Hepatomegaly and hernias are common. Ligamentous laxity of large joints is common and atlantoaxial dislocation can be life threatening. Paralysis from myelopathy, cardiac valvular disease, and restrictive chest wall movement are additional factors contributing to a shortened lifespan in MPS-IV patients.[4,17] Patients with the severe form rarely survive beyond the second or third decade of life.[24]

Radiologic changes include mild scaphocephaly, dwarfism with short trunk, platyspondyly, odontoid hypoplasia, kyphosis, scoliosis, deformities of the vertebrae, inclinations of distal ends of the radius and ulna toward each other, deformities of metacarpals and short phalanges, epiphyseal deformities of tubular bones, widened metaphyses, and osteoporosis.[10,24]

### Otolaryngological manifestations

Coarse facies with prognathism, small teeth with enamel hypoplasia, wide mouth, and deafness are common.

### Etiology

The deficiency of one of the two enzymes necessary for the degradation of keratan sulfate can cause MPS-IV types A or B. The deficient enzymes are N-acetylgalactosamine 6–sulfatase (galactose 6–sulfatase) in MPS-IVA and $\beta$-galactosidase in MPS-IVB.[24,40]

The gene for MPS-IVA has been localized by in situ hybridization to 16q24.[1,23] A number of deletions and mutations have been characterized.

## MPS-VI (Maroteaux-Lamy syndrome)

(MIM Nos. *253200; POSSUM No. 3313)

### General manifestations

MPS-VI is a Hurler-like syndrome with a wide range of clinical variability and normal intelligence. The somatic involvement is severe. Macrocephaly and chest deformity may be present at birth. Growth may be normal early in life but cessation of growth becomes evident between the ages of 6 and 8 years.[19,24] Features include coarse facies, corneal opacities, umbilical and inguinal hernias, hepatosplenomegaly, restricted movement of large joints, claw-hand deformities, nerve entrapment syndromes—particularly the carpal-tunnel syndrome—aortic and mitral valvular dysfunction, cardiomyopathy, tight skin with hirsutism, hydrocephalus, and shortened trunk with protuberant abdomen and prominent lumbar lordosis.[9,12,35] Atlantoaxial dislocation may occur. Spinal cord compression with resultant myelopathy is frequent in patients with milder forms.[45] Most patients with the severe form die of heart failure in the second and third decades. Radiologic changes associated with severe MPS-VI are similar to those of Hurler syndrome. Mental development is usually normal in most patients, although physical and visual handicaps may affect their psychomotor performance.

### Otolaryngological manifestations

Macroglossia, mixed deafness, and noisy breathing are common features.

### Etiology

Patients have a deficiency of the enzyme N-acetylgalactosamine 4 sulfatase (arylsulfatase B) and excrete mainly dermatan sulfate.

The gene for MPS-VI has been localized to 5q13–q14 by in situ hybridization.[22] Analysis of residual enzyme activity has not allowed precise correlation with the clinical phenotype.[5] The availability of a cDNA sequence has allowed the identification of mutations that correlate with the severity of manifestations.[24]

## MPS-VII (Sly syndrome)

(MIM No. *253220; POSSUM No. 3314)

### General manifestations

The clinical features are somewhat similar to MPS-IH or MPS-II and include unusual facies, variable corneal clouding, pigeon chest, hepatosplenomegaly, hernias, thoracolumbar kyphosis, short stature, and moderate mental deficiency.[16,24,28] Neurologic impairment and psychomotor retardation appear to be nonprogressive. Severe and milder forms exist. A severe neonatal form has been reported in association with fetal deaths and hydrops fetalis with clinical and pathological findings of a lysosomal storage disorder, including dysostosis multiplex.[19,41] A less severe form presents in the first years of life with repeated episodes of pneumonia, hernias, and hepatosplenomegaly. A milder form, with onset after 4 years of age, is characterized by mild to severe dysostosis multiplex changes and normal intelligence.[24]

### Etiology

MPS-VII is caused by a deficiency in $\beta$-glucuronidase enzyme and is characterized by excessive glycosaminoglycan excretion and coarse granulocyte inclusions.

The gene for MPS-VII has been localized on 7q21.11.[30a,36] Several mutations have been found.[36]

### References

1. Baker E, Guo XH, Orsborn AM, Sutherland GR, Callen DF, Hopwood JJ, Morris CP: The Morquio A syndrome (mucopolysaccharidosis IVA) gene maps to 16q24.3. Am J Hum Genet 52:96–98, 1993.
2. Beck M, Cole G: Disc oedema in association with Hunter's syndrome: ocular histopathological findings. Br J Ophthalmol 68:590, 1984.
3. Beck M, Glossl J, Grubisic A, Spranger J: Heterogeneity of Morquio syndrome. Clin Genet 29:325–331, 1986.
4. Blaw ME, Langer LO: Spinal cord compression in Morquio-Brailsford's disease. J Pediatr 74:593–600, 1969.
5. Brooks DA, McCourt PAG, Gibson GJ, Ashton LJ, Shutter M, Hopwood JJ: Analysis of N-acetylgalactosamine-4-sulfatase protein and kinetics in mucopolysaccharidosis type VI patients. Am J Hum Genet 48:710–719, 1991.
6. Butman SM, Karl L, Copelands JG: Combined aortic and mitral valve replacement in an adult with Scheie's disease. Chest 96:209–210, 1989.
7. Cawson RA: The oral changes in gargoylism. Proc R Soc Med 55:1066–1070, 1962.
8. Donaldson MDC, Pennock CA, Berry PJ, Duncan AW, Cawdery JE, Leonard JV: Hurler syndrome with cardiomyopathy in infancy. J Pediatr 114:430–432, 1989.
9. Goldberg MF, Scott CI, McKusick VA: Hydrocephalus and papilledema in the Maroteaux-Lamy syndrome. Am J Ophthalmol 69:969–974, 1970.
10. Gorlin RJ, Cohen MM Jr, Levin LS: Syndromes of the Head and Neck, 3rd ed. Oxford University Press, New York, 1990, pp 99–117.
11. Grossman H, Dorst JP: The mucopolysaccharidoses and mucoli-

pidoses. In: Progress in Pediatric Radiology, Vol 4, HJ Kaufman, ed. Karger, Basel, 1973, pp 495.
12. Hayflick S, Rowe S, Kavanaugh-McHugh A, Olson JL, Valle D: Acute infantile cardiomyopathy as a presenting feature of mucopolysaccharidosis VI. J Pediatr 120:269–272, 1992.
13. Hecht JT, Scott CI, Smith TK, Williams JC: Mild manifestations of the Morquio syndrome. Am J Med Genet 18:369–371, 1984.
14. Holzgreve W, Grobe H, von Figura K, Kresse H, Beck H, Mattei JF: Morquio syndrome: clinical findings in 11 patients with MPS IVA and 2 patients with MPS IV B. Hum Genet 57:360–365, 1981.
15. Hopwood JJ, Bunge S, Morris CP, Wilson PJ, Steglich C, Beck M, Schwinger E, Gal A: Molecular basis of mucopolysaccharidosis type II: mutations in the iduronate-2-sulphatase gene. Hum Mutat 2:435–442, 1993.
16. Hoyme HE, Jones KL, Higginbottom MC, O'Brien JS: Presentation of mucopolysaccharidosis VII (beta-glucuronidase deficiency) in infancy. J Med Genet 18:237–239, 1981.
17. John RM, Hunter D, Swanton RH: Echocardiographic abnormalities in type IV mucopolysaccharidosis. Arch Dis Child 65:746–749, 1990.
18. Jonsson JJ, Aronovich EL, Braun SE, Whitley CB: Molecular diagnosis of mucopolysaccharidosis type II (Hunter syndrome) by automated sequencing and computer-assisted interpretation: toward mutation mapping of the iduronate-2-sulfatase gene. Am J Hum Genet 56:597–607, 1995.
19. Kagie MJ, Kleijer WJ, Huijmans JGM, Maaswinkel-Mooy P, Kanhai HHH: Beta-glucuronidase deficiency as a cause of fetal hydrops. Am J Med Genet 42:693–695, 1992.
20. Kaplan P, Wolfe LS: Sanfilippo syndrome type D. J Pediatr 110:267–271, 1987.
21. Le Guern E, Couillin P, Oberle I, Ravise N, Boue J: More precise localization of the gene for Hunter syndrome. Genomics 7:358–362, 1990.
22. Litjens T, Baker EG, Beckmann KR, Morris CP, Hopwood JJ, Callen DF: Chromosomal localization of ARSB, the gene for human N-acetylgalactosamine-4-sulphatase. Hum Genet 82:67–68, 1989.
23. Masuno M, Tomatsu S, Nakashima Y, Hori T, Fukuda S, Masue M, Sukegawa K, Takahashi E, Hori T, Orii T: Assignment of the human N-acetylgalactosamine-6-sulfate sulfatase gene (GALNS) to chromosome 16q24. Genomics 16:777–778, 1993.
24. Neufeld EF, Muenzer J: The mucopolysaccharidoses. In: The Metabolic and Molecular Bases of Inherited Disease, Vol 2, 7th ed, CR Scriver, AL Beaudet, WS Sly, D Valle, eds. McGraw-Hill, New York, 1995, pp 2465–2495.
25. Nidiffer FD, Kelly TE: Developmental and degenerative patterns associated with cognitive, behavioral and motor difficulties in the Sanfilippo syndrome: an epidemiological study. J Ment Defic Res 27:185–203, 1983.
26. O'Brien JS, Gugler E, Giedion A, Wiesmann U, Herschkowitz N, Meier C, Leroy J: Spondyloepiphyseal dysplasia, corneal clouding, normal intelligence and acid $\beta$-galactosidase deficiency. Clin Genet 9:495–504, 1976.
27. Peck JE: Hearing loss in Hunter syndrome—mucopolysaccaaridosis II. Ear Hear 5:243–246, 1984.
28. Pizzutillo PD, Osterkamp JA, Scott CI Jr, Lee MS: Atlantoaxial instability in mucopolysaccharidosis type VII. J Pediatr Orthop 9:76–78, 1989.
29. Pyeritz RE: Cardiovascular manifestations of heritable disorders of connective tissue. In: Progress in Medical Genetics, Vol 5, AG Steinberg, AG Bearn, AG Motulsky, B Childs, eds. WB Saunders, Philadelphia, 1983, pp 191–302.
30. Robertson DA, Callen DF, Baker EG, Morris CP, Hopwood JJ: Chromosomal localization of the gene for human glucosamine 6-sulphatase to 12q14. Hum Genet 79:175–178, 1988.
30a. Schwartz C, Stanislovitis P, Phelan MC, Klinger K, Taylor HA, Stevenson RE: Deletion mapping of plasminogen activator inhibitor, type I (PLANH 1) and beta-glucuronidase (GUSB) in 7q21–q22. Cytogenet Cell Genet 51:152–153, 1991.
31. Scott HS, Ashton LJ, Eyre HJ, Baker E, Brooks DA, Callen DG, Sutherland GR, Morris CP, Hopwood JJ: Chromosomal localization of the human $\alpha$-L-iduronidase gene (IDUA) to 4p16.3. Am J Hum Genet 47:802–807, 1990.
32. Scott HS, Litjens T, Nelson PV, Thompson PR, Brooks DA, Hopwood JJ, Morris CP: Identification of mutations in the alpha-L-iduronidase gene (IDUA) that cause Hurler and Scheie syndrome. Am J Hum Genet 53:973–986, 1993.
33. Shapiro J, Strome M, Crocker AC: Airway obstruction and sleep apnea in Hurler and Hunter syndromes. Ann Otol Rhinol Laryngol 94:458–461, 1985.
34. Stephan MJ, Stevens EL Jr, Wenstrup RJ, Greenberg CR, Gritter HL, Hodges GF, Guller B: Mucopolysaccharidosis I presenting with endocardial fibroelastosis of infancy. Am J Dis Child 143:782–784, 1989.
35. Tan CT, Schaff HV, Miller FA J, Edwards WD, Karnes PS: Valvular heart disease in four patients with Maroteaux-Lamy syndrome. Circulation 85:188–195, 1992.
36. Tsui L-C, Farrall M, Donis-Keller H: Report of the committee on the genetic constitution of chromosomes 7 and 8. Interim human gene mapping workshop 9.5. Cytogenet Cell Genet 51:166–201, 1989.
37. Upadhyaya M, Sarfarazi M, Bamforth JS, Thomas NST, Oberle I, Young I, Harper PS: Localization of the gene for Hunter syndrome on the long arm of X-chromosome. Hum Genet 74:391–398, 1986.
38. Van Aerde J, Plets C, van der Hauwert L: Hydrocephalus in Hunter syndrome. Acta Paediatr Belg 34:93–96, 1981.
39. Van de Kamp JJP, Niermeijer MF, von Figura K, Giesberts MA: Genetic heterogeneity and clinical variability in the Sanfilippo syndrome (types A, B, and C). Clin Genet 20:152–160, 1981.
40. Van der Horst GTJ, Kleijer WJ, Hoogeveen AT, Huijman JGM, Blom W, van Diggelen OP: Morquio B syndrome: A primary defect in $\beta$-galactosidase. Am J Med Genet 16:261–275, 1983.
41. Wilson D, Melnik E, Sly W, Makesbery WR: Neonatal $\beta$-glucuronidase-deficiency mucopolysaccharidosis (MPS VII): autopsy findings. J Neuropathol Exp Neurol 41:344–351, 1982.
42. Young ID, Harper PS: Mild form of Hunter's syndrome: clinical delineation based on 31 cases. Arch Dis Child 57:828–836, 1982.
43. Young ID, Harper PS: The natural history of the severe form of Hunter's syndrome: a study based on 52 cases. Dev Med Child Neurol 25:481–489, 1983.
44. Young ID, Harper PS, Archer IM, Newcombe RG: A clinical and genetic study of Hunter's syndrome. 1. Heterogeneity. J Med Genet 19:401–407, 1982.
45. Young R, Kleinman G, Ojemann RG, Kolodny E, Davis K, Halperin J, Zalneraitis E, Delong GR: Compressive myelopathy in Maroteaux-Lamy syndrome: clinical and pathological findings. Ann Neurol 8:336–340, 1980.

## Multiple mucosal neuroma syndrome

### Multiple endocrine neoplasia type IIB (MEN-IIB)

(MIM No. #162300; POSSUM No. 3319)

#### General manifestations

These include failure to thrive and a Marfanoid habitus in 75% of patients with excessive wasting and weakness. Gastrointestinal anomalies such as megacolon with defects of autonomic innervation, diverticulum, and intestinal ganglioneuromatoses have been documented. Pheochromocytoma is diagnosed in half of the patients. Ophthalmological findings include pedun-

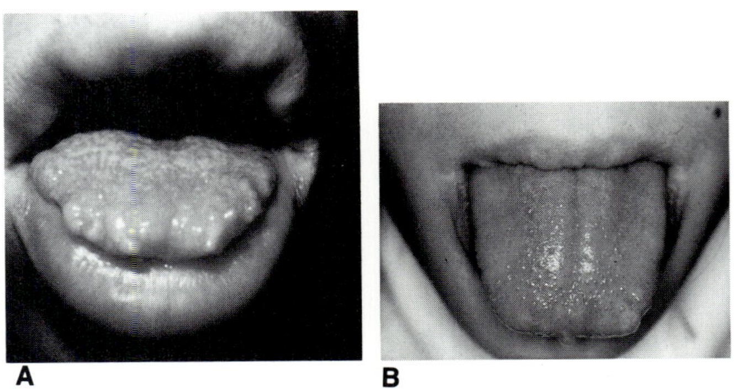

**Fig. 45.** Multiple mucosal neuroma syndrome. A: Multiple neuromas of the tongue; B: A milder form. (Courtesy of Dr. C Polychronakos.)

culated neuromas of the palpebral conjunctiva. Occasional abnormalities include parathyroid hyperplasia, developmental delay, and carcinoid tumors of the rectum.[1–10]

### Otolaryngological manifestations

Multiple neuromas of the tongue and lips associated with medullary carcinoma of the thyroid are very common. The diagnosis is usually made after the age of 12 years.

### Etiology

This syndrome is of autosomal dominant inheritance. More than half of the cases represent new mutations. The gene is mapped to 10q11.2.[1a,7] It is possible that MEN-IIA and MEN-IIB are allelic disorders.[7,8]

### References


1. Block MB, Roberts JP, Kadair RG, Seifer AE, Hull SF, Nofeld EFD: Multiple endocrine adenomatosis type IIB. JAMA 234:710–714, 1975.
1a. Brooks-Wilson AR, Lichter JB, Ward DC, Kidd KK, Goodfellow PJ: Genomic and yeast artificial chromosome long-range physical maps linking six loci in 10q11.2 and spanning the multiple endocrine neoplasia type 2A (MEN 2A) region. Genomics 17:611–617, 1993.
2. Carney JA, Bianco AJ Jr, Sizemore GW, Hayles AV: Multiple endocrine neoplasia with skeletal manifestations. J Bone Joint Surg 63:405–410, 1981.
3. Carney JA, Sizemore GW, Hayles AV: Multiple endocrine neoplasia, type 2b. Pathobiol Annual 8:105–153, 1978.
4. Casino AJ, Sciubba JJ, Ohri GL, Roshner F, Winston J, Yunis M, Wolk D: Oral-facial manifestations of the multiple endocrine neoplasia syndrome. Oral Surg Oral Med Oral Pathol 51:516–523, 1981.
5. Dunn EL, Nishiyama RH, Thompson NW: Medullary carcinoma of the thyroid gland. Surgery 73:848–858, 1973.
6. Gorlin RJ, Vickers RA: Multiple mucosal neuromas, pheochromocytoma, medullary carcinoma of the thyroid and marfanoid body build


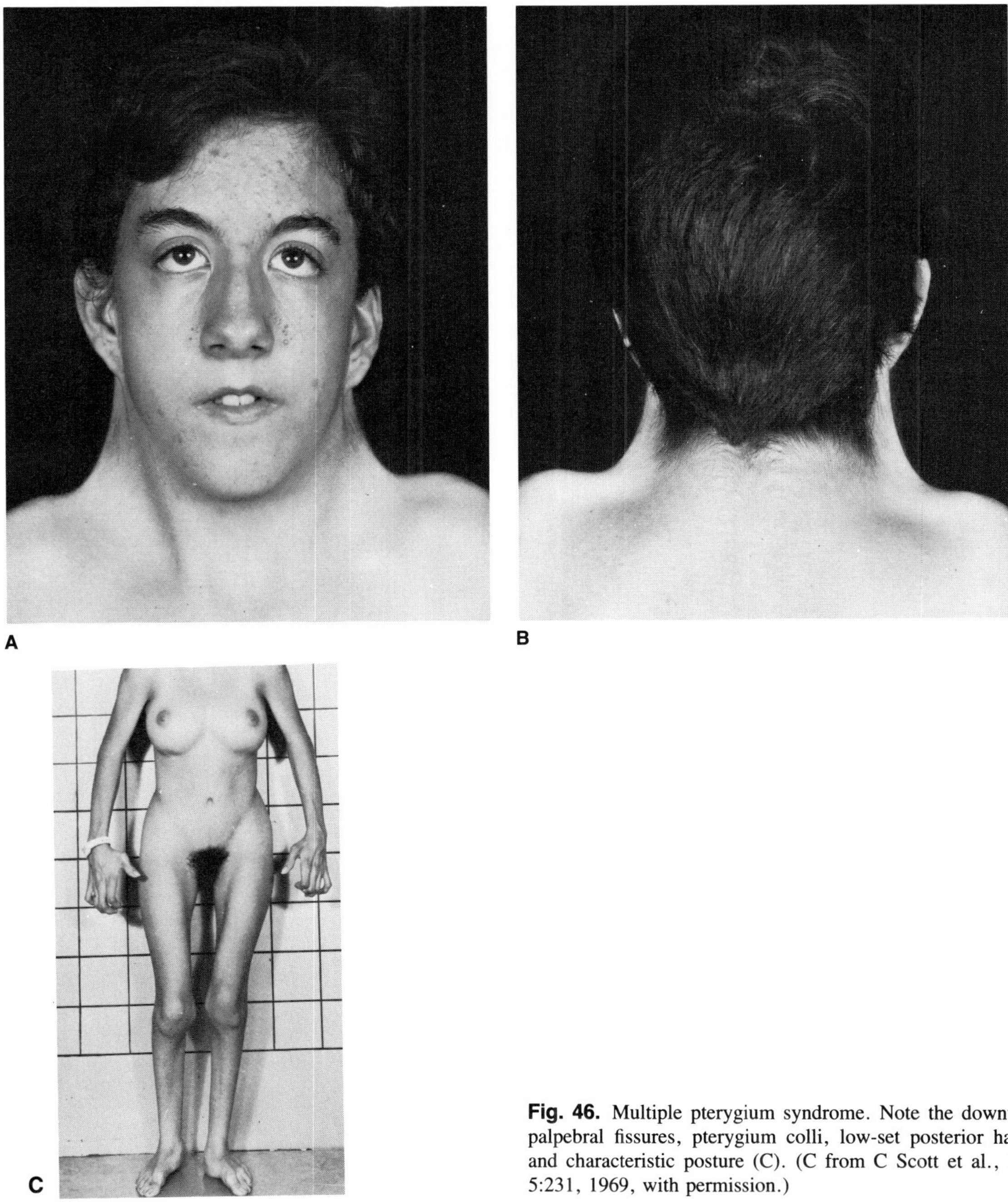

A B C

**Fig. 46.** Multiple pterygium syndrome. Note the downward slanting palpebral fissures, pterygium colli, low-set posterior hairline (A,B), and characteristic posture (C). (C from C Scott et al., Birth Defects 5:231, 1969, with permission.)

with muscle wasting: reexamination of a syndrome of neural crest malmigration. Birth Defects 7:69–72, 1971.

7. Lairmore TC, Howe JR, Korte JA, Dilley WG, Aine L, Aine E, Wells SA Jr, Donis-Keller H: Familial medullary thyroid carcinoma and multiple endocrine neoplasia type 2B map to the same region of chromosome 10 as multiple endocrine neoplasia type 2A. Genomics 9:181–192, 1991.
8. Pryse JC, Kuftinec MM, Buszynski NJ: A dento-craniofacial study of the multiple endocrine neoplasia (MEN) type 3 syndrome. J Oral Med 34:85–88, 1979.
9. Schimke RN: Multiple endocrine adenomatosis syndromes. Adv Intern Med 21:249–266, 1974.
10. Weidmer N, Flanders DJ, Mitros FA: Mucosal ganglioneuromatosis associated with multiple colonic polyps. Am J Surg Pathol 8:779–786, 1989.

## Multiple pterygium syndrome

### Escobar syndrome
(MIM No. *265000; POSSUM No. 3472)

#### General manifestations

This syndrome is characterized by growth retardation (100%), and webbing that involves the popliteal (90%), antecubital (90%), and intercrural areas (60%), preventing full extension of the extremities. Multiple joint contracture, syndactyly, and camptodactyly of the fingers. Foot deformities are common.

Kyphoscoliosis, posterior fusion of the vertebrae, is seen in 60% of cases. Cryptorchidism, absent labia majora, and inguinal hernia are occasional findings.[1,3,4,7]

#### Otolaryngological manifestations

The face is described as flat, sad, and emotionless. Eyelid ptosis and puffiness with a downward slant (85%) and epicanthal folds (75%) characterize this syndrome. The angles of the mouth are downturned, the mouth and mandible are small. Webbing of the neck occurs in all patients. The philtrum is long. Conductive hearing loss is reported. Cleft lip occurs in 35% of cases.[4,5,7]

#### Etiology

Multiple pterygium syndrome is of autosomal recessive inheritance. The origin of the pterygia is unknown. Biopsy of the involved muscles shows degeneration and disorganization of the myofibrils. This syndrome is relatively common among Arabs.[3,6]

#### Differential diagnosis

Multiple pterygium syndrome should be differentiated from Klippel-Feil anomaly, Turner, Noonan and LEOPARD syndromes, which have cervical pterygia. Gorlin et al.[2] distinguished four types of lethal multiple pterygium syndromes that are different from multiple pterygium syndrome.

#### References

1. Chen H, Chang CH, Misra RP, Peters HA, Grijalva NS, Opitz JM: Multiple pterygium syndrome. Am J Med Genet 7:91–102, 1980.
2. Gorlin RJ, Cohen MM Jr, Levin LS: Syndromes of the Head and Neck, 3rd ed. Oxford University Press, New York, 1990, p 627.
3. Naguib KK, Teebi AS, al-Awadi SA, Moosa A, Ali NR: Multiple pterygium syndrome in five Arab sibs. Ann Genet 30:122–125, 1987.
4. Ramer JC, Ladda RL, Demuth WW: Multiple pterygium syndrome: an overview. Am J Dis Child 142:794–798, 1988.
5. Scott CI: Pterygium syndrome. Birth Defects 5:231–232, 1969.
6. Teebi AS, Daoud AS: Multiple pterygium syndrome: a relatively common disorder among Arabs. J Med Genet 27:791, 1990.
7. Thompson EM, Donnai D, Baraitser M, Hall CM, Pembrey ME, Fixsen J: Multiple pterygium syndrome: evolution of the phenotype. J Med Genet 24:733–749, 1987.

## Nager acrofacial dysostosis syndrome

### Mandibulofacial dysostosis, limb anomalies, or Preaxial acrofacial dysostosis
(MIM No. 154400; POSSUM No. 3143)

This syndrome was first recognized by Nager and de Reynier.[10]

#### General manifestations

Ocular manifestations include lower lid colobomas (20%) and a reduced number of cilia in 60% of patients.[8] Hypoplastic thumbs are characteristic of the syndrome. Duplication or triphalangy has been seen occasionally.[3] Deformities of the toes and radioulnar synostosis are seen in one-third of the patients. Other limb deformities include shortened humerus, dislocated hips, and rib anomalies.[2,7,9] Uncommon deformities such as dystopic kidneys, pectus excavatum, lentigenes of the face, atrophy of the thymus, and cardiac murmur have also been reported.[2,4,11]

#### Otolaryngological manifestations

Bilateral mandibular and malar hypoplasia, downward slanting palpebral fissures, absence of the soft palate, a high-arched palate, external auditory canal abnormalities, and middle ear deformities are the most common features.[1,2]

The pinnae are posteriorly angulated in most patients. Preauricular dimples or tags are seen in 15% of patients. Absence of middle ear ossicles and/or absence of the tympanic membrane are also described.[2,5,6] Abnormalities of the larynx and speech

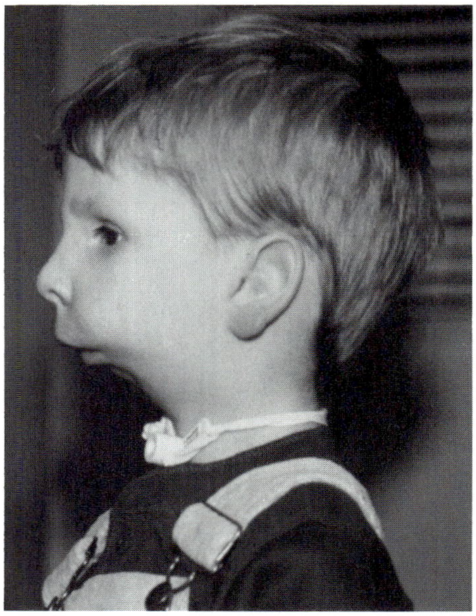

**Fig. 47.** Nager syndrome. Note the severe micrognathia in a 5-year-old patient. (Courtesy of Dr. C. Scott, from RE Stevenson et al., *Human Malformations and Related Anomalies,* Vol. 2, Oxford University Press, 1993, p. 648.)

are known.[7,9] Hearing loss is conductive and an airborne gap of 50 to 60 dB is not uncommon.[2]

### Etiology

The cause of this syndrome is unknown. Most cases are sporadic. Autosomal dominant transmission has been suggested in some cases.[4,10] Sulik et al.[12] suggested that the pathogenesis is related to the apical ectoderm of the limb buds. The condition has been associated with an inherited and apparently balanced X;9 translocation.[13]

### Differential diagnosis

Nager acrofacial dysostosis syndrome should be differentiated from Treacher Collins syndrome and other types of acrofacial dysostosis such as Richieri-Costa-Gollop-Coletto syndrome, Rodriguez type and Weyers type (MIM Nos. 154400, 201170, and 193530, respectively).

### References


1. Bowen P, Harley F: Mandibulofacial dysostosis with limb malformations (Nager's acrofacial dysostosis). Birth Defects 10:109–115, 1974.
2. Danziger I, Brodsky L, Perry R, Nusbaum S, Bernat J, Robinson L: Nager's acrofacial dysostosis. Case report and review of the literature. Int J Pediatr Otorhinol 20:225–240, 1990.
3. Giugliana R, Pereira CH: Nager's acrofacial dysostosis with thumb duplication: report of a case. Clin Genet 26:228–230, 1984.
4. Halal F, Herrmann J, Pallister PD, Opitz JM, Desgranges MF, Grenier G: Differential diagnosis of Nager acrofacial dysostosis syndrome: Report of four patients with Nager syndrome and discussion of other related syndromes. Am J Med Genet 14:209–224, 1983.
5. Jones RG: Mandibulofacial dysostosis. Cent Afr J Med 14:193–200, 1968.
6. Kawira EL, Weaver DD, Bender HA: Acrofacial dysostosis with severe facial clefting and limb reduction. Am J Med Genet 17:641–647, 1984.
7. Krauss CM, Hassell LA, Jang DL: Anomalies in an infant with Nager acrofacial dysostosis. Am J Med Genet 21:761–764, 1985.
8. Lowry B: The Nager syndrome (acrofacial dysostosis): Evidence of autosomal dominant inheritance. Birth Defects 13:195–202, 1977.
9. Meyerson MD, Jensen KM, Meyers JM, Hall BD: Nager acrofacial dysostosis: early intervention and long-term planning. Cleft Palate J 14:35–40, 1977.
10. Nager FR, de Reynier JP: Das Gehörorgan bei den angeborenen Kopfmissbildungen. Pract Otorhinolaryngol 10:1–128, 1948.
11. Pfeiffer RA, Stoess H: Acrofacial dysostosis (Nager syndrome). Synopsis and report of a case. Am J Med Genet 15:255–260, 1993.
12. Sulik KK, Smiley SJ, Turvey TA, Speight HS, Johnston MC: Pathogenesis of cleft palate in Treacher Collins, Nager and Miller syndromes. Cleft Palate J 126:209–216, 1989.
13. Zori RT, Gray BA, Bent-Williams A, Driscoll DJ, Williams CA, Zackowski JL: Preaxial orofacial dysostosis (Nager syndrome) associated with an inherited and apparently balanced X;9 translocation: prenatal and postnatal late replication studies. Am J Med Genet 46:379–383, 1993.


## Neurofibromatosis I (NF1)

**Von Recklinghausen disease**
(MIM Nos. *162220, 162240, 162260, 162270; POSSUM No. 3332)

### General manifestations

The criteria for diagnosis include two or more of the following: more than five café-au-lait spots (0.5cm in diameter before puberty, 1.5 cm after), axillary or inguinal freckling, multiple cutaneous neurofibromas, or at least one plexiform neurofibroma, optic glioma, iris Lisch nodule, a distinct bony lesion such as tibial bowing or pseudoarthrosis, sphenoid wing dysplasia, and an affected first-degree relative.[14,16,18a]

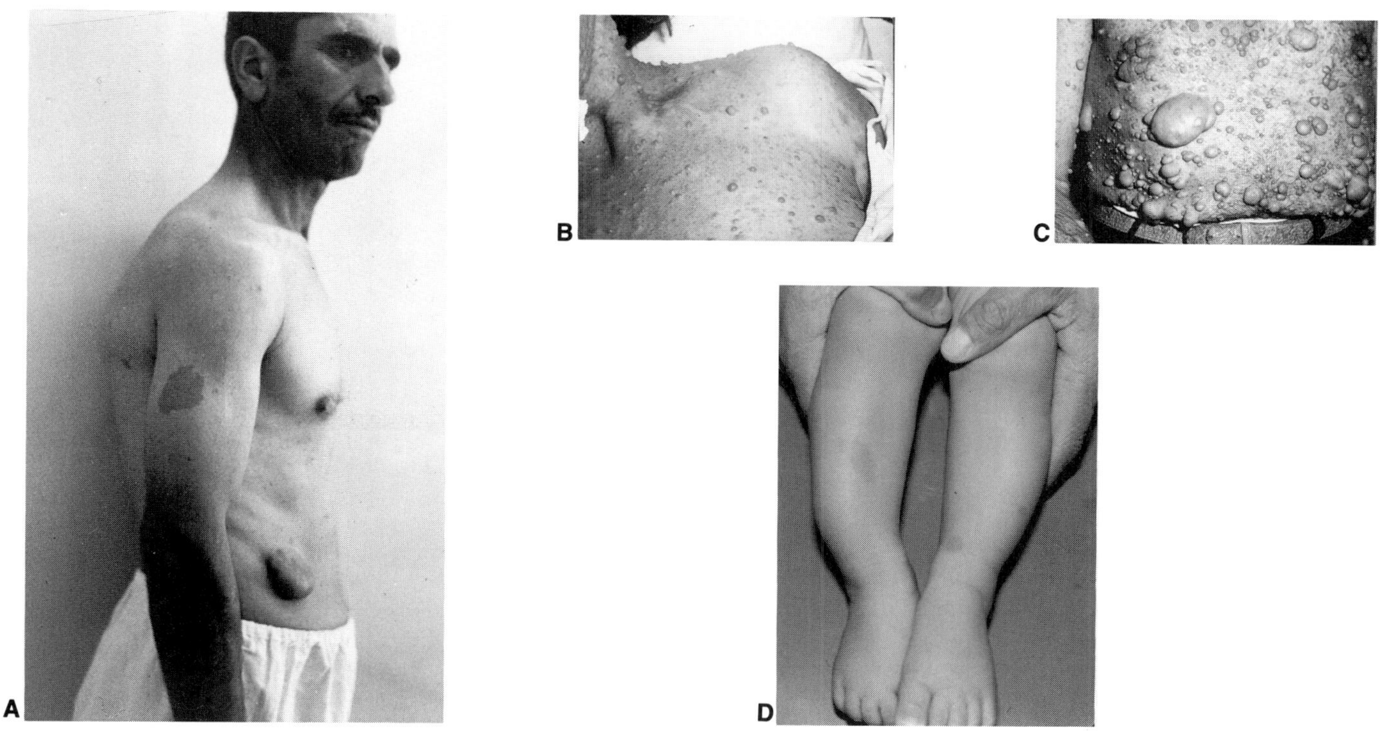

**Fig. 48.** Neurofibromatosis 1. A: Note caté-au-lait spot on the right arm and cutaneous fibroma in the right upper abdominal region. B, C: Numerous cutaneous and subcutaneous tumors. D: Pseudarthrosis of the tibia and café-au-lait spots. (A–C from VM DerKaloustian, AK Kurban, *Genetic Diseases of the Skin,* Springer-Verlag, Berlin, 1979, p. 256, with permission.)

The café-au-lait spots and axillary freckling may be present at birth and become more evident with age. Cutaneous neurofibromas may be sessile or pedunculated. These develop around the second decade and increase with age. Plexiform neurofibroma occurs in one-third of the patients. Malignant degeneration is estimated to be 5%–15%.

Mental retardation, learning disabilities, and speech defects are not uncommon. Macrocephaly, hydrocephalus, aqueductal stenosis, and seizures may occur.[7,8,10,15,19]

Lisch iris nodules are present in 90% of patients. They cause no clinical impairment. Other ocular findings include optic glioma (15%), optic nerve meningioma and congenital glaucoma (1%).[2,16,19]

Multiple organ involvement may cause serious complications. Paraspinal, retroperitoneal, mediastinal, renal, laryngeal, and cardiac tumors are reported. Acoustic neuromas do not occur in NF1. Scoliosis, kyphosis, and cervical spine anomalies may develop.

Precocious puberty, hypopituitarism, gigantism, hypogonadism, and diabetes insipidus have been described, as well as intracranial calcifications.[3,11,13,18]

### Otolaryngological manifestations

Velopharyngeal insufficiency, macroglossia, jaw lesions, hypoplasia of the facial bones, enamel and dentine defects may be seen.[4,15,17]

### Etiology

NF1 is of autosomal dominant inheritance. NF1 gene location is in the 17q11.2 region. Fresh mutations represent about 50% of cases. The prevalence is 1:3,000. NF1 is caused by deletions, insertions, translocations, and point mutations in the NF1 gene, which spans 350 kb.[12]

### Differential diagnosis

NF1 should be differentiated from neurofibromatosis types 2 through 7,[16] as well as types 8 and 9 (added by Gorlin et al.[5]). Other syndromes with café-au-lait spots, include McCune-Albright, Watson, multiple mucosal neuroma (MEN type 2) and LEOPARD syndromes.[1,6,9]

### References


1. Allanson JE, Hall JG, Van Allen MI: Noonan phenotype associated with neurofibromatosis. Am J Med Genet 21:457–462, 1985.
2. Cunliffe IA, Moffat DA, Hardy DG, Moore AT: Bilateral optic nerve sheath meningiomas in a patient with neurofibromatosis type 2. Br J Ophthalmol 76:310–312, 1992.
3. Egelhoff JC, Bates DJ, Ross JS, Rotner AD, Cohen BH: Spinal MR findings in neurofibromatosis types 1 and 2. Am J Neuroradiol 13:1071–1077, 1992.
4. Freeman MJ, Standish SM: Facial and oral manifestations of familial disseminated neurofibromatosis. Oral Surg 19:52–59, 1965.
5. Gorlin RJ, Cohen MM Jr, Levin LS: Syndromes of the Head and Neck, 3rd ed. Oxford University Press, New York, 1990, pp 392–399.
6. Heimann R, Verhest A, Verschraegen J, Grosjean W, Drops JP, Hecht F: Hereditary intestinal neurofibromatosis I. A distinctive genetic disease. Neurofibromatosis 1:26–32, 1988.
7. Horwich A, Riccardi VM, Francke U: Aqueductal stenosis leading to hydrocephalus—an unusual manifestation of neurofibromatosis. J Med Genet 14:577–581, 1983.
8. Huson SM: The different forms of neurofibromatosis. Br Med J 294:1113–1114, 1987.
9. Kaplan P, Rosenblatt B: A distinctive facial appearance in neurofibromatosis von Recklinghausen. Am J Med Genet 21:463–470, 1985.
10. Knight WA, Murphy WK, Gottlieb JA: Neurofibromatosis associated with malignant neurofibromas. Arch Dermatol 107:747–750, 1973.
11. Laue L, Comite F, Hench K, Loriaux DL, Cutter GB Jr, Pescovitz OH: Precocious puberty associated with neurofibromatosis and optic gliomas. Am J Dis Child 139:1097–1100, 1985.
12. Lázaro C, Gaona A, Lynch M, Kruyer H, Ravella A, Estivill X: Molecular characterization of the breakpoints of a 12–kb deletion in the *NF1* gene in a family showing germ-line mosaicism. Am J Hum Genet 57:1044–1049, 1995.
13. Mayfrank L, Mohadjer M, Wullich B: Intracranial calcified deposits in neurofibromatosis type 2—A CT study of 11 cases. Neuroradiology 32:33–37, 1990.
14. Neary WJ, Newton VE, Vilder M, Ramsden RT, Lye RH, Dulton JE, Richardson PL, Harris R, Evans DG, Strachan T: A clinical, genetic and audiological study of patients and families with bilateral acoustic neurofibromatosis. J Laryngol Otol 107:6–11, 1993.
15. Pollack MA, Shprintzen RJ: Velopharyngeal insufficiency in neurofibromatosis. Int J Pediatr Otorhinolaryngol 3:257–262, 1981.
16. Riccardi VM: Von Recklinghausen neurofibromatosis. N Engl J Med 305:1617–1627, 1981.
17. Rittersma J, Kate LT, Westerink P: Neurofibromatosis with mandibular deformities. Oral Surg 33:718–727, 1972.
18. Saxema K: Endocrine manifestations of neurofibromatosis in children. Am J Dis Child 120:265–271, 1970.
18a. Sobol S, Tewfik TL, Ortenberg J: Otolaryngologic manifestations of neurofibromatosis in children. J Otolaryngol (in press).
19. Zehavi C, Romano A, Goodman RM: Iris (Lisch) nodules in neurofibromatosis. Clin Genet 29:51–55, 1986.


## Neurofibromatosis II (NF2)

(MIM No. *101000; POSSUM No. 4256)

### General manifestations

Café-au-lait spots and cutaneous neurofibromas are not consistent findings of NF2. Axillary freckling is uncommon. Other neurogenic tumors are common. These include schwannomas, intracranial or spinal meningiomas, or astrocytomas. Increased symptoms may be noted during late pregnancy. Posterior capsular cataracts are common (80%). Lisch nodules are absent in NF2.[1a,2,4,7,9]

Symptoms usually develop unilaterally and involvement of the other side occurs within 2 years.

Diagnostic criteria include bilateral acoustic neuroma, which can be seen with appropriate imaging technique (CT or MRI), or a first-degree relative with NF2 and either unilateral VIII nerve mass, or two of the following: neurofibroma, meningioma, glioma, schwannoma, or juvenile posterior subcapsular lenticular opacity.[5] The incidence is estimated to be 1: 50,000.

### Otolaryngological manifestations

Symptoms are usually the result of pressure on the vestibulocochlear (VIIIth nerve) and facial nerve complex. Hearing loss is often the first symptom, which occurs in the teens or early twenties, the average age being 20. Tinnitus, imbalance, and vertigo accompany the deafness. Small acoustic neuromas of less than 8 mm have been detected in asymptomatic children (aged 7 and 11) with the use of gadolinium-enhanced MRI.

Other symptoms of facial pain, numbness, or weakness and paralysis, headache, diplopia, nausea, and vomiting may develop. Cervical kyphoscoliosis may be related to a paraspinal neurofibroma.[6,7]

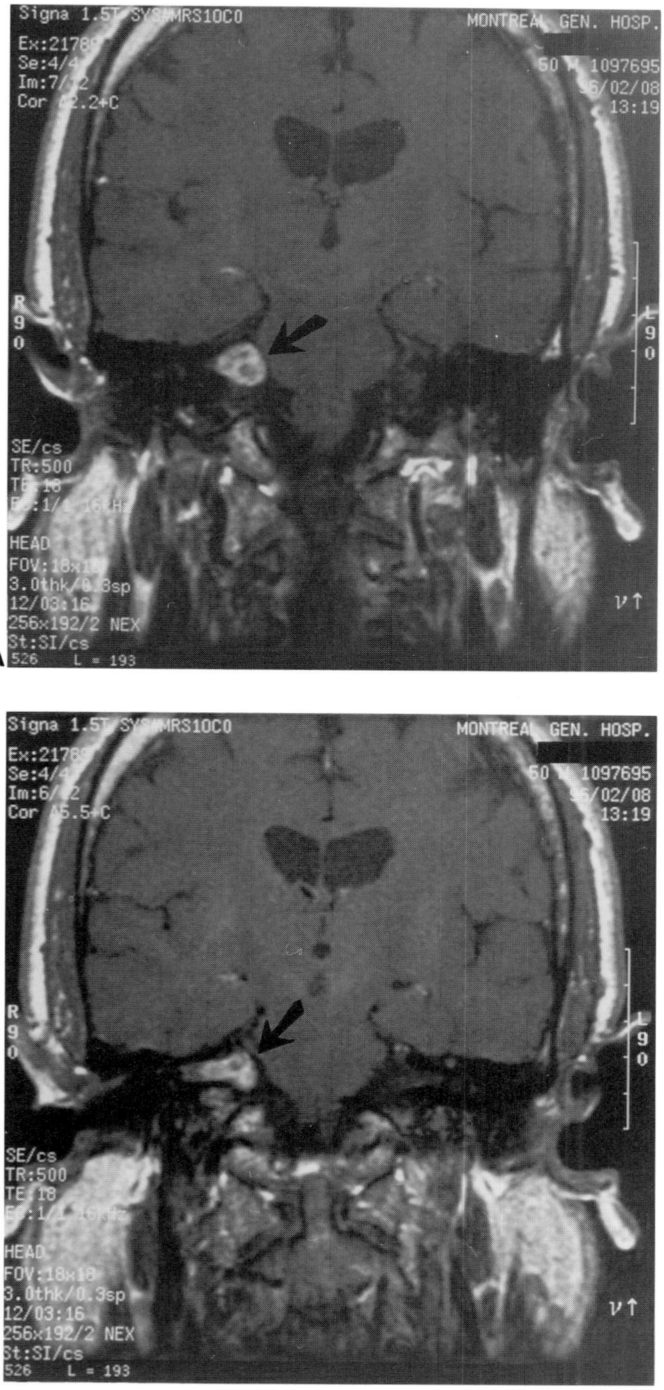


**Fig. 49.** Neurofibromatosis 2. A,B: T1 weighted MRI (gadolinium enhanced) of acoustic neuroma. (Courtesy of Dr. H. Remy.)

### Etiology

NF2 is of autosomal dominant inheritance, with 95% penetrance and mapping to 22q11.2.[1,8] The NF2 gene has been isolated. It encodes a protein named *merlin*. Mutational analysis of patients has been done.[3]

### Differential diagnosis

NF2 should be differentiated from NF1 and multiple schwannomatosis.

### References


1. Arai E, Ikeuch T, Karasawa S, Tamura A, Yamamoto K, Kida M, Ichimura K, Yuasa Y, Tonomura A: Constitutional translocation t(4;22)(q12;q12.2) associated with neurofibromatosis type 2. Am J Med Genet 44:163–167, 1992.

1a. Glasscock ME 3d, Kveton JF, Jackson CG, Levine SC, McKennan K: A systemic approach to the surgical management of acoustic neuroma. Laryngoscope 96:1088–1094, 1986.

2. Huson SM: The different forms of neurofibromatosis. Br Med J 294:1113–1114, 1987.
3. MacCollin M, Ramesh V, Jacoby LB, Louis DN, Rubio M-P, Pulaski K, Trofatter JA, Short MP, Bove C, Eldridge R, et al: Mutational analysis of patients with neurofibromatosis 2. Am J Hum Genet 55:314–320, 1994.
4. Martuza RL, Eldridge R: Neurofibromatosis 2 (bilateral acoustic neurofibromatosis). N Engl J Med 318:684–688, 1988.
5. NIH Consensus Development Conference: Neurofibromatosis: conference statement. Arch Neurol 45:475–578, 1988.
6. Parry DM, Kaiser-Kupfer MI, Sherman JL, Pikus A, Eldridge R: Neurofibromatosis 2 (bilateral acoustic or central neurofibromatosis), a treatable cause of deafness. Recommendations for screening and follow up based on study of large kindred. Ann NY Acad Sci 630:305–307, 1991.
7. Pastores GM, Michels VV, Jack CR Jr: Early childhood diagnosis of acoustic neuromas in presymptomatic individuals at risk for neurofibromatosis 2. Am J Med Genet 41:325–329, 1991.
8. Seizinger BR, Martuza RL, Gusella JF: Loss of genes in chromosome 22 in tumorigenesis of human acoustic neuroma. Nature 322:644–647, 1986.
9. Wertelecki W, Rouleau GA, Superneau DW, Forehand LW, Williams JP, Haines JL, Gusella JF: Neurofibromatosis 2: clinical and DNA linkage studies of a large kindred. N Engl J Med 319:278–283, 1988.


## Noonan syndrome

### Ullrich-Noonan syndrome
(MIM No. *163950; POSSUM No. 3335)

### General manifestations

Birth weight is usually within normal limits. It may be increased due to subcutaneous tissue swelling. Prepubertal growth is slow, and the pubertal spurt is reduced or absent, which leads to short stature.[14] Congenital heart anomalies occur in two-thirds of the patients. Left axis deviation and pulmonary valve stenosis are relatively common. Atrial septal defect and septal hypertrophy are less common. Congestive heart failure and pulmonary edema are not rare complications. Pectus deformity occurs in 70% of cases with characteristic pectus carinatum occurring superiorly and pectus excavatum inferiorly. Cubitus valgus (50%), vertebral anomalies, and blunt fingertips may be present. The irises may be blue or blue-green. Bleeding tendencies are present in 20% of cases and include Von Willebrand disease, platelet dysfunction, and factor XI deficiency.

Hypoplastic or aplastic lymphatic vessels, lymphangiectasia, and cystic hygromas also occur in a significant proportion of cases.

Other uncommon manifestations include pheochromocytoma, malignant hyperthermia, odontogenic keratocysts, vasculitis, arthrogryposis, thyroiditis, and sterility.[3,4,8,12,15] Mild mental retardation occurs in one-third of patients.[9] IQ ranges between 64 and 127 with a median of 102.

### Otolaryngological manifestations

During the newborn period, this syndrome is characterized by downward slanting palpebral fissures and hypertelorism (95%), low-set, posteriorly-angulated ears (90%), a deep and elongated

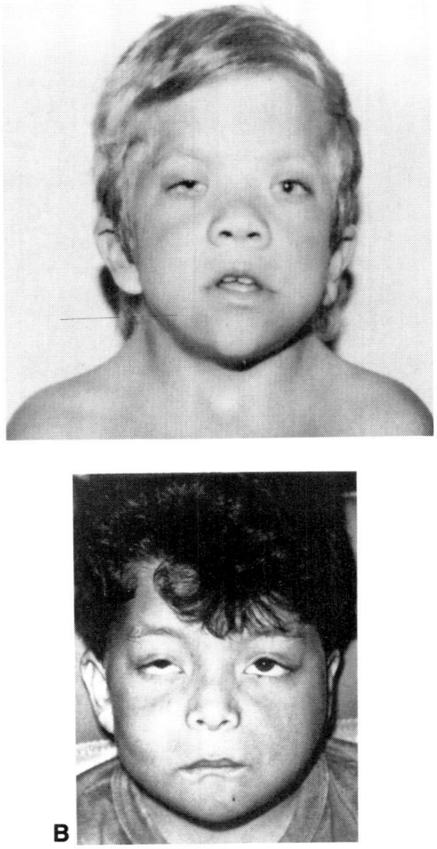

A

B

**Fig. 50.** Noonan syndrome. Note the pterygium colli and low-set ears (A), and the hypertelorism and ptosis (B). (From J Dunlap et al., *Oral Surg Oral Med Oral Pathol* 67:698, 1989, with permission.)

philtrum (95%), excess nuchal skin with a low nuchal hairline (55%), a high-arched palate and a small mouth.[1]

In infancy the head is relatively large, with hypertelorism and thick-hooded eyelids. The nose has a bulbous tip and the facies appears coarse later in childhood.

With advanced age, the face assumes a triangular shape and the neck appears webbed due to the accentuated trapezius (90%). The nasolabial folds are prominent and the anterior hairline is high. The skin is transparent and wrinkled. Malocclusion occurs in one-third of the patients. Sensorineural and conductive hearing loss may occur. Language delay may be present in 20% of cases. Congenital anomalies of the ossicular chain, such as absence of the long process of the incus, have been described.[1,2,5,6]

### Etiology and pathogenesis

Inheritance of Noonan syndrome is autosomal dominant with variable expression. The gene has been mapped to chromosome 12q (12q22–qter).[10] Transmission from parent to child occurs in 30 to 75% of cases. The lymphedema hypothesis explains the disruption of the normal tissue migration that results in pterygium colli, widely spaced nipples, cryptorchidism, hypertelorism, and low-set ears.[11]

### Differential diagnosis

Noonan syndrome should be differentiated from Turner syndrome. The absence of chromosomal abnormality and family history should differentiate the two conditions. Williams syndrome, cardio-facio-cutaneous syndrome, and Costello syndrome,[7] as well as several Noonan-like syndromes and neurofibromatosis—Noonan syndrome should be included in the differential diagnosis. The latter entity could be a variant of neurofibromatosis type 1 or could be a separate neurocristopathy.[13]

### References


1. Allanson JE: Noonan syndrome. J Med Genet 24:9–13, 1987.
2. Allanson JE: Time and natural history: the changing face. J Craniofac Genet Develop Biol 9:21–28, 1989.
3. Bawle EV, Black V: Nonimmune hydrops fetalis in Noonan's syndrome. Am J Dis Child 140:758–760, 1986.
4. Berberich MS, Hall JG: Noonan syndrome in an unusual family with above average intelligence, a high incidence of cancer and rare type of vasculitis. Birth Defects 12:181–186, 1976.
5. Char F, Rodriguez-Fernandez HL, Scott CI Jr, Borgaonkar DS, Bell BB, Rowe RD: The Noonan syndrome—a clinical study of forty-five cases. Birth Defects 8:110–118, 1972.
6. Cremers CW, van der Burgt CJ: Hearing loss in Noonan syndrome. Int J Pediatr Otorhinolaryngol 23:81–84, 1992.
7. Der Kaloustian YM, Moroz B, McIntosh N, Watters AK, Blaichman S: Costello syndrome. Am J Med Genet 41:69–73, 1991.
8. Dunlap C, Neville B, Vickers RA, O'Neil D, Barker B: The Noonan syndrome/cherubism association. Oral Surg Oral Med Oral Pathol 67:698–705, 1989.
9. Gorlin RJ, Cohen MM Jr, Levin LS: Syndromes of the Head and Neck, 3rd ed. Oxford University Press, New York, 1990, pp 803–806.
10. Jamieson CR, van der Burgt I, Brady AF, van Reen M, Elsawi MM, Hol F, Jeffery S, Patton MA, Mariman E: Mapping a gene for Noonan syndrome to the long arm of chromosome 12. Nat Genet 8:357–360, 1994.
11. Mendez HM, Opitz JM: Noonan syndrome. A review. Am J Med Genet 21:493–506, 1985.
12. Nelson JF, Tsaknis PJ, Jouzelman JL: Noonan's syndrome: report of a case with oral findings. J Oral Med 33:94–96, 1978.
13. Sharland M, Taylor R, Patton MA, Jeffrey S: Absence of linkage of Noonan syndrome to the neurofibromatosis type I locus. J Med Genet 29:188–190, 1992.
14. Thientz G, Savage MO: Growth and pubertal development in five boys with Noonan's syndrome. Arch Dis Child 57:13–17, 1982.
15. Witt DR, McGillivray BC, Allanson JE, Hughes HE, Hathaway WE, Zipinsky A, Hall JG: Bleeding diathesis in Noonan syndrome. A common association. Am J Med Genet 31:305–317, 1988.


## Norrie disease

### (MIM No. *310600; POSSUM No. 3336)

A report on a new hereditary bilateral pseudotumor of the retina was published by Warburg in 1961, who described the disease in 7 generations of a Danish family.[9] Gordon Norrie was credited for describing this syndrome earlier.[6] A confusion exists in the literature between pseudoglioma, Norrie disease, and microphthalmos. *Leukocoria* is a term that includes retinal dysplasia, congenital retinal folds, primary hyperplastic vitreous, metastatic endophthalmitis, toxoplasmosis, or granulomatosis.[6,9]

### General manifestations

The anterior chamber of the eye is shallow, the pupils are dilated, and the light reflex is absent. Other ocular findings include posterior synechiae, a gray-yellow membrane behind the lens, and elongated ciliary processes. The affected patients are totally blind. Phthisis bulbi occurs by age 10. Up to 40% of patients become mentally retarded. Other findings include cryptorchidism, hypogonadism, and psychoses. A variant of Norrie disease that has been associated with microcephaly, has been described. A pedigree of 16 affected males in 5 generations

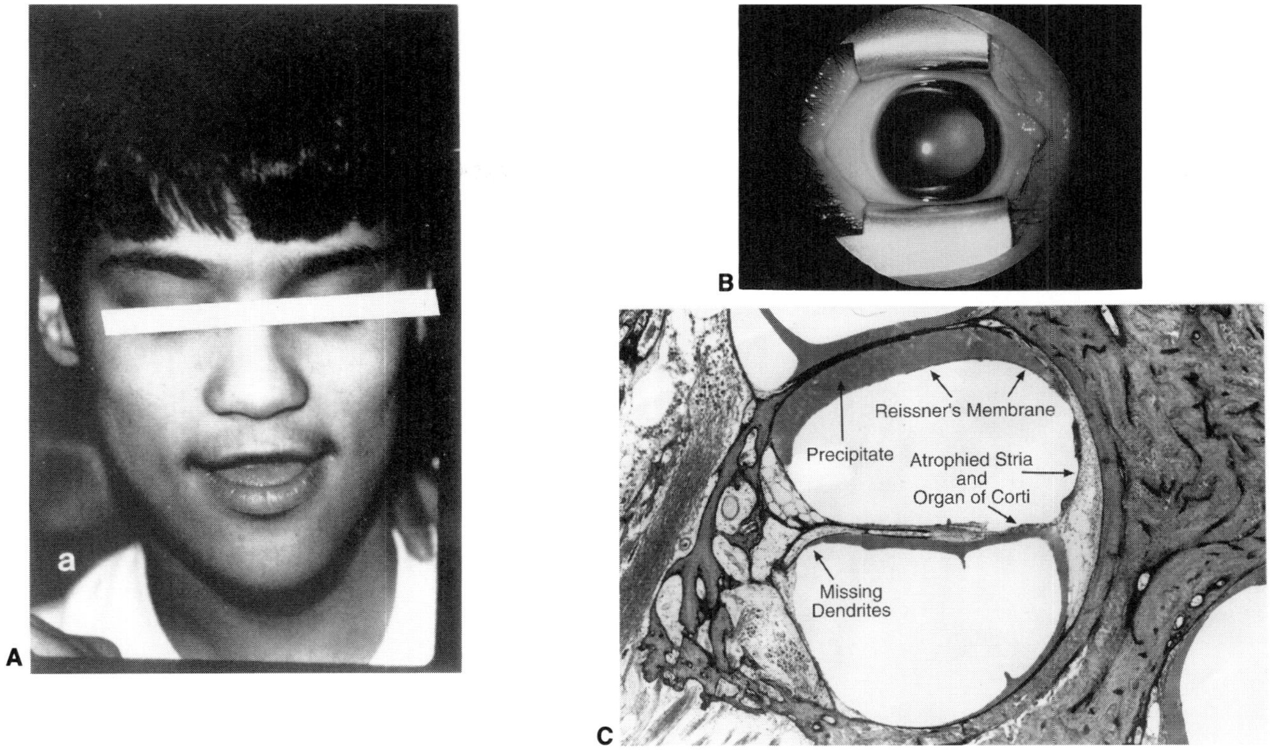


**Fig. 51.** Norrie disease. A: Patient with Norrie disease. (From S Antonarakis, Am J Med Genet 42:127, 1992, with permission.) B: Eye in Norrie disease. (Courtesy of Dr. J. Little.) C: Histology of the temporal bone. Torn and atrophied Reissner's membrane is caused by a protein clot. It appears that the genetic influence is on the ectodermal derivatives of the cochlear duct and that the neuronal losses are attributable to retrograde neuronal degeneration. (From HF Schuknecht, *Pathology of the Ear,* 2nd ed., Lea & Febiger, Philadelphia, 1993, p. 140 with permission.)

from Episkopi in Cyprus was published by Taylor et al.[8] Since then, the condition has also been known as Episkopi blindness. Early ocular intervention, such as cataract extraction, vitrectomy, and repair of retinal detachment, may prevent phthisis bulbi but does not improve visual acuity. Hearing aids and/or rehabilitation are needed for the hearing loss.[1,2,4,8]

### Otolaryngological manifestations

Sensorineural hearing loss of a progressive nature beginning in the second decade develops in 25%–30% of patients. Brainstem evoked potentials suggest that deafness is of a cochlear nature.[7] Congenital nystagmus may be seen.

### Etiology

The condition follows the X-linked recessive pattern of inheritance and is mapped to Xp11.4-p11.3.[2] Norrie disease is caused by mutations in an extracellular protein resembling the C-terminal globular domain of mucins.[3,5]

### Differential diagnosis

Norrie disease should be differentiated from pseudoglioma syndrome and microphthalmia.

### References

1. Apple DJ, Fishman GA, Goldberg MF: Ocular histopathology of Norrie's disease. Am J Ophthalmol 78:196–203, 1974.
2. Collins FA, Murphy DL, Reiss AL, Sims KB, Lewis JG, Freund L, Karoum F, Zhu D, Maumenee IH, Antonarakis SE: Clinical, biochemical and neuropsychiatric evaluation of a patient with a contiguous gene syndrome due to a microdeletion Xp11.3 including the Norrie disease locus and monamine oxidase (MAOA & MAOB) genes. Am J Med Genet 42:127–134, 1992.
3. Fuchs S, Zu SY, Caballero M, Salcedo M, La OA, Wedemann H, Gal A: A missense point mutation (Leu 13 Arg) of the Norrie disease gene in a large Cuban kindred with Norrie disease. Hum Mol Genet 3:655–656, 1994.
4. Moreira-Filho CA, Neustein I: A presumptive new variant of Norrie's disease. J Med Genet 16:125–128, 1979.
5. Meindl A, Berger W, Meitinger T, van de Pol D, Achatz H, Dorner C, Hassemann M, Hellebrand H, Gal A, Cremers F, et al: Norrie disease is caused by mutations in an extracellular protein resembling C-terminal globular domain of mucins. Nat Genet 2:139–143, 1992.
6. Norrie G: Nogle Blindhedsaarsager: en oversigt. Hospitalsidende 76:141–147, 1933.
7. Parving A, Elberling C, Warburg M: Electrophysiological study of Norrie's disease. Audiology 17:293–298, 1978.
8. Taylor PJ, Coates T, Newhouse ML: Episkopi blindness: hereditary blindness in a Greek Cypriot family. Br J Ophthalmol 43:340–344, 1959.
9. Warburg M: Norrie's disease: a new hereditary bilateral pseudotumor of the retina. Acta Ophthalmol 39:757–772, 1961.

## Opitz (BBB/G) Syndrome

### G syndrome, Opitz oculo-genito-laryngeal syndrome, type 2

(MIM No. *145410; POSSUM No. 3239)

This syndrome is characterized by hypertelorism, hypospadias, dysphagia, and anal anomalies.

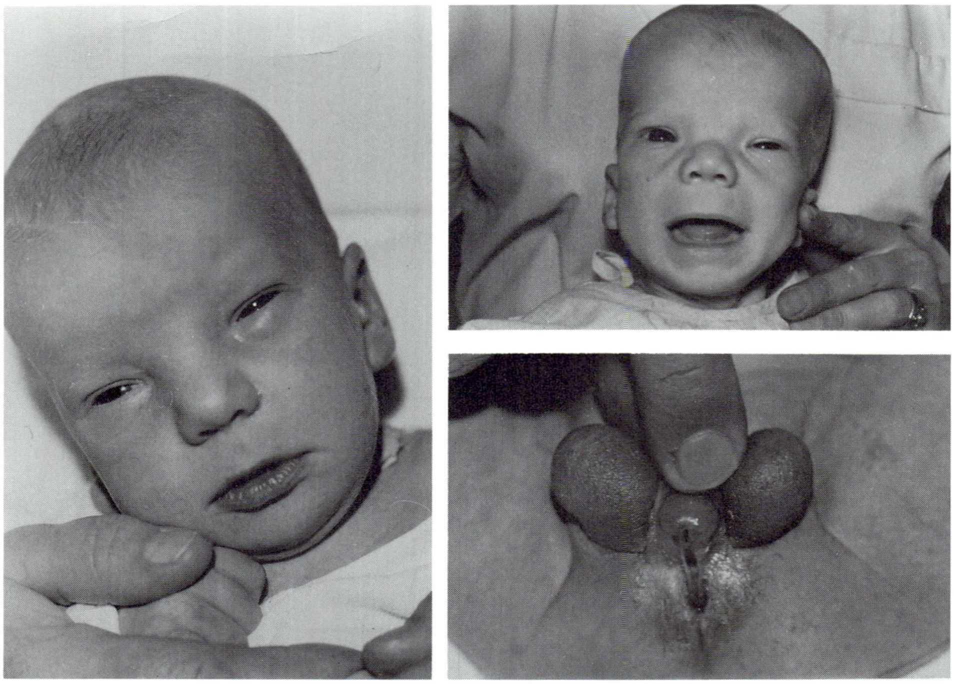

**Fig. 52.** Opitz BBB/G syndrome. A,B: Note the flat nose with anteverted nostrils and posteriorly angulated ears. C: Hypospadias. (From J Opitz et al., Birth Defects 5:95, 1969, with permission.)

### General manifestations

Patients have normal intelligence, but mild mental retardation may be seen.[1,16] Corpus callosum agenesis was reported in one patient.[8] Hypospadias of varying degree is present in most cases. Cryptorchidism and cleft scrotum are documented.[5] Renoureteral malformations and inguinal hernia also occur in a high percentage of cases.[4,9,10] Affected females have normal genitalia.[13] Ectopic and imperforate anus have been reported.[3,10,15]

Cardiovascular anomalies such as patent ductus arteriosus and abnormal position of the heart have been described.[14] Other anomalies include Meckel's diverticulum, duodenal stricture, and agenesis of the gall bladder.[6] Absent lung fissures, multiple lipomas, and hyperextensible joints are uncommon occurrences.[3,11]

### Otolaryngological manifestations

The nose is flat with anteverted nostrils, the philtrum is flattened and inapparent.[4] Cleft palate/lip is seen in 25% of cases.[1,13,16] Bifid uvula, ankyloglossia, or tongue tie[8] may also occur. The ears are posteriorly angulated and micrognathia is present and usually mild.[2] The parietal and occipital eminences are prominent. The cry is usually hoarse and infants have difficulty in swallowing. Various anomalies of the upper respiratory tract are described: laryngotracheoesophageal cleft,[18] vocal cord/epiglottis hypoplasia, short trachea, and absent tracheal rings. Two-thirds of the patients have abnormal esophageal motility. Gastroesophageal reflux has been reported by Wilson and Oliver.[19]

### Etiology

Inheritance of this syndrome is marked by an autosomal dominant trait, with male preponderance.[7] Opitz syndrome is heterogeneous, with one locus on Xp22 and a second locus on 22q11.2.[12]

### Differential diagnosis

Opitz syndrome should be differentiated from the following:

1. BBB syndrome or Opitz oculo-genital-laryngeal syndrome type 1, which is not associated with laryngo-tracheo-esophageal defects. This is considered to be in the spectrum of G syndrome and may be indistinguishable from it. The term *BBBG syndrome* has been suggested for the amalgamated condition.[17]
2. Other syndromes with hypertelorism.
3. Other syndromes with hypospadias.

### References


1. Cappa M, Borrelli P, Marini R, Neri G: The Opitz syndrome: A new designation for the clinically indistinguishable BBB and G syndrome. Am J Med Genet 28:303–309, 1987.
2. Coté GB, Katsantoni A, Papadakou-Lagoyannis, Costalos C, Timotheou, Skordalakis A, Deligeorgis D, Pantelakis S: The G syndrome of dysphagia, ocular hypertelorism and hypospadias. Clin Genet 19:473–478, 1981.
3. Forndon PA, Donnai D: Male to male transmission of the G syndrome. Clin Genet 24:446–448, 1983.
4. Gonzalez CH, Herrmann J, Opitz JM: Studies of malformation syndromes of man VB: the hypertelorism-hypospadias (BBB) syndrome. Eur J Pediatr 125:1–3, 1977.
5. Jones KL: Smith's Recognizable Patterns of Human Malformation, 5th ed. WB Saunders, Philadelphia, 1996, p 133.
6. Kasner J, Gilbert EF, Viseskul C: Studies of malformation syndrome VID: the G Syndrome—further observations. Z Kinderheilkunde 118:81–85, 1974.
7. Kimmelman CP, Denneny JC: Opitz (G) syndrome. Int J Pediatr Otorhinolaryngol 4:343–347, 1982.
8. Neri G, Genuardi M, Natoli G, Costa P, Maggioni G: A girl with G syndrome and agenesis of the corpus collosum. Am J Med Genet 28:287–291, 1987.
9. Noe HN, Peeden JN, Jerkins GR, Wilroy RS Jr: Hypertelorism-hypospadias syndrome. J Urol 132:951–952, 1984.

10. Opitz JM, Frias JL, Gutenberger JE, Pellett JR: The G syndrome of multiple congenital anomalies. Birth Defects 5:95–101, 1969.
11. Opitz JM, Summitt RL, Smith DW: The BBB Syndrome. Familial telecanthus with associated congenital anomalies. Birth Defects 5:86–94, 1969.
12. Robin NH, Feldman GJ, Aronson AL, Mitchell HF, Weksberg R, Leonard CO, Burton BK, Josephson KD, Laxová R, Aleck KA, et al: Opitz syndrome is genetically heterogeneous, with one locus on Xp22, and a second locus on 22q11.2. Nat Genet 11:459–461, 1995.
13. Stevens CA, Wilroy RS: The telecanthus-hypospadias syndrome. J Med Genet 25:536–552, 1988.
14. Stoll C, Gerandel A, Berland H, Roth MP, Dott B: Male-to-male transmission of the hypertelorism-hypospadias (BBB) syndrome. Am J Med Genet 20:221–225, 1985.
15. Tolmie JL, Coutts N, Drainer IK: Congenital anal anomalies in two families with the Opitz G syndrome. J Med Genet 24:688–691, 1987.
16. Van Biervlict JP, Van Hemel JO: Familial occurrence of the G syndrome. Clin Genet 7:238–244, 1975.
17. Verloes A, Merrer ML, Briard ML: BBBG syndrome or Opitz syndrome: new family. Am J Med Genet 34:313–316, 1989.
18. Williams CA, Frias JL: Apparent G syndrome presenting as neck and upper limb dystonia and severe gastroesophageal reflux. Am J Med Genet 28:297–302, 1987.
19. Wilson GN, Oliver WJ: Further delineation of the G syndrome: a manageable genetic cause of infantile dysphagia. J Med Genet 25:157–163, 1988.

## Orofaciodigital syndrome, type I (OFD I)

### Papillon-Léage-Psaume syndrome
(MIM No. *311200; POSSUM No. 3347)

This syndrome was characterized by Papillon-Léage and Psaume in 1954.[6] It comprises oral frenulae and clefts, absent lateral incisors, hypoplastic alae nasi, bifid hallux, digital asymmetry, and mental deficiency.

### General manifestations

Mild mental deficiency is seen in 60% of cases. The average IQ is 70. Precocious puberty, cerebral atrophy, hydrocephalus, agenesis of the corpus collosum, heterotopia of gray matter, and hamartoma of the hypothalamus have all been described.[1,3,4,8]

Shortening and asymmetry of the digits, syndactyly, bifid or duplicated hallux, and polydactyly of the foot occur.[7,9] Polycystic kidneys develop later in life.[1,10]

### Otolaryngological manifestations

Oral hyperplastic frenulae occur in 75% of patients. This is associated with clefts. Webbing occurs between the alveolar ridge and the buccal mucous membrane, making retraction of the upper lip difficult. The soft palate is cleft in most cases. The tongue may be bilobed or trilobed, and may display hamartomas. Diffuse tongue-tie is seen in over one-third of the patients. Absent lateral incisors and other dental anomalies usually exist. The mandible is hypoplastic. The face and ears display evanescent milia. These usually disappear by the third year. The alar cartilages are hypoplastic and the nostrils may be asymmetric. The small zygomatic bones give the face a flat appearance. Choanal atresia is occasionally seen. Dry scalp hair with alopecia has also been reported. The nasosellar-basion angle is increased.[3,4,5,7]

### Etiology

Inheritance follows the X-linked dominant pattern, and is lethal in the hemizygous male. The incidence is 1:50,000 live births.[2,3,4]

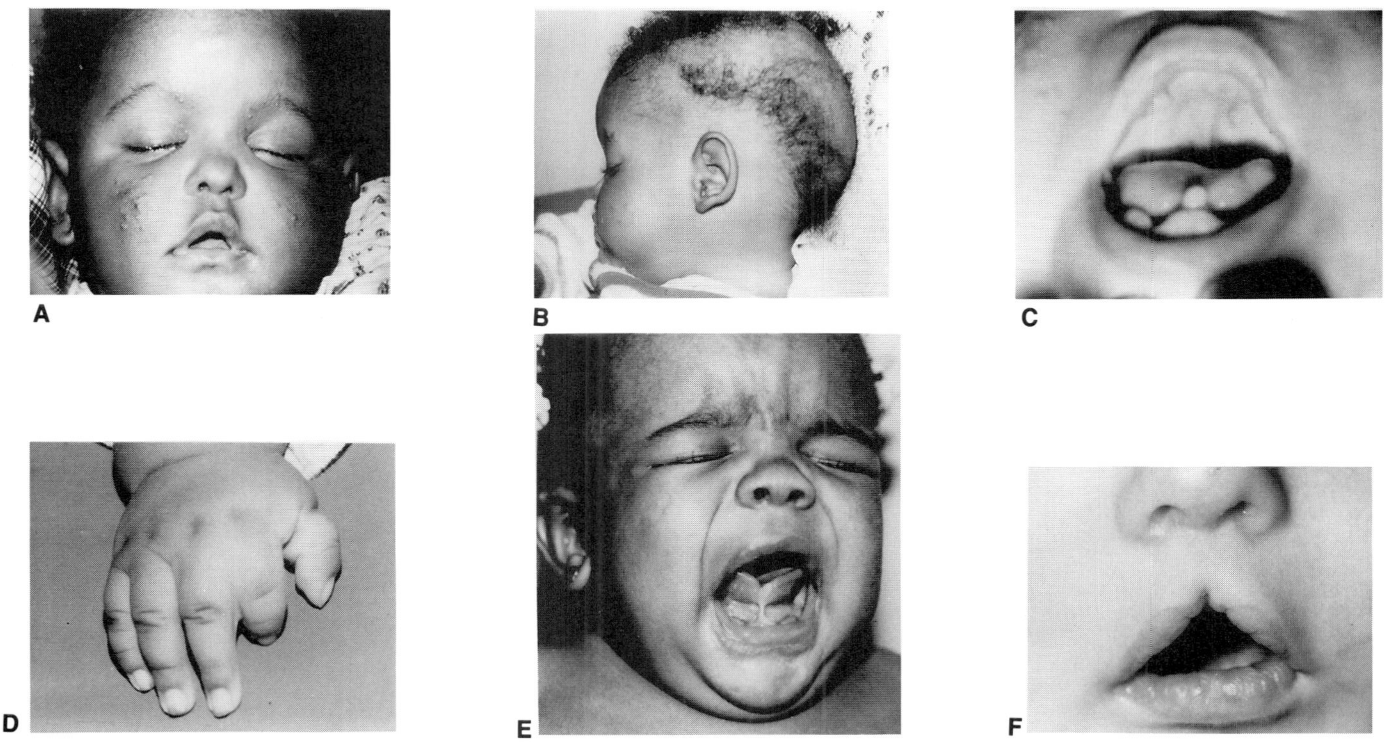

**Fig. 53.** Orofaciodigital syndrome, type I. A: Lethargic child, with high forehead, broad nasal bridge, and abundant milia. B: Hypotrichosis and fine hair. C: Palatal grooves, alveolar notching, and bifid tongue hamartomas. D: Brachydactyly and syndactyly of second and third digits. E: Patient with flat nasal bridge, bifid tongue, and ankyloglossia. F. Median cleft of the upper lip. (A–E from CF Salinas et al., Am J Med Genet 38:574, 1991; F from M Baraitser, J Med Genet 23:116, 1986, with permission.)

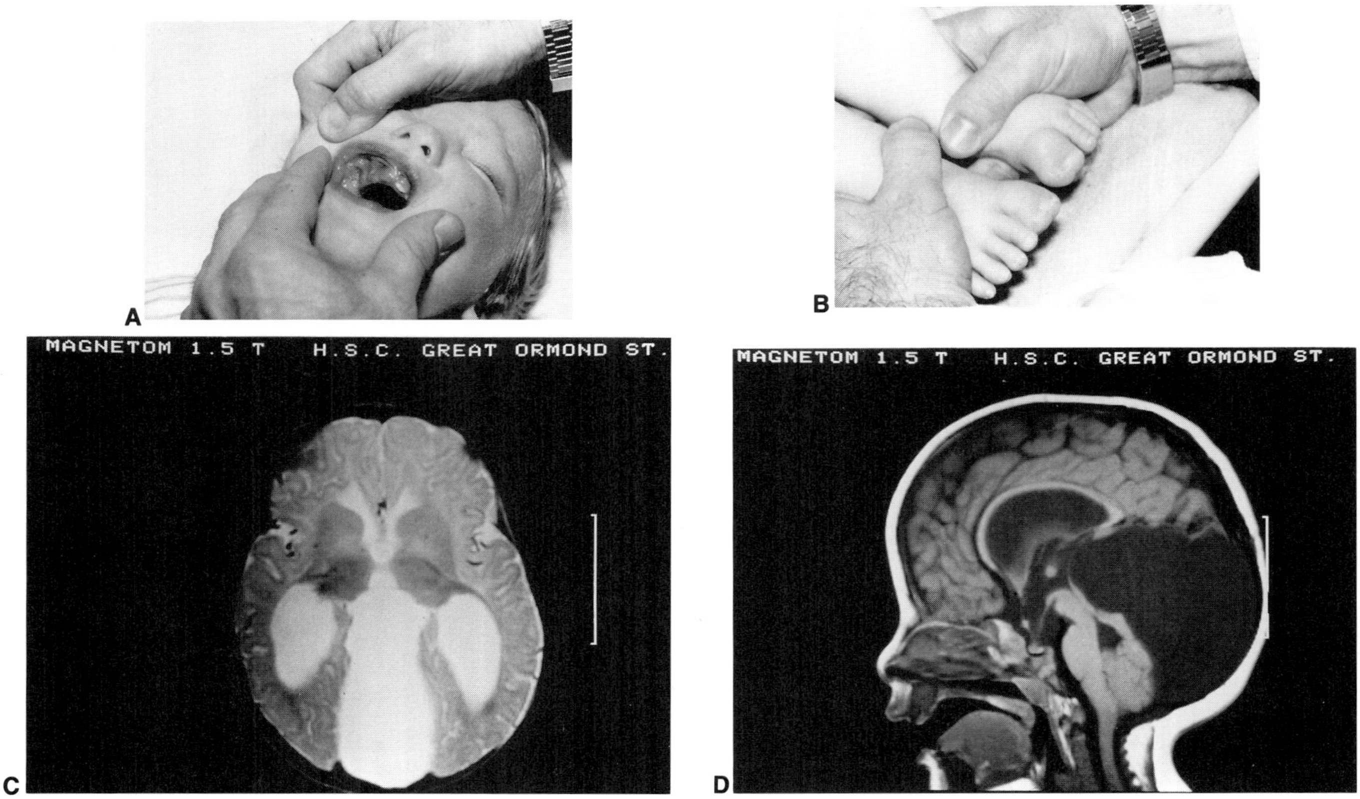


**Fig. 54.** Orofaciodigital syndrome, type II. A: Accessory alveolar frenulae. B: Bilateral hallucal duplication and syndactyly. C: Axial T2 weighted MRI showing dilated lateral and third ventricles. D: Sagittal T1 weighted MRI showing a large arachnoid cyst compressing the cerebellum and brain stem anteriorly. (A–D from W Reardon et al., J Med Genet 26:659, 1989, with permission.)

### Differential diagnosis

OFD, type I should be differentiated from other OFD syndromes, Ellis-van Creveld syndrome, and syndromes with hallucal polydactyly, such as Pfeiffer syndrome, Saethre-Chotzen syndrome, and Rubinstein-Taybi syndrome.

### References

1. Connacher AA, Forsyth Cc, Stewart WK: Orofaciodigital syndrome type I associated with polycystic kidneys and agenesis of the corpus callosum. J Med Genet 24:116–122, 1987.
2. Doege TC, Thuline HC, Priest JH, Norby DE, Bryant JS: Studies of a family with the oral-facial-digital syndrome. N Engl J Med 271:1073–1080, 1964.
3. Gorlin RJ: The oral-facial-digital (OFD) syndrome. Cutis 4:1345–1349, 1968.
4. Majewski F, Lenz W, Pfeiffer RA, Tunte W, Müller H: Das oro-facio-digitale Syndrom. Z Kinderheilkd 112:89–112, 1972.
5. Melnick M, Shields ED: Oro-facio-digital syndrome, type I: a phenotypic and genetic analysis. Oral Surg 40:590–610, 1975.
6. Papillon-Léage M, Psaume J: Une malformation héréditaire de la muqueuse buccale: brides et freins anormaux. Rev Stomatol 55:209–227, 1954.
7. Solomon L, Fretzin DF, Pruzansky S: Pilosebaceous dysplasia in OFD syndrome. Arch Dermatol 102:598–602, 1970.
8. Somer M, Lindahl E, Perheentupa J: Precocious puberty associated with oral-facial-digital syndrome, type I. Acta Paediatr Scand 75:672–675, 1986.
9. Stahl A, Fuhrmann W: Oro-facio-digitales Syndrom. Dtsch Med Wochenschr 93:1224–1228, 1968.
10. Stapleton FB, Bernstein J, Koh G, Roy S 3d, Wilroy RS: Cystic kidneys in a patient with oral-facial-digital syndrome, type I. Am J Kidney Dis 1:288–293, 1982.

## Orofaciodigital syndrome, Type II (OFD II)

**Mohr syndrome**
(MIM No. *252100; POSSUM No. 3348)

The first description of OFD II was by Mohr in 1941.[7] This syndrome is characterized by cleft or lobulated tongue, absent central incisors, polysyndactyly, partial duplication of the hallux, and conductive deafness.

### General manifestations

Polydactyly of the hands, duplicated thumbs, and post-minimus digitis have been described. Partial duplication of the hallux, first metatarsal, cuneiform, and cuboid occur in the foot.[1,5,6,8] Other occasional features include wormian cranial bones, cleft palate, pectus excavatum, scoliosis, and mental deficiency. Choroid colobomas, microcephaly, porencephaly, and cerebellar atrophy are rare occurences.[2,6,8] Failure to thrive and respiratory complications are the main causes of mortality.

Treatment includes surgical repair of the lip and tongue. A hearing aid or exploratory tympanotomy with a prosthesis to replace the deformed ossicles may be needed.

### Otolaryngological manifestations

A cleft or lobulated tongue is common to all cases. Ankyloglossia and fatty hamartomatous nodules are also described in most patients. A cleft or pseudocleft of the upper lip with multiple frenulae are also present. Hypertelorism, micrognathia, and hypoplastic mandibular body usually exist. Dystopia canthorum and a broad nasal bridge may be seen.[3,9]

The ears are posteriorly angulated, and hearing loss is conductive in nature. The incus was described in one case as short and malformed, the long process did not articulate with the stapes, and the lenticular process was absent.[4,9] Laryngeal anomalies have been described in 2 patients.[10]

### Etiology

OFD II is of autosomal recessive inheritance. The frequency is 1:300,000 live births.[1]

### Differential diagnosis

OFD II should be differentiated from other OFD syndromes, short rib–polydactyly syndrome (II), and Majewski-Joubert syndrome.

#### References


1. Ajacques JC: Le syndrome de Mohr. Syndrome orofaciodigital type II. Rev Stomatol Chir Maxillofacial 82:234–240, 1981.
2. Annazen G, Gastarson K, Jozwiak S, Kjartansson S, Stromberg B: Abnormalities of the cerebellum in oro-facio-digital syndrome II (Mohr syndrome). Clin Genet 38:69–73, 1990.
3. Baraitser M: The orofacial digital (OFD) syndromes. J Med Genet 23:116–119, 1986.
4. Goldstein E, Medina JL: Mohr syndrome or oral-facial-digital II: report of two cases. J Am Dent Assoc 89:377–382, 1974.
5. Levy EP, Fletcher BD, Fraser FC: Mohr syndrome with subclinical expression of the bifid great toe. Am J Dis Child 128:531–533, 1974.
6. Mayer UM, Schnidder AC: Les symptômes oculaires dans le syndrome oro-facio-digital type II de Mohr-Claussen. Bull Mem SFO 95:520–524, 1984.
7. Mohr O: A hereditary sublethal syndrome in man. Avh Utgitt 14:1–18, 1941.
8. Kushnick T, Massa TP, Baukema R: A case report: oro-facio-digital syndrome in a male. J Pediatr 63:1130–1134, 1963.
9. Rimoin DL, Edgerton MT: Genetic and clinical heterogeneity in the oral-facial-digital syndromes. J Pediatr 71:94–102, 1967.
10. Silengo MC, Bell GL, Biagioli M, Franceschini P: Oro-facial-digital syndrome II: transitional type between the Mohr and the Majewski syndromes: report of 2 new cases. Clin Genet 31:331–336, 1987.


## Osteogenesis imperfecta spectrum

(Type I: MIM No. #166200; POSSUM No. 3349)
(Type II: MIM No. #166210; POSSUM No. 3366)
(Type III: MIM No. #259420; POSSUM No. 4350)
(Type IV: MIM No. #166220; POSSUM No. 4351)

Osteogenesis imperfecta (OI) is a group of disorders characterized by bone fragility. At least four types of OI exist. Type III is the only recessive disorder of the group. The incidence of all types is 0.5 per 10,000 births.[17]

### General manifestations

The blue sclera is a hallmark of OI. This is due to an increase in noncollagenous matrix and molecular disorganization. In type III OI, the blue color fades away after the first year of life. Patients with type IV OI usually have normal sclerae.[8] Other ocular anomalies seen in type I are embryotoxon (circular opacities in the periphery of the cornea), keratoconus, and megalocornea. The long bones display bowing and angulation due to the sparse trabeculae and thin cortices. About 20% of adult patients with OI type I have kyphosis with or without scoliosis. Macrocephaly and wormian bones are also reported. A higher incidence of fractures occurs between ages 5 and 20 years. According to Sillence et al.,[14,15] 10% of type I OI patients do not have fractures. The limbs are short and thick in type II OI, with multiple fractures and callus formation present at birth. Fifty percent of type III OI patients demonstrate fractures at birth. The placement of intramedullary rods is required to prevent excessive bowing deformities. Some patients with OI type IV may not have fractures. Many authors have demonstrated that approximately 25% of patients with this type may have fractures at birth.[4,8,14–16,18]

The cardiovascular manifestations in OI have been studied by Hortop et al.[6] About 12% of patients suffer from aortic dilatation. Others have demonstrated mitral regurgitation and medial necrosis of the aorta.[1,10] Type II patients have many more cardiovascular anomalies, but no significant anomalies have been described for types III or IV. Manifestations involving the central nervous system include an abnormal electroencephalogram, diffuse dilatation of the ventricles, and cortical atrophy.[20]

### Otolaryngological manifestations

Deafness, usually of the conductive variety, is detected at the end of the first decade. By the seventh decade, most patients lose their hearing. The hearing loss may be sensorineural or mixed.[9,11]

The stapes is the most affected ossicle. The foot plate is thickened, and the crura demonstrate an abnormal ossification pattern with thinning or fractures. The temporal bone also exhibits deficient ossification in the facial canal and cochlear lamina. The internal auditory canal is grossly widened. Histologically, the stria vascularis may show calcified deposits and the utricle displays abnormal structures. Hearing loss is more prominent in type I OI patients. Type IV patients experience deafness 30% of the time. Deafness has not been well documented in types II and III.[2,11,13]

Dental anomalies include opalescent teeth, due to the hypoplastic dentine and pulp. There is an increased susceptibility toward caries and malocclusion. Radiologically, the coronal-radicular junctions demonstrate increased constriction. Histologically, the dental enamel junction is flatter than normal. One study pointed out that teeth are biochemically abnormal in OI patients even if dental abnormalities were not clinically or histologically obvious.[5,7,12]

Normal dentition has been described for OI types IA, II, and III. In type IB and IVB dental abnormalities are much more common. The maxilla is usually hypoplastic, exhibiting mandibular prognathism, and the facies is triangular, with bulging temples in types I and IV.[3]

### Etiology and pathogenesis

OI type I has an autosomal dominant inheritance and extremely variable expressivity. In some families the penetrance is reduced and skipping of generations may occur. OI type II is also an autosomal dominant condition where most of the cases are new mutations. The inheritance of OI type III is clearly autosomal recessive in most cases, especially among Black individu-

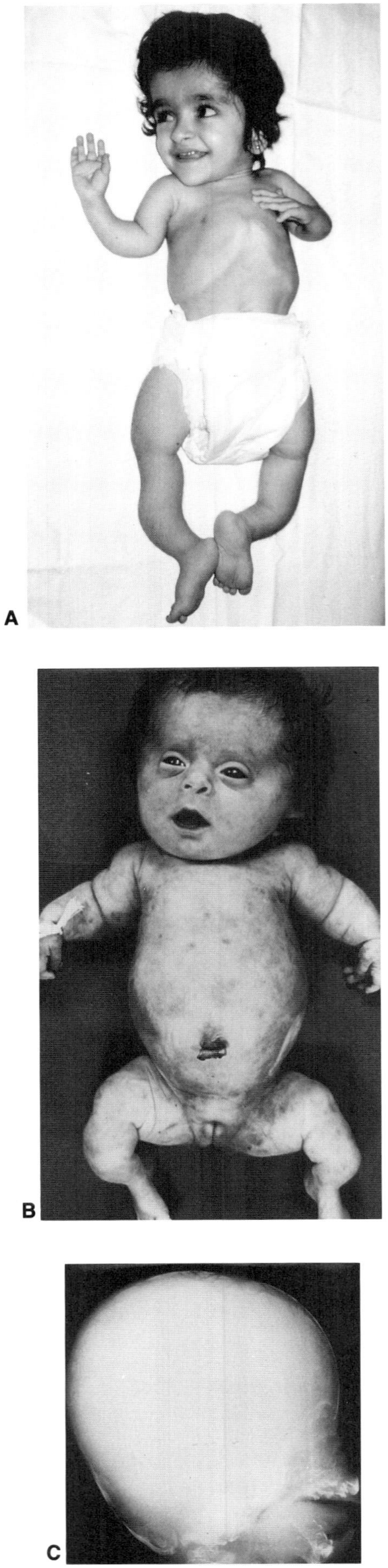

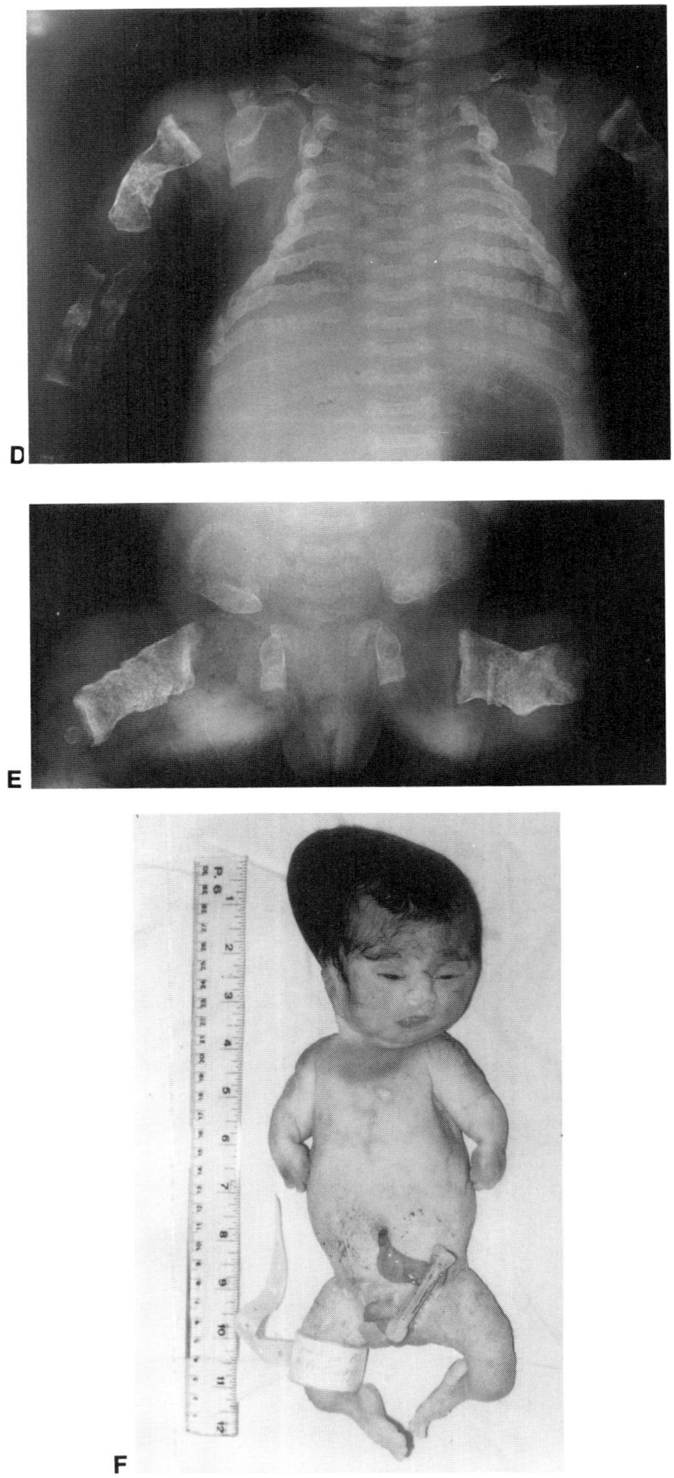

**Fig. 55.** Osteogenesis imperfecta (OI). A: OI type I. Note macrocephaly, and bowing and angulation of the upper and lower limbs. B: OI type II. Perinatal death with frontal bossing, limb shortening, andducted thighs. C: OI type II. Skull X-ray. Note extreme osteopenia and wormian bones in areas of the forehead and vertex. D: OI type II. Chest X-ray. Note beading of the ribs and short humeri. E: OI type II X-ray of the pelvis; note abnormal femora. F: Another patient with osteogenesis imperfecta type II (B–E from DO Sillence et al., Am J Med Genet 17:407, 1984, with permission.)

als in Southern Africa. Autosomal dominant inheritance has been documented also, although infrequently. OI type IV is inherited as an autosomal dominant trait.[19]

Most individuals with the OI type I phenotype have mutations linked to the *COL1A1* gene (17q21.31–q22.05). In some families, however, a similar phenotype is thought to result from mutations in the *COL1A2* gene (7q22.1).

OI type II phenotype is produced by a wide array of mutations: point mutations in the triple helical domain that result in substitutions for glycine (largely in COL1A1 gene); multiexon rearrangements; small deletions in the triple-helical domain of either collagen chain; and mutations in the carboxyterminal propeptide that interfere with molecular assembly.

Patients affected with OI type III have mutations in the genes that encode the chains of procollagen I.

Mutations at both *COL1A1* and *COL1A2* may lead to the OI type IV phenotype.

### References


1. Acar J, Breil B, Lavabre J, Chomette G, Roland J, Dewilde J, Hospitel S: Osteogénèse imparfaite et insuffisance aortique. Ann Med Interne (Paris) 8:514–518, 1980.
2. Bretlau, P, Jorgensen MG, Johansen H: Osteogenesis imperfecta. Light and electron microscopic studies of the stapes. Acta Otolaryngol 69:172–184, 1970.
3. Cole NL, Goldberg MH, Loftus M, Kwok V: Surgical management of patients with osteogenesis imperfecta. J Oral Maxillofac Surg 40:578–584, 1982.
4. Eichholtz W, Müller D: Electron microscopic findings on the cornea and sclera in osteogenesis imperfecta. Klin Monatsbl Augenkheilkd 161:646–653, 1972.
5. Gage JP, Francis MJ, Whitaker GE, Smith R: Dentine is biochemically abnormal in osteogenesis imperfecta. Clin Sci 70:339–346, 1986.
6. Hortop J, Tsipouras P, Hanley JA, Maron BJ, Shapiro JR: Cardiovascular involvement in osteogenesis imperfecta. Circulation 73:54–61, 1986.
7. Levin LS: The dentition in the osteogenesis imperfecta syndromes. Clin Orthop Rel Res 159:64–74, 1981.
8. Paterson CR, McAllion S, Miller R: Osteogenesis imperfecta with dominant inheritance and normal sclerae. J Bone Joint Surg 65:35–39, 1983.
9. Pedersen U: Osteogenesis imperfecta. Clinical features. Hearing loss and stapedectomy. Acta Otolaryngol 145 (Suppl):1–36, 1985.
10. Pyeritz RE, Levin LS: Aortic root dilatation and valvular dysfunction in osteogenesis imperfecta. Circulation 64:1193, 1981.
11. Riedner ED, Levin LS, Holliday MJ: Hearing patterns in dominant osteogenesis imperfecta. Arch Otolaryngol 106:737–740, 1980.
12. Schwartz S, Tsipouras P: Oral findings in osteogenesis imperfecta. Oral Surg Oral Med Oral Path 57:161–167, 1984.
13. Shapiro JR, Pikus A, Weiss G, Rowe DW: Hearing and middle ear function in osteogenesis imperfecta. JAMA 247:2120–2126, 1982.
14. Sillence DO, Barlow KK, Cole WG, Ditrich G, Garber AP, Rimoin DL: Osteogenesis imperfecta type III. Delineation of the phenotype with reference to genetic heterogeneity. Am J Med Genet 23:821–832, 1986.
15. Sillence DO, Lenn A, Danks DM: Genetic heterogeneity in osteogenesis imperfecta. J Med Genet 16:101–116, 1979.
16. Smith R, Francis MJ, Sykes B: The eye and collagen in osteogenesis imperfecta. Birth Defects 12:563–568, 1976.
17. Stoll C, Dott B, Roth MP, Alembik Y: Birth prevalence rates of skeletal dysplasias. Clin Genet 35:88–92, 1989.
18. Thompson EM, Young ID, Hall CM, Pembrey ME: Recurrence risks and prognosis in severe sporadic osteogenesis imperfecta. J Med Genet 24:390–405, 1987.
19. Tsipouras P: Osteogenesis imperfecta. In: McKusick's Heritable Disorders of Connective Tissue, P Beighton, ed. CF Mosby, St. Louis, 1993, pp 281–314.
20. Tsipouras P, Barabas G, Matthews WS: Neurologic correlates of osteogenesis imperfecta. Arch Neurol 43:150–152, 1986.


## Otopalatodigital syndrome, type I (OPD I)

### Taybi syndrome
(MIM No. *311300; POSSUM No. 3352)

OPD I was first reported in 1962 by Taybi.[9] Subsequently, Dudding et al.[3] and Langer[5] supported evidence of the X-

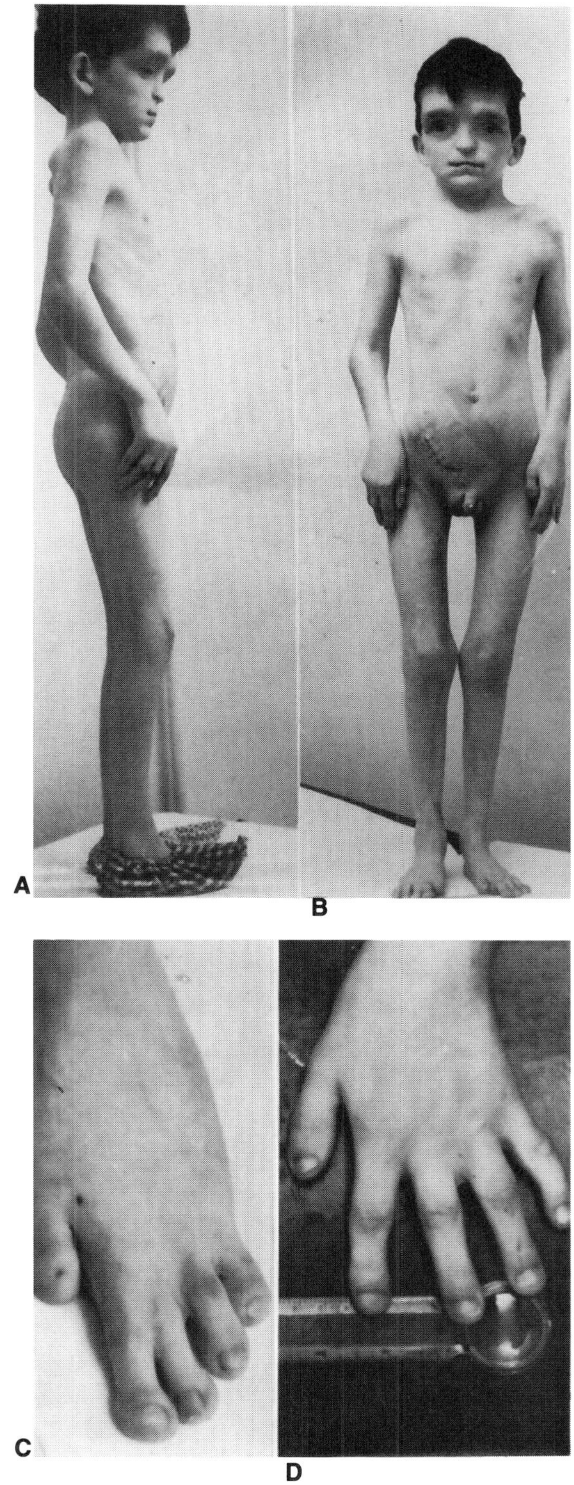

Fig. 56. Otopalatodigital syndrome, type I. Note the pugilistic facies (prominent supraorbital ridges and wide, depressed nasal bridge) (A,B), and abnormal toes and fingers (C,D). (From H Taybi, Am J Roentgenol 88:450, 1962, with permission.)

linked inheritance. This syndrome is characterized by cleft palate, moderate conductive hearing loss, short stature, short terminal phalanges, and characteristic facies.

### General manifestations

IQ ranges from 75 to 90. Most patients are below the 10th percentile in height. Mild coxa vara occurs and the iliac bones are less flared than normal. Various anomalies are noted in the feet. The second and third metatarsals fuse with the cuneiform bones. Tarsal fusion is also found. Anomalies of the upper limbs include subluxation of the radial head, clinodactyly, short middle phalanx of the fifth finger, accessory ossification center in the second metacarpal, and bowing of the femurs and lower tibias. The toes are broad and curved, often with webbing, resembling feet of a tree frog. The nails are short and dystrophic. The skull base is thickened, the nasion-sella-basion angle is reduced. The skull has a mushroom appearance due to frontal and occipital thickening.[4,8] Severe scoliosis has ocasionally been described.[6]

### Otolaryngological manifestations

The pugilistic facies are characterized by prominent supraorbital ridges, hypertelorism, and a broad nasal root. The midface is flat, the palpebral fissures slant downward, and the occiput is prominent. Female patients have a milder facial appearance.[2] Cleft palate is a common finding. Conductive hearing loss varies between 30 and 90 db. A variety of ossicular anomalies have also been described: thickened incus, unstable incudostapedial joints, short anterior crus, or wide head of the stapes. Retarded speech occurs due to hearing loss. The paranasal sinuses and mastoids are poorly pneumatized. The mandibular angle is more obtuse than normal.[2,7]

### Etiology

Inheritance of this syndrome has an X-linked semidominant pattern; the OPD I gene has been mapped to Xq28.[1] An autosomal dominant inheritance has also been proposed.

### Differential diagnosis

OPD I should be differentiated from Larsen's syndrome and OPD II.

### References


1. Biancalana V, Le Marec B, Odent S, Van den Hurk JA, Hanauer A: Oto-palato-digital syndrome type I: further evidence for assignment of the locus to Xq28. Hum Genet 88:228–230, 1991.
2. Buran DJ, Duvall AJ 3d. The oto-palato-digital (OPD) syndrome. Arch Otolaryngol 85:394–399, 1967.
3. Dudding BA, Gorlin RJ, Langer LO: The oto-palato-digital syndrome. A new symptom-complex consisting of deafness, dwarfism, cleft palate, characteristic facies, and a generalized bone dysplasia. Am J Dis Child 113:214–221, 1967.
4. Gall JC Jr, Stern AM, Poznanski AK, Garn SM, Weinstein DC, Hargward JR: Oto-palato-digital syndrome: comparison of clinical and radiological manifestations in males and females. Am J Hum Genet 24:24–36, 1972.
5. Langer LO: The roentgenographic features of the oto-palato-digital (OPD) syndrome. Am J Roentgenol 100:63–70, 1967.
6. Pazzaglia UE, Beluffi G: Oto-palato-digital syndrome in four generations of a large family. Clin Genet 30:338–344, 1986.
7. Podoshin L, Heymans HS, Fradis M: The oto-palato-digital syndrome. J Laryngol Otol 90:407–411, 1976.
8. Poznanski AK, Macpherson RI, Dijkman DJ, Gorlin RJ, Gall JC Jr, Stern AM Jr, Garn SM, Nagy JM: Oto-palato-digital syndrome: radiological findings in the hand and foot. Birth Defects 10:125–139, 1974.
9. Taybi H: Generalized skeletal dysplasia with multiple anomalies. Am J Roentgenol 88:450–457, 1962.


## Otopalatodigital syndrome, type II (OPD II)

(MIM No. 304120; POSSUM No. 3710)

The first description of OPD II was by Fitch et al.[4] in 1976 and later by Kozlowski et al.[5]

This syndrome is characterized by cleft palate, broad forehead, unusual facies, low-set ears, short stature, and multiple anomalies of the skeleton.

### General manifestations

Death may occur in the neonatal period due to feeding and respiratory difficulties.[4,7] In early life, the long bones are bowed and tend to improve with advanced age. The fibulae may be absent or small. The acetabulae and vertebral bodies are usually flat. Malformed wrists, ankles and absent metacarpals or metatarsals are also frequent, as well as abnormal ribs and pectus excavatum.[3] The skeletal features are much more severe in this syndrome as compared with those of OPD type I. Psychomotor development may be normal or retarded.[2,7]

### Otolaryngological manifestations

The forehead is prominent with large anterior fontanelle, a flat nasal bridge, low-set ears, and a cleft palate. The palpebral fissures slant downward. Hearing loss is conductive. Ossicular deformities include malformed ankylosed stapes and abnormal incus. The mandible is hypoplastic,the facial bones are small and the skull base is thickened.[1,2,7]

### Etiology

OPD II is of X-linked recessive inheritance. The main abnormality is defective intramembranous ossification.[6]

### Differential diagnosis

OPD II should be differentiated from OPD type I and campomelic dysplasia.

### References


1. André M, Cigneron J, Didier F: Abnormal facies, cleft palate and generalized dysostosis: a lethal X-linked syndrome. J Pediatr 98:747–752, 1981.
2. Brewster TG, Lochman RS, Kushner DC, Holmes LB, Isler RJ, Rimouin DL: Oto-palato-digital syndrome type II—an X-linked skeletal dysplasia. Am J Med Genet 20:249–254, 1985.
3. Fitch N, Jéquier S, Gorlin R: The oto-palato-digital syndrome, proposed type II. Am J Med Genet 15:655–664, 1983.
4. Fitch N, Jéquier S, Papageorgiou A: A familial syndrome of cranial, facial, oral and limb anomalies. Clin Genet 10:226–231, 1976.
5. Kozlowski K, Turner G, Scougall J, Harrington J: Oto-palato-digital syndrome with severe X-ray changes in two half brothers. Pediatr Radiol 6:97–102, 1977.
6. Ogata T, Matsuo N, Nichimira G, Hajikano H: Oto-palato-digital syn-

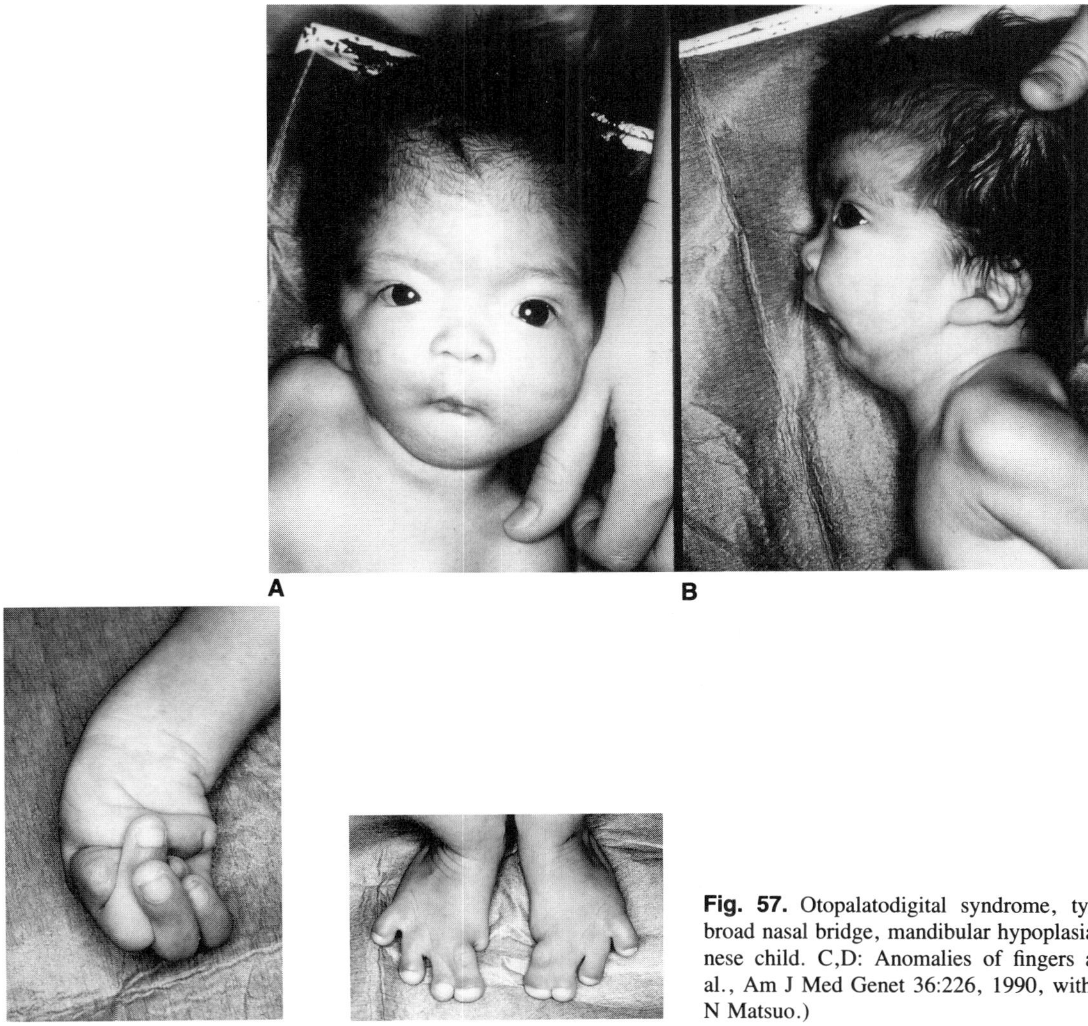

A B C D

**Fig. 57.** Otopalatodigital syndrome, type II. A,B: Hypertelorism, broad nasal bridge, mandibular hypoplasia, and low-set ears in a Japanese child. C,D: Anomalies of fingers and toes. (From T Ogata et al., Am J Med Genet 36:226, 1990, with permission; courtesy of Dr. N Matsuo.)

drome, type II: evidence for defective intramembranous ossification. Am J Med Genet 36:226–231, 1990.
7. Shi SR: Temporal bone findings in a case of oto-palato-digital syndrome. Arch Otolaryngol 111:119–121, 1985.

## Pallister-Hall syndrome

### Hypothalamic hamartoblastoma syndrome
(MIM No. *146510; POSSUM No. 3471)

This syndrome is characterized by hypothalamic hamartoblastoma, hypopituitarism, postaxial polydactyly, variable skeletal defects, congenital anomalies, and early death.

#### General manifestations

The most striking systemic manifestation is the congenital hypothalamic hamartoblastoma on the inferior surface of the cerebrum that replaces the hypothalamus and extends from the optic chiasma to the interpeduncular fossa. Limb abnormalities include postaxial polydactyly, syndactyly, and nail dysplasia. Distal shortening of the limbs, particularly the arms, is noted. Endocrine abnormalities include pituitary aplasia or hypoplasia with hypopituitarism, adrenal aplasia or hypoplasia with hypoadrenalism, and thyroid aplasia or hypoplasia with hypothyroidism. Other frequent anomalies include an imperforate or anteriorly placed anus, renal dysplasia, and congenital heart defects. Occasional anomalies include microphthalmia, holoprosencephaly, hemiverebrae, narrow cervical vertebrae, congenital dislocation of the hip, subluxation of the knee, a hypoplastic pancreas, and a micropenis.[1–5,7–11]

#### Otolaryngological manifestations

These include a flat midface with a capillary hemangioma in the midline. A short nose with anterveted nostrils and a flat nasal bridge, posteriorly angulated and low-set ears with small ear lobules, microglossia, micrognathia, multiple buccal frenulae, gingival cysts, a cleft palate, and occasionally, a cleft uvula have been documented. A laryngeal cleft and a hypoplastic or bifid epiglottis with tracheomalacia are common.[1–5,7–10,12]

#### Etiology

The cause of this syndrome is unknown. Most cases have been sporadic.[3,4,7] However, familial cases have also been reported.[8–10] One patient has been described with a chromosomal anomaly involving 3p and 7q.[6]

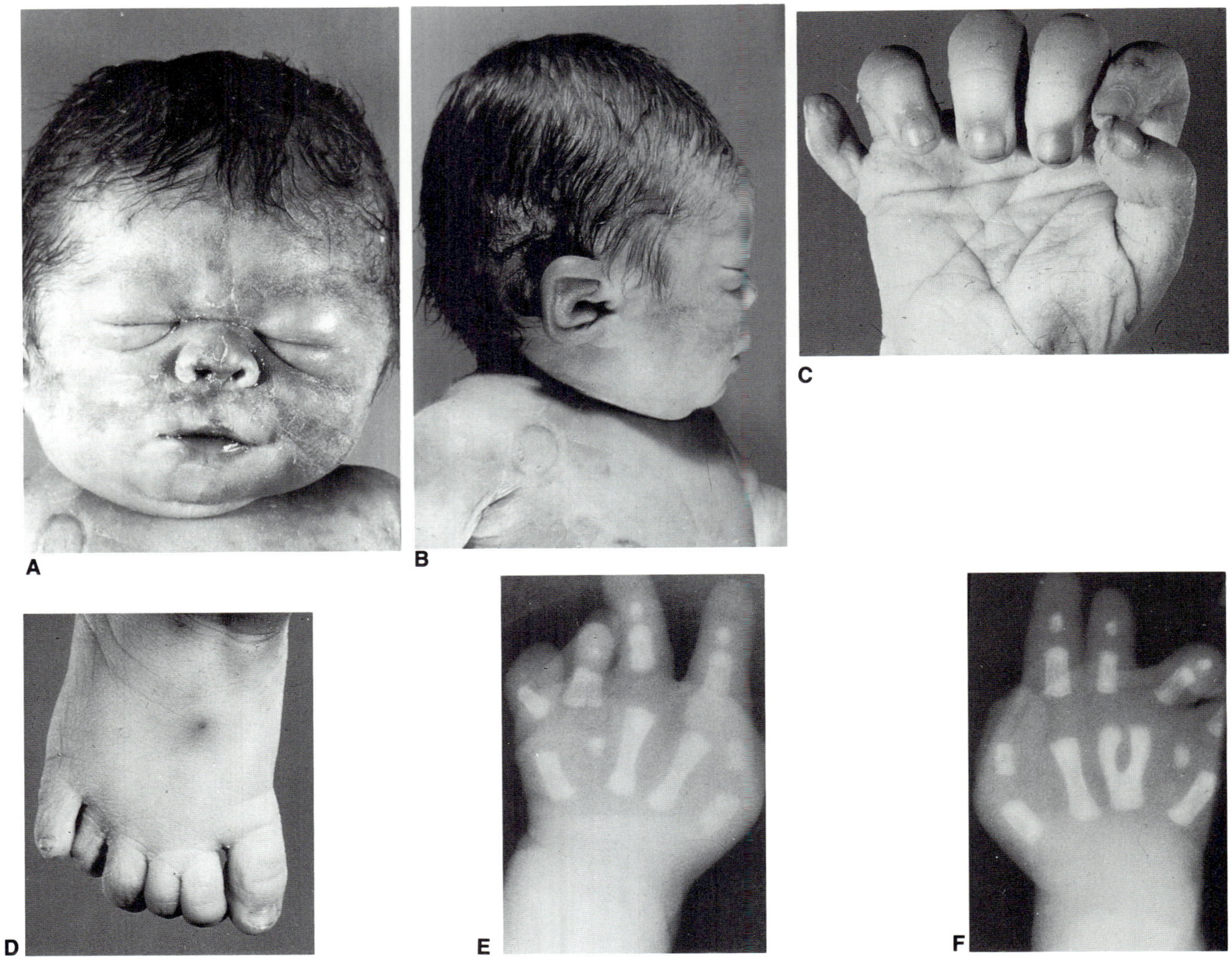

**Fig. 58.** Pallister-Hall syndrome. A: Short nose with anteverted nostrils and flat nasal bridge. B: Low-set and abnormally-shaped ears. C: Polydactyly of the right hand. D: Polydactyly of the right foot. E,F: X-rays of the hands; note various bone anomalies. (From J Hall et al., Am J Med Genet 4:47, 1980, with permission.)

### Differential diagnosis

Pallister-Hall syndrome should be differentiated from nonlethal hypopituitarism and polydactyly syndrome, Meckel syndrome, and Smith-Lemli-Opitz syndrome.

### References


1. Clarren SK, Alvord EC Jr, Hall JG: Congenital hypothalamic hamartoblastoma, hypopituitarism, imperforate anus, and postaxial polydactyly in a new syndrome? II. Neuropathological considerations. Am J Med Genet 7:75–83, 1980.
2. Culler FL, Jones KL: Hypopituitarism in assocation with postaxial polydactyly. J Pediatr 104:881–884, 1984.
3. Graham JM Jr, Saunders R, Fratkin J, Spiegel P, Harris M, Klein RZ: A cluster of Pallister-Hall syndrome cases (congenital hypothalamic hamartoblastoma syndrome). Am J Med Genet (Suppl) 2:53–63, 1986.
4. Hall JG, Pallister PD, Clarren SK, Beckwith JB, Wiglesworth FW, Fraser FC, Cho S, Benke PJ, Reed SD: Congenital hypothalamic hamartoblastoma, hypopituitarism, imperforate anus, and postaxial polydactyly—a new syndrome? Clinical, causal and pathogenetic considerations. Am J Med Genet 7:47–74, 1980.
5. Iafolla K, Fratkin JD, Spiegel PK, Cohen MM Jr, Graham JM Jr: Case report and delineation of the congenital hypothalamic hamartoblastoma syndrome (Pallister-Hall syndrome). Am J Med Genet 33:489–499, 1989.
6. Kuller JA, Cox VA, Schonberg SA, Golabi M: Pallister-Hall syndrome associated with an unbalanced chromosome translocation. Am J Med Genet 43:647–650, 1992.
7. Pallister PD, Hecht F, Herrman J: Three additional cases of congenital hypothalamic "hamartoblastoma" (Pallister-Hall) syndrome. Am J Med Genet 33:500–501, 1989.
8. Sills IN, Rapaport R, Desposito F, Lieber C: Familial Pallister-Hall syndrome. Three affected offspring. Am J Med Genet 52:251, 1994.
9. Thomas HM, Todd PJ, Heaf D, Fryer AE: Recurrence of Pallister-Hall syndrome in two sibs. J Med Genet 31:145–147, 1994.
10. Topf KF, Kletter GB, Kelch RP, Brunberg JA, Biesecker LG: Autosomal dominant transmission of Pallister-Hall syndrome. J Pediatr 123:943–946, 1993.
11. Unsinn KM, Neu N, Krejci A, Posch A, Menardi G, Gassner I: Pallister-Hall syndrome and McKusick-Kaufmann syndrome: one entity? J Med Genet 32:125–128, 1995.
12. Winter WE, Rosenbloom AL, MacLaren NK, Mickle JP: Solitary central maxillary incisor associated with precocious puberty and hypothalamic hamartoma. J Pediatr 101:965–967, 1982.

## Pendred syndrome

(MIM No. *274600; POSSUM No. 3910)

Pendred described two sibs with goiter and deafmutism in 1896.[16] In 1927 Brain described the syndrome in greater detail.[4] Five percent of all genetic deafness is attributed to Pendred's syndrome. It is among the most frequent syndromes involving hereditary deafness.[1,13,14] Fraser et al.[8] estimate the frequency of the syndrome to be 0.000075 in the British Isles.

### General manifestations

Goiter usually appears during puberty or later. In some cases, it may be observed at birth. Most patients are euthyroid, but hypothyroidism may develop during childhood.[1,2] Longstanding goiters, especially in females, tend to be nodular. The recurrence rate after thyroidectomy is high, unless thyroid therapy is instituted.[3,11] The amount of retinol-binding protein in the plasma is in the lower range of normal.[5] Thyroid carcinoma has been reported.[7,18] Suffocation may occur sporadically in neonates, due to the size of the thyroid.[9]

There is an unusual deposition of retinal pigment. This has been described in three sibs.[10] Most patients are normal mentally and psychologically, with a few exceptions.[8,13]

### Otolaryngological manifestations

Hearing loss is congenital and sensorineural. Audiograms show a severe to profound high-tone loss. Caloric stimulation reveals hypofunction of the vestibular labyrinth in most patients.[2,12,13,19] Temporal bone changes involve the bony and membraneous inner ear. They correspond to the Mondini defect. The semicircular canals are larger than normal and the cochlea has only two turns. Occasionally there are no hair cells in the organ of Corti. The tectorial membrane may be absent. Other otological changes include hyperostosis of the promontory and round window.[10,12,13]

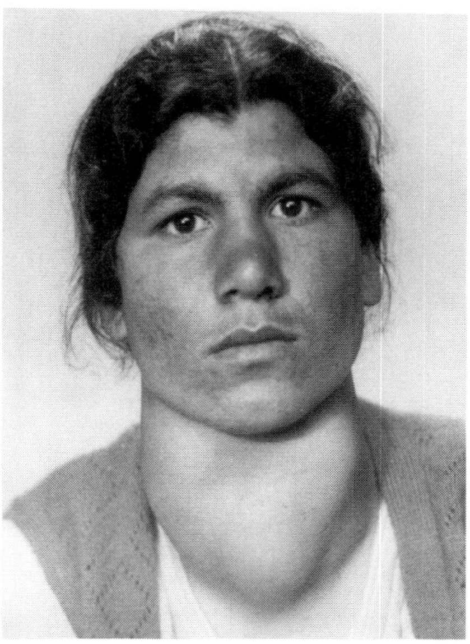

**Fig. 59.** Pendred syndrome. Patient with goiter and hearing loss. (From Y Kabakkaya et al., Ann Otol Rhinol Laryngol 102:285, 1993, with permission.)

### Etiology

Pendred syndrome is of autosomal recessive inheritance. The cause is an intrinsic defect of thyroid organification.[8] Pendred syndrome maps to chromosome 7q21–q34, in the region containing the nonsyndromic deafness gene *DFNB4*.[6,17]

### Differential diagnosis

Pendred syndrome should be differentiated from endemic cretinism with deafness, and hearing loss with hypothyroidism.[15]

### References


1. Batsakis JG, Nishiyama RH: Deafness with sporadic goitre: Pendred's syndrome. Arch Otolaryngol 76:401–406, 1962.
2. Bergstom L: Congenital deafness. In: Otolaryngology, Vol 1, GM English, ed. v 1, JB Lippincott, Philadelphia, 1988, p 17.
3. Bouchard R, Gaedeney J, Mazet P, Castaing N: Discussion d'un syndrome de Pendred. Arch Fr Pediatr 25:453–464, 1968.
4. Brain WR: Heredity in simple goitre. J Med 20:203–303, 1927.
5. Biesalski HK, Gross M, Ehrenthal W, Harth O: The diagnosis of Vitamin A (retinol) and retinol-binding protein (RBP) in serum of hearing impaired children. Laryngol Rhinol Otol 60:631–635, 1981.
6. Coyle B, Coffey R, Armour JAL, Gausden E, Hochberg Z, Grossman A, Britton K, Pembrey M, Reardon W, Trembath R: Pendred syndrome (goitre and sensorineural hearing loss) maps to chromosome 7 in the region containing the nonsyndromic deafness gene *DFNB4*. Nat Genet 12:421–423, 1996.
7. Elman DS: Familial associaton of nerve deafness with nodular goiter and thyroid carcinoma. N Engl J Med 259:219–223, 1958.
8. Fraser GR, Morgan ME, Trotten WR: The syndrome of sporadic goitre and congenital deafness. J Med 114:279–295, 1960.
9. Fritsch MH, Sommer A: Handbook of Congenital and Early Onset Hearing Loss. Igaku-Shoin, New York, 1990, pp 103–105.
10. Gomez-Pan A, Evered DC, Hall R: Pituitary-thyroid function in Pendred's syndrome. Br Med J 2:152–153, 1974.
11. Gorlin RJ, Toriello HV, Cohen MM Jr: Hereditary Hearing Loss and Its Syndromes, Oxford University Press, New York, 1995, pp 337–339.
12. Hvidberg-Hansen J, Jorgensen MB: The inner ear in Pendred's syndrome. Acta Otolaryngol 66:129–135, 1968.
13. Kabakkaya Y, Bakan E, Yigitoglu MR, Gokce G, Dogan M: Pendred's syndrome. Ann Otol Rhinol Laryngol 102:285–288, 1993.
14. Meyerhoff WL, Liston SL: Metabolic hearing loss. In: Otolaryngology, Vol 2, MM Paparella, DA Shumrick, JL Gluckman, WL Meyerhoff eds. WB Saunders, Philadelphia, 1991, pp 1677–1678.
15. Nilsson LR, Borgors N, Gamstorp L, Holst H, Liden G: Non-endemic goitre and deafness. Acta Paediatr Scand 53:117–131, 1964.
16. Pendred V: Deafmutism and goitre. Lancet 2:532, 1896.
17. Sheffield VC, Kraiem Z, Beck JC, Nishimura D, Stone EM, Salameh M, Sadeh O, Glaser B: Pendred syndrome maps to chromosome 7q21–34 and is caused by an intrinsic defect in thyroid organification. Nat Genet 12:424–426, 1996.
18. Thompson J, Maguire WC, Hurwitz LJ: A family with deafness, goitre, epilepsy and low intelligence segregating independently. Ir J Med Sci 3:427–431, 1970.
19. von Deuster C: Horschädigung nach Pockenschutzimpfung oder Pendred Syndrom. HNO. 24:122–126, 1976.


## Pfeiffer syndrome

(MIM No. *101600; POSSUM No. 3010)

The diagnostic criteria for this syndrome are craniosynostosis, broad thumbs and great toes, and variable soft tissue syndactyly of the hands.

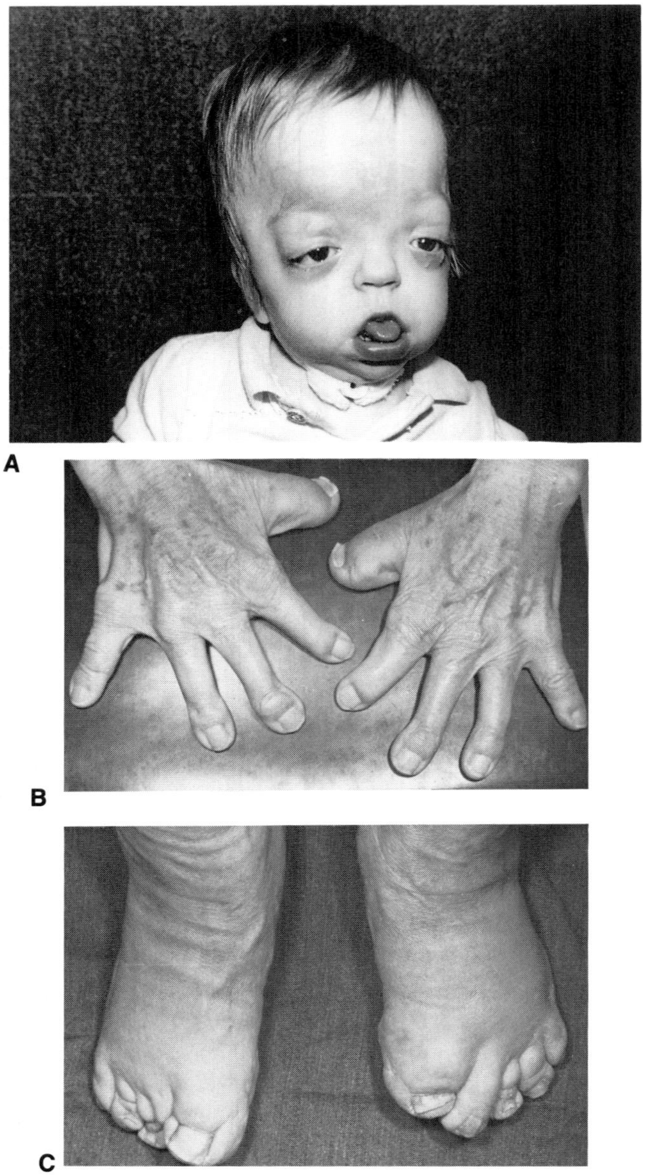

**Fig. 60.** Pfeiffer syndrome. A: Note flat nasal bridge, maxillary hypoplasia, and mandibular prognathism. B: Note broad, deviated thumbs and abnormal fingers. C: Note broad halluces and abnormal toes. (A: courtesy of Dr. JL Frias. B,C from RJ Gorlin et al., *Syndromes of the Head and Neck,* 3rd ed., Oxford University Press, New York, 1990, p. 526.)

### General manifestations

The degree of craniosynostosis varies from turribrachycephaly to minimal or no synostosis. Other anomalies include broad, short thumbs with radial deviation and soft tissue syndactyly. The hands show brachymesophalangy and synphalangism. Similar abnormalities are found in the feet. The proximal phalanges of the great toes are malformed, trapezoid shaped, duplicated, or absent. Hallux varus and cutaneous syndactyly involving the second and third toes are common. Accessory epiphyses of the first and second metatarsals, fusion of the carpals, and synostosis of the radioulnar and radiohumeral joints have been described. Intelligence is usually normal. However, poor mental development has been described. Seizures, hydrocephaly, Arnold-Chiari malformation, spina bifida, and cloverleaf skull have been reported.[1–3,6] In the form associated with cloverleaf skull, early demise is common.[3]

### Otolaryngological manifestations

These include craniofacial asymmetry, a flattened nasal bridge, beaked nose, high-arched palate, crowded teeth, maxillary hypoplasia, and mandibular prognathism. Hypertelorism with downward slanting palpebral fissures and strabismus are common findings. Conductive hearing loss with ossicular fixation and ankylosed stapes have been reported. Absence of the auditory canals has also been documented.[2,4] Occasional manifestations include preauricular tags, gingival hypertrophy, and fused cervical and lumbar vertebrae.

### Etiology

Pfeiffer syndrome is of autosomal dominant inheritance with complete penetrance and variable expressivity. Genetic heterogeneity has been demonstrated, as mutations of *FGFR1* (fibroblast growth factor receptor 1) and *FGFR2* genes were found to cause familial and sporadic cases of Pfeiffer syndrome.[5,7,8] *FGFR1* and *FGFR2* have been mapped to chromosomes 8p11.2–p12 and 10q25.3–q26 respectively.

### Differential diagnosis

Pfeiffer syndrome should be differentiated from Apert, Crouzon, and Saethre-Chotzen syndromes.

### References


1. Cohen MM Jr: An etiologic and nosologic view of craniosynostosis syndromes. Birth Defects 11:137–189, 1975.
2. Cohen MM Jr: Craniosynostosis: Diagnosis, Evaluation and Management. Raven Press, New York, 1986.
3. Cohen MM Jr: Pfeiffer syndrome update, clinical subtypes and guidelines for differential diagnosis. Am J Med Genet 45:300–307, 1993.
4. Cremers CWRJ: Hearing loss in Pfeiffer syndrome. Int J Pediatr Otorhinol 3:343–353, 1987.
5. Lajeunie E, Ma HW, Bonaventure J, Munnich A, Le Merrer M, Renier D: FGFR2 mutations in Pfeiffer syndrome. Nat Genet 9:108, 1995.
6. Martsolf JT, Cracco JB, Carpenter GG, O'Hara AE: Pfeiffer syndrome (An unusual type of acrocephalosyndactyly with broad thumbs and great toes). Am J Dis Child 121:257–262, 1971.
7. Saldino RM, Steinbach HL, Epstein CJ: Familial acrocephalosyndactyly (Pfeiffer syndrome). Am J Roentgenol 116:609–622, 1972.
8. Schell U, Hehr A, Feldman GJ, Robin NH, Zackai EH, de Die-Smulders C, Viskochil DH, Stewart JM, Wolff G, Ohashi H, Price RA, Cohen MM Jr, Muenke M: Mutations in FGFR 1 and FGFR 2 cause familial and sporadic Pfeiffer syndrome. Hum Mol Genet 4:323–328, 1995.


## Progeria

### Hutchinson-Gilford syndrome
(MIM No. 176670; POSSUM No. 3362)

### General manifestations

Growth failure begins after the first year. The subsequent growth rate is one-third to one-half of the normal rate. There is no sexual maturation. The absence of subcutaneous fat and restricted growth of the long bones result in the characteristic

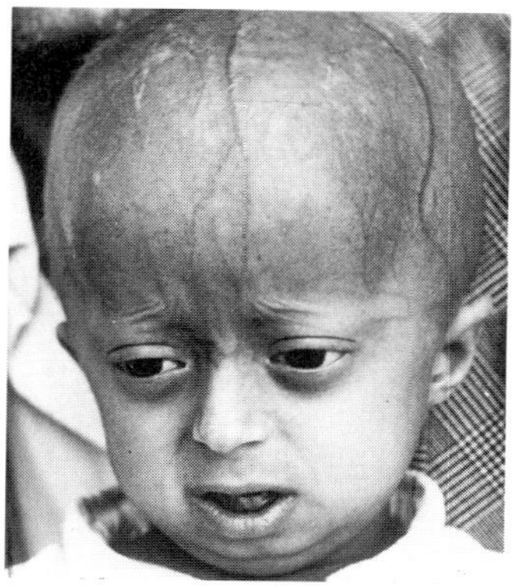

**Fig. 61.** Progeria. Note alopecia and prominent scalp veins. (VM Der Kaloustian, AK Kurban, *Genetic Diseases of the Skin,* Springer-Verlag, Berlin, 1979, p. 117, with permission.)

spindly limbs, prominent joints, and coxa vara. The shoulders are narrow, the clavicles are short, and the thorax assumes a pyriform shape. The nails are hypoplastic, brittle, and yellowish. Atherosclerosis and cardiovascular accidents may result in death. The average life span is 14 years. Death is usually due to myocardial infarction.[2]

### Otolaryngological manifestations

Children appear to be normal at birth and develop the characteristics of the syndrome during the second year of life. Alopecia, prominent scalp veins, and frontal and parietal bossing develop. Micrognathia is due to slow growth of the mandible. Delayed eruption of deciduous and permanent dentition is common. The teeth are often crowded. Senile microscopic changes have been documented in the dental pulp.[4,7] The ears are small and lack a lobule. Mild to moderate hearing loss of the conductive variety has been observed. Fixation of the ossicular chain was confirmed surgically. Brain stem–response audiometry suggests possible auditory central nervous system involvement.[5,8] The nose is small and beaked, and the cartilagenous frame is visible under the thin skin. The paranasal sinuses and mastoids are poorly pneumatized. The voice is high pitched.

### Etiology and pathogenesis

Progeria may be of autosomal dominant inheritance. Increased paternal age is noted. Autosomal recessive inheritance has also been suggested. Abnormal metabolism of glycosaminoglycans has been hypothesized due to elevated hyaluronic acid excretion. A fault in vitamin E metabolism has been suggested, and vitamin E therapy is recommended for its antioxidant effect. The estimated incidence is 1:250,000 births.[1,3,4,6]

### Differential diagnosis

Progeria should be differentiated from Hallermann-Streiff, Cockayne, and Ehler-Danlos syndromes.

### References


1. Ayres S, Mihan R: Progeria: a possible therapeutic approach. JAMA 227:1381–1382, 1974.
2. Baker PB, Baba N, Boesel CP: Cardiovascular abnormalities in Progeria. Arch Pathol Lab Med 105:384–386, 1981.
3. Brown WT: Human mutations affecting aging—a review. Mech Ageing Dev 9:325–336, 1979.
4. Gabr M, Hashem N, Hashem M, Fahmi A, Safouh M: Progeria, a pathologic study. J Pediatr 57:70–77, 1960.
5. Hall JW 3d, Denneny JC 3d: Audiologic and otolaryngologic findings in progeria: case report. J Am Acad Audiol 4:116–121, 1993.
6. Maciel AT: Evidence for autosomal recessive inheritance of progeria (Hutchinson Gilford). Am J Med Genet 31:483–487, 1988.
7. Manschot W: A case of progeronanism (progeria of Gilford). Acta Pediatr Scand 39:158–164, 1950.
8. Nelson M: Progeria, audiologic aspects. Ann Otol Rhinol Laryngol 74:376–385, 1965.


## Proteus syndrome

(MIM No. 176920; POSSUM No. 3515)

This disorder was presented as a clinical entity in 1983 by Wiedemann. The syndrome is named after the Greek god Proteus to characterize the changing manifestations of this condition.

### General manifestations

Growth may be asymmetric because of overgrowth of any part of the body. The skin is generally thickened. Patients may have lipomata, lymphangiomata, or hemangiomata. Macrodactyly may be present, along with gyriform changes, particularly over the plantar surfaces of the feet. Strabismus, enlarged eyes, lung abnormality, muscle atrophy, pelvic lipomatosis and café-au-lait spots may also be part of the syndrome.[4,7,8]

### Otolaryngological manifestations

A broad and depressed nasal bridge, hyperostosis of the external auditory canals and alveolar ridges, along with different nonspecific deformities of the skull and face may occur.[3,8]

### Etiology and pathogenesis

The cause of this syndrome is unkown. All cases have been sporadic. Somatic mutation has been detected by DNA fingerprinting.[5 6]

### Differential diagnosis

Proteus syndrome should be differentiated from Klippel-Trenaunay-Weber syndrome and Proteus-like syndromes with mental retardation and eye defects.[1,2]

### References


1. Baskerville PA, Ackroyd JS, Lea Thomas M, Browse NL: The Klippel-Trenaunay syndrome: clinical, radiological and haemodynamic features and management. Br J Surg 72:232–236, 1985.
2. Cohen MM, Hayden PW: A newly recognized hamartomatous syndrome. Birth Defects 15:291–296, 1979.
3. Kreiborg S, Cohen MM Jr, Skovby F: Craniofacial characteristics of Proteus syndrome: two modes of abnormal growth. Proc Finn Dent Soc 87:183–188, 1991.
4. Mayatepek E, Kurczynski TW, Ruppert ES, Hennessy JR, Brinker RA, French BN: Expanding the phenotype of the Proteus syndrome: a severely affected patient with new findings. Am J Med Genet 32:402–406, 1989.
5. Schwartz CE, Brown AM, Der Kaloustian VM, McGill JJ, Saul RA: DNA fingerprinting: the utilization of minisatellite probes to detect a somatic mutation in the Proteus syndrome. In: DNA Fingerprinting: Ap-

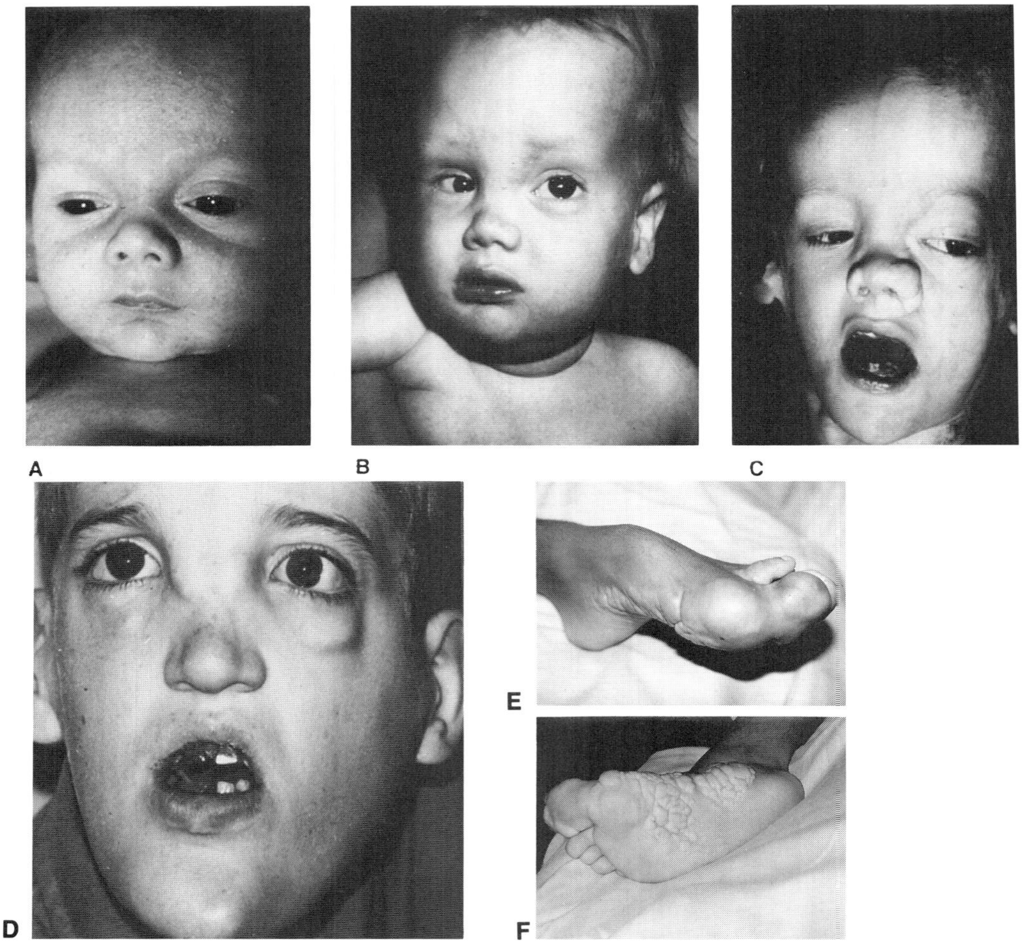


**Fig. 62.** Proteus syndrome. C: Patient at the age of 1 month, 5 months, and 5½ years. D: Another patient with hyperostoses of the nose, left infraorbital region, and mandible. E,F: Note abnormally enlarged toe and typical lesions of the sole. (A–C from JAR Tibbles, MM Cohen Jr, Br Med J 293:683, 1986; D from MM Cohen Jr, PW Hayden, Birth Defects 15:291, 1979, with permission.)

proaches and Applications, T Burke, G Dolf, AJ Jeffreys, R Wolff, eds. Springer-Verlag, New York, 1991, pp 95–105.
6. Smeets E, Fryns J-P, Cohen MM Jr: Regional Proteus syndrome and somatic mosaicism. Am J Med Genet 51:29–31, 1994.
7. Vaughn RY, Selinger AD, Howell CG, Parrish RA, Edgerton MT: Proteus syndrome: diagnosis and surgical management. J Pediatr Surg 28:5–10, 1993.
8. Viljoen DL, Nelson MM, de Jong G, Beighton P: Proteus syndrome in Southern Africa: natural history and clinical manifestations in six individuals. Am J Med Genet 27:87–97, 1987.

## Refsum disease

### Heredopathia atactica polyneuritiformis
(MIM No. *266500; POSSUM No. 3463)

This condition was described by Refsum in 1946.[7]

#### General manifestations

Progressive muscle wasting and loss of vision occur in the second decade of life. The ocular manifestations start gradually as night blindness with narrowing of the visual field. On fundus examination, there is a marked increase in retinal pigmentation with optic disk pallor and a narrowing of the retinal vessels. Miosis, hemeralopia, posterior cataracts, and nystagmus are also common. The gait is ataxic in early adulthood, muscle weakness affecting the legs first, then the arms. Skeletal changes are also described in most cases (75%), e.g., exostoses of the sternum, kyphoscoliosis, pes cavus, and spondylitis. Cardiovascular manifestations such as tachycardia, systolic murmur, and cardiac insufficiency and enlargement have been noted in 80% of reported patients. Ichthyosis of the skin may also be present. Dietary restriction of phytanic acid is recommended.[3,8,9]

#### Otolaryngological manifestations

Sensorineural hearing loss occurs and one ear is usually affected more than the other. In one series, 70% of the patients were affected. No abnormalities were detected in the vestibular system.[2] Anosmia has been also noted in some patients.

Studies of pathology of the ear have shown collapse of Reissner's membrane, degeneration of the stria vascularis, atrophy of the organ of Corti, and loss of spiral ganglion cells.[4]

#### Etiology

Refsum disease is an autosomal recessive condition. The syndrome results from an error in phytanic acid metabolism.[3,9] Due to phytanic acid oxidase deficiency, phytanic acid is not degraded to hydroxyphytanic acid.[8] Heterozygotes can be identified easily. Peroxisomes are not decreased in number.[1] Antenatal diagnosis is possible.[5] Refsum disease with increased pipecolic acidemia was localized to chromosome 10p by homozygosity mapping and carrier testing.[4a]

### Differential diagnosis

Refsum disease should be differentiated from Usher syndrome, Kearns-Sayre syndrome, and infantile Refsum disease.

## Infantile Refsum disease
(MIM No. *266510)

This disease is manifested by retinitis pigmentosa, sensorineural hearing loss, and phytanic acid oxidase deficiency. In contrast to adult or classic Refsum disease, it is characterized by microcephaly, severe developmental delay, hypotonia, hepatomegaly, and flat facies. The biochemical findings include elevated pipecolic acid, increased very long chain fatty acids in serum and cultured fibroblasts, and markedly decreased peroxisomal function.[6,10]

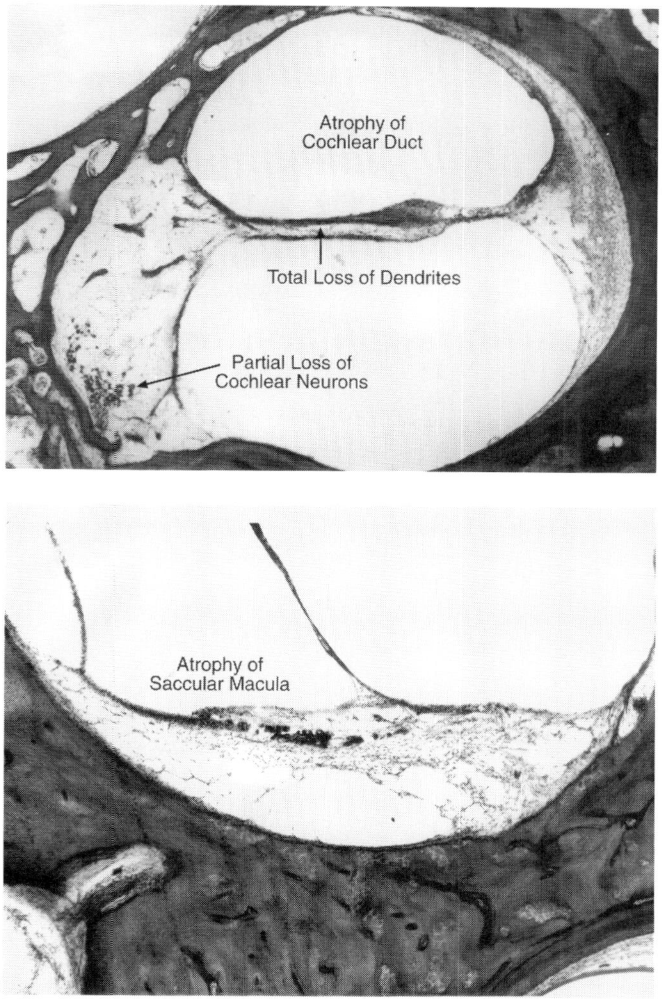


**Fig. 63.** Refsum disease. A: Histological section of temporal bone showing severe atrophy of the organ of Corti, tectorial membrane, and striae vasculares. A few hair cells remain. B: Temporal bone showing atrophy of the saccular macula. (From HF Schuknecht, *Pathology of the Ear*, 2nd ed., Lea & Febiger, Philadelphia, 1993, p. 136, with permission; courtesy of DG Davis and R Williams.)

### References

1. Beard ME, Sapirstein V, Kolodny EH, Holtzman E: Peroxisomes in fibroblasts from skin of Refsum's disease patients. J Histochem Cytochem 33:480–484, 1985.
2. Bergsmark J, Djupesland G: Heredopathia atactica polyneuritiformis (Refsum's disease). An audiological examination of two patients. Eur Neurol 1:122–130, 1968.
3. Djupesland G, Flottorp G, Refsum S: Phytanic acid storage disease: hearing maintained after 15 years of dietary treatment. Neurology 33:237–240, 1983.
4. Hallpike CS: Observations on the structural basis of two varieties of hereditary deafness. In: Myotatic, Kinesthetic and Vestibular Mechanisms, CIBA Foundation Symposium, AVS de Reuch, and J Knight, eds. Little, Brown, Boston, 1967, pp 285–294.

4a. Nadal N, Rolland MO, Tranchant C, Reutenauer L, Gyapay G, Warter JM, Mandel JL, Koenig M: Localization of Refsum disease with increased pipecolic acidaemia to chromosome 10p by homozygosity mapping and carrier testing in a single nuclear family. Hum Mol Genet 4:1963–1966, 1995.

5. Poll-Thé BT, Poulos A, Sharp P, Boué J, Ogier H, Odièvre M, Saudubray JM: Antenatal diagnosis of infantile Refsum's disease. Clin Genet 27:524–526, 1985.
6. Poulos A, Sharp P, Whiting M: Infantile Refsum's disease (phytanic acid storage disease). A variant of Zellweger's syndrome? Clin Genet 26:579–586, 1984.
7. Refsum S: Heredopathia atactica polyneuritiformis. Acta Psychiatr Neurol Scand 38:1–303, 1946.
8. Richterich R, Moser H, Rossi E: Refsum's disease (heredopathia atactica polyneuritiformis) Humangenetik 1:324–332, 1965.
9. Robertson EF, Poulos A, Sharp P, Manson J, Wise G, Jaunzems A, Carter R: Treatment of infantile phytanic acid storage disease: clinical, biochemical and ultrastructural findings in two children treated for 2 years. Eur J Pediatr 147:133–142, 1988.
10. Steinberg D: Refsum disease. In: The Metabolic and Molecular Bases of Inherited Diseases, 7th ed, CR Scriver, AL Beaudet, WS Sly, D Valle, eds. McGraw-Hill, New York, 1995, pp 2351–2369.

## Roberts syndrome

### Pseudothalidomide syndrome
(MIM No. *268300; POSSUM No. 3378)

Roberts[8] in 1919 described a syndrome with a bilateral cleft lip, imperfect development of the four extremities, and abnormal facies. Later it was established that Roberts syndrome and SC phocomelia syndrome are the same.[9,10]

### General manifestations

Birth weight is below normal with a tendency toward microcephaly. Skeletal defects involve all limbs. The long bones are shortened. Absence or severe hypoplasia of the radius, ulna, tibia, fibula and femur is commonly seen. The number of digits is less than normal, especially on the hands; the thumbs may be missing. Talipes, polydactyly, and syndactyly are observed. Humeroradial or humeroulnar synostosis and femorotibial fusion have been described. Wormian bones are frequent.

The cornea may be vascularized (Peters anomaly); there may also be cataracts leading to blindness if the patient survives. Urogenital anomalies are common and include an enlarged penis, hypospadias, and cryptorchidism in the male, and an enlarged clitoris and labia minora and vaginal septum in the female.[5,8,10] Polycystic and horseshoe kidneys occur. Mental retardation, hydrocephalus, encephaloceles, olfactory hypoplasia, and malignant melanoma are documented.[1,5,6] Cardiovascular anomalies and thrombocytopenia are occasional occurrences. Feeding difficulties and respiratory infections lead to failure to thrive and death in infancy.

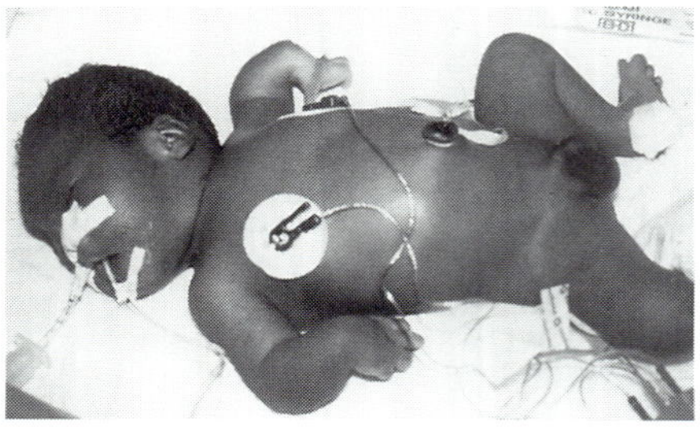

A

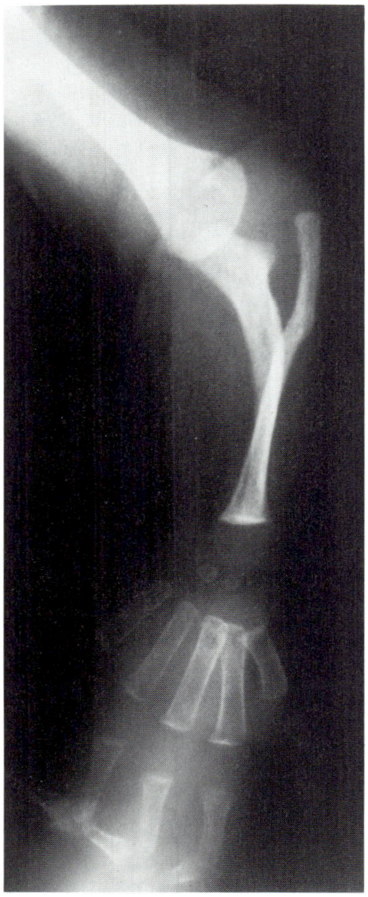

B

**Fig. 64.** Roberts syndrome. A: Note cleft lip; short, curved, abnormal left forearm, and elongated phallus. B: X-ray of the limb showing hypoplasia with bowing of ulna and radius and dislocation of radial head. From L Keppen et al., Am J Med Genet 38:21, 1991, with permission.)

### Otolaryngological manifestations

The facies includes severe midfacial clefts, agenesis of the nostrils, hypertelorism, and micrognathia. The ears are abnormal, lobeless, and posteriorly angulated. Bilateral cleft lip/palate is more common than an isolated cleft palate. Facial hemangiomas are also seen in patients who survive infancy.[3,7,10]

### Etiology

An autosomal recessive gene defect is quite certain. Chromosomal changes occur in 50% of cases. These involve the heterochromatic, C-banding regions of most chromosomes and appear as puffing around the centromeres and nuclear organizers. This leads to premature separation of chromatids during prophase and metaphase.[2,4,10]

### Differential diagnosis

Roberts syndrome should be differentiated from thalidomide embryopathy, trisomy 18, TAR (**T**hromocytopenia, **A**bsent **R**adius) syndrome, and VACTERL association.

#### References


1. Fryns J, Goddeeris P, Moerman F, Herman F, van den Berghe H: The tetraphocomelia-cleft palate syndrome in identical twins. Hum Genet 53:279–281, 1980.
2. German J: Roberts syndrome. I. Cytological evidence for a disturbance in chromosome pairing. Clin Genet 16:441–447, 1979.
3. Grosse FR, Pandel C, Wiedemann HR: The tetraphocomelia-cleft palate syndrome. Humangenetik 28:353–356, 1975.
4. Louie E, German J: Robert's syndrome. II. Aberrant Y-chromosome behavior. Clin Genet 19:71–74, 1981.
5. Mann NP, Fitzsimmons J, Fitzsimmons E, Cooke P: Roberts syndrome. Clinical and cytogenetic aspects. J Med Genet 19:116–119, 1982.
6. Parry DM, Mulvihill JJ, Tsai SE, Kaiser-Kupfer MI, Cowan JM: SC phocomelia syndrome, premature centromere separation, and congenital cranial nerve paralysis in two sisters, one with malignant melanoma. Am J Med Genet 24:653–672, 1986.
7. Pfeiffer RA, Zwerner H: Das Roberts-Syndrom. Bericht über eine Beobachtung (ohne Anomalie der Centromerregion). Monatsschr Kinderheilkd 130:296–298, 1982.
8. Roberts JB: A child with double cleft of lip and palate, protrusion of the intermaxillary portion of the upper jaw and imperfect development of the bones of the four extremities. Ann Surg 70:252, 1919.
9. Romke C, Froster-Iskenius U, Heyne K, Hohn W, Hof M, Grzejszczyk G, Rauskolb R, Rehder H, Schwinger E: Roberts syndrome and SC phocomelia: A single genetic entity. Clin Genet 31:170–177, 1987.
10. Zergollern L, Hitrec V: Four siblings with Roberts syndrome. Clin Genet 21 1–6, 1982.


## Robin sequence

(MIM Nos. 261800, 311900; POSSUM No. 3371)

The major diagnostic criteria for this condition are micrognathia, glossoptosis, and an inverted U–shaped cleft palate.

### General manifestations

Congenital heart defects are associated with Robin sequence in 14% of cases. Limb anomalies, ocular malformations, and rib and sternal abnormalities are described. Management of the newborn depends on the severity of the clinical diagnosis. The infant is kept in a prone position and respiration is monitored. Repair of the cleft palate is done at a later age.[5,8,10]

### Otolaryngological manifestations

Micrognathia, glossoptosis, and an inverted U–shaped palate are the main otolaryngological anomalies. Respiratory difficulty with periodic cyanotic attacks are associated with sternal retraction and are more apparent when the baby is in a supine position.

Radiologically, the mandibular ramus and body are smaller than normal and the mandibular angle is obtuse.

### Etiology and pathogenesis

Robin sequence is a very heterogeneous condition with birth prevalence of 1:8,500. The initial defect is thought to be hypoplasia of the mandible, occurring before 8 weeks of gestation. This would result in the posterior location of the tongue, thereby preventing closure of the posterior palatal shelves. The Robin sequence cleft is different from the usual, inverted V–shaped cleft, which is not formed by mandibular involvement. Oligohydramnios is thought to play a role in the pathogenesis. The reduced amount of amniotic fluid results in compression of the chin and impaction of the tongue between the palatal shelves. Other hypotheses include neurogenic hypotonia and connective tissue disorder.[2,3,7]

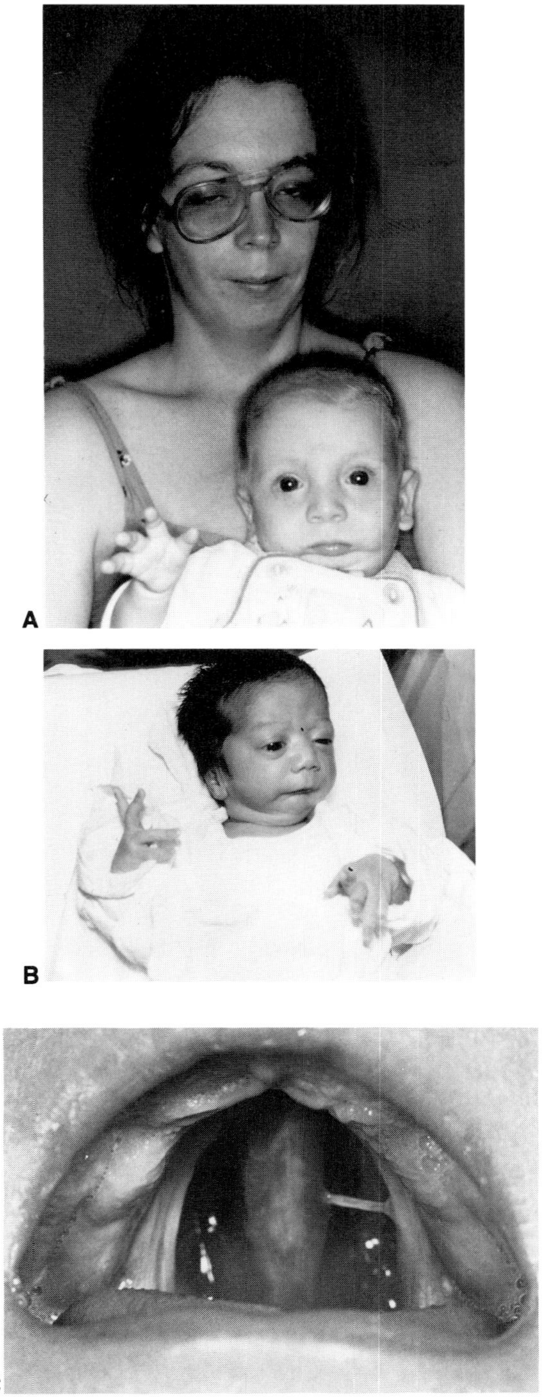

**Fig. 65.** Robin sequence. A: Child with mother. Note the small, receded mandible and oligodactyly. (From M Robinow, Am J Med Genet 25:293, 1986, with permission.) B: 5-month-old baby. Note severe micrognathia. C: Note characteristic inverted U–shaped cleft palate. (From RJ Gorlin et al., *Syndromes of the Head and Neck,* 3rd ed., Oxford University Press, New York, 1990, p. 703.)

### Differential diagnosis

Robin sequence may occur as an isolated anomaly, but may also be a feature of a malformation syndrome. Examples are diastrophic dysplasia, Nager acrofacial dysostosis, Otopalatodigital syndrome II, popliteal pterygium, Stickler, Shprintzen, del 6q, Möbius, and other syndromes, as well as CHARGE association.[1,3,4,6,9]

#### References


1. André M, Vigneron J, Didier F: Abnormal facies, cleft palate, and generalized dysostosis: a lethal X-linked syndrome. J Pediatr 98:747–752, 1981.
2. Bush PG, Williams AJ: Incidence of the Robin anomalad (Pierre Robin syndrome). Br J Plast Surg 36:434–437, 1983.
3. Carey JC, Fineman RN, Ziter FA: The Robin sequence as a consequence of malformation, dysplasia, and neuromuscular syndromes. J Pediatr 101:858–864, 1982.
4. Cohen MM Jr: The Robin anomalad—its specificity and associated syndromes. J Oral Surg 34:586–593, 1976.
5. Figueroa AA, Glupker TJ, Fitz MG, Begole EA: Mandible, tongue and airway in Pierre Robin sequence: a longitudinal cephalometric study. Cleft Palate Craniofac J 28:425–434, 1991.
6. Pagon RA, Graham JM Jr, Zonana J, Yong SL: Coloboma, congenital heart disease and choanal atresia with multiple anomalies: CHARGE association. J Pediatr 99:223–227, 1981.
7. Poswillo D: The etiology and surgery of cleft palate with micrognathia. Ann R Coll Surg Engl 43:61–88, 1968.
8. Robinow M, Johnson GF, Apesos J: Robin sequence and oligodactyly in mother and son. Am J Med Genet 25:293–297, 1986.
9. Shprintzen RJ: Pierre Robin micrognathia and airway obstruction: The dependency of treatment on accurate diagnosis. Int Anesthesiol Clin 26:64–71, 1988.
10. Smith JL, Stowe FR: The Pierre Robin syndrome (glossoptosis, micrognathia, cleft palate): a review of 39 cases with emphasis on associated ocular lesions. Pediatrics 27:128–133, 1961.


## Robinow syndrome

#### Fetal face syndrome
(MIM No. *180700; POSSUM No. 3379)

### General manifestations

Most patients with this syndrome have three or more of the following: a fetal face, genital hypoplasia, limb shortness, and moderate dwarfism. Mesomelic shortness of the lower limbs is less marked. A micropenis and cryptorchidism are present in 65% of patients or more. During puberty the glans penis attains normal size but the shaft remains small. The clitoris and labia minora are hypoplastic in female patients.

Vertebral anomalies (65%), scoliosis, and abnormal ribs are seen (35%–50%). Hand and finger anomalies occur in 85% of cases. Radial head dislocation is common in the recessive form. The umbilicus is higher than usual.[2,3,5] Intelligence is usually normal; however, mental and developmental retardation occurs in 20% of patients. Ambiguous genitalia, persistent Müllerian ducts and partial deficiency of androgen receptors

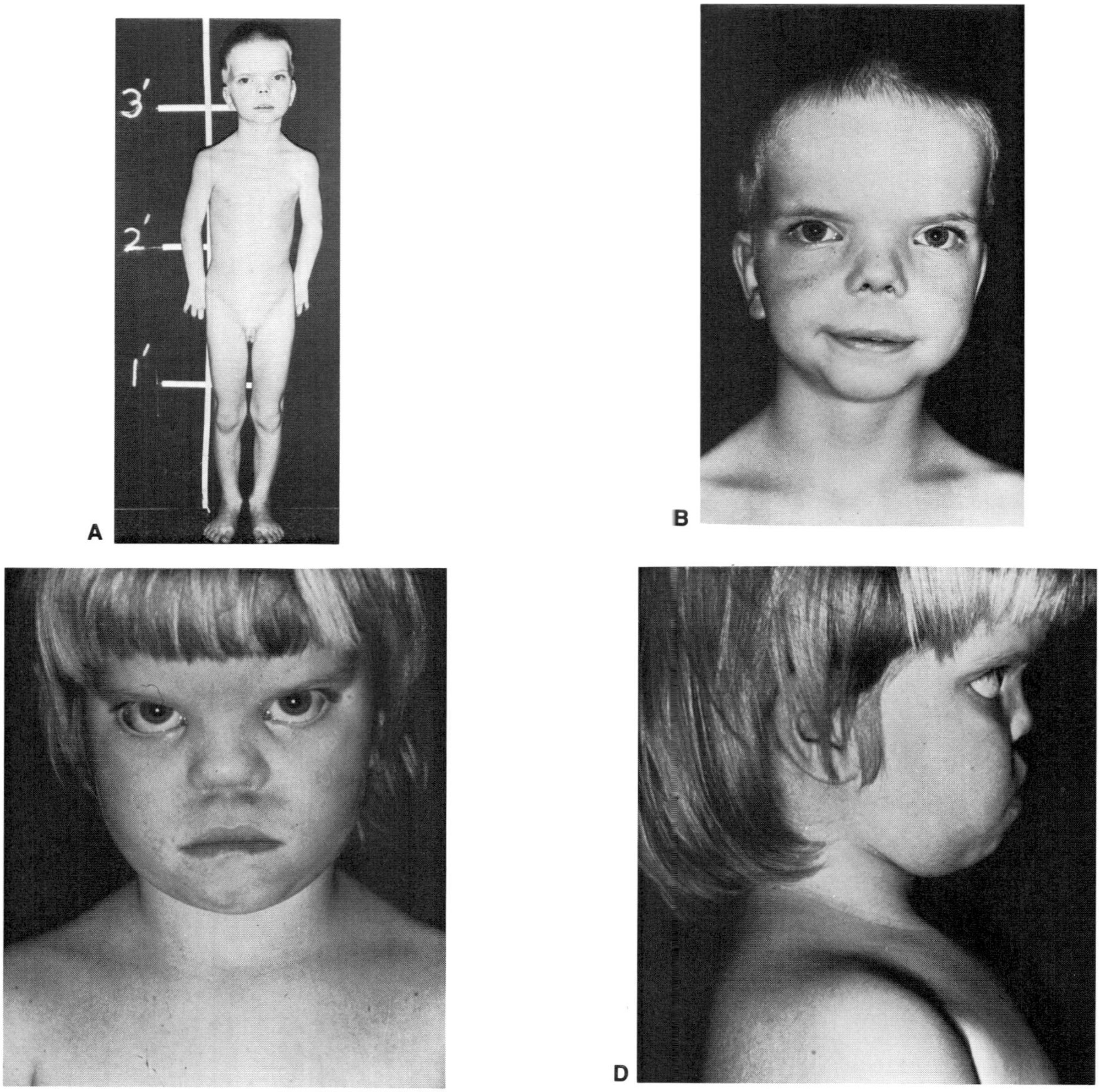

**Fig. 66.** Robinow syndrome. Note mesomelic shortening of extremities and micropenis (A), fetal proportions of the face (B), and characteristic ocular hypertelorism and midfacial hypoplasia (C). (From RJ Gorlin et al., *Syndromes of the Head and Neck,* 3rd ed., Oxford University Press, 1990, p. 797; courtesy of Dr. M Robinow.)

have been documented. Occasional anomalies include seizures, pilonidal dimple, pectus excavatum, nevus flammeus, and ventricular septal defects.[6,7,10,11]

## Otolaryngological manifestations

The facies are similar to those of a fetus of 8–10 weeks. The skull is disproportionately large, the face is relatively small, with a bulging forehead, hypertelorism and wide palpebral fissures. The nose is upturned and short, with anteverted nostrils. The philtrum is long. The mouth is triangular with down-turned angles and a small upper lip shaped like an inverted V. The alveolar ridges are hyperplastic. Cleft lip/palate and short uvula are noted in 10%–20% of cases.

The ears have folded-over helices. The facial characteristics become less striking at puberty.[1,2,4,5]

## Etiology

Robinow syndrome is of autosomal dominant inheritance; autosomal recessive forms also exist.[1,8,9]

## Differential diagnosis

Robinow syndrome should be differentiated from Aarskog syndrome, achondroplasia, and pseudohyoparathyroidism.

## References


1. Butter MG, Wadlington WB: Robinow syndrome: report of two patients and review of the literature. Clin Genet 31:77–85, 1987.
2. Israel H, Johnson G: Craniofacial pattern similarities, additional orofacial findings in siblings with Robinow syndrome. J Craniofac Genet Dev Biol 8:63–73, 1988.

3. Kelly TE, Benson R, Temtamy S, Plotnick L, Levin S: The Robinow syndrome: an isolated case with a detailed study of the phenotype. Am J Dis Child 129:383–386, 1975.
4. Khayat D, Szpirglas H, Lemonnier MP, Laufer J, Schaison G: Syndrome de Robinow. Rev Stomatol 84:222–224, 1983.
5. Pfeiffer RA, Müller H: Ein komplex multipler Missbildungen bei zwei nicht verwandten Kindern. Pädiatr Padol 6:262–267, 1971.
6. Schonau E, Pfeiffer RA, Schweikert HU, Bowing B, Schott G: Robinow or "fetal face syndrome" in a male infant with ambiguous genitalia and androgen receptor deficiency. Eur J Pediatr 149:615–617, 1990.
7. Shprintzen RJ, Goldberg RB, Saenger P, Disoti EJ: Male-male transmission of Robinow's syndrome. Its occurrence in association to cleft lip and palate. Am J Dis Child 136:594–597, 1982.
8. Teebi AS: Autosomal recessive Robinow syndrome. Am J Med Genet 35:64–68, 1990.
9. Vallée L, Van Nerom P, Ferraz F, Delecour M, Maroteaux P, Farriaux JP, Fontaine G: Syndrome de Robinow à transmission dominante. Arch Fr Pediatr 39:447–448, 1982.
10. Wadlington WB, Tucker VL, Schimke RN: Mesomelic dwarfism with hemivertebrae and small genitalia (The Robinow syndrome). Am J Dis Child 126:202–205, 1973.
11. Webber SA, Wargowski DS, Chitayat D, Sandor GG: Congenital heart disease and Robinow syndrome: coincidence or an additional component of the syndrome? Am J Med Genet 37:519–521, 1990.

## Rubinstein-Taybi syndrome

(MIM No. *180849; POSSUM No. 3384)

This is a rare multiple congenital anomaly syndrome that comprises mental and growth retardation, broad big toes and thumbs, and microcephaly with an unusual face.

### General manifestations

Head circumference, length, and weight are within normal range at birth. With advancing age, microcephaly and short stature become evident. It is estimated that 1:300–500 persons institutionalized for mental retardation over age 5 suffer from this syndrome. IQ ranges between 17 and 86, with an average of 51 and no behavioral problems. Broad thumbs and great toes are reported in over 95% of cases. Clinodactyly of the fifth finger and overlapping toes are present in over half of the cases. The gait is unsteady and stiff. Seizures and EEG abnormalities are reported in 60% of patients.

Vertebral anomalies, cryptorchidism (80%), ventricular septal defect, hypoplastic kidneys, and duplicated ureters are also reported.[3,9,13]

Excess keloid formation and neoplasms have been documented. Leukemia, intraspinal neurilemmoma, meningioma, and nasopharyngeal rhabdomyosarcoma are documented.[10,11]

### Otolaryngological manifestations

The facies is characterized by a prominent forehead, downward slanting palpebral fissures, epicanthal folds, and ptosis. The maxilla is hypoplastic with a narrow palate (100%). The nose is beaked and the septum extends below the alae nasi. The columella is short and broad (70%). The ears are posteriorly angulated, low set, and have thick helices (84%). Hearing loss and recurrent otitis media are also reported.[1,3,7] Occasional findings include submucous cleft palate, bifid uvula, bifid tongue, macroglossia, tongue-tie, a thin upper lip, and laryngomalacia.[5,12]

### Etiology

Causation of this syndrome is unknown. Some families show an apparent autosomal dominant inheritance. The recurrence rate is 1%. Parental consanguinity was noted in more than one instance. The incidence is 1:300,000 to 1:720,000. It is associated with submicroscopic interstitial deletions within 16p13.3 in approximately 25% of cases.[2,4,7] It has been proposed that the loss of one functional copy of the *CBP* (human CREB binding protein) gene underlies the developmental abnormalities in the Rubinstein-Taybi syndrome and possibly the propensity for malignancy.[8]

### Differential diagnosis

Rubinstein-Taybi syndrome should be differentiated from Saethre-Chotzen, Apert, Pfeiffer, and Cornelia-de-Lange syndromes.[6]

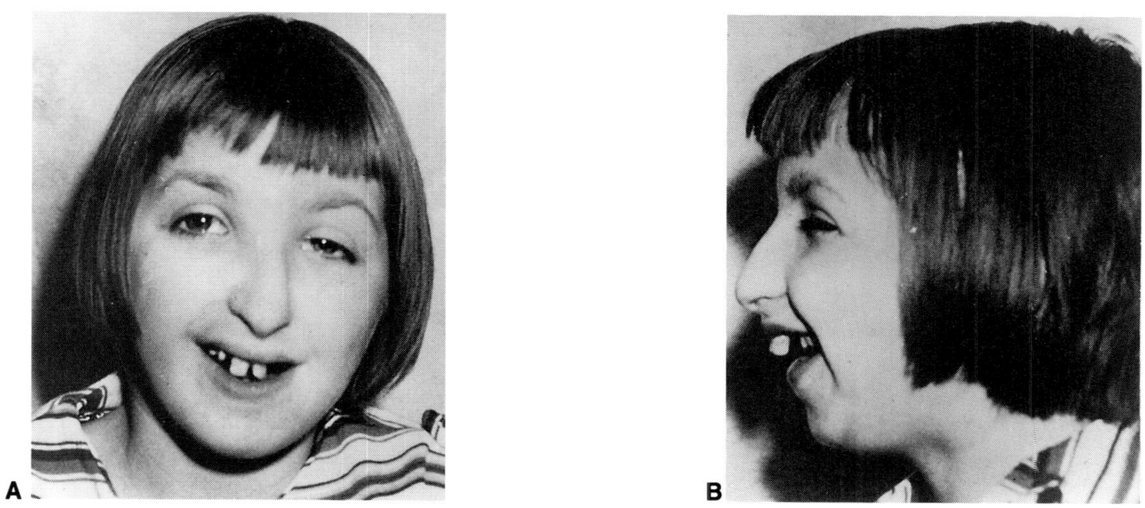

**Fig. 67.** Rubinstein-Taybi syndrome. A,B: Typical facies with antimongoloid slant of the eyes, beaked nose and micrognathia. (From JH Rubinstein, in *The Clinical Delineation of Birth Defects,* D Bergsma, ed., vol. V, no. 2, pt. II, Williams & Wilkins, 1969, p. 25, with permission.)

### References

1. Allanson JE: Rubinstein-Taybi syndrome: the changing face. Am J Med Genet 6:38–41, 1990.
2. Breuning MH, Dauwerse HG, Fugazza G, Saris JJ, Spruit L, Wijnen H, Tommerup N, van der Hagen CG, Imaizumi K, Kuroki Y, et al: Rubinstein-Taybi syndrome caused by submicroscopic deletions with 16p13.3. Am J Hum Genet 52:249–254, 1993.
3. Filippi G: The Rubinstein-Taybi syndrome. Report of 7 cases. Clin Genet 3:303–319, 1972.
4. Hennekam RCM, Lommen EJP, Strengers JLM, Van Spijker HG, Jansen Kokx TMG. Rubinstein-Taybi syndrome in a mother and son. Eur J Pediatr 148:439–441, 1989.
5. Kinirons MJ: Oral aspects of Rubinstein-Taybi syndrome. Br Dent J 154:46–47, 1983.
6. Lowry RB: Overlap between Rubinstein-Taybi and Saethre-Chotzen syndromes: a case report. Am J Med Genet 6:73–76, 1990.
7. Padfield CJ, Partington MW, Simpson NE: The Rubinstein-Taybi syndrome. Arch Dis Child 43:94–101, 1968.
8. Petrij F, Giles RH, Dauwerse HB, Saris JJ, Hennekam RCM, Masuno M, Tommerup N, van Ommen G-JB, Goodman RH, Peters DJM et al: Rubinstein-Taybi syndrome caused by mutations in the transcriptional co-activator CBP. Nature 376:348–351, 1995.
9. Robson MJ, Brown LM, Sharrad WJ: Cervical spondylolisthesis and other skeletal abnormalities in Rubinstein-Taybi syndrome. J Bone Joint Surg 62:297–299, 1980.
10. Siraganian PA, Rubinstein JH, Miller RW: Keloids and neoplasms in the Rubinstein-Taybi syndrome. Med Pediatr Oncol 17:485–491, 1989.
11. Sobel RA, Woerner S: Rubinstein-Taybi syndrome and nasopharyngeal rhabdomyosarcoma. J Pediatr 99:1000–1001, 1981.
12. Stevens CA, Corey JC, Blackburn BL: Rubinstein-Taybi syndrome: a natural history study. Am J Med Genet 6:30–37, 1990.
13. Taybi H, Rubinstein JH: Broad thumbs and toes, and unusual facial features: a probable mental retardation syndrome. Am J Roentgenol 93:362–366, 1965.

## Russell-Silver syndrome

### Silver syndrome
(MIM No. *180860, 312780; POSSUM No. 3385)

Russell[9] and Silver[11] described this syndrome independent of each other. It is characterized by short stature of prenatal onset, lateral asymmetry, and a small fifth finger curved inward.

#### General manifestations

The average birth weight is 2200 gm and the placenta is small. The body displays asymmetry in 65% to 80% of cases.[1] The asymmetry may only involve the skull, spine, and part of a limb.

Limb abnormalities include clinodactyly of the fifth finger (75%), soft tissue syndactyly between the second and the third toes, and disproportionate toes. Single transverse palmar creases are not uncommon.

Various urogenital anomalies can occur. Delayed sexual development has been reported in 36% of cases.[10]

Ambiguous genitalia and renal and ureteral malformations have also been reported.[6,12] Mild mental retardation is described in 35% of cases. Testicular tumors as well as craniopharyngioma may occur.[3,15] Café-au-lait spots occur in about 25% of cases.[5] These may vary in size and are usually well circumscribed and not raised. Hepatocellular carcinoma has been described in one patient.[2]

#### Otolaryngological manifestations

The face is small and triangular, with corners of the mouth turned down (shark-mouth) while the upper lip appears thin. The forehead is somewhat prominent and there is delayed closure of the anterior fontanelle.[5] The head is relatively large, with its craniofacial disproportion referred to as *pseudohydro-cephaly*. The palate is high and narrow and the ears are prominent.[14]

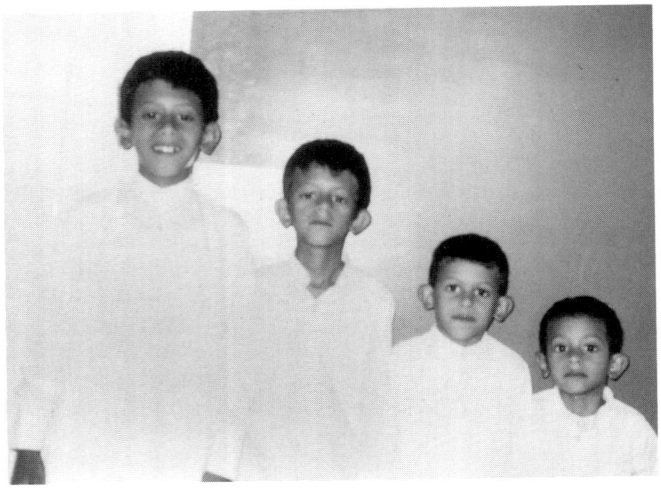

**Fig. 68.** Russell-Silver syndrome. Four brothers with triangular facies, prominent ears, and relatively large crania.

#### Etiology

Most cases are sporadic. However, several autosomal-dominant[4] and autosomal-recessive[14] pedigrees have been published. The possibility of an X-linked form was raised by Partington.[7a] A patient with Russell-Silver syndrome had a ring chromosome 15 involving deletion of the insulin-like growth factor receptor gene.[13] Two other cases have been reported with chromosomal anomalies involving 17q25.[7,8]

#### Differential diagnosis

Russell-Silver syndrome should be differentiated from disorders with intrauterine growth retardation as well as syndromes manifesting proportionate short stature, such as the 3-M syndrome and Dubowitz syndrome.

### References

1. Anoussakis C, Karpathios T, Zervos N, Liakakos D: Les nanismes congénitaux avec dysmorphie. 1. Le nanisme congénital avec dysmorphie cranio-faciale et asymétrie corporelle (type Silver-Russell). Pediatrie 29:249–259, 1974.
2. Chitayat D, Friedman JM, Anderson L, Dimmick JE: Hepatocellular carcinoma in a child with familial Russell-Silver syndrome. Am J Med Genet 31:909–914, 1988.
3. Draznin MB, Stelling MW, Johanson AJ: Russell-Silver syndrome and craniopharyngioma. J Pediatr 96:887–889, 1980.
4. Duncan PA, Hall JG, Shapiro LR, Vibert BK: Three generation dominant transmission of Silver-Russell syndrome. Am J Med Genet 35:245–250, 1990.
5. Escobar V, Gleiser S, Weaver DD: Phenotypic and genetic analysis of the Silver-Russell syndrome. Clin Genet 13:278–288, 1978.
6. Haslam RH, Berman W, Heller RM: Renal abnormalities in the Russell-Silver syndrome. Pediatrics 51:216–222, 1973.
7. Midro AT, Debek K, Sawicka A, Marcinkiewicz D, Rogowska M: Second observation of Silver-Russel syndrome in a carrier of a reciprocal translocation with one breakpoint at site 17q25 [Letter] Clin Genet 44:53–55, 1993.

7a. Partington MW: X-linked short stature with skin pigmentation: evidence for heterogeneity of the Russell-Silver syndrome. Clin Genet 29:151–156, 1986.
8. Ramirez-Duenas ML, Medina C, Ocampo-Campos R, Rivera H: Severe Silver-Russell syndrome and translocation (17;20)(q25;q13). Clin Genet 41:51–53, 1992.
9. Russell A: A syndrome of "intrauterine" dwarfism recognizable at birth with craniofacial dysostosis, disproportionately short arms and other anomalies. Proc R Soc Med 47:1040–1044, 1954.
10. Silver HK: Asymmetry, short stature and variations in sexual development. A syndrome of congenital malformations. Am J Dis Child 107:495–515, 1964.
11. Silver HK, Kiyasu W, George J, Deamer WC: Syndrome of congenital hemihypertrophy, shortness of stature and elevated urinary gonadotrophins. Pediatrics 12:368–376, 1953.
12. Spirer Z, Soferman R, Bogair N: Renal abnormalities in the Russell-Silver syndrome. Pediatrics 54:120, 1974.
13. Tamura T, Tohma T, Ohta T, Soejima H, Harada N, Abe K, Niikawa N: Ring chromosome 15 involving deletion of the insulin growth factor/receptor gene in a patient with features of Silver-Russell syndrome. Clin Dysmorphol 2:106–113, 1993.
14. Teebi AS: Autosomal recessive Silver-Russell syndrome. Clin Dysmorphol 1:151–156, 1992.
15. Weiss GR, Garnick MB: Testicular cancer in a Russell-Silver dwarf. J Urol 126:836–837, 1981.


## Saethre-Chotzen syndrome

### Acrocephalosyndactyly type III
### (MIM No. *101400; POSSUM No. 3009)

This syndrome was first described by Saethre in 1931[10] and later by Chotzen in 1932.[3]

#### General manifestations

Low anterior hairline and ptosis are common. Syndactyly (between the second and third fingers) is a consistent finding. The most common trait is craniosynostosis, which is usually variable and often involves the coronal sutures. Clinodactyly of the fifth finger and hypoplasia of the distal phalanges are sometimes found. Single palmar creases were noted in over 50% of patients.[2,9]

Most of the individuals who have this syndrome have normal intelligence. In some instances, mild to moderate mental retardation may be found. Occasional findings include epilepsy, schizophrenia,[2,10] synostosis of the radio ulnar joints,[9] cryptorchidism, and renal and cardiovascular defects.[1,2]

Short stature, cervical and lumbar vertebral abnormalities, and short clavicles have also been reported.[7] Muliple malignancies are described in one family.[8]

#### Otolaryngological manifestations

The nose is parrot beaked, the nasal septum is commonly deviated, the maxilla is often hypoplastic, and the palate is high arched. Anomalies of the teeth, such as peg-shaped and supernumerary teeth, may be present. Anomalies of the ears, such as posterior angulation, prominent crus, or low-set pinnae, are common. About 15% of patients have congenital hearing loss.[4,9] Mixed hearing loss has been reported by Dolivo and Gillieron.[6]

#### Etiology

This syndrome is of autosomal dominant inheritance with a high degree of variability in expressivity and penetrance. There is cytogenetic evidence that the Saethre-Chotzen gene maps to 7p21.2.[5] However, there may be genetic heterogeneity, with a locus outside the candidate regions on 7p.[11]

#### Differential diagnosis

Saethre-Chotzen syndrome should be differentiated from Apert, Pfeiffer, and Crouzon syndromes. It should also be ruled out in cases of isolated craniosynostosis.

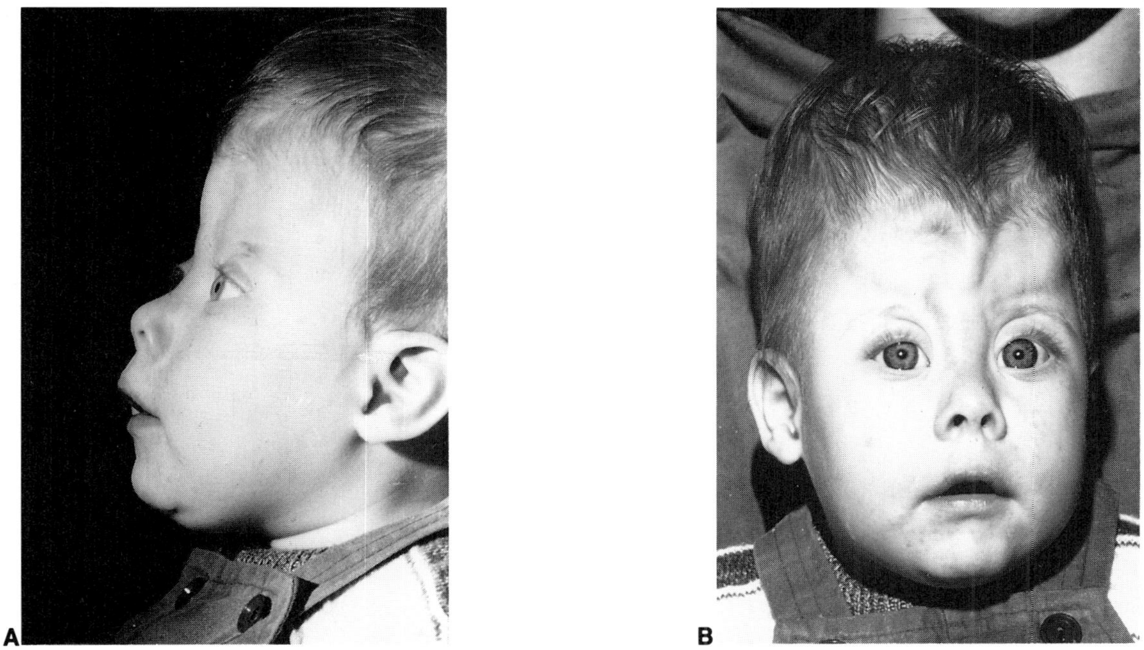


**Fig. 69.** Saethre-Chotzen syndrome. A,B: Note acrocephaly, facial asymmetry, and low hairline. (From S. Niemann-Seyde et al., Clin Genet 40:271, 1991, with permission.)

#### References

1. Aase JM, Smith DW: Facial asymmetry and abnormalities of palms and ears: a dominantly inherited developmental syndrome. J Pediatr 76:928–930, 1970.
2. Bartsocas CS, Weber Al, Crawford JD: Acrocephalosyndactyly type 3: Chotzen's syndrome. J Pediatr 77:267–272, 1970.
3. Chotzen F: Fine eigenartige familiäre Entwicklungsstörung. (Akrocephalosyndaktylie, synostosis craniofacialis und Hyperextalorismus), Monatsschr Kinderheilkd 55:97–122, 1932.
4. Cohen MM Jr: Craniosynostosis and syndromes with craniosynostosis: incidence, genetics, penetrance, variability and new syndrome updating. Birth Defects 15:85–89, 1979.
5. Cohen MM Jr: Craniosynostoses: phenotypic/molecular correlations. Am J Med Genet 56:334–339, 1995.
6. Dolivo G, Gillieron JD: Une famille de "Crouzon-fruste" ou "pseudo-Crouzon". J Genet Hum 4:88–101, 1955.
7. Friedman JM, Hanson JW, Graham CB, Smith DW: Saethre-Chotzen syndrome: a broad and variable pattern of skeletal malformations. J Pediatr 91:929–933, 1977.
8. McKeen EA, Mulvihill JJ, Levine PH, Dean JH, Howley PM: The concurrence of Saethre-Chotzen syndrome and malignancy in a family with in vitro immune dysfunction. Cancer 54: 2946–2951, 1984.
9. Pantke OA, Cohen MM Jr, Witcop CJ Jr, Feingold M, Schaumann B, Pantke HC, Gorlin RJ: The Saethre-Chotzen syndrome. Birth Defects 11:190–225, 1975.
10. Saethre H: Ein Beitrag zum Turmschadälproblem. (Pathogenese, Erblichkeit und Symptomologie). Dtsch Z Nervenheilkd 117:533–555, 1931.
11. von Gernet S, Schuffenhauer S, Golla A, Lichtner P. Balg S, Mühlbauer W, Murken J, Fairley J, Meitinger T: Craniosynostosis suggestive of Saethre-Chotzen syndrome: clinical description of a large kindred and exclusion of candidate regions on 7p. Am J Med Genet 63:177–184, 1996.

## Schinzel-Giedion syndrome

(MIM No. 269150; POSSUM No. 3025)

### General manifestations

The forehead is prominent with large fontanels and wide cranial sutures.

Skeletal defects include wide occipital synchondrosis, hypoplastic distal phalanges, moderate shortening of forearms and legs, hypoplastic first ribs, broad ribs, and hypoplasia of the pubic bone.[2]

Congenital hydronephrosis, hydroureter, and a short penis with hypospadias and cryptorchidism or deep interlabial sulcus have been reported. Congenital cardiac defects, hypoplastic nipples, hypoplastic dermal ridges, brain anomalies, embryonal tumors, and facial telangiectases are not rare.[1–5] Growth retardation, failure to thrive, and profound mental deficiency accompanied by seizures and spasticity have been documented. Early death is common.

### Otolaryngological manifestations

Midface hypoplasia, a short nose with a high nasal bridge, choanal stenosis, macroglossia, low-set ears, hearing loss, and a broad neck with abundant skin folds are all characteristics of this syndrome.

### Etiology

Schinzel-Giedion syndrome is of autosomal recessive inheritance. Autosomal dominant inheritance with parental gonadal mosaicism cannot be excluded.[3]

#### References

1. Al-Gazali LI, Farndon P, Burn J, Flannery DB, Davison C, Mueller RF: The Schinzel-Giedion syndrome: clinical features and natural history. J Med Genet 27:42–47, 1990.
2. Kelley RI, Zackai EH, Charney EB: Congenital hydronephrosis, skeletal dysplasia and severe developmental retardation: the Schinzel-Giedion syndrome. J Pediatr 100:943–946, 1982.
3. Labrune P, Lyonnet S, Zupan V, Imbert MC, Gautieres F, Hubert P, Le Merrer M: Three new cases of the Schinzel-Giedion syndrome and review of the literature. Am J Med Genet 50:90–93, 1994.
4. Rodriguez JI, Jimenez-Hefferman JA, Leal J: Schinzel-Giedion syndrome: autopsy report and additional clinical findings. Am J Med Genet 53:374–377, 1994.

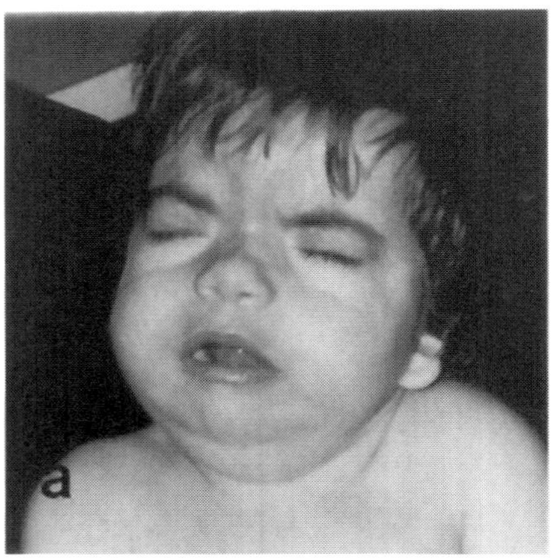


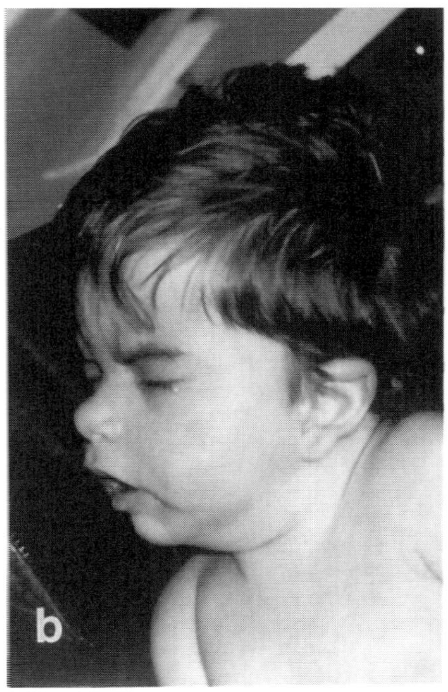


**Fig. 70.** Schinzel-Giedion syndrome. a,b: Note the midfacial hypoplasia, short nose, and low-set ears. (From NH Robin, Am J Med Genet 47:852, 1993, with permission.)

5. Schinzel A, Giedion A: A syndrome of severe midface retraction, multiple skull anomalies, club feet, and cardiac and renal malformations in sibs. Am J Med Genet 1:361–375, 1978.

## Schwartz-Jampel syndrome

### Chondrodystrophic myotonia
(MIM No. *255800; POSSUM No. 3403)

#### General manifestations

Continuous muscle contracture at rest, short stature, pectus carinatum, kyphoscoliosis, and lumbar lordosis all characterize this syndrome. Joint contractures result in an inability to ambulate.

Ocular abnormalities include ptosis, microcornea, blepharophimosis, severe myopia, juvenile cataract, microphthalmos, and impaired vision.

Umbilical and inguinal herniae, abnormally small testes, a patent anal sphincter, and bilateral carpal tunnel are occasionally reported.

Psychological abnormalities develop after prolonged and repeated hospitalization.[1,4] Mental retardation has been observed in 25% of cases. Malignant hyperpyrexia is also documented.[6,10]

#### Otolaryngological manifestations

Symptoms appear during the second year of life and are progressive in nature. The face is relatively flat with a fixed facial expression. Progressive contraction of the facial muscles results in puckered lips and contraction of the orbicularis oris. The palate is high arched and the pinnae are unusual. The voice is high pitched and the neck is short. Dysphagia and choking on cold liquids has been observed.[1,3,4]

#### Etiology and pathogenesis

This syndrome is of autosomal recessive inheritance. Dominant inheritance has been also suggested.[10] Based on findings from muscle and bone biopsies, electromyography (EMG) and other studies, several hypotheses on the pathogenesis of Schwartz-Jampel syndrome have been suggested.[2,3,5,7–9] The Schwartz-Jampel syndrome (SJS) locus has been mapped to chromosome 1p34–p36.1 by homozygosity mapping.[1a,2a]

#### Differential diagnosis

Marden-Walker syndrome has similar facies but presents at birth.

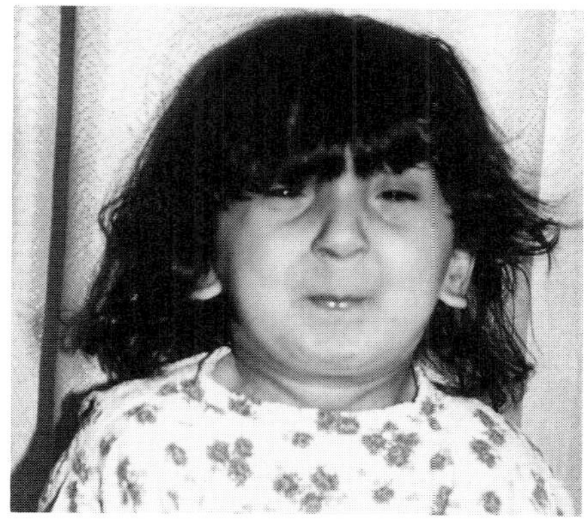

**Fig. 71.** Schwartz-Jampel syndrome. Note the contracted facial muscles and puckered lips.

#### References

1. Edwards WC, Root AW: Chondrodystrophic myotonia (Schwartz-Jampel syndrome). Am J Med Genet 13:51–56, 1982.
1a. Fontaine B, Nicole S, Topaloglu H, Ben Hamida C, Beighton P, Spaans F, Cantù JMA, Bakouri S, Romero N, Ricker K et al.: Recessive Schwartz-Jampel syndrome (SJS): confirmation of linkage to chromosome lp, evidence of genetic homogeneity and reduction of the SJS locus to a 3-cM interval. Hum Genet 98:380–385, 1996.
2. Fowler WM Jr, Layzer RB, Taylor RG, Eberle ED, Sims GE, Munsat TL, Philippart M, Wilson BW: The Schwartz-Jampel syndrome. Its clinical, physiological and histological expressions. J Neuro Sci 22:127–146, 1974.
2a. Nicole S, Ben Hamida C, Beighton P, Bakouri S, Belal S, Romero N, Viljoen D, Ponsot G, Sammoud A, Weissenbach J et al.: Localization of the Schwartz-Jampel syndrome (SJS) locus to chromosome lp34–p36.1 by homozygosity mapping. Hum Mol Genet 4:1633–1636, 1995.
3. Parone L, Mollica F, Grasso A, Cao A, Gullota F: Schwartz-Jampel syndrome in two daughters of first cousins. J Neurol Neurosurg Psychiatr 41:161–169, 1978.
4. Saadat M, Mokfi H, Vakil H, Ziai M: Schwartz syndrome: myotonia with blepharophimosis and limitation of joints. J Pediatr 81:348–350, 1972.
5. Scribanu N, Ionanescu V: Schwartz-Jampel syndrome: a case report. Stimulating effect of calcium and A23187 calcium ionophore for protein synthesis in muscle cell cultures. Eur Neurol 20:46–51, 1981.
6. Seay AR, Ziter FA: Malignant hyperpyrexia in a patient with Schwartz-Jampel syndrome. J Pediatr 93:83–84, 1983.
7. Spaans F: Schwartz-Jampel syndrome with dominant inheritance. Muscle Nerve 14:1142–1144, 1991.
8. Spaans, F, Theunissen P, Reekers AD, Smit L, Veldman H: Schwartz-Jampel syndrome I. Clinical, electromyographic and histologic studies. Muscle Nerve 13:516–527, 1990.
9. Taylor RG, Layzer RB, Davis HS, Fowler WM Jr: Continuous muscle fiber activity in the Schwartz syndrome. Electroencephalogr Clin Neurophysiol 33:497–509, 1972.
10. Viljoen D, Beighton P: Schwartz-Jampel syndrome (chondrodystrophic myotonia). J Med Genet 29:58–62, 1992.

## Shprintzen syndrome

### Velo-cardio-facial syndrome
(MIM No. #192430; POSSUM No. 3132)

Shprintzen et al.[9] described the syndrome in 1978. Previous reports describing patients with similar features can be found in the literature.[7]

#### General manifestations

Ocular findings include retinal vascular tortuosity, posterior embryotoxon, narrow palbebral fissures, suborbital discoloration, small optic nerves, iris nodules, and cataracts.[5]

Cardiothoracic anomalies include pulmonary atresia, ventricular septal defects, and hypoplastic pulmonary arteries. Severe abnormalities of the arborization of the pulmonary arterial tree were reported by Jedele et al.[2] Fallot tetralogy, aberrant subclavian arteries, and right-sided aortic arch are common. The fingers are tapered and slender in most cases. Most children experience learning disability and difficulty with abstraction and reading comprehension.[3a] Verbal IQ score ranged between 69 and 87 in one study. Other less common traits include herniae (inguinal or umbilical), hypocalcemia, and an absent thymus.[1,2,10,12]

### Otolaryngological manifestations

The nose is prominent and tubular, the alae nasi and nasal cavities are hypoplastic. The mandible is retrognathic and the vertical diameter of the maxilla is increased. The upper lip and the philtrum are elongated. Over 80% of cases have adenoid hypoplasia, which contributes to nasal speech. Velopharyngeal insufficiency and hypernasal speech are the main presenting symptoms. Approximately 15% of patients have a Robin sequence and 35% have a cleft palate. Obstructive sleep apnea is common. Some authors classify the facial features as humerous or nervous, based on the pursed lips versus the upward slanting palbebral fissures. Conductive hearing loss is more frequent than sensorineural hearing loss. The pinnae are usually small.[3,4,8,11]

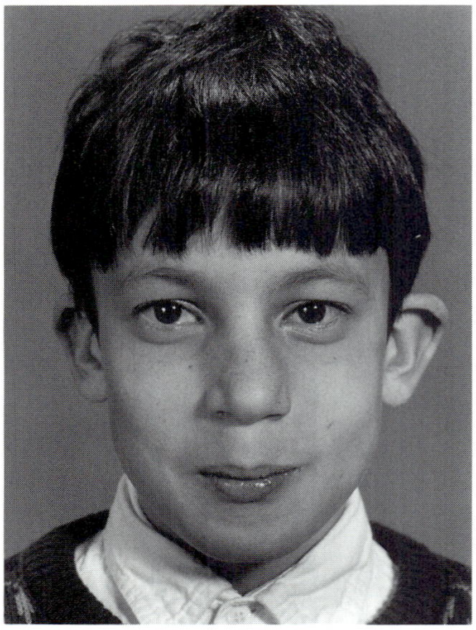

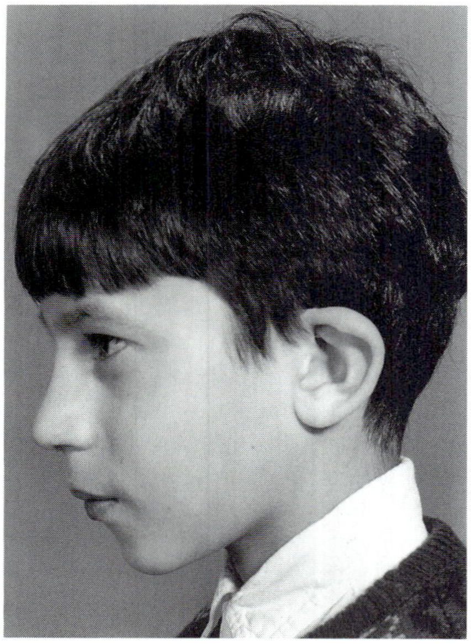

**Fig. 72.** Shprintzen syndrome. A,B: Patient with prominent tubular nose, long philtrum, and small and cupped pinnae.

### Etiology

This syndrome is of autosomal dominant inheritance. Scambler et al.[6] suggested an etiological connection between velo-cardio-facial syndrome and DiGeorge syndrome and hypothesize that both represent part of a spectrum seen with monosomy for 22q11. Precise definition of molecular aspects is available.[5a]

### Differential diagnosis

Shprintzen syndrome should be differentiated from disorders with velopharyngeal insufficiency and the nonsyndromic entity of velopharyngeal incompetence (MIM No. 167500).

### References


1. Colding-Kushner KJ, Weller G, Shprintzen RJ: Velo-cardio-facial syndrome: Language and psychological profiles. J Craniofac Genet Dev Biol 5:259–264, 1985.
2. Jedele KB, Michels VV, Puga FJ, Feldt RH: Velo-cardio-facial syndrome associated with ventricular septal defects, pulmonary atresia and hypoplastic pulmonary arteries. Pediatrics 89:915–919, 1992.
3. Kimura A: Congenital velopharyngeal insufficiency without cleft palate, involving typical facies. Presented at Proc Congr Int Assoc Logopediatr Phoniatr, 3–7 August 1986, Tokyo, Japan.

3a. Kok LL, Solman RT: Velocardiofacial syndrome: Learning difficulties and intervention. J Med Genet 32:612–618, 1995.

4. Lipson AH, Yuille D, Angel M, Thompson PG, Vandervoord JG, Beckerham EJ: Velocardiofacial (Shprintzen) syndrome: an important syndrome for the dysmorphologist to recognize. J Med Genet 28:596–604, 1991.
5. Mansour AM, Goldberg RB, Wang FM, Shprintzen RJ: Ocular findings in the velo-cardio-facial syndrome. J Pediatr Ophthalmol Strabismus 24:263–266, 1987.

5a. Morrow B, Goldberg R, Carlson C, Das Gupta R, Sirotkin H, Collins J, Dunham I, O'Donnell H, Scambler P, Shprintzen R et al.: Molecular definition of the 22q11 deletions in velo-cardio-facial syndrome. Am J Hum Genet 56:1391–1403, 1995.

6. Scambler PJ, Kelly D, Lindsay E, Williamson R, Goldberg R, Shprintzen R, Wilson DI, Goodship JA, Cross IE, Burn J: Velocardiofacial syndrome associated with chromosome 22 deletions encompassing the DiGeorge locus. Lancet 339:1138–1139, 1992.
7. Sedlacková E: The syndrome of the congenitally short velum. The dual innervation of the soft palate. Folia Phoniatr 19:441–443, 1967.
8. Shprintzen RJ: The velo-cardio-facial syndrome: a clinical and genetic analysis. Pediatrics 67:167–172, 1981.
9. Shprintzen RJ, Goldberg RB, Lewin ML, Sidoti EJ, Berkman MD: A new syndrome involving cleft palate, cardiac anomalies, typical facies and learning disabilities: velo-cardio-facial syndrome. Cleft Palate J 5:56–62, 1978.
10. Williams MA, Shprintzen RJ, Goldberg RB: Male-to-male transmission of the velo-cardio-facial syndrome: a case report and review of 60 cases. J Craniofac Genet Dev Biol 5:175–180, 1985.
11. Williams MA, Shprintzen RJ, Rakoff SJ: Adenoid hypoplasia in the velo-cardio-facial syndrome. J Craniofac Genet Dev Biol 7:23–26, 1987.
12. Young D: Cardiac malformations in the velo-cardio-facial syndrome. Am J Cardiol 46:643–648, 1980.


## Simpson-Golabi-Behmel syndrome

### Golabi-Rosen syndrome
(MIM No. *312870; POSSUM No. 3325)

Simpson et al.[8] reported on a previously unrecognized X-linked syndrome of dysmorphia in 1975. Later Golabi and Rosen[2] de-

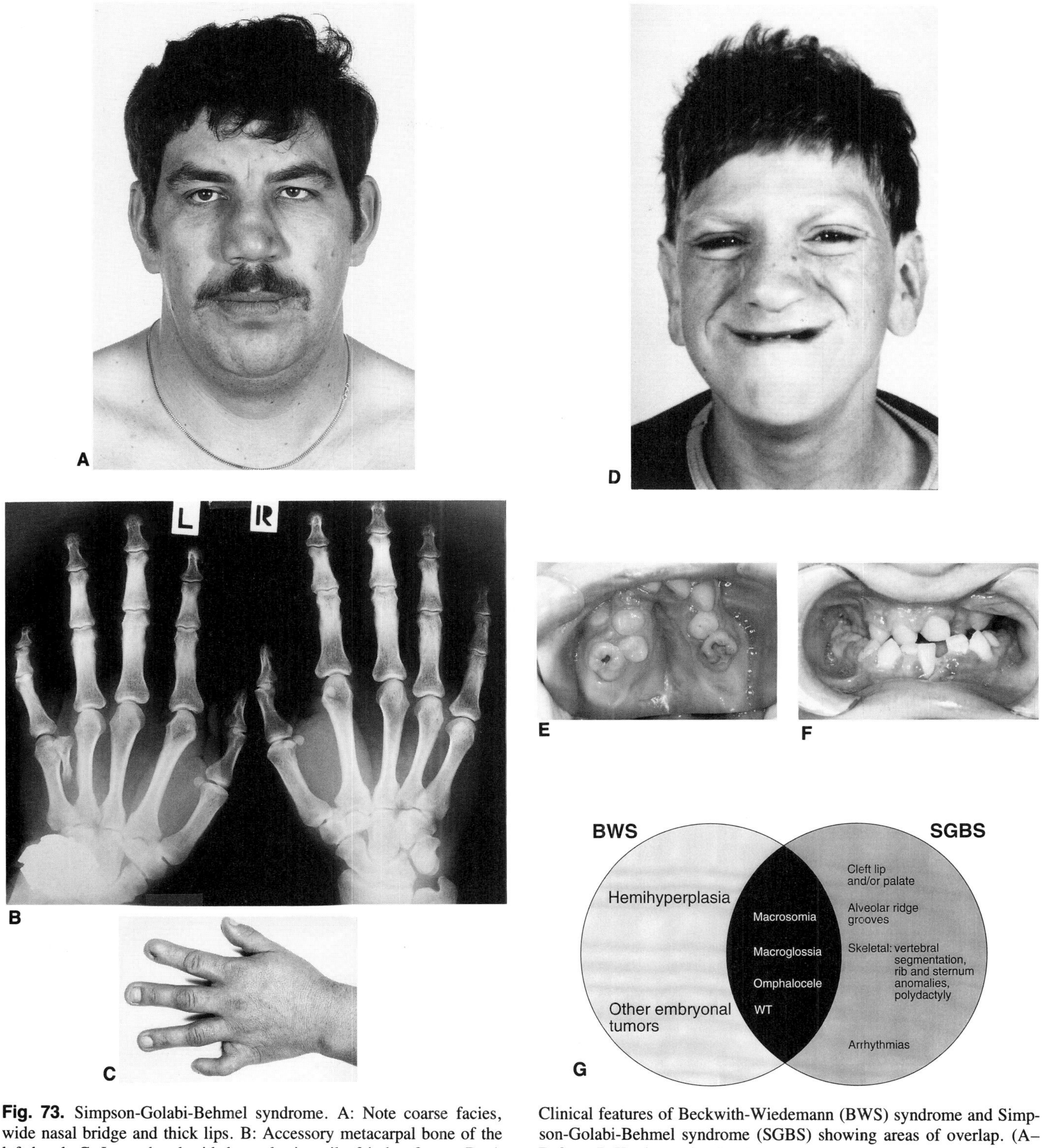


**Fig. 73.** Simpson-Golabi-Behmel syndrome. A: Note coarse facies, wide nasal bridge and thick lips. B: Accessory metacarpal bone of the left hand. C: Large hand with hypoplastic nail of index finger. D: A young patient with the syndrome. E,F: Note the high, narrow-arched palate and abnormalities of the teeth resulting in malocclusion. G: Clinical features of Beckwith-Wiedemann (BWS) syndrome and Simpson-Golabi-Behmel syndrome (SGBS) showing areas of overlap. (A–D from R König et al., Am J Med Genet 38:244, 1991; E–G from R Weksberg et al., Nat Genet 12:225, 1996, with permission.)

scribed 4 male patients with peculiar facies, mental retardation, and overgrowth.

## General manifestations

Large hands, postaxial polydactyly, broad thumbs and halluces, hypoplasia of the nails, and single palmar creases are seen. Cryptorchidism, large cystic kidneys, coccygeal skin tag and bony appendages, segmentation defects of the vertebrae, and advanced bone age have been described. Skeletal growth is generally advanced.[1,4]

Other defects include cardiovascular conduction defects, Meckel's diverticulum, inguinal hernia, pectus excavatum, skin hyperpigmentation, hyperinsulinemia, and spongiform degeneration of the cerebrum and brain stem.[3,5,6] There is predisposition toward development of Wilms tumor.

### Otolaryngological manifestations

These include coarse facies, hypertelorism, wide nasal bridge, macroglossia, and macrostoma with thick lips. The palate is high arched and narrow. The lower lip may be cleft. The external ears are cup shaped and may demonstrate preauricular pits or tags.[1,9] The syndrome has also been called *Bulldog syndrome.*[7]

### Etiology

This syndrome is of X-linked recessive inheritance. It is caused by mutations in *GPC3,* a glypican gene.[7,10] *GPC3* encodes a putative extracellular proteoglycan, glypican 3, that is thought to play an important role in growth control in embryonic mesodermal tissues in which it is selectively expressed.[7,10] One study claims that glypican 3 forms a complex with insulin-like growth factor 2 (IGF2), thereby modulating IGF2 action.[7]

### Differential diagnosis

Simpson-Golabi-Behmel syndrome should be differentiated from other overgrowth syndromes, e.g., Weaver syndrome, and Marshall-Smith and Beckwith-Wiedemann syndromes.

#### References


1. Behmel A, Plochl E, Rosenkranz W: A new X-linked dysplasia gigantism syndrome: follow up in the first family and report on a second Austrian family. Am J Med Genet 30: 275–285, 1988.
2. Golabi M, Rosen L: A new X-linked mental retardation overgrowth syndrome. Am J Med Genet 17:345–358, 1984.
3. Konig R, Fuchs S, Kern C, Langebeck U: Simpson-Golabi-Behmel syndrome with severe cardiac arrhythmias. Am J Med Genet 38:244–247, 1991.
4. Neri G, Marini R, Cappa M, Barrelli P, Opitz JM: Simpson-Golabi-Behmel syndrome: an X-linked encephalo-tropho-schisis syndrome. Am J Med Genet 30:287–299, 1988.
5. Opitz JM: The Golabi-Rosen syndrome: report of a second family. Am J Med Genet 17:359–366, 1984.
6. Opitz JM, Herrmann J, Gilbert EF, Matalon R: Simpson-Golabi-Behmel syndrome: follow up of the Michigan family. Am J Med Genet 30:301–308, 1988.
7. Pilia G, Hughes-Benzie RM, MacKenzie A, Baybayan P, Chen EY, Huber R, Neri G, Cao A, Forabosco A, Schlessinger D: Mutations in *GPC3,* a glypican gene, cause the Simpson-Golabi-Behmel overgrowth syndrome. Nat Genet 12:241–247, 1996.
8. Simpson JL, Landey S, New M, German J: A previously unrecognized X-linked syndrome of dysmorphia. Birth Defects 11:18–24, 1975.
9. Tsukahara M, Tanaka S, Kajii T: A Weaver-like syndrome in a Japanese boy. Clin Genet 25:73–78, 1984.
10. Weksberg R, Squire JA, Templeton DM: Glypicans: a growing trend. Nat Genet 12:225–227, 1996.


## Smith-Lemli-Opitz (SLO) syndrome

### (MIM No. *270400; POSSUM No. 3391)

This syndrome was first described in 1964 by Smith et al.[9] It is characterized by growth and mental retardation, microcephaly, cleft palate, facial and genital anomalies associated with syndactyly of the second and third toes, and postaxial polydactyly of the hands.

### General manifestations

Mental retardation and failure to thrive occur in most cases (over 90%). Poor sucking, gastroesophageal reflux, hypotonia during the newborn period with resultant bronchopneumonia are frequent features of Smith-Lemli-Opitz (SLO) syndrome. Other features include microcephaly with a high, square forehead, ptosis, epicanthic folds, cataracts, and strabismus. Around 70% of males have abnormal external genitalia, including hypospadias, cryptorchidism, microphallus, and/or cordae.

Various cardiac defects have been reported, such as PDA, tetralogy of Fallot, and aberrant subclavian artery. Renal defects (ureteral constriction, hydronephrosis, cystic renal disease) and incomplete lobation of the lungs have also been described.

Soft tissue syndactyly between the second and third toes, single palmar creases, polydactyly, and dislocated hips are examples of limb anomalies.[1a–4,6–8] Occasional findings include a hypoplastic thymus, pyloric stenosis, pancreatic giant cells, and a deep sacral dimple.[2–7]

### Otolaryngological manifestations

These include a short nose, a broad nasal bridge, anteverted nostrils, broad maxillary and alveolar ridges, a cleft palate, and low-set ears.[3,8]

### Etiology

Smith-Lemli-Opitz syndrome is of autosomal recessive inheritance. Recently a defect in cholesterol synthesis was suggested by the abnormally low plasma cholesterol level and the accumulation of 7–dehydrocholesterol.[5,10] The defect presumably resides in 7–dehydrocholesterol reductase or in an associated protein necessary for its activity.[10] The gene maps to 7q32.[1]

#### References


1. Alley TL, Gray BA, Lee S-H, Scherer SW, Tsui L-C, Tint GS, Williams CA, Zori R, Wallace MR: Identification of a yeast artificial clone spanning a translocation breakpoint at 7q32 in a Smith-Lemli-Opitz syndrome patient. Am J Hum Genet 56:1411–1416, 1995.

1a. Cherstvcy ED, Lazjuk GI, Lurie IW, Nedzved MK, Usoev SS: The pathological anatomy of the Smith-Lemli-Opitz syndrome. Clin Genet 7:382–387, 1975.

2. Cotlier E, Rice P: Cataracts in the Smith-Lemli-Opitz syndrome. Am J Ophthalmol 72:955–959, 1971.
3. Curry CJR, Carey JC, Holland JS, Chopra D, Fineman R, Golabi M, Sherman S, Pagon RA, Allanson J, Shulman S, et al: Smith-Lemli-Opitz syndrome type II: multiple congenital anomalies with male pseudohermaphroditism and frequent early lethality. Am J Med Genet 26:45–57, 1987.
4. Dallaire L: Syndrome of retardation with urogenital and skeletal anomalies (Smith-Lemli-Opitz syndrome): clinical features and mode of inheritance. J Med Genet 6:113–120, 1969.
5. Irons M, Elias ER, Tint GS, Salen G, Frieden R, Buie TM, Ampola M: Abnormal cholesterol metabolism in the Smith-Lemli-Opitz syndrome: report of clinical and biochemical findings in four patients and treatment in one patient. Am J Med Genet 50:347–352, 1994.
6. Johnson VP: Smith-Lemli-Opitz syndrome: review and report of two affected siblings. Z Kinderheilkd 119:221–234, 1975.
7. Joseph DB, Uehling DT, Gilbert E, Laxova R: Genitourinary abnormalities associated with Smith-Lemli-Opitz syndrome. J Urol 137:719–721, 1987.
8. Opitz JM, Penchaszadeh VB, Holt MC, Spano LM: Smith-Lemli-Opitz (RSH) syndrome bibliography. Am J Med Genet 28:745–750, 1987.

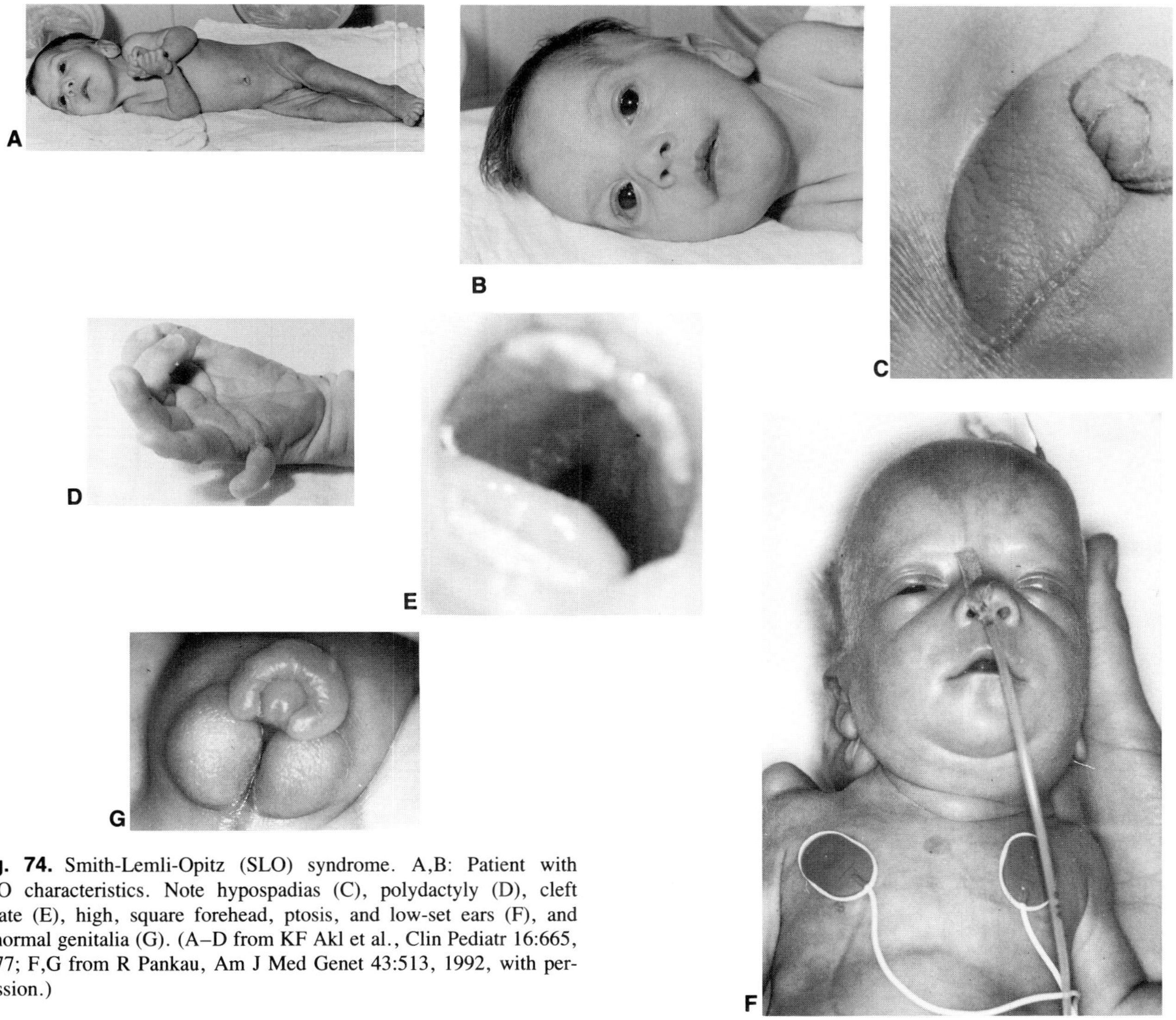

**Fig. 74.** Smith-Lemli-Opitz (SLO) syndrome. A,B: Patient with SLO characteristics. Note hypospadias (C), polydactyly (D), cleft palate (E), high, square forehead, ptosis, and low-set ears (F), and abnormal genitalia (G). (A–D from KF Akl et al., Clin Pediatr 16:665, 1977; F,G from R Pankau, Am J Med Genet 43:513, 1992, with permission.)

9. Smith DW, Lemli L, Opitz JM: A newly recognized syndrome of multiple congenital anomalies. J Pediatr 64:210–217, 1964.
10. Tint GS, Irons M, Elias ER, Batta AK, Frieden R, Chen TS, Salen G: Defective cholesterol biosynthesis associated with the Smith-Lemli-Opitz syndrome. N Engl J Med 330:107–113, 1994.

## Stickler syndrome

### Hereditary arthro-ophthalmopathy
(MIM No. #108300, *184840; POSSUM No. 3030)

Stickler et al. in 1965 reported a syndrome with eye anomalies, hearing loss, cleft palate, and osseous changes in patients with marfanoid habitus.[10] The syndrome was further characterized in 1975 by Herrmann.[5]

#### General manifestations

Ocular anomalies occur in 80% of patients and include high myopia (8–18 diopters) presenting before 10 years of age, retinal detachment, and cataracts.[4,6,8] Other eye manifestations are vitreous degeneration, astigmatism, strabismus, and glaucoma. It is important to schedule all patients diagnosed with Robin sequence for ophthalmological periodic visits since a high percentage of them have Stickler syndrome and may have ophthalmological complications. Cardiovascular manifestations have also been reported as part of this condition.[7] The joints are often hyperextensible and prominent. The vertebrae show anterior wedging. The long bones display narrow shafts relative to the wide metaphyses. Some patients have a marfanoid habitus and tend to be short. At least 25% of patients have short stature.[9]

#### Otolaryngological manifestations

The facies are characteristially flat, due to midfacial hypoplasia, short maxilla, a depressed nasal bridge, and an elongated philtrum. Fifteen to twenty percent of patients have a normal face. Cleft palate/lip occurs in about 20% of patients.[4] Hearing loss (progressive sensorineural or conductive) has been reported in 10 to 80% of patients.[3,9]

#### Etiology

Stickler syndrome is of autosomal dominant inheritance. Even though there have been controversial reports, it is now well

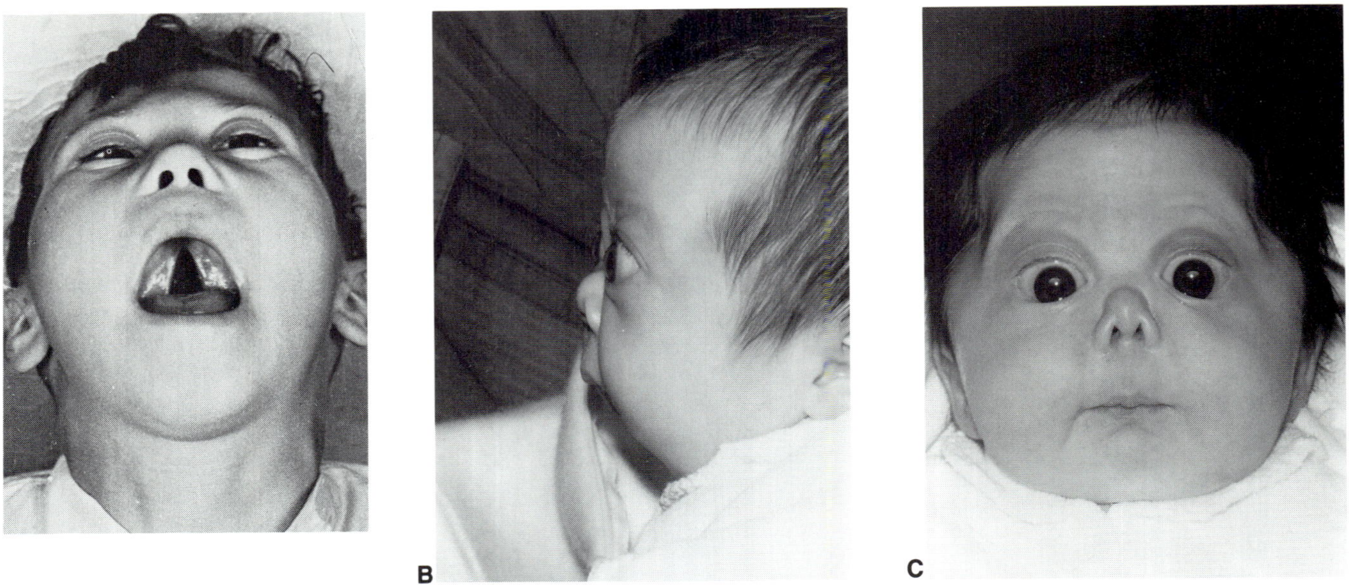

**Fig. 75.** Stickler syndrome. A: Patient with cleft palate. (From RJ Gorlin et al., *Syndromes of the Head and Neck,* 3rd ed., Oxford University Press, New York, 1990, p. 290.) B,C: Note the midfacial flattening and small mandible. (From K Temple et al., J Med Genet 26:119, 1989, with permission; courtesy of Dr. M Baraitser.)

established that there is clinical and locus heterogeneity. The condition can be sub-classified on the basis of vitreo-retinal phenotype. Type 1 families have a characteristic congenital vitreous anomaly, showing linkage without recombination to markers at the *COL2A1* locus (12q13.11–q13.2).[1,2] Type 2 families with different congenital vitreo-retinal phenotypes are linked to the *COL11A1* gene (1p21).[9a,9b] In a large Dutch kindred with a Stickler syndrome phenotype, close linkage was demonstrated to the *COL11A2* gene (6p21.3).[1a]

#### References


1. Brown DM, Vandenburgh K, Kimura AE, Weingeist TA, Sheffield VC, Stone EM: Novel frameshift mutations in the procollagen 2 gene (COL2A1) associated with Stickler syndrome (hereditary arthro-ophthalmopathy). Hum Mol Genet 4:141–142, 1995.

1a. Brunner HG, van Beersam SE, Warman ML, Olsen BR, Ropers HH, Mariman EC: A Stickler syndrome gene is linked to chromosome 6 near the COL11A2 gene. Hum Mol Genet 3:1561–1564, 1994.

2. Francomano CA, Liberfarb RM, Hirose T, Maumenee IH, Streeten EA, Myers DA, Pyeritz RE: The Stickler syndrome: evidence for close linkage to the structural gene for type II collagen. Genomics 1:293–296, 1987.

3. Gorlin RJ, Cohen MM Jr, Levin LS: Syndromes of the Head and Neck, 3rd ed. Oxford University Press, New York, 1990, pp 288–289.

4. Hall JC, Herrod H: The Stickler syndrome presenting as a dominantly inherited cleft palate and blindness. J Med Genet 12:397–404, 1975.

5. Herrmann J, France TD, Spranger JW, Opitz JM, Wiffler C: The Stickler syndrome (hereditary arthroophthalmopathy). Birth Defects 11:76–103,1975.

6. Knobloch WH: Inherited hyaloideo-retinopathy and skeletal dysplasia. Trans Am Ophthalmol Soc 73:417–429, 1975.

7. Liberfarb RM, Goldblatt A: Prevalence of mitral valve prolapse in the Stickler syndrome. Am J Med Genet 24:387–392, 1986.

8. Nielsen CE: Stickler syndrome. Acta Ophthalmol 59:286–295, 1981.

9. Popkin JS, Polomeno RC: Stickler's syndrome (hereditary progressive arthro-ophthalmopathy). Can Med Assoc J 111:1071–1076, 1974.

9a. Richards AJ, Yates JRW, Williams R, Payne SJ, Pope FM, Scott JD, Snead MP: A family with Stickler syndrome type 2 has a mutation in the *COL11A1* gene resulting in the substitution of glycine 97 by valine in $\alpha$1 (XI) collagen. Hum Mol Genet 5:1339–1343, 1996.

9b. Snead MP, Payne SJ, Barton DE, Yates JRW, al-Imara L, Pope FM, Scott JD: Stickler syndrome: Correlation between vitreo-retinal phenotypes and linkage to COL2A1. Eye 8:609–614, 1994.

10. Stickler GB, Belau PG, Farrell FJ, Jones JD, Puch DG, Steinberg AG, Ward LE: Hereditary progressive arthro-ophthalmopathy. Mayo Clin Proc 40:433–455, 1965.


## Sturge-Weber syndrome

(MIM No. 185300; POSSUM No. 3397)

This syndrome is characterized by port-wine facial angioma taking the course of the ophthalmic division of the trigeminal nerve. It is accompanied by intracranial calcifications and seizures in over 90% of cases. Mental deficiency occurs in one-third of the patients.[1]

### General manifestations

Venous angiomas of the leptomeninges are quite characteristic of Sturge-Weber syndrome and occur in the temporal, occipital, or parietal regions. Arteriovenous malformations or arterial thrombosis may be encountered.

With age, the intracranial calcifications mature and detection of vascular angiomas becomes difficult radiologically.[1,9] The calcifications are usually gyriform and form double-contoured parallel lines.[2–4] Ocular findings include angiomas of the choroid, congenital glaucoma, and hemianopsia.[7]

Angiomas may be observed in other organs such as the thyroid, pituitary, gastrointestinal tract, or ovaries.[5,12]

### Otolaryngological manifestations

Capillary angioma of a pink to purplish-red color are seen in almost all patients. It may extend to the back or neck. Angiomatosis also occurs on the buccal mucosa or lips and hypertrophy of the tongue may develop. The gingiva may show enlargement and the teeth may display irregular positioning, premature eruptions, and malocclusion.[1,8,10,11] Blue nevus around the trigeminal territory (Ota's nevus) and the blue nevus around the shoulder girdle (Ito's nevus) may also be observed.[6]

### Etiology

This condition is sporadic. It probably results from the failure of regression of the vascular plexus around the neural tube during the ninth week of gestation.[3]

A

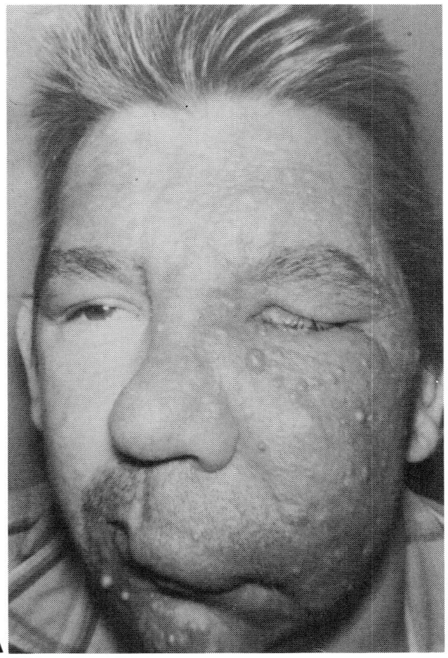

B

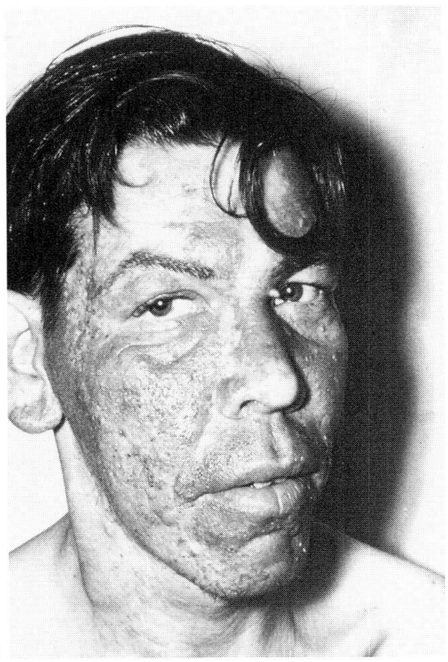

**Fig. 76.** Sturge-Weber syndrome. A: Unilateral cutaneous angioma with involvement of the eye. B: Hemangioma involving the whole face. (From VM Der Kaloustian, AK Kurban, *Genetic Diseases of the Skin,* Springer-Verlag, Berlin, p. 257, with permission; courtesy of Dr. I Zeligman.)

### Differential diagnosis

Sturge-Weber syndrome should be differentiated from other syndromes with angiomatosis, e.g., Beckwith-Wiedemann syndrome, neurofibromatosis 1, Klippel-Trenaunay-Weber syndrome, and Coat's disease (telangiectasia of the retinal vessels).[2,6]

### References


1. Alexander Gl, Normal RM: The Sturge-Weber Syndrome. John Wright and Sons, Bristol, 1960.
2. Allen HB, Parlett HL: Coat's disease. Arch Dermatol 108:413–415, 1973.
3. Andriola M, Stolfi J: Sturge-Weber syndrome. Am J Dis Child 123:507–510, 1972.
4. Arendt A: Sturge-Weberishe Erkrankung. Dtsch Gesundheitsw 8:137–41, 1953.
5. Bentz M, Towfighi J, Greenwood S, Zaino R: Sturge-Weber syndrome. A case with thyroid and choroid plexus hemangiomas and leptomeningeal melanosis. Arch Pathol Lab Med 106:75–78, 1982.
6. Fuzukawa T: Sturge-Weber and Klippel-Trenaunay syndrome with nevus of Ota and Ito. Arch Dermatol 102:640–645, 1970.
7. Miller SJN: Ophthalmic aspects of the Sturge-Weber syndrome. Proc R Soc Med 56:419–421, 1965.
8. Myle G: Sémiologie de l'angiomatose encéphalo-trigéminée ou encéphalo-cranio-faciale. Acta Neurol Belg 50:713–785, 1950.
9. Poser CM, Tavaras JM: Cerebral angiography in encephalo-trigeminal angiomatosis. Radiology 68:237–336, 1957.
10. Schuermann H: Krankheiten des Mundschleimhaut und der Lippen, 2nd ed. Urban and Schwarzenberg, Berlin, 1958.
11. Sujansky E, Conradi S: Outcome of Sturge-Weber syndrome in 52 adults. Am J Med Genet 57:35–45, 1995.
12. Wohlwill FJ, Yakovlev PI: Histopathology of meningo-facial angiomatosis (Sturge-Weber's disease): report of four cases. J Neuropathol Exp Neurol 16:341–364, 1957.


## Treacher Collins syndrome

**Fraceschetti-Zwahlen-Klein syndrome**
**Mandibulofacial dysostosis**
(MIM No. *154500; POSSUM No. 3283)

Treacher Collins described the essential traits of this syndrome in 1900.[19] Diagnostic criteria include microtia and malformed ears, hypoplastic midface, downward slanting of the palpebral fissures, coloboma of the outer third of the lower eyelids, and micrognathia.

### General manifestations

Most patients have normal intelligence. Developmental retardation is reported in only 5% of cases. Delays are probably secondary to undetected hearing loss. The most common ocular findings are lower lid colobomas (77%) with absence of cilia medial to the coloboma. Microphthalmia and coloboma of the iris may occasionally be seen.[2] Other uncommon anomalies include congenital heart defects and cryptorchidism.

### Otolaryngological manifestations

The facies is characteristic: the supraorbital ridges are flat, the nose appears large because of the depressed malar bones, the lower nasal cartilages are underdeveloped and the bridge of the nose is often high. The auricles are malformed and microtia is reported in 60 to 77% of cases.[6] The external auditory canals are stenosed or absent. In the middle ear, different anomalies

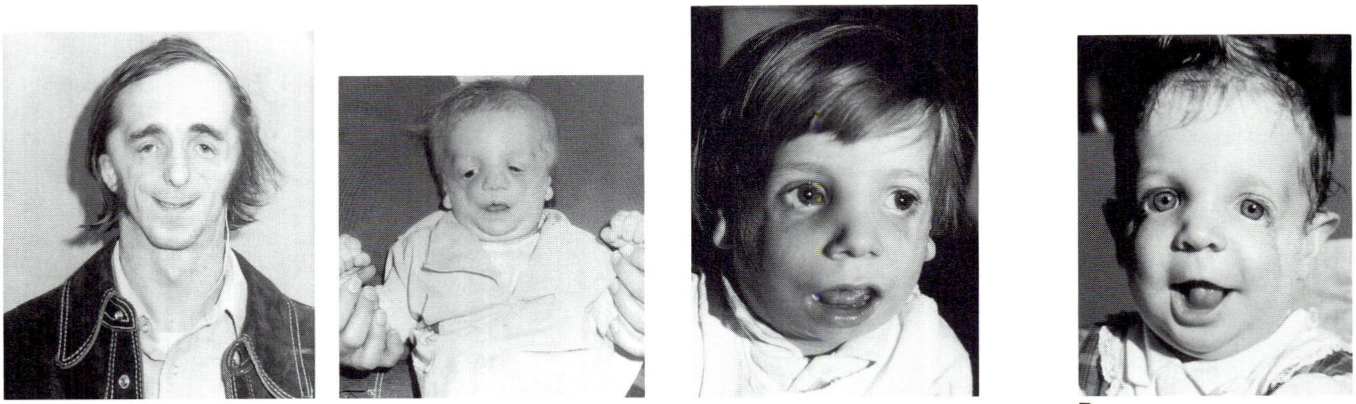

A B C D

**Fig. 77.** Treacher Collins syndrome. A,B: Father and child. Note the downward palpebral slant, hypoplasia of the malar and zygomatic areas, and abnormal pinnae. The father wears a hearing aid (left ear). C,D: Milder form of the syndrome. (From GG Nora, FC Fraser, *Medical Genetics*, Lea & Febiger, Philadelphia, 1974, p. 123, with permission.)

are described, such as monopodal stapes, ankylosed foot plate, bony bridge to the fallopian canal, and malformed incus. The tympanum may be filled with connective tissue and the epitympanum and mastoid show different degrees of hypoplasia or agenesis.[4,7,10,12] The cochlea and vestibule may show abnormalities.[16] Hearing loss is usually conductive, although a sensorineural component has also been described.[5] One-third of the patients have cleft palate or velopharyngeal insufficiency.[11] Macrostoma and hypoplasia of the parotid glands are also seen. The coronoid process of the mandible is flat and the condyles may be malformed.[15] Blind fistula between the auricle and angle of the mouth, choanal atresia, and pharyngeal hypoplasia are occasional abnormalities.[17]

## Etiology

Treacher Collins syndrome is of autosomal dominant inheritance with variable expressivity and high penetrance. A recessive form has also been described.[7,8] Experimental embryological studies[13,14,18,20] using vitamin A and isotretinoin produced similar changes in rats, hamsters, and mice. Hypersensitivity of the mother to vitamin A has also been suggested.[9] The gene location is 5q32–q33.1. Dixon et al. have found mutations in a novel gene, *Treacle,* leading to premature termination of the coded protein.[1] Five different mutations have been identified so far. The mutations that have been characterized are unique to each family. This gene appears to be widely expressed in fetal and adult tissues. A clear understanding of why haploinsufficiency causes the specific craniofacial abnormalities observed is still needed.[1,21]

The precise function of *Treacle* is currently unknown. On the basis of the clinical phenotype, the gene likely plays a fundamental role in early embryonic development, particularly of the craniofacial complex.[1]

## Differential diagnosis

Treacher Collins syndrome should be differentiated from oculoauriculovertebral spectrum (Goldenhar syndrome), Nager acrofacial dysostosis, and other types of acrofacial dysostosis.[2,3]

## References


1. Dixon J, Edwards SJ, Glawdin AJ, Dixon MJ, Loftus SK, Bonner CA, Koprivnikar K, Wasmuth JJ: Positional cloning of a gene involved in the pathogenesis of Treacher Collins syndrome. Nat Genet 12:130–136, 1996.
2. Franceschetti A, Klein D, Brocher JE: La dysostose mandibulofaciale dans le cadre des syndromes du premier arc branchial. Schweiz Med Wochenschr 89:478–483, 1959.
3. Halal F, Hermann J, Pallister PD, Opitz JM, Desgrange MF: Differential diagnosis of Nager acrofacial dysostosis syndrome: report of four patients with Nager syndrome and discussion of other related syndromes. Am J Med Genet 14:209–224, 1983.
4. Hutchinson JC Jr, Caldarelli DD, Valvassori GE, Pruzansky S, Parris PJ: The otologic manifestations of mandibulofacial dysostosis. Trans Am Ophthalmol Soc 84:520–528, 1977.
5. Kittel G, Fleisher-Peters A: Das Ohr bie Dysostosesyndromen des Schädels. Laryngol Rhin Otol 42:384–397, 1963.
6. Kolar JC, Farkas LG, Munro IR: Surface morphology in Treacher Collins syndrome: an Anthropometric Study. Cleft Palate J 22:266–274, 1985.
7. Lloyd GA, Phelps PD: Radiology of the ear in mandibulofacial dysostosis-Treacher Collins syndrome. Acta Radiol Diagn 20:233–240, 1979.
8. Lowry RB, Morgan K, Holmes TM, Metcalf PJ, Stauffer GF: Mandibulofacial dysostosis in Hutterite sibs: a possible recessive trait. Am J Med Genet 22:501–512, 1985.
9. Lungarotti MS, Marinelli D, Mariani T, Calabro A: Multiple congenital anomalies associated with apparently normal maternal intake of vitamin A: a phenocopy of the isoretinoin syndrome? Am J Med Genet 27:245–248, 1987.
10. McKenzie J, Craig J: Mandibulo-facial dysostosis (Treacher Collins syndrome). Arch Dis Child 30:391–395, 1955.
11. Peterson-Falzone S, Pruzansky S: Cleft palate and congenital palatopharyngeal incompetency in mandibulo-facial dysostosis: Frequency and problems in treatment. Cleft Palate J 13:354–360, 1976.
12. Phelps PD, Poswillo D, Lloyd GA: The ear deformities in mandibulofacial dysostosis (Treacher Collins syndrome). Clin Otolaryngol 6:15–28, 1981.
13. Poswillo D: The pathogenesis of the Treacher Collins syndrome (mandibulo-facial dysostosis). Br J Oral Surg 13:1–26, 1975.
14. Poswillo D: Pathogenesis of craniofacial syndromes exhibiting colobomata. Trans Ophthalmol Soc UK 96:69, 1976.

15. Roberts FG, Pruzansky S, Aduss H: An X-radiocephalometric study of mandibulofacial dysostosis in man. Arch Oral Biol 20:265–282, 1975.
16. Sands I, Hemenway WG, Morgan WR: Histopathology of the temporal bones in mandibulofacial dysostosis. Trans Am Acad Ophthalmol Otol 72:913–924, 1968.
17. Shprintzen RJ, Croft C, Berkman MD, Rakoff SJ: Pharyngeal hypoplasia in Treacher Collins syndrome. Arch Otolaryngol 105:127–131, 1979.
18. Sulik KK, Johnston MC, Smiley SJ, Speight HS, Jarvis BE: Mandibulofacial dysostosis (Treacher Collins syndrome): a new proposal for its pathogenesis. Am J Med Genet 27:359–372, 1987.
19. Treacher Collins E: Cases with symmetrical congenital notches in the outer part of each lid and defective development of the malar bones. *Trans Ophthalmol Soc UK* 20:190–192, 1900.
20. Wiley MJ, Cawenbergs P, Taylor IM: Effects of retinoic acid on the development of the facial skeleton. Early changes involving neural crest cells. Acta Anat 116:180–192, 1983.
21. Winter RM: What's in a face? Nat Genet 12:124–129, 1996.

## Trisomy 13

### Patau syndrome
(POSSUM No. 3090)

#### General manifestations

Microcephaly and holoprosencephaly are common. Common ocular findings include microphthalmia, hypertelorism, and epicanthal folds. Iris colobomas are seen in only one-third of the cases. Cardiovascular anomalies, in decreasing order of frequency, include atrial septal defect, patent ductus arteriosus, ventricular septal defect, dextrocardia, and an abnormal great vessel. Frequent urogenital anomalies include polycystic kidneys and cryptorchidism. Hydronephrosis, bicornuate uterus, hydroureter, and horseshoe kidney may also occur. Severe developmental retardation is the rule.[6]

Polydactyly (75%), dystrophic nails (70%), single palmar crease (65%), hypotonia (40%–50%), and prominent calcaneus (30%) are also found in this condition.[3–5]

#### Otolaryngological manifestations

The forehead slopes and the nose is prominent. Scalp defects and ulceration occur in the vertex area. Cleft palate and/or lip and micrognathia are present in over 50% of patients. The pinnae are malformed and the inner ear may show Mondini or Scheibe's dysplasia. Cochleosaccular degeneration, thickened middle ear mucosa due to unresolved mesenchyme, a small tympanic membrane, thick manubrium of the malleus, distorted incudostapedial joint, deformed stapes, and absent stapedial muscle have also been reported. The stapedial artery may persist. The facial canal may display wide dehiscences. Vestibular anomalies include anomalies of the superior and posterior semicircular canals and the internal auditory canals may be wider than normal.[7,8] The neck is short and the skin is loose over the nape region. Capillary hemangiomas occur in over 70% of patients. Apneic episodes are described in approximately 60% of patients.[1,9]

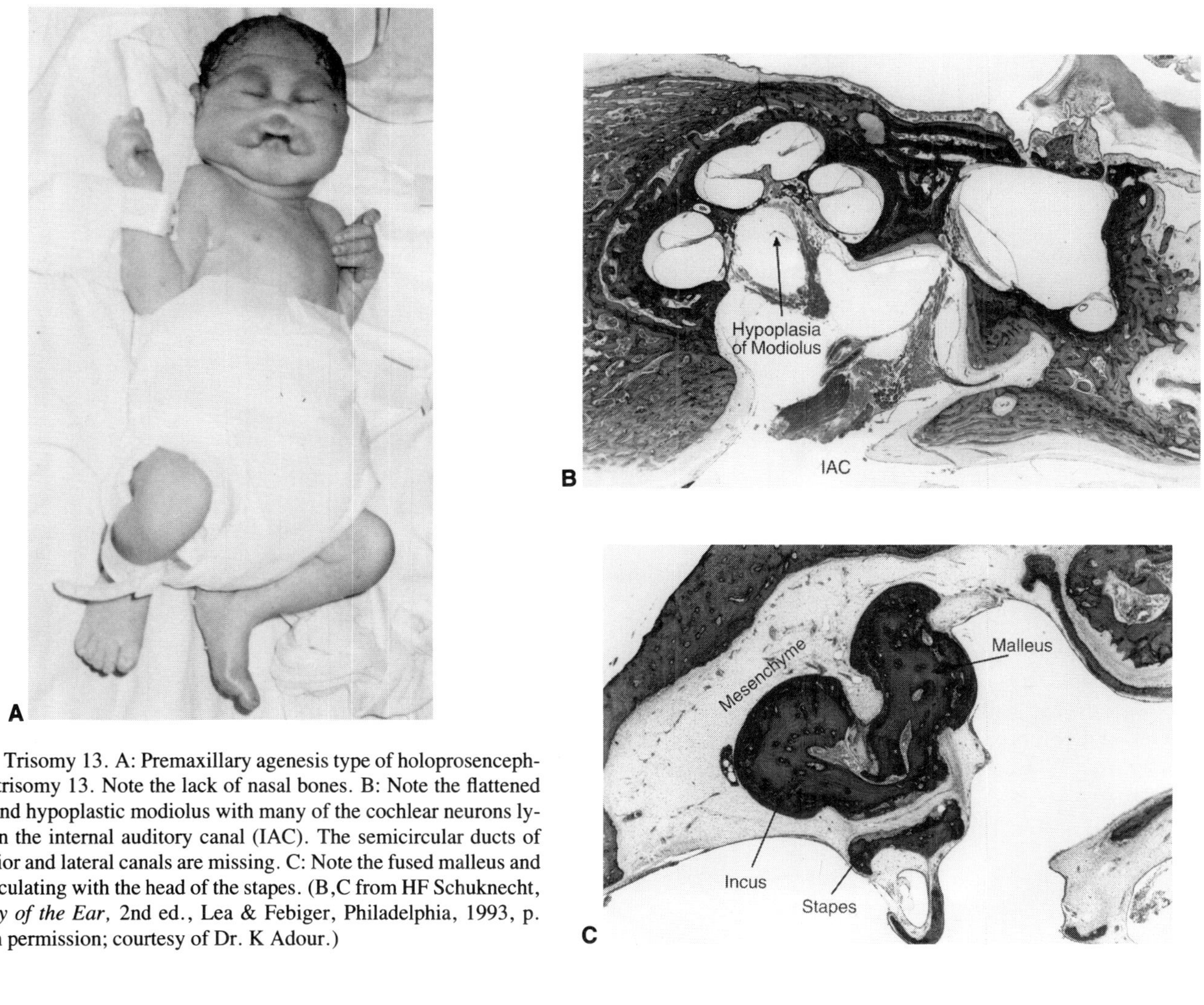


**Fig. 78.** Trisomy 13. A: Premaxillary agenesis type of holoprosencephaly with trisomy 13. Note the lack of nasal bones. B: Note the flattened cochlea and hypoplastic modiolus with many of the cochlear neurons lying within the internal auditory canal (IAC). The semicircular ducts of the superior and lateral canals are missing. C: Note the fused malleus and incus articulating with the head of the stapes. (B,C from HF Schuknecht, *Pathology of the Ear,* 2nd ed., Lea & Febiger, Philadelphia, 1993, p. 184, with permission; courtesy of Dr. K Adour.)

### Etiology

Older maternal age is a factor in the occurrence of trisomy 13 because nondisjunction during meiosis occurs. The frequency of free trisomy 13 is approximately 1:12,000. The frequency of the translocation is 1:56,000 to 1:80,000. Half of all patients die during the first month of life, and the survivors rarely reach the age of 1 year.

### Differential diagnosis

Pseudotrisomy 13 (McKusick No. 264480, POSSUM No. 3982) resembles trisomy 13 but the former has a normal karyotype. Features of pseudotrisomy 13 include holoprosencephaly, midline cleft lip, polydactyly and multiple visceral anomalies.[2] Trisomy 13 should also be differentiated from Smith-Lemli-Opitz syndrome and trisomy 18.

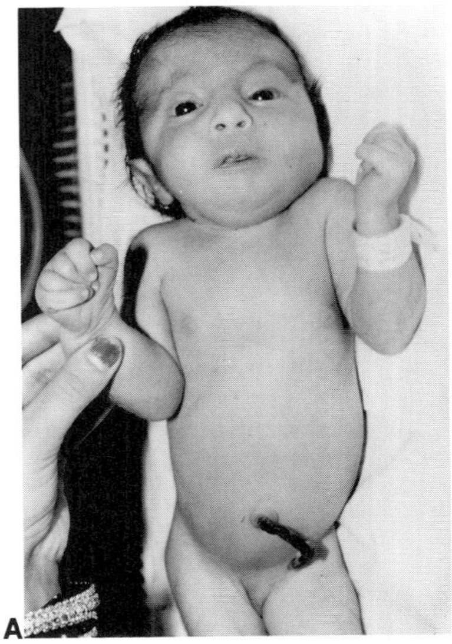

A

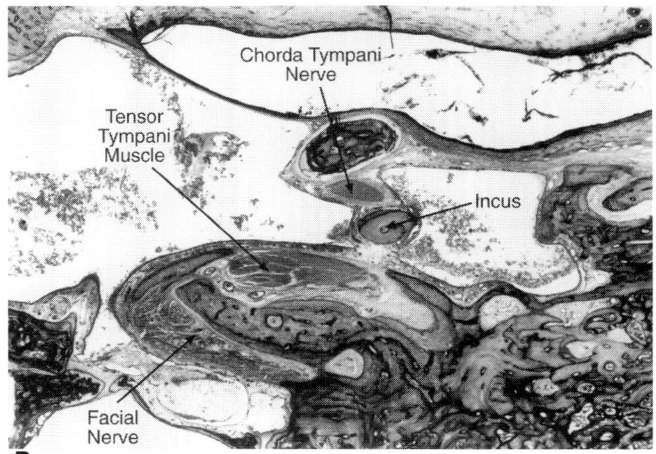


B

**Fig. 79.** Trisomy 18. A: Note micrognathia, low-set ears, and overlapping fingers. B: Middle ear anomalies consist of a large cochleariform process, abnormal course of the facial nerve, bifurcated tensor tympani muscle, and ossicular deformities. (B from HF Schuknecht, *Pathology of the Ear,* 2nd ed., Lea & Febiger, Philadelphia, 1993, p. 186, with permission.)

#### References

1. Addor C, Cox J, Cabrol C, Crippa L: Patau's syndrome. A pathological and cytogenetic study of two cases. J Genet Hum 23:83–109, 1975.
2. Boles RG, Teebi AS, Neilson KA, Meyn MS: Pseudotrisomy 13 with upper limb shortness and radial hypoplasia. Am J Med Genet 50:381–382, 1994.
3. Cohen MM Jr: Perspectives on holoprosencephaly. Part I. Epidemiology, genetics and syndromology. Teratology 40:211–235, 1989.
4. Fujinaga M, Shepard TH, Fitzsimmons J: Trisomy 13 in the fetus. Teratology 41:233–238, 1990.
5. Hodes ME, Cole J, Palmer CG, Reed T: Clinical experience with trisomies 18 and 13. Am J Med Genet 15:48–60, 1978.
6. Patau K, Smith DW, Therman E, Inhorn SL, Wagner HP: Multiple congenital anomalies caused by an extra autosome. Lancet 1:790–793, 1960.
7. Saito H, Okano Y, Furuta M, Asamoto H, Fujita H: Temporal bone findings in trisomy D. Arch Otolaryngol 100:386–389, 1974.
8. Sando I, Leiberman A, Bergstrom L, Isumi S, Wood RP: Temporal bone histopathological findings in trisomy 13 syndrome. Ann Otol Rhinol Laryngol Suppl 84:1–20, 1975.
9. Taylor AI: Autosomal trisomy syndromes: a detailed study of 27 cases of Edwards syndrome and 27 cases of Patau's syndrome. J Med Genet 5:227–252, 1968.

## Trisomy 18

#### Edwards syndrome
(POSSUM No. 3094)

### General manifestations

Growth deficiency is the rule. The nipples are widely spaced and the sternum is short. Microcephaly is common. The occiput is prominent. Overlapping fingers are characteristic (clenched hand). Cardiovascular anomalies occur in 85% of cases (polyvalvular disease, ventricular septal defect, patent ductus arteriosus, and coarctation of the aorta), cryptorchidism in 100% and small pelvis in 68% of cases. Occasional anomalies include tracheoesophageal fistula, Meckel's diverticulum, diaphragmatic hernia, absent corpus callosum, abnormal gyri and short frontal lobe.[2]

Syndactyly (10%–50%), club feet (89%), and hypoplastic nails (100%) are documented. Wilms tumor, hepatoblastoma, and neurogenic neoplasia have been described.[1,7,10] Ocular manifestations include corneal opacities, microphthalmia, blue sclera, and the persistent hyaloid artery. The skin of the neck is loose.[4,7,11]

### Otolaryngological manifestations

Micrognathia and microstoma occur in most cases and the palate is narrow. The ears are low set, the external auditory canals may be stenotic, and the ossicles are abnormal. An abnormal course of the seventh nerve and the chorda tympani have been described. Absent semicircular canals, hypoplasia of the spiral ganglion, a widened cochlear aqueduct, underdeveloped cystic stria vascularis, absent utriculoendolymphatic valve, and enlarged endolymphatic duct all occur in this syndrome. Various other anomalies in the organ of Corti have been described.[2,6,8,9]

### Etiology

The vast majority of trisomy 18 cases originate as a result of nondisjunction during meiosis. Translocation and mosaicism may also occur. The frequency of the condition is approximately 1:5,000 to 1:7,000. Ninety percent of affected patients die before the age of 1 year. The mean age of death is 48 days.[3,5]

### Differential diagnosis

Trisomy 18 should be differentiated from trisomy 13 and Pena-Shokeir syndrome.

### References


1. Dasouki M, Barr M Jr: Brief clinical report. Trisomy 18 and hepatic neoplasia. Am J Med Genet 27:203–205, 1987.
2. Edwards JH, Harnden DG, Cameron AH, Crosse VM, Wolff OH: A new trisomic syndrome. Lancet 1:787–790, 1960.
3. Goldstein H, Gjerum Nielsen K: Rates and survival of individuals with trisomy 13 and 18. Clin Genet 34:366–372, 1988.
4. Hodes ME, Cole J, Palmer CG, Reed T: Clinical experience with trisomies 18 and 13. J Med Genet 15:48–60, 1978.
5. Hook EB, Woodbury DF, Albright SG: Rates of trisomy 18 in live births, stillbirths, and at amniocentesis. Birth Defects 15:81–93, 1979.
6. Keleman G, Hooft C, Kluystkeu P: The inner ear in autosomal trisomy syndromes. Pract Otorhinolaryngol 30:251–258, 1968.
7. Matsuoka R, Misugi K, Goto A, Gilbert EF, Ando M: Congenital heart anomalies in the trisomy 18 syndrome, with reference to congenital polyvalvular disease. Am J Med Genet 14:657–668, 1983.
8. Miglets AW, Schuller D, Rupert E, Lim DJ: Trisomy 18. A temporal bone report. Arch Otolaryngol 101:433–437, 1975.
9. Sando I, Bergstrom L, Wood RP II: Temporal bone findings in trisomy 18 syndrome. Arch Otolaryngol 91:552–559, 1970.
10. Taylor AI: Autosomal trisomy syndromes: a detailed study of 27 cases of Edward's syndrome and 27 cases of Patau's syndrome. J Med Genet 5:227–252, 1968.
11. Wright CG, Brown OE, Meyerhoff WL, Rutledge JC: Inner ear anomalies in two cases of trisomy 18. Am J Otolaryngol 6:392–404, 1985.


## Turner syndrome

(POSSUM No. 3104)

Turner[14] is credited with describing the syndrome of small stature, sexual infantilism, webbed neck, and cubitus valgus.

### General manifestations

Growth is stunted and the birth weight is lower than normal. Patients tend to be obese. Cubitus valgus (70%), medial exostosis of the knees, and short metatarsals and metacarpals occur in over 50% of cases. A coarse trabecular pattern is observed on X-rays of the long bones and osteoporosis is observed in older patients. Craniosynostosis was also described. The chest is usually broad with widely spaced nipples. Mild pectus excavatum is also observed. Edema of the hands and feet, usually resolving in childhood, and dystrophic or deep-set nails are also characteristic.[2,9] Coarctation of the aorta, hypertension, ventricular septal defects, and other cardiovascular malformations occur in 20% of cases.[16] Ocular anomalies include epicanthic folds, ptosis, and myopia. Ovarian dysgenesis with absent germinal elements is characteristic of this syndrome. Amenorrhea and sterilitiy are the rule. However, in rare instances, fertility has been reported. Renal anomalies such as horseshoe kidney, duplicated renal pelvis, duplicated ureters, or unilateral renal aplasia may exist. Visual-spacial and memory impairment are usually described, due to the right hemisphere hypofunction. Learning disabilities, speech delay, hyperactivity, and anorexia nervosa are documented.[10]

Occasional abnormalities include hemangioma of the intestine, diabetes mellitus, Crohn's disease, thyroid disease, brachial plexus neuropathy, and giant cell arteritis.[4] Gonadoblastoma, leukemia, pituitary tumors, and other brain tumors are also reported.[12,15]

### Otolaryngological manifestations

Anomalies of the ear are common (60%–80%). These include prominent auricles, an abnormal ear canal, underdeveloped mastoids, and an abnormal stapes.[13] Otitis media is frequent (82%). Conductive or sensorineural hearing loss is documented.[1] In their review, Sculerati et al.[11] described 22 patients with this syndrome, 37% of whom had nerve loss and 45% had

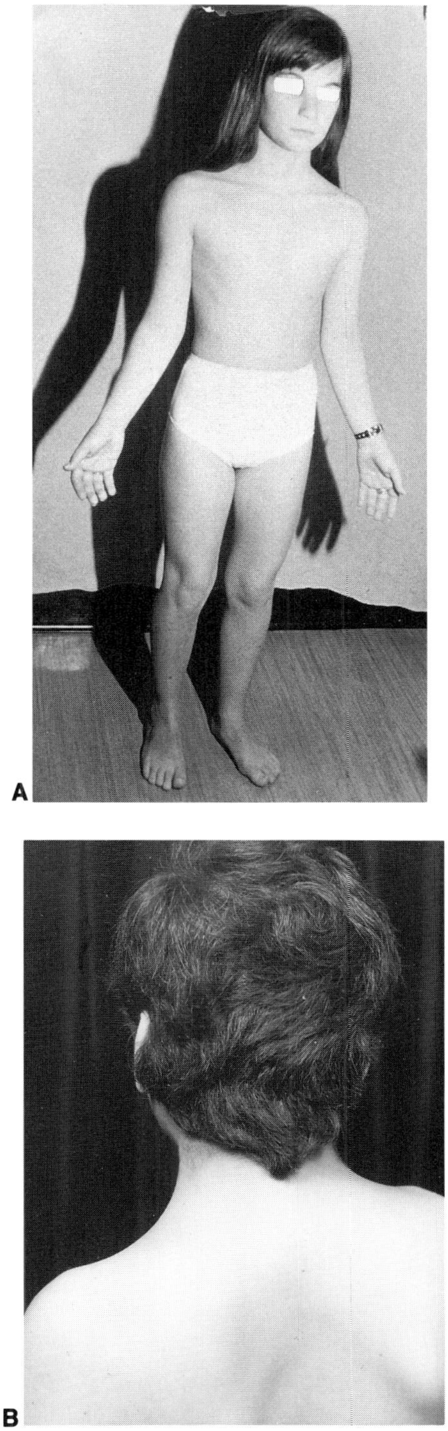

**Fig. 80.** Turner syndrome. A: Webbed neck, shield chest, and increased carrying angle. (Courtesy of Dr. FC Fraser.) B: Posterior hairline and webbed neck. (A,B from VM DerKaloustian, AK Kurban, *Genetic Diseases of the Skin,* Springer-Verlag, Berlin, 1979, p. 292, with permission.)

serous effusion. The neck is short and webbed with excessive skin in 80% of cases. Cystic hygroma has also been reported.[8] Micrognathia, high-arched palate, abnormal dentition, and premature eruptions are frequent occurrences.[5,6]

### Etiology

Approximately 50% of patients have one missing sex chromosome (45X). Other karyotypes also occur, e.g., 46,Xi(Xq), 45,XO/46XX, and 45,X/47,XXX. The frequency is estimated at 1:5,700 live female births. It is also estimated that 20% of miscarried fetuses have 45,X karyotypes.[3,7]

### Differential diagnosis

Turner syndrome should be differentiated from Klippel-Feil syndrome, Noonan syndrome, and multiple pterygium syndrome.

### References


1. Anderson H, Filipson R, Fleur E: Hearing impairment in Turner syndrome. Acta Otolaryngol 247:1–26, 1969.
2. Cohen MM Jr: Craniosynostosis in the Turner syndrome. Am J Med Genet 35:289–290, 1990.
3. De La Chapelle A: Sex chromosome abnormalities. In: Principles and Practice of Medical Genetics, EH Emery, DL Rimoin, eds. Churchill Livingstone, Edinburgh, 1983, pp 193–215.
4. Dierckx RA, Ebinger G, Herregodts P, Michotte A, Carly B, Schmedding E, Maillet B: Recurrent brachial plexus neuropathy and giant cell arteritis. Clin Neurol Neurosurg 92:71–74, 1990.
5. Horowitz SL, Morishima A: Palatal abnormalities in the syndrome of gonadal dysgenesis and its variants and in Noonan's syndrome. Oral Surg 38:839–844, 1974.
6. Jensen BL: Craniofacial morphology in Turner syndrome. J Craniofac Genet Dev Biol 5:327–340, 1985.
7. Kafu T, Ferrier A, Niikawa N, Takahara H, Ohama K, Avirachan S: Anatomic and chromosomal anomalies in 639 spontaneous abortuses. Hum Genet 55:87–98, 1980.
8. Kassanos D, Botsis D, Pyrgiotis E, Solarnalekis E, Giannaki F, Zourla PA: Cystic hygroma associated with Turner syndrome. Clin Exp Obstet Gynecol 19:222–225, 1992.
9. Risch WD, Bauzer DH, Moltz L, Schneider U, Rudloff R: Bone mineral content in patients with gonadal dysfunction. Am J Radiol 126:1302–1309, 1976.
10. Rovet JP: The psychoeducational characteristics of children with Turner syndrome. J Learn Disabil 26:333–341, 1993.
11. Sculerati N, Ledesma-Medina J, Finegold DN, Stool SE: Otitis media and hearing loss in Turner syndrome. Arch Otolaryngol Head Neck Surg 116:704–707, 1990.
12. Simpson JL: Gonadal dysgenesis and abnormalities of the human sex chromosomes: current status of phenotypic-karyotypic correlation. Birth Defects 11:23–59, 1975.
13. Szpunar J, Rybak M: Middle ear disease in Turner's syndrome. Arch Otolaryngol 87:34–40, 1968.
14. Turner HH: A syndrome of infantilism, congenital webbed neck and cubitus valgus. Endocrinology 23:566–578, 1938.
15. Wertelecki W, Fraumeni JF Jr, Mulvihill JJ: Nongonadal neoplasia in Turner's syndrome. Cancer 26:485–488, 1970.


## Usher syndrome

**Type IA:** MIM No. *276900; **Type IB:** (MIM No. *276903); **Type IC:** (MIM No. *276904); **Type II:** (MIM No. *276901);**Type III:** (MIM No. 276902; POSSUM No. 3421)

Von Graefe and Leibreich were the first to recognize the association between deafness and retinitis pigmentosa (RP). Usher subsequently emphasized its genetic nature.[11] The incidence of

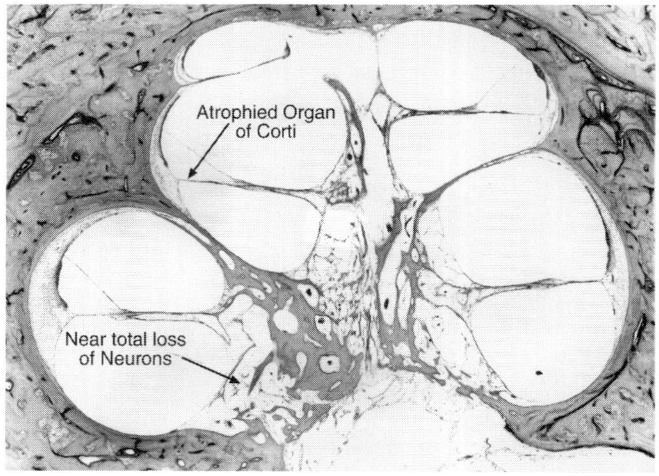


**Fig. 81.** Usher syndrome. Histological picture showing missing organ of Corti in the basal 15 mm and elsewhere, consists of a flat mound of undifferentiated cells. Reissner's membrane is thin and atrophic. The striae vasculares show patchy atrophy in the different turns. (From HF Schuknecht, *Pathology of the Ear,* 2nd ed., Lea & Febiger, Philadelphia, 1993, p. 135, with permission.)

Usher syndrome is estimated to be 3 to 5 per 100,000 in the general population and 1 to 10% among profoundly deaf children.[3,5,6]

### General manifestations

Clinical manifestations are deafness and retinitis pigmentosa. Ocular findings include cataracts in 50% of patients by age 40[8,9] and occasionally, glaucoma. Mental deficiency, psychosis, ataxia, and cataracts are sometimes associated with retinitis pigmentosa and deafness and are termed *Hallgren syndrome.*[7] Abnormalities of nasal cilia and sperm axonemes have been described.[8]

The life span is normal. Social and vocational preparation as deaf and blind adults is required.

### Otolaryngological manifestations

Deafness and vestibular dysfunction are important features and their assessment makes type classification possible.

### Clinical types[4,9]

*Usher, type I* (USH1). Profound congenital deafness and loss of vestibular functions characterize type I. Onset of retinitis pigmentosa is before puberty (around the age of 10 years). This constitutes 90% of patients.

*Usher, type II* (USH2). Hearing loss is moderate to severe from birth, and the vestibular functions are normal. Onset of retinitis pigmentosa is in the late teens.

*Usher, type III* (USH3). Progressive hearing loss occurs, and retinitis pigmentosa begins at puberty.

*Usher, type IV* (USH4). This type is clinically similar to type II, but in addition has X-linked recessive inheritance.

Types III and IV constitute less than 1% of patients. The changes in the temporal bone involve the cochlea.[2] Marked atrophy of the organ of Corti in the basal turn is associated with spiral ganglion degeneration.[1,10] These cochlear changes are similar to Scheibe inner ear dysplasia.

### Etiology

Usher syndrome is of autosomal recessive inheritance in most cases. X-linked recessive inheritance occurs in rare instances. Ush 1 is heterogeneous, with loci on chromosomes 14 (USH1A),[8a] 11q (USH1B),[8b,10a] 11p (USH1C)[10a] and 10q (USH1D).[12] USH2A and USH3 have been mapped to chromosomes 1q and 3q respectively.[9a,9b] The USH1B encodes myosin VII A.[13] Those individuals with Usher syndrome who are of Acadian heritage, most of whom live in Louisiana have the USH1C type. At least one additional Usher syndrome exists with an unidentified gene. Nearly 10% of USH2 families have been excluded from chromosome 1q linkage.[12]

### Differential diagnosis

Usher syndrome should be differentiated from syndromes involving retinal degeneration and hearing loss. These include the following autosomal recessive disorders:

1. Cockayne syndrome (retinitis pigmentosa [RP], optic atrophy, deafness, premature senility, dwarfism, and mental retardation)
2. Alström syndrome (RP, nystagmus, hearing loss, obesity, diabetes mellitus, nephropathy, and acanthosis nigricans)
3. Friedreich ataxia (RP, optic atrophy, nystagmus, deafness, spinocerebellar dystrophy, and dysarthria)
4. Refsum disease (pigmentary retinopathy, chronic polyneuritis, cerebellar signs, ECG changes, ichthyosis, and excess of phytanic acid)

Autosomal dominant disorders that should be considered include

1. Alport syndrome (nephropathy, myopia, anterior lenticonus, cataracts, occasional retinal pigmentary changes, and deafness)
2. Congenital spondyloepiphyseal dysplasia (retinal degeneration, high myopia, dwarfism, cleft palate, cataract, congenital glaucoma, and mild deafness)
3. Flynn Aird syndrome (RP, cataract, myopia, ataxia, peripheral neuritis, dementia, epilepsy, skin atrophy, baldness, dental caries, cystic bone changes, and deafness)

### References


1. Belal A: Usher's syndrome: a temporal bone report. J Laryngol Otol 89:175–181, 1975.
2. Cremers CWRJ, Delleman WJW: Usher's syndrome: temporal bone pathology. Int J Pediatr Otolaryngol 16:23–30, 1988.
3. Fritsch M, Sommer A: Handbook of Congenital and Early Onset Hearing Loss. Igaku-Shoin, New York, 1990, pp 133–137.
4. Gorlin RJ: Usher's syndrome, type III. Arch Otolaryngol 105:353–354, 1979.
5. Gorlin RJ, Toriello HV, Cohen MM Jr: Hereditary Hearing Loss and Its Syndromes. Oxford University Press, New York, 1995, pp 105–108.
6. Grondahl J: Estimation of prognosis and prevalence of retinitis pigmentosa and Usher syndrome in Norway. Clin Genet 31:225–264, 1987.
7. Hallgren V: Retinitis pigmentosa combined with congenital deafness, with vestibulo-cerebellar ataxia and mental abnormality in a proportion of cases. A clinical and geneticostatistical study. Acta Psychiatr Scand 18:1–101, 1959.
8. Hunter DG: Abnormal sperm and photoreceptor axonemes in Usher's syndrome. Arch Ophthalmol 141:600–604, 1986.

8a. Kaplan J, Gerber S, Bonneau D, Rozet JM, Delrieu O, Briard ML, Dollfus H, Ghazi I, Durier JL, Frézal J, Munnich A: A gene for Usher syndrome type I (USH1A) maps to chromosome 14q. Genomics 14:979–987, 1992.

8b. Kimberling WJ, Möller CG, Davenport S, Priluck IA, Beighton PH, Greenberg J, Reardon W, Weston MD, Kenyon JB, Grunkemeyer JA et al.: Linkage of Usher syndrome type I gene (USH1B) to the long arm of chromosome 11. Genomics 14:988–994, 1992.

9. Kimberling W, Smith RJ: Gene mapping of the Usher syndromes. Otolaryngol Clin North Am 25:923–935, 1992.

9a. Kimberling WJ, Weston MD, Möller C, Davenport SLH, Shugart YY, Priluck IA, Martini A, Milani M, Smith R: Localization of Usher syndrome type II to chromosome 1q. Genomics 7:245–249, 1990.

9b. Sankila EM, Pakarinen L, Kääriäinen H, Aittomäki K, Karjalainen S, Sistonen P, de la Chapelle A: Assignment of an Usher syndrome type III (USH3) gene to chromosome 3q. Hum Mol Genet 4:93–98, 1995.

10. Shinkawa H, Nadol JB Jr: Histopathology of the inner ear in Usher's syndrome as observed by light and electron microscopy. Ann Otol Rhinol Laryngol 95:313–318, 1986.

10a. Smith RJH, Lee EC, Kimberling WJ, Daiger SP, Pelias MZ, Keats BJB, Jay M, Bird A, Reardon W, Guest M et al.: Localization of two genes for Usher syndrome type I to chromosome 11. Genomics 14:995–1002, 1992.

11. Usher CH: On the inheritance of retinitis pigmentosa with notes of cases. R Lond Ophthalmol Hosp Rep XIX:130–236, 1914.

12. Wayne S, Der Kaloustian VM, Schloss M, Polomeno R, Scott DA, Hejtmancik JF, Sheffield VC, Smith RJH: Localization of the Usher syndrome type ID (USH1D) to chromosome 10. Hum Mol Genet 5:1689–1692, 1996.

13. Weil D, Blanchard S, Kaplan J, Guilford P, Gibson F, Walsh J, Mburu P, Varela V, Levilliers J, Weston MD et al.: Defective myosin VII A gene responsible for Usher syndrome type 1B. Nature 374:60–61, 1995.


## Van Buchem disease

**Hyperostosis corticalis generalisata**
(MIM No. 239100; POSSUM No. 3256)

This disease was first described by Van Buchem et al. in 1962[5] and is characterized by osteosclerosis of the skull, mandible, clavicles, and ribs. The long and short bones display hyperplasia of the diaphyseal cortex.

### General manifestations

These include mild exophthalmos, headaches, and optic atrophy preceded by papilledema which leads to blindness after age 30.

The radiological features rarely include obliteration of the medullary cavities. The serum alkaline phosphatase is usually elevated. Anemia and spontaneous fractures do not occur.

### Otolaryngological manifestations

Van Buchem disease usually presents in late childhood as a widened chin and thickened mandible similar to acromegaly. X-ray studies reveal thickening of the skull roof and base without increase in the circumference. The facial changes develop slowly. The osteosclerosis of the skull results in facial paralysis and sensorineural hearing loss, usually progressive in nature.[3]

### Etiology

This syndrome is of autosomal recessive inheritance.

### Differential diagnosis

A recessive form of the disease has been described by Beighton et al.,[1] where syndactyly of the second and third fingers occur.

A sporadic case was described by Gorlin et al.,[3] where the mandible was huge and the scapula and tarsal bones were in-

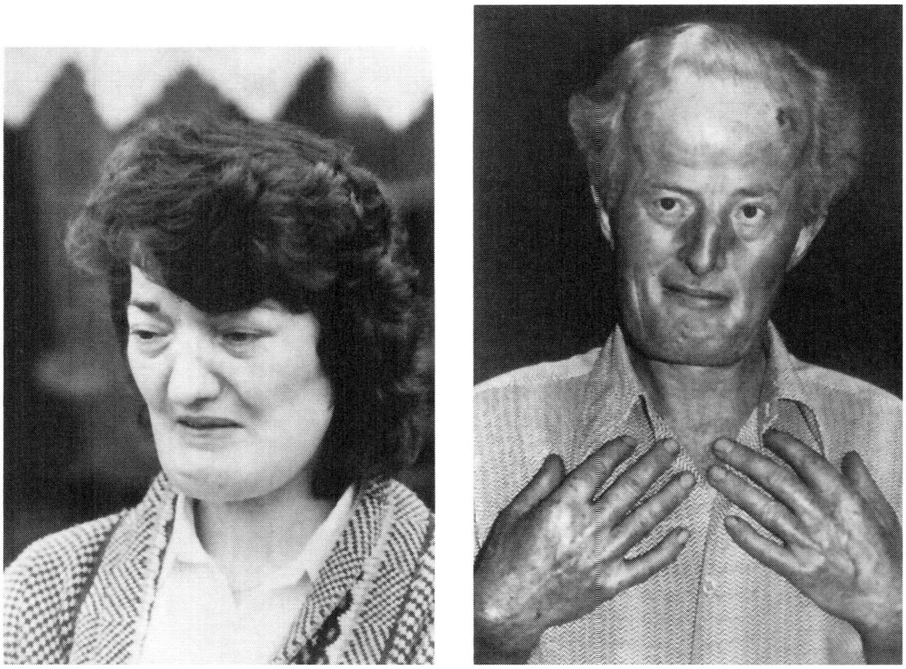

A B

**Fig. 82.** Van Buchem disease. A,B: Note the wide and thick mandible in both patients. (From P Beightonet et al., Clin Genet 25:175, 1984, with permission.)

volved but the ribs were not sclerosed. It was termed *pseudo-Van Buchem disease.*

A dominant form has also been reported[2,4] in which the medullary cavity of the long bones is filiform and their growth is reduced.

### References


1. Beighton P, Barnard A, Hamersma H, van der Wouden A: The syndromic status of sclerosteosis and Van Buchem disease. Clin Genet 25:175–81, 1984.
2. Caffey JP: Congenital stenosis of medullary spaces in tubular bones and calvaria in two proportionate dwarfs. Am J Roentgenol 100:1–14, 1967.
3. Gorlin RJ, Cohen MM, Levin LS: Syndromes of the Head and Neck, 3rd ed. Oxford University Press, New York, 1990, p 240.
4. Kenny FM, Linarelli L: Dwarfism and cortical thickening of tubular bones: transient hypocalcemia in mother and son. Am J Dis Child 111:201–207, 1966.
5. Van Buchem FSP, Hadders HN, Hansen JF, Woldring MG: Hyperostosis corticalis generalisata: report of seven cases. Am J Med 33:387–397, 1962.


## Van der Woude syndrome

### Cleft lip/palate with lip pits
(MIM NO. *119300; POSSUM No. 3140)

Congenital lip pits were described as early as 1845.[5] Van der Woude is credited with describing the clinical features of the syndrome that bears his name.[14]

#### General manifestations

Fusion of the eyelids has been described.[12] Accessory nipples, talipes equinovarus, syndactyly, aganglionic megacolon, and congenital heart anomalies have also been reported.[7,8,11]

#### Otolaryngological manifestations

Paramedian lip pits are usually bilateral. Occasionally, they are asymmetric. They vary in depth from a few mm to 3 cm or more. They usually occur on the vermilion border of the lower lip. The depth may reach 10 to 15 mm and they may secrete mucus. A communication with the minor salivary glands of the lower lip may exist. Midline pits or grooves are rarely seen. Hypodontia and missing second premolars and/or bicuspids may occur. The association of cleft lip/palate with lip pits is estimated to be 66%. Submucous cleft palate is not rare. Adhesions between the maxilla and mandible have been noted.[2,10,12]

#### Etiology and pathogenesis

Van der Woude syndrome is of autosomal dominant inheritance, with 90% or higher penetrance. New mutations account for 30%–50% of cases.

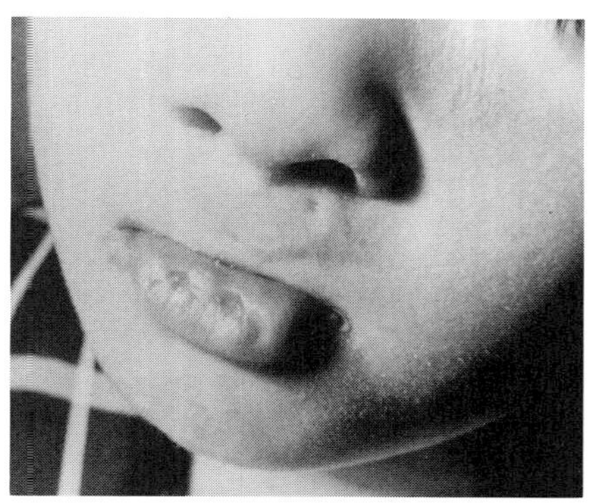

**Fig. 83.** Van der Woude syndrome. Note the paired depressions of the lower lips, or lip pits. (From GG Nora, FC Fraser, *Medical Genetics,* Lea & Febiger, Philadelphia, 1974, p. 113, with permission.)

The lip pits represent vestigeal remnants of the lateral sulci of the mandible at the 7.5 to 12.5 mm stage embryo.[3,9,13]

A patient was described with an interstitial deletion of chromosome 1q,del(1q32–q41).[1] Linkage found to loci on chromosome 1q.[6,9a]

A locus for orofacial clefting has also been found on chromosome 6p24.[4]

### Differential diagnosis

Commissural lip pits in the corner of the mouth occur more frequently and do not relate to this syndrome. Their incidence is approximately 1:300 among Caucasians and 1:48 in the American black population. Lip pits occur in the popliteal pterygium syndrome and in the entity of aganglionic megacolon with cleft lip/palate.

### References


1. Bocian M, Walker AP: Lip pits and deletion 1q32–q41. Am J Med Genet 26:437–443, 1987.
2. Burdick AB: Genetic epidemiology and control of genetic expression in Van der Woude syndrome. J Craniofac Genet Dev Biol Suppl 2:99–105, 1986.
3. Cervenka J, Gorlin RJ, Anderson VE: The syndrome of pits of the lower lip and cleft lip and/or palate. Genetic considerations. Am J Hum Genet 19:416–432, 1967.
4. Davies AF, Stephens RJ, Olavesen MG, Heather L, Dixon MJ, Magee A, Flinter F, Ragoussis J: Evidence of a locus for orofacial clefting on human chromosome 6p24 and STS content map of the region. Hum Mol Genet 4:121–128, 1995.
5. Demorquay JN: Quelques considérations sur le bec-de-lièvre. Gazette Med (Paris) 13:52–54, 1845.
6. Murray JC, Nishimura DY, Buetow KH, Ardinger HH, Spence MA, Sparkes RS, Falk RE, Falk PM, Gardner RJM, Harkness EM, et al: Linkage of an autosomal dominant clefting syndrome (Van der Woude) to loci on chromosome 1q. Am J Hum Genet 46:486–491, 1990.
7. Pauli RM, Hall JG: Lip pits, cleft lip and/or palate and congenital heart disease. Am J Dis Child 134:293–295, 1980.
8. Pohl L: Letter to the editor. Dent Pract Dent Rec 7:112, 1956.
9. Rintala AE, Ranta R: Lower lip sinuses. Epidemiology, microforms and transverse sulci. Br J Plast Surg 34:25–30, 1980

9a. Sander A, Murray JC, Scherpbier-Heddema T, Bueton KH, Weissenbach J, Zingg M, Ludwig K, Schmelzle R: Microsatellite-based fine mapping of the Van der Woude syndrome locus to an interval of 4.1 cM between D1S245 and D1S414. Am J Hum Genet 56:310–318, 1995.

10. Schinzel A, Klausler M: The Van der Woude syndrome (dominantly inherited lip pits and cleft). J Med Genet 23:291–294, 1986.
11. Schwartz KB: Congenital lip pits and Hirschsprung disease. J Pediatr Surg 14:162–164, 1979.
12. Shaw WC, Simpson JP: Oral adhesions associated with cleft lip and palate and lip fistulae. Cleft Palate J A:127–131, 1980.
13. Shprintzen RJ, Goldberg RB, Sidoti EJ: The penetrance and variable expression of the Van der Woude syndrome: implications for genetic counselling. Cleft Palate J 17:52–57, 1980.
14. Van der Woude A: Fistula labii inferioris congenita and its association with cleft lip and palate. Am J Hum Genet 6:224–256, 1954.


## VATER association

(MIM No. 192350; POSSUM No. 3425)

### General and otolaryngological manifestations:

*VATER* is an acronym used for **V**ertebral defects, **A**nal atresia, **T**racheoesophageal fistula with **E**sophageal atresia and **R**adial dysplasia. The diagnosis is made if three of the above are present. The association is presently expanded to the term *VACTERL*. The *C* stands for Cardiac malformations, the *R* for **R**enal anomalies, and the *L* for **L**imb anomalies, such as hexadactyly, humeral hypoplasia, radial aplasia, and a proximally placed thumb. Others use the acronym *VATERS,* with the *V* standing for **V**ertebral defects and **V**entricular septal defect and the *S* for **S**ingle umbilical artery.[3,5]

It is uncommon to see seven or eight anomalies in one patient. Mental retardation is an occasional problem.

Vertebral anomalies are seen in 70% of cases, cardiovascular defects in 50%, anal atresia with or without fistula in 80%, tracheoesophageal fistula with esophageal atresia in 70%, limb abnormalities in 65%, renal anomalies in 50%, and single umbilical artery in 35% of cases.[3–5] The prognosis depends on the particular combination and severity of the anomalies. An overall survival of 72% was reported for 46 patients.[6]

### Etiology

The etiology is unknown. The occurrence is sporadic. It is more frequently seen in children of diabetic mothers.[1,2]

### References


1. Auchterlonie IA, White MP: Recurrence of the VATER association within a sibship. Clin Genet 21:122–124, 1982.
2. Khoury MJ, Cordero JF, Greenberg F, James LM, Rickson JD: A population study of VACTERL association: evidence for its etiologic heterogeneity. Pediatrics 71:815–820, 1983.
3. Quan L, Smith DW: The VATER association, vertebral defects, anal atresia, T-E fistula with esophageal atresia, radial and renal dysplasia: a spectrum of associated defects. J Pediatr 82:104–107, 1973.
4. Say B, Balci S, Pirnar T, Tuncbilek E: A new syndrome of dysmorphogenesis: imperforate-anus associated with poly-oligodactyly and skeletal (mainly vertebral) anomalies. Acta Paediatr Scand 60:197–202, 1971.
5. Temtamy SA, Miller JD: Extending the scope of VATER association: definition of a VATER syndrome. 85:345–349, 1974.
6. Weaver DD, Mapstone CL, Yu P: The VATER association: analysis of 46 patients. Am J Dis Child 140:225–229, 1986.


## Waardenburg syndrome

(Type I: MIM No. *193500; POSSUM No. 3426
Type II: MIM No. *193510; POSSUM No. 4100)

Van der Hoeve and Mende described certain aspects of this syndrome but Waardenburg was the first to define it in 1951.[12,22]

### General manifestations

Along with congenital sensorineural deafness there are multiple congenital anomalies. The widely spaced medial canthi (dystopia canthorum) is characteristic of type I. Lack of penetrance of this sign occurs in no more than 1% of cases. Confluent eyebrows with hypertrichosis of their medial portions (synophyrs) is present in 85% of type I and 25% of type II. White forelock (poliosis) occurs 20 to 40% of the time in type I or II and heterochromia irides occurs in 30% of patients of both types.

Other findings include craniosynostosis, blepharophimosis, glaucoma, mild prognathic mandible,[15] Hirschsprung megacolon, premature graying of hair, anophthalmia with limb malformations, VSD, meningocele, spina bifida, hypoplasia of the shoulder girdle, and axillary webbing.[10]

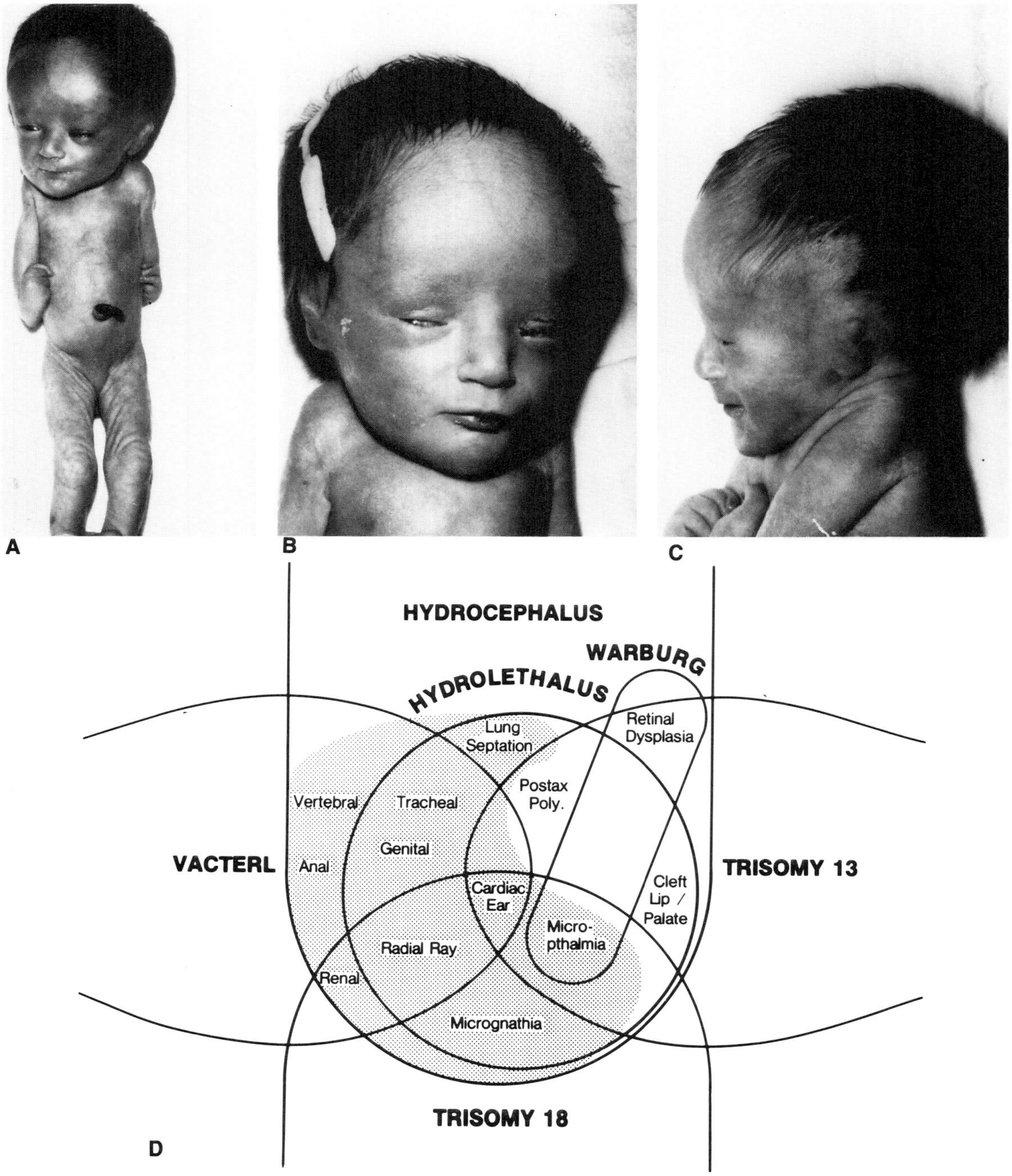


**Fig. 84.** VACTERL association. A–C: VACTERL association (with hydrocephalus). D: Diagram illustrating the overlap between VACTERL and hydrocephalus (shaded area), and other syndromes with similar findings. (From JA Evans et al., Am J Med Genet 34:177, 1989, with permission.)

## Clinical types

In type I dystopia canthorum is present. This condition is 20 times more common in type I than in type II.

In type II dystopia canthorum is not present. Hearing loss is more common in this type (50%), as are pigmentary disorders.

Type III: Klein-Waardenburg syndrome or pseudo-Waardenburg: no dystopia canthorum, but instead a one-sided ptosis of the upper eyelid and upper limb anomalies.[1]

A Waardenburg-Hirschsprung disease association has also been described as a clinical type.[13]

## Otolaryngological manifestations

Deafness, a broad nasal bridge, hypoplastic alae nasi, a high-arched or cleft palate, abnormal vestibular function,[11] and hypoplastic ear cartilage all characterize Waardenburg syndrome.

Sensorineural hearing loss is either unilateral (15% incidence in type I and 5% in type II) or more commonly bilateral (20% incidence in type I and 55% in type II).[4,7] The loss is usually in the low and middle frequencies and in normal hearing of 6,000 to 8000 Hz. Abnormal vestibular functions are noted in type II but not in type I.[8]

Temporal bone studies showed an absence of the organ of Corti with thickening of the basal membrane and degeneration of the spiral ganglion.[4,17]

## Etiology

Inheritance follows the autosomal dominant pattern with variable penetrance. Three percent of all congenitally deaf children have Waardenburg syndrome. Its incidence is estimated to be 1 in 20,000 to 1 in 40,000 of the population.

Waardenburg syndrome, types I (WSI) and III (WSIII) have been mapped to 2q35 and found to be associated with *PAX3* mutations.[3,5,21] They are considered to be allelic.[19] Waardenburg syndrome type II (WSII) is heterogeneous, with about 20% of cases caused by mutations in the human microphthalmia *(MITF)* gene mapped at 3p14.1–p12.3.[18a,19,20] Individuals with auditory, pigmetary, or neural crest syndromes which do not fit stringent definitions of Waardenburg syndrome are unlikely to have mutations in either *PAX3* or *MITF* genes.[19]

Families carrying substitutions in the same codon do not necessarily reveal conspicuous clinical similarities. Intrafamilial variation may not be explained by mutational heterogeneity. The possibility of modifier genes or a polygenic background must be taken into consideration.[14]

A mutation of the endothelin-receptor B *(EDNRB)* gene has been reported in Waardenburg-Hirschprung disease.[2] This is a homozygous missense mutation in exon 2 of the *EDNRB* gene, lending support to the involvement of an endothelin-mediated pathway in the development of neural crest derivatives during early embryonic stages.

## Differential diagnosis

Dystopia canthorum and hypertelorism, could be identified in a variety of syndromes.[16] In Vogt-Koyanagi syndrome patients display poliosis, vitiligo, and dysacousia associated with alopecia and uveitis.[9] De Lange syndrome patients have synophyrs associated with pilonidal cyst.[18] Other syndromes may be asso-

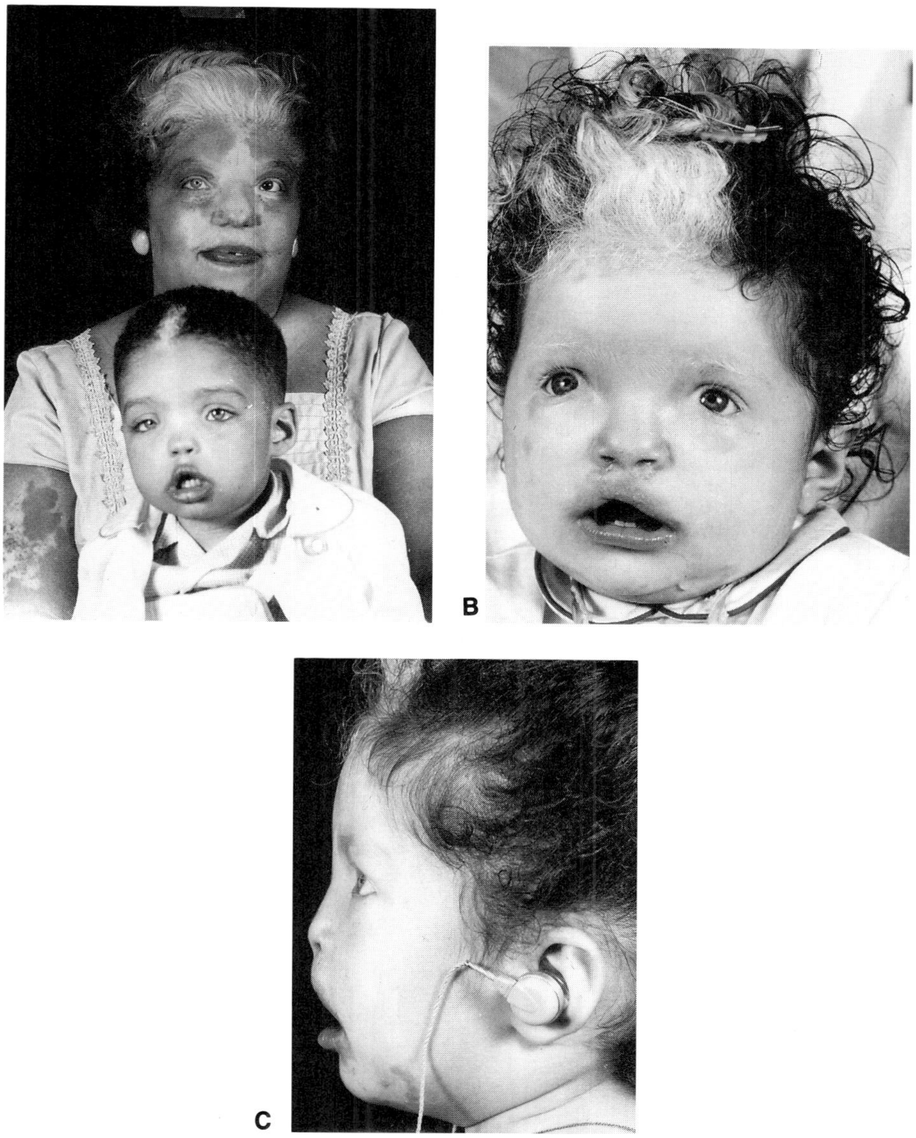

**Fig. 85.** Waardenburg syndrome. A–C: Mother and children with Waardenburg syndrome. Note heterochromia of the iris (in the mother), broad nasal bridge, dystopia canthorum, and synophyrs (child in B). (From VM Der Kaloustian, AK Kurban, *Genetic Diseases of the Skin,* Springer-Verlag, Berlin, 1979, p. 66, with permission; courtesy of Dr. VA McKusick.)

ciated with heterochromia irides, poliosis, or hypoplastic alar cartilages.[6]

## References


1. Arias S: Genetic heterogeneity in the Waardenburg syndrome. Birth Defects 7:87–101, 1971.
2. Attié T, Till M, Pelet A, Amiel J, Edery P, Boutrand L, Munnich A, Lyonnet S: Mutation of the endothelin-receptor B gene in Waardenburg-Hirschsprung disease. Hum Mol Genet 4:2407–2409, 1995.
3. Baldwin CT, Hoth CF, Macina RA, Milunsky A: Mutations in PAX3 that cause Waardenburg syndrome Type I: ten new mutations and review of the literature. Am J Med Genet 58:115–122, 1995.
4. Fisch L: Deafness as part of a hereditary syndrome. J Laryngol Otolaryngol 73:355–383, 1959.
5. Foy C, Newton V, Wellesley D, Harris R, Read AP: Assignment of the locus for Waardenburg Syndrome type I to human chromosome 2q37 and possible homology of the Splotch mouse. Am J Hum Genet 46:1017–1023, 1990.
6. Gorlin RJ, Cohen MM Jr, Levin LS: Syndromes of the Head and Neck, 3rd ed. Oxford University Press, New York, 1990, pp 466–469.
7. Hageman MJ, Delleman JW: Heterogeneity in Waardenburg syndrome. Am J Hum Genet 29:468–485, 1977.
8. Hageman MJ, Oosterveld WJ: Vestibular findings in 25 patients with Waardenburg's syndrome. Arch Otolaryngol 103:648–652, 1977.
9. Hague EB: Uveitis, dysacousia, alopecia, poliosis and vitiligo. Arch Ophthalmol 31:520–538, 1944.
10. Klein D: Albinisme partiel (leucisme) accompagné de surdimutité, d'ostéomyodysplasie, de raideurs articulaires congénitales multiples et d'autres malformations congénitales, Arch Klaus Stift Vererbungs forsch Sozialanthropol Rassenhyg 22:336–342, 1947.
11. Marcus RE: Vestibular function and additional findings in Waardenburg's syndrome. Acta Otolaryngol (Suppl) 229:1–30, 1968.
12. Mende I: Über eine Familie hereditär—degenerativer Taubstummer mit mongoladem Einschlag und teilweisen Leukismus der Haut und Haare. Arch Kinderheilkd 79:214–222, 1926.
13. Omenn GS, McKusick VA: The association of Waardenburg syndrome and Hirschsprung megacolon. Am J Med Genet 3:217–223, 1979.
14. Pandya A, Xia X-J, Landa BL, Arnos KS, Israel J, Lloyd J, James AL, Diehl SR, Blanton SH, Nance WE: Phenotypic variation in Waardenburg syndrome: mutational heterogeneity, modifier genes or polygenic background? Hum Mol Genet 5:497–502, 1996.
15. Pantke OA, Cohen MM Jr: The Waardenburg syndrome. Birth Defects 7:147–152, 1971.
16. Peterson MQ, Cohen MM Jr, Sedano HO, Frerichs CT: Comments on frontonasal dysplasia, ocular hypertelorism and dystopia canthorum. Birth Defects 7:120–124, 1971.
17. Rarey KE, Davis LE: Inner ear anomalies in Waardenburg's syndrome with Hirschsprung's disease. Int J Pediatr Otorhinolaryngol 8:181–189, 1984.
18. Sebrechts PH: A significant sign of pilonidal cyst. Dis Colon Rectum 4:56–59, 1961.

18a. Tachibana M, Takeda K, Nobukuni Y, Urabe K, Long JE, Meyers KA, Aaronson SA, Miki T: Ectopic expression of *MITF,* a gene for Waardenburg syndrome type 2, converts fibroblasts to cells with melanocyte characteristics. Nat Genet 14:50–54, 1996.

19. Tassabehji M, Newton VE, Liu X-Z, Brady A, Donnai D, Krajeswka-Walasek M, Murday V, Norman A, Obersztyn E, Reardon W, et al: The mutational spectrum in Waardenburg syndrome. Hum Mol Genet 4:2131–2137, 1995.
20. Tassabehji M, Newton VE, Read AP: Waardenburg syndrome type 2 caused by mutations in the human microphtalmia (MITF) gene. Nature Genet 8:251–255, 1994.
21. Tassabehji M, Read AP, Newton VE, Harris R, Balling R, Gruss P, Strachan T: Waardenburg's syndrome patients have mutations in the human homologue of the PAX-3 paired box gene. Nature 355:635–636, 1992.
22. Waardenburg PJ: A new syndrome combining developmental anomalies of the eyelids, eyebrows, and nose root with pigmentary defects of the iris and head, hair and congenital deafness. Am J Hum Genet 3:195–253, 1951.


## Weaver syndrome

### Camptodactyly, overgrowth, and unusual facies syndrome
### (MIM No. 277590; POSSUM No. 3429)

This syndrome was first reported by Weaver et al. in 1974.[5] It is characterized by overgrowth, unusual facies, broad distal splaying of the femurs, camptodactyly, and atlantoaxial instability.

#### General manifestations

Postnatal excessive growth is seen in most patients. Motor and developmental delay are also common. Most cases have excessive appetite, hypertonia, and occasional seizures. The extremities show prominent finger pads, limited extension of the big joints, and hyperextensibility of the digits.[1,2,5]

The carpal bone age is generally increased. Talipes equinovarus, scoliosis or kyphosis, and umbilical herniae are features in over half of the reports.[1]

Less common traits are thin scalp hair, short ribs, epicanthal folds, ventricular dilatation, and cerebral atrophy.

#### Otolaryngological manifestations

Micrognathia, hypertelorism, and large ears occur in almost all cases. The palate is high arched. The nasal bridge is depressed, palpebral fissures slant downward, the occiput is flat, and the neck displays redundant skin folds.[1,3] The voice and cry are low pitched. Dysphagia also occurs.[6]

#### Etiology

The etiology is unknown. Almost all cases have been sporadic.

#### Differential diagnosis

This should include other overgrowth syndromes, e.g., Soto's, Marshall-Smith, and Teebi overgrowth syndrome.[4]

#### References


1. Ardinger HH, Hanson JW, Harros MJ, Cohen MM JR, Tibbles JA, Welch JP, Young-Wee T, Sommer A, Goldberg R, Shprintzen RJ, et al: Further delineation of Weaver syndrome. J Pediatr 108:228–235, 1986.
2. Farrell SA, Hughes HE: Weaver syndrome with pes cavus. Am J Med Genet 21:737–739, 1985.
3. Fitch N: Update on the Marshall-Smith-Weaver controversy. Am J Med Genet 20:559–562, 1985.
4. Teebi AS, Sundareshan TS, Hammouri MY, al-Awadi SA, al-Saleh QA: A new autosomal recessive disorder resembling Weaver syndrome. Am J Med Genet 33:479–482, 1989.
5. Weaver PD, Graham CB, Thomas IT, Smith DW: A new overgrowth syndrome with accelerated skeletal maturation, unusual facies and camptodactyly. J Pediatr 84:547–552, 1974.
6. Weisschichert PH, Knapp G, Willich E: Accelerated bone maturation syndrome of the Weaver type. Eur J Pediatr 137:329–333, 1981.

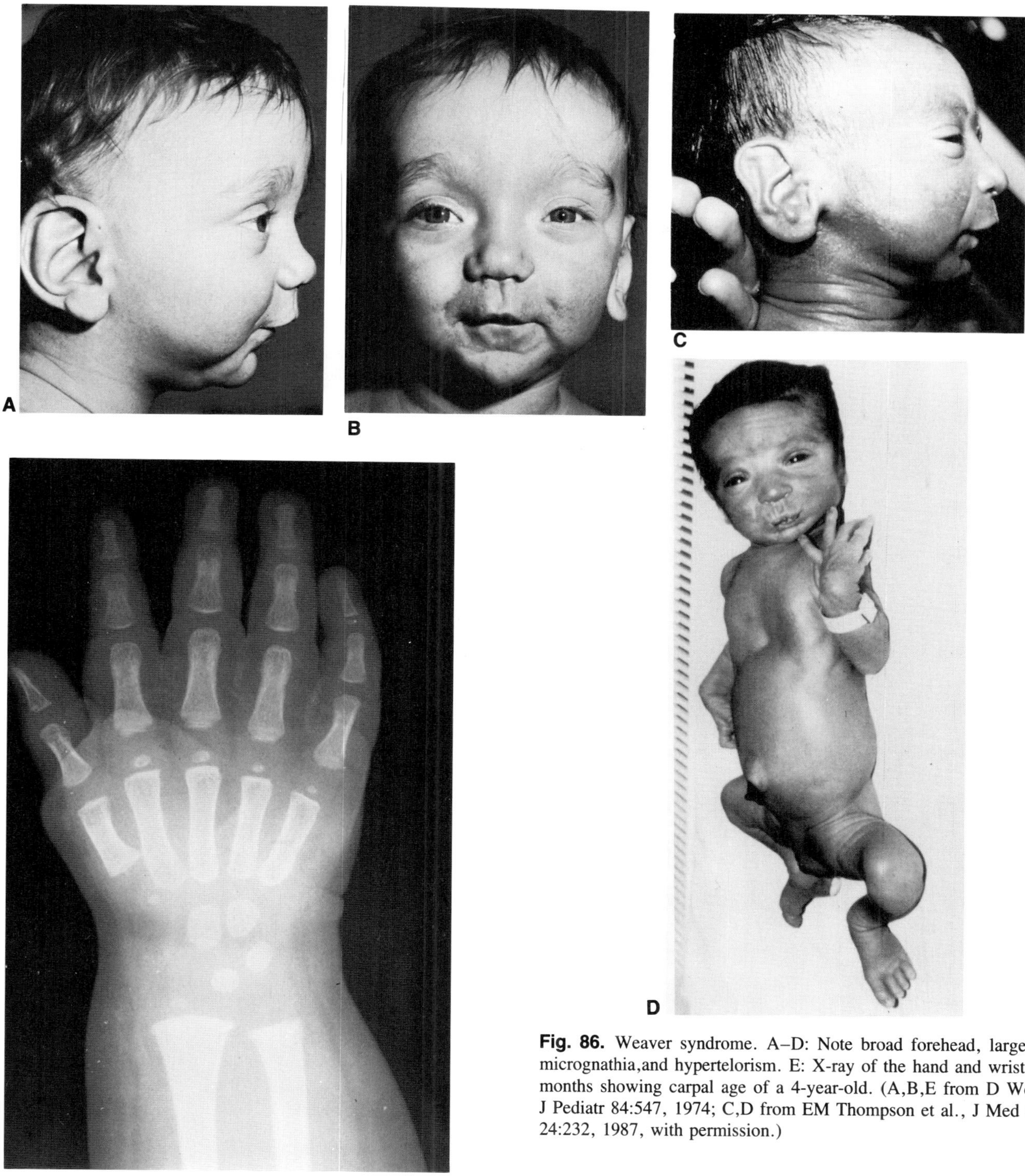

**Fig. 86.** Weaver syndrome. A–D: Note broad forehead, large ears, micrognathia,and hypertelorism. E: X-ray of the hand and wrist at 11 months showing carpal age of a 4-year-old. (A,B,E from D Weaver, J Pediatr 84:547, 1974; C,D from EM Thompson et al., J Med Genet 24:232, 1987, with permission.)

## Whistling face syndrome

### Freeman-Sheldon syndrome or Cranio-carpo-tarsal dysplasia

(MIM No. *193700; POSSUM No. 3156)

This syndrome was first described by Freeman and Sheldon[6] in 1938. It is characterized by the puckered appearance of the mouth, microstoma, flat facies, camptodactyly with ulnar deviation of the hands and talipes equinovarus. Burian[2] in 1963 coined the term *whistling face syndrome*.

#### General manifestations

The ulnar deviation of the hands is described as congenital windmill vane position.[8] Flexion contractures of fingers is common. The thumbs may be adducted at the metacarpophalangeal joint. The skin is thick over the flexor surface of the hands.

Talipes equinovarus is mostly unilateral and occurs in most patients. The neck is usually short; spina bifida occulta is a less frequent anomaly. Growth retardation, below the third percentile, is often described.[7] Bronchopneumonia is mentioned as the cause of death.[10]

### Otolaryngological manifestations

The face is immobile with microstomia and hypertelorism. An H- or V-shaped crease is usually seen extending from the lower lip to the chin in one-third of the cases.[4] The eyes are sunken and strabismus and/or epicanthus may be present. The palate is high arched, the tongue and mandible are hypoplastic. The nose and nostrils are small. Speech is usually nasal. The philtrum is elongated and the cheeks bulge. Radiologically, the anterior cranial fossa is steep.[11,13]

Typical facies are seen in approximately half of the cases.[1] Marasovich et al. described conductive hearing loss and serous otitis media in two patients and Burzynski et al. had one patient with sensorineural hearing loss.[3,9]

### Etiology

Whistling face syndrome is of autosomal dominant inheritance. Autosomal recessive forms are also reported.[5] Some others suggest that the syndrome is a form of congenital myopathy.[12]

### Differential diagnosis

Whistling face syndrome should be differentiated from Schwartz-Jampel syndrome, Burton syndrome, and Kniest syndrome.

### References

1. Antley RM, Uga N, Burzynski NJ, Baum RS, Bixler D: Diagnostic criteria for the Whistling Face syndrome. Birth Defects 11:161–168, 1975.
2. Burian F: The "whistling face" characteristic in a compound cranio-facio-carpotarsal syndrome. Br J Plast Surg 16:140–143, 1963.
3. Burzynski NJ, Podruch PE, Howell J, Snawder K: Cranio-carpo-tarsal dysplasia syndrome (Whistling Face syndrome). Oral Surg Oral Med Oral Pathol 39:893–900, 1975.

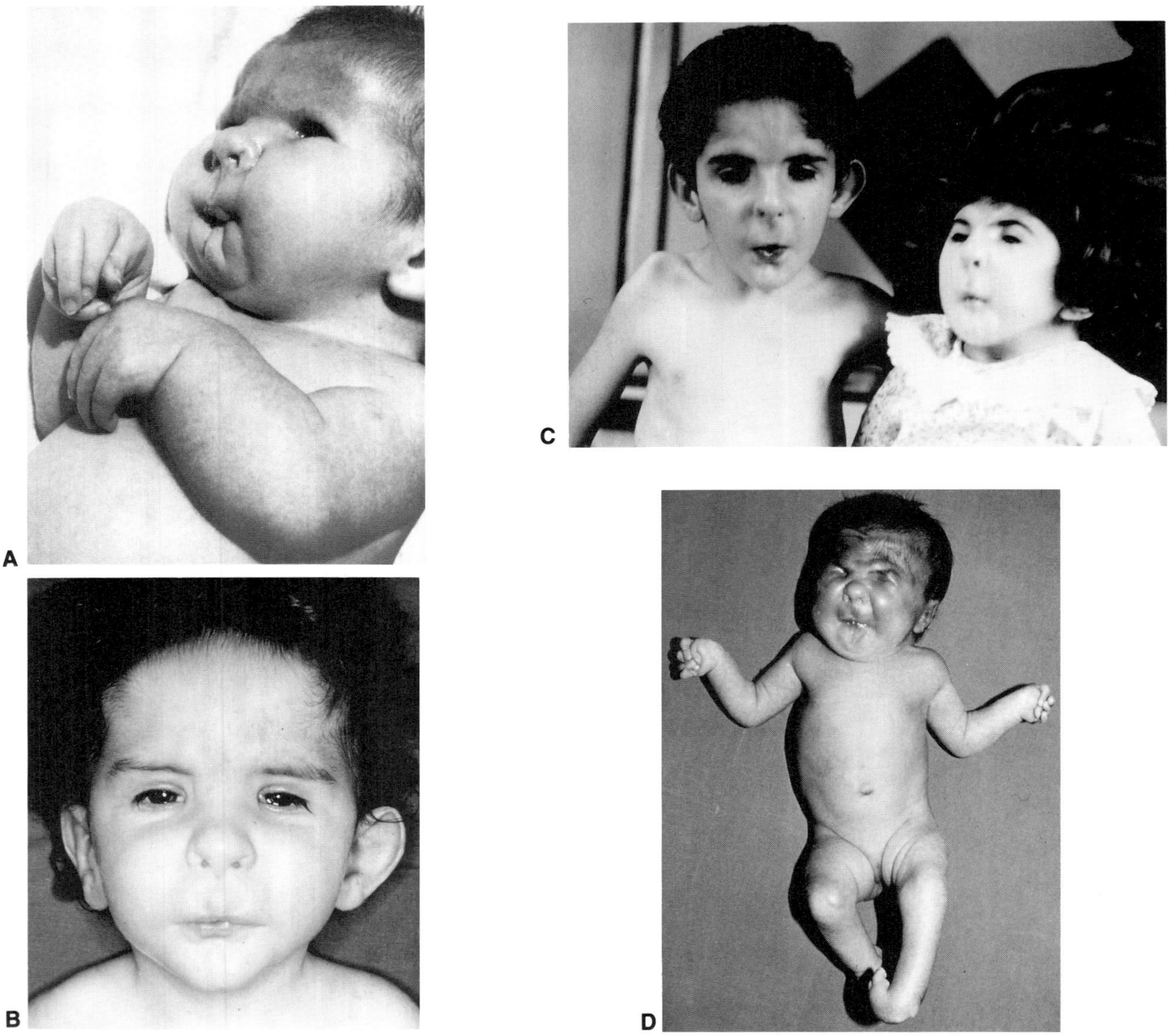

**Fig. 87.** Whistling face syndrome. A: Child with sunken eyes, pursed lips, long philtrum, band from lower lip to chin demarcated by grooves. (From VM Der Kaloustian, AK Kurban, *Genetic Diseases of the Skin,* Springer-Verlag, Gerlin, 1979, p. 96, with permission; courtesy of Dr. FC Fraser.) B: Another patient with characteristic facies. Note abnormal left ear. C: Brother and sister with the syndrome. D: Note the adducted thumbs and talipes equinovarus. (B–D from B Dallapiccola et al., Am J Med Genet 33:542, 1989, with permission, courtesy of Dr. L Zelante.)

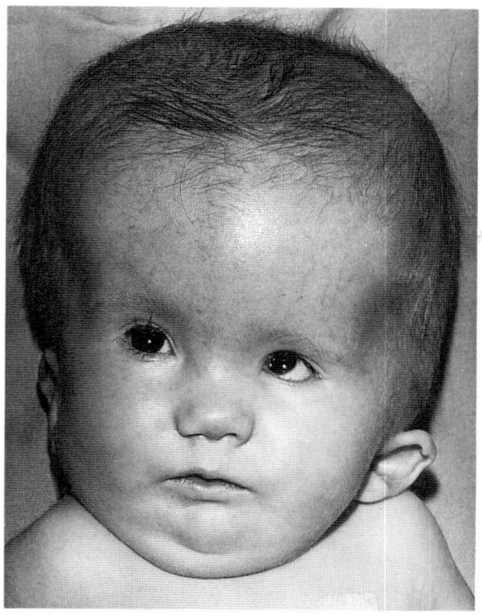

A

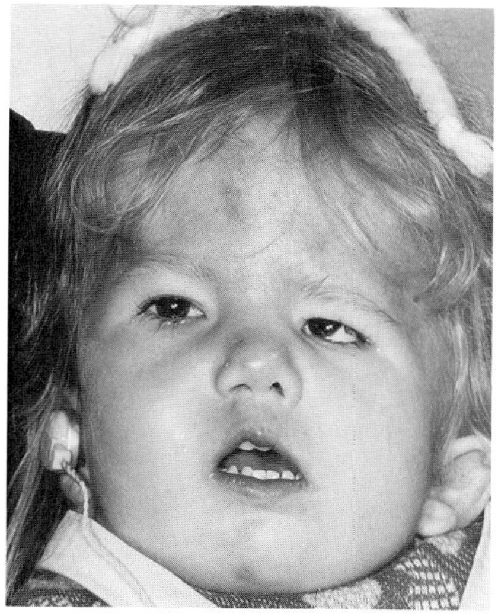

B

**Fig. 88.** Wildervanck syndrome. A,B: Same patient at different ages. Note the hydrocephaly, strabismus, and right hearing aid. (From RJ Gorlin et al., *Syndromes of the Head and Neck,* 3rd ed., Oxford University Press, New York, 1990, p. 660.)


4. Cervenka J, Gorlin RJ, Figalova P, Farkasova J: Craniocarpotarsal dysplasia or Whistling Face syndrome. Arch Otolaryngol 91:183–187, 1970.
5. Dallapiccola B, Giavinotti A, Lembo, A, Sagui L: Autosomal recessive form of Whistling Face syndrome in sibs. Am J Med Genet 33:542–544, 1989.
6. Freeman EA, Sheldon JH: Cranio-carpotarsal dystrophy: undescribed congenital malformation. Arch Dis Child 13:227–283, 1938.
7. Hall JG, Reed SD, Greene G: The distal arthrogryposes: delineation of new entities—review and nosologic discussion. Am J Med Genet 11:185–239, 1982.
8. Jacquemain B: Die angeborene Windmuhlenflugelstellung als erbliche Kombinationsmissbildung. Z Orthop 102:146–154, 1966.
9. Masarovich WA, Mazaheri M, Stool SE: Otolaryngologic findings in Whistling Face syndrome. Arch Otolaryngol Head Neck Surg 115:1373–1380, 1989.
10. Millner MM, Mutz ID, Rosenkranz W: Whistling Face syndrome: a case report and literature review. Acta Paediatr 31:279–289, 1991.
11. Otto FM: Die cranio-carpo-tarsale Dystrophie (Freeman und Sheldon): Ein casuistischer Beitrag. Z Kinderheilkd 73:240–250, 1953.
12. Vanek J, Janda J, Amblerova V, Losan F: Freeman-Sheldon syndrome: a disorder of congenital myopathic origin? J Med Genet 23:231–236, 1986.
13. Weinstein S, Gorlin RJ: Cranio-carpo-tarsal dysplasia or the Whistling Face syndrome. I. Clinical considerations. Am J Dis Child 117:427–423, 1969.


## Wildervanck syndrome

### Cervico-oculo-acoustic syndrome
(MIM No. 314600; POSSUM No. 3059)

This syndrome is characterized by congenital nerve deafness with Klippel-Feil and Duane anomalies.

#### General manifestations

These include abducens paralysis and globe retraction with narrowing of the palpebral fissures on attempted adduction (Duane anomaly). This may be unilateral or bilateral. Other ocular findings include ectopia lentis and epibulbar dermoids. Cervical or dorsal vertebral fusion and a short neck with restricted mobility are quite characteristic of the syndrome. Torticollis, kyphosis, winged scapulae, fused or absent ribs, and short stature have been reported.[1,4,7,10]

#### Otolaryngological manifestations

According to McKusick,[9] this syndrome is responsible for 1% of profound deafness in females. The loss may be unilateral or bilateral, sensorineural[6,7,10] or conductive.[2] Severe inner ear anomalies are noted on CT scans.[6] Mondini dysplasia and abnormal semicircular canals are also described.[13,14] Abnormalities of the pinnae, atresia of the external auditory canals, and middle ear anomalies, such as absent or dysplastic ossicles, fixed foot plate, and small internal auditory meatus, are documented.[3,7,8] Vestibular symptoms are rare.

#### Etiology

Polygenic inheritance with limitation to females,[12] multifactorial inheritance,[5] and X-linked dominant inheritance with lethality in males have been suggested.[11]

#### Differential diagnosis

Wildervank syndrome should be differentiated from Klippel-Feil anomaly and oculo-auriculo-vertebral spectrum.

#### References


1. Cross HE, Pfaffenbach DD: Duane's retraction syndrome and associated congenital malformations. Am J Ophthalmol 73:442–449, 1972.
2. Eismann ML, Sharma GK: The Wildervanck syndrome: Cervico-oculo-acoustic dysplasia. Otolaryngol Head Neck Surg 87:892–897, 1979.
3. Everberg G, Ratzen E, Sorensen H: Wildervanck's syndrome. Klippel-Feil's syndrome associated with deafness and retraction of the eyeball. Br J Radiol 36:562–567, 1963.
4. Frazer WI, MacGilivray RC: Cervico-oculo-acoustic dysplasia ("The syndrome of Wildervanck"). J Ment Defic Res 12:322–329, 1968.
5. Gorlin RJ, Toriello HV, Cohen MM Jr: Hereditary Hearing Loss and Its Syndromes. Oxford University Press, New York, 1995, pp 204–207.

6. Keeney G, Gebarski SS, Brunberg JA: CT of severe inner ear anomalies including aplasia in a case of Wildervanck syndrome. Am J Neuroradiol 13:201–202, 1992.
7. Kirkham TH: Cervico-oculo-acusticus syndrome with pseudopapilloedema. Arch Dis Child 44:504–508, 1969.
8. Lindsay JR: Inner ear histopathology in genetically determined congenital deafness. Birth Defects 7:21–32, 1971.
9. McKusick VA: Mendelian Inheritance in Man, A Catalog of Human Genes and Genetic Disorders, 11th ed. The Johns Hopkins University Press, Baltimore, 1992, p 2552.
10. Strisciuglio P, Raia V, Di Meo A, Rinaldi E, Andria G: Wildervanck's syndrome with bilateral subluxation of lens and facial paralysis. J Med Genet 20:72–73, 1983.
11. Wettke-Schaffer R, Kautner G: X-linked dominant inherited diseases with lethality in hemizygous males. Hum Genet 64:1–23, 1983.
12. Wildervanck LS: The cervico-oculo-acusticus syndrome. In: Handbook of Clinical Neurology, Vol 32, PJ Vinken, GW Bruyn, NC Myranthopoulos, eds. North-Holland, Amsterdam, 1978, pp 123–30.
13. Wildervanck LS, Hoeksema PE, Penning L: Radiological examination of the inner ear of deaf mutes presenting the cervico-oculo-acousticus syndrome with a summary of roentgenologic and pathologico-anatomical findings in other endogenous forms of deafness. Acta Otolaryngol 61:445–453, 1966.
14. Windle-Taylor PC, Emery PJ, Phelps PD: Ear deformities associated with the Klippel-Feil syndrome. Ann Otol Rhinol Laryngol 90:210–246, 1981.

## Williams syndrome

(MIM No. #194050; POSSUM No. 3427)

### General manifestations

Mental retardation (IQ 40–80), reduced motor and perceptual functions, and moderate growth deficiency characterize this syndrome. During childhood most patients are described as friendly, with a characteristic psychological and emotional profile and an echolalic speech.[11] Autism has also been observed. Cardiovascular malformations include supravalvular aortic stenosis, pulmonary stenosis, aortic hypoplasia, bicuspid aortic valves, coarctation of the aorta, and coronary artery stenosis.[3,4,6] Renal and carotid arteries may also be involved.[10,11] Hypercalcemia, nephrocalcinosis, small kidneys, and renal failure are not uncommon.[2,8,13] Other anomalies include blue eyes with a stellate pattern of the iris, fifth finger clinodactyly, a small penis, pectus excavatum, inguinal and/or umbilical hernia, bladder diverticulae, myopathy, and progressive joint limitation.[1,10]

### Otolaryngological manifestations

These include a depressed nasal bridge, short palpebral fissures, epicanthal folds, periorbital fullness, prominent lips with open mouth, anteverted nares, hypertelorism, and strabismus. The voice is often brassy and hoarse. Abnormal teeth (hypodontia or microdontia and hypoplastic deciduous second molars and permanent first molars) have also been described. Delayed mineralization of the teeth and prominent accessory labial frenulae have been reported.[2,7,8]

### Etiology

Sporadic. About 90% of the patients have deletions of the elastin gene region at 7q11.2. The condition is considered to be a contiguous gene syndrome.[5,9,12]

### References

1. Babbit DP, Dobbs J, Boedecker RA: Multiple bladder diverticulation in Williams "elfin facies" syndrome. Pediatr Radiol 8:29–31, 1979.
2. Borghraef PL, Volcke PH, van den Berghe H, Fryns JP: Adults in

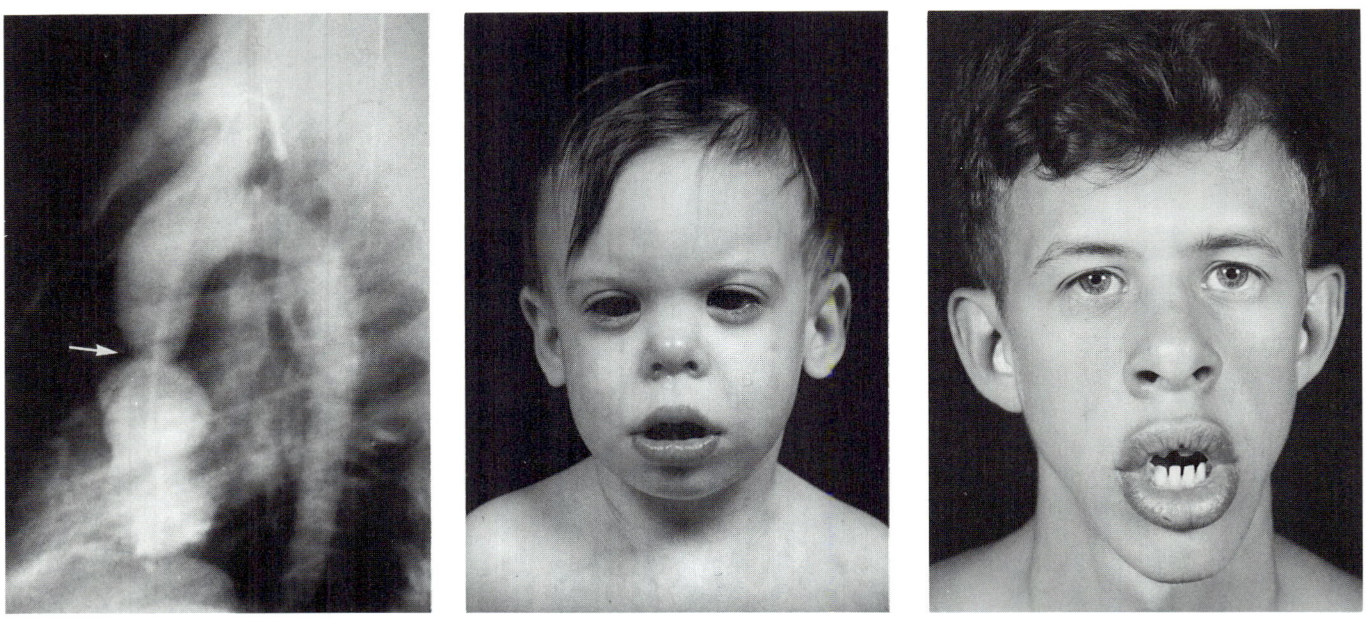

A B C

**Fig. 89.** Williams syndrome. A: Aortography in a patient with Williams syndrome showing supravalvar aortic stenosis (arrow). B,C: Typical facial features in males at 19 months and 22 years. Note epicanthus, anteverted nares, and prominent lips. (From R Stevenson et al., *Human Malformations and Related Anomalies,* Oxford University Press, New York, 1993, A: p. 336, courtesy of Dr. J Opitz; B,C: p. 247, courtesy of Dr. CI Scott Jr.)

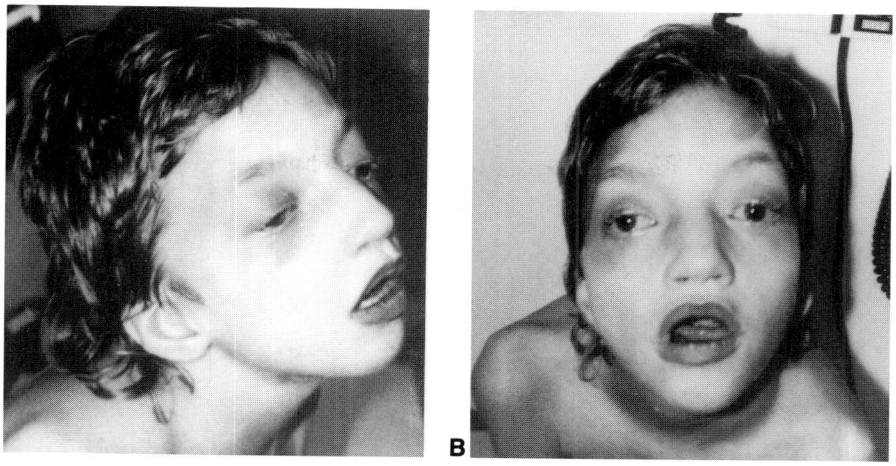

A B

**Fig. 90.** Wolf-Hirschhorn syndrome. A,B: Note the broad nasal bridge, high forehead, hypertelorism, and missing ear lobule.

Williams-Beuren syndrome: evaluation of medical, psychological and behavioural aspects. Clin Genet 46:161–167, 1994.
3. Daniels SR, Loggie JM, Schwarts DC, Strife JL, Kaplan S: Systematic hypertonia secondary to peripheral vascular anomalies in patients with Williams syndrome. J Pediatr 106:249–251, 1985.
4. Eie H, Semb G, Muller O, Bramness G: Localized supravalvular aortic stenosis combined with mental retardation and peculiar facial appearance. Acta Med Scand 191:517–520, 1972.
5. Ewart AK, Morris CA, Atkinson D, Jin W, Sternes K, Spallone P, Stock AD, Leppert M, Keating MT: Hemizygosity at the elastin locus in a developmental disorder, Williams syndrome. Nat Genet 5:11–16, 1993.
6. Feigl A, Feigl D, Yahini JH, Deutsch V, Neufeld HN: Supravalvular aortic and peripheral pulmonary stenosis. A report of eight cases in 2 generations. Isr J Med Sci 16:496–502, 1980.
7. Kelly JR, Barr ES: The elfin facies syndrome. Oral Surg 40:205–218, 1995.
8. Lopez-Rangel E, Maurice M, McGillivray B, Friedman JM: Williams syndrome in adults. Am J Med Genet 44:720–729, 1992.
9. Lowery MC, Morris CA, Ewart A, Brothman LJ, Zhu XL, Leonard CO, Carey JC, Keating M, Brothman AR: Strong correlation of elastin deletions detected by FISH, with Williams syndrome: evaluation of 235 patients. Am J Hum Genet 57:49–53, 1995.
10. Martin NDT, Snodgrass GJ, Cohen RD: Idiopathic infantile hypercalcemia—a continuing enigma. Arch Dis Child 59:605–613, 1984.
11. Meyerson MD, Frank RA: Language, speech and hearing in Williams syndrome: intervention approach and research needs. Dev Med Child Neurol 29:258–262, 1987.
12. Nickerson E, Greenberg F, Keating MT, McCaskill C, Shaffer LG: Deletions of the elastin gene at 7q11.23 occur in approximately 90% of patients with Williams syndrome. Am J Hum Genet 56:1156–1161, 1995.
13. Pober BR, Lacro RV, Rice C, Mandell V, Teele RL: Renal findings in 40 individuals with Williams syndrome. Am J Med Genet 46:271–274, 1993.

## Wolf-Hirschhorn syndrome

### 4p- syndrome
(POSSUM No. 3069)

#### General manifestations

The birth weight is approximately 2,000 gm. Microcephaly, severe psychomotor retardation, grand mal and petit mal seizures are frequent. Midline scalp defects are seen in 10% of cases.[2,4,6] The eyebrows are high arched, ptosis, and strabismus exist. Coloboma of the iris is seen in half of the cases, exophthalmos is an occasional finding. Hypospadias, hypoplastic müllerian derivatives, and kidney abnormalities are common urogenital anomalies. Cardiovascular defects are noted in 50% of cases. Absence of the pubic rami, vertebral fusion, and dislocated hips are occasionally documented.[1,3,4]

#### Otolaryngological manifestations

The facies is characteristic. The forehead is high with prominent glabella, hypertelorism, a broad nasal bridge, and a beaked nose (Greek-helmet appearance). The ears are low set, have preauricular pits, are poorly differentiated, lack a lobule, and have a narrow external auditory canal. The mouth is small with down-turned corners (carp-shaped) and a small chin. Cleft palate is documented in approximately half of the cases.

#### Etiology

Partial deletion of the short arm of chromosome 4 takes place in this syndrome. Deletion of band 4p16 is essential for the full expression of the syndrome. Such deletion could be submicroscopic and arise de novo. Translocation is responsible for about 15% of cases. Most cases are sporadic. The frequency is 1 in 50,000 births, the female-to-male ratio is 2:1.[5]

#### References

1. Gonzales CH: Pathologic findings in the Wolf-Hirschhorn (4p-) syndrome. Am J Med Genet 9:183–187, 1981.
2. Johnson VP, Mulder RD and Hosen R: The Wolf-Hirschhorn (4p-) syndrome. Clin Genet 10:104–112, 1976.
3. Lurie IW, Lazjuk GI, Ussova YI, Pressman EB, Gurevich DB: The Wolf-Hirschhorn syndrome. Clin Genet 17:375–384, 1980.
4. Morishita M, Shiba R, Chiyo H, Furuyama J, Fujita H, Atsumi Y: The oral manifestations of 4p- syndrome. J Oral Maxillofac Surg 41:601–605, 1983.
5. Rivas F, Hernandez A, Nazara Z, Fragoso R, Olivares N, Rolon A, Cantu JM: On the deletion 4p16 Wolf-Hirschhorn syndrome. Ann Genet 22:228–231, 1979.
6. Zellweger H, Bardach J, Bordwell J, Williams K: The short arm deletion syndrome of chromosome 4 (4p- syndrome). Arch Otolaryngol 101:29–32, 1975.

# Addendum

## Chromosomal Map of Syndromes and Conditions with Congenital Anomalies of the Ear, Nose, and Throat

The mapping of genes and their characterization is progressing at a fast pace. This process helps to better understand the biological and developmental basis of clinical conditions in general, and their genetic heterogeneity, in particular. It also allows prenatal and postnatal diagnosis with molecular methods.

The graphic representation of mapped genes provides an easily accessible source of reference. In this Addendum, we present the chromosomal location of syndromes and conditions with congenital and/or hereditary anomalies of the ear, nose, and throat cited in this book.

Each condition or syndrome is first identified by its most commonly used name, followed by the abbreviation(s) of the gene, Mendelian Inheritance in Man (MIM) or McKusick's catalog number, and finally, the chromosomal location. We have the chromosomal diagrams at the level of 550 bands. This gives enough detail without overly crowding the maps.

We have presented the mitochondrial loci as a list because the graphic representation of the mitochondrial DNA does not offer a particular advantage for the understanding of, or the clinical approach to, these conditions.

We have used a modification of the chromosomal diagrams published by ISCN (An International System for Human Cytogenetic Nomenclature, F Mitelman, ed. S Karger Publishers Inc, Farmington, 1995, pp 14–21) with permission.

Information on the gene sites was obtained from GDB(TM) Genome Database, Baltimore (Maryland, USA): Johns Hopkins University, 1990. Updated daily, available from Internet http://gdbwww.gdb.org/

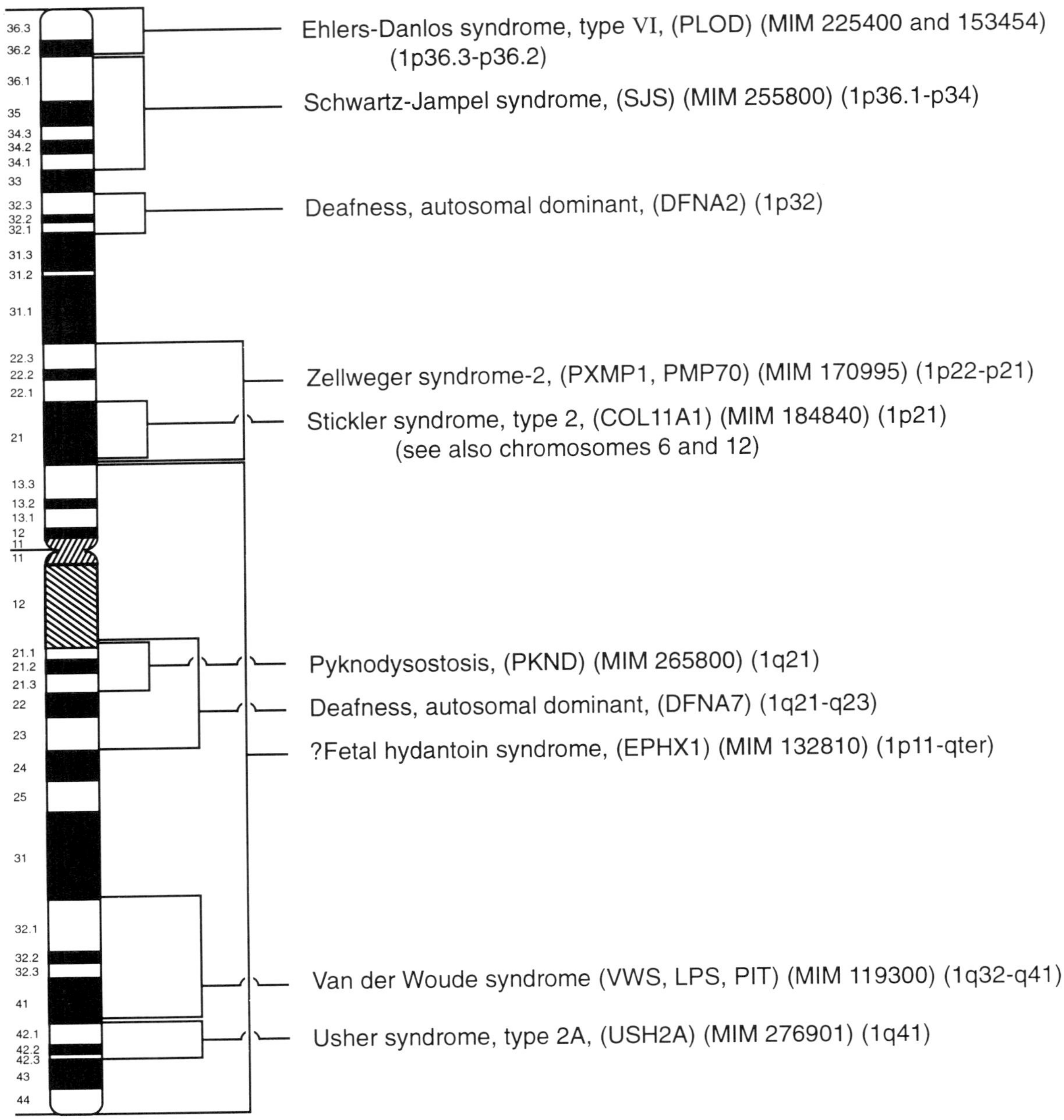
Ehlers-Danlos syndrome, type VI, (PLOD) (MIM 225400 and 153454) (1p36.3-p36.2)
Schwartz-Jampel syndrome, (SJS) (MIM 255800) (1p36.1-p34)
Deafness, autosomal dominant, (DFNA2) (1p32)
Zellweger syndrome-2, (PXMP1, PMP70) (MIM 170995) (1p22-p21)
Stickler syndrome, type 2, (COL11A1) (MIM 184840) (1p21) (see also chromosomes 6 and 12)
Pyknodysostosis, (PKND) (MIM 265800) (1q21)
Deafness, autosomal dominant, (DFNA7) (1q21-q23)
?Fetal hydantoin syndrome, (EPHX1) (MIM 132810) (1p11-qter)
Van der Woude syndrome (VWS, LPS, PIT) (MIM 119300) (1q32-q41)
Usher syndrome, type 2A, (USH2A) (MIM 276901) (1q41)

**1**

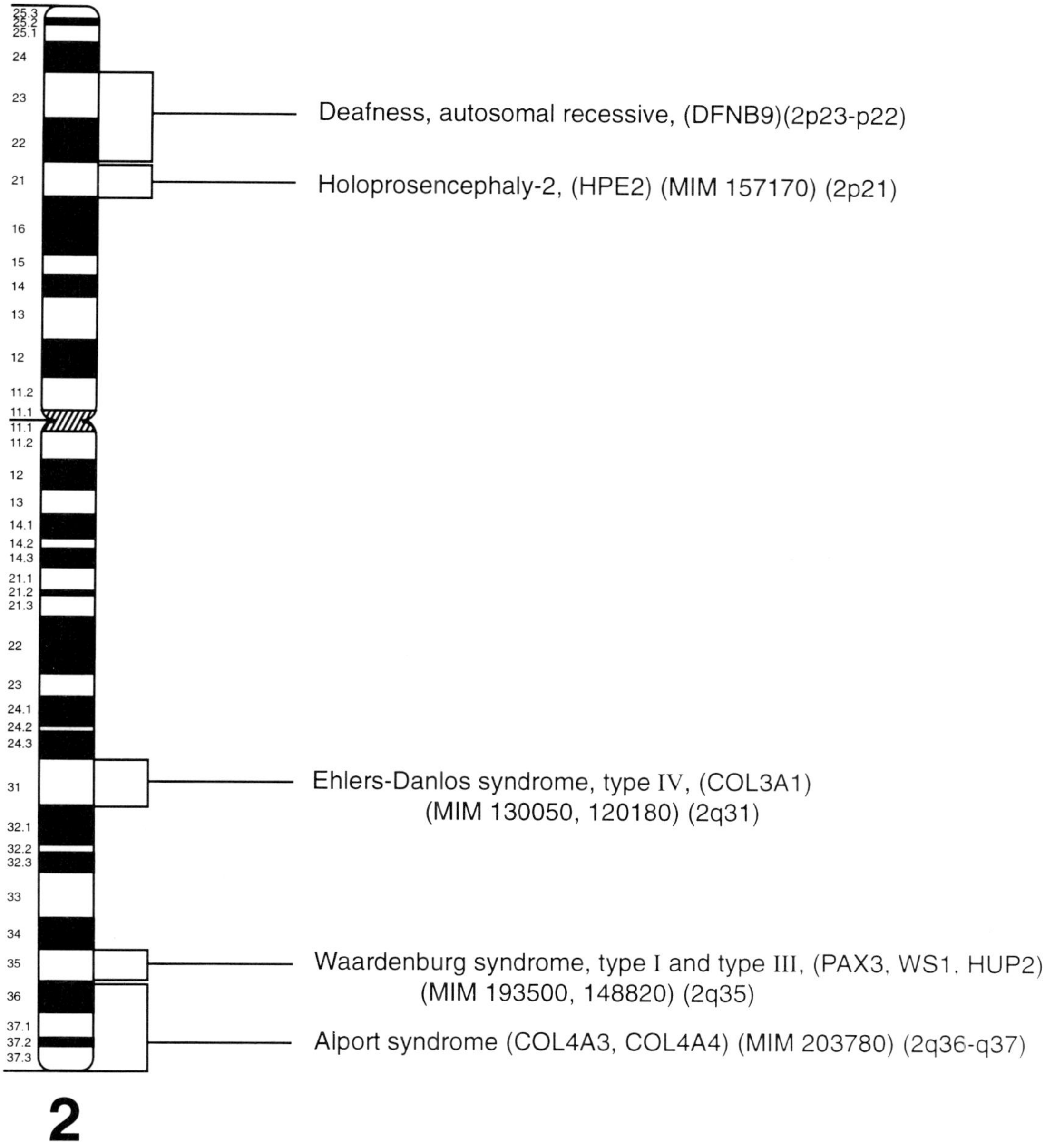
25.3
25.2
25.1
24
23
22
21
16
15
14
13
12
11.2
11.1
11.1
11.2
12
13
14.1
14.2
14.3
21.1
21.2
21.3
22
23
24.1
24.2
24.3
31
32.1
32.2
32.3
33
34
35
36
37.1
37.2
37.3
Deafness, autosomal recessive, (DFNB9)(2p23-p22)
Holoprosencephaly-2, (HPE2) (MIM 157170) (2p21)
Ehlers-Danlos syndrome, type IV, (COL3A1) (MIM 130050, 120180) (2q31)
Waardenburg syndrome, type I and type III, (PAX3, WS1, HUP2) (MIM 193500, 148820) (2q35)
Alport syndrome (COL4A3, COL4A4) (MIM 203780) (2q36-q37)
2

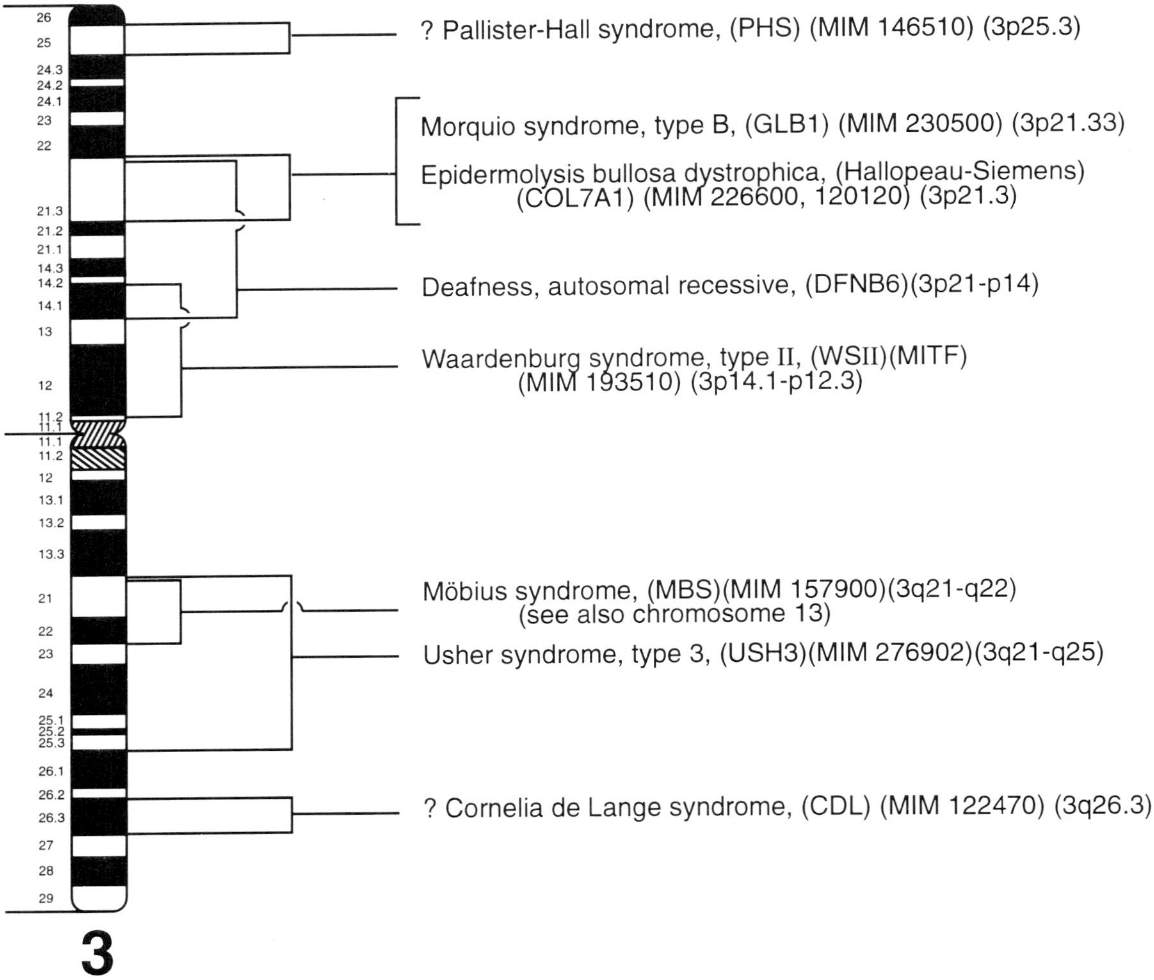
? Pallister-Hall syndrome, (PHS) (MIM 146510) (3p25.3)
Morquio syndrome, type B, (GLB1) (MIM 230500) (3p21.33)
Epidermolysis bullosa dystrophica, (Hallopeau-Siemens) (COL7A1) (MIM 226600, 120120) (3p21.3)
Deafness, autosomal recessive, (DFNB6)(3p21-p14)
Waardenburg syndrome, type II, (WSII)(MITF) (MIM 193510) (3p14.1-p12.3)
Möbius syndrome, (MBS)(MIM 157900)(3q21-q22) (see also chromosome 13)
Usher syndrome, type 3, (USH3)(MIM 276902)(3q21-q25)
? Cornelia de Lange syndrome, (CDL) (MIM 122470) (3q26.3)
3

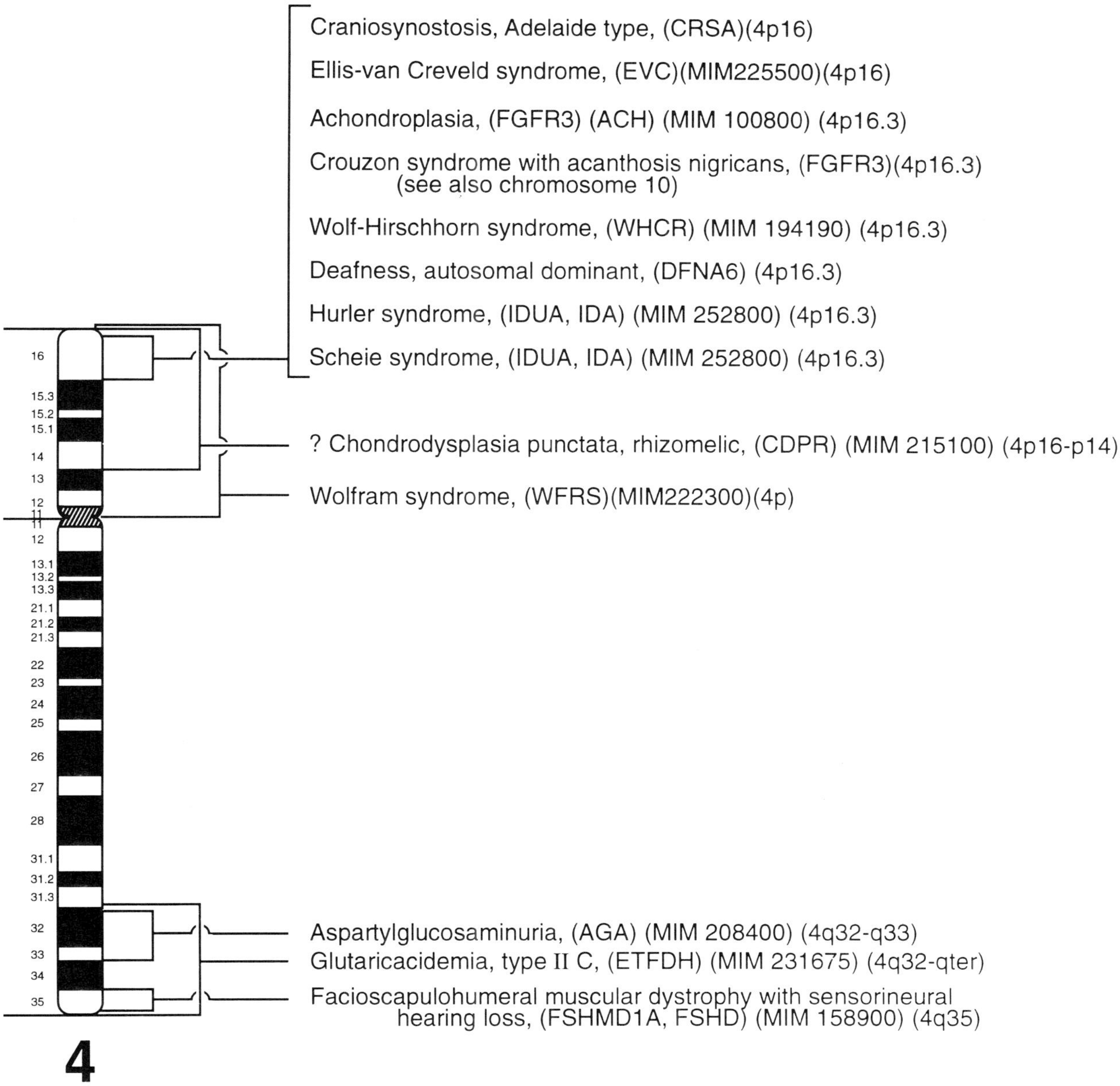

Craniosynostosis, Adelaide type, (CRSA)(4p16)
Ellis-van Creveld syndrome, (EVC)(MIM225500)(4p16)
Achondroplasia, (FGFR3) (ACH) (MIM 100800) (4p16.3)
Crouzon syndrome with acanthosis nigricans, (FGFR3)(4p16.3) (see also chromosome 10)
Wolf-Hirschhorn syndrome, (WHCR) (MIM 194190) (4p16.3)
Deafness, autosomal dominant, (DFNA6) (4p16.3)
Hurler syndrome, (IDUA, IDA) (MIM 252800) (4p16.3)
Scheie syndrome, (IDUA, IDA) (MIM 252800) (4p16.3)
? Chondrodysplasia punctata, rhizomelic, (CDPR) (MIM 215100) (4p16-p14)
Wolfram syndrome, (WFRS)(MIM222300)(4p)
Aspartylglucosaminuria, (AGA) (MIM 208400) (4q32-q33)
Glutaricacidemia, type II C, (ETFDH) (MIM 231675) (4q32-qter)
Facioscapulohumeral muscular dystrophy with sensorineural hearing loss, (FSHMD1A, FSHD) (MIM 158900) (4q35)
16
15.3
15.2
15.1
14
13
12
11
11
12
13.1
13.2
13.3
21.1
21.2
21.3
22
23
24
25
26
27
28
31.1
31.2
31.3
32
33
34
35
4

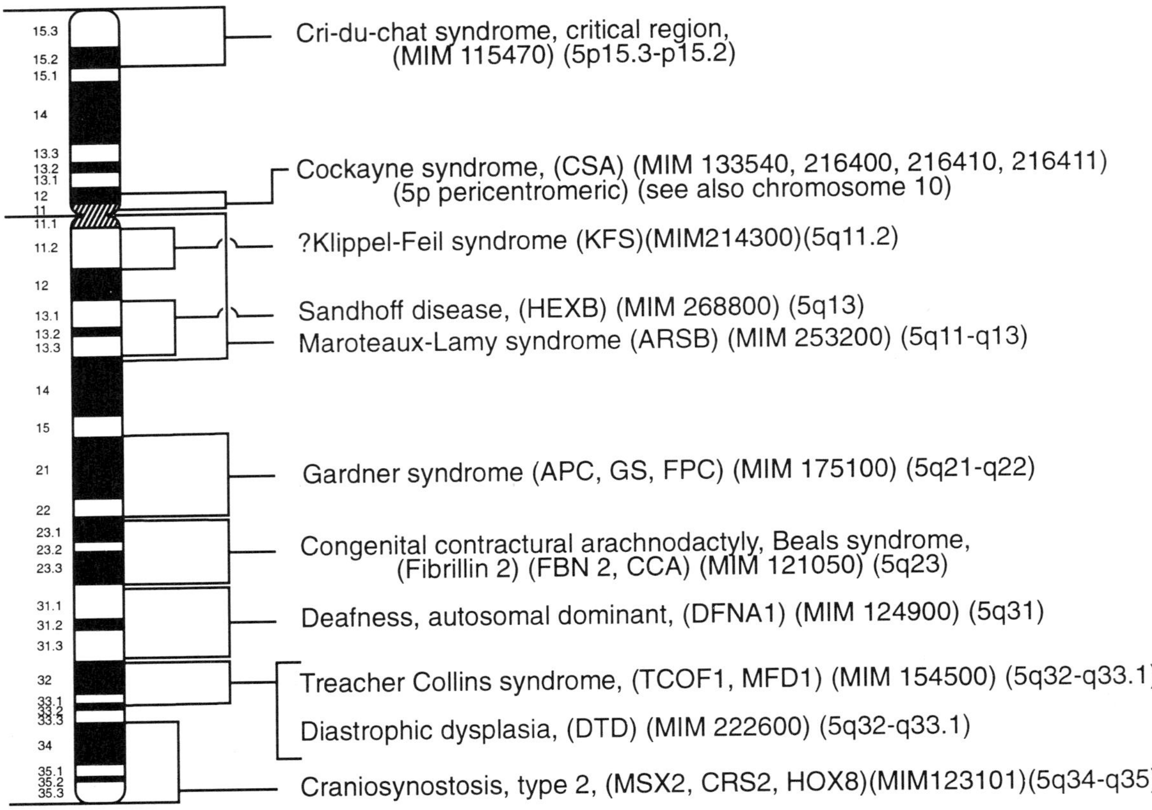
Cri-du-chat syndrome, critical region, (MIM 115470) (5p15.3-p15.2)
Cockayne syndrome, (CSA) (MIM 133540, 216400, 216410, 216411) (5p pericentromeric) (see also chromosome 10)
?Klippel-Feil syndrome (KFS)(MIM214300)(5q11.2)
Sandhoff disease, (HEXB) (MIM 268800) (5q13)
Maroteaux-Lamy syndrome (ARSB) (MIM 253200) (5q11-q13)
Gardner syndrome (APC, GS, FPC) (MIM 175100) (5q21-q22)
Congenital contractural arachnodactyly, Beals syndrome, (Fibrillin 2) (FBN 2, CCA) (MIM 121050) (5q23)
Deafness, autosomal dominant, (DFNA1) (MIM 124900) (5q31)
Treacher Collins syndrome, (TCOF1, MFD1) (MIM 154500) (5q32-q33.1)
Diastrophic dysplasia, (DTD) (MIM 222600) (5q32-q33.1)
Craniosynostosis, type 2, (MSX2, CRS2, HOX8)(MIM123101)(5q34-q35)

**5**

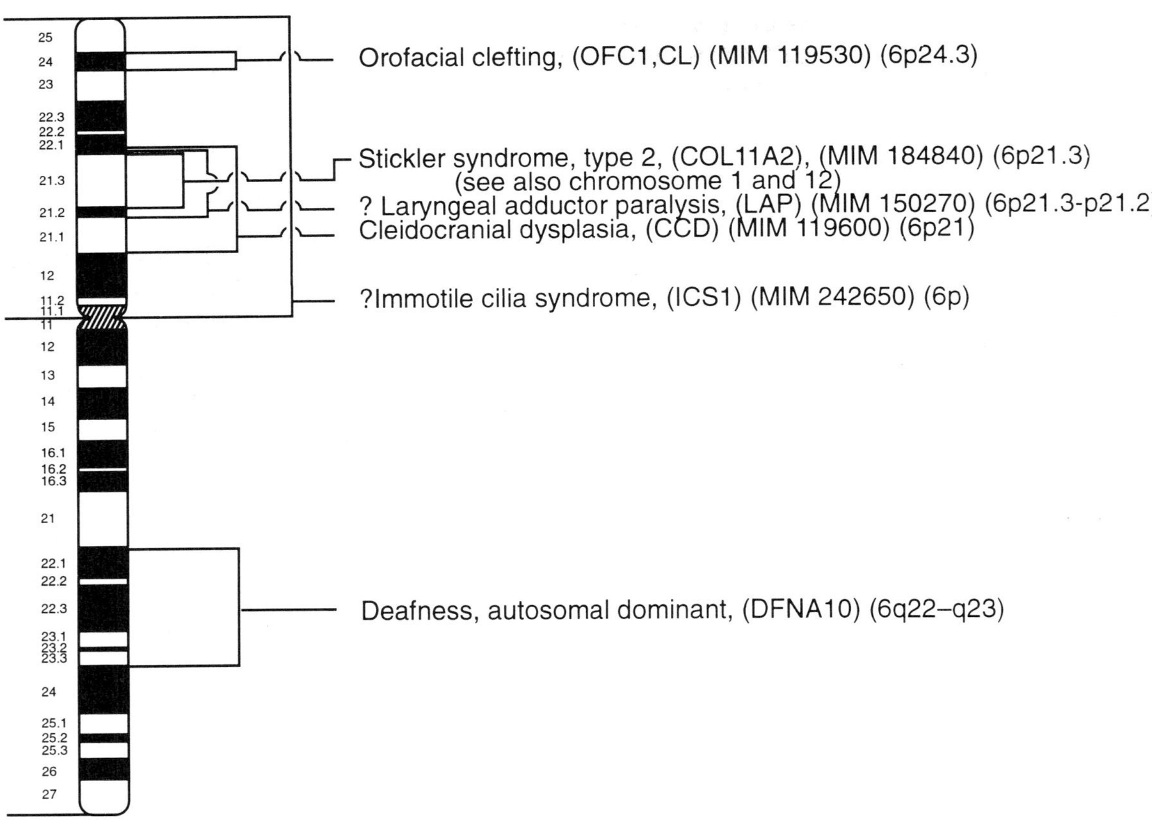
Orofacial clefting, (OFC1,CL) (MIM 119530) (6p24.3)
Stickler syndrome, type 2, (COL11A2), (MIM 184840) (6p21.3) (see also chromosome 1 and 12)
? Laryngeal adductor paralysis, (LAP) (MIM 150270) (6p21.3-p21.2)
Cleidocranial dysplasia, (CCD) (MIM 119600) (6p21)
?Immotile cilia syndrome, (ICS1) (MIM 242650) (6p)
Deafness, autosomal dominant, (DFNA10) (6q22–q23)

**6**

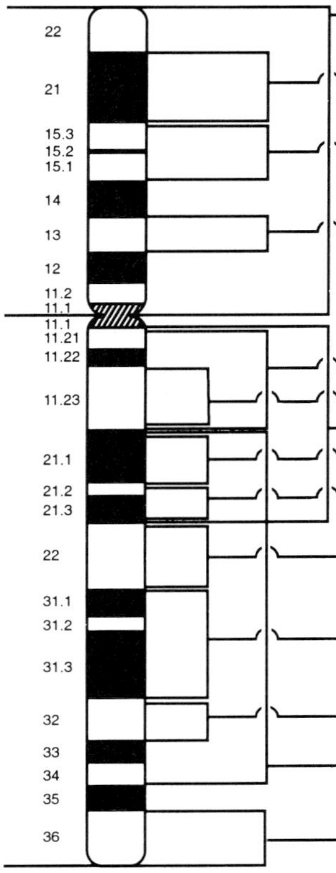


? Goldenhar syndrome, (GHS) (MIM 141400) (7p)

Saethre-Chotzen syndrome, (ACS3, SCS) (MIM 101400) (7p21.2)
Craniosynostosis, type 1, (CRS, CSO) (123100) (7p21.3-p21.2)

Deafness, autosomal dominant, (DFNA5)(7p15)

Greig cephalopolysyndactyly syndrome, (GLI3) (MIM 175700) (7p13)

Williams syndrome, (Elastin) (ELN) (MIM 130160) (7q11.2)

Zellweger syndrome-1, (ZWS1) (MIM 214100) (7q11.23)

? EEC syndrome, (EEC) (MIM 129900) (7q11.2–q21.3)

Sly syndrome, (MPS VII, GUSB) (MIM 253220) (7q21.11)

Split-hand/split-foot deformity, type 1, (SHFD1) (MIM 183600) (7q21.2-q21.3)

Osteogenesis imperfecta (COL1A2) (MIM 120160, 166200, 166210, 166220, 259420) (7q22.1) (see also chromosome 17)

Deafness, autosomal recessive, (DFNB4)(7q31)

Smith-Lemli-Opitz syndrome, (SLOS) (MIM 270400) (7q32)

Pendred syndrome, (PDS) (MIM 274600) (7q21-q34)

Holoprosencephaly-3, (HLP3) (MIM142945) (7q36)

**7**

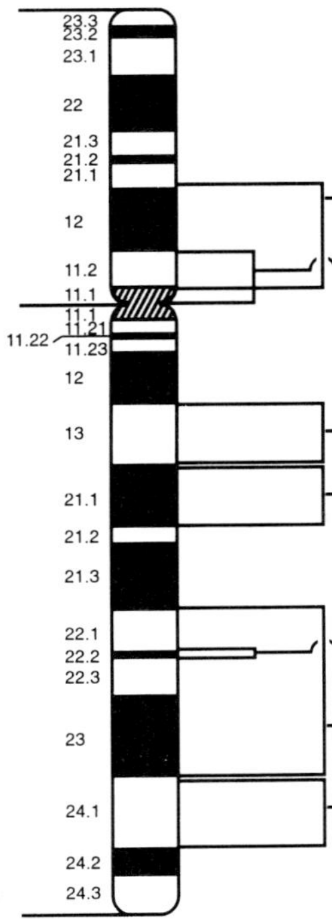


Werner syndrome, (WRN) (MIM 277700) (8p12-p11.2)

Pfeiffer syndrome, (FGFR1)(ACSV) (MIM 101600) (8p11.2-p11.1) (see also chromosome 10)

Branchiootorenal dysplasia, (BOR) (MIM 113650) (8q13.3)

Zellweger syndrome-3, (Peroxisomal assembly factor-1) (PAF1, PMP35) (170993) (8q21.1)

Klippel-Feil syndrome with laryngeal malformation, (KFSL) (MIM 148900) (8q22.2)

Cohen syndrome, (CSH1) (MIM 216550) (8q22-q23)

Trichorhinophalangeal syndrome, type I, (TRPSI) (MIM 190350) (8q24.12)

Langer-Giedion syndrome, trichorhinophalangeal syndrome, type II, (LGCR, LGS, TRPS2) (MIM 150230) (8q24.11-q24.13)

**8**

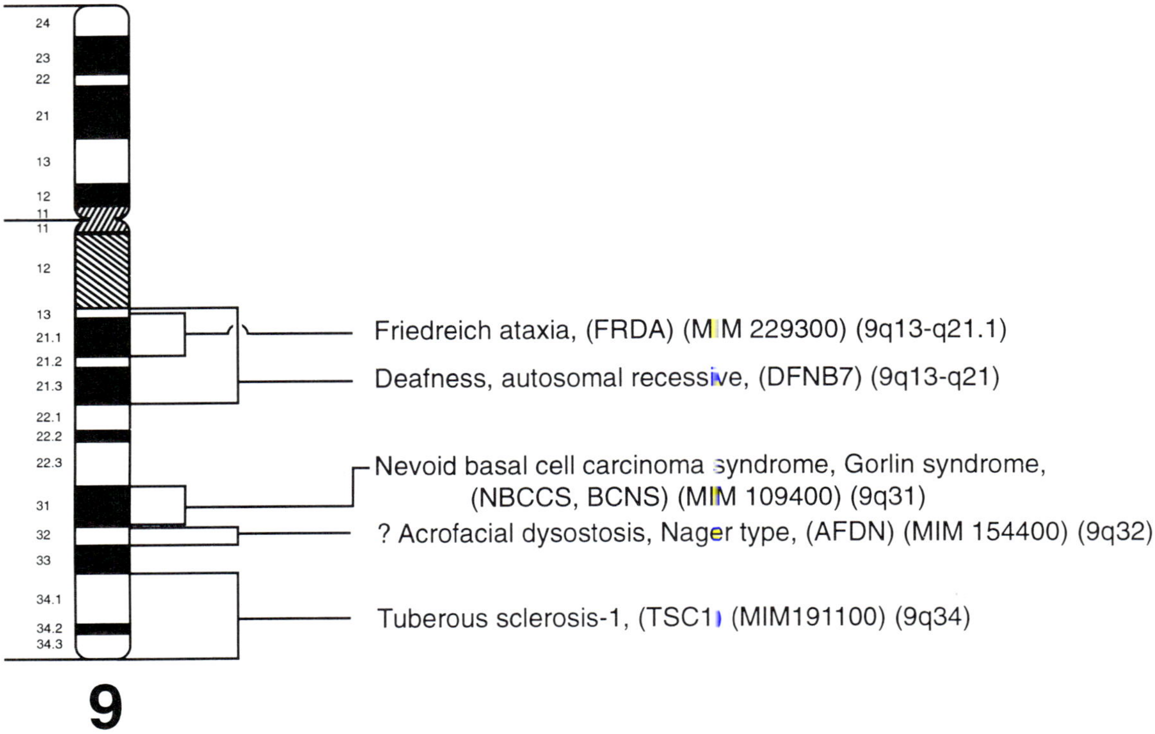
Friedreich ataxia, (FRDA) (MIM 229300) (9q13-q21.1)
Deafness, autosomal recessive, (DFNB7) (9q13-q21)
Nevoid basal cell carcinoma syndrome, Gorlin syndrome, (NBCCS, BCNS) (MIM 109400) (9q31)
? Acrofacial dysostosis, Nager type, (AFDN) (MIM 154400) (9q32)
Tuberous sclerosis-1, (TSC1) (MIM191100) (9q34)
9

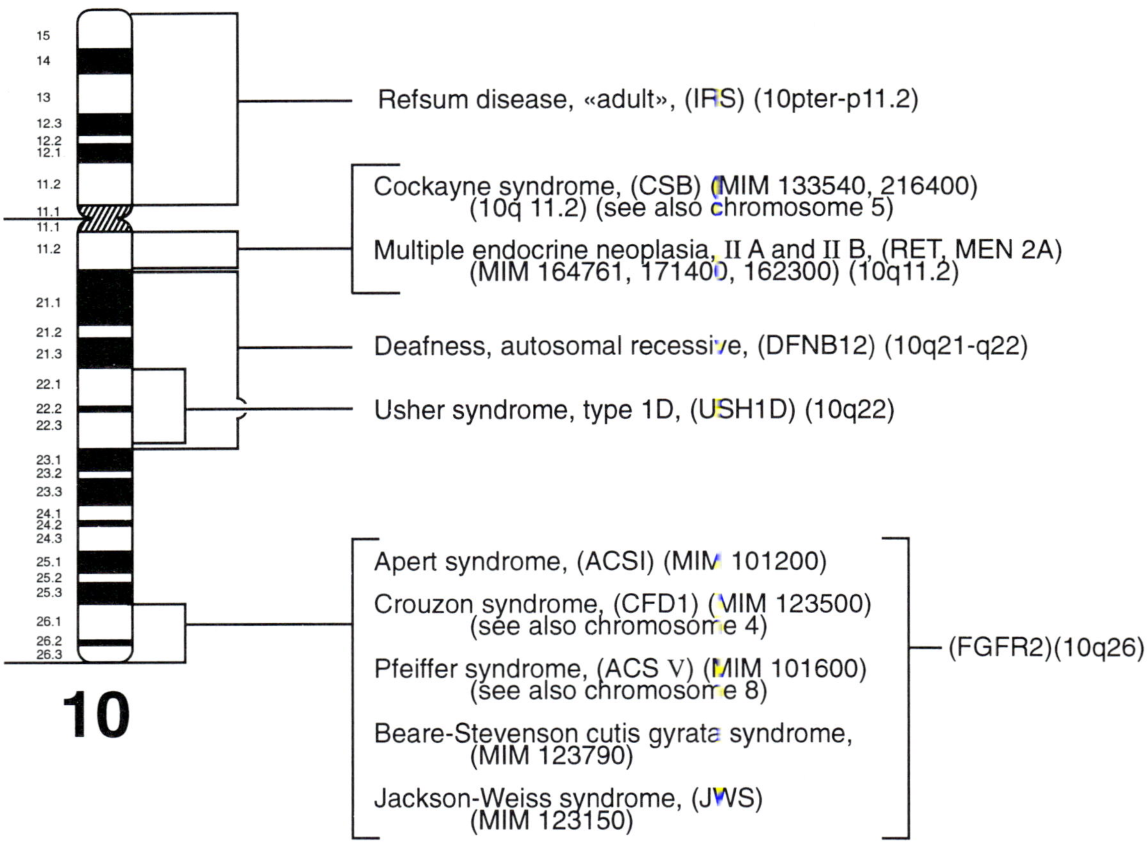
Refsum disease, «adult», (IRS) (10pter-p11.2)
Cockayne syndrome, (CSB) (MIM 133540, 216400) (10q 11.2) (see also chromosome 5)
Multiple endocrine neoplasia, II A and II B, (RET, MEN 2A) (MIM 164761, 171400, 162300) (10q11.2)
Deafness, autosomal recessive, (DFNB12) (10q21-q22)
Usher syndrome, type 1D, (USH1D) (10q22)
Apert syndrome, (ACSI) (MIM 101200)
Crouzon syndrome, (CFD1) (MIM 123500) (see also chromosome 4)
Pfeiffer syndrome, (ACS V) (MIM 101600) (see also chromosome 8)
Beare-Stevenson cutis gyrata syndrome, (MIM 123790)
Jackson-Weiss syndrome, (JWS) (MIM 123150)
(FGFR2)(10q26)
10

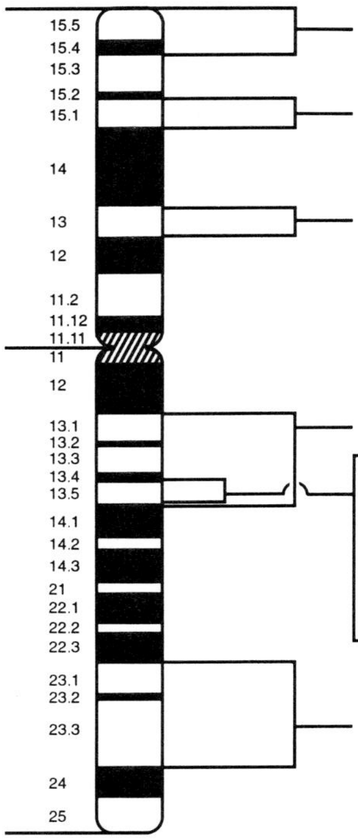


Beckwith-Wiedemann syndrome, (BWS) (MIM 130650) (11pter-p15.4)

Usher syndrome, type 1C, (USH1C) (MIM 276904) (11p15.1)

Aniridia, Peters anomaly, (PAX6, AN2) (MIM 106210) (11p13)

Multiple endocrine neoplasia I, (MEN I) (MIM 131100) (11q13)

Usher syndrome, type 1B, (MYO7A, USH1B) (MIM 276903) (11q13.5)

Deafness, autosomal dominant, (DFNA11) (11q13.5)

Deafness, autosomal recessive, (DFNB2) (11q13.5)

Amyloidosis, Iowa type, (APOA1) (MIM 107680) (11q23)

**11**

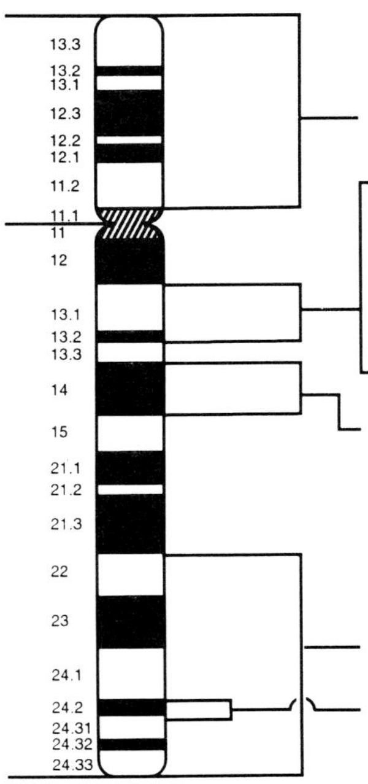


? Acrocallosal syndrome, (ACLS) (MIM 200990) (12p13.3–p11.2)

Spondyloepiphyseal dysplasia, (SED) (MIM 120140)

Kniest dysplasia, (MIM 120140)

Stickler syndrome, type 1, (MIM 108300, 120140) (see also chromosomes 1 and 6)

(COL2A1)(12q13.11-q13.2)

Sanfilippo syndrome D, (GNS, G6S) (MIM 252940) (12q14)

Noonan syndrome, (NS1) (MIM 163950) (12q22-qter)

? Fetal alcohol syndrome, (ALDH 2) (MIM 100650) (12q24.2)

**12**

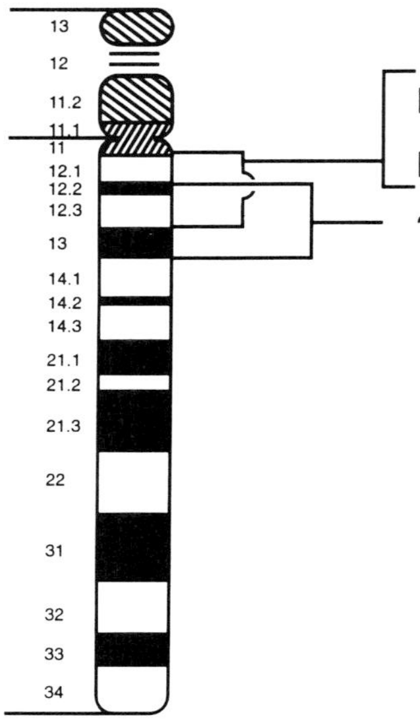

Deafness, autosomal dominant, (DFNA3) (13q12)

Deafness, autosomal recessive, (DFNB1) (MIM 220290) (13q12)

? Möbius syndrome, (MBS) (MIM 157900) (13q12.2-q13) (see chromosome 3)

**13**

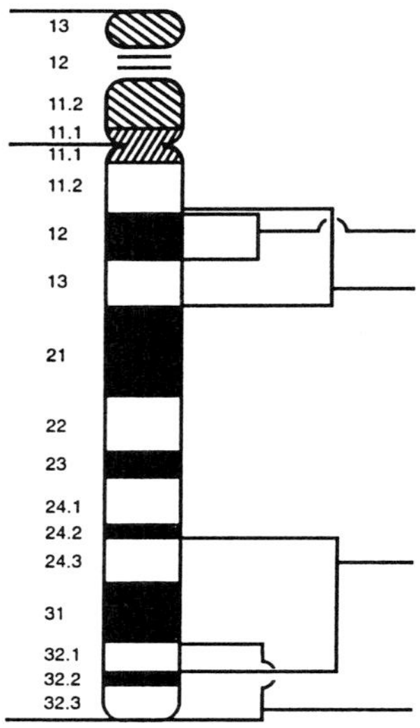

Deafness, autosomal recessive, (DFNB5) (14q12)

Deafness, autosomal dominant, (DFNA9) (14q12-q13)

Krabbe disease, (GALC) (MIM 245200) (14q24.3-q32.1)

Usher syndrome, type 1A (USH1A, USH1) (MIM 276900) (14q32)

**14**

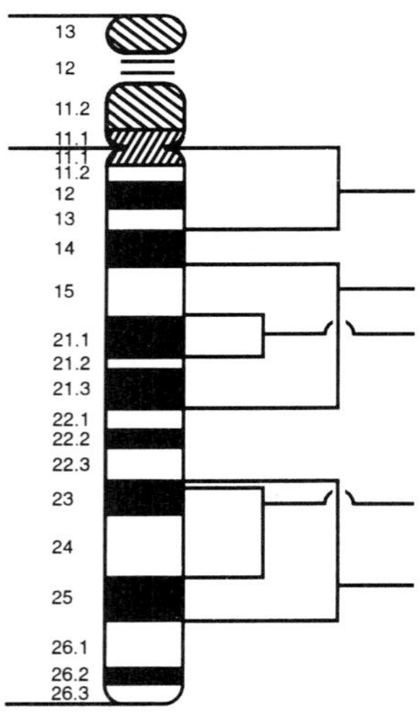

? Albright hereditary osteodystrophy - 2, (AHO2) (MIM 103581) (15q11-q13)

Deafness, autosomal dominant, (DFNA8) (15q15-q21)

Marfan syndrome, (Fibrillin 1)(FBN1) (MIM 134797, 154700) (15q21.1)

Tay-Sachs disease, (HEXA, TSD) (MIM 272800) (15q23-q24)

Glutaricacidemia, type II A, (ETFA, GA2) (MIM 231680) (15q23-q25)

**15**

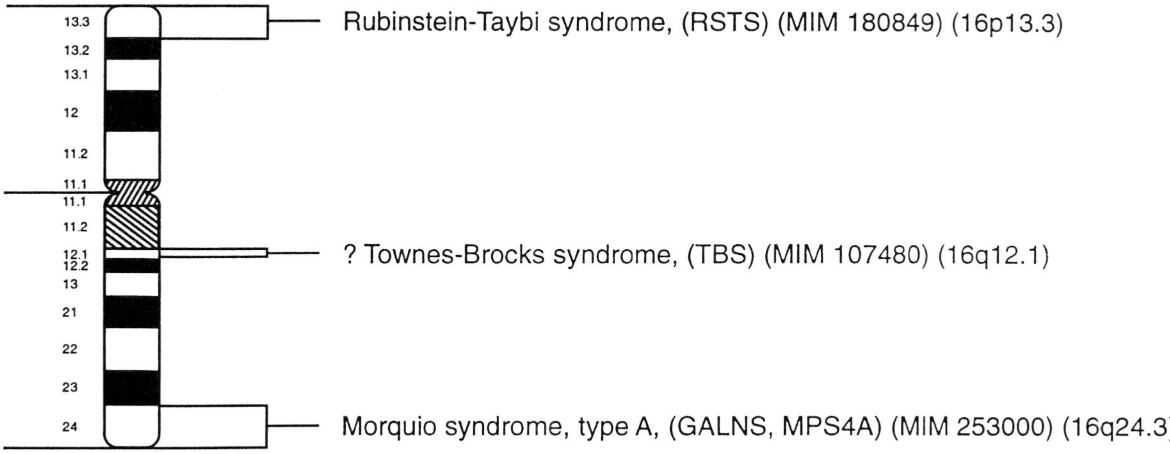
13.3
13.2
13.1
12
11.2
11.1
11.1
11.2
12.1
12.2
13
21
22
23
24
Rubinstein-Taybi syndrome, (RSTS) (MIM 180849) (16p13.3)
? Townes-Brocks syndrome, (TBS) (MIM 107480) (16q12.1)
Morquio syndrome, type A, (GALNS, MPS4A) (MIM 253000) (16q24.3)

**16**

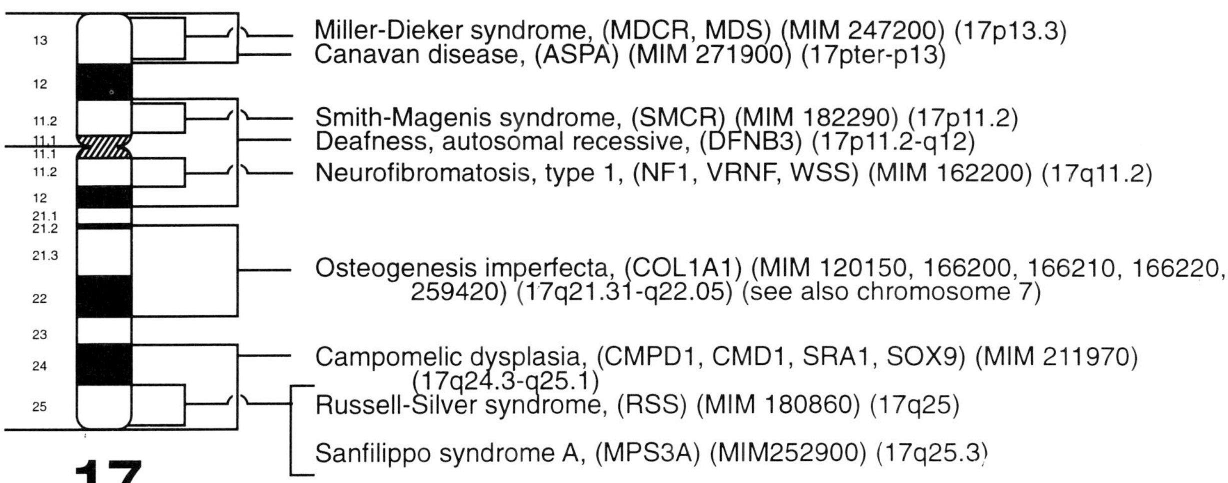
13
12
11.2
11.1
11.1
11.2
12
21.1
21.2
21.3
22
23
24
25
Miller-Dieker syndrome, (MDCR, MDS) (MIM 247200) (17p13.3)
Canavan disease, (ASPA) (MIM 271900) (17pter-p13)
Smith-Magenis syndrome, (SMCR) (MIM 182290) (17p11.2)
Deafness, autosomal recessive, (DFNB3) (17p11.2-q12)
Neurofibromatosis, type 1, (NF1, VRNF, WSS) (MIM 162200) (17q11.2)
Osteogenesis imperfecta, (COL1A1) (MIM 120150, 166200, 166210, 166220, 259420) (17q21.31-q22.05) (see also chromosome 7)
Campomelic dysplasia, (CMPD1, CMD1, SRA1, SOX9) (MIM 211970) (17q24.3-q25.1)
Russell-Silver syndrome, (RSS) (MIM 180860) (17q25)
Sanfilippo syndrome A, (MPS3A) (MIM252900) (17q25.3)

**17**

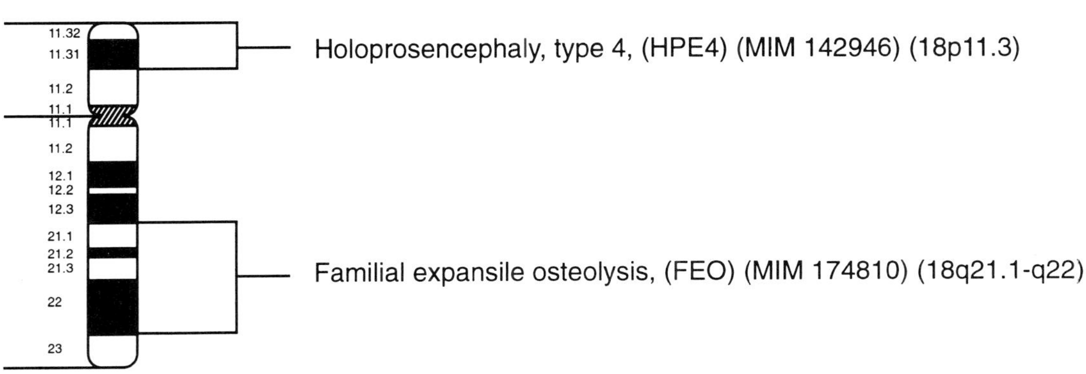
11.32
11.31
11.2
11.1
11.1
11.2
12.1
12.2
12.3
21.1
21.2
21.3
22
23
Holoprosencephaly, type 4, (HPE4) (MIM 142946) (18p11.3)
Familial expansile osteolysis, (FEO) (MIM 174810) (18q21.1-q22)

**18**

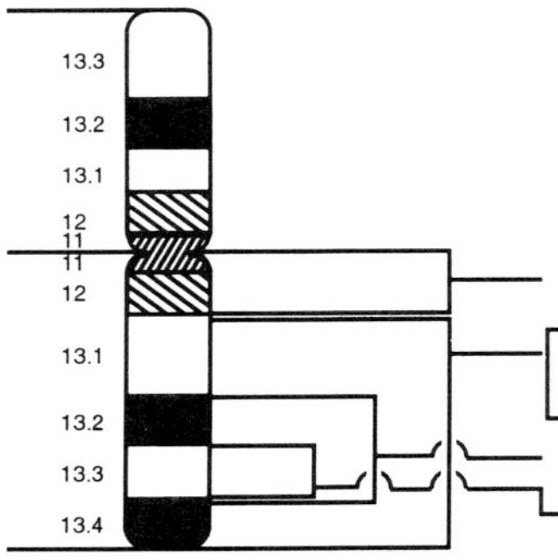


Mannosidosis, (MANB) (MIM 248500) (19 cen-q12)

Deafness, autosomal dominant, (DFNA4) (19q13)
Orofacial cleft 3 (OFC3) (19q13)

Myotonic dystrophy, (DM) (MIM 160900) (19q13.2-q13.3)

Glutaricaciduria, type II B, (ETFB) (MIM 130410) (19q13.3)

**19**

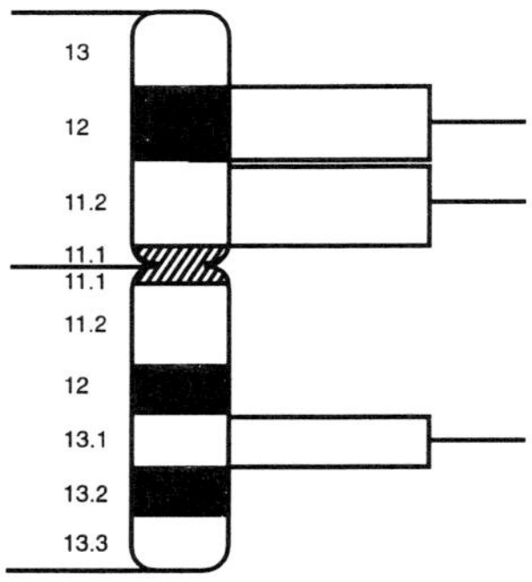


? Fibrodysplasia ossificans progressiva, (BMP2A) (MIM 112261) (20p12)

Alagille syndrome, (AGS, AHD) (MIM 118450) (20p11.2)

Galactosialidosis, (GSL) (MIM 256540) (20q13.1)

**20**

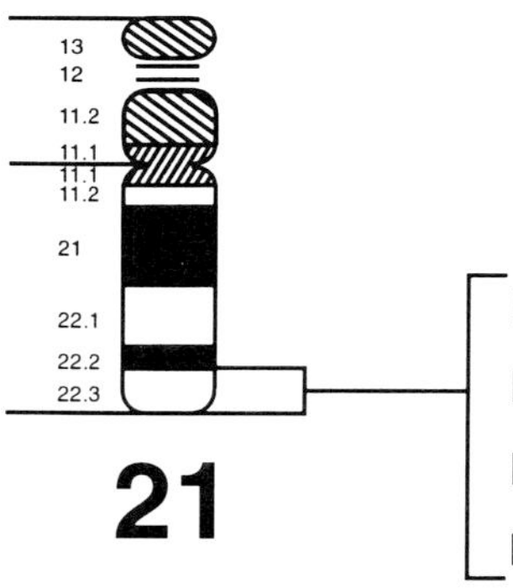


Deafness, autosomal recessive, (DFNB8)(21q22.3)

Deafness, autosomal recessive, (DFNB10)(21q22.3)

Down syndrome, critical region, (DSCR) (MIM 190685) (21q22.3)

Holoprosencephaly-1, (HPE1) (MIM236100) (21q22.3)

**21**

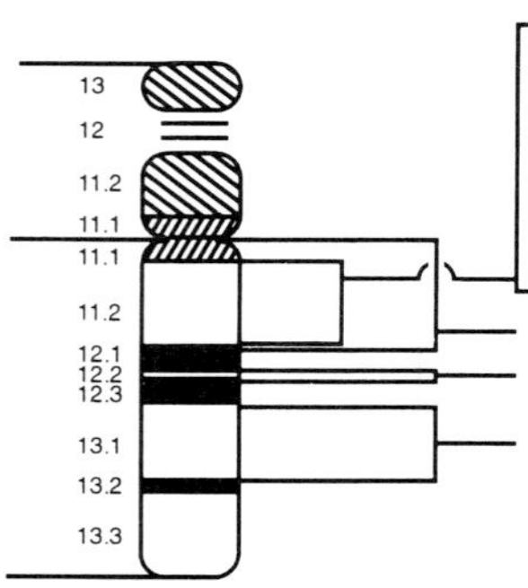


DiGeorge/Velocardiofacial-Shprintzen syndrome, (DGCR, DGS, VCF) (MIM 188400) (22q11.2)

Opitz G/BBB syndrome, (OGS2) (MIM 145410) (22q 11.2) (see also chromosome X)

Cat-eye syndrome, (CECR, CES) (MIM 115470) (22q11)

Neurofibromatosis, type 2, (NF2) (MIM 101000) (22q12.2)

Sorsby syndrome, (SFD) (MIM 136900) (22q 13.1)

**22**

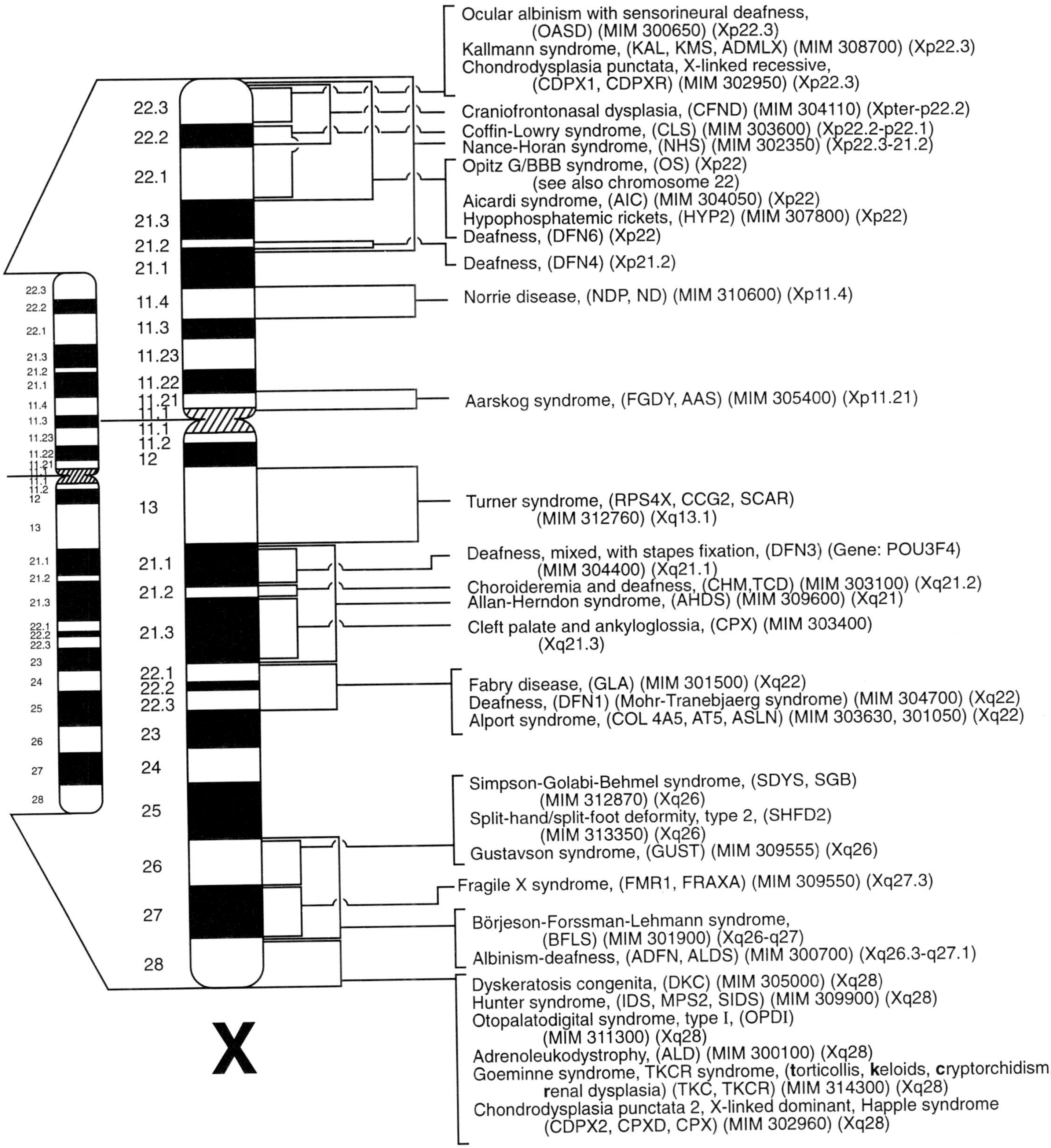

Ocular albinism with sensorineural deafness, (OASD) (MIM 300650) (Xp22.3)
Kallmann syndrome, (KAL, KMS, ADMLX) (MIM 308700) (Xp22.3)
Chondrodysplasia punctata, X-linked recessive, (CDPX1, CDPXR) (MIM 302950) (Xp22.3)
Craniofrontonasal dysplasia, (CFND) (MIM 304110) (Xpter-p22.2)
Coffin-Lowry syndrome, (CLS) (MIM 303600) (Xp22.2-p22.1)
Nance-Horan syndrome, (NHS) (MIM 302350) (Xp22.3-21.2)
Opitz G/BBB syndrome, (OS) (Xp22) (see also chromosome 22)
Aicardi syndrome, (AIC) (MIM 304050) (Xp22)
Hypophosphatemic rickets, (HYP2) (MIM 307800) (Xp22)
Deafness, (DFN6) (Xp22)
Deafness, (DFN4) (Xp21.2)
Norrie disease, (NDP, ND) (MIM 310600) (Xp11.4)
Aarskog syndrome, (FGDY, AAS) (MIM 305400) (Xp11.21)
Turner syndrome, (RPS4X, CCG2, SCAR) (MIM 312760) (Xq13.1)
Deafness, mixed, with stapes fixation, (DFN3) (Gene: POU3F4) (MIM 304400) (Xq21.1)
Choroideremia and deafness, (CHM,TCD) (MIM 303100) (Xq21.2)
Allan-Herndon syndrome, (AHDS) (MIM 309600) (Xq21)
Cleft palate and ankyloglossia, (CPX) (MIM 303400) (Xq21.3)
Fabry disease, (GLA) (MIM 301500) (Xq22)
Deafness, (DFN1) (Mohr-Tranebjaerg syndrome) (MIM 304700) (Xq22)
Alport syndrome, (COL 4A5, AT5, ASLN) (MIM 303630, 301050) (Xq22)
Simpson-Golabi-Behmel syndrome, (SDYS, SGB) (MIM 312870) (Xq26)
Split-hand/split-foot deformity, type 2, (SHFD2) (MIM 313350) (Xq26)
Gustavson syndrome, (GUST) (MIM 309555) (Xq26)
Fragile X syndrome, (FMR1, FRAXA) (MIM 309550) (Xq27.3)
Börjeson-Forssman-Lehmann syndrome, (BFLS) (MIM 301900) (Xq26-q27)
Albinism-deafness, (ADFN, ALDS) (MIM 300700) (Xq26.3-q27.1)
Dyskeratosis congenita, (DKC) (MIM 305000) (Xq28)
Hunter syndrome, (IDS, MPS2, SIDS) (MIM 309900) (Xq28)
Otopalatodigital syndrome, type I, (OPDI) (MIM 311300) (Xq28)
Adrenoleukodystrophy, (ALD) (MIM 300100) (Xq28)
Goeminne syndrome, TKCR syndrome, (torticollis, keloids, cryptorchidism, renal dysplasia) (TKC, TKCR) (MIM 314300) (Xq28)
Chondrodysplasia punctata 2, X-linked dominant, Happle syndrome (CDPX2, CPXD, CPX) (MIM 302960) (Xq28)
X

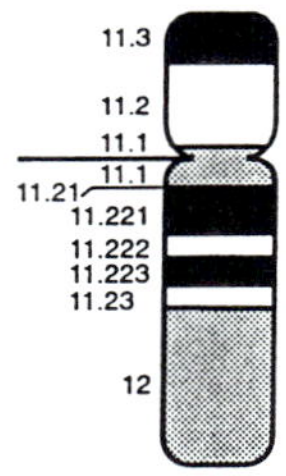


# Y

- Negative or pale staining Q and G bands
- Positive Q and G bands
- Variable bands
- Centromeric area (except for Y chromosome)
- Heterochromatin

Ideogram corresponds to ISCH (1995) nomenclature (550 band level)

The relative sizes of the different chromosomes are kept. The X chromosome is enlarged on the right side of the page to accommodate the multiple loci.

## Mitochondrial Chromosome

- Deafness, aminoglycoside–induced (MTRNR1) (MIM 561001) (Mutation at nucleotide 1555 in mitochondrial 12S rRNA gene)
- Deafness, late in life (Mutation at nucleotide 1555)
- Deafness, non-syndromic, (Mutation at nucleotide 7445 on one strand and cytochrome oxidase I gene on other strand) ($tRNA^{ser(ucn)}$ gene)
- Deafness, two locus disorder, (autosomal recessive and mitochondrial at nucleotide 1555)
- Diabetes mellitus–deafness syndrome (MIM 520000) (Heteroplasmic nucleotide 3243 mutation)
- Kearns–Sayre syndrome (KSS) (MIM 530000)
- MELAS syndrome (*M*itochondrial *E*ncephalopathy, *L*actic *A*cidosis, *S*troke-like episodes) (MIM 590051) (A-G transition mutation at nucleotide 3243 in mitochondrial gene for $tRNA^{leu(uur)}$)
- MERRF syndrome (*M*yoclonic *E*pilepsy with *R*agged *R*ed *F*ibers) (MIM 545000, 590061, 590062)
- Myoneurogastrointestinal encephalopathy syndrome (MNGIE syndrome) (MIM 550900)

# Index

*Italic* type for page numbers indicates illustrative material or tables.